Midwifery

Preparation for Practice

Sally Pairman
Jan Pincombe
Carol Thorogood
Sally Tracy

Publisher's note

Knowledge and best practice in this field are constantly changing. As research and clinical experience broaden our knowledge, changes in practice, treatment and drug therapy may become necessary or appropriate. Readers are advised to check the most current information available (i) on procedures featured, (ii) on the reader's individual practice obligations, or (iii) from the manufacturer of any product to be administered to verify the recommended dose, the method and duration of administration, and contraindications. It is the responsibility of the treating person, relying on experience and knowledge of the patient, to determine dosages and to take all appropriate safety precautions. Neither the Publisher nor the editors assume any responsibility for any injury and/or damage to persons or property. The Publisher

ELSEVIER

Churchill Livingstone
is an imprint of Elsevier

Elsevier Australia
(a division of Reed International Books Australia Pty Ltd)
30–52 Smidmore Street, Marrickville, NSW 2204
ABN 70 001 002 357

© 2006 Elsevier Australia

National Library of Australia Cataloguing-in-Publication Data

Midwifery : preparation for practice.

Bibliography.
Includes index.

ISBN-10: 0-7295-3756-0
ISBN-13: 978-0-7295-3756-8

1. Midwifery — Australia. 2. Midwifery — New Zealand. 3. Maternity nursing — Australia. 4. Maternity nursing — New Zealand. I. Pairman, Sally.

618.20231

Contents

Preface

This new midwifery textbook is the first to reflect Australasian historical and socio-political contexts for midwifery practice and the first to frame content within the philosophy and standards of the New Zealand and Australian Colleges of Midwives. This text is intended to provide an up-to-date evidence- and practice-based resource for midwives who work in partnership with women in women-centred models of midwife-led care.

As such this text is designed for midwifery students and practising midwives in New Zealand and Australia, and will also be relevant to midwives in other parts of the world where midwifery autonomy is acknowledged and emerging, such as Canada, Europe, Scandinavia, Japan and the United Kingdom.

We acknowledge that not all contexts in Australia and elsewhere currently support midwifery autonomy as we have described it. However, the primary purpose of this text is to equip midwives to practise autonomously and in partnership with women once contextual constraints to midwifery autonomy have been removed through political action. This text provides a model of midwifery to which midwives can aspire and for which they can be prepared. We hope that this knowledge will strengthen midwives' determination to find ways to work with women and with each other that will enhance midwifery autonomy and women-centred midwifery practice.

Philosophical framework

The philosophical framework of this text is shaped by our vision for maternity services: that each woman should have access to a midwife of her choice and that each midwife should be able to work within the full scope of midwifery practice. The context within which midwives practise may either support or limit the individual midwife's ability to practise in a way that is congruent with this philosophy. A primary purpose of this textbook is to articulate and exemplify the way in which midwifery partnership is, or can be, actualised in practice.

We believe that midwifery is both an art and a science. It occurs within historical, social, cultural, political and legal contexts. Midwifery knowledge is derived from the wisdom of women and experienced midwives, and from scientific research. The individual midwife's knowledge develops by scholarship and praxis.

A midwife forms a partnership with a woman as she experiences the life process of childbearing and early parenting.

Midwifery care is woman-centred; however, care of the woman includes those she considers to be her family. The midwife shares knowledge, experience and wisdom reciprocally with the woman and her family. The midwife protects and promotes the dignity of each woman and accepts her culture, beliefs, values, expectations and previous experiences. The midwife and the woman make decisions together through a process of negotiation.

Midwives are autonomous health practitioners who, like other health practitioners, have a social mandate to practise within legally defined professional boundaries. The scope of midwifery practice involves care of the woman and her family pre-pregnancy and during all phases of childbearing and early parenting up until six weeks after the birth. The midwife works on her own responsibility, but in partnership with the woman, as long as the woman and her baby remain well and healthy.

When there is an indication that the woman or the baby requires the service of another healthcare provider, the midwife works collaboratively with the other healthcare provider. The midwife maintains her relationship with the woman and her family even if referral to another health provider is needed, and in most cases continues to provide care in collaboration with the other provider.

Structure of the textbook

Aim

The overall aim of this textbook is to support the development of competent and confident midwifery practitioners who are able to make professional judgements, in partnership with women, on their own responsibility. These practitioners will:

- have a women-centred approach
- work in partnership with women as autonomous practitioners in all settings
- have a sound knowledge base
- be critical thinkers
- be reflective practitioners
- be ethical decision-makers
- critically appraise the literature and provide evidence-based midwifery care
- be accountable and responsible for their practice
- contribute to the development of midwifery knowledge and the profession.

Structuring concepts

The text is broadly structured around the following concepts derived from its philosophical framework:

- *Context*—a reflection of the history of colonisation and the impact on the Indigenous peoples of Australia and New Zealand, our current bicultural and multicultural societies, our laws and legal systems, our political structures and processes, our healthcare systems, the organisation of maternity services and payment of maternity care providers. Childbirth and midwifery practice have been constructed within these different contexts. Each person involved in childbearing is affected by the context from which they have emerged and brings with them their individual life histories and culturally moulded attitudes, values and beliefs.
- *Woman*—includes the self of each woman and encompasses the baby that each woman carries within her body and to which she gives birth. This concept also includes each woman's partner, family/whanau, and cultural and subcultural group, and incorporates each woman's experience(s) of childbearing.
- *Midwife*—includes the self of each midwife, her knowledge, attitudes and beliefs, her partner and/or family/whanau, her cultural or subcultural group and her professional role as midwife. A midwife cares for and supports a woman as she grows and nurtures her baby, and strengthens the woman in her role as a mother.
- *Partnership*—implies a relationship of trust, reciprocity and equity through which both partners are strengthened. Each midwife strives to ensure that she does not impose her professional and personal power onto women; rather, through negotiation a midwife seeks to establish relationships in which each woman is the primary decision-maker. (*Note*: because most midwives are women we have chosen to use the feminine pronoun throughout this text.)
- *Autonomous practice*—occurs when a midwife provides care to a woman and her baby on her own responsibility. As autonomous practitioners, midwives have the knowledge and skills to provide care independently without a requirement to refer to another health professional. This does not mean that midwives practise alone; rather, midwives work in partnership with midwifery colleague(s). Nor are midwives independent of women, because all midwifery professional judgements emerge from midwife/women relationships.
- *Collaborative practice*—means working with other healthcare professionals/providers when the health of a woman or baby is outside the scope of midwifery practice. The relationship and responsibilities of each woman, each midwife and other health professionals needs to be negotiated.

Sections of the textbook

These structuring concepts are reflected in the ordering of the chapters. Part A focuses on the two partners within a midwifery partnership—the woman and the midwife, and the context within which their partnership relationship establishes and develops.

Part B focuses on midwifery practice. Section one explores the notion of midwifery partnership, while sections two and three explore midwifery practice from the perspectives of midwifery autonomy and collaborative practice.

Because midwifery practice is an integration of knowledge, skills and attitudes, the following strands are articulated within each of the three sections in Part B:

- physiology
- assessment
- evidence for practice
- professional judgements and decision-making.

We acknowledge that a number of disciplines contribute to the knowledge, attitudes and skills that a midwife needs, but the focus of this book is on midwifery-specific knowledge and the application of knowledge from other disciplines where it directly relates to the scope of midwifery practice. Where additional depth is required, readers are referred to more specific texts from other disciplines.

Each chapter provides:

- learning outcomes
- clinical scenarios to contextualise practice issues
- reflective and critical thinking exercises
- questions for review
- a list of online resources.

This text provides a new approach to midwifery education. In focusing on the midwife as an autonomous practitioner with a specific scope of practice, we have endeavoured to show how professional judgements and practice decisions rely on strong assessment skills, knowledge and understanding of physiology, application of evidence-based practice knowledge, and integration of attitudes and philosophy within a professional framework for practice. Midwives who approach practice in this way will be able to provide individualised and women-centred care. They will be able to identify when they have reached their level of expertise and when it is necessary to consult and collaborate with others to ensure that the needs of women and their babies are met. It is this awareness and midwifery 'thinking' that ensures midwives are competent and safe practitioners.

We hope you enjoy using this textbook.

Sally Pairman
Jan Pincombe
Carol Thorogood
Sally Tracy

About the editors

Sally Pairman

DMid, MA, BA, RM, RGON is Head of School of Midwifery and Health Group Manager at Otago Polytechnic, Dunedin, New Zealand. Actively involved in the New Zealand College of Midwives in various roles, including President, and currently inaugural Chairperson of the Midwifery Council of New Zealand, Sally has been at the forefront of establishing midwifery autonomy and degree-level direct-entry midwifery education in New Zealand.

Sally is co-author with Karen Guilliland of *The Midwifery Partnership: A Model for Practice*, a monograph describing a theoretical model of midwifery as a partnership between a woman and a midwife. Sally's master's research resulted in refinement of the model. Her professional doctorate in midwifery further analysed midwifery partnership in relation to midwifery leadership, midwifery education and midwifery regulation in her exploration of New Zealand midwifery's professionalising strategies from 1986 to 2005. Sally has published and presented extensively on these topics.

Sally is married to Michael Lucas and they have two sons, Oscar and Felix.

Jan Pincombe

PhD, MAppSc, PGDipEd, BA, RM, RIN, RN, FACMI is Professor of Midwifery, University of South Australia, Adelaide, and has extensive teaching and research experience. Over the past three years she held the position of Joint Professor of Midwifery between the University of South Australia and the Women's and Children's Hospital, Adelaide, where she has clinical teaching privileges.

More recently Jan was appointed Program Director of Midwifery for undergraduate and postgraduate programs at the University of South Australia, where she has taught and researched since 1992. She has successfully supervised PhD, masters and honours students in midwifery, alternative therapies and maternal and childcare topics over the past ten years and has taught a variety of courses in the midwifery programs.

Jan is a member of the Australian College of Midwives and the Australian National Education Standards Taskforce. She is married to Adrian, has two children, Brandon and Shauna, and two grandchildren, Will and Emma.

Carol Thorogood

PhD, MPhil, BAppSc, DipEd, PGDipArts, RN, RM, FACMI is the coordinator of midwifery programs in the School of Nursing, Midwifery and Postgraduate Medicine at Edith Cowan University in Perth, Western Australia. She is a Fellow of the Australian College of Midwives and a member of the Education Committee and Instructor for the Australian chapter of the Advanced Life Support in Obstetrics© programs. A member of the Board of Community Midwives Western Australia, the State's only publicly funded caseload, home birth program, Carol has a long-term research and clinical interest in home birth and autonomous midwifery practice.

Carol has considerable expertise in curriculum development, implementation and evaluation, including the design and evaluation of competency standards in midwifery. Her current research is concerned with the design of midwifery education programs for qualified midwives beginning tertiary study that embed generic skills such as critical thinking, reflection and written expression into clinically focused curricula.

Sally K Tracy

DMid, MA, BNurs, ADN, RM, RGON was appointed Associate Professor of Midwifery Practice Development at Northern Sydney and Central Coast Area Health Service in 2003. During that year she led the implementation and evaluation of one of the first Australian free-standing caseload midwifery units, the Ryde Midwifery Group Practice. In 2004, as part of her research program, she became a postdoctoral Research Fellow on the NH&MRC-funded Health Research and Outcomes Network (HERON), a collaborative program of the Institute for Health Research and the University of Sydney, the University of New South Wales, University of Technology Sydney, the Cancer Council NSW and NSW Health. She is based at the Australian Institute of Health and Welfare National Perinatal Statistics Unit at the University of New South Wales, where she is Associate Professor (Conjoint) in the School of Women's and Children's Health.

Sally was educated as a midwife in New Zealand and the United Kingdom, and has extensive community and hospital experience in New Zealand and Australia.

Sally was awarded the world's first professional doctorate in midwifery at the University of Technology Sydney in 2003 and has published widely on the epidemiology of obstetric intervention in labour and birth. She is married to Mark and has four children, Gabriel, Raphael, Amy and Imogen.

Foreword

'Midwifery knowledge is derived from the wisdom of women'—these words, contained in the preface, take us to the heart of this wonderful, useful, groundbreaking book. The words contain a world of meaning. The essence is crucial. In countries like New Zealand and Australia (and Canada too), midwifery is being transformed in a way that contains the ancient meaning and traditional ways of working of midwifery, being with the woman, while meeting the needs of modern-day health services and society.

It is no accident, I believe, that fresh approaches not only to practice but also to developing knowledge and skills are finding fertile soil in countries that are conscious not only of the general effect of colonisation on their societies, but also of the effect that colonisation has had on the midwifery profession. Awareness of the powerlessness that arises among the colonised is finding translation into an awareness of the effect of unequal power structures in the health services and the way that this affects childbearing women. The conscious intention to work in partnership with women, through a relationship that seeks to redress the power imbalance between each midwife and each woman, changes every aspect of midwifery practice, and calls for new knowledge and skills, and a new perspective on life and the world.

This is the first textbook to be written to reflect Australasian historical and socio-political contexts for midwifery practice and the first to frame content within the philosophy and standards of the New Zealand and Australian Colleges of Midwives. It will be invaluable to midwives and students in Australasia. However, it will also be invaluable to any midwife wherever she lives and practises. The kind of midwifery that is defined by this book, working in partnership, practising autonomously, in a way that gives mothers and their families the best start in life, requires deep knowledge and skills. It requires the ability to think critically and creatively, to be able to practise not only in partnership with women but also with a passion for developing skill, intellect and knowledge.

Midwifery is the partnership between the woman and her midwife, and the midwife in practice draws on the childbearing woman's knowledge. Working with the woman, rather than working with the institution, which is where many midwives find themselves in today's world, gives us an entirely new view, and requires an entirely new way of developing, using and transmitting knowledge. This book is the kind of rich resource that midwives need when they face the world from a position alongside a woman and her family, rather than from the institution looking on.

The position of 'being with' rather than 'doing to', of working in partnership, requires much of us but brings huge rewards. We need good resources to practise midwifery well in this way. This book is a goldmine for the modern midwife wherever she may be.

Lesley Page
Joint Head of Midwifery Guy's and St Thomas' NHS Trust and
Visiting Professor of Midwifery
Nightingale School of Nursing and Midwifery
King's College London

Foreword

It is not often that one comes across a midwifery textbook like this one. This volume brings together a team of midwives from both Australia and New Zealand who are leaders in their field and who share in these pages a wealth of knowledge and expertise in midwifery practice, education, research and regulation.

Yet the credentials of the authors, while impressive, are not the only reason this book is a 'must have' for every student of midwifery. This book's unique contribution is its focus on both the universal principle that underpins midwifery philosophy and practice—that of partnership with women—and midwifery autonomy in practice.

The midwifery partnership between a woman and midwife working together to achieve the best outcome for that mother and baby differentiates it from other models of care, where the health professional assumes expertise over the mother. It is this point of difference that gives society the body of knowledge called midwifery.

Drawing on midwifery partnership, this book approaches midwifery care from the perspective of a midwife as a primary health practitioner, based in the community but interfacing with hospitals and specialists as necessary to meet the needs of individual women. It explores both autonomous practice and collaborative practice, and is the first textbook to discuss midwifery practice in the context of community and primary health rather than hospital-based maternity services.

Just as childbirth is far more than a physiological process, the art and science of midwifery is more than a study of the female human body and its reproductive powers. Like childbirth, midwifery occurs in a social, political and historical context that shapes the practice of midwifery in any given time and place. It is therefore essential that all would-be midwives have a sound understanding of this context, and an awareness of how it may influence their own practice in providing care to women. This book provides a clear and accessible introduction to the historical and contemporary context of midwifery practice in Australia and New Zealand, and examines practice within the professional frameworks of the philosophy and standards of both the Australian and New Zealand Colleges of Midwives.

Midwifery care in Australia and New Zealand is currently provided to women in very different maternity care systems. In Australia, most midwives work in public or private hospitals, providing professional care to women as best they can without the benefit of being able to get to know the women they care for. Lacking prescribing rights, independent access to public funding, and professional indemnity insurance, midwives are mostly obliged to work within services that segment women and their midwives into antenatal, labour and postnatal wards and limit the opportunities for relationship building. Midwives in New Zealand, by contrast, are free to practise in either hospitals or the community. All can access public funding for their professional services, have prescribing rights, and work in partnership with women and with each other if they choose to.

The freedom to practise in partnership with women cannot be taken for granted. Policy and legislative change in New Zealand has been achieved through twenty years of sustained political advocacy by midwives and women in partnership.

Even so, twenty years ago, when New Zealand midwives and women were in the heart of their 'save the midwife campaign', they could hardly have envisaged how successful the reinstatement of the midwifery profession would be in today's health system. In focusing on midwifery autonomy and midwifery partnership, this textbook reinforces for all midwives the achievements of women and midwives in giving childbirth back to women and their whanau. It reminds us of what a struggle it was, and still is, to keep women central to the birthing process, and each chapter provides valuable knowledge and guidance to both experienced and new midwives that will help ensure that midwifery continues to keep women and their babies safely at the centre of practice decisions.

Similarly, advocacy by midwives and women has also been under way in Australia for the past decade, and is beginning to bear fruit in creating greater freedom for midwives to practise and for women to choose their own midwife. However, there remains much to be done before midwifery in Australia achieves the level of professional autonomy and responsibility that is commonplace in New Zealand and other developed nations.

Yet for all the differences between maternity services in these two countries, midwifery remains universally constant, guided by the same theoretical and practice knowledge and skills that combine to make midwifery such a vital profession for women and babies. The commonalities far outweigh the differences, and this book is rich with up-to-date and relevant information aimed at supporting all midwives to practise autonomously and ever with an eye on the needs of the women they care for.

Dr Barbara Vernon
Executive Officer, Australian College of Midwives

Karen Guilliland
Chief Executive, New Zealand College of Midwives

Contributors

Jacqui Anderson MMid candidate, PGradDipMid, RM, RGON; co-Head of Midwifery, School of Midwifery, Christchurch Polytechnic Institute of Technology, Christchurch; Member National Perinatal and Maternal Mortality Committee, New Zealand; self-employed homebirth midwife and antenatal educator, New Zealand

Lynley Anderson MHealSci, Chair Ethics Committee NZSP; member of Ethics Committee Assisted Reproductive Technology (ECART); Lecturer, Bioethics Centre, Dunedin School of Medicine, University of Otago, New Zealand

Sally Baddock PhD, BSc(Physiology), DipTchg; Associate Head of School, Principal Lecturer, School of Midwifery, Otago Polytechnic, Dunedin, New Zealand

Helen Calabretto PhD, MEd St, BEd, DipTchg, RM, RN, FRCNA; Senior Lecturer, School of Nursing and Midwifery, University of South Australia, Adelaide, Australia

Shea Caplice MA, PGradDipIndPract, FPNP, RM; self-employed midwife; Clinical Midwifery Consultant, South Eastern Sydney and Illawarra Health Service; Honorary Associate, University of Technology Sydney, Australia

Debra Creedy PhD, MEd, BA(Hons), RN, FANZCMHN; Dean, Griffith Health, Griffith University, Gold Coast Campus, Southport, Australia

Rhondda Davies MA(Appl) Midwifery, BA, RM, ADN, RCpN; self-employed midwife, Dunedin, New Zealand

Lesley Dixon RN, RM, BA(Hons), IBCLC; Charge Midwife, Burwood Birthing Unit, Christchurch, New Zealand

Catherine Donaldson MSc (AdvMidPractice), ADM, RM, RGON; independent midwifery educator and self-employed midwife, Motueka, New Zealand

Roslyn Donnellan-Fernandez RM, RMHN, RN, BN, MN (Women's Hlth), Jt Midwifery Unit Head, Midwifery Group Practice; Women's and Children's Hospital, Children, Youth and Women's Health Service, Adelaide, Australia; Deputy Chair, Nurse's Board of South Australia, Australia

Sandra L Elias MSc; Senior Lecturer, School of Midwifery, Otago Polytechnic, Dunedin, New Zealand

Maralyn Foureur PhD, BA, GradDipClinEpidem, RM, RGON; Clinical Professor, Midwifery, Graduate School of Nursing and Midwifery, Victoria University of Wellington; Director, Collaborating Centre for Midwifery and Nursing Education, Practice and Research, Capital and Coast District Health Board; self-employed midwife, Wellington

Jenny Gamble PhD, MHlth, BN, RM; Convenor, Master of Midwifery Program, School of Nursing and Midwifery, Griffith University, Queensland, Australia

Christine Griffiths MA(Hons), DipSocSci(Dist), RM, RGON; self-employed midwife, Wellington, New Zealand

Celia Grigg MM, BM, BA(Ed), RM; self-employed midwife, Christchurch, New Zealand

Karen Guilliland MNZM, MA, ADN (Maternal & Child Health), RM, RGON; Chief Executive, New Zealand College of Midwives; Director, NZ Pharmaceutical Management Agency (PHARMAC); Member, Canterbury District Health Board

Jackie Gunn MA, BHSc(Ng), AdvDipN(Maternal & Child Health), RM, RGON; Head of Midwifery, School of Midwifery, Auckland University of Technology, Auckland; Education Consultant, New Zealand College of Midwives; Member, Health Practitioner's Disciplinary Tribunal, New Zealand

Ann Henderson PhD, MEdStudies, BEd, DipTchg, IBCLC, DipBus, RN, RM; Midwifery Educator, Centre for Continuing Education, Children, Youth and Women's Health Service, Adelaide, Australia

Sue Hendy MM, RN, RM (UK) ADM; Midwifery Consultant, NSW Aboriginal Maternal and Infant Health Strategy, NSW Pregnancy and Newborn Service Network, Sydney, Australia

Caroline Homer PhD, RM; Professor of Midwifery, Centre for Midwifery and Family Health, Faculty of Nursing, Midwifery and Health, University of Technology Sydney, Australia

Marion Hunter MA(Hons), BA, RM, RGON, AdvDipNg, Senior Lecturer, School of Midwifery, Auckland University of Technology; self-employed midwife, South Auckland, New Zealand

Linda Jones PhD, MNA, GradDipEd, BAppSc, RM, RN, FACM, FRCNA, FCN; Midwifery Programs Leader, Division of Nursing and Midwifery, RMIT University, Melbourne, Australia

Karen Lane PhD, BA(Hons); Lecturer, School of History, Heritage and Society, Deakin University, Melbourne, Australia

Nicky Leap DMid, MSc, RM; Director of Midwifery Practice, South Eastern Sydney and Illawarra Area Health Service; Associate Professor of Midwifery, University of Technology Sydney, Australia

Judith McAra-Couper Doctoral candidate (Auckland University of Technology), PGradCert(Ed), BA, RM, RGON; Senior Lecturer Midwifery, Auckland University of Technology; Clinical Midwifery Educator, Delivery Unit, Middlemore Hospital, Counties Manukau, South Auckland, New Zealand

Robyn Maude PhD candidate, MA(Appl) Midwifery, BN, RM, RN; Midwifery Advisor, Capital and Coast District Health Board, Wellington; Director, Midwifery and Maternity Provider Organization (MMPO); External Clinical Advisor to ACC; member of New Zealand Health Practitioners' Disciplinary Tribunal

Suzanne Miller PGradCert(Mid), RM, RCompN, MMid candidate, Normal Birth Research Unit, Victoria University, Wellington; self-employed midwife, Wellington, New Zealand

Helen Newnham MSc, LLB, BAppSc, RN, RM, FRCNA; Lecturer, School of Nursing, Midwifery and Postgraduate Medicine, Edith Cowan University, Perth, Australia

Sally Pairman DMid, MA, BA, RM, RGON; Head of School, School of Midwifery and Group Manager Health, Otago Polytechnic, Dunedin, New Zealand; Chair, Midwifery Council of New Zealand; honorary member and founder member, New Zealand College of Midwives

Jackie Pearse MBHL(Dist), LLB(Hons), ADN, RM, RN; HR Advisor, Transfield Services Ltd; legal advisor to Te Pihopatanga O Aotearoa, Chair of Te Kotahitanga Scholarship Committee; member of NZ Social Worker's Disciplinary Tribunal; member of Auckland Medico Legal Society; member of Statutes and Canons Committee (ACANZP); life member, New Zealand College of Midwives

Bronwen Pelvin RM, RGON; Professional Development Advisor, New Zealand College of Midwives; Professional Midwifery Advisor, Nelson Marlborough District Health Board, Nelson, New Zealand; life member and founder member, New Zealand College of Midwives; Associate Member, Australia and New Zealand Psychodrama Association

Jan Pincombe PhD, MAppSc, PGradDipEd, BA, RM, RN, RIN, FACMI; Professor of Midwifery, Program Director, School of Nursing and Midwifery, University of South Australia, Adelaide, Australia

Marlene Scobbie PGradCertHlthSc (Midwifery), BHlthSc(Midwifery), IBCLC, RGON, RM; Clinical Midwife Manager, Birthcare, Auckland, New Zealand

Joan Skinner PhD, MA(Appl), RM, RN(Comp); Lecturer, Graduate School of Nursing and Midwifery, Victoria University of Wellington, New Zealand

Chris Stanbridge ADN, NZRN, NZRM; self-employed midwife and grief counsellor; advisor, New Zealand College of Midwives, Christchurch, New Zealand

Carol Thorogood PhD, MPhil, BAppSc Psych, PGradDipArts, DipEd, RN, RM, FACM; School of Nursing, Midwifery and Postgraduate Medicine; Coordinator Midwifery Studies, Edith Cowan University, Perth, Australia

Juliet Thorpe MMid, DipMid, RM, RCompN; self-employed homebirth midwife and antenatal class educator, Christchurch, New Zealand

Sally K Tracy DMid, MA, BNurs, ADN, RM, RGON; Research Fellow (NH&MRC), HERON Project, AIHW National Perinatal Statistics Unit; Associate Professor (conjoint), School of Women's and Children's Health, Faculty of Medicine, University of New South Wales, Sydney, Australia

Stephanie Vague MHlthSc(Midwifery)(Hons), RM, RGON; self-employed midwife, Auckland, New Zealand

Jill White PhD, MEd, RN, RM; Dean, Faculty of Nursing, Midwifery and Health, University of Technology, Sydney, Australia

Annette Wright BHlthSc(Nursing), NICC, RM, RN; Nurse Educator, Newborn Care Centre, Royal Hospital for Women, Sydney, Australia

Acknowledgements

This textbook has taken many months to prepare and would not have been completed without the support of many people. We give heartfelt thanks to the following:

- all the authors who worked so hard to complete their chapters on time despite their very busy lives and personal challenges
- our employers—Otago Polytechnic, University of South Australia, Edith Cowan University and the Australian National Perinatal Statistics Unit—who have supported us with time to write
- the manuscript reviewers, in conjunction with Elsevier Australia, for their insightful comments, including: Jenny Browne (University of Newcastle), Margaret Duff (Waikato Institute of Technology), Joanne Gray (University of Technology Sydney), Virginia King (Southern Cross University), Jan Robinson (Jan Robinson Midwifery Education Services) and Rachel Smith (University of Technology, Sydney). We would also like to thank those contributors who kindly provided valuable feedback to their peers on selected chapters, including Sally Baddock, Shea Caplice and Roslyn Donnellan-Fernandez.
- colleagues who provided particular expertise and advice: Bronwyn Hegarty, Patrice Hickey, Karen Guilliland and Hannah Dahlen
- David Vernon for use of a birth story from the book titled *Having a Good Birth in Australia*
- David Hancock for the photographs in Chapter 24
- the New Zealand College of Midwives, Archives New Zealand and the Alexander Turnbull Library (NZ) for the photographs in Chapters 6 and 20
- our professional organisations—the New Zealand College of Midwives and the Australian College of Midwives—for their support of our vision for this book
- our hard-working team from Elsevier Australia: Helena Klijn, Suzanne Hall, Amanda Simons and Kay Waters, for their diligence, perseverance and endless patience
- and, finally, our families and friends, who supported us in so many ways over the long months of writing and reviewing, and who encouraged us when the end seemed nowhere in sight.

Sally Pairman, Jan Pincombe, Carol Thorogood, Sally Tracy

Publisher's acknowledgements

Ch 1: p 12, Maternity Services: Notice pursuant to section 88 of the New Zealand Public Health and Disability Act 2000, New Zealand Health and Information Services (NZHIS), Ministry of Health, Wellington; Box 1.1, Blackwell Publishing; Box 1.3, Community Midwifery WA (Inc.); p 17, Clinical Point, New Zealand Health and Information Services (NZHIS), Ministry of Health, Wellington; Fig 1.6, BMJ Publishing Group; Fig 1.9, New Zealand Health and Information Services (NZHIS), Ministry of Health, Wellington. Ch 2: p 37, Broome (2001, 92–93), Aboriginal Australians (3rd edn), Allen & Unwin, Sydney (www.allenandunwin.com.au); p 40, used with permission from End of Equality (Random House, Australia) © 2003 by Anne Summers; p 45, (Michael King 2003, pp 519–20) Penguin Group, New Zealand. Ch 3: Fig 3.1, reproduced by permission of Oxford University Press Australia, from Second Opinion (3rd edn) by Germov © Oxford University Press, www.oup.com.au. Ch 5: Box 5.1, Blackwell Publishing; Boxes 5.2, 5.3, 5.12, BMJ Publishing Group. Ch 6: p 97, photo, Alexander Turnbull Library, National Library of New Zealand; p 98, photo, Archives New Zealand/Te Rua Mahara o te Kawanatanga, Wellington Office. Ch 7: Tables 7.1, 7.2, 7.3, Medical Journal of Australia; Fig 7.4, reproduced from Alcohol consumption in pregnancy, Guideline no. 9, December 1999, with permission of the Royal College of Obstetricians and Gynaecologists; Table 7.5, UNAIDS www.unaids.org; Box 7.3, New Zealand College of Midwives (Inc); Table 7.9 WHO (1997) A joint WHO/UNICEF/UNFPA statement. Geneva, World Health Organisation. Ch 8: Fig 8.1, © 2004, Heffner, Advanced Maternal Age—How Old Is Too Old? Vol 351, pp 1927–1929, Massachusetts Medical Society. All Rights Reserved; Table 8.1, United Nations Population Fund; Figs 8.2, 8.3, New Zealand Health and Information Services (NZHIS), Ministry of Health, Wellington. Ch 10: Box 10.1, Fig 10.1, New Zealand College of Midwives (Inc); Box 10.2, ACMI Role and Functions, January 2005, Australian College of Midwives (ACMI), www.acmi.org.au; Fig 10.2, Australian College of Midwives Framework for Midwifery (ACMI 2004), www.acmi.org.au; Box 10.6, Australian Midwives Act Lobby Group. Ch 12: Boxes 12.1, 12.3, New Zealand College of Midwives (Inc). Ch 25: Figs 25.1–25.5, redrawn from Gunn, J., Maintaining the Integrity of the Pelvic Floor, David and Geck Education Centre, Table 35.1, American Academy of Family Physicians (AAFP). Ch 27: Table 27.4, New Zealand College of Midwives (Inc); Fig 27.10g, Dr AMM Oakley; Box 27.1, New Zealand College of Midwives (Inc); Box 27.2, New Zealand Health and Information Services (NZHIS), Ministry of Health, Wellington. Ch 28: Fig 28.1, Jones and Bartlett Publishers, MA; Figs 28.2, 28.3, 28.4, Australian Breastfeeding Association. Ch 30: Fig 30.1,

New Zealand Health and Information Services (NZHIS), Ministry of Health, Wellington, Appendix A, Ministry of Health 2005, WellChild Tamariki Ora Health Book, Wellington, New Zealand Ministry of Health, Appendix B, New Zealand Health and Information Services (NZHIS), Ministry of Health, Wellington. Ch 31: Table 31.2, ABS data used with permission from the Australian Bureau of Statistics, www. abs.gov.au. Ch 33: Table 33.3, © The Board of Management and Trustees of the British Journal of Anaesthesia, reproduced by permission of Oxford University Press/British Journal of Anaesthesia. Ch 35: Table 35.1, American Academy of Family Physicians (AAFP), Manning, FA; Box 35.15, Canadian Association of Midwives/Association Canadienne des sage-femmes; Table 35.6, New Zealand Health Information Service, 2002, Report on Maternity: Maternal and Newborn Information 2002, Wellington, Ministry of Health. Ch 36: Box 36.13, Confidential Enquiry into Maternal and Child Health (CEMACH)

PART A
Partners

CHAPTER 1

Australian and New Zealand health and maternity services

Karen Guilliland, Sally K Tracy and Carol Thorogood

Key terms

Annual Salary Agreements, federal health, funding models, health, lead maternity carer (LMC), Maternal and Newborn Information Service (MNIS), Medicare, midwifery models, Mothers and Babies Report/NPDC, New Zealand District Health Boards, primary health, public health, Section 88 funding

Chapter overview

This chapter provides an overview and explanation of the development and current structure of the New Zealand and Australian maternity systems. It discusses the role that midwives and women have played in that development and identifies how the maternity service structure in each country supports, or does not support, the provision of midwife-led maternity care. The chapter begins with an introduction to primary healthcare and makes the case that maternity care is a primary health service and needs to be recognised as such if it is to best meet the needs of women and their families.

Learning outcomes

Learning outcomes for this chapter are:

1 To define primary, secondary and tertiary healthcare

2 To explore why maternity services need to be recognised as primary healthcare rather than secondary and tertiary services

3 To describe the structure and funding of New Zealand's maternity services

4 To describe the structure and funding of Australia's maternity services

5 To explain how funding models affect the provision of services and outcomes of care

6 To discuss the role of midwives within New Zealand and Australian maternity services.

What is health?

Health is not merely the absence of disease or infirmity; it is a social phenomenon, the determinants of which cannot be separated from the social world in which we live. Health does not necessarily relate to the availability of health services. Indeed, even in industrialised nations such as Australia and New Zealand, rich in knowledge, technology and expertise, and with relatively equal access to health services, the health of some members of society remains poor. Geoffrey Rose, in his influential book, *The Strategy of Preventive Medicine* (1992), goes some way to explaining this phenomenon when he argues that 'the primary determinants of disease are mainly economic and social, and therefore its remedies must also be economic and social. Medicine and politics cannot and should not be kept apart' (p 129). Consequently, the only way to tackle health inequalities and improve health for all is to take a multipronged approach that addresses the social and economic factors in which health and illness are generated, while also providing appropriate, affordable and accessible health services aimed at ameliorating risk factors, promoting health, and combating and curing disease.

The provision of such health services involves complex social and political processes that require political decision-making not only at the sectorial level but also by the state. Health cannot be the responsibility of any single bureaucratic–administrative sector of the state; nor can it be owned by specific groups. Health is everyone's responsibility—individuals, social groups and the state.

Adequate healthcare services will only be achieved when all members of society have access to healthcare services that meet their specific needs. Access is not possible if healthcare providers, facilities and supporting healthcare system infra-structure are not in place. Even when essential health services are available, they may not be accessible. Barriers to access include language, ethnicity, culture, geography, weather, or a lack of affordable public or medical transportation services.

The traditional Western, biomedical approach to health service provision has focused on identifying those at risk of disease, diagnosis, providing treatment for individuals who request care, and assessing outcomes of these treatments. In contrast, primary healthcare takes a broader approach to supporting individuals' health and wellness through community-based services and health promotion. Primary healthcare is not the same as public health, although there are similarities. Where primary health focuses on individuals, public health is concerned with the health of populations. It focuses on protecting and improving the health of entire populations through health promotion and education, disease prevention, control of communicable diseases, and provision of the fundamental conditions and resources required for health, such as peace, shelter, education, food, income, a stable ecosystem, sustainable resources, social justice and equity. Public healthcare addresses the factors that underpin health and illness, such as income, social status, education, employment, working conditions, social and physical environments, biology and genetics, personal health practices and coping skills, child development, health services, gender and culture.

Definitions of healthcare services

Healthcare services can be loosely categorised as primary healthcare, primary medical care, secondary care, tertiary care and public healthcare.

Primary healthcare is both a philosophy and an approach to providing health services. According to the Alma-Ata Declaration of 1978, primary healthcare:

- is a practical approach to making essential healthcare universally accessible to individuals and families in the community in an acceptable and affordable way and with their full participation
- means much more than the mere extension of basic health services
- aims to use only those technologies that have really proved their worth and can be afforded
- is delivered by community health providers who understand the real health needs of the communities they serve and have the confidence of the people.

Primary healthcare is the first level of service provision. It is usually the initial point of contact that people have with the healthcare system. Primary healthcare aims to be universally accessible to individuals and families in the community. Services are coordinated, accessible to all, and accessed through a variety of providers (not all of whom are healthcare professionals) who possess the appropriate skills to meet the needs of individuals and the community they serve.

Although the terms 'primary medical care' and 'primary healthcare' are often used interchangeably they are not the same, and it is important to distinguish between the two. Primary medical care is concerned with the initial management of an individual's health problem and, in New Zealand and Australia, is mostly provided by general practitioners (GPs) supported by nurses in community practices. Primary healthcare is supporting and improving individual wellness and promoting prevention of individual health problems through community-based care. Public health is the application of similar principles to the population or community as a whole.

Secondary healthcare is healthcare to which people do not have direct access and for which they must be referred from some other part of the health system, such as a primary health practitioner. It is a specialty service that is generally provided from hospitals.

Tertiary healthcare encompasses highly specialised, complex and costly inpatient treatment services such as neonatal intensive care. Tertiary healthcare providers are highly specialised and their equipment is usually expensive. Moreover, tertiary healthcare requires a multidisciplinary team, and high levels of organisation and coordination between providers are required.

Midwifery and primary healthcare

Midwives are uniquely positioned to provide a combination of primary, public and secondary/tertiary services. As primary health practitioners, midwives provide community-based midwifery care for individual women where care is provided in women's homes or community clinics and the focus is on enhancing and supporting the normal life process of pregnancy and childbirth. Midwives provide initial responses to problems or needs and can intervene and treat conditions within their scope of practice. They also work in collaboration with obstetric and other specialists to provide secondary and tertiary care, and can provide continuous midwifery care to women even when secondary and tertiary care specialists are involved. Midwives utilise a social justice approach to service provision. In partnership with women and each other, midwives work to empower women and their families towards self-health and self-determination so they can make the best decisions for themselves, but also for their families and the wider community. In so doing they utilise public health methodologies.

This model of midwifery care requires a strong foundation of community-based services if it is to enable women and families to maintain and strengthen their own health status and enjoyment. New Zealand midwifery provides a clear example of midwifery as primary healthcare.

New Zealand midwifery's partnership model is based on the premise that primary healthcare is the cornerstone of the maternity service. Together with the government's overall primary and public health strategies, it has been accepted as the central strategy for improving the health and wellbeing of mothers and babies. A unique aspect of New Zealand's primary health model of maternity care is that primary services are seamlessly integrated with secondary and tertiary services. Secondary maternity care encompasses the provision of comprehensive specialist services which may or may not require hospitalisation. Tertiary maternity care encompasses multidisciplinary care for women and babies with complex needs such as co-morbidities. Women who experience complications during the antenatal, labour, birth and postnatal periods are referred to secondary or tertiary specialist services for either consultation or transfer on a planned or emergency basis.

While New Zealand has a well functioning and integrated model of maternity care based in primary midwifery care, Australian maternity services are still based largely in secondary care hospital facilities and in the primary medical care arena. However, many states are moving towards community and primary health models to provide maternity services, including primary midwifery care. Both countries have developed mechanisms for linkages between primary, secondary and tertiary maternity services and these services and referral guidelines are described in the relevant service specifications issued by the Ministry of Health in New Zealand or Australian state and federal departments of health.

Internationally, midwifery is increasingly being recognised as a primary health service that can operate effectively in the community and away from medical facilities and hospitals. Community interventions have the potential to improve preventive care in isolated communities, reduce delays in seeking and obtaining care, and support primary care services and referral systems (Barnett et al 2005).

As Kaufman (2002) puts it:

> public health is a natural territory for midwives . . . Midwifery sees each woman holistically, taking into account her social, psychological and emotional needs as well as her physiological status. Midwifery understands that a woman's confidence and sense of control, her relationships with those who are important to her and her home situation are as important as the clinical interventions provided her in determining her overall well-being throughout pregnancy and early motherhood.

Midwifery, then, is of fundamental importance to the enhancement and maintenance of health. Its ideological framework and holistic agenda provide a platform for community empowerment, potentially ranging along a continuum from individual development through to the collective ability to influence external policy development, legislation and an equitable distribution of resources. Midwives understand that primary healthcare is not merely about moving resources out of the hospitals and into the community; it is also concerned with equity, access, power and politics. Maternal health does not simply mean providing more obstetric services in hospitals; it is more likely achieved through community-based care directly accessed by women and appropriate to their specific needs.

The following sections identify some basic primary health principles in more depth and provide examples from New Zealand, Australia and internationally of how—and whether—these principles have been implemented.

Principles of primary healthcare

Care should be aimed at the most needy

This principle espouses the notion of equity—resources should be distributed fairly according to need, with more directed at those who require it most. The World Bank estimates that, worldwide, 1.1 billion people live in extreme poverty; that is, they survive on less than a $1 a day. Recently, Sachs (2005), writing in *Time* magazine, said:

> Households [of people living in extreme poverty] cannot meet basic needs for survival. They are chronically hungry, unable to get healthcare, lack safe drinking water and sanitation, cannot afford education for their children and perhaps lack rudimentary shelter—a roof to keep rain out of the hut—and basic articles of clothing like shoes . . . [This is called] the poverty that kills (p 47).

In 2005, even in comparatively rich countries there are still gaping inequities and social injustice between individuals, communities and states that leave large segments of the population without basic healthcare. Poverty is on the rise (Sachs 2005) and the few resources that societies can allocate to education and health are sometimes invested and spent in misguided and inequitable ways, so that those who need support the most do not get it.

This principle is also about reaching groups who are denied equitable access to services. In some cases, services are available but for some reason are not accessed as often or as well as they might be. In others, some population groups live so far below the poverty line that they simply cannot pay for the services they need or pay for the transport they require to get there.

Significant changes in neonatal mortality in New Zealand since 1990

Although there are still some gaps between birth outcomes for Maori, Pacific Island and Pakeha (non-Maori) babies in New Zealand, the gap is considerably less than that for Australian Aboriginal women. Examination of neonatal and perinatal

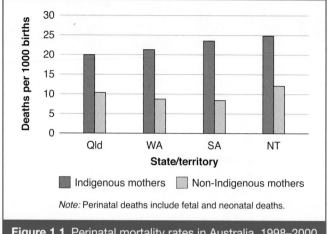

Figure 1.1 Perinatal mortality rates in Australia, 1998–2000 (based on AIHW 2004)

Research

According to the Australian Bureau of Statistics (2004), the perinatal mortality rate for Aboriginal or Torres Strait Island infants is more than twice that of the non-Indigenous population. On average, a baby of Aboriginal or Torres Strait Island descent weighs 200 g less (low birthweight) than one from another Australian background. Between 2001 and 2003, the infant death rate in both Western Australia and the Northern Territory was 16 in 1000. In contrast, the mortality rate for non-Indigenous babies was 5 in 1000 (Australian Bureau of Statistics 2004).

Lack of antenatal care is associated with a significant number of poor pregnancy outcomes. Humphrey and Keating (2004), exploring the reasons that women living in far north Queensland do not access antenatal care and their subsequent pregnancy outcomes, discovered that non-attenders were more likely to be highly parous or young Indigenous women and users of alcohol than those who did access antenatal care. Women who lived in remote communities and women with significant medical conditions complicating their pregnancies were more likely not to attend. Poor attenders had higher incidences of preterm birth and postpartum haemorrhage, and their babies were more likely to be of low birthweight, to be born with five-minute Apgar scores less than five, and had a higher incidence of perinatal death. The authors concluded that lack of antenatal care is associated with a significant number of poor outcomes, but this cannot be explained solely by the women's epidemiological characteristics. Non-attenders tended to be from the most disadvantaged or marginalised groups in society.

statistics in Australia and New Zealand provides one indicator of the success or otherwise of maternity services in meeting the needs of those in most need of care.

In New Zealand in 2000, the neonatal death rate (3.8 per 1000 live births) was 9.5% lower than in 1990. The total post-neonatal death rate (2.5 per 1000 live births) was 40.5% lower than in 1990. The total infant death rate (6.3 per 1000 live births) was 25.0% lower than in 1990 (Ministry of Health 2004).

The Sudden Infant Death Syndrome (SIDS) death rate (1.1 per 1000 live births) was 63.4% lower than in 1990 and was the lowest rate recorded since SIDS became a separate category in the International Classification of Diseases in 1979. There were 64 infant deaths under one year of age attributed to SIDS in 2000. In 2000, 40.6% of post-neonatal deaths and 17.5% of all infant deaths were attributed to SIDS (Ministry of Health 2004). It is important to note that the rate of stillbirth among Maori babies continues to fall significantly, from 7.1 per 1000 births in 1996 to 5.8 per 1000 births in 2000. For the total population this rate fell from 7.2 to 6.4 (Ministry of Health 2004).

Other outcomes measures where Maori figures are the same as or better than Pakeha include birthweight and gestational age. While 71% of Pakeha babies are fully breastfed at two weeks, Maori babies (63%) do better than Pacific (59%) or Asian babies (57%) (Ministry of Health 2004). In 2003 some 85% of Maori women had a midwife Lead Maternity Carer to provide one-on-one care (Ministry of Health 2004). Maori women are also more likely to access primary maternity units than any other ethnic group. It is reasonable to conclude that primary midwifery and maternity care does meet the needs of Maori women and that resulting improvements in health outcomes are beginning to be seen.

Primary healthcare should include essential, appropriate activities

A common concern worldwide is the lack of communication between funding bodies and consequent failure to coordinate

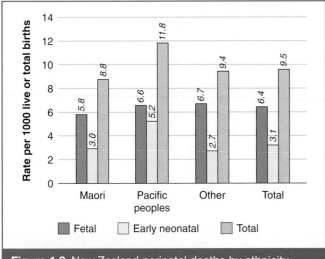

Figure 1.2 New Zealand perinatal deaths by ethnicity, 2000 (based on Ministry of Health 2004)

programs. Vertical programs may be introduced to combat a particular problem but often they are not integrated with other services. For example, immunisation programs have been introduced to reduce the number of deaths from childhood diseases. However, although this initiative has stopped infants dying from infectious diseases, in developing countries children still die of malaria or gastroenteritis from drinking contaminated water.

> In sub-Saharan Africa, malaria is estimated to cause 400,000 cases of severe maternal anaemia and between 75,000–200,000 infant deaths per year. Pregnant women in south eastern Ghana are protecting themselves and their newborns against malaria, thanks to a project funded by the Department of International Development which relies on the skills and influencing power of local midwives. The midwives provide insecticide-treated nets to women attending local clinics and encourage women to use them (Department for International Development, n.d.).

In New Zealand, midwives are the main providers responsible for referring mothers to the well child services for their babies to start their immunisation program at six weeks. Some 95% of babies receive their first vaccination, indicating an effective integration from maternity care into the next primary health service, the well child service (Ministry of Health 2004). Regretfully this level of vaccination in infants is not maintained in the well child service. Nevertheless this example demonstrates that integration from service to service is a possible consequence of a well organised one-on-one primary health maternity service.

Care should be accessible and acceptable to everybody

In general, societies dominated by one social group create health services to meet the cultural needs of that group. In Australia and New Zealand the dominant stakeholders are primarily urban-dwelling people from Anglo-European backgrounds. This means that some Australians and New Zealanders are alienated from these services because their specific cultural needs and values are not recognised. Feelings of alienation may lead to health services not being used even if they are accessible.

Dr Lowitja O'Donoghue (1999), a prominent Australian Aboriginal activist, told her audience at a rural health conference that members of remote Aboriginal communities who are ill experience triple jeopardy. First, they are Aboriginal with all the socioeconomic disadvantages that go with that; secondly, many live far from medical services. And finally, in rural and remote areas in particular, Indigenous people have little involvement in the health services they can access; and even if they do, they feel alienated from mainstream facilities.

Although the distances are much smaller in New Zealand than in Australia, the principle of establishing services within communities rather than moving women out to access services is an important consideration. New Zealand's maternity service is women-centred and aims to meet the individual needs of women and their families. Midwives visit women in their homes if necessary and state support for home birth and primary maternity unit birthing means that women can generally access services in their local community.

Primary healthcare should be affordable

Unlike countries such as the United States, all Australians and New Zealanders have access to 'free' healthcare. However, in

---

Reflective exercise

Imagine you are visiting a foreign country for the first time. You do not speak the language and you do not have an interpreter. You know nothing about the country's health system and very little about its culture. Imagine how it would be for you if you develop a severe urinary tract infection when you are 30 weeks pregnant and begin to have uterine contractions. You know you need urgent medical care but do not have the means to pay for it. What will you do?

Clinical point

Maternity services are often most needed by those who cannot access them. Over 12% of Aboriginal people have to travel more than 100 kilometres to get to a hospital. More than half of Indigenous people living in rural Australia have to travel more than 50 kilometres to a hospital (O'Donoghue 1999). Many do not own or have access to vehicles. It is little wonder then that Aboriginal women are 'poor attendees' at antenatal clinics; they have no means of getting there. A hallmark of quality maternity care is a good transportation system to enable referrals to a higher level of care.

Australia in particular, differences in the quality and quantity of these services, especially with regard to community-based midwifery, hospital waiting times and outpatient services, mean that many must pay extra for services that are better able to meet their needs. For example, until very recently, Western Australia was the only state to offer a publicly funded midwife-led home birth service. In other states, women who prefer this model of care are expected to pay for it, although some insurance companies will offset some of the costs associated with these services.

The picture is very different in New Zealand, where all maternity care is free. All women expect to have their own lead maternity carer (LMC) and 78% choose a midwife LMC (Ministry of Health 2004). Women can choose where they give birth and home birth is also fully funded. Women who do not require referral to specialist care can still choose a private obstetrician to be their LMC instead of the public obstetric service, although the private obstetrician is likely to charge a fee.

Primary healthcare should contribute to the self-reliance and self-determination of communities

Health bureaucrats and funding bodies often pay lip-service to the ideal of community participation in decision-making. Although structures for consultation may exist, stakeholders are rarely delegated any serious power or decision-making authority. Hence the wishes and priorities of the community are often buried in many layers of the consultation process. Moreover, a token 'consumer' on a Board of Health usually has little say in proceedings. For example, the West Australian Government consistently invites the community to join it in the identification of priority issues and to have input into the creation and implementation of programs to solve them (Thorogood 2001). However, the wishes of the community are often overruled if they are not in alignment with the needs of the powerful medical lobby.

There is good evidence (Barnett et al 2005) that community-based initiatives aimed at lowering maternal and perinatal morbidity and mortality are effective, sustainable and more likely to achieve high coverage in the poorest communities than secondary or tertiary hospital-based approaches. The Strong Women, Strong Babies, Strong Culture (SWSBSC) program (see Box 1.1) is a good example of such an approach. The SWSBSC program provides health promotion through local women's groups. This social intervention harnesses the creativity and self-organising skills of Indigenous women living in the Top End of Australia.

New Zealand has established Primary Health Organisations (PHOs) which are required to have strong community governance. However, most have struggled to overcome the dominance of GPs, and primary healthcare remains largely primary medical care. It is for this reason that the midwifery profession has recommended that maternity services remain outside PHO structures until they can demonstrate a more integrated, community-based, multidisciplinary approach.

Some non-government organisations (NGOs) that emerged from the Union health clinics and Maori provider organisations have succeeded in developing a more primary health model, and midwives have been successfully incorporated into their services without losing the midwifery/primary health focus. In 2005 the New Zealand College of Midwives initiated a proposal to the Minister of Health for a joint venture between primary health provider NGOs, Plunket (well child), the Family Planning Association, the Midwifery and Maternity Provider Organisation (MMPO) and Parents Centres (childbirth education) This joint venture is investigating the provision of an integrated well women and child health service for women, pregnant women and children up to five years old (NZCOM 2005). The joint venture would sit parallel to the PHOs and work collaboratively with them, and in this way build their understanding around the provision of primary healthcare.

Primary healthcare should be integrated with other health programs and sectors

If it is to be successful, primary healthcare has to involve horizontal, symmetrical and participatory relationships and direct, active and effective participation of the population it serves. Primary healthcare is multipronged, interdisciplinary, participatory and decentralised. Change will inevitably be slow and it will never come about by the efforts of a single sector or institution, isolated programs or specific services. As O'Donoghue (1999) remarks, none of the factors that lead to ill health, be they geographic, environmental or socio-economic, can be treated in isolation from one another. Nor can they be seen as problems of the here and now, divorced from their history (O'Donoghue 1999).

Midwifery is a primary health workforce

For the vast majority of the world's women, childbearing is a normal, physiological process influenced by culture, family traditions, religion, economics and psychosocial factors. It is a family event that requires a health-oriented approach, even in the presence of co-morbidities. In New Zealand, as in many other countries, midwifery is the primary health workforce whose specific role is to facilitate the transition to parenthood for women and their families regardless of their choices of service provider or place of birth. Australian midwifery is also working to achieve this model of care.

The underlying principles of primary healthcare provision apply to maternity services. That is, services should be provided equitably and at the most accessible level of the healthcare system capable of performing them adequately. It is considered internationally that the person best equipped to provide community-based, appropriate technology, and safe and cost-effective care to women during their reproductive lives, is the person with midwifery skills who lives in the community alongside the women she attends (WHO 1994, 2004).

Maternal health is not simply a question of providing access to technologically oriented biomedical services. It is a public

---

BOX 1.1 Strong women, strong babies

The Strong Women, Strong Babies, Strong Culture Program

In the 1990s the Northern Territory Department of Health and Community Services developed the first community-based intervention initiative, the Strong Women, Strong Babies, Strong Culture Program (SWSBSC). Its aim was for senior women from Aboriginal communities to help younger women prepare for pregnancy and to support pregnant Aboriginal women, by encouraging them to visit clinics for antenatal care early in pregnancy, by providing advice and encouragement about healthy pregnancy management in relation to nutrition (including bush foods), by promoting the adoption of safe practices such as refraining from alcohol and not smoking, and by reinforcing the need to seek adequate, timely medical help. Senior women delivered the program because they were better able to lead a culturally appropriate and attuned package of supporting care and education. The program's structure and content was fluid and altered according to the personal and social circumstances of the women, the available health and social services and the skill level of the SWSBSC women. An independent evaluation of the SWSBSC showed a marked increase in birthweight of the babies whose mothers attended the program. Apart from the benefits for pregnant women and their babies, the SWSBSC has had a social and economic impact in the wider community, providing opportunities for gainful and useful employment, earnings and recognition of the skills of Australian Aboriginal people tackling their own issues (d'Espaignet et al 2003).

Critical thinking exercise

Identify the strengths, weaknesses, opportunities and threats to midwifery services based on a philosophy of primary healthcare in your area. Think about acceptable solutions to problems you identify and the strategic initiatives you would put in place if the primary health midwifery service is to be sustained.

---

health issue, for which community interventions that are cost-effective, woman-focused, appropriate, affordable and sustainable must be implemented. In keeping with primary healthcare's philosophy of self-determination, community-controlled primary healthcare services are initiated, planned and managed by local communities. They aim to deliver high-quality, holistic and culturally appropriate healthcare and have the potential to improve health and wellbeing and reduce delays in seeking and obtaining secondary and tertiary medical services.

The next sections of this chapter provide an overview of the structure and funding of maternity services in New Zealand and Australia.

Midwifery and maternity services in New Zealand

New Zealand has a similar history to other Commonwealth colonies in the development of its maternity services. In the absence of an easily accessible health service due to a scattered, isolated geographic environment, the maternity system was built from personal experience and women helping other women. Maori had a similar history of family or whanau-centred attendance at birth. As with Pakeha, the nature and style of Maori birth attendance differed with each hapu/iwi (family or tribe), depending on their experience and belief systems. In the 1800s and early 1900s there were women (or men for some iwi) who were considered midwives, although few had structured or formal education specific to midwifery. The introduction of midwifery regulation in 1904 was an attempt to provide a more formal framework for midwifery and to give women a better standard of maternity care. This support for midwifery was not to last. A fuller discussion on the early maternity systems can be read in the historical accounts provided by Philippa Mein-Smith (1986), Joan Donley (1986), Elaine Papps and Mark Olssen (1997), Jane Stojanovich (2004) and Sally Pairman (2005).

Legislative and social changes over several decades increasingly diluted the midwifery identity to a point in the early 1980s where it was difficult to distinguish the role of midwifery from that of nursing. Parallel to the demise of midwifery was the loss of society's perception of birth as a normal life process largely belonging to the woman and her family. The struggle to reclaim both the role of midwives and birth as a family event saw women and midwives on a similar journey. This journey shaped the philosophical basis for the development of New Zealand's contemporary women-centred and midwife-led maternity services.

Historical background

As discussed earlier in this chapter, any maternity system must always be seen in the social and political context of the time, and then in the context of the health system overall. In New Zealand the 1990s was a decade notable for economic reforms and considerable changes in the health sector (Gauld 2001). These changes provided a context that was favourable to the development of the current maternity services model, and politically aware women and midwives were able to capitalise on these health sector changes or 'reforms' to create the successful maternity service that New Zealand enjoys today (Pairman & Guilliland 2003).

The health reforms were largely economically driven as New Zealand, along with most Western democracies, considered the level of demand and the spiralling costs of health services unsustainable. However, there were also other drivers for change. These included a competitive (or market model) government economic ideology, health workforce shortages and concern about the growing and largely uncontrolled use of technology. In the maternity services another driver was the presence of a long-established and strong women's health network and consumer rights movement. It was these consumer advocates who initiated and drove the impetus that eventually brought about change in the midwifery and maternity services.

Consumer voice

From the 1920s through the 1980s, women in consumer advocacy organisations voiced their concerns over maternity care. They did not like the impersonal, hospital-controlled birthing culture and they lobbied hard over many years for a more women- and family-centred maternity service (Dobbie 1990). They identified a need for the midwife to be more visible, and demanded that she take a stronger role in providing maternity care (Tully 1999).

For most of these years the midwifery profession was submerged within the nursing profession and not well organised to use its collective voice. While some individual midwives, in particular the home birth midwives, were very clear about what midwifery was and had solid links to the consumer movement, the profession overall was slow to align itself with women. However, as women's organisations became stronger and more universal, midwives also became more organised, and by the late 1980s had become part of this women-led movement. Once politicised, women's groups and the midwifery profession worked together to make birthing services a political issue that could not be ignored (Guilliland & Pairman 1995). Helen Clark, the then Minister of Health, not only understood the foundation of the women's health movement but was also strongly focused on the essential role of primary healthcare. She was sympathetic to the view that birth was a normal life event that should be controlled by each woman and her family in their own community. She understood that in order for this to happen women would need midwives who were educated and resourced in a way that would make this care available and effective.

Maternity choices pre-1990

Prior to 1990, maternity services were almost entirely hospital based. Less than 1% of women had their babies at home, and there were a handful of domiciliary or home birth midwives and general medical practitioners who provided services for these women. General practitioners were able to claim fees from the Maternity Benefit Schedule without any cap for every service they provided, at considerably higher rates than domiciliary midwives, who were funded separately. Domiciliary midwives received funding from the Department of Health for three antenatal visits, labour and birth care, and 12–14 postnatal visits in the first two weeks post partum. As for all women and midwives at the time, they were required by law to be 'supervised' by a medical practitioner, but as home birth was frowned upon it took a brave doctor and a brave midwife to offer a home birth service, as they continually faced hostility from other health professionals.

Women accessed the maternity service mostly through the GP, who confirmed pregnancy and then directed the care in a variety of ways. Some provided the care themselves, although (according to the New Zealand Medical Association's submissions to the Maternity Benefit Tribunal in 1993) at best only about 20% ever offered a full maternity service. A larger number offered antenatal services to 28 weeks gestation before referring the woman to the hospital clinic, private obstetric specialist or a GP colleague who did provide full care.

'Teams' provided the hospital antenatal clinic service. An obstetrician, who delegated the majority of care to registrars or house surgeon trainees, led the teams. Midwives provided support to the medical team. There were very few instances of midwife-led clinics. Antenatal clinics were crowded and women waited hours to be seen. As was the case in most of the Western world, a woman could be seen by as many as 50 health professionals during pregnancy, labour, birth and the postpartum period (Flint 1986). Fathers and other family members struggled to be involved, and the information provided was heavily risk-averse and based on hospital and medical priorities.

Care was also delegated when a woman was in labour. If women were 'normal', midwives conducted the births regardless of who the client was booked under, and this was considered the midwife's role. Doctors could still claim the $300 'delivery' fee even though they were not present. In 1986, midwives, rather than GPs, medical trainees or obstetricians, conducted between 66% and 90% of normal births (NZCOM 1986). However, the rate and type of midwife-managed care depended on hospital protocols, the type of midwifery leadership, the number and availability of obstetricians and the influence that obstetrics had over service delivery. It seldom relied on women's wishes.

All midwifery care, regardless of whether it was for well, compromised or seriously sick women, was organised on a nursing framework, with midwives on rostered shifts for labour and birth and postnatal inpatient care. There was no postpartum midwifery care for women once they left the hospital. Midwives were not known to women and women had no way to access a known midwife. The exception was home birth, but only in the few areas where there was a midwife willing to provide a home-based service. However, in rural or small towns with primary maternity hospitals the care was more personalised, as the community were more likely to know each other. Women who wanted primary care from an obstetrician usually paid for that service and this remains the case today.

Secondary-level services—that is, services for complicated pregnancy, labour and birth or the postnatal period—were provided to women under the care of a hospital-based obstetrician. Although in all major cities and many provincial cities there was a parallel private obstetric system, once in the state-funded service a woman could not choose a known obstetrician, and in fact most women never saw the obstetrician who was deemed to be providing their care. Obstetric medical care was provided mostly by registrars and house surgeons in training. The obstetrician leading the 'team' was not routinely present in the hospital, but 'on call' for registrars to contact if required. This continues in many hospitals today, although it is changing.

Medical education

By the late 1980s, many GPs had a postgraduate diploma in obstetrics, although that was not a legal requirement at the time, and some had no specific education in relation to normal birth, obstetrics or maternity care. The Diploma of Obstetrics was then a six-month course at a tertiary (teaching or base) hospital that focused on acute obstetrics, neonatal care and gynaecological services.

As the medical specialty of obstetrics developed and grew during the 1970s and 1980s, obstetricians slowly displaced the GP in maternity care, particularly in urban hospitals. By 1990 most GPs referred to obstetricians for operative procedures such as forceps and other specialised interventions, as did midwives. Rural GPs kept their obstetric skills for longer but they too eventually dropped out of intrapartum care. A 1990 report to the Canterbury Area Health Board found that GPs in Canterbury provided maternity care to an average of 10 women per year (Canterbury Area Health Board, unpublished minutes of meetings, 1990). While the style and method of service delivery may have been different, the scope of practice of most GPs was essentially the same as that of midwives by 1990. General practitioners have been reluctant to acknowledge this. Furthermore, general practice struggled to attract new graduates to maternity service provision. From 1990 onwards there was a decrease in the number of GPs providing maternity services. This exit of GPs from providing intrapartum care was a worldwide phenomenon and had similar causes in each country. Causes included doctors being less willing to provide 24-hour care (also manifested in the establishment of arrangements to provide care outside of 9 am to 5 pm, such as after-hours clinics and sports clinics) and the perception that general practice was a low-income, lower-status choice than some of the highly specialised options in medicine.

Midwifery education

Midwives' education prior to 1990 was based on a general and obstetric nursing qualification followed by the Advanced Diploma of Nursing (ADN) in which midwifery was a 12-week module. The ADN was theoretically focused on primary health and midwifery philosophy but struggled to provide clinical experience outside the tertiary hospital system (Pairman 2002). Most midwives were unhappy with their training and in 1986 an overwhelming 88% trained overseas (Guilliland 1994). Registered midwives were also disillusioned with their limited role, and increasing numbers left midwifery practice (Department of Education 1987). It had been clear to midwives for decades that midwifery education required a major review, and Sally Pairman's chapter in Papps (Pairman 2002) explains how midwifery education developed and responded to the consumer challenges and legal opportunities provided by the *Nurses Amendment Act 1990*.

The *Nurses Amendment Act 1990*

The environment in the late 1980s was therefore one of increasingly inappropriate education of the primary maternity providers (midwives and GPs), job dissatisfaction, hospitalisation or medicalisation of normal birth services, fragmented and impersonal care for the majority of women, and vociferous consumer dissatisfaction.

The first step the government of the day took to improve the situation was to strengthen the midwifery profession's ability to provide continuity of care. The *Nurses Amendment Act 1990* enabled midwives to practise all the competencies within a midwifery scope of practice. This meant that midwives could offer women the full range of antenatal, labour, birth and postnatal services from conception to six weeks post partum on their own responsibility and without the supervision of a doctor.

The Act also enabled midwives to access hospital beds—that is, to have admission rights for their clients, to prescribe if necessary and to claim for their services from the same government-funded Maternity Benefit Schedule (MBS) that funded medical practitioners. Importantly, the Act also established a pathway for an experimental education program to prepare midwives without first requiring them to undertake a nursing qualification.

Midwifery's right to claim from the MBS was challenged by the New Zealand Medical Association in 1993. The Minister of Health convened the Maternity Benefits Tribunal, and after a week-long legal hearing the Tribunal confirmed that midwives provided the same or similar services and outcomes for pregnant and birthing women as GPs. The Tribunal accepted the principle that if the work was the same then it must be of equal value and therefore midwives were entitled to claim the same payment as medical practitioners from the Maternity Benefit Schedule.

Professionalism

The 1990 Nurses Amendment Act (NAA) was the legislative vehicle for change, but importantly for midwifery its achievement enabled midwives to recognise that real change would only come if practice reflected the wish of consumers to have control over their birthing experiences. If the potential the NAA gave midwifery to develop as a profession was to be realised, fundamental change was required in the way midwifery education and practice was organised.

Midwifery had started to reclaim its identity from nursing in 1989 by separating from the Nurses Association and forming the New Zealand College of Midwives (the College). The College provided a specific focus for both midwives and women who wanted to influence the maternity services to be more women-centred and less medicalised. The College's foundation and its philosophy is that of partnership between midwives and the women for whom they provide services. Women consumers were welcomed as members of the College and were a part of all the College's decision-making structures from the beginning. The aim of the College was to replicate this partnership model within the maternity services, and consequently it was to become a major player in the reformation of the maternity service.

The New Zealand College of Midwives

The College has a unique structure that reflects its beginnings in the women's health movement and its commitment to a partnership way of working. It is the professional organisation for midwives but it is also organised in a way that protects its professional standards and its place in ensuring that women have a safe and enabling maternity experience, without undermining its important roles as the voice of and support for midwives and midwifery. It does this by separating the professional, business and industrial functions into separate but parallel organisations. It is in effect an organisation of structural partnerships, each with their own autonomy and purpose but with midwifery in common. The College is the umbrella under which individual midwives and the profession as a whole are guided. It retains its primary functions of setting and maintaining professional standards, providing professional indemnity cover for practising midwives, and promoting to and providing New Zealand women with an effective and women-responsive midwifery service. It brings its professional voice to its other arms through representation on each structure. A midwife must be a member of the College in order to be able to access membership of the midwifery union (MERAS) or the business arm (MMPO) of the College.

Contemporary maternity services in New Zealand

The New Zealand health system

It is important to understand how the maternity system fits into the overall health services. Health services for New Zealanders are the portfolio of the Minister of Health. The minister is served by a Ministry of Health, which sets strategy and makes policy and funding decisions, which are in turn implemented by the 21 District Health Boards (DHBs) spread throughout New Zealand. Each DHB is funded on a population basis—that is, its funding reflects the numbers and make-up of its community of people, and each Board is responsible for ensuring that the population receives the best possible range, mix and types of services their funding allows. Each DHB must have Primary Health Organisations (PHOs) to manage primary care and coordinate appropriate referrals to the hospital services. People enrol with a PHO in their area if they wish to take advantage of the benefits a PHO can offer, such as subsidised prescriptions and doctors' fees, and coordinated care. Currently most PHOs are centred on GP and practice nurse services but it is envisaged that eventually all primary medical and health services, including maternity, will be coordinated through community-governed PHOs. At the time of writing, community (primary) maternity and well child services remain outside the management of the regional DHBs and the PHOs, and are funded nationally by the Ministry of Health. Other nationally operated services that affect maternity services in general include: the National Screening Unit, which directs policy for all the national screening programs (such as cervical, breast, HIV and antenatal screening); the New Zealand Health Information Service, which manages the health data provided by hospitals and health professionals (such as midwives and GPs); HealthPac, the payment arm of the Ministry, which pays health providers for services; the National Health Committee and the Health Workforce Advisory Committee, which advise the Minister on policy and workforce issues.

The maternity service

The maternity service in New Zealand takes an integrated and women-centred partnership approach. The service is placed within the primary health arena in recognition that birth is a normal life event and that women and their families should direct the care. The service specifications are explicit and within a set budget per woman. Standardised referral guidelines give the framework for consultation and transfer of care to hospital specialists if necessary.

Vision for the maternity service

The government has a vision for the maternity service. The Ministry of Health sets this vision out under Section 88 of the *Public Health and Disability Act 2000*.

> Each woman, and her whanau, will have every opportunity to have a fulfilling outcome to her pregnancy and childbirth, through the provision of services that are safe and based on partnership, information and choice. Pregnancy and childbirth are a normal life-stage for most women, with appropriate additional care available to those women who require it. A Lead Maternity Carer chosen by the woman with responsibility for assessment of her needs, planning her care with her and the care of her baby and being responsible for ensuring provision of Maternity Services, is the cornerstone of maternity care in New Zealand (Ministry of Health 2000, p 11).

The influence of New Zealand's pioneering women and midwives is obvious in this statement. The health system, including maternity, is overseen by a strong code of patient's rights and a culture of informed consent. In 2005 New Zealand has a free maternity service, with equity of access for women to all the levels of care required. These levels of care cover primary care in the community and hospital-based specialist or secondary and tertiary care. All levels of service cross the geographic boundaries of 21 different DHBs and numerous PHOs. See Figure 1.3 for the funding mechanisms of New Zealand's maternity services.

All women can have an LMC to provide and coordinate their maternity care, develop a care plan with them and attend their labour, birth and postpartum period of up to six weeks. The LMC service is a primary health one and therefore is provided mainly in the community. Most antenatal care is in women's homes or in community clinics. If not birthing at home, the majority of women in the first 12 to 48 hours following birth have their postnatal care in the hospital or birthing unit but then receive care at home for four to six weeks. This primary health service is centrally funded by the Ministry of Health, and LMCs claim directly from the Ministry for their service fees. When a woman requires additional medical or hospital care her LMC can choose to provide the care herself, arrange additional medical or other specialist carers but continue to provide midwifery care, or transfer the care to a hospital team including obstetricians, midwives and paediatricians.

Place of birth

New Zealand women have a variety of options as to where they can give birth. Although there are no universal booking criteria for place of birth, the national consultation and referral guidelines provide a screening tool to assist women to make appropriate choices. The maternity facilities or hospitals and their associated services are funded separately from the primary LMC budget and this funding is managed by the DHBs rather than the Ministry.

Birth at home is a mainstream government-supported and funded option. The LMC is almost always a midwife. While many women are supported by consumer-led home birth associations, the majority of women today who choose home birth do so as a natural matter of course and no longer view it as a 'fringe' option. Some 6% to 10% of women have their babies at home.

There are 64 primary birthing or maternity units throughout New Zealand, most located in rural or provincial towns, although women in most big cities also have access to a primary birthing unit either via a DHB or at a privately owned but publicly funded enterprise. A primary unit provides in-house midwifery services for labour, birth and immediate postpartum care. They have no access to on-site obstetric and medical specialists. Approximately 15% of births in 2003 were in primary units. There is an ethnic difference in usage of primary, secondary and tertiary facilities, with 40% of Maori women giving birth in primary facilities—twice the national average (Ministry of Health 2004).

Secondary facilities or hospitals are generally in provincial towns or the smaller cities. The secondary service provides some additional specialist obstetric and midwifery services for women experiencing complications, but transfers women and babies with intensive care needs to tertiary facilities.

There are five tertiary facilities in New Zealand. While all services are provided, the tertiary hospitals are specialists in high-technological services such as neonatal intensive care, infertility and high-dependency obstetric care.

Section 88, *Public Health and Disability Act 2000*

As discussed above, the maternity service framework in New Zealand follows a women-centred continuity of care model. Section 88 of the *New Zealand Public Health and Disability Act 2000* is the legislative framework that outlines the model of care and gives notice of the terms and conditions for the provision of maternity services. The Ministry of Health sets these terms, conditions and fees after consultation with the New Zealand College of Midwives and the New Zealand Medical Association.

The Maternity Advice Notice, or Section 88 as it is referred to, provides a nationally consistent set of service specifications and is the practice framework for midwives, GPs, obstetricians, paediatricians, anaesthetists and radiologists. It includes 20 items that cover issues such as arrangements for antenatal care, health promotion, personal and cultural safety, education, referral, screening and planning. It does not detail or describe specific aspects of care or practice but provides a generic blueprint for service delivery. The New Zealand College of Midwives provides a detailed framework for midwifery practice (NZCOM 2005a). This includes a statement of philosophy, definition of midwifery scope of practice, a code of ethics, detailed standards of practice and decision points for midwifery care.

The Maternity Advice Notice in general:

● specifies all aspects of services to be provided by LMCs— it outlines all expected services from the woman's first contact with the maternity services until discharge and referral of her baby to the well child services. If the LMC cannot provide any aspect of care, they must ensure that others provide the care.

● identifies quality indicators and processes—the notice expects all LMCs to take part in professional quality assurance mechanisms such as NZCOM's Midwifery Standards Review.

● sets out prices and payment rates—the Notice has a comprehensive and integrated pricing structure that recognises such things as miscarriage, referral, transfer of care, place of birth, and rural and travel requirements.

● provides a set of referral guidelines—these guidelines were drawn up by all maternity providers and professionals in 1996 and are a comprehensive set of guidelines on conditions/circumstances that require referral based on a three-way conversation between the woman and her family, the LMC and the obstetrician or specialist to whom she is being referred or transferred. A Level One referral is optional; a Level Two referral requires the LMC to recommend to the woman that she consult a specialist; and a Level Three referral requires an LMC to recommend to a woman that her care be transferred to the secondary or tertiary service.

● specifies a generic access to hospital facilities agreement—this is an agreement between the hospital facility and the LMC on the conditions under which the LMC can access the hospital for their clients.

● provides claim form templates—LMCs must provide information on the service they provided, including outcomes, in order to claim their fees.

Women and their families have a range of LMC choices, including the following:

1 *Self-employed or independent midwife*—midwives specialise in attending women and their family for 'normal' or physiological pregnancy and birth. They can provide all care during pregnancy, labour, birth and post partum. Care may be in the woman's home or in the midwife's clinic rooms. Midwives can also provide care for women with complicated maternity conditions alongside a specialist in either the public or the private health system.

2 *Family doctor or GP*—GPs also provide care for normal pregnancy and birth and for some existing medical

---

BOX 1.2 Section 88 specifications

The service specifications of the Section 88 Notice provide that:

▶ LMCs receive written authorisation from the Ministry of Health to provide maternity services, as authorised practitioners, in order to be able to work under the conditions of the notice.

▶ Payment is made to authorised practitioners via Healthpac, the business unit of the Ministry of Health, which administers payment for primary care services.

▶ Each women chooses an LMC, who works with the woman to assess, plan and provide her primary maternity care, coordinate and arrange access to additional care as required. This allows for continuity of carer throughout the maternity care episode.

▶ An LMC can be either a midwife, a GP with a diploma in obstetrics, or an obstetrician.

▶ Care is from the woman's registration with an LMC to four to six weeks post partum according to clinical need. There are four modules of care, with the expectation that all four will be provided by the same carer.

▶ In the first trimester prior to registration with an LMC and for all consultations with obstetric specialists, the service is funded on a fee-for-service basis.

▶ After the first trimester, the payment structure is modular and based on: the second and third pregnancy trimester; labour and birth; and postnatal care. Each module of care is capped at a set price but there are a variety of mechanisms to enable LMC work to be recompensed if it falls outside these module definitions.

▶ Childbirth education other than the usual information provided by the woman's individual LMC also has a separate budget, and a variety of educators contract with the Ministry to provide this service.

▶ A woman can only have one LMC at a time but there is provision for her to change at any time.

The choice of LMC depends to some extent on where a woman lives, as the full range of options is not available in all areas. There is a nationwide government-funded telephone service that provides women with information on LMCs available in their area. This is the 0800 MUM2BE number. The College also provides this service nationally. A full copy of the Maternity Advice Notice is accessible from the Ministry of Health website (www.moh.govt.nz) and more information about midwifery practice in New Zealand is available from the NZCOM website (www.midwife.org.nz).

---

provide medical care for women experiencing a normal pregnancy. They attend labour as needed and are present for the birth with a core/staff or self-employed midwife. They share care with hospital or self-employed midwives. Care provided by private obstetricians usually involves a cost to the woman.

4 *Hospital LMC midwives*—some maternity hospitals offer primary LMC services. They do this in a variety of ways, including:

● 'Know Your Midwife', sometimes referred to as KYM, Domino, continuity of care, or one-on-one, schemes. All or most visits will be with the same midwife, who will also attend the labour, birth and postpartum visits in hospital and at home.

● midwifery teams, where women receive care from a small team of midwives, generally no more than three or four, but possibly up to six. The woman usually gets to meet them all. Team care has decreased over the years as women have become accustomed to one-on-one care from a known LMC.

5 *Hospital specialists*—hospital specialists provide care for women whose pregnancies and births involve complications. Other hospital staff (such as midwives, registrars and house surgeons) will be involved in the care. Pregnancy care is usually provided by the hospital team at hospital antenatal clinics but is often also in collaboration or a shared care arrangement with the LMC midwife or GPs in the community, particularly if the woman lives rurally. Care during labour and birth is provided by hospital staff or an independent midwife under the supervision of the specialist who is on duty at the time.

6 *Core or hospital staff midwives*—if women are having their babies in a hospital with their own LMC, their LMCs all rely on the core midwife to facilitate the experience for them as they move from a community to hospital service. The core midwife is on rostered duties for either 8 or 12 hours depending on hospital employment practices. She provides support and back-up for the LMC midwife and full midwifery care for the women with doctor LMCs.

LMCs have a range of experience. Some will continue to provide care in all situations and some will transfer the care of the women to the hospital obstetric team because of the women's need for more intensive obstetric care. The core midwife can then provide the secondary or tertiary midwifery services for those women, with the LMC midwife remaining in a support role.

Midwives have for several years consistently represented over 78% of the LMCs in New Zealand. As LMCs they have a contractual relationship not only with the women for whom they provide care, but also with the Ministry of Health, which provides payment for the services provided under the Notice.

In order for midwives to provide care as LMCs within the continuity-of-care model, and meet the conditions of the Section 88 Notice, most choose to work as self-employed

problems that may complicate pregnancy, such as diabetes or asthma. General practitioners provide care in their practice rooms/surgery, attend labour when needed and are present for the birth with an independent midwife or a core/staff midwife. They share postnatal care with hospital- or self-employed midwives.

3 *Private obstetrician*—obstetricians specialise in complications during pregnancy and birth but can also

practitioners. Midwives generally work in with a midwife partner who provides back-up, and these pairs of midwives often work within larger group practices for further collegial support.

Midwifery practice management systems

Because the maternity service in New Zealand is fully funded by the government, the midwives and doctors who provide the service require a system to claim their fees. The Ministry of Health, via Health Pac, provides a system for all medical benefits claims, including maternity. However, it is a very big organisation and claiming is complex. As a result the midwifery profession and some individual businesses have developed a more midwifery-focused payment system. The College practice management system, the Midwifery and Maternity Provider Organisation (MMPO), is the largest of these and is underpinned by the belief that payment systems should be integrated with quality control mechanisms.

The Midwifery and Maternity Provider Organisation (MMPO)

The concept of the MMPO was initiated by the College and formed in 1997 as a separate limited liability company with its own governance structure. The purpose of the MMPO is to support the business side of midwifery and it is essentially a practice management system for midwives who carry caseloads and provide continuity of care based in the community. In 2005 there were 550 midwives throughout New Zealand using this service and it is now the largest non-government maternity provider in the country. Some midwife members are employed by District Health Boards or Community Trusts and the MMPO also manages the midwife claims for these employers. However, most members are self-employed and the MMPO manages all their fee claims from the MBS and deals with Health Pac directly on their behalf.

The claiming system works from a set of maternity notes held by each woman that the midwife uses for day-to-day care. All data is in triplicate, so one copy remains with the woman as her birth story, one is kept by the midwife as her clinical and legal record and the third is sent to the MMPO for fee-claiming purposes and for clinical data entry into the NZCOM

midwifery database. Increasingly, midwives are choosing to enter their own data electronically. Midwives receive their fee payment together with a report on their clinical outcomes and statistics, which they take to their annual Midwifery Standards Review.

The New Zealand College of Midwives contracts the MMPO to enter the clinical data for its midwifery database. It then uses the database to produce a national report on midwife practice outcomes. Any themes or issues that result from the analysis of the aggregated and anonymous data form the basis of the College's continuing education program.

Other practice management or fee-claiming systems

There are other midwifery or maternity provider organisations that provide business services to self-employed midwives. In Auckland, New Zealand's largest city, there are alternative options. The Mothers and Midwives Association (MAMA) is a consumer and midwife organisation that also provides the College with midwife outcome data for the national database. South Auckland Maternity Collective Association Ltd (SAMCAL) is a business organisation directed by midwives and obstetricians providing their members with payment management services. River Ridge and Waterford Birthing Centres in Hamilton are midwifery owned and run businesses that also operate maternity birthing units. There are also privately owned but government-funded maternity-led birthing units scattered throughout the country that both employ midwives and give access to self-employed LMCs. Birthcare in Auckland, and Huntley and Charlotte Jean in Alexandra, are examples of early entrepreneurial thinking that established midwifery-led units for women to access midwifery care in a primary health setting.

Midwifery workforce

The midwife of today can choose a range of working roles. She (over 99% of midwives are women) can use her full scope of practice and accompany the woman into whatever service she requires wherever she requires it. As an LMC she can provide primary, secondary and tertiary midwifery services (often to the same woman) if she feels she has the capability.

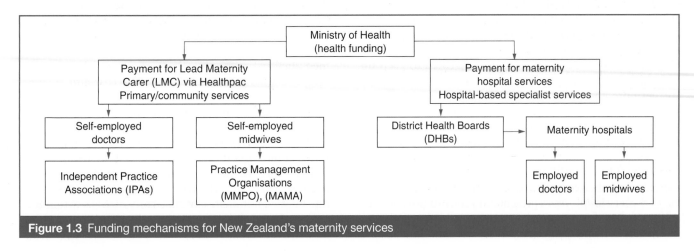

Figure 1.3 Funding mechanisms for New Zealand's maternity services

However, she has the choice of which level of care she provides, and can transfer care or ask for support if necessary. She can provide birthing support to women in hospital and/or home births across DHB and PHO boundaries. The hospital or core midwife is the essential link between the primary and secondary interface and in the LMC partnership with women clients. The core midwife provides advice and consultation to midwife LMCs when extra care is required, and full midwifery services for women with medical LMCs and secondary care needs.

This integrated service is the result not only of the professional changes enabled by the NAA as discussed above, but also the health reforms and the way in which services were funded. Understanding the funding and contractual nature of the service is essential to understanding why midwives succeeded in giving women and midwives the service they have today.

Midwifery was New Zealand's first workforce 'redesign'—that is, the first non-medical discipline in New Zealand to get practice autonomy, full prescribing rights, referral to diagnostics and access to hospital facilities and government fees for services. Midwives have many work options. In 2002, Nursing Council (which regulated midwifery prior to 2004) workforce statistics stated that 52.9% of midwives reported working in core midwifery, 39.9% in caseload midwifery, 2.9% in administration and management, 3.3% in education, 0.6% in professional advice/policy development, and 0.4% in research (Nursing Council of New Zealand 2004). There were 2107 actively practising in midwifery in total for that year. Although only 24% of midwives identified as self-employed to the Nursing Council, claiming patterns in 2002 to the Ministry of Health's payment organisation (Health Pac) for service fees identify that some 42% of the midwifery workforce were self-employed for at least some of their working time (NZCOM 2005b).

These 42% of midwives provided LMC services for 73% of birthing women in that same year. General practitioners provided LMC services for 9% of women and obstetricians provided 14% (NZHIS 2004). This is a complete reversal of the workforce picture since the 1980s, where doctors were reported as the main provider of maternity care. In 2003 the workforce picture was still changing and midwives were 78% of LMCs, GPs 7.9% and obstetricians 7.8% (NZHIS 2005). In 2005 the impression was that even more midwives are now the LMC, and as a result midwifery is under considerable stress, as midwife numbers have not increased to keep up with this phenomenal growth in demand (NZCOM 2005b). Furthermore, the fees and structure in Section 88 have not been reviewed for three years and therefore none of this changing pattern of workloads has received remuneration or recognition.

Industrial representation

Since 2003 midwives have had their own midwifery union, the Midwifery Employee Representation and Advisory Service (MERAS). The formation of the union enabled negotiation specifically for midwifery-centred services and in 2005 the union had its own collective agreement for midwives only. This agreement was a national multi-employer collective agreement (MECA) involving all DHBs. Prior to this, employed midwives relied on the Nurses Organisation to negotiate on their behalf under a variance to the collective nursing agreement. The MERAS presence in negotiations immediately influenced the way in which the midwifery workforce was seen and described, as it insisted on a more professionally based agreement reflecting standards of practice and quality assurance policies.

Outcomes of midwifery care in New Zealand

For 15 years, tens of thousands of New Zealand women have had a midwife as their primary caregiver. Contrary to the expected view and much to the dismay of midwives, this continuity of midwifery care model doesn't appear, on the face of it, to have stopped the increasing caesarean rates experienced throughout the Western world. It is not clear why this is so but there are several theories. Six possibilities are proposed below.

1 In 1996, just five years after midwives had gained autonomy, the model of maternity care was changed at a national level to introduce the LMC model. These changes were introduced without any supportive structures provided to the midwives, who were expected to completely change their way of practice from a tertiary/secondary facility-based service to a community-based, women-centred model. Consequently, some midwives simply moved their hospital practice habits into the women's homes.

2 The public was given very little information or education on the new systems—both the implications of midwifery autonomy and the structure and functioning of the LMC system—which would have boosted public confidence in the changes.

3 While midwifery was given access to claiming fees for service from the same schedule as doctors, unlike general medical practice (a similar model of practice with which it is reasonable to compare) midwifery did not receive postgraduate or continuing education funding, information technology (IT) grants or practice management system support. Nor were there any subsidies for locum relief or allowances for rural inequities.

4 Hospitals used the new LMC system to cost shift expensive secondary care services onto the community LMC without any supportive systems for collaborative care.

5 As more midwives in the community took on normal births at the request of women, the obstetrician's private source of income from these women started to decrease. Even GPs, who had previously enjoyed largely uncontested dominance of maternity care, particularly antenatal care, also started to lose clients as women chose midwives as their LMCs.

6 Probably most importantly, relationships between GPs, obstetricians and midwives were deliberately set up to be in competition under the newly competitive health environment of that time, and without any thought about the effect this would have on service delivery. Hostility from doctors was directed at midwives as the 'newcomers'. This had the effect of compromising doctors' trust in midwives' opinions and referrals. There was an obvious conflict of interest when, on the one hand, obstetricians lost clients to midwives and on the other hand, midwives consulted with obstetricians over some of those same women. This made working relationships stressful. Stressful environments influence decision-making and clinical judgement, so it is not surprising that all practitioners resorted to the use of technology (Degeling et al 1998).

In addition, the way in which outcome data are published in New Zealand does not allow for examination of the long-term impact of midwifery's primary and public health focus. Intervention rates are presented as rising annually but trends over several years are not explored. When all data are examined together, a different picture emerges. For example, there was a 5.2% increase in caesarean sections between 1988 and 1996 and before the advent of LMC care. Following the introduction of LMC care, the rise to 2003 (the latest data available) is slightly higher at 6.2%. However, the largest percentage increase in caesareans was likely to have been even earlier, between the 1970s and the 1980s. St Helens Hospital in Auckland published its caesarean section rates for the Jubilee celebrations in 1981, and these showed that from 1970 to 1981 there was an increase of 11.2% (Donley 1986). Obviously this rise had nothing to do with midwife LMCs, since there were none.

It is reasonable to assume from New Zealand's history that the rising caesarean rate cannot be laid at midwifery's door alone. It is also reasonable to assume that midwifery today may have had an influence in keeping intervention rates contained. In the debate on rising rates of caesarean section, commentators have failed to notice that over the past few years intervention rates in other areas have been contained or decreased (Ministry of Health 1999a,b; NZHIS 2005). Instrumental vaginal births have decreased from 11.8% in 1988 to 9.9% in 2003; inductions have decreased from 22.1% in 1997 to 20.1% in 2003; and epidurals have only marginally increased from 23.3% in 1997 to 24.4% in 2003 (MOH 1999a,b; NZHIS 2005). As discussed previously, exclusive breastfeeding continues to improve and immunisation rates at six weeks are high.

The Maternal and Newborn Information System (MNIS) has been collecting data on LMC provider type since 1999 (Ministry of Health 2001; NZHIS 2003, 2004, 2005). The data show that where New Zealand's intervention rate has increased, it has increased for all provider types. Furthermore, the outcome data are highly variable from region to region— further evidence that birth outcomes have multifactorial influences (NZHIS 2005). All published data where LMCs are identified by profession both prior to and post 1996 confirm that midwifery outcomes are similar to or better than those of GPs (Ministry of Health 1999, 2001; NZHIS 2003, 2004, 2005; National Women's Hospital 2000; Wellington Women's Hospital 1998).

Ministry of Health and DHB data on outcomes also indicate continuing improvement in the following:

- decrease in perinatal mortality
- significant decrease in SIDS
- decreased antenatal admissions for serious complications
- sustained decrease in admissions of very sick babies to neonatal intensive care.

Furthermore, recent trend research from 1980 to 2001 confirmed markedly decreased rates of small for gestational age babies for Maori, Pacific Island and lower socio-economic groups of women (Mantell et al 2004). Although the gap between Maori and Pakeha baby outcomes in relation to prematurity remain unacceptably large, it appears that Maori rates have improved. Teenage pregnancy is slowly decreasing, and outcomes for young Maori women have improved over

Clinical point

In 2003, birth rates in New Zealand were as follows:

Type of birth/procedure	Rate (%)		
	LMC midwife	LMC GP	LMC obstetrician
Normal birth	73.5	70.5	52.7
Stillbirth	(identical rates)		
Total caesarean	16.8	17.6	31.4
Forceps ventouse	8.6	11.4	15.1
Epidural	22.9	31.3	43.4
Episiotomy	9.5	17.0	18.0
(Source: NZHIS 2005)			

TABLE 1.1 Comparative rates of caesarean section and unassisted vaginal birth between primary units in New Zealand and overall hospital rates for New Zealand and Australia, 2002

Hospitals	Unassisted vaginal birth (%)	Caesarean section (%)
New Zealand primary* (15% of births 2002)	71.0	8.03
Overall national hospital rates		
New Zealand (*n* = 53,039)	67.7	22.7
Australia (*n* = 250,758)	61.7	27.0

* Excluded St George Private Hospital New Zealand.
(Sources: AIHW 2004; NZHIS 2004)

Critical thinking exercise

1   How can women's voices be heard within the maternity service in general and by the midwifery profession specifically? What influences do you think society itself brings to bear on the way birth is experienced and midwifery is practised?

2   Do you think the way maternity services are funded can influence the practice of midwifery? If so, how can we ensure this influence is used in a positive way? Imagine you are a self-employed midwife about to set up practice. What can you do to ensure you utilise your income potential while providing optimal care?

these years also. Maori, young women and women from lower socio-economic groups are more likely to choose a midwife for their LMC (NZHIS 2003). Women's satisfaction with maternity services has increased over three national surveys (MOH 1999b, 2003), as has the intensity of that satisfaction.

The intangible effects of these positive experiences on women are hard to quantify. It is not unreasonable to postulate that healthy, informed and happy women are also empowered women and that empowerment has a positive influence on both women's mothering and society in general (Guilliland 2005).

Health funding: Australia and New Zealand

Some similarities exist today between the health systems of Australia and New Zealand. For example, both countries meet the cost of publicly funded health through taxation rather than social insurance; government provides for both secondary and tertiary care. General practitioners act as 'gatekeepers' to control access to general medical secondary services, and specialist staff work in both the public and the private sphere (Davies & Hindle 1999). However, major differences have also emerged between Australia and New Zealand in the funding of the health systems, and these have influenced the way in which maternity services can be provided.

New Zealand has a unique constitutional relationship between the Crown and the Maori people—the Treaty of Waitangi, signed in 1840. No such treaty exists in Australia between the Aboriginal and Torres Strait Island people and the Crown. The Treaty of Waitangi has, over time, fostered innovative approaches to healthcare, resulting in greater autonomy for Indigenous people over their own healthcare and lowering disparities in health status (Davies & Hindle 1999). Davies and Hindle (1999) outline five other important differences:

● New Zealand has a unitary national system of funding, whereas Australia divides responsibilities between the state and Commonwealth governments.
● From 1993 New Zealand distinguished between purchaser and provider agencies but this changed in 2000, when removing this split between purchaser and provider was one of the focal points of that year (Devlin et al 2001).
● Private health insurance in New Zealand is not subsidised or regulated by government, as it is in Australia.
● New Zealand makes greater use of co-payments, in particular with respect to GPs. However, there is no provision for co-payments in maternity, except for private obstetricians, who can charge women in addition to the government maternity payment.
● New Zealand's publicly owned hospitals are constrained in their ability to deliver services to private patients.

Whether by virtue of its isolation, or the fact that it has a smaller, less cumbersome economy than Australia without the two-tier confusion of state and Commonwealth divisions in funding, New Zealand embarked on cutting-edge health reform 20 years ago. It led the charge in forging market-based health reforms in the 1980s, and also led the way in rejecting the same model of economic rationalism in health (Ham 1997b; Hornblow 1997; Malcolm 1998). Over the past decade, New Zealand's health sector has undergone a series of structural reforms and rollbacks: first an area health board system, then a competitive internal market system with regional health authorities and crown health enterprises (1993–96), a centralised purchasing system (1997–2000), and from 2002, a system of DHBs.

Health funding in Australia

A 1999 World Health Organization (WHO) report suggested that Australia was going the wrong way by limiting government funding of healthcare in favour of 'user pays', by retaining fee-for-service payment of providers, and by promoting markets in the private sector (WHO 1999b). Many of the leaders in health policy in Australia are also highly critical of Australia's stance on health funding (Baum et al 1998; Deeble 2002; Duckett 1997; Gray 2004; Leeder 1998; Nelson 1998; Smith 1998a, b).

According to one well-known health economist, Australia's health sector is characterised by government intervention limiting and constraining, through regulation, the size and behaviour of the market. Transactions are characterised by asymmetrical information, and asymmetrical power. Service provision is dominated by politically effective individuals and organisations, and private health insurance is 'bizarre' (Richardson 2002, p 10). The former Dean of Australia's largest medical faculty agrees when he claims that: 'The decision to subsidise all private health insurance may have other negative effects. It is plausible that the Commonwealth will seek to recover the billions it pays for private health insurance by decreasing the support it offers public hospitals' (Leeder 2002, p 7).

In addition to undermining the extent to which Medicare covers the costs of services, the system has generated significant health inflation since 1999, and the policies that are in place ensure a continuation of this trend. The indications are that Australia is on the road to becoming one of the higher spenders among OECD countries, compared with being an average spender a decade ago (Gray 2004).

Medicare is an insurance system. It is not a health delivery system. Over time Medicare has come to be seen by the public, politicians and providers as encompassing *everything* in relation to Australian healthcare—in other words, that it *is* the whole healthcare system. It is a financial arrangement for ensuring universal access to services on equitable terms. It does not *provide* those services—that is the job of the health services themselves and the health professionals (Deeble 2002).

In single-payer systems, governments generally have the capacity and the will to regulate and control budget outlays and to keep overall costs under control. In multi-payer systems, no one is in charge and no single agency has the power to control total expenditures. Funders are usually interested in their own costs, not the costs of the system as a whole. Under these circumstances, the easiest way of reducing costs is to shift them to other payers. Cost shifting replaces cost control, with expensive and regressive results (Gray 2004).

The situation in 2005 is continuing to cause concern, as illustrated on the front cover of the *Australian Doctors Reform Society Journal* 2005 (see Fig 1.4).

A national review of the role of primary healthcare in health promotion in Australia concluded that in areas of effectiveness, efficiency and equity of disease prevention and health promotion in Australia, there have been significant limitations caused by the lack of a more coherent, adequately resourced primary healthcare sector (NCEPH 1992). The same review found the 'four basic principles of primary health (collaborative networking; consumer and community involvement; a balancing of healthcare priorities between the micro and immediate on one hand, and the macro and

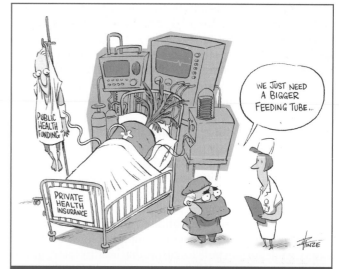

Figure 1.4 Cartoon depicting the state of health funding in favour of private health in Australia, 2005 (Doctors Reform Society 2005) © Hinze/Scratch! Media (www.scratch.com.au)

long term on the other; a partnership relationship with the secondary and tertiary sectors)' to be seriously lacking in primary care in Australia (Baum et al 1998).

The problems facing Australia in the new millennium were outlined by the Director General for Health in New South Wales in Sydney in July 1999 (Reid 1999), who stressed that his views applied to Australia in a general sense. The eight major issues in his address are summarised below in an effort to give an overview of the extent of the problems facing Australia today. Seven years later these issues are as important and as urgent as they were in 1999:

● providing a better balance between acute care, community care and prevention. In changing the focus from supply issues to demand benefits, a long-term efficiency in health spending would be guaranteed.

● addressing the neglect of three groups within the population, namely Aboriginal people, people with mental illness, and rural and regional communities. This would involve trying to decrease the widening gap in health status between the Indigenous and non-Indigenous populations, reducing the rate of suicide of the young, and funding and a level of commitment by the public sector to give a degree of certainty to the continuation of appropriate services to rural and regional areas.

● integrating healthcare services. This can be improved by linking various service providers.

● refocusing attention on the effectiveness of care and assessing the most effective way of providing quality in healthcare. This involves the development and use of clinical indicators, clinical governance, and credentialling and accreditation processes.

● improving the funding arrangements in Australia. Currently, funds are spent more on the basis of functional responsibility than true need. To address the problem of cost shifting between states and Commonwealth, a single pool of dollars for health is called for.

● clarifying the role of private health insurance, taking account of the increased Commonwealth investment, the real ability of people to choose within the system, and the increasing demands being placed on public hospitals

● improving workforce planning, addressing in particular restrictive trade practices, and the undersupply and multiskilling of health professionals

● managing the location, range and mix of tertiary services, and the management and monitoring of the introduction of technology (Reid 1999).

In 2005 declining bulk billing through Medicare and increasing user charges had serious implications for access and equity, while current policies ensure that health costs continue to outpace inflation. While Australian policy makers and interest groups argue counterproductively about financing channels, overseas debates have moved to the question of long-term sustainability. The central challenge for the health systems of all OECD countries is how to provide high-quality, appropriate healthcare to all citizens at an affordable price in the face of rapid technological advance. Radical reforms, involving much higher levels of public management and control, are being suggested (Gray 2004).

The split between Commonwealth and state and territory health funding

In 1946 the Australian Constitution was amended to enable the Commonwealth to provide health services and benefits without changing the status of the states and territories in

this regard. Consequently, two levels of government have overlapping responsibilities in the area of funding healthcare. The states and territories are responsible for: delivering public health services; regulating health professionals; public acute and psychiatric hospital services and community services such as school health, dental health, maternal and child health, and environmental health programs. The Commonwealth funds most medical services out of hospital via the Medical Benefits Schedule (MBS) and Medicare, and the Pharmaceutical Benefits Schedule (PBS) in addition to most health research. It also finances and regulates care for older people and the disabled.

In 1999 a non-means-tested rebate of 30% of the cost of private health insurance premiums was introduced in Australia. The initial cost to the public was $1.6 billion, an amount that could have financed approximately 10,000 new public hospital beds. Unfortunately, this measure failed to significantly increase private health insurance coverage. In fact, by March 2000, the insured population had increased by only 2.1% (Gray 2004). (Private health insurance can cover private and public hospital charges and a portion of medical costs for inpatient services. Private insurance can also cover allied health and paramedical services as well as some aids and appliances.)

In July 2000, the Commonwealth Government made a further bid to encourage Australians to take out private health insurance, running a public publicity campaign called *Run for Cover*, at a cost of $8.7 million. It was suggested that people joined up because they were afraid their access to healthcare would be jeopardised if they did not have private insurance (Deeble 2002). Also, there was to be an economic incentive of a 2% tax penalty for those who did not join. This campaign for Lifetime Health Cover (LHC) increased private insurance

TABLE 1.2 Medicare spending increases from 2003–2004 after the introduction of the Commonwealth Government's Medicare 'safety net'		
	Spending Jul–Sep 2004 ($ m)	**Rise on same quarter 2003 (%)**
TOTAL Medicare	2,440.0	12.8
Professional attendances		
General practice	1,120.0	6.1
Therapeutic procedures		
Specialist doctors	411.0	15.1
Radiology	373.0	9.7
Pathology	380.0	11.4
Obstetrics	32.1	71.1
Ophthalmology	28.5	14.8
Orthopaedics	26.4	6.9
(Source: Quinlivan 2004, *BRW*, 11–17 November, p 26; based on Australian HIC data.)		

coverage by 50% to 45.8% of the population by September 2000 (Gray 2004).

In an effort to increase the public uptake of private health insurance and promote bulk billing rates in Australia, the Commonwealth Government introduced a series of policy changes beginning in 2000. (Bulk billing is a foundational pillar of Medicare because it is the mechanism through which citizens can access services without being required to pay at the point of service.)

In August 2000, 'Gap' insurance for in-hospital medical services was reintroduced. And in March 2004 the Medicare 'safety net' came into being. This was designed to protect the public from heavy non-hospital out-of-pocket health costs after these costs had reached $300 per annum for low- and middle-income families and $700 per annum for high-income earners. It was also intended to increase the rate of bulk billing. When yearly costs had reached the levels stated above, the government was to pay 80% of the gap between the normal Medicare rebate refund and the actual medical care fee. This 'safety net' policy was so badly designed and so severely misused by doctors that in November 2004 the Health Insurance Commission (HIC) reported the blowout in expenditure shown in Table 1.2. Note the extraordinary increases in Medicare spending in relation to obstetrics.

Health funding in Australia is a very complex business, due to several factors. There is a level of Commonwealth funding and a level of state funding. Within these two funding systems there is the partial funding of private health services, as described above. Figure 1.5 is a simplified representation of the current Australian model for health funding.

Funding midwifery

Midwifery in Australia is similar to midwifery in New Zealand pre-1990, although a few 'cracks' are beginning to appear and small examples of system change are beginning to emerge. Australia's funding model, outlined above, affects the development of midwifery services in the following ways:

- The only access to funding for midwifery is through each state acute health services budget (except the WACMP; Thiele & Thorogood 1998, 2001 (see below), and the Northern Women's Community Midwifery Program, Adelaide, SA (Church & Nixon 2002)). This means that women don't have the opportunity to choose a midwife as their LMC as they do in New Zealand. Where continuity-of-care models have been implemented in Australia, the area health services may draw up an annualised salary agreement for the midwives in the Midwifery Group Practices and their funding continues to come out of the acute services budget for public hospitals. In addition to this, there is not an agreed 'salary' for midwives offering these midwifery models of care, and even within states the salary package differs in terms of 'on call' costs between 25% and 29% both between and within states (SA and NSW and within NSW). There are also different levels of base rates, again between and within states. For example, some Midwifery Group Practitioners are paid a base rate for Level 8 midwifery and others a Clinical Midwifery Consultant base rate (NSWNA 2005, personal communication).

- The governments in Australia do not recognise women's choice of home birth and therefore there is no rebate or subsidy that these women can access. In general, this service saves the government at least $3000 per birth; however, women who wish to have a home birth pay

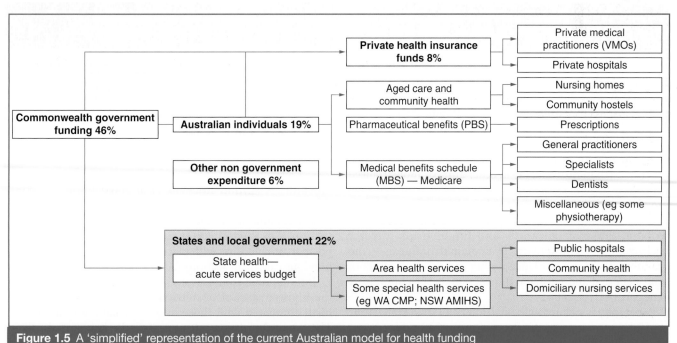

Figure 1.5 A 'simplified' representation of the current Australian model for health funding

for the privilege out of their own pockets. Some private health insurance companies are currently reviewing their policies to possibly include home birth within the next couple of years (private health insurance companies 2005, personal communication).

- Professional indemnity cover for independently practising midwives was lost in July 2001. This means that home birth is offered by midwives who do not have access to professional indemnity cover. This situation may change with the introduction of home birth within publicly funded Midwifery Group Practice Models. (There are a small number of home birth services available in the Northern Territory, Western Australia and South Australia, and a publicly funded home birth service commenced in Sydney at the time of writing in 2005.)

The Community Midwifery Program in Western Australia (WACMP) and the Northern Women's Midwifery Program in Adelaide, South Australia, have both struggled to cement a secure funding source with the health departments who fund them in those respective states.

Urgent reform is required in Australia to allow midwives to access Medicare provider numbers, so that women can choose for themselves to have a midwife caregiver for pregnancy, labour and birth. So far the negotiations for Medicare provider numbers have hit huge resistance from all sectors of the Australian medical profession. Until midwives in Australia have the same status as their medical counterparts offering the same service in maternity care, they will not achieve equal pay for equal work.

The success of the South Australian Midwifery Group Practices within the Women's and Children's Hospital in Adelaide, and the Ryde and Belmont Midwifery Group Practices in New South Wales, offer a ray of hope in the bid to offer women the opportunity to book with a midwife and have more continuity of midwifery care in Australia (at the time this book goes to press).

The impact of funding on maternal and infant outcomes

Medicare is the universal taxpayer-funded health insurance system that offers subsidised private medical services and free public hospital care for all Australians. Its guiding principles are equal access to equal care for equal need.

Having a baby in Australia is by any standards a safe event.[1] Consequently, the measure of a safe and effective outcome for childbirth in Australia (as in other affluent industrialised countries) has shifted its focus from a measure of maternal mortality to measures of maternal morbidity.

Notwithstanding, there are some women—Indigenous women, those of culturally and linguistically diverse backgrounds, and those living in remote and rural areas—who are more likely to experience poorer outcomes in terms of both maternal and perinatal mortality than the community generally (AIHW 2004).

Morbidity associated with birth interventions (Waterstone et al 2001) and long-term effects of operative and caesarean birth include increased risk of hospitalisation with infective

---

> **BOX 1.3 Community midwifery**
>
> **The WA Community Midwifery Program, 1996–2005**
>
> In terms of a national strategy, the Community Midwifery Program in Western Australia (WACMP) provides a proven template of excellence in maternity care, and is a readily adaptable model for duplication in both urban and regional/rural locations. The WACMP was specifically established to provide a publicly funded home birth service.
>
> The Community Midwifery Program (CMP) has been providing one-to-one continuous care from community midwives since 1996, primarily for women who meet the criteria for home birthing.
>
> Two evaluations so far have shown it to be both a successful model of care with good outcomes, and highly valued by the women who utilise the service.
>
> The CMP's guiding philosophy is that childbirth is, in the majority of cases, a normal life event, which, left to nature, will proceed to an uncomplicated outcome. This is underpinned by providing expert midwifery care that respects the individual needs of women and their families by supporting their emotional, social and cultural needs.
>
> The CMP is fully government funded and offers primary community midwifery care to women in the Perth metropolitan area. The service provides women with the option of continuity of care and carer throughout their pregnancy, labour/birth and postnatal phases. Currently funding allows for the service to be offered to 150 women per annum; demand for 'places', however, exceeds this number.
>
> The CMP is managed by Community Midwifery WA Inc, a not-for-profit community organisation that aims to improve the availability of choices in childbirth. The success of the CMP is assisted by the close working relationship between the Program's management and the Department of Health. For example, in response to the withdrawal of professional indemnity insurance, the Department of Health took over employment of the midwives to ensure their access to indemnity cover.
>
> The fact that the program is based in the community, i.e. is community managed, has contributed to its flexibility, appropriateness, ongoing success and growth.
>
> (Source: Thiele & Thorogood 1998, 2001)

---

morbidities (Lydon-Rochelle et al 2000; Lui et al 2005), increased risk of unexplained stillbirth in a subsequent pregnancy among women who have had a previous caesarean section (Smith et al 2003), and increased rates of severe postpartum bleeding with placental complications following previous caesarean sections (Armstrong et al 2004).

International comparisons show Australia to have among the highest rates of obstetric intervention in labour and birth compared with those in other resource-rich nations. The caesarean section rate appears to be rising markedly in comparison with the New Zealand rate, which appears to have reached a plateau over the past five years. Future research will determine whether we are at last seeing the positive results of 15 years of midwifery-led maternity care on the population outcomes in New Zealand.

Interestingly, no midwifery-led care appears to be able to withstand the seduction of opiates offered during labour in tertiary hospital care, and the only places where women seem to be able to escape the seduction of drugs is in the stand-alone and primary-level birth units and home birth in both Australia and New Zealand.

Data from the Australian Institute of Health and Welfare (AIHW 2004) reported that more than one in four women in Australia gave birth by caesarean section and that nearly 80% of mothers with a history of caesarean section were likely to have another caesarean section, while less than 20% had a spontaneous vaginal birth in the next pregnancy (AIHW 2004). The report also showed that labour was induced in 25% of births and augmented in a further 19.2% of births, and that almost one in five women had an elective caesarean section with no labour at all (AIHW 2004).

Obstetric intervention is life-saving when serious complications arise during pregnancy or labour. However, previous population-based research from Australia (Roberts et al 2000) showed that private obstetric care in Australia was a stronger risk factor for intervention in childbirth than either age or risk status (Roberts et al 2000). When women are offered interventions in labour, such as induction and epidurals, they may not be informed of the cascade of interventions in birth that inevitably follow. There is a possibility that if women have information on the extent of the association between interventions in labour and birth this may ultimately influence their choice of caregiver and place of birth. Morbidity is costly in monetary, social and emotional health terms, for both families and funders of healthcare.

Research by Tracy and Tracy (2003) into the antecedents of operative birth showed through cost modelling that the introduction of interventions during labour for women who were otherwise 'low risk' increased the expenditure incrementally in association with the introduction of each labour intervention (see Fig 1.6).

In 1996 and 1997, the rate of normal birth in low-risk primiparous women studied by Roberts et al (2000) was 66%, with 36% of women having private health insurance. The hypothetical model suggests that as the proportion of low-risk primiparous women with private health insurance increases, the rate of normal birth decreases.

This was also demonstrated by Homer (2002) in her paper commenting on the increased levels of private health insurance rates in Australia. She argued that recent Australian government policy has encouraged large numbers of women of childbearing age to enter private health insurance and that this increased uptake of private health insurance affects the rate of normal birth, caesarean section and the costs of providing maternity care for low-risk primiparous women in New South Wales. Private providers and hospitals are heavily subsidised by government and so the additional costs are costs to the Australian community, not merely additional costs to women and their families (Homer 2002, p 36).

Homer and colleagues (2000) randomised 1089 women into 'standard' hospital-based care at St George Hospital in Sydney and community-based collaborative care involving a small team of midwives and hospital obstetricians. The emphasis of the study was on continuity. They found a significant reduction in caesarean rates, their primary outcome of interest (OR 0.6, CI 0.4–0.9).

A later paper reviewed the costs achieved in this reduction in caesarean rates and found a saving of at least $1000 in the community midwifery (STOMP) group. Overall, the mean cost of providing care per woman was lower in the STOMP group than in the control group ($2579 vs. $3483) (Homer et al 2001).

Recent history

Variations in government funding schemes in the past 15 years in Australia have had a serious impact on the provision of midwifery services.

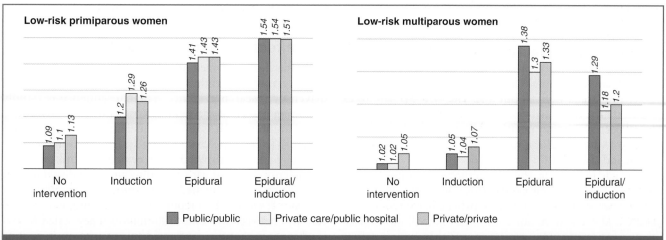

Figure 1.6 Costing the cascade: a model of the cost units per woman that are incurred with the introduction of interventions in labour, Australia 1996–97 (based on Tracy & Tracy 2003)

TABLE 1.3   Type of hospital (private or public) where women in Australia gave birth, by state and territory, 2002

Hospital sector	NSW	Vic	Qld	WA	SA	Tas	ACT	NT	Australia
Number									
Public	60,052	40,708	32,335	14,268	11,453	3,354	2,735	2,905	167,810
Private	22,096	19,477	15,280	9,645	4,865	2,174	1,692	686	75,915
Not stated	1	–	–	–	–	–	–	2	3
Total	82,149	60,185	47,615	23,913	16,318	5,528	4,427	3,593	243,728
Per cent									
Public	73.1	67.6	67.9	59.7	70.2	60.7	61.8	80.9	68.9
Private	26.9	32.4	32.1	40.3	29.8	39.3	38.2	19.1	31.1
Not stated	0.0	–	–	–	–	–	–	0.1	0.0
Total	100.0	100.0	100.0	100.0	100.0	100.0	100.0	100.0	100.0

(Source: AIHW 2004b)

In September 2000 the Hunter Valley Team Midwifery Project was closed due to inadequate funding levels. This was a public hospital funded team midwifery service that had been operating successfully for 10 years and had been found to be safe and accessible to women. At the John Hunter Hospital in Newcastle, NSW, continuity of care provided by midwives was evaluated by Rowley et al (1995) through a randomised, controlled study with 814 women, and found to be as safe as routine care. It also reduced the need for medical interventions including induction of labour, analgesia use, and need for neonatal resuscitation. Women receiving team care were significantly more satisfied with their experience and there was a significant reduction in cost (Rowley et al 1995).

The Alternative Birthing Program introduced as a Labor Government incentive in the 1990s was lost to Australian women when that party was elected out of government. Other midwifery models of care similarly face a bleak future as targeted funds run out and they remain, in general, 'on the edge' rather than integrated into routine services. For example, the Alternative Birthing Service funded models of care in Western Australia were all but lost. The WACMP still faces an uncertain future (Reibel 2005, personal communication). The project evaluation unanimously supported midwifery models of care for all the women who took part (Thiele & Thorogood 1998, 2001).

Similarly in Victoria, the six alternative birthing services funded by the Commonwealth, and found to offer all women from a range of socioeconomic groups benefit from continuity of care and carer, were not continued and will not replace the current fragmented arrangements that exploit rather than protect women's vulnerability during childbirth (Lane 1999). Despite the proven safety, high levels of satisfaction and reduced costs, these services have remained marginal to the mainstream services offered within most institutions and separate from their funding base. An important exception is the St George Hospital Sydney, where a community midwifery team service was developed out of regular funding and became a normal part of options available for women.

A report from the Centre for the Study of Mothers' and Children's Health in Victoria found that the constraints in budget expenditure in public hospitals in Victoria had a very real impact on the quality of care for women during labour and birth. The research also found that recommendations from previous research in 1993 calling for the introduction of team midwifery care and multidisciplinary team care for women 'at risk' had not been implemented and in fact had been reduced in some instances (Brown & Lumley 1998).

The effect of fee-for-service

Australia has developed an ad hoc 'fee-for-service' model of maternity care rather than one led by outcomes and driven by research evidence. The consequence is rapidly escalating costs and accelerating cost shifting between state and Commonwealth as the consequences are felt within both systems. There is no overarching system to monitor these costs, align them with best practice evidence, or link outcomes of current models of care according to morbidity data. For example, an editorial in the *Medical Journal of Australia* in 2002 (Wallace & Oates 2002) reported that spending in antenatal care was between $75 and $100 million. They stated that 'it is of concern that there is considerable variation in routine antenatal testing in our hospitals, and that practice is often at odds with available evidence. These inconsistencies are not only indicative of inequalities in care, but also suggest wastage of precious and limited resources' (Wallace & Oates 2002, p 468).

The Senate Inquiry in 1999 (Rocking the Cradle, Commonwealth of Australia 1999) heard that the total Medicare benefit paid for obstetric ultrasound (MBS category 5, diagnostic imaging, item numbers 55040 and 55041) for the financial year 1997/98 was $34,888,421. This accounted for more than half of the entire obstetric Medicare rebate, $54,865,447 for the same financial year (Medicare tables 1999).

One of the unfortunate legacies of the funding system's bias towards bed day funding is the relative underdevelopment of non-inpatient services. The challenge, in attempting to provide evidence-based improvement in maternity care within the 'casemix' model, is to fund services that extend beyond the hospital bed and provide effective services in the community. At present there are disincentives for hospital services to provide what research evidence shows to be 'best care'. Midwives, most often salaried hospital staff, not only cost less on an hourly rate, but the indirect costs attached to interventionist care such as increased bed days and use of equipment and tests are reduced when they provide care to healthy women.

Current research into the high rates of obstetric intervention for otherwise 'low-risk' women indicates a very large commitment of Commonwealth and state budgets to tertiary-level maternity care among those who might least need such expensive medical support. These rates have an impact across all levels of the system, affecting resource usage at state-funded hospital level and fee-for-service costs at Commonwealth level.

The most recent research by one of the authors of this chapter (ST) shows that paying for a private obstetrician and giving birth in a private hospital is still the greatest risk factor among low-risk women for having an operative or instrumental birth with an episiotomy. Given the number of women who think that having private maternity care is desirable, this information should be more accessible in the public domain.

Within the Medicare funding system, public hospital expenditure is capped. Although prices are controlled for general and specialist services, there is less limitation on volume and hence a 'perverse incentive to over service'. The generally uncoordinated nature of the system allows for major deficiencies at this level, with patients moving from one professional to another (Leeder 1998).

One area of absolute certainty, however, is the model for home birth. Home birth saves the taxpayer money in that it uses none of the resources funded by state or Commonwealth health funds. In this respect the woman and her family are disadvantaged in that they do not qualify for any of the benefits of the health system. The onus falls entirely on the woman and her family to engage and pay the midwives who attend the birth. Some private health funds have agreed to privately insure women for home birth, because they can see the cost saving when compared to an elective caesarean birth, for example (Sprague 1999).

Options for change to general funding mechanisms

According to one of the co-founders of the original Medicare agreement, part of the strategic response to the long-term solution to the funding of Australia's health will be found in structural reform rather than incremental change (Scotton 1999). He advocates a model of managed competition that is specifically designed to induce profound changes in provider arrangements, in the way they are paid, what they deliver and how they are structured (Scotton 1999). The equity objective remains a government function and is even more apparent today due to growing health costs, and widening gaps between those with income and those without, and requires governments to subsidise both health status and income. The structural problems, according to Scotton and others, are: fragmentation of programs; payment incentives which not only lack incentives but in many cases involve perverse incentives; jurisdictional and functional overlap; and conflict between levels of government and between the private and public sectors (Leeder 1998; Owens 1999; Scotton 1999).

Having turned their backs on competition, countries such as the United Kingdom, Sweden, the Netherlands and New Zealand have stressed the need to focus on achieving health outcomes and improving the health status of the population, developing an approach based on family health teams for delivering some primary care services. 'The importance of integrated care is being emphasised as both politicians and health professionals recognise the need for team working and coordination of delivery of services after a period in which competition has militated against such an approach' (Ham 1997c, p 1845).

Increasingly, funding bodies and consumers are calling for evidence to demonstrate the effectiveness of health services, and the need for healthcare is both increasing and changing. Organisations and people need to become increasingly interdependent, willing to question existing values and beliefs in order to adapt to change. Public sector healthcare organisations have a particular need for an external orientation to identify new ways of doing more with less while maintaining quality standards (Perkins & Powell 1999).

New models of maternity care will eventually require cooperation between Commonwealth and state funding systems. At the moment, however, the new stand-alone units do not have access to Commonwealth monies because they are funded within existing area health services (state budgets), and therefore within the existing funding patterns. It is imperative that Commonwealth funding be accessed in the future, otherwise this will impinge on the ability and enthusiasm of area health services to introduce such models. The consequence of not collaborating is the extensive cost shifting that is occurring now and reducing the quality of care for women.

Data retrieval

Maternity systems in Australia and New Zealand rely on adequate and appropriate data retrieval and analysis in order to evaluate processes, outcomes and costs in relation to maternity care. Systems for the collection of a minimum dataset are in place in both countries, although the data retrieved is not uniform across all states and territories in Australia and complete data was not available in New Zealand until 2003 and is not yet reported (Sullivan 2005, personal communication; NZHIS 2005).

A National Minimum Dataset (NMDS) is a core set of data elements agreed to and endorsed by the health departments of each country for mandatory collection and reporting at a national population level. An NMDS depends on national agreements to collect uniform data. A perinatal NMDS includes data items relating to the mother, including demographic characteristics and factors relating to the pregnancy, labour and birth, and data items relating to the baby including birth status, sex and birth weight.

The Australian National Perinatal Data collection (NPDC) is a collection of national data based on notifications to the perinatal data collection in each state and territory. Midwives and other staff using information obtained from mothers and from hospital and other records complete notification forms for each birth in each state and territory. Information is included in the NPDC for all births of at least 400 grams birthweight or at least 20 weeks gestation. Each year the Australian Institute of Health and Welfare National Perinatal Statistics Unit (AIHW NPSU) produces a report using the NPDC known as the Mothers and Babies Report.

National maternity data has been collected in New Zealand for some years but reports have been limited and data incomplete. The Maternal and Newborn Information System (MNIS) was established to collect perinatal information amalgamating data from both the Lead Maternity Carer payment claims through HealthPac and the data collected at hospital discharge through the NMDS. Now that all LMCs work under the Section 88 Notice, effective from July 2002, data for all births will be available for the first time in the report on the 2003 data. When New Zealand established its NMDS it was based on the Australian NPDC in order to facilitate comparison between both countries; it also includes data for all births of at least 400 grams birthweight or at least 20 weeks gestation. The quality relies on data being accurately entered by LMC practitioners and hospital coders. The New Zealand Health Information Service (NZHIS) is responsible for producing the Report on Maternity.

In both countries it takes approximately two years to analyse each year's data and therefore the most recent report available in Australia is based on data collected in 2003 (Laws & Sullivan 2005). At the time of writing, the 2003 report is still in draft form in New Zealand (NZHIS 2005).

New Zealand midwives also contribute to another data collection developed by the New Zealand College of Midwives and administered through the Midwifery and Maternity Provider Organisation (MMPO). Collected directly from a standard set of Maternity Notes, midwives report on the clinical outcomes of their care as part of the process of making claims for payment for midwifery care. The data from this practice management system provides information in relation to the health of mothers and babies—including pregnancy and birth conditions, procedures and outcomes, and neonatal morbidity—relating to every episode of care undertaken by midwife members. The proposed reports from the MMPO database will provide a benchmark for individual midwife LMCs against which they can measure their own activities and care outcomes. It will also provide the midwifery profession with valuable data to guide planning and the improvement of care outcomes.

Evaluation of maternity care in particular needs to consider both the value of health interventions to the wider population, and the value of the expected outcomes of the intervention to the individual. Data fields for economic evaluation can be designed to respond to the growing need to recognise the value of the intervention both to the individual and to society at large (Viney 1999).

Each perinatal data collection has the potential to inform both women and practitioners about the results of practice.

Conclusion

In Western societies such as Australia and New Zealand, all women should have access to a publicly funded and integrated maternity service that meets their individual needs.[2] Such a service begins with strengthening its community-based primary care provisions while also ensuring easy access to secondary and tertiary care when required. There is strong evidence that a midwife-led maternity service and stand-alone primary units provide a safe service and meet the needs of women and their families (Walsh & Downe 2004; Sandall et al 2001).

In 1990, the New Zealand Government took an unprecedented lead in making women the central focus of its maternity services reform. A comparison of the rates of access to midwifery care between Australia and New Zealand (see Fig 1.7) demonstrates the potential of such reform.

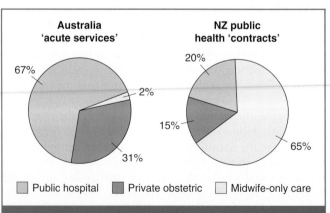

Figure 1.7 Percentage of women who access midwives under the funding models for New Zealand and Australia, 2002 (based on Ministry of Health 1999b; Roberts et al 2000; Laws & Sullivan 2004)

For 10 to 15 years now, midwives in New Zealand have been funded to provide a primary care service, to provide care for the entire maternity experience, and provide the majority of care by being present during labour and birth. In 2005 at least 78% of women booked with a midwife, compared with Australia's 1.0% of women (Tracy et al 2006, unpublished data).

The funding mechanisms that govern the provision of maternity care in Australia are in urgent need of reform. Current funding that is costed solely on acute hospital casemix models does not fund care to be undertaken in the community. Where caseload midwifery models have been implemented in Australia, and evaluated, the outcomes show they are of benefit to women and babies (Homer et al 2000; Kenny et al 1994; Rowley et al 1995; Thiele & Thorogood 1998, 2001; Tracy & Hartz 2005). Until funding encourages non-intervention by providers, probably through some form of capped prospective allowance for each woman attended, mothers and babies will continue to be disadvantaged by not having access to proven practices of safety and comfort in childbirth. Such a system is based on 'collaboration' and 'cooperation' across all levels of service provision.

The service itself must cross both acute hospital and community boundaries to achieve a balance between hospital-based and community-based care. This, coupled with funding a lead maternity carer through a capped maternity allowance allocated in terms of a maternity benefit for every pregnant woman, is known to contribute significantly to the welfare of childbearing populations.

Review questions

1 What is the difference between public, primary, secondary and tertiary healthcare?

2 List six reasons why midwifery can be defined as primary healthcare.

3 Identify four principles of primary healthcare.

4 Define the terms 'lead maternity carer' and 'continuity of care'.

5 Identify the key mechanism by which New Zealand's maternity service funding supports midwifery professional autonomy.

6 Identify four main differences between the maternity services and maternity service funding mechanisms in Australian and New Zealand.

7 How do funding mechanisms affect maternity outcomes for mothers and babies?

8 How does private obstetric care pose a risk to women and babies?

9 Why is the collection of data important for midwifery and what is the best way to collect information about birth outcomes?

10 How would you describe the most cost-effective maternity services in New Zealand and Australia?

Notes

1 However, the latest maternal mortality report for the triennium 1994–1996 shows a worrying change in rates (AIHW 2001; NHMRC 2001).

2 As this chapter highlights, there is no universally agreed model of maternity care. Most health systems in most countries have not achieved a model of care that fully recognises and adapts to the needs of women and their babies in a way that allows all women and their babies to meet their health and wellbeing potential. Nor is there a model that completely enables midwives to practise in an environment that strengthens their potential to keep birth normal.
Scrutiny of the antecedents of normal birth will possibly reveal that women should be encouraged to birth in units where intrathecal and epidural opioids and other invasive technology is not routinely on hand and is not used unless the condition of the mother and baby require intervention.

Online resources

Commonwealth of Australia 1999, Senate Community Affairs References Committee. Rocking the Cradle: a report into childbirth procedures. Commonwealth of Australia, Canberra, December 1999, http://www.aph.gov.au/senate/committee/history/index.htm#Community

Enkin M, Keirse JNC, Neilson J et al 2000 A guide to effective care in pregnancy and childbirth (3rd edn). Oxford University Press, Oxford, http://maternitywise.org/guide/about.html

House of Commons Health Committee 2003 Choice in maternity services. Ninth Report of Session 2002–03. Volume I. http://www.parliament.the-stationery-office.co.uk/pa/cm200203/cmselect/cmhealth/796/796.pdf

Ministry of Health 1999 Obstetric procedures 1998/99–1997/8 and Report on maternity, both available online, http://www.moh.govt.nz

National Health & Medical Research Council (NHMRC) (1999) A review of services offered by midwives, http://www.health.gov.au/nhmrc/gov.au

National Health Insurance Board of the Netherlands 1998 Obstetric manual: final report of the Obstetric Working Group (abridged version). Amstelveen, December 1998, http://europe.obgyn.net/nederland/richtlijnen/vademecum_eng.htm

National Maternity Action Plan 2002, http://www.maternitycoalition.org.au

New South Wales Health Department 2000 Maternity Services Advisory Committee, The NSW framework for maternity services, http://www.health.nsw.gov.au/pubs/f/pdf/msreport148.pdf

New Zealand Health Information Service 2000 Maternity services: a reference document, http://www.moh.govt.nz

New Zealand Health Information Service 2004 Report on maternity 2002, http://www.moh.govt.nz/moh. nsf/ea6005dc347e7bd44c2566a40079ae6f/ 57d46cd598be7e06cc256ecf000a00dc?OpenDocument

New Zealand Ministry of Health 2002 Section 88 Maternity Notice, http://www.moh.govt.nz/moh.nsf/

NICE 2004 National Collaborating Centre for Women's and Children's Health. Caesarean section. Clinical guidelines 13 (commissioned by the National Institute for Clinical Excellence), 2004. RCOG Press, London, http://www.rcog.org.uk

Scottish Executive Health Department 2001, The report of the Expert Advisory Group on Caesarean section in Scotland, http://www. show.scot.nhs.uk/crag

Select Committee on Health of the House of Commons 2001 Second Report. Public Health 2001. Vol. 1. http://www. publications.parliament.uk/pa/cm200001/cmselect/ cmhealth/30/3011.htm#n93

WHO 1999 Care in normal birth: a practical guide. WHO/FRH/ MSM/96.24. http://www.who.int/rht/documents/MSM96-24/ msm9624.htm

References

AHA 1997 The Australian Healthcare Agreements 1998–2003: Submission to the Federal Minister of Health: cited in Australian Health Review 21(2):3–8

Armstrong CA, Harding S, Matthews T et al 2004 Is placenta accreta catching up with us? The Australian and New Zealand Journal of Obstetrics and Gynaecology 44:210–213

Australian Bureau of Statistics 2004a Australian Birth Statistics 2003. ABS, Canberra

Australian Bureau of Statistics 2004b Deaths in Australia 2003. Cat. No. 3302.0. ABS, Canberra

Australian Institute of Health and Welfare (AIHW) 2001 Cat. No. PER 13. Commonwealth of Australia Online: http://www.nhmrc.gov. au/publications/pdf/wh32.pdf

Australian Institute of Health and Welfare (AIHW) 2004a Australia's health 2004. AIHW, Canberra

Australian Institute of Health and Welfare (AIHW) 2004b Australia's Mothers and Babies 2002. AIHW, Canberra

Barnett S, Nair N, Lewycka S et al 2005 Commentary: community interventions for maternal and perinatal health. British Journal of Obstetrics and Gynaecology 112:1170–1173

Baum F, Kalucy E, Lawless A et al 1998 Health promotion in different medical settings: women's health, community health and private practice. Australian and New Zealand Journal of Public Health 22:200–205

Brown S, Lumley J 1998 Are cuts to health expenditure in Victoria compromising quality of care? Australian and New Zealand Journal of Public Health 22(2):279–281

Church A, Nixon A 2002 An evaluation of the Northern Suburbs Community Midwifery Program, Adelaide. Department of Human Services, SA

Davies P, Hindle D 1999 Editorial. Health policy and management across the Tasman. Australian Health Review 22(4):3–7

Davis P 2002 Editorial. Health policy: drawing on a 'global laboratory'. Social Science and Medicine 54:323–324

Deeble J 2002 Funding the essentials: the Australian Health Care Agreements 2003–2008. Australian Health Review 25(6): 1–7

Degeling P, Kennedy J, Carnegie M et al 1998 Professional subcultures and hospital reform—a study of the attitudes and beliefs of staff of Australian and English hospitals. The Centre for Hospital and Information Systems Research, University of New South Wales, Sydney

Department for International Development (n.d.) Midwives help deliver malaria prevention in Ghana. Online: http://www.dfid.gov. uk/casestudies/files/africa/ghana/ghana-malaria.asp, accessed 23 August 2005

Department of Education 1987 Report on the Advanced Diploma of Nursing. Department of Education, Wellington

d'Espaignet ET, Measey M, Carnegie M et al 2003 Monitoring the 'Strong Women, Strong Babies, Strong Culture' Program: the first eight years. Journal of Paediatrics and Child Health 39(9):668–672

Devlin N, Maynard A, Mays N 2001 New Zealand's new health sector reforms: back to the future? British Medical Journal 322: 1171–1174

Dobbie, M 1990 The trouble with women: the story of Parents Centre New Zealand. Cape Cately, Whatamongo Bay, Queen Charlotte Sound.

Donley, J 1986 Save the midwife. New Women's Press, Auckland

Walsh D, Downe SM 2004 Outcomes of free-standing, midwifery-led birth centres: a structured review. Birth 31(3):222–229

Duckett S 1997 Internal and external challenges for hospitals in the future. Med J Aust 166(1):20–22

Flint C 1986 Sensitive midwifery. Heineman Midwifery, London

Gauld R 2001 Revolving doors: New Zealand's health reforms. Victoria University of Wellington, Wellington

Gray G 2004 The politics of Medicare. UNSW Press, Sydney

Guilliland KM 2005 Do women want midwives? Midwives and the New Zealand maternity system in 2005. Proceedings, International Confederation of Midwives Conference, Brisbane (CD-ROM)

Guilliland KM, Pairman S 1995 The midwifery partnership: a model for practice. Monograph Series 95/1. Department of Nursing and Midwifery, Victoria University of Wellington

Ham C 1997a Primary managed care in Europe: innovation by doctors is creating European health maintenance organisations. British Medical Journal 314(7079):457

Ham C 1997b Reforming New Zealand health reforms: big bang gives way to incrementalism as competition is abandoned. British Medical Journal 314 (7098): 1844–1845

Ham C 1997c Replacing the NHS market: the white paper should focus on incentives as well as directives. British Medical Journal 315(7117): 1175–1176

Healthcare Insurance Commission (HIC) 1999 Online: http://www. hic.gov.au/index.htm. Australian Government, Medicare Australia

Homer C 2002 Private health insurance uptake and the impact on normal birth and costs: a hypothetical model. Australian Health Review 25(2):32–37

Homer CSE, Davis GK, Brodie P et al 2000 Collaboration in maternity care: a randomised controlled trial comparing community-based continuity of care with standard hospital care. British Journal of Obstetrics and Gynaecology 108:16–22

Homer C, Matha D, Jordan L et al 2001 Community-based continuity of midwifery care versus standard hospital care: a cost analysis. Australian Health Review 24(1):85–93

Hornblow A 1997 New Zealand's health reforms: a clash of cultures. British Medical Journal 314:1892

Humphrey M, Keating S 2004 Lack of antenatal care in far north Queensland. Australian and New Zealand Journal of Obstetrics and Gynaecology 44:10–13

Kaufman T 2002 Midwifery and public health. MIDIRS: Midwifery Digest 12(supp): S23–S26

Kenny P, Brodie P, Eckermann S et al 1994 Westmead Hospital Team Midwifery Project Evaluation. Final Report. Centre for Health Economics Research and Evaluation, Westmead, NSW

Lane K 1999 Continuity of care: the birthing services transition project. Conference abstracts: Australian and New Zealand Health Services Research Conference, p. 90. Sydney, 8–11 August 1999

Laws PJ, Sullivan EA 2004 Australian's mothers and babies 2002. Australian Institute of Health and Welfare, Canberra. AIHW Cat. No. PER 28, Perinatal Statistics Series No. 151

Leeder SR 1998 We have come to raise Medicare, not to bury it. Australian Health Review 21(2):28–33

Lui S, Heaman M, Joseph KS et al 2005 Risk of maternal postpartum readmission associated with mode of delivery. Obstetrics and Gynecology 105:836–842

Lydon-Rochelle M, Holt VL, Martin DP et al 2000 Association between method of delivery and maternal rehospitalization. Journal of the American Medical Association 283:2411–2416

Malcolm L 1998 Towards general practice-led integrated healthcare in New Zealand. Medical Journal of Australia 69(3):48

Mantell CD, Craig ED, Stewart AW et al 2004 Ethnicity and birth outcome: New Zealand trends 1980–2001. Part 2, Pregnancy outcomes for Maori women. Australian and New Zealand Journal of Obstetrics and Gynaecology 44:537–540

Mein-Smith P 1986 Maternity in dispute. New Zealand 1920–1939. Historical Publications Branch, Department of Internal Affairs, Wellington

Ministry of Health 1999a Obstetric procedures, 1998/99–1997/8. Ministry of Health, Wellington

Ministry of Health 1999b Report on maternity: maternal and newborn information. Online: http://www.moh.govt.nz

Ministry of Health 2000 Maternity services. Notice pursuant to Section 88 of the *New Zealand Public Health and Disability Act 2000*

Ministry of Health 2001 Report on maternity 1999. Ministry of Health, Wellington

Ministry of Health 2003 Media release, 21 January 2003. Ministry releases maternity services consumer survey. Online: http://www.moh.govt.nz/moh.nsf/30ad137c772c883e4c25665c002c4198/aff55e5ea7fb6b8bcc256cbf0013a036?OpenDocument

Ministry of Health 2004 Fetal and infant deaths 2000. Ministry of Health, Wellington

National Health & Medical Research Council (NHMRC) 2001 Report on maternal deaths in Australia 1994–96. Cat. No. 0145246

National Women's Hospital 2000 Annual reports, 1996–2000. National Women's Hospital, Auckland.

NCEPH 1992 Improving Australia's health: the role of primary care / summary of the final report of the review of the role of primary healthcare in health promotion in Australia. National Centre for Epidemiology and Population Health, ANU, and National Better Health Program 1992

New Zealand College of Midwives (NZCOM) 2005a Handbook for Practice. NZCOM, Christchurch

New Zealand College of Midwives (NZCOM) 2005b Workforce Report to the Ministry of Health. NZCOM, Christchurch

New Zealand Health Information Service (NZHIS) 2003 Report on maternity 2000 and 2001. Ministry of Health, Wellington

New Zealand Health Information Service (NZHIS) 2004 Report on maternity 2002. Ministry of Health, Wellington

New Zealand Health Information Service (NZHIS) 2005 Draft report on maternity: maternal and newborn information, 2003. Ministry of Health, Wellington

NSW Health Department 1998 New South Wales mothers and babies 1997. Number 2, December 1998

NSW Health Department 1999 The NSW Framework for Maternity Services. A discussion paper for comment. Maternity Services Advisory Committee

Nursing Council of New Zealand 2004 New Zealand registered nurses, midwives and enrolled nurses: workforce statistics 2002. Nursing Council of New Zealand, Wellington

O'Donoghue L 1999 Towards a culture of improving indigenous health in Australia. Australian Journal of Rural Health 7:64–69

Owens H 1999 Scotton's proposal worth a serious look in quest for best 'mixed system'. Healthcover 9(4):24–26

Pairman S 2002 Towards self-determination: the separation of the midwifery and nursing professions in New Zealand. In: E Papps (Ed) Nursing in New Zealand: critical issues, different perspectives. Pearson Education, Auckland

Pairman S 2005 Workforce to profession: an exploration of New Zealand midwifery's professionalising strategies from 1986 to 2005. Unpublished doctoral thesis, University of Technology, Sydney

Pairman S, Guilliland K 2003 Developing a midwife-led maternity service: the New Zealand experience. In: M Kirkham (Ed) Birth centres. A social model for maternity care. Books for Midwives, London

Papps E, Olssen M 1997 Doctoring childbirth and regulating midwifery in New Zealand. A Foucauldian perspective. Dunmore Press, Palmerston North, NZ

Paterson RJ 1999 Regulating for quality: patient's rights in the US and New Zealand. Conference Abstracts: Australian and New Zealand Health Services Research Conference. Sydney, 8–11 August 1999, p 105

Perkins RJ, Powell M 1999 Scenarios and future challenges for health management in New Zealand. Health Manager 6(3):15–18

Pringle M, Heath I 1997 Primary care: opportunities and threats. Distributing primary care fairly. British Medical Journal 314:595–599

Quinlivan B 2004 Medicare cuts an artery. BRW, November 11–17, p 26

Reid M 1999 NSW health chief lists his national reform agenda. Healthcover 9(5):59–63

Roberts CL, Tracy S, Peat B 2000 Rates for obstetric intervention among private and public patients in Australia: a population based descriptive study. British Medical Journal 321:137–141. Online: http://British Medical Journal.com/cgi/content/abstract/321/7254/137

Rose G 1992 The strategy of preventive medicine. Oxford University Press, Oxford

Rowley M, Hensley M, Brinsmead M et al 1995 Continuity of care by a midwife team versus routine care during pregnancy and birth: a randomised trial. Medical Journal of Australia 163(9):289–293

Sachs J 2005 The end of poverty in a world of plenty. Time March 14:42–55

Sandall J, Davies J, Warwick C 2001 Evaluation of the Albany Midwifery Practice: final report. March 2001. Florence Nightingale School of Nursing and Midwifery, London

Scally G, Donaldson J 1998 Clinical governance and the drive for quality improvement in the new NHS in England. British Medical Journal 317:61–65

Scotton D 1999 The contribution of research evidence to health policy. Healthcover 9(4):21–24

Smith J 1998 A simplified representation of the current financing model, the Australian Healthcare Association. Australian Health Review 21(2):38–64

Sprague A 1999 Senate Inquiry into Childbirth Procedures. Senate references. Community Affairs Hansard, Melbourne, 6 September 1999: CA 137. Online: http://www.aph.gov.au/hansard

Stonavich J 2004 'Leaving your dignity at the door' maternity in Wellington 1950–1970. New Zealand College of Midwives Journal 31:12–18

Thiele B, Thorogood C 1998a Evaluation of the Community Based Midwifery Program. Community Midwifery WA Inc, Fremantle WA

Thiele B, Thorogood C 1998b Evaluation of the Community Midwifery Program. Report to Community Midwifery WA Inc.

Thiele B, Thorogood C 2001 Evaluation of the Community Midwifery Program. Preliminary report to Community Midwifery WA Inc

Thorogood C 2001 Politics and the professions: homebirth in Western Australia. School of Social Sciences, Humanities and Education. Murdoch University, Perth

Tracy SK, Tracy MB 2003 Costing the cascade: estimating the cost of increased intervention in childbirth using population data. British Journal of Obstetrics and Gynaecology 110(8): 717–724

Tracy SK, Hartz D 2005 Final report: the quality review of Ryde Midwifery Group Practice, September 2004 to October 2005. Northern Sydney and Central Coast Health, December 2005

Tully E 1999 Doing professionalism differently: negotiating midwifery autonomy in Aoteoroa/New Zealand. Unpublished doctoral thesis. University of Canterbury, New Zealand

Viney R 1999 Risk and uncertainty in healthcare: issues for economic evaluation. Conference abstracts: Australian and New Zealand Health Services Research Conference. Sydney, 8–11 August 1999, p 121

Wallace E, Oates J 2002 National guidelines for antenatal testing (Editorial). Medical Journal of Australia 177(9):468

Waterstone M, Bewley S, Wolfe C 2001 Incidence and predictors of severe obstetric morbidity: case-control study. British Medical Journal 322:1089–1093

Weigers T 1997 Home or hospital birth. A prospective study of midwifery in the Netherlands. Thesis. Rijksuniversiteit te Leiden

Wellington Women's Hospital 1998 Annual Report 1998. WWH, Wellington

World Health Organization (WHO) 1994 Care in normal birth: a practical guide. Report of a technical working group. Online: http://www.who.int/reproductive-health/publications/MSM_96_24/MSM_96_24_Chapter1.en.html. Maternal and Newborn Health/Safe Motherhood, Division of Reproductive Health. WHO, Geneva

World Health Organization (WHO) 1999a Care in normal birth: a practical guide. WHO/FRH/MSM/96.24. Online: www.who.int/rht/documents/MSM96-24/msm9624.htm

World Health Organization (WHO) 1999b Making a difference. WHO, Geneva

Further reading

Australian Consumer Focus Collaboration: Strategic Plan 1998

AMWAC Report 1998 The Obstetrics and Gynaecology Workforce in Australia; Australian Medical Workforce Advisory Committee. NSW Department of Health, June 1998

Angell M, Kassirer JP 1996 Quality and the medical market place—following elephants. New England Journal of Medicine 335:883–885

Baker R, Lakhani M, Fraser R et al 1999 A model for clinical governance in primary care groups. British Medical Journal 318:779–783

Barclay L, Brodie P 1999 A report on low risk birthing services for metropolitan Adelaide. Prepared for the South Australian Department of Human Services and submitted to the Birthing Services Review Committee, 28 June 1999

Bero L, Grilli R, Grimshaw J et al 1998 Closing the gap between research and practice: an overview of systematic reviews of interventions to promote the implementation of research findings British Medical Journal 317:465–468

Bigg I, Azmi S, Maskell-Knight C 1998 The Commonwealth's proposal for the 1998–2003 Healthcare Agreements. Australian Health Review 21(2):8–19

Bodenheimer T 1999 The movement for improved quality in healthcare. New England Journal of Medicine 340:488–492

Bovbjerg RR, Miller RH, Shapiro DW 2001 Paths to reducing medical injury: professional liability and disciplines vs patient safety—and the need for a third way. Journal of Law, Medicine and Ethics 2:369–383

Braithwaite J, Hindle D, Degeling PJ 1998 Rebuilding the English National Health Service: doctors in the driving seat? Medical Journal of Australia 169(2):71–73

Brennan TA, Leape LL, Laird NM et al 1991 Incidence of adverse events and negligence in hospitalised patients. New England Journal of Medicine 324:370–376

Burroughs T 2002 New Statesman 131(4573):32–34

Cary AJ 1990 Intervention rates in spontaneous term labour in low risk nulliparous women. Australian and New Zealand Journal of Obstetrics and Gynaecology 30:46–51

CHERE, Centre for Health Economics Research and Evaluation 2000 Funding of Public Hospitals. Centre for Health Economics Research and Evaluation. Issue 16, November

Chernichovsky D 1995 Health system reforms in industrialised democracies: an emerging paradigm. Millbank Quarterly 73(3):339–372

Chernichovsky D 2002 Pluralism, public choice, and the state in the emerging paradigm in health systems. Millbank Quarterly 80(1):5–39

Commonwealth of Australia 2000 Senate Community Affairs References Committee. First Report—Public Hospital Funding And Options For Reform. Online: http://www.aph.gov.au/senate/committee/clac_ctte/phealth_first/index.htm

Coulter A 1995 Shifting the balance from secondary to primary care. British Medical Journal 311:1447–1448

Coulter A 1998 Managing demand at the interface between primary and secondary care. British Medical Journal 316:1974–1976

Coulter A, Mays N 1997 Primary care: opportunities and threats. Deregulating primary care. British Medical Journal 314:506

Creedy D 1999 Unpublished doctoral thesis.

Cuff C 2002 Long term care costs. 1st speaker at the Australian Health Ministers Advisory Council medical litigation workshop to discuss opportunities for legal change and administrative reform, Canberra, 22 April 2002

Cumming J, Scott C 1998 The role of outputs and outcomes in purchaser accountability: reflecting on the New Zealand experience. Health Policy December

Dawson W, Brown S, Gunn J et al 1999 Shared obstetric care: challenges for hospitals and care providers. Conference abstracts: Australian and New Zealand Health Services Research Conference. Sydney, 8–11 August 1999, p 68

Day P, Sullivan E, Lancaster P 1999 Australian mothers and babies 1996. AIHW Cat. No. PER 4. Sydney: Australian Institute of Health & Welfare National Perinatal Statistics Unit (Perinatal Statistics Series No. 7)

Department of Health 1997 The new NHS. Department of Health, London

Department of Health 2000 NHS plan: a plan for investment, a plan for reform. Department of Health, London

DiMatteo MR, Morton SC, Lepper HS et al 1996 Caesarean childbirth and psychosocial outcomes: a meta-analysis. Health Psychology 15(4):303–314

Dixon J, Holland P, Mays N 1998 Primary care: core values developing primary care: gatekeeping, commissioning and managed care. British Medical Journal 317:125–128

Duggan JM 1997 The Australian healthcare system: John Hunter's long shadow. Med J Aust 167(9):481–483

Eisenberg L 2001 Good technical outcome, poor service experience: a verdict on contemporary medical care? Journal of the American Medical Association 285(20):2639–41

Elwyn G, Edwards A, Gwyn R et al 1999 Towards a feasible model for shared decision making: focus group study with general practice registrars. British Medical Journal 319:753–756

Evans RG 1997 Going for the gold: the redistributive agenda behind market based healthcare reform. Journal of Health Politics, Policy and Law 22(2):427–465

Fairfield G, Hunter D, Mechanic D et al 1997a Managed care: implications of managed care for health systems, clinicians and patients. British Medical Journal 314:1895–1898

Fairfield G, Hunter D, Mechanic D et al 1997b Managed care: origins, principles and evolution. British Medical Journal 314:1823–1826

Fisher J 1999 Senate Inquiry into Childbirth Procedures. Senate references, Community Affairs Hansard, Melbourne, 6 September 1999: CA85-99. Online: http://www.aph.gov.au/hansard

Fisher J, Smith A, Astbury J 1995 Private health insurance and a healthy personality: new risk factors for obstetric intervention? Journal of Psychosometrics, Obstetrics and Gynecology 16:1–9

Flint C, Poulengeris P 1989 The 'Know Your Midwife' scheme—a randomized trial of continuity of care by a team of midwives. Midwifery 5:11–16

Gabel J, Levitt L, Pickreign J et al 2001 Job-based health insurance in 2001: inflation hits double digits, managed care retreats. Health Affairs 20(5):180–186

Greenfield S, Nelson EC, Zubkoff M 1992 Variations in resource utilization among medical specialties and systems of care. Results from the medical outcomes study. Journal of the American Medical Association 267:1624–1630

Grembowski DE, Cook KS, Patrick DL et al 2002 Managed care and the US healthcare system: a social exchange perspective. Social Science and Medicine 54:1167–1180

Gress S, Groenewegen P, Kerssens J et al 2002 Free choice of sickness funds in regulated competition: evidence from Germany and the Netherlands. Health Policy 60:235–254

Grol R 1997 Personal paper: beliefs and evidence in changing clinical practice. British Medical Journal 315:418–421

Grol R, Dalhuijsen J, Thomas S et al 1998 Attributes of clinical guidelines that influence use of guidelines in general practice: observational study. British Medical Journal 317:858–861

Guilliland KM 1998 Demographic profile of self-employed/independent midwives in New Zealand and their birth outcomes. MA thesis. Victoria University of Wellington, Wellington

Guilliland KM 1999a Autonomous midwifery in New Zealand: the highs and lows. Birth Issues 8(1):14–20

Guilliland KM 1999b Shared care in maternity services: with whom and how? Health Manager 6(2):4–8

Ham C 1996 Contestability: a middle path for healthcare. British Medical Journal 312:70–71

Ham C 1998a Financing the NHS. British Medical Journal 316: 212–213

Ham C 1998b Retracing the Oregon trail: the experience of rationing and the Oregon health plan. British Medical Journal 316 (7149):1965–1969

Ham C 1999 Improving NHS performance: human behaviour and health policy. British Medical Journal 319:1490–1492

Hancock L 1999 Health, public sector restructuring and the market state. In: L Hancock (Ed) Health Policy in the Market State. Allen & Unwin, Sydney, pp 48–68

Harvey S, Jarrell J, Brant R et al 1996 A randomized, controlled trial of nurse-midwifery care. Birth 23(3):128–135

HCUP Net 1999 Healthcare cost and utilization project. Agency for healthcare Policy and Research, Rockville, MD. Online: http://www.ahcpr.gov/data/hcup/hcupnet.htm

Heath I 1997 Threat to social justice. British Medical Journal 314:598–599

Hendry C 2001 Riding the waves of change: the development of modern midwifery within the New Zealand health sector. New Zealand College of Midwives Journal 25:10–15

Hensher M, Fulop N, Coast J et al 1999 The hospital of the future: better out than in? Alternatives to acute hospital care. British Medical Journal 319:1127–1130

Hillan EM 1995 Postoperative morbidity following Caesarean delivery. Journal of Advanced Nursing 26(6):1035–1042

Hillman KM 1998 Restructuring hospital services. Medical Journal of Australia 169:239

Hodnett ED 1999 Caregiver support for women during childbirth (Cochrane Review). Cochrane Library (3). John Wiley & Sons, Oxford

Hofmeyr GJ, Kulier R 1999 Operative versus conservative management for 'fetal distress' in labour (Cochrane Review). Cochrane Library (2). John Wiley & Sons, Oxford

Homer C 1999 The St George Outreach Maternity Project (STOMP) in current research projects. Family Health Research Unit Business Plan 1999–2000, February 1999, p 7

Howell CJ 1999 Epidural versus non-epidural analgesia for pain relief in labour (Cochrane Review). Cochrane Library (2). John Wiley & Sons, Oxford

Hueston WJ, Rudy M 1993 A comparison of labour and delivery management between nurse midwives and family physicians. Journal of Family Practice 37(5):449–453

Hundley V, Cruickshank F, Lang G et al 1994 Midwife managed delivery unit: a randomised controlled comparison with consultant led care. British Medical Journal 309(11):1400–1404

Inglehart JK 1994 Physicians and the growth of managed care: health policy report. New England Journal of Medicine 331: 1167–1171

Kildea S 1999 And the women said. . . . . reporting on birthing services for Aboriginal Women from remote Top End communities. Women's Health Strategy Unit, Northern Territory Health Services, Australia

King's Fund 2001 Every voice counts: primary care organisations and public involvement. King's Fund bookshop, London

Kmietowicz Z 2002 Primary care trusts should give local people a voice. British Medical Journal 324(7338):633

Kohn LT, Corrigan JM, Donaldson (Eds) 2000 (IOM Report) Committee on Quality of Healthcare in America, Institute of Medicine. To err is human: building a safer health system. National Academy Press, Washington DC. Online: http://books.nap.edu/books

Labonte R 1999 Globalism and health: threats and opportunities. Health Promotion Journal of Australia 9(2):126–132

Laing BA 1990 Error in medicine: legal impediments to US reform. Journal of Health Politics, Policy and Law 24:27–58

Lancaster P 1999 Senate Inquiry into Childbirth Procedures; Senate references Community Affairs Hansard, Canberra, 27 August 1999: CA 1-36. Online: http://www.aph.gov.au/hansard

Law R 2000 'Do all things practicable to reduce risk' should apply in the health system. (Letters) British Medical Journal 321:505

Leap N 1999 Defining midwifery as we develop woman-centred practice. ACMI Conference proceedings, Hobart, 2–4 September 1999

Leape LL, Lawthers AG, Brennan TA et al 1993 Preventing medical injury. Qualitative Review Bulletin 19:144–149

Leatherman S, Berwick DM 2000 The NHS through American eyes. It has an enviable goal and constancy of purpose: build on it. British Medical Journal 321(7276):1545–1546

Leeder SR 2002 The 'health insurance' furphy that the public can't afford. In Touch. Newsletter of the Public Health Association of Australia Inc. 19(3):7–12

Light D 1997 From managed competition to managed cooperation: theory and lessons from the British experience. Millbank Quarterly 75(3):297–341

Light D 1999 Good managed care needs National Health Insurance. Annals of Internal Medicine 130:686–689

Light D 2000 Fostering a justice-based health care system. Contemporary Sociology. A Journal of Reviews 29(1):62–74

Loombia Ania 1998 Colonialism/postcolonialism: the new critical idiom. Routledge, London

MacDorman M, Singh G 1998 Midwifery care, social and medical risk factors and birth outcomes in the USA. Journal of Epidemiology and Community Health 52(5):310–317

MacFarlane AJ, Chamberlain GVPC 1993 What is happening to Caesarean section rates? Lancet 342:1005–1006

Majeed A 1996 Allocating budgets for fundholding and prescribing. British Medical Journal 313:1274–1275

Majeed A, Malcolm L 1999 Unified budgets for primary care groups. British Medical Journal 318:772–776

Malcolm L 1997 GP budget holding in New Zealand: lessons for Britain and elsewhere? British Medical Journal 314:1890–1892

Malcolm L, Barnett P, Wright L 1999 Towards integrated primary care in New Zealand: contrasts with Australia. Conference abstracts: Australian and New Zealand Health Services Research Conference. Sydney, 8–11 August 1999, p 97

Malcolm L, Mays N 1999 New Zealand's independent practitioner associations: a working model of clinical governance in primary care? British Medical Journal 319:1340–1342

Marmot M 1999 The solid facts: the social determinants of health. Health Promotion Journal of Australia 9(2):133–139

Martin Emily 1989 The woman in the body. Open University Press, Milton Keynes

McCourt C, Page L 1996 Report on the evaluation of one-to-one midwifery practice. Wolfson School of Health Sciences, Thames Valley University

McWhinney I 1998 Core values in a changing world. British Medical Journal 316:1807–1809

Mechanic D 1975 The comparative study of healthcare delivery systems. Annual Review of Sociology 1:43–65

Mechanic D 1997 The dilemmas of managed care. Letters in response. Journal of the American Medical Association 287(10):820

Mechanic D 1998 The functions and limitations of trust in the provision of medical care. Journal of Health Politics, Policy and Law 23(4):661–686

Mechanic D, Rochefort DA 1996 Comparative medical systems. Annual Review of Sociology 22:239–270

Middle C, MacFarlane A 1995 Labour and delivery of 'normal' primiparous women: analysis of routinely collected data. British Journal of Obstetrics and Gynaecology 102:970–977

Mooney G, Scotton R 2000 Economics and Australian health policy. Allen & Unwin, Sydney

Murray J 2002 Refining the process of Litigation. 2nd speaker at the Australian Health Ministers Advisory Council Medical Litigation Workshop to Discuss Opportunities for Legal Change and Administrative Reform, Canberra 22 April 2002

Nancarrow SA 1999 An outcomes framework for community healthcare. Conference abstracts: Australian and New Zealand Health Services Research Conference. Sydney, 8–11 August 1999, p 102

Nassar N, Sullivan E 2001 Australia's mothers and babies 1999. AIHW National Perinatal Statistics Unit, Sydney. AIHW Cat. No. PER 19, p 48. Online: http://www.aihw.gov.au/npsu/

National Health & Medical Research Council (NHMRC) 1996 Options for effective care in childbirth. AGPS, Canberra

National Health & Medical Research Council (NHMRC) 1999 WH26. A review of services offered by midwives. Online: http://www.health.gov.au/nhmrc/publicat/wh-home.htm

Neilson JP 1999 Ultrasound for fetal assessment in early pregnancy (Cochrane Review). Cochrane Library (2). John Wiley & Sons, Oxford

New Zealand College of Midwives (NZCOM) 1986 Records of labour ward log books (unpublished)

New Zealand College of Midwives (NZCOM) 2005 Joint venture proposal to The Minister of Health, New Zealand College of Midwives, Christchurch

Noble AA, Troyen BA 2001 Managing care in the new era of 'systems think': the implications for managed care organizational liability and patient safety. Journal of Law, Medicine and Ethics 16(4):290–297

Olsen O 1997 Meta-analysis of the safety of home birth. Birth 24(10):4–13

Olsen O, Jewell MD 1999 Home versus hospital birth (Cochrane Review). Cochrane Library (3). John Wiley & Sons, Oxford

Orellana C 2002 Reform in German hospital funding system concerns doctors. Lancet 359(9303): 328

Palmer G 1994 New Zealand's accident compensation scheme twenty years on. University of Toronto Law Journal 44:223–273

Parloff R 2002 Tortageddon: why the September 11 victims' fund could become a template for mass tort reform. (September 11 Victims Compensation Fund) American Lawyer 24(3):106–108

Pearson V 1994 Antenatal ultrasound scanning. University of Bristol, Healthcare Evaluation Uni, 26

Pena-Dolhun E, Grumbach K, Vranizan K et al 2001 Unlocking specialists attitudes toward primary care gatekeepers. Journal of Family Practice 50:1032–1037

Pollack H, Zeckhauser R 1996 Budgets as dynamic gatekeepers. Management Science 42:642–658

Rajan L 1994 The impact of obstetric procedures and analgesia/anaesthesia during labour and delivery on breast feeding. Midwifery 10(2):87–103

Reibel T 1999 Senate Inquiry into Childbirth Procedures. Senate references. Community Affairs Hansard, Perth, 8 September 1999: CA 314–320. Online: http://www.aph.gov.au/hansard

Reynolds JL 1997 Post-traumatic stress disorder after childbirth: the phenomenon of traumatic birth. CMAJ 156(6):831–835

Richards T 1996 European health policy: must redefine its raison d'etre. British Medical Journal 312:1622–1623

Richards T 1998 Partnership with patients: patients want more than simply information; they need involvement too. British Medical Journal 316:85–86

Richardson J 2002 What are the objectives of the health system? Healthcover 12(1):15–17

Robinson JC 2002 The end of managed care. Journal of the American Medical Association 285:2622–2628

Rockner G, Fianu-Jonasson A 1999 Changed pattern in the use of episiotomy in Sweden. British Journal of Obstetrics and Gynaecology 106:95–101

Ryding EL, Wijma K, Wijma B 1998 Psychological impact of emergency Cesarean section in comparison with elective Cesarean section, instrumental and normal vaginal delivery. Journal of Psychosomatic Obstetrics and Gynecology 19(3):135–144

Shorten A, Shorten B 1999 Episiotomy in NSW hospitals 1993–1996: towards understanding variations between public and private hospitals. Australian Health Review 22(1): 19–32

Sleep J, Grant AM 1987 West Berkshire perineal management trial: three year follow up. British Medical Journal 295:749–751

Sleep J, Grant AM, Garcia J et al 1984 West Berkshire perineal management trial. British Medical Journal 289: 587–590

Smith J 1998a On complexities of health systems, journals and associations. Australian Health Review 21(1):3–7

Smith J 1998b The AHA's ideas on health policies for Australia. Australian Health Review 21(2):38–65

Smith PC 1999 Setting budgets for general practice in the new NHS. British Medical Journal 318:776–779

Starfield B 1994 Is primary care essential? Lancet 344:1129–1133

Starfield B 2001 New paradigms for quality in primary care. British Journal of General Practice 51:303–310

Surender R, Bradlow J, Coulter A et al 1995 Prospective study of trends in referral patterns in fundholding and non-fundholding practices in the Oxford region, 1990–4. British Medical Journal 311:1205–1208

Tew M & Damstra-Wijmenga S 1991 Safest birth attendants: recent Dutch evidence. Midwifery 7(2):55–63

The Ljubljana Charter on Reforming Healthcare 1996. British Medical Journal 312:1664–1665

Tito F 1996 Review of professional indemnity arrangements for healthcare professionals: Final Report. AGPS, Canberra

Toop L 1998 Primary care: core values. Patient centred primary care. British Medical Journal 316:1882–1883

Tracy SK 1997 Midwifery care for women in pregnancy and childbirth: a systematic review of the literature. MA Midwifery Practice thesis. Thames Valley University & Wolfson School of Health Sciences, London

Turnbull D, Holmes A, Shields N et al 1996 Randomised controlled trial of efficacy of midwife-managed care. Lancet 348(9022):213–218

UK Department of Health 1997 The New NHS. Department of Health, London

Waldenstrom U, Turnbull D 1998 A systematic review comparing continuity of midwifery care with standard maternity services. British Journal of Obstetrics and Gynaecology 105(11): 1160–1170

Westin S 1998 The NHS's 50th anniversary. A great leap for humankind? British Medical Journal 317:49–51

White J 2002 Nursing: a health services management crisis amenable to health services research? Plenary speaker's address New Zealand—Australian Health Services and Policy Research Conference, December 2–4, Wellington New Zealand. Reported in Healthcover 12(1):30–33

Wilson RM, Runciman WR, Gibberd RW et al 1995 The Quality in Australian Healthcare Study. Medical Journal of Australia 163:458–471

Wilson T, Sheikh A 2002 Enhancing public safety in primary care. British Medical Journal 324(7337): 584–588

World Health Organization (WHO) 1998 The Solid Facts. WHO, Copenhagen Regional Office. Online: http://www.who.dk.document/e59555.pdf

World Health Organization (WHO) 2000 The WHO Report 2000: Health Systems Performance. WHO, Geneva

CHAPTER 2

The Australian and New Zealand context

Jill White

Key terms

Anglo-Celtic, Australian Aboriginal, Indigenous, mana, Maori, multiculturalism, Pakeha, tapu, Treaty of Waitangi, utu

Chapter overview

Other chapters of this book introduce the philosophical contexts of midwifery and maternity services generally, and the specific contexts of women in the world. This chapter seeks to situate this understanding of women, mothers and their babies, and maternity services within the social, historical and cultural contexts of Australia and New Zealand.

Having lived as woman, mother, midwife and nurse in both countries I am approaching this chapter as I lived in these countries. My approach was to accept that despite their geographic closeness they are as different as France and Germany, or the United States and Mexico. It is, I believe, important to try to understand their separateness and then to be surprised by the similarities rather than, as many do, think of them as the same and only gradually, after episodes that can only be seen as culturally insensitive, come to understand the differences. Appreciating such difference, this chapter will look at each country in turn.

In exploring the social, historical and cultural contexts of any country, looking first at the history provides an explanatory backdrop for the current relationships

and attitudes as played out socially and culturally. The brief histories presented here are by no means historians' histories. The social and cultural comments are those of neither sociologists nor anthropologists. They are practitioner histories, and social and cultural commentaries, stories that highlight some salient social and historical events that give colour to a picture of a past that inevitably influences the present and the people with whom we work as midwives, and the values the women and their families express in our interactions with them in practice.

Learning outcomes

Learning outcomes for this chapter are:

1   To describe the cardinal elements of the histories of Australia and New Zealand

2   To analyse the effects of European colonisation on the Indigenous peoples of both countries

3   To discuss the importance of the Treaty of Waitangi to Maori and Pakeha in contemporary New Zealand society

4   To discuss the place of women in contemporary New Zealand and Australian societies, and the influence of history on this positioning

5   To explain the key social and cultural similarities and differences between Australia and New Zealand.

Australia

Early Australia

Australia has been home to its Aboriginal population for more than 50,000 years, and to Europeans for a mere 200 years. For Aborigines this represents 2000 generations of living, hunting and gathering in this often harsh environment. There are estimated to have been about 300,000 Aborigines living in Australia in 1788 when Europeans arrived. This population was spread across over 500 tribes, each with its own dialect, history, culture and territory. While all tribes were semi-nomadic hunters and gatherers moving across their specific territory with seasonal purpose, the size of their tribal grounds varied from 500 square kilometres in generous coastal areas to 100,000 square kilometres in desert areas (Broome 2001). Land connection was and is fundamental to Aboriginal being and features in their stories, songs and paintings. In particular, 'the lives of the Aborigines were shaped by their Dreamtime stories which were both an explanation of how the world came to be, and how people must conduct their behaviour and social relations' (Broome 2001, p 19).

From the time the Dutch navigated to what is now known as Indonesia in the sixteenth century there had been tales of rich southern lands, and ships from many countries sought these lands. A Spaniard, de Torres, navigated the straits between northern Australia and New Guinea in 1606. In 1616 the Dutch commander Hartog found the western Australian coast. There followed many more ships from Holland finding and naming land along the southern Australian coast. Tasman found what was to become Tasmania and named it van Dieman's Land after the Governor of the East Indies in Java, then a Dutch colony. Then, rather than travelling north along the Australian coast, Tasman sailed further east and found the coast of New Zealand. But as these ships were in search of gold and spices, their discoveries of land that appeared undeveloped and lacking in riches was not valued by their home countries.

At the end of the seventeenth century an Englishman, Dampier, voyaged to western Australia but again reported he had found little of value, little water and little available food. Some signs of European life were found on the edges of the continent but were the flotsam and jetsam of wrecked ships and sailors who had perished.

So Australia became known to the European world piece by piece in multiple voyages from many different countries, but was coveted mainly by the British. When the British government sent Captain Cook to the South Seas, ostensibly to study an eclipse from the oceans near Tahiti in order to help problems of navigation, the opportunity presented itself to search for the southern land and to take possession of it for Britain. International law at the time required a 'new' country to be taken only after permission was sought from the 'natives', that is, unless the land was either uninhabited or inhabited by a people who did not appear to use the land. In 1770 James Cook 'discovered' Australia's eastern coast and he and his party landed in what has become known as Botany Bay. The ship's name and date were carved on a tree and the British flag planted on the soil. After many reported attempts to engage peacefully with the 'natives' Cook recorded in his diary, 'All they seem'd to want was for us to be gone' (Clark et al 2000, p 20). He recorded the lack of interest of the Aborigines in the trinkets, ribbons and cloth that he had left for them, and their lack of clothing, organised housing or land usage, thus attempting to justify, according to the law of the time, his taking of the land, as it had no organised system of government with whom to negotiate. Cook arrived back in England in 1771 and the government, far from being uninterested in his 'discovery', began to make plans to use this new land as a penal colony as England's gaols were overcrowded and they could no longer sell their prisoners to America, as had been their most recent solution to their social problem (Clark et al 2000).

Here we have the first of many of the significant differences in the development of Australia and New Zealand as neighbouring but distinctly different countries. The organised system of Maori living, recognised by the Europeans as familiar, led to the development and signing of a treaty, rather than just a taking of 'empty' lands.

In January 1788 the eleven ships of the First Fleet entered the harbour in Botany Bay carrying 759 convicts and 200 marine guards, the chaplain and the captain who was to govern them, Captain Arthur Phillip. This was the place Cook had detailed in his week-long visit in a wet autumn eighteen years earlier. But as any antipodean knows, Sydney in January is quite a different picture to the cool of autumn, and the harsh reality of what they had before them in setting up a colony must have been a terrifying thought. They quickly realised the place they had landed would not support them and moved just north to Sydney Cove with its fresh water source and more fertile plains. But accidents of history are amazing. Within days of the English landing, a French ship under Captain La Perouse landed. What would have happened had storms or winds delayed the First Fleet and La Perouse attempted to claim the land for France we will never know. How different might the outcome for the Indigenous population have been? Again we cannot know, but given the similar patterns of constructing European communities one can imagine a contest would still have occurred for the best and most productive lands and for sources of fresh water.

Accounts of the early days of the settlement are of Aborigines being frightened off their lands by musket-discharging soldiers, and convicts and soldiers being frightened by spear-throwing 'natives'. Two groups of people thrust together in a harsh environment, with no understanding of the way of life of the other, no common language and each with a determination and need to survive. The early 1800s saw the senior members of the European colony discussing the 'native problem' and seeing 'civilising' the natives as the only solution. But these discussions concerned a relatively small colony around the area of Sydney. The rest of Australia remained relatively untouched by European settlement. That is, until the stroke of a pen on the other side of the world resulted in the slashing of duty for Australian wool compared to that of European wool producers. By 1850 200,000 migrants had moved from the United Kingdom to fell trees, clear land and graze sheep.

By 1860 4000 Europeans with 20 million sheep occupied the prime river-fed land from southern Queensland to South Australia (Broome 2001). An itinerant male workforce working in rough country with a male to female ratio of 40 men to every woman framed the beginnings of the nation that 'grew on the sheep's back' as it was colloquially described. A nation of burly men, of mateship and of women being seen as 'damned whores and God's police', a situation so colourfully captured by Anne Summers (1994) in the title of her book chronicling women's lives in early Australia. The small number of women compared to men throughout the early days of European settlement had predictable consequences for the Aboriginal people, as the Indigenous women became 'useful' to white men as domestic servants and at times in sexual relationships, both consensual and non-consensual.

As white men moved further away from the coast, they increasingly disrupted the tribal grounds of individual Aboriginal groupings and forced them onto the traditional grounds of others. This progressively disrupted the seasonal movements across the lands and brought Aboriginal tribal groups into conflict with each other as well as with the white 'settlers'. But far more devastatingly it disturbed a way of life that had existed for thousands of years, with rules of kinship and community and spirituality that were difficult to sustain out of the more nomadic lifestyle. Nutrition and infection control in the form of sanitation were adversely affected by a static form of living and resulted in poor diet, ear, eye and chest infections and diarrhoea. Also negatively affected was the sense of purpose in what were the daily rituals associated with hunting and gathering. European infections of smallpox, influenza, measles and even the common cold also damaged the Indigenous communities, who had no resistance to these new and foreign organisms. Fighting was particularly intense on the frontiers, with many deaths on both sides, but the balance of musket and spear was irrevocably disturbed by the introduction of the repeating rifle in 1870.

Aborigines were forced to live either in distant government-controlled reserves, on church-run 'missions' or close to but on the edges of white settlements in order to provide their families with safety, food and shelter. It is estimated that by the early 1900s, the population was only a quarter of that of 1788.

Variations on the New South Wales experience were repeated throughout the country. In 1829 Captain Fremantle annexed 7000 kilometres of the western Australian coast for Britain and settlement began. By 1830 over 1500 British immigrants had landed in the Swan River region of western Australia. However, unlike the beginnings in New South Wales, the Western Australian experience was of young people and families coming to start new lives, not of convicts and soldiers and a virtually all-male environment. In 1836 a further colony was begun, this time in South Australia at a site close to the mouth of the river Murray. This too was a settlement of 'free settlers'. Settlement by families had the potential to create very different societies to those dominated by men and may hold some explanation of the more 'cultured' reputation of Adelaide.

Other settlements that were to become state capitals grew at around the same time. They all experienced similar hardships and conflicts with those Aboriginal tribes who had also valued the land where rivers meet the sea and which are the most fertile. But there are stories of settlements with better race relations than others. Captain George Grey, for example, had developed a genuine respect for and understanding of the Aborigines after having experienced an accident in the north of Western Australia. He had been sheltered and fed by the 'natives' there and had come to hold them in higher esteem than his predecessor British colonial officers. Captain George Grey's 'success' with the natives resulted in several of his subsequent government postings, first to Adelaide as Governor and then to New Zealand, as the Maori Wars were causing British nervousness about the stability of the new country. We will meet up with Governor Grey later, in New Zealand, as he was to very nearly play an interesting role in Maori health and wellbeing post colonisation.

Darwin's 1859 *On the Origin of Species* and his notion of 'survival of the fittest' was well known in Australia by the late 1800s and provided what was at the time an acceptable, 'logical' and 'scientific' explanation for the racism that had come to dominate Australian attitudes to its Indigenous people by the latter part of the 1800s and early 1900s.

Broome (2001, pp 92–93) paints this picture of misunderstanding:

> The cultural and physical differences between the Aborigines and the Europeans created basic misunderstandings and a lack of sympathy between the two groups. Racism thrived on this gulf of ignorance. The first Europeans viewed Aboriginal society in terms of European values and thus saw it negatively. They stressed Aborigines did not wear clothes, build houses, till the soil or have recognizable religions, kings or forms of government. It never occurred to them that a hunter-gatherer society in a warm climate had no use for clothes, permanent houses or agriculture. The Europeans were also clearly wrong when they thought the Aborigines had no religion, law, leaders or forms of government. Seeing the world as they did, the Europeans rated their own society as the highest on the scale of human development and Aboriginal society as one of the lowest. Yet Aboriginal society was not 'primitive' as Europeans claimed, but simply different. There is no doubt that Aborigines in turn did not understand why the Europeans wore heavy clothing in a warm climate or bothered to build homes or grow crops when there were hundreds of varieties of food in the bush for the taking. Aboriginal philosophers would have rated European society low, and much European activity as valueless.
>
> Also both groups were generally unimpressed by the physical appearance of the other. The Aborigines were shocked by the pale eyes, thin noses, fair hair and white skins of the European, so much so that they first thought them to be spirits of the dead. The Europeans in turn were startled by the ritual ornamentation … applied to Aboriginal bodies, their flat noses, their black skin and their nakedness. Not all on both sides were repulsed as the frequent sexual contacts between the two groups revealed.

The paternalistic attitude and the overt racism that such attitudes brought forth were a feature of Australian society until the 1970s, and many would say are still present.

Federation of the colonies into a nation: a Commonwealth of Australia

On 1 January 1901 the six colonies that had developed around the coastline of Australia became a federated nation: the Commonwealth of Australia. Its population was recorded at the time as 3.75 million. Aborigines were not counted as part of this census; nor, when the parliament was set up, were they permitted to vote. Indeed it was not until 1962 that Aborigines were allowed to vote.

The perception of many Australians is of politics as having been male-dominated from its inception but a study of the political history of Australia tells a different story. From the beginning of Federation, women nominated for parliament, with three women nominating for the senate as early as 1903, although it was 41 years before a woman was elected to federal parliament (Sawer & Simms 1993). Clearly, women were anxious for the role but not elected into it. Thus parliament may have been male-dominated but politics was not—women used the elections as opportunities to voice their concerns and lobby for change.

The new Australia was seen as full of promise and potential wealth, and as the dominant view was that the Aborigines would soon die out, it was seen to be a country for and of white people. Two of the first pieces of legislation passed in the new federal parliament were restricting immigration to white people (the language used at the time to describe what is now referred to as Anglo-Celtic or European). Unofficially this legislation became known as the 'White Australia Policy'. This was not the first legislation to keep out or restrict the rights of those who were not white. In the mid-1800s, gold had been found in New South Wales and the gold rush began, doubling the population in less than 10 years. With wool and gold, Australia looked like the land of opportunity. People began to come not only from Europe—Chinese people flooded in, in their tens of thousands, for gold. Consequently, legislation was passed to limit Chinese immigration; those who were already here were not permitted to be naturalised and were to be regarded for generations as 'foreigners'. This dismissal of the Chinese as legitimate citizens occurred in spite of the fact that in the Northern Territory by 1879 there were only 400 Europeans but 3500 Chinese.

Federation was seen as a mechanism for integrating the whole of Australia under a British parliamentary structure and hence ensuring its 'white' future. This situation is perplexing when one looks at the already existing ethnic mix. Manning Clark et al (2000, p 127) quote the following demographics at the time of Federation:

> Three-quarters had been born in Australia, the greatest majority were of English, Irish or Scottish descent. But there were also 30,000 people born in China, 4,000 in Japan, 7,600 in India, 38,400 in Germany, 10,000 in Sweden, 5,600 in Italy, 6,300 in Denmark, 7,500 in the United States and 5,200 born at sea.

The World Wars

The First World War was important in the formation of a sense of a national Australian identity and an identity separate from

Reflective exercise

Imagine yourself a convict woman arriving on one of the early ships to settle in Port Jackson. What would be your hopes and fears?

Imagine yourself as an Aboriginal woman and mother in the early 1800s in south-eastern Australia. What would be your hopes and fears?

Britain. By 1914 more than 20,000 men had joined the armed forces and had landed in Egypt for training. The Australians landed at the same time as the troops from New Zealand and collectively they became known as the ANZACs (the Australian and New Zealand Army Corps). Together they met some of the most ferocious fighting, particularly at Gallipoli, in Turkey. The way in which these men dealt with their dire and tragic situation led to the development of what became known as the ANZAC spirit; more than 26,000 Australians and over 7500 New Zealanders died at Gallipoli, but the stories of the determination, mateship and bravery are now legend. Following the debacle of Gallipoli, many of the survivors were taken to Europe to fight at the Western Front against the German army in different but equally atrocious conditions. The conditions faced on the Western Front are graphically represented by Sebastian Faulks (1993) in his book *Birdsong: A Novel of Love and War*, a harrowing but accessible account of the kinds of hardships the Australians and New Zealanders would have faced.

Many Australian women joined the war effort as nurses, but women were not allowed to be part of the war in any other formal capacity. They were left to undertake all the everyday jobs that had previously been the province of men, particularly in the country, with fencing, shearing and heavy farm work.

As we have seen, Australia, while choosing to see itself as racially Anglo-Celtic, was already a very multicultural country. Many Germans had settled in the areas around Adelaide and had begun Australia's winemaking industry as early as the 1840s. With Australia, through its ties to Britain, now at war with Germany, internment camps were set up to house the over 6000 German, Austrian and Turkish people living in Australia in 1916–17 (Eshuys et al 1996). Yet again, racial divisions across the country raised their ugly heads as people were rounded up and placed behind barbed wire in guarded compounds, many miles away from homes, work and friends.

Following the war, the 1920s were prosperous and exciting. Women began to enter state parliaments, with Western Australia first in 1921, New South Wales in 1925, Queensland in 1929 and South Australia last in 1959. But the joys of the post-war twenties were followed quickly by the depression of the 1930s. People were evicted from their houses and many men went 'on the long road with their swag'—in other words, walked from town to town in search of whatever work they could find and sleeping in the open on bedding carried rolled on their backs.

In 1939 Australia was once more at war. This time the immediate threat to Australia was from the Japanese. Internment camps were again set up, this time for Italians, Germans and Japanese. Women moved again out of the home and into industry and were relied upon to keep not only the 'home fires burning' but also the furnaces of industry.

Unlike the First World War, the Second World War was also fought in the Pacific, and therefore posed a significant threat to Australia directly. This war was more about fighting for Australia than for any notion of the 'Mother Land'.

The 1950s and beyond

The situation following the Second World War was different from that of the previous post-war experience. The direct threat to Australia had made politicians acutely aware of the vastness of the country, its small population and the potential threat this presented from the 'teeming hordes from Asia', a popular phrase at the time. This time the government knew there was a need for workers for factories, farms and service industries. Government policy was 'populate or perish' and the first waves of post-war immigration began. British immigrated on a very heavily assisted passage for a mere ten pounds. These people became known as the 'ten quid Poms'. Italians, Greeks, Germans and Dutch were also encouraged to come to Australia.

In the 1950s the economy grew, unemployment was low and the birth rate soared as a result of the 'baby boomers', babies born between the end of the war and 1960. Women's place was again seen as predominantly in the home, and outside work returned to being the province of the men. Australia experienced a period of domestic 'harmony' through the 1950s and 1960s as a 'miniature England', with beginning influences of the United States, following its interaction with Australia in the Second World War. It was a time reminiscent of scenes in the movie of *The Stepford Wives*—domestic bliss with men as Men and women as their contented domestic servants.

Australia was to change profoundly with the international winds of change of the early seventies, with the growing peace movement, calls for the end of war and nuclear weapons, demands for civil rights for all citizens, demands for equal rights for women by groups like the newly formed Women's Electoral Lobby, and a questioning of traditional 'family values'. The Whitlam government came to power in 1972 and quickly Australia was challenged with respect to its racist and sexist complacency. In its first fortnight in power, Whitlam's government abolished conscription, moved towards equal pay for women, increased spending on Aboriginals, abolished British knighthoods and introduced Australian honours, increased spending on education, the arts and health; race was no longer a consideration in immigration, and sporting teams who selected on colour or race were banned from Australia. Unfortunately, a slump in the world economy, rising oil prices and a hostile Senate led to the curtailment of these radical changes.

Whitlam's changes to foreign policy and immigration policy changed Australia's ethnic mix forever. The Whitlam government was dismissed by the governor-general, John Kerr, and the leader of the opposition was installed as caretaker prime minister until an election could be called. Whitlam lost in a Liberal landslide. By then, Australia had changed. There was now a different understanding of the place of women, Aborigines, land rights, and attitudes to non-European immigrants.

The next significant immigration wave was of South-East Asian people after the Vietnam War, followed in the 1970s and 1980s by an influx from Middle-Eastern countries and South America. By the end of the 1980s Australia was one of the most multicultural countries in the world.

Australian 'identity'

The Australian 'identity' has long been a contradictory one. Described by Ward in *The Australian Legend* nearly 50 years ago as 'the rough, honest, easy-going bushman, laconic, resourceful, loyal to his mates, uncomfortable with parsons and women, facing adversity with a stoical joke' (summarised in Hudson & Bolton 1997, p 1), to which could be added 'Anglo-Celtic bloke', this view still permeates society despite the multicultural nature of the population and the fact that more than three-quarters of the population live an urban life in coastal cities.

Hudson and Bolton (1997) exhort us to look to Australia's multiple personalities rather than find attachment in a single, perhaps only briefly existing, 'rural ideal' and to be cognisant of the amazing diversity that is the essence of the different regions within Australia. What it is to be Australian and live in Australia is very different if one is in inner-city Sydney or in Bourke or Broken Hill, and different again if one is in Perth or Broome. Even within the large cities there are now suburbs with such ethnic homogeneity that the shop signs are in Vietnamese or Arabic or Greek, and the norms of behaviour and identity vary in each.

The single Australian story may have been male, with the female either absent or as the shadow behind the man, but the women's history is a varied one too. Early attempts to tell a women's story, such as Miriam Dixon's (1976) *The Real Matilda*, paint a picture of an oppressed group. The introduction to Dixon's book begins, 'In this exploratory book I propose that Australian women, women in the land of mateship, "the Ocker", keg-culture, come pretty close to top rating as the "Doormats of the Western World"' (Dixon 1993, p 11). But the women's story is populated also by gutsy feminists at the turn of the century standing for parliament, fighting for peace, for pensions for the aged and invalided.

These women broke down the barriers to women's entry to medicine (1897), law (1903) and architecture (1889), but had to wait until after the Second World War to enter the other male bastions of the Church, the armed forces and engineering. Vida Goldstein in 1902 went to Washington to the founding conference of what was to become the International Women's Suffrage Alliance and served as its secretary. Women were also internationally published authors, such as Miles Franklin, who gives us a glimpse into a gutsy heroine in Sybylla Melvyn in *My Brilliant Career*. Jesse Street in 1946 was the Australian delegate to the United Nations. These women were part of the first wave of feminism. The second wave was to come in the 1970s.

But if there was one constant in the interruption to the development of women and their voices in Australian history, it is war. War created the ANZAC legend, reinforcing the mateship ethic as central to being 'dinky-di' Australian. It gave women the unsung role of keeping the urban and rural productivity going while the men were overseas, but they were expected to relinquish these positions when the men returned and to adjust to living with a generation of men brutalised by their experiences of the inhumanity of war. Following the Second World War, women again left the jobs they had managed but this time they were not only child-bearing but were also expected to join the workforce without the advantage of the same educational, occupational and economic opportunities as men.

The need for the country to have a single common image to relate to is seen by White (1981, 1997) to be a construction of a market that had products to sell. He writes of the relationship between the market and a sense of being a nation, citing as examples the Heidelberg school of painting's need to be iconic, as they had to be saleable to galleries rather than private collectors, the *Bulletin*'s need for a single popular market, and latterly in the 1980s and 1990s, the advertising agencies' need to sell beer, collectively contributing to over a hundred years of image reinforcement. Women did not control the spending power and were thus rendered invisible in all but domestic commercials and image portrayals.

So the quintessential Australian became a construction that was male, of mateship, exhibiting a laconic sense of humour, and while predominantly white, of 'tolerance' to others. The Anglo-Celtic Australian notion of multicultural tolerance is questioned by Curthoys (1997, p 35). 'Tolerance' suggests two elements: the tolerators and the tolerated.

> Tolerance may be better than intolerance but it does not guarantee equality. Anglo-Celtic Australians, in their enthusiasm for multiculturalism and thereby the new inclusive Australian identity, are, then, still expressing power relations, still speaking from a self-confident centre, the Australian nation. They are doing the including, not being included. The politics of inclusion, based on notions of community and identity absorbs difference within a pre-given and predefined space.

Taking the argument a step further, Curthoys says: 'Everyone in Australia who is non-Indigenous, the "tolerators" and the "tolerated" alike, still share in and are advantaged by a history of colonialism'. In speaking also of tolerance and diversity, Don Watson, in his now famous speech, 'A Toast to the Postmodern Republic', said:

> I'm only just game enough to say it: it might be the first postmodern republic, and I mean that in the nicest possible way. I mean a republic that exalts the nation less than the way of life. Whose principal value is tolerance rather than conformity, difference rather than uniformity (quoted in Wark 1997, p 152).

Watson's 1997 speech pre-dated the move to the Right and the resurgence of sexism and racism in Australian society that has occurred under the Liberal Howard government.

A very interesting and easily readable book that traverses Australia from the 1950s to the beginning of the twenty-first century is the autobiography of Wendy McCarthy (2000), *Don't Fence Me In*.

Anne Summers (2003) again became the conscience of Australia with her powerful recent book *The End of Equality: Work, Babies and Women's Choices in 21st Century Australia*. In the introduction, Summers (2003, pp 2–3) says:

> Yet although the language of equality is still used, and despite the successes of so many individual women, the actual experience of far too many women in Australia today suggests that the promise of equality has not been met. Sadly, we are actually going in the opposite direction. If we look at the economic, physical and social markers of women's well-being, the picture that is revealed is in grim contrast to the rhetoric of equality and accomplishment … Despite appearances to the contrary, the proportion of women in full-time employment has not increased in thirty years. More Australian women work part-time than in any other country in the industrialized world . . . not from choice . . . but because of a lack of childcare or other support . . . Equal pay is a myth . . . The number of women totally dependent on welfare has increased to an unprecedented degree . . . As a result of all these factors, there are more women living at the economic margin, or actual poverty than ever before.

In contradiction to a self-image of tolerance, the plight of refugees and asylum seekers in Australia has shocked many in the Australian community. The Australian government's agreement to assist the United States in a war 'against terrorism' in Iraq again divided the nation. Any notion of being a nation with a single voice has recently been seriously challenged. Australia's stance on both these issues is in stark contrast to the stance of New Zealand, again reinforcing the separateness of the two countries.

Modern Aboriginal society

I position myself in writing this section as a middle-class Anglo-Celtic, fifth-generation Australian woman and do not presume to be able to authentically tell an Aboriginal and

---

Reflective exercise

What are the issues that affect you as a woman in contemporary Australian society, and in what way have these issues been influenced by the history of this country?

Torres Strait Islander story. I will distill some of what writers have seen as the cardinal events in Aboriginal society for you here so you can form a schema from which to do your own further reading.

No version of modern Australian Aboriginal and Torres Strait Islander society can make sense without an understanding of the effects of European colonisation. We were briefly introduced to this earlier in the chapter. What we did not focus on at that time is the collision of paternalistic intentions to try to 'save a dying race' and the removal of children from their parents and families, to become known in Australian history as 'The Stolen Generation'.

In 1906 Bishop Frodsman was reported to have said:

> The Aborigines are disappearing. In the course of a generation or two, at the most, the last Australian blackfellow will have turned his face to warm mother earth . . . Missionary work then may be only smoothing the pillow of a dying race, but I think if the Lord Jesus came to Australia he would be moved with great compassion for these poor outcasts, living by the wayside, robbed of their land, wounded by the lust and passion of a stronger race, and dying (Broome 2001, p 105).

Thinking of the adults as 'lost causes', the missionaries and the government determined to 'save the children'. The main strategy used was to separate the children from their parents. Some parents agreed to this separation as they saw it as a means to enhance and protect their children's health and wellbeing, despite the grief of separation; some children were forcibly removed from their parents. The children were removed to either government reserves or church missions.

Mission or reserve schooling and life left the children between two worlds, belonging to neither. Restricting the children and young adults to life on the missions or reserves not only introduced them to European foods and language but disturbed their learning of bush ways and independence in being able to hunt and gather their own foods, increasing their dependency and depriving them of traditional rituals such as initiations, which were often banned. Most missions introduced the notion of matrimonial monogamy and marriage without respect for traditional relationship rules that had stood for generations. In 1953 the Australian Government financed the provision of medical and educational facilities on the missions, further entrenching their function in the assimilation of Aboriginal children into the lifestyle of white Australia.

But such a loss can remain submerged for only so long. The stories of the lives dislodged began to be recorded and the cry for self-determination for Aboriginal people became louder through the 1960s and 1970s, with several government inquiries into the treatment received on the missions and reserves, which had at times included severe physical punishment as well as family dislocation. To generalise on the experience of all missions and reserves is to do an injustice to some who valued and upheld the traditional language and customs but they do appear to have been in the minority.

The mission story and experience dominated the northern Aboriginal settlements but the story of south-eastern Aboriginals was of fringe settlement around the edges of the towns and cities or on government reserves, of which there were 49 in 1960 (Broome 2001). The people on the reserves were rigidly controlled under the *Aboriginal Protection Act* of 1909 and later amendments. In 1936, amendments to the Act gave the Aboriginal Protection Board powers to carry out compulsory medical checks and remove people to government settlements. Aboriginal children were not permitted in state schools until 1949.

Discrimination and racism caused poverty and lack of political power, which reinforced the cycle of poverty and discrimination. The flow-on effects of poverty, being of course poorer health and education status, led to further cycles of alienation and despair, confusion and loss of purpose, but with growing defiance for some. Alcohol became an increasing problem for some old enough to obtain it, and, for some younger Aborigines, glue and petrol sniffing. Although local group identity was strong, there had not been a history of a broader sense of national Aboriginal solidarity. Sport and art were two of the few areas in which Aboriginal young people had had opportunities to excel, as they did in boxing, football, tennis, dance and painting.

Movements for Aboriginal rights had existed sporadically since the 1920s. One of the most public and decisive movements came from William Cooper, who in 1937 led a campaign for the 150th anniversary of the landing of the First Fleet to be proclaimed a day of mourning, commemorating instead the 150th anniversary of misery and degradation of the original inhabitants by white invaders (Broome 2001). This was to resurface 50 years later, when the Bicentennial created a focus for national Aboriginal cohesion, and a questioning of Australia Day as a cause for celebration as opposed to a recognition of it as a day of mourning for the Indigenous people of Australia.

In 1961 the Federal Council for the Advancement of Aborigines was formed, changing its name in 1964 to include Torres Strait Islanders. In 1967, 89% of voters voted for Aboriginal citizenship, and the federal government, rather than the states, was given power to legislate on Aboriginal affairs, and the Department of Aboriginal Affairs was created. In 1972 the first Aboriginal tent embassy was set up on the lawns of Parliament House and was a symbol of a new Aboriginal determination. In 1973 a federal inquiry into Aboriginal land rights was established. Aboriginal stories began to be recorded and in the 1980s there was an explosion of oral history recording.

But it was not until 1992 that the fiction of the empty land, *terra nullius*, was overturned by the Mabo High Court decision after 222 years of European colonisation. Native title was enshrined in the *Native Title Act 1993* and required proof of continuous relationship to the land. The national focus of the 1990s and into the early 2000s is on Aboriginal and Torres Strait Islander health—physical, mental and spiritual.

The Human Rights and Equal Opportunity Commission in 1995 explored, amongst other matters, the removal of children from their parents and families. The inquiry heard that since 1911 in Queensland alone, over 6000 children had been removed. Some thought this to be a gross underestimation. The Stolen Generation and its sequelae are now an acknowledged part of Australian history, and their impact on current social and cultural life are recognised. The Commission's report, *Bringing Them Home*, estimated that 40,000 Aboriginal children had been removed from their families in the 1900s (HREOC 1997). In the decade from 1919, up to one-third of children were taken in the southern states.

The complex and troublesome issue for a generation of European Australians in attempting to come to terms with the consequences of the actions of their forebears has been explored in a highly readable book, *Being Whitefella*, edited by Duncan Graham (1994). This book is a compilation of 16 well-known and respected 'whitefellas' exploring their relationship with Aboriginal Australia.

In 1996 the Premier of New South Wales, Bob Carr, formally apologised in parliament, saying:

> I affirm in this place, formally and solemnly as Premier, on behalf of the government and people of New South Wales, our apology to Aboriginal people.

The federal government is yet to say 'Sorry', the word called for by Indigenous Australians. It has, however, committed to the 'process of reconciliation with Aboriginal and Torres Strait Islander people, in the context of redressing their profound social and economic disadvantage'. It appeared that Australia was beginning to take the necessary steps to atone for its past injustices. However, the 1996 federal election saw the election of Queensland Senator Pauline Hanson. Her maiden speech in parliament was a blatant attack on Aboriginal people and ignited racism again in Australia.

Poor health in the form of diabetes, renal disease, mental health problems, violence, alcoholism and domestic violence are difficulties still facing many Aboriginal families, for whom poverty is still the fundamental issue of discrimination. Half the deaths of Aboriginal men occur before they are 50, compared to only 13% in non-Indigenous men. The 1997 Census revealed that a smaller proportion of Aboriginal people than non-Aboriginal Australians drink alcohol—33% compared to 45%—but those Aborigines who drink do so more publicly and heavily than their non-Aboriginal counterparts. Twelve per cent of all drinkers drank harmful levels of alcohol; 80% of Aboriginal drinkers did so (Broome 2001). The Aboriginal

health statistics still show an unacceptable discrepancy in life expectancy and maternal and perinatal mortality. This will be addressed in detail later in the text.

This section would not, however, be complete without acknowledgement of the extraordinary accomplishment of many Aboriginal and Torres Strait Islander people, in business, parliament, sport, art, academia and indeed all aspects of life in Australia, in spite of two hundred years of colonisation.

New Zealand

Early New Zealand

New Zealand too is an ancient land, separating as its own land mass 80 million years ago. Yet, even in their geological and ecological foundations, Australia and New Zealand are profoundly different. The New Zealand land mass is turbulent and shaky, with large earthquakes a constant possibility and small tremors part of everyday life. The vegetation looks different, to an Australian eye, and vice versa—different green, different scrub or bush; and as flat and solid as Australia is, New Zealand is mountainous and forever shifting its footing.

By the time of British settlement in New Zealand, Maori had been living in New Zealand for at least a thousand years, having come from Polynesia in canoes ('waka'). Belich (1996, p 18) suggests that three cardinal features of Maori society that are still prized today were strongly present even at this time: mana, utu and tapu.

> Mana was a kind of spiritual capital, often translated as prestige or authority, inherited, acquired and lost by both individuals and groups. Utu was not simply revenge, but reciprocity, obliging one to return gifts as well as a blow. It was particularly important in relations between groups: the exchange of gifts and hospitality were positive utu. Tapu, a system of sanctity, social constraint and sacred laws, was complemented by its opposite—noa, which can be translated as normal, ordinary or unrestricted.

Maori were and are a tribal people with specific land affiliation. These lands they cultivated for root crops, supplementing their diet through fishing and hunting. Belich (1986, p 19) describes the first Maori–European interaction thus: 'The first Maori reaction to contact with Europeans was, unambiguously enough, to kill and eat them'. Tasman, the Dutch explorer spoken of earlier, visited the New Zealand coast in 1642, and his boats were attacked and several of his crew killed. When Cook visited in 1769, similarly violent incidents occurred. However, there is evidence of trade with Pakeha (non-Maori New Zealanders, a name already in use by 1814), particularly in whaling, sealing and as missionaries (King 2003). And there is evidence of significant movement between Port Jackson, the New South Wales colony, and the Maori world, particularly in trade for timber and flax (King 2003). The return trade was in metals and tools and, devastatingly, muskets. Belich (1986, p 19) summarised the interactions in the following way:

> If Europeans mistreated Maori(s), they would be killed. If Maori(s) mistreated Europeans, trade would stop.

Reflective exercise

If you were an Aboriginal woman whose child was taken to a mission, how might you have consoled yourself and what effect might this have had on your life?

If you were a young Aboriginal woman brought up on a mission with little contact with your family, how might this have affected your life physically, socially, culturally and spiritually? What are the positives, what are the negatives, and how do you heal and move forward?

King puts a slightly different complexion on these interactions:

> Where Europeans took the trouble to try to understand Maori codes of behaviour and to identify Maori expectations Maori–Pakeha relations in the nineteenth century were generally harmonious … Where they did not, there were severe disappointments on the European side, accusations of Maori unreliability and treachery, and bloodshed (King 1988, p 205).

The key to successful interaction clearly was the effort or ability to understand the importance and place of mana, utu and tapu.

As indicated above, from the early 1800s there had been small numbers of Europeans in New Zealand as missionaries, whalers and traders. Missionaries began to teach the writing of Maori languages, which until that time had been exclusively oral, as well, of course, as trying to convert the 'natives' to their God. Prior to 1840, the time of the establishment of the Treaty of Waitangi, there were only approximately 2000 non-Maori living in New Zealand.

Tribal warfare was part of New Zealand history, with the North Island in internal warfare from 1818 to 1833. This inter-tribal warfare was made worse by the phenomenon of the musket brought to them by Europeans, giving rise to the naming of these as the Musket Wars.

The interactions of Maori with the British colonies in eastern Australia brought them into increasing contact with Europeans and eventually to the attention of London. In 1832 a formal link was established, with James Busby being sent to New Zealand as a representative of the British Crown. This appointment was to protect the interests of New Zealand trade with the Australian colonies. According to King (2003), Busby's instruction from London, via the NSW Governor, 'was to protect "well disposed" settlers and traders, guard against the exploitation of Maori by Europeans and outrages committed against them, and recapture escaped convicts' (King 2003, p 153).

The British, keen to prevent expansion of the French in the southern oceans and to control the sale of land to Europeans, planned to annex and then colonise parts of New Zealand. Given that the country was clearly 'owned, governed and used' by its Indigenous people, unlike Australia, some form of negotiated settlement was required by international law. Relationships with Maori chiefs had been cultivated for about 50 years of contact through New South Wales and Busby had moved these further since coming to live in New Zealand. In 1839 William Hobson was sent from London to take the constitutional steps necessary to establish a British colony. This was to be in the form of a treaty.

The original plan was to annex small portions of land only. However, the behaviour of the New Zealand Company, a British company set up to establish trading colonies, together with the threat of the French, who had set up a colony on the South Island at Akaroa and who were planning further colonisation of the rich pastoral lands of the Canterbury plains, and Baron de Thierry's attempts to establish himself at Hokianga, caused Hobson to proclaim sovereignty over the whole country in the Treaty of Waitangi, discussed more fully later.

In everyday life, British annexation had relatively little obvious effect outside the towns of Auckland, Wellington, Wanganui, New Plymouth and Nelson. Although Maori dominated the country areas, the way in which Maori tribes interacted with each other had been irrevocably disturbed by European contact and resulted in what are known as the New Zealand Wars of 1845 to 1872 (until the 1980s these were referred to as the Maori Wars). These were wars of Maori tribes against each other and the British, and resulted in an enormous influx of British military. These wars are well documented in the book *The New Zealand Wars* by James Belich (1988), if you are interested in further reading, or Chapter 15 of King's (2003) *The Penguin History of New Zealand*.

Governor George Grey was sent to New Zealand as Governor in 1845 at a time of great unrest between Maori and Maori, and Maori and Pakeha. He had had contact with Australian Aborigines and was seen as 'good with natives'. He was particularly influential in New Zealand, attempting to ensure that the Treaty conditions were observed and Maori land rights respected. Governor Grey learned the Maori language and assisted in having Maori legends and traditions written down. His papers eventually became one of the most important repositories of Maori language in the country. Governor Grey was also concerned with Maori health and built several hospitals, and also wrote to Florence Nightingale asking how to improve the deteriorating health of the Maori people. Unfortunately, Florence Nightingale's response was not received until shortly before Grey left for South Africa and was never to be influential in New Zealand. The document that influenced health and education policy at the time was a book by Dr AS Thompson, who advocated separation of Maori into English housing and compulsory attendance at European schools. The advice was completely contrary to that suggested by Nightingale, whose letter was eventually found decades later in Grey's South African papers. Nightingale warned against too quickly seeking to educate Maori, to increase the separations between beds in Marae and not to remove the people to individual English-style houses. The advice was not dissimilar to public health advice that may be given today, and if attended to at the time may have changed the course of Maori health history (Keith 1988). Grey also left a legacy of a draft of the constitution that was to become the foundation for governance for 150 years. Under this constitution, Maori men were given the vote in 1867 and all women given the vote in 1893.

The 1860s were dominated by further flare-ups of the New Zealand Wars and by the gold rush with discoveries on both Islands, in the Coromandel Peninsula and in the south, in Nelson and Otago. By 1860 the European population had surpassed that of Maori.

In the towns, European development continued as if a subset of England, or, in the south, Scotland. In 1848, Dunedin was established as a Scottish Free Church settlement and Christchurch in 1850 as a Canterbury Association (Church of England) settlement, both based on New Zealand Company settlement models. Dunedin and Christchurch today display visible signs of their respective Scottish and English heritages. In 1874 Dunedin had a population of 29,832, Auckland 27,840, Wellington 15,941 and Christchurch 14,270 (King 2003, p 209). But the landscape of the South Island was dominated not by people, but by sheep, of which there were 13 million by 1878.

Again, unlike the experience in Australia, the coexistence of the two dominant cultures moved in a virtually parallel existence until after the Second World War, when the numbers of Maori seeking to live an urban lifestyle grew exponentially.

The Treaty of Waitangi and British 'annexation' in 1840

The Treaty of Waitangi is a foundational document for all New Zealanders and is the basis for the claim that New Zealand is a bicultural country. It is a statement of intent by two very different groups to live equitably and harmoniously together. It was, however, drawn up hastily and by non-lawyers, and translated into Maori by people other than the original authors. On 5 February 1840, copies of the Treaty in both languages were put before a gathering of Northern Chiefs at Busby's house near Waitangi.

There were three articles to the Treaty. The first declared that the chiefs would 'cede to her Majesty the Queen of England absolutely and without reservation all rights and powers of Sovereignty . . . over their respective Territories' (as quoted in King 2003, p 159).

The second article in English held a guarantee from the Queen to the chiefs and tribes and their families 'full exclusive and undisturbed possession of their lands and Estates Forests Fisheries and other properties . . . So long as it is their wish and desire to retain the same in their possession' (as quoted in King 2003, p 159). In return, chiefs would give exclusive right of any sale to the Crown.

The third article extends to the 'Natives of New Zealand Her royal protection and imparts to them all the Rights and Privileges of British Subjects' (as quoted in King 2003, p 153). How one explained to different groups of people with different languages and cultural background the subtle meaning of these words, especially a word such as 'sovereignty', leaves significant questions of informed consent, which have been played out in courts over the past three decades. These misunderstandings were further complicated by the translation into Maori, where the word 'sovereignty' was translated as 'kawanatanga', which to Maori means 'governorship'—vastly different from sovereignty. This misunderstanding was to be reinforced in the wording of article two, which assured the retention of 'the unqualified exercise of their chieftainship over their lands, villages and all their treasures' (King 2003, p 160). These discrepancies were, however, not obvious to anyone at the signing of the Treaty. As part of the Treaty negotiations there was a commitment also that all land transactions that had taken place prior to 1840 were to be investigated by a Land Claims Commissioner.

The Treaty of Waitangi was signed on 6 February 1840 by Hobson and by many, but not all, of the Maori chiefs. Hobson then travelled the country, acquiring the signatures of most of the remaining chiefs, and the document was completed on 3 September that year. Five hundred chiefs signed the Treaty, although a number of important chiefs would not, including Te Wherewhero of Waikato, Tairaia of Thames, Tupaea of Tauranga, the Te Arawa of Rotorua, and the Ngati Tuwharetoa of Taupo. Land purchases began, with land in the South Island becoming readily available as Te Rauparaha and his warring tribe had seriously depleted the number of Maori in the south. This included the purchase by the New Zealand Company of the Canterbury Plains, the most fertile pastoral land in New Zealand. The gold rush also led to the European settlement of the South Island, with gold found in Nelson and large finds on Otago, leading to a doubling of the Otago population in six months in the 1860s.

From 1840 to 1914, 90% of those migrating to New Zealand were from Britain or Ireland, most on assisted passage either from the five New Zealand Company settlements, by assisted passage to the South Island to settle Canterbury or Otago, or as military persons brought in in their thousands to protect the colony.

Despite the existence of the treaty, the mechanisms for purchasing land were by no means straightforward, as often several different chiefs were involved and negotiation with one did not mean permission of the other. These complicated land contestations led to what have become known as the New Zealand Land Wars. Following these wars there was significant confiscation of lands in the North Island and even though this was deemed unjust by a Royal Commission 60 years later, the return of the lands was by then impossible. Maori retreated to their rural communities and Pakeha lived predominantly in the towns, and this segregation continued until the Second World War, when rural economic difficulties and growing job availability in the cities lured young Maori to the towns.

War and beyond

The New Zealand and Australian experiences were often shared experiences in the First World War, and this has already been explored. A major part of New Zealand's Second World War campaign took place in Greece and in Crete. As noted by King (2003, p 398), 'Of all the New Zealand battles in World War II, none engraved itself more deeply on the national consciousness than that for Crete. It was the Gallipoli of its era'. The other major theatre of war was North Africa and included the well known battle of El Alamein in 1942. The New Zealand armed forces also moved to Italy to continue the fight with the Germans. With the fall of Singapore to the Japanese in 1942, New Zealand also dispatched troops to the Pacific. As with the Australian experience, war appeared to unify the nation. But the post-war time was the catalyst for a disruption of the seemingly cohesive nation of parallel lives of Maori and Pakeha. The movement of Maori from the rural areas to the city grew from a 'trickle to a torrent' (King 2003, p 417).

In the 1920s, New Zealand's Pakeha population was 95% 'British'. Those not British but European fitted quickly into the dominant culture. Those who did not, like the Chinese who had migrated with the gold rush, suffered similar discrimination as they had in Australia, relegated to market gardening and never really seen as part of the identity of the nation. It took until the 1990s for an apology to be offered by Helen Clark to the New Zealand Chinese for the discrimination shown towards them for over a century.

For women, both Maori and Pakeha, freedom was much more limited than for men. Having moved on abruptly from its anachronistic British civilisation of the period up until the 1980s, when shops had shut early and never opened on weekends, and the cars looked like they belonged in the 1950s and 1960s, New Zealand in the 1980s caught up three decades in a very short period once international travel became faster and affordable, and when tariffs and industrial relations policies changed to bring New Zealand business into closer alignment with other OECD countries. New Zealand's small size as a country had ensured a history of intellectuals, artists and writers going overseas to further their talents and creativity. From the 1970s it became possible to remain in New Zealand and still participate actively in the international community. Painters such as McCahon, Woolaston and Hotere stayed in New Zealand to work.

Contemporary New Zealand society

The beginnings of change to the steady and time-warped New Zealand Britishness began in the latter part of the 1960s, with the coming together of television, the Vietnam War, to which New Zealand had committed troops, and the collapse of wool prices with its flow-on effect on the economy. The late 1960s and 1970s saw protests related to land, women's issues, Maori issues and issues of sexuality. These immediately became national issues because they could be played out on television. Perhaps the most insightful and accessible writing on the change in the life of Pakeha growing up in the 1940s and 1950s in New Zealand and living through the turbulence of the 1970s and 1980s is the book by Michael King (1985), *Being Pakeha*.

New Zealand women began organising themselves through the early 1970s, having had their consciousness raised by the US women's movement and the growing movements in Australia, of which Germaine Greer's book *The Female Eunuch* was influential. One advantage of the smallness of New Zealand is that change can happen quickly and critical mass is relatively easily reached. New Zealand had a group of articulate, well-educated women who, when they began to speak and write, tilled the soil for New Zealand to become a world force in Women's Studies. Sandra Coney, Phillida Bunkle and Marilyn Waring became household names for several decades. In some ways this is not surprising, as New Zealand European settlement was by families, and New Zealand women appear to have been more equal participants in public life than their eastern coast Australian sisters. They have a history of working with and beside, rather than in service to, the men since colonisation.

Between 1984 and 1990 the Labour government of the time was sympathetic to women's issues and in 1984 it established the Ministry of Women's Affairs. It passed legislation important to raising women's status, including the *Parental Leave and Employment Protection Act 1987*, the *State Sector Act 1988*, which required equal employment opportunities, and the *Employment Equity Act 1990*. Under Helen Clark, the then Minister for Health, the *Nurse Amendment Act 1990* was passed with the full support of all women in parliament of both parties. This Act separated midwifery from nursing and hence from direct control of doctors. It enabled midwives to practise as independent practitioners and has changed the face of childbirth in New Zealand in less than a decade.

Much of the political awareness of women's issues had been raised through the Cartwright Inquiry of 1987–89. The inquiry exposed the mistreatment of women's cervical cancer in Auckland for 20 years from 1966. The experience was captured in the book by Sandra Coney (1988), *The Unfortunate Experiment*. The inquiry resulted in a strong and vocal consumer movement in New Zealand, a disillusionment with the medical profession and a call for cultural sensitivity in healthcare (Guilliland & Pairman 1995).

The late 1980s to the mid-1990s saw an economic revolution in New Zealand that disturbed the whole country. It was economic rationalism on a scale not witnessed anywhere in the world. All understandings of New Zealand's caring, socialist society were shed and a user-pays, individualistic, contractually based, privatised society dominated. Introduced by the Labour government but taken to an increased pitch by the Nationals, the country's assets were restructured and many jobs were lost. Many would contend that this revolution was necessary for New Zealand's economic survival; others would say there was no need for the haste or brutality of what occurred. This tumultuous time has since subsided and a new era of 'collaboration, cooperation and consultation' has taken over as 'the New Zealand way of doing business'.

The progress of women in New Zealand is demonstrated in an unparalleled way with, at the beginning of the twenty-first century, a woman governor-general, woman prime minister and woman minister for health, attorney-general and chief justice.

Michael King (2003, pp 519–20) ends *The Penguin History of New Zealand* with the following words:

> The Maori culture of the twenty-first century is not Maori culture frozen at 1769, nor at 1840. Nor should it be. It changed and grew dynamically according to changing needs and circumstances prior to the eighteenth century, and it continues to do so in the twenty-first century.
>
> Similarly, Pakeha culture continues to borrow and to learn from Maori. That was one of the features that made it different from its European cultures of origin. It took words and concepts (mana, tapu, whanau, taonga, haka, turangawaewae), attitudes (the traditional hospitality which, in the early nineteenth century, was so much more visible from the Maori side of the frontier than the Pakeha), ways of doing business (an increasing willingness to talk issues through to consensus in preference to dividing groups 'for' and 'against' a given motion), and rites of passage

(loosening up of formerly formal and highly structured funeral services)...

And most New Zealanders, whatever their cultural backgrounds, are good-hearted, practical, commonsensical and tolerant. Those qualities are part of the national cultural capital that has in the past saved the country from the worst excesses of chauvinism and racism seen in other parts of the world. They are as sound a basis as any for optimism about the country's future.

Modern Maori society

The caveat with which I introduced the section on modern Aboriginal society holds even more deeply for this section. I had the privilege of living in New Zealand for four years in the 1990s and travel frequently to that country, but I do not presume to do more here than highlight some respected texts and again attempt to assist in the development of a conceptual framework from which to further develop your personal understanding.

Unlike the circumstance of the Australian Aboriginal and Torres Strait Islander people, New Zealand Maori had, as we have seen, the benefit of having had a system of living recognisable to the European colonisers, leading to the existence of a founding document of living together, the Treaty of Waitangi, and until after the Second World War there was a prevailing sense of racial harmony, mainly related to the separation of Maori, predominantly to rural areas of the North Island. Post-war industrial development brought young Maori to the cities. In little over a generation, Maori had became a predominantly urban people.

> For the first time since the nineteenth century, the country's two major cultural traditions collided and generated the white water of confusion and hostility. Nobody was prepared for this outcome. Maori experienced discrimination in accommodation, employment and hotel bars. They were confronted with a world that was aggressively European in orientation at the very time that they had severed bonds with many sources of their own culture—traditional marae, hapu and extended families. Many of them became marginal people, weakened both by what they had relinquished and what confronted them. They were soon disproportionately represented in the ranks of convicted criminals, problem drinkers and the unemployed (King 1988, p 12).

In 1936, 11.2% of Maori were urban; in 1945, 25.7% and in 1996 over 81% (King 2003, p 473). Distress and dislocation of urban Maori grew, Maori protest groups formed, and with the assistance of media attention their claims that the Treaty had not been honoured were heard. Maori were insisting on and gaining major changes in government departmental operations, and language nests—'Kohanga reo'—were set up to teach preschoolers Maori language. A Maori renaissance was being witnessed. The difficulties emerging from the dislocation of people and culture was graphically depicted in Alan Duff's novel *Once Were Warriors*, later made into a harrowing but illuminative film. This brought the issues of alcohol abuse and domestic violence into the open to be addressed by Maori themselves. Perhaps the most momentous of all the changes was the establishment of the Waitangi Tribunal in 1975, which over the next decade explored breaches of the Treaty retrospectively to 1840.

The 1980s resurgence of Maori pride and power has resulted in New Zealand being, and being seen to be, a bicultural country. Maori language infuses the national public communication. A recent film, *Whale Rider*, provides a compelling contemporary view of New Zealand Maori and their challenges.

Pacific Islands people in New Zealand

No snapshot of New Zealand would be complete without acknowledgement of the dramatic increase in the number of Pacific Islands people who have made their home in New Zealand since the 1960s and 1970s. Sitting somewhere outside the bicultural notions of either Maori or Pakeha, the Pacific Islands people have become an integral part of New Zealand identity, art, music and culture. By 2001 there were 232,000 Pacific Islands people in New Zealand, representing 6.5% of the population, 58% of whom are New Zealand born. They have predominantly settled in South Auckland and North-west Wellington, and while they have made a significant contribution to rugby, they are disproportionately represented in manual labouring jobs. They experience significant health problems related to obesity and its sequelae. The six major cultural groups represented are Samoan, Cook Islanders, Tongan, Niuean, Tokalauan and Fijian.

In celebration of similarity and difference

As we have seen, there are similarities between Australia and New Zealand in that their non-Indigenous antecedents were predominantly British. This inevitably brings some

Reflective exercise

You are a Pacific Islands woman living in South Auckland. You are asked by your teenage child how you see yourself in relation to New Zealand and your Pacific Island country of origin. How would you respond?

commonality of culture. These bonds provide a facade of sameness in the countries but, as we have seen, the differences are significant.

The difference, for me, is symbolised in the flatness and solidity of one compared to the mountainous and unstable nature of the other, where green in one country is a very different colour to the green in the other. These differences are paralleled in the differing histories. New Zealand is a bicultural country with a recent history of immigration bringing it very much into the Pacific. This compares to Australia's recent history of immigration and trade, which positions it clearly as part of Asia.

The relationship between the Indigenous and non-Indigenous people is also a strong contrast, and the modern impacts of the Indigenous cultures have been played out in very different ways. Australia describes itself as multicultural, New Zealand as bicultural. New Zealand everyday language is infused with Maori words; the Australian vernacular is barely touched by Aboriginal languages.

Perhaps the two countries are at this time at a point further away from each other than at any time since European colonisation. Australia faces Asia, New Zealand faces the Pacific; metaphorically they stand with their backs to each other. Australia has taken an international position aligned with the United States, New Zealand an independent stance. The temptation of Australians to view New Zealand as a ninth state or territory of Australia could never be more deceptive. The richness of the multiple cultures in both countries is a cause for celebration and exploration, and for practitioners is essential if cultural inappropriateness is to be avoided and culturally appropriate and safe practice is to be achieved. I hope this chapter has helped your understanding of these two countries, their similarities and differences.

Review questions

1   Summarise the impact that history and culture have on health in general and maternity services in particular.

2   Identify strategies that will improve the health and wellbeing of either Australian Aboriginal or Maori women and their babies.

3   Why is the health of Australian Aboriginals and Maori generally poorer than that of non-Indigenous peoples? What can you, as a midwife, do about this situation?

4   Indigenous women in Australia and New Zealand begin childbearing at a much younger age than their non-Indigenous peers. Once socio-economic status has been taken into account, teenage pregnancy is not a risk factor for poor obstetric outcomes. How can midwives provide a culturally safe environment for young mothers while they prepare for parenting and at the same time continue their education?

5   What impact does history have on the conduct of midwifery in New Zealand and Australia?

6   In what ways has the Treaty of Waitangi affected policy development and midwifery in New Zealand?

7   How can midwives work in partnership with Indigenous women to develop strategies for health gain and appropriate health and maternity services?

8   Compared to women from European backgrounds, Maori and Australian Indigenous women do not have the same levels of participation in decision-making, planning, development and delivery of health and maternity services. How can midwives work in partnership with Indigenous women to remedy these inequities?

9   Do midwives have a responsibility to work with women to help safeguard their nations' heritage, cultural concepts, values and practices? If so, how should they go about this and why is it important?

10   From the 1800s to 1969, part-Australian Aboriginal babies and children were taken from their mothers and families and placed into government-run institutions or fostered or adopted by white families. Should all midwifery education programs include compulsory units of study aimed at increasing midwives' understanding of the effects of the Stolen Generation on Aboriginal culture, history and health? If so, why?

Online resources

Australian Government Department of Health and Ageing, http://www.health.gov.au

Ministry of Culture and Heritage, http://www.nzhistory.net.nz

Ministry of Health New Zealand, http://www.maorihealth.govt.nz

Ministry of Pacific Island Affairs, http://www.minpac.govt.nz

Ministry of Women's Affairs, http://www.mwa.govt.nz

National Library of Australia, http://www.nla.gov.au/oz/histsite.html

Treaty of Waitangi, http://www.treatyofwaitangi.govt.nz; also http://www.archives.govt.nz/exhibitions/permanentexhibitions/treaty.php

References

Belich J 1988 The New Zealand Wars and the Victorian interpretation of racial conflict. Penguin, Auckland

Belich J 1996 Making peoples: a history of New Zealanders from Polynesian settlement to the end of the nineteenth century. Penguin, Auckland

Broome R 2001 Aboriginal Australians (3rd edn). Allen & Unwin, Sydney

Clark M, Hooper M, Ferrier S 2000 History of Australia. Scholastic Books, Sydney

Coney S 1988 The unfortunate experiment. Penguin, Auckland

Curthoys A 1997 History and identity. In: W Hudson, G Bolton (Eds) Creating Australia. Allen & Unwin, Sydney, pp 23–36

Dixon M 1993 The real Matilda (3rd edn). Penguin, Melbourne

Duff A 1990 Once were warriors. Tandem Press, Auckland

Eshuys J, Guest V, Lawrence J 1996 Australia emerges. Macmillan, Melbourne

Faulks S 1993 Birdsong: a novel of love and war. Random House, London

Franklin M 1965 My brilliant career. Angus and Robertson, Sydney

Graham D (Ed) 1994 Being whitefella. Fremantle Arts Centre Press, Fremantle

Greer G 1970 The female eunuch. MacGibbon & Kee, London

Guilliland K, Pairman S 1995 The midwifery partnership. Department of Nursing and Midwifery, Victoria University of Wellington, Wellington

Hudson W, Bolton G (Eds) 1997 Creating Australia. Allen & Unwin, Sydney

Human Rights and Equal Opportunity Commission (HREOC) 1997 Bringing them home—a guide to the findings and recommendations of the National Inquiry into the Separation of Aboriginal and Torres Strait Islander Children from Their Families. HREOC, Sydney

Keith J 1988 Florence Nightingale: statistician and consultant epidemiologist. International Nursing Review 35(5):147–150

King M 1985 Being Pakeha. Hodder & Stoughton, Auckland

King M 2003 The Penguin History of New Zealand. Penguin, Auckland

McCarthy W 2000 Don't fence me in. Random House, Sydney

Sawer M, Simms M 1993 A woman's place: women and politics in Australia (2nd edn). Allen & Unwin, Sydney

Summers A 1994 Damned whores and God's police (rev. edn). Penguin, Melbourne

Ward R 1958 The Australian legend. Oxford University Press, Melbourne

White R 1981 Inventing Australia: images and identity 1688–1980. Allen & Unwin, Sydney

White R 1997 Inventing Australia, revisited. In: W Hudson, G Bolton (Eds) Creating Australia. Allen & Unwin, Sydney

Further reading/viewing

Belich J 1988 The New Zealand Wars and the Victorian interpretation of racial conflict. Penguin, Auckland

James B, Saville-Smith K 1999 Critical issues in New Zealand society 2: gender, culture and power (2nd edn). Oxford University Press, Auckland

Kawharu I (Ed) 1989 Waitangi—Maori and Pakeha perspectives of the Treaty of Waitangi. Oxford University Press, Auckland

King M 2003 The Penguin History of New Zealand. Penguin, Auckland

Films

Caddie 1976 Dir. Douglas Crombie. A woman's life in Australia in the depression

Muriel's Wedding 1994 Dir. PJ Hogan. A humorous look at contemporary Australia

Once Were Warriors 1994 Dir. Lee Tamahori. Maori poverty and domestic violence in Auckland in the 1980s

Rabbit Proof Fence 2002 Dir. Phillip Noyce. Children of the Stolen Generation finding their way back home

Sunday Too Far Away 1976 Dir. Ken Hannam. Australian rural life in the early 1970s

The Piano 1993 Dir. Jane Campion. Early New Zealand settlement by Europeans

They're a Weird Mob 1966 Dir. Michael Powell. Australia in the 1950s with Mediterranean migration

Whale Rider 2002 Dir. Niki Caro. Intergenerational cultural clashes and resolution, a gentler and more hopeful Once Were Warriors.

Novels

Grace, Patricia 1998 Baby no-eyes. Penguin (NZ), Auckland

Hulme, Kerrie 1984 The bone people. Picador, London

Morgan, Sally 1988 My place. Fremantle Arts Centre Press, Fremantle

Winton, Tim 2001 Dirt music. Picador, Sydney

Poets

Banjo Paterson – Early Australian life

Les Murray – Contemporary Australian life

Sam Hunt – Contemporary New Zealand life

Wilfred Owen – on WWI

CHAPTER 3

Understanding world views for midwifery

Karen Lane

Key terms

biological-reductionist theory, biomechanical/biomedical model of disease, discourse, essentialism, foundationalism, generativity, individualism, interpretive theories, materialism, medical dominance, medicalisation, micro-capillaries of power, narratology, objectivist, partnership, positivism, post-structuralism, professionalisation, psychologism, reflexive self, self, self-narrative, social model of health, sociological imagination, structuralism

Chapter overview

Midwifery entails:

> working with women throughout the continuum of childbirth, which extends from preconception to early parenting. In the provision of care, which ideally is provided within a continuity of care model, the midwife is cognisant of the woman's physical, psychological, social, cultural, spiritual needs and expectation . . . The philosophy for this care is women-centred . . . (Victorian Midwifery Code of Practice, Nurses Board of Victoria 1999)

Midwives understand that in order to sustain the health of the woman through pregnancy and birth, they need to look at the social context and to factor in the distinct identity of the woman—that is, her particular orientation to herself and broader society. Like the WHO (1946) definition of health as 'a state of complete physical, mental and social well-being and not merely the absence of disease or infirmity', midwifery has stepped outside the boundaries of conventional healthcare, or the *biomechanical/biomedical model of disease*. I argue in this chapter that midwifery practised in the above mode will be instrumental in facilitating a positive self-identity or self-narrative for the woman and that this, in turn, is pivotal in creating the intergenerational health of women and babies.

Learning outcomes

Learning outcomes for this chapter are:

1 To explain the difference between the biomechanical or medical model of illness and disease, and the social model of health

2 To describe the relationship between the individual and their social context

3 To differentiate structuralist theories of health from social constructionist theories of health

4 To examine the relationship between discourses and resistance

5 To discuss discourses of the self

6 To highlight the relevance of 'professional generativity' in securing the intergenerational health of women and their babies.

The biomechanical model of medicine and disease

According to the biomechanical model:

- Disease is an organic condition—psychological or social conditions are ignored on the assumption that the causes of disease or illness can be found within the body or biology.
- Disease makes individuals sick; they then report their malaise and take on the sick role (Parsons 1951), while the medical practitioner assumes the role of expert whose object of practice is the sick body.
- The diseased state can be cured by medical intervention.
- The medical intervention is reactive; it treats symptoms of the disease.
- Disease is treated in a medical setting (Bilton et al 2002, p 356).

In the traditional medical model, the 'patient' submits patiently to the expertise of the practitioner, whose exclusive knowledge authorises her or him to judge the causes and treatment of the diseased part of the body without recourse to the social milieu or interior status of the patient. For doctors, the relationship is one of subject/object. The patient becomes the object of the professional medical 'gaze'; there is no reason for the patient to be drawn into more than a formative and cursory discussion of the treatment or its causes, because the expert possesses knowledge about the body independently of the knowledge conveyed by the patient. Although the patient may be able to describe their symptoms accurately, they cannot know the causes because the causes have a pathological origin within the body. The model is inherently expansionary in that it constantly recruits new domains for exclusive jurisdiction. This is what is meant by medicalisation or a situation where ordinary social problems are turned into medical problems and then quarantined as the province of accredited medical practitioners who control the entry, practice and use of equipment and treatment regimes through strategies of professionalisation (Foucault 1973). Examples include homosexuality, alcoholism and childbirth. The outcome is broad-based medical dominance. For example, midwives often argue that birth has been medicalised—that a normal physiological event in the social lives of many Western women in different cultures has been reconceptualised as a dangerous event best undertaken in an acute-care setting under the care of specialist obstetricians. They then claim exclusive legal authority over women by virtue of their exclusive use of special equipment (forceps, scalpels or drugs) or accredited skills to undertake special procedures (surgical, chemical and physiological).

In summary, we could call this model of care 'objectivist' because it assumes that there is an objective reality that can be studied, learned and applied to solving problems, like disease (Rothfield 1995, pp. 174–80). This is sometimes called positivism (reality is posited rather than constructed). It does not accept that the world is a socially constructed world—that reality is culturally mediated. In other words, the medical model fails to acknowledge that how we understand ourselves (including our diseases and our health) cannot be separated from the social, political, historical and cultural contexts in which we live. These social forces form us (our 'self'/our identity/our bodies/our diseases/our health) and our knowledge about the world, including our knowledge about diseases, how we define them and what we label as 'disease'.

The biomechanical model remains the dominant model of the body in the twenty-first century and it is acknowledged here that the above outline is a rather stylised and wooden version. In reality, medical practitioners do attend to factors in the patient's social environment, they do elicit information from the patient about their preferences, and they do share information about the disease. However, the basic premise is sustained—the biomechanical model may be categorised as a biological-reductionist theory that seeks causes primarily within the body and treats the symptoms rather than the larger social causes. An illustration of the causation of disease may be seen in the following:

social conditions → psychological state → biological condition

Obviously the further back we go, the earlier we can prevent the condition (Eckerman 2000, p 55).

There are substantial critiques that challenge the efficacy of the biomechanical model. First, if social forces did not affect physical health, then placebo drugs would not work, yet there is substantial evidence that they do. Second, non-Western health practices are often very effective even though the principle and philosophy behind them are antipathetic to the Western medical model. Third, there is macro statistical evidence that every major health problem, including cancer, coronary heart disease, stroke and diabetes (and we can include birth) varies with the physical, social, economic and physical environments (AIHW 2001; Synnott 1992, p 102).

A social model of health, illness and the body

Such evidence is persuasive that our health status is sensitive to issues of social identity such as gender, ethnicity, education, occupational status, wealth and geographical location. Therefore, explaining why people are healthy or unhealthy demands a social model of the body.

> A social model of the body is one that can incorporate social, cultural, political and economic factors (both micro and macro) that impinge upon health status. This model does not reject the importance of pathogens as causes of disturbance of the efficient functioning of the body but it does enlarge the landscape of causative factors. Further, this model adds another layer of complexity in recognising the interaction of social factors in either causing ill-health or in alleviating or deepening the effects of an existing malaise or disease (Brown 1996, pp 302–3).

Going back to the definition of midwifery quoted earlier, it is evident that the midwifery definition stands as the antithesis of the biomechanical model, at least as it is related to birth. For professional midwives, midwifery is more than just providing skills. The midwifery profession and midwifery practice are defined in relation to the woman. Further, this relationship is not a distant, objective one but 'a partnership' (Davis-Floyd 1992; Guilliland & Pairman 1995; Wagner 1994). In short, it is a dialogic relationship characterised by trust, reciprocity and integrity (Lane 2000). Further, unlike conventional medical practice, midwives attribute to the woman 'needs and expectations'. In other words, midwifery recognises that the woman possesses agency—she harbours 'physical, psychological, social, cultural, spiritual needs and expectations' and it is the midwife's role to assist her to achieve them. Thus, the woman has a self that has been fashioned by the sum total of the social forces she has experienced and negotiated. Giddens (1987, p 11) calls this the 'double involvement of individuals and institutions' ('institutions' here means patterns of human action over time). What he implies is that human beings create social systems or institutions and those institutions (social, economic, political and historical forces including scientific and medical knowledge) are constantly being changed by the ongoing actions of social individuals—individuals who have themselves been formed and re-formed over time by those very forces. This is a dynamic model of social life and social knowledge. It asserts that the ideas, beliefs, values and institutions we engage with are constantly undergoing reinterpretation in the light of ongoing social changes.

Taking pregnancy and birth as cases in point, we can argue that how a woman progresses in her pregnancy and how she gives birth will reflect the way she processes those social forces. This is what it means to have a 'self'.

> Having a self refers to 'a person's *own* understandings, opinions, stocks of knowledge, cognition and . . . practical knowledge or consciousness' (Elliott 2001, p 5; Taylor 1989). Since every woman has a self, she is entitled to be treated as the final authority on how to proceed and how to achieve outcomes for herself and her baby. (my italics)

We can say, therefore, that professional midwifery (read 'midwifery practice that eclipses the subsidiary role of medical assistant') stands in contradistinction to the conventional biomechanical model of disease in every important way—ways that will affect the progress and outcomes of pregnancy and birth. Comparative trials of midwifery and obstetric models of care typically reflect better outcomes for midwifery care precisely because women are given due recognition for the uniqueness of the self in addition to the usual medical concerns.

In an ideal sense, midwifery embraces a social model of health, one that recognises the social bases of health and illness. In so doing, midwives recognise that in order to achieve competence in their professional practice they must attend carefully to the ways in which the complexity of the social forces in the environment has a variable effect on the woman's/consumer's health status. The diagram in Figure 3.1 (Germov 1998, p 11) depicts a schema whereby the social model of health may be applied to women-centred midwifery care.

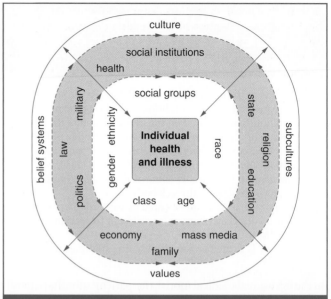

Figure 3.1 Social structure: the links between personal health and social factors (based on Germov 1998, p 11)

We need to stress that the individual is not a pre-social, 'natural' or isolated subject but one that is irreducibly social and must therefore be seen in a given social and cultural context. Individual values are socially acquired values. They change according to different cultures, within subcultures and over time.

C. Wright Mills (1970) called this 'the sociological imagination'. It refers to the idea that we should see the individual as being socialised by the multiplicity of social forces, or the product of interactions within primary social groups such as friends and family as well as major institutions including cultural groups, the education system, health system, political system, the media and economic system, including global political and economic forces. The term 'socialisation' is not used here to imply that social forces are all-determining or that we learn the rules and then placidly obey them. Wrong (1998) called this 'the oversocialised conception of man'. Rather, we want to see individuals as self-reflexive—they have the ability to reflect on their lives, their actions, their own values and where they come from, and with this knowledge are able to reinterpret the world, change their own actions, values and the 'self' and, ultimately, even to change institutions and dominant prevailing attitudes or values.

While professional midwifery practice embraces a social model of birth—since it begins with complex needs and expectations of the woman—there remain substantial questions about how to conceptualise the 'woman' and the 'self' in relation to the social milieu. Failure to be clear about these concepts will ultimately compromise the 'needs and expectations' of the woman and, therefore, the very practice of midwifery itself and its claim to provide a service different from the 'objectivist' model of medical care. An example of this would be ignoring the substantial disadvantages borne by Aboriginal women who travel long distances from their family, cultural traditions and social supports to deliver their babies without incident in Western hospitals. Another example would be asking a woman within her own culture to deliver a baby without impediment without soliciting her preferences for procedures and support. The questions we need to ask ourselves relate to the diagram in Figure 3.1. How do we understand the impact of all of the social forces upon the woman? Do we prioritise some social forces, like gender, class or ethnicity, as being more important in their effects than others and generalise these to all women? How do we gauge the responses of the woman to those social forces, bearing in mind the 'double involvement of individuals and institutions' outlined by Giddens (above). This means that we understand social individuals as not merely passive recipients of the forces in the social universe. Rather, we actively negotiate their effects upon us according to our sense of who we are—our 'self' or identity. In the diagram, the 'double involvement of individuals and institutions' is depicted by the movement of the arrows outwards as well as inwards.

Structuralism and health

Theories of health that deny the ability of the individual to negotiate structures are called structuralist. These assume that people are victims of their historical and social circumstances. Structuralist theories give exclusive weight to social forces or institutions in determining health status, individual identity and social actions. The person is accorded little or no power to impose their own interpretation on events or to resist a dominant ethos. Structuralism is a form of positivism within the social sciences.

Like natural science, these theories tend to view reality as static and as external to the actor. In research terms they refer to the respondent as the 'subject'. In clinical settings, the person becomes the 'patient'. Positivism changes the person into an object of analysis that is transparent to the (elitist) gaze of the researcher/clinician. Under a positivist framework, the task of the researcher/obstetrician/midwife is to develop better and more sophisticated tools to discover what this reality is. Scientists might develop more powerful telescopes or more sophisticated technological apparatus to uncover DNA. Clinicians/midwives might apply apparatus to the woman's body to obtain a tracing of the baby's and woman's heart rates. Let me hasten to say that this is not a dictum to avoid technological aids. Rather, it is a caution that to rely only on technologies without inquiring into the ways in which women make sense of their social world through their own value framework would be considered positivist or objectivist. Positivism assumes that one can reveal the truth by delving deeper and deeper until you find the smallest and most basic element, which will then reveal the causes of the larger

whole. These explanations are then extrapolated to social events, behaviours and patterns. For example, the Human Genome Project currently seeks to discover the relevant gene associated with every labelled biological and social 'disorder' or behaviour, including sexual preferences. Natural science may also try to establish macro causal relationships, such as the relationship between genetic inheritance and criminality, or the relationship between gender and personality traits. Social scientists who subscribe to this view of social reality also try to develop more sophisticated methods of revealing the essence of the world, or the 'natural' or the 'normal'. Their principal methodologies include covert and overt observational techniques, data analysis, large-scale surveys and laboratory experiments.

Consider the theories of health devised by structuralist sociologists and feminists. All assume that one can locate a major explanatory cause to explain the entire course of human history. Structuralist theories assume that knowledge can be posed in terms of a series of dualisms (structure/agency, social structure/culture, social/psychological, family/society, individual/society, subjective/objective, reason/emotion), and that power relations comprise hierarchical orderings such as state/civil, individual/society, men/women, management/worker. We also call this view of history 'modernism'. All modernist theories reflect a yearning to find a single source of power and authority—a 'truth' that is posited outside the everyday social intercourse of humans, a point of reference from which all other things may be measured or assessed or valued. In this sense they follow the path of Enlightenment theorists of the sixteenth century onwards, who courageously challenged the traditional, pre-modernist notion of the absolute authority of God channelled through the King and his minions. Modernists discharged the authority of God, but not the idea of a single authority (Yeatman 1990, pp 286–9). The significant part of their theories for understanding individuals and individual health is that the major source of reference for the truth was a single vantage point from which structuralist/modernist theorists rewrote human history and from which they deduced individual thoughts, beliefs, values and actions. It was assumed that individuals (the 'self' or subjectivity) could be understood according to a single, unitary identity like class (Marx), rationalisation (Weber) or sex/gender (modernist feminisms). From now on I will call this foundationalism. In the following theories we find either biological or social foundationalism. They are not exhaustive of structuralist theories of health, but they are included to demonstrate the nature and range of application and to provide a point of comparison with interpretive explanations of social life. I will deal with this approach later. Interpretive theories assume that there are no such reference points because social individuals construct meaning through interactions with each other. Meanings change over time and across cultures. We may share some commonality of meanings within the same culture perhaps but we cannot predict how social individuals will employ meanings to construct their own identity or to make sense of the external world.

Marxist theories of class and health

Theories of health using a conflict Marxist perspective assume that one's location within the capitalist labour market will largely determine one's health status.

Capitalism is a system of class conflict between the property-owning class and the class of wage-labourers. These differential social locations confer different advantages and disadvantages in terms of education, housing, wealth, cultural attributes (manners and individual aspirations), social networks and health. White collar workers enjoy better health generally because they enjoy higher incomes and can afford better education, food, holidays, safer cars and better healthcare. Several studies comparing perinatal mortality rates of working-class and middle-class areas of Melbourne, Sydney and Adelaide confirm that class is a major factor in health outcomes. For example, one study found that low birthweight infants were born 1.6 times more frequently to women who were considered to be 'socially disadvantaged' (working-class women). Social factors pertaining to low birthweight and perinatal morbidity and mortality include smoking, drug and alcohol consumption and diet, factors that are more prevalent in working-class populations. Other studies have found that mortality rates from diseases such as heart disease, cancers, strokes, bronchitis, pneumonia, cirrhosis, suicide and accidents are higher in some socially disadvantaged local government areas than others (George & Davis 1998, pp 58–61). Other sites of conflict may include ethnicity. Indeed, studies have forged a close correlation between ethnicity, class and mortality rates. In Australia, Aboriginal and Torres Strait Islander people suffer lower life expectancies, higher age-specific death rates at every age, and higher rates of mortality from circulatory diseases, infections, injuries, diabetes and mental illness. In 1991, Aboriginal women were twice as likely to produce low birthweight babies as white women. Aboriginal maternal deaths accounted for 30% of the overall maternal mortality rate in Australia even though their childbirth rates are only 3% of total births (George & Davis 1998, p 63). Within the conflict perspective also, theorists are likely to point to the crucial role of the capitalist state in legislating for individualist models of healthcare—in accrediting doctors as small businesspeople serving their own economic interests on a fee-for-service basis rather than allocating scarce resources to a public infrastructure, including public housing and public health. It also means that small practices are increasingly open to corporatisation, where profit-seeking takes precedence over universal systems of access to healthcare and health becomes a commodity to be sold on a market like any other good or service (Germov 1998, pp 15, 34).

Weberian theories of health

For theorists taking a Weberian perspective on health, the major thread running through their analyses of health systems is the increasing tendency of industrialised societies to be bureaucratised, or governed by rules (Germov 1998, pp 15–18). This approach tends to focus on professions and rules governing practice, to the detriment of patient-centred care.

For example, casemix funding focuses on categorising health conditions in order to rationalise costs. Critics argue that this may compromise the type of care that a provider is willing to offer a patient. This might occur when a woman is encouraged to return home from hospital sooner than she should because the hospital is only funded by the state for a certain number of bed-days for parturient women. (The opposite would be a process-dominated approach, where individual parts of the health service are not measured in terms of comparative cost (Leeder 1999, p 76). It would be accepted that some benefits cannot be measured accurately, like the importance to a woman of having continuity of care from one midwife. The service is provided because it is of immense benefit to the woman and her family.) Weberian approaches also use class as a macro social indicator of health status but, unlike Marxian analyses, classes are not seen as necessarily in conflict. Different classes (upper, middle, lower and the self-employed) experience differential access to the health system premised on property ownership or non property ownership and also according to their marketable skills. That is, some workers may not own property but still enjoy high incomes, social status and expansive life chances because they possess valuable skills. Examples would be an airline pilot, an accountant or a scientist.

Feminist theories of health

For modernist feminists, the major social division in society is based on gender differences (as opposed to class in the case of Marx, or class and rationality in the case of Weber). The larger, structural framework that is invoked to explain power differences between men and women is not capitalism (at least in the first instance) but patriarchy, or the dominance of some men over other men and all women.

Much has now been written about structuralist feminisms and I will not attempt to reproduce all the theories in detail. A clear and basic overview of all theories may be found in Wearing (1996, pp 3–30). A more challenging text is Weedon (1992) and a more difficult but exhilarating text is Nicholson (1999), especially Chapter 4. I will deal with structuralist theories here in terms of how they may be distinguished from interpretive or social constructionist theories of gender. Basically, modernist and postmodernist/poststructuralist (meaning 'after the structures') theories diverge in how they conceive of the sex/gender distinction. For modernist feminists, the body was a biological given (the basic point of reference) and 'gender' was the cultural layering that formed on top of the biological foundation (Nicholson 1999, pp 53–55). They therefore recognised some degree of social constructionism in the concept of 'gender' (the social construction of biological sex differences) but the backbone of the theory was foundationalist. That is, like the (male) classical theorists from which they drew much of their theory, they did not question the law-like property of the body as a foundation for theorising about women's consciousness or subjectivity (the self). I will now review some of the major streams of modernist feminisms and offer critiques of each, before moving on to social constructionist theories of health.

Liberal feminism

Liberal feminists argued that women should be able to choose to forgo domesticity in favour of competing fairly with men for public sector roles. Given equal opportunities guaranteed through law, individual women could achieve equally with men. Domestic tasks could be contracted out on a commercial basis, freeing women for the more interesting and demanding tasks in the full-time public sphere workforce. The problems with this theory are as follows:

- It conceptualises women as free-floating individuals divorced from domestic ties and traditional responsibilities and relationships with dependants. It does not recognise that men and women are located within different relationships within the family as a result of socialisation, particularly with regard to the bearing, rearing and socialisation of children. These are not entirely optional relationships because some women construct their own identities primarily in relation to intimate relationships and family life, while many men seem to perceive a robust masculine identity as based on competing successfully against others in the public sphere. The 'stickiness' of cultural identities explains why women working full-time in the public sphere continue to shoulder 70% of all domestic tasks (Bittman & Pixley 1997).
- It fails to appreciate that gender distinctions are reconstructed constantly in the public sphere, to the detriment of women's ascendancy (Wearing 1996, pp 9–11). The 'glass ceiling' is the obvious example.
- It therefore gives no credence to the importance of the differential effects of cultural understandings on the self-identification of women. For example, some women do not wish to take the corporate road and those who do so often report a residual angst about straddling two realms and managing competently in both, especially in relation to their families.

Marxist feminism

Marxist feminists do acknowledge the wider social, political and economic parameters that shape women's identities. Women are structured by their relationship to the means of production. Women exchanged sexual and reproductive services in return for economic subsistence from their husbands. Under socialism, women would be free to produce their own living in the wider public sphere. Gender inequality was a symptom of class oppression that made women slaves within the family, where they became the proletariat to the bourgeoisie status of their husbands. The criticisms of this approach are that:

- gender inequality precedes capitalism. In so-called socialist countries in Eastern Europe before the fall of the Berlin wall, there was ample evidence that women remain clustered in the low-income, low-status jobs that mimicked their domestic lives.
- although gender is accepted as a social construction of biological sex differences, there is an assumption that

the larger social forces affect men and women uniformly (Wearing 1996, pp 11–14). It is, therefore, a form of social foundationalism.

Radical feminism

Radical feminists did address the sex–gender nexus, arguing either that women's oppression was rooted in the biological capacity for reproduction or that male aggression accounted for the subordination of women. The proposition that women have an essential creativity that is threatened by male jealousy and resolved through violence and economic, social and political domination is the mantra of radical feminism. The only solution for this kind of cultural imperialism was for women to separate from men and wrest control of technology away from male-dominated institutions. The major problem here is biological reductionism/biological foundationalism—the assumption that female and male identity are linked to biology and that biological differences between men and women yield universal behaviours, one being an aggressive quest for power and domination by men, and the other an essential procreative ability in women (Weedon 1992, p 17). The problems here are that:

- it assumes that sex and gender are merged, producing universal behaviours for men and women, one of which is essentially positive and the other essentially negative
- it fails to appreciate cultural and social differences among women and among men.

Social feminism

Socialist feminists also adopt a Marxist framework of capitalist class relations but add the importance of understanding patriarchy and racism in the oppression of women. They accept that these intersections are variable throughout history. Thus gender (female or male identity) is not reduced directly to biology. On the other hand, all institutions, including the family, the workplace and leisure, are patriarchal and produce an acceptance among men and women of the naturalness of patriarchy. How we think about our relationships must change and all existing institutions must be abolished because they are the expression of male domination (Weedon 1992, pp 18–19). Ultimately, then, socialist feminists do not resort to biological reductionism/foundationalism but they do resort to sociological foundationalism—a framework that subscribes to the idea of the overwhelming pressure of social forces having a uniform impact upon all women. They give no credence to individual self-reflexivity in both accepting and rejecting male-dominated structures at work and home or to the notion that the female psyche is formed by women's conscious and unconscious sifting through the mass of social influences to form their own position in relation to their intimate and formal relationships.

The summary so far

In summary, structuralist or foundationalist theories posit a fundamental point of departure that can be used to explain the wider social world. For Marx it was class, for Weber it was class and rationalisation. The classical theorists ignored the body or biology but earlier feminists, particularly radical feminists, turned to biology as a way of explaining the widespread exclusion of women from structures of power. However, in so doing they denied 'the reflexive self' or the ability of women (and men) to actively interpret and negotiate the complex social forces circulating and interacting in the social milieu and, in this way, to create and re-create their own identities.

For midwives and other health practitioners who make a leap from sexual, biological foundations to gender or cultural overlay, this same critique would apply. We need, therefore, a theory that allows for differences among women and among men, and between men and women, so that in considering any health treatment regimen, practitioners take into account individual constructions of the social world. Indeed, any treatment regimen that ignored the ways in which individuals idiosyncratically negotiate their social world in order to construct a 'self' would almost certainly fail or at least earn the disrespect and ire of those at the receiving end.

A final postscript to this discussion is necessary, to acknowledge the validity of some aspects of structuralist theories of health. For example, statistical evidence attests to the causal importance of gender and class as determining variables in the uneven distribution of health and illness. However, the overriding shortcoming of such theories is their biological or sociological foundationalism (Nicholson 1999, p 56). They deny the capacity of individuals for self-reflexivity, which means a conscious awareness of what we do and why we do it (Giddens 1995). Individuals in contemporary societies constantly examine and monitor their daily practices in the light of knowledge available to them, and in so doing create and re-create the self as an ongoing project (Elliott 2001, p 154). By contrast, in eschewing the existence of a robust self, the modernist theorists discussed above (excluding Weber, who did accept some form of reflexivity in his concept of *Verstehen*) explained social action by recourse to the concept of a false consciousness, either due to the suffocating power of a dominant class ideology or, for feminists, a patriarchal ideology. People were unable to know what their 'true' interests were, and so the charter of a revolutionary social movement (feminism, socialism) was to liberate the victim of history from the oppressor (capitalism, the capitalist state, men or the capitalist class).

Interpretive theories of health

Phenomenology, symbolic interactionism and post-structuralism/postmodernism fall under the rubric of interpretive sociologies because they deny that macrostructures solely cause and explain the actions of individuals. They assume that individuals are meaning-conferring, or impose their own meaning on events. All focus upon:
- microsocial relations, or interactions between individuals, rather than macro structural relations

- multiple, local knowledges rather than grand theorising or grand narratives (social forces such as gender, class or rationality or a physical basis, such as biology) as a way of explaining the entire course of human history and action.

Postmodern and poststructuralist interpretative sociologies introduce the idea of:
- complex, multiple identities rather than the autonomous, rational and unitary individual of Western individualism (the idea that you can understand the social world by reference to single individuals)
- power relations as a resource available to everyone, not just single or peak institutions of power like the 'state', 'biology' or 'class struggle'.

The objective here is to provide an explanatory framework that can grasp who it is that midwives (and obstetricians) are dealing with when they engage with the 'woman'. To assume that 'woman' may be defined by her biological capacities alone, or by gender (the social construction of biological sex characteristics), would be to fall into the same essentialist trap (the assumption that human action can be explained by reference to one cause, such as biology or genetic inheritance) as the structuralist feminists. The woman's sense of self would be derived solely from her surrounding political influences or from a biological essence. The self would be a kind of blotting paper where, for example, women would all share the same experiences because they share the same biological characteristics. This would ignore the importance of differences between women based on intersecting social influences (namely class, gender, ethnicity and subculture) as well as biological differences. Note that here we are using biology not as a fact but as a culturally variable entity. In other words, biology is itself a social construction. Under interpretive or social constructionist theories, biology ceases to be a point of departure, or an indisputable fact of analysis, to explain social behaviour (notably gender differences between men and women). This does not mean that the body is unimportant; quite the reverse. It does mean that the body and sexuality may be fashioned and changed in order to construct a self. The body becomes a cultural resource. Gallagher and Laqueur (cited in Lupton 1995, p 21) have noted that throughout history the body has 'been perceived, interpreted, and represented differently in different epochs, but it has also been lived differently, brought into being within widely dissimilar material cultures, subjected to various technologies and means of control and incorporated into different rhythms of production and consumption, pleasure and pain'. The body is thus a mixture of a materialism (the physical sentient base) and discourses (the way it has been moulded by social discourses). As Grosz (1994) says, the body is 'plastic'— it bends and forms according to the discourses that shape it. For example, the performance of the body during childbirth is closely related to the way in which women construct ideas about birth and mothering from a range of competing discourses, as well as how they perceive the immediate social environment. If they are fearful of birth and lack confidence in their body and then encounter practitioners in a high-technology setting who endorse their feelings of incompetence through their language and actions, women are much more likely to experience delays and obstructions, which then demand increasing types of intervention. The outcome is the now well-documented 'cascade of intervention' charted in hospital births.

To take a social constructionist approach to the body and sexual identity would be to point out that over time different cultures do recognise genital differences as the basis of similar or different identities (Nicholson 1999, p 74), but this feature does not guarantee similar social experiences. Nor does it determine sexuality. For example, people in dominant heterosexual cultures may adopt homosexual behaviours because of their circumstances (men in prison), but consider themselves and identify to others as predominantly heterosexual. Formerly heterosexual women and men may also change their sexual identity in the course of a lifetime, even after having been married for years and having children. Sometimes they change back again. Sexual preference is better conceptualised as a matter of identity, rather than a biological imperative ruled by genetic or any other anatomical causes. This identity may take many years to take coherent form. For example, Plummer (1995, p 54) describes the construction of a homosexual identity as being 'a journey, engaging in a contest, enduring suffering, pursuing consummation, establishing a home'. It is a difficult journey because it takes place in a homophobic and dominant heterosexual culture. For most homosexuals it is a process (of 'coming out') taking varying amounts of time, sometimes years, to admit to themselves and to others that they are homosexual. Within dominant heterosexual cultures, there is also variation over generations about what is considered 'normal' sexual behaviour (Rubin, cited in Giddens 1995, pp 9–16). If there are no solid foundations such as genetic material, sexual impulses, social conflict between classes or between men and women or social harmony to explain human behaviour and social history, then what is there? How can we have a political agenda if the very cement that pulls it together and defines its cause (in our case, the universal category 'woman') disappears as a solid conceptual grounding for clinical decision-making and collective political action?

Nicholson (1999, pp 74–75) suggests we use the word 'game' originally coined by the philosopher Wittgenstein to depict a social entity that shares some characteristics but also differs within cultures over time and between different cultures. As Nicholson says, having a vagina may be one of the similar characteristics but there are exceptions, like the person who identifies as a woman before a sex-change operation. 'Woman' can also mean different kinds of behaviours and preferences or orientations depending on the intersection of other social influences, or discourses, about reality. For example, a black, working-class woman from a rural area will have different experiences of what it is to be a woman than a white, middle-class female executive. Neither can speak for the experiences of the other about what it is like to be a woman.

'Woman', then, is 'a map of intersecting similarities and differences' where the body becomes socially variable according to the discourses that are used to describe it (Nicholson 1999, p 74). Political action need not discard the term 'woman' as

the organising principle but it would need to be cognisant of the diverse needs of women, and their complex and shifting identities, and couch their political claims in sufficiently abstract terms to encompass diversity (Nicholson 1999, p 75).

For example, no one is ever just a woman or a man. I would describe myself as a Western, middle-aged, heterosexual mother and lecturer with a small physical build. All of these parts of the identity or the self come from categories which themselves arise from different ideas about social reality, or discourses. The different parts of my 'self' are not equally dominant all of the time. Different characteristics become more or less significant depending on my interpretation of the social context, my own objectives and how I perceive the response from my audience.

The point about the diversity of the self and its fluid nature is important for health practitioners because large-scale research surveys often claim to know 'what women want'. For example, macro surveys of women's needs and expectations during pregnancy and birth (Darcy et al 2001) have been charted to arrive at a set of dictums that privilege some models of maternity care over others. At best this kind of exercise produces a set of aggregate figures that reflect an ambiguous and fairly arbitrary response to a question that would have been interpreted in a number of ways by respondents and where the results may be interpreted in a number of ways by researchers and other readers. We need to accept that women have diverse identities or selves and that to know what they want demands asking each and every one of them not once but constantly. As Nicholson (1999, p 76) says:

> it is time that we explicitly acknowledge that our claims about 'women' are not based on some given reality but emerge from our own places within history and culture; they are political acts that reflect the contexts out of which we emerge and the futures we would like to see.

For midwives, whose own political and professional identities are based on being 'with women', it is vital that they are clear about individual idiosyncrasy. First, it means they need to be in constant dialogue with each woman at each point of her pregnancy and stage of birth because her needs may well change, depending on the circumstances in which she finds herself, including additional knowledge, surprising events and other pressures. We need to put all of this on a viable theoretical basis. That is, to avoid the pitfalls outlined in the foregoing discussion of structuralism, we need to employ a social constructionist framework that does not slip into biological or social foundationalism, that institutes a self that is capable of changing over time in relation to the wider social milieu, that is complex in its constitution and cannot be 'read off' a single social, biological or psychic base, and, importantly, that recognises the power of individuals to negotiate their social world.

Discourses of the self

Individuals negotiate complex social influences from their own unique social location to form a unique self. Yet, in saying this, I am not arguing for a completely different social universe for everyone because a great deal of our social environment is shared in common. We need to understand, however, how culture is forged and modified. What are the transmission mechanisms? For post-structuralists and postmodernists, the starting point for a 'politics of transformative recognition'[1] is language and discourse. To my mind, Foucault's (1981) determination of 'discourse' is preferable to Lacan's use of the term. As it has been interpreted, Lacan's meaning of 'discourse' commonly devolves into structuralism in assuming that gender identity is determined by a pre-existing, male-dominated symbolic order, where women's subordination is inevitable. This symbolic order is conveyed through a particular view of language as a system of static meanings.[2] Lacan's theory therefore succumbs to 'psychologism'—a causal explanation that relies upon a single, underlying reference point (in this case a psychology of male domination) from which the course of human history may be explained. Its insistence on a static symbolic order of male domination cannot account for shifts in the self over time, the challenge to male domination or other forms of domination, alternative and multiple perspectives and struggles over social meanings (Fraser 1997, p 159).

We need a theory that links language with society and social change. In this way we can see how power is maintained but also how it may be challenged, that is, how to account for resistance at the macro level (including collective social struggles and social movements) as well as at the micro level of the self. Importantly, discourse provides this link to understanding how we confer meaning on social and non-social physical events and how meanings change over time.

Discourse is defined as:

> a pattern of words, figures of speech, concepts, values and symbols. A discourse is a coherent way of describing and categorizing the social and physical worlds. Discourses gather around an object, person, social group or event of interest, providing a means of 'making sense' of that object, person and so on. All discourses are textual, or expressed in texts, inter-textual, drawing upon other texts and their discourses to achieve meanings, and contextual, embedded in historical, political and cultural settings (Lupton 1995, p 18).

Discourses convey knowledge of the world through language. They influence us to see the world in one way rather than another. Thus language is never neutral; it would be a mistake to see language as just a transparent tool for describing the world. It is a mechanism for constructing reality. This is why it is disempowering to say to women that 'their cervix has failed to dilate', or to say, even innocently, 'I can't find the baby's heartbeat'. These words create a reality. This is why Foucault calls the power of discourse 'constitutive power'—it constitutes realities, subjectivities (how we see ourselves and others). Discourses are thus inevitably bound up with the exercise of power. It is not that knowledge produces power, but that power produces knowledge. This is why the medical discourse is powerful—because the institutionalised power

of medicine in law, via government policy and in systems of knowledge, conveys an aura of truth. Yet medicine is only a discourse. It is accepted within medical circles that all concepts are contested, often vigorously, among researchers, clinicians and across different specialties. For poststructuralists also there is no undisputed or singular 'truth', only competing discourses. Their juxtaposition allows us to challenge the authenticity of any discourse and thereby to resist social dominance (Weedon 1992, p 111). Note that exercising power will be an uneven process across individuals and across events: not all people will feel powerful all the time in all situations, but the point remains that individuals do possess some power at all times, even if it is just the power to silently disagree. Repressive political regimes inherently know this, which is why the Berlin Wall was constructed and why it had to be pulled down.

This puts the concept of power in a very different light than a structuralist theory of power, where power is conceptualised as a system of top-down domination on the part of, say, a capitalist ideology (Marx) or a patriarchal ideology (feminism). For Foucault, power is exercised at all levels—within institutions at the macro level but also at the level of interpersonal relations. Foucault refers to this as the micro-capillaries of power. Take, for example, the discourse that birth is a dangerous event and that women should deliver in a high-technology, acute-care unit in a hospital with access to obstetric care. This is a dominant medical discourse that exercises power over many individuals because it meshes with other discursive networks, such as the idea that science is only ever conducted in the benign interests of progress and the benefit of patients. Some discourses are suppressed, such as the discourse that obstetrics is at least partially conducted in the economic interests of obstetricians to secure a viable financial base against competitors. We could include the fact that, historically, science and medicine have constituted the body in ways that allow for few alternative constructions, or at least render alternatives as dangerous or foolish or 'unscientific' (for example, homeopathy, naturopathy, midwifery and home birth). Historically also, medical practices have colluded with other institutions such as governments, prisons, hospitals, the military and schools in monitoring, regulating and disciplining bodies (Lupton 1995, p 23).

The body may be conceived, therefore, as the site of competing discourses of sexuality, health, disease and childbirth. The political effects of these discourses include the co-opting of people into their mesh-like nature. For example, people begin to extend the 'medical gaze' to monitor and discipline themselves through dietary practices, health regimens and forms of abstinence. Foucault called this 'docile bodies'. It resonates with the current fashion for the perfect body and the popular cult of the 'extreme makeover'. However, taken on its own, this view is far too structuralist—it presents a view of the self that is passive and reactive, rather than proactive in constructing alternative discourses to challenge the status quo, including dominant medical discourses.

Discourses and resistance

Foucault's theory of power proposes that power is not top-down, as discussed above, and nor is it exercised in a binary fashion, as in a zero-sum game where if one person has power another must lose it. As Foucault (1981, p 101) says:

> There is not, on the one side, a discourse of power, and opposite it another discourse that runs counter to it. Discourses are tactical elements or blocks operating in the field of force relations; there can run different and even contradictory discourses within the same strategy; they can, on the contrary, circulate without changing their form from one strategy to another, opposing strategy.

Although not fully developed as a tool of resistance, Foucault's concept of 'constitutive power' is promising because it conceives of power as creating subjectivities or social positions, which could include resistant positions. Thus, Foucault (1981, p 101) proposes that:

> Discourse transmits and produces power; it reinforces it *but it also undermines and exposes it, renders it fragile and makes it possible to thwart it*. In like manner, silence and secrecy are a shelter for power, anchoring its prohibitions, but they also loosen its hold and provide for relatively obscure areas of tolerance. (italics mine)

In his later work, Foucault (1985) shifted his focus from 'technologies of domination' to 'technologies of the self' that declared a parallel shift in his thinking about the body. Bodies were no longer docile effects of dominant discourses but potentially reflexive in the shaping of the self. However, Foucault did not provide a solid foundation for understanding exactly how resistance may occur, because he was mainly concerned with emphasising the political effects of changes in social organisations (Turner 1990, p 222). We do need to theorise resistance, however, because it looms large in understanding changes in maternity arrangements. For example, the consumer movement of the 1980s is an example of a broadly based rejection of a very powerful medical discourse. So too the professionalisation of midwifery as the guardianship of the 'normal' (Kent 2000, p 28) may be interpreted as a critique of the abstract, scientific and dehumanising practices of obstetrics epitomised by 'the Dublin method'.

The idea of midwifery partnership is the implicit recognition that the consumer possesses power to make decisions and that they may do this by weighing up various discourses from a range of sources, including the midwife and the obstetrician. They will undoubtedly, given adequate information, sift through others circulating via the popular media, their friends, their families and other literature to come to a final decision. I argued earlier that this is how the self emerges. We need to understand the self and the creative ability of the individual to resist dominant discourses, because midwives would want to challenge Foucault's claim that as members of the 'helping professions' they are acting as instruments of social control.

The postmodern self

At this point it is important to qualify the concept of individual autonomy or 'voluntarism' in relation to self-identity and thus the power of resistance. Postmodernists insist that the self in the post-industrial, postmodern, consumption-oriented, communication society of global capitalism produces a highly reflexive self, but one that is also highly fragmented and fluid. How is it then that women could manage to resist dominant discourses when the self is so malleable? Many explanations of the self turn to psychoanalysis but, as argued earlier, these typically resort to rigid symbolic orders where individual resistance and social change is theoretically negated or becomes an incidental outcome of the slippage of meanings between signifiers (words, pictures or sounds) over time. I am suggesting that the self is produced and reproduced much more proactively through engagement with various discourses over time. Thus the self is always shifting according to one's position historically and socially, but to do this the individual needs a sense of consistency and continuity, especially at the level of emotion. The way in which individuals do this is by harvesting elements from sometimes competing discourses where the outcome is a coherent self-narrative. This allows them to act in the world in a relatively autonomous fashion. Theoretically, poststructuralism (the construction of reality through language) is married with narratology (the way in which people give meaning to their lives by constructing stories about their experiences) (Gergen 1994) to provide a solid theoretical grounding to explain women's agency. Let me provide an example of how one woman reported her home birth to construct a narrative of good mothering in the future:

Q So how was home birth for you?

A Extremely good. I am a very strong believer as well that a positive launch into motherhood, into parenthood, into the world for the baby is like the crest of a wave that helps to carry you along for quite a long time. And I think if you don't have that, for those who've had difficult and traumatic births, I think they are struggling. They haven't got that crest of a wave and they are struggling for a long time afterwards, sometimes forever. It colours their whole attitude towards their child or children and parenthood. And I think that I had that crest of a wave. OK, I had ups and downs afterwards, but I really feel that on the crest of the wave I was launched.

Self-narrative represents the outcome of a process of imposing order on a random set of events in the external world over which people have limited or no control. People construct a life history through embellishing and promoting some aspects of their lived experience in order to forge coherence between the past, present and future. This is an interesting strategy because it intuitively balances the uncertainty and risk that defines contemporary social existence. It grounds the postmodern self, not from a universal vantage point (as in structuralist theorising) but from the individual author's own lived, embodied experience and interpretive practice (Gubrium & Holstein 1994). In the example above, the woman decided to claim some events over others that happened in her birth to conclude that it had been successful and that this was an auspicious beginning to motherhood. In so doing, the woman's self-narrative depended on a range of other discourses from which she also drew. Hers was what Gergen (1994) terms a progressive narrative—'Life is in every way getting better'. The regressive narrative is where life goes backwards or downwards—'Life is just one damned thing after another'. The stability narrative links events in such a way that things go on the same. All recount the past in terms of how to make decisions to steer the future. Constructing a self-narrative is what it means to be self-reflexive. However, our choice of events to harvest is not arbitrary but draws upon certain culturally sanctioned archetypes appropriate for one's age, gender, social class and so on. For example, a 'getting older' narrative for women means dressing and acting in a certain way. Women want to avoid being perceived as 'mutton dressed as lamb', whatever that means to them. Some teenagers want to avoid being perceived as 'nerds', whatever that means to their subcultural group. We are sensitive, then, to the prevailing discourses around us that position professionals as key figures in the construction of either progressive or regressive narratives. It would be helpful, therefore, to think about how professionals can position themselves so that women may more readily construct a progressive self-narrative.

Generativity

Generativity is a term coined by Erikson (1963) to refer to a life-stage in the middle post-marriage years when people are ready to orient their energies to others and to the larger social sphere. The opposite is self-absorption. Multidisciplinary scholarship has spawned variants on the original concept but all refer to social practices that are intended to contribute to the wellbeing of the next generation and the common good. If a woman has experienced a lack of power in many dimensions of her past life (and many feminists would argue that women typically do experience political subordination in a range of spheres), a birth that mimics loss of control and respect is likely to reinforce a regressive self-narrative. Conversely, a maternity career that is interpreted by the woman as positive and life-enhancing for herself and her baby will galvanise a positive self-narrative and this narrative will re-form the self and be projected onto the future relationship with her child and onto other aspects of her life and other relationships.

Clinical generativity

Clinical generativity is described as:

> a way of conceiving of and conducting the clinical process such that emphasis is given to community and temporal context, choice and capability, and spiritual and moral dimensions in relation to sustaining and strengthening intergenerational relationships. Generative counselling explicitly and systematically seeks to transcend the medical model in these contexts (Dollahite et al 1998, p 453).

We might see generativity as revitalising Foucauldian and sociological critiques of professionalism defined by power and pecuniary self-interest, market domination of competitors through limitation, subordination and exclusion and the infantilisation of clients to ensure their ignorance and ongoing need for the service (Turner 1990; Willis 1983). Clinical generativity may go some way to neutralising the market competitiveness and cultural dominance that has in the past characterised obstetrics, and it may prevail over the clinical timidity of some midwives. It would underpin a genuine partnership approach to the care of pregnant woman by highlighting the 'spiritual and moral dimensions in relation to sustaining and strengthening intergenerational relationships' by focusing on the woman's needs rather than the narrow professional needs of either midwifery or obstetrics. Clinical generativity challenges a medical model of determinism; that is, that events could not have happened otherwise because of some pathology of the mind or body. Clinical generativity does accept a quasi-determinism—that people's actions are embedded in their history and family dynamics—but it does not dwell on deficiencies. It assumes that people may choose generative actions given sufficient individual self-reflexivity about the past to redirect the future. Events are not entirely outside the individual's control (Dollahite et al 1998, pp 464–5). For example, a person who has been the victim of child abuse need not necessarily repeat that behaviour with their own children, and a person who has been a perpetrator of violence may, with sufficient professional help and self-determination, be able to reform their behaviour.

Professional generativity

However, we need to go one step further. Because clinical generativity has been applied to individual counsellors it is less applicable to situations such as childbirth, where women may see different kinds of professional carers over the period of their maternity career. Under these conditions, generativity needs to be institutionalised into a social model of care that systematically recognises the importance of women's agency and self-reflexivity.

We could call this professional generativity. This model of care would also endorse the importance of providing appropriate care for women, that is, care that may require more than one professional. It follows that the professionals involved would be focusing on the woman's needs. A collaborative model of care is indicated here, one in which professionals genuinely value the respective skills and competencies of the other and minimise traditional tensions and anxieties. Like generative counselling (Dollahite et al 1998, p 471), it could encompass a spiritual dimension in transcending a limited concern with professional self-interest and placing a premium upon affirming the values and beliefs of women and their families.

The following self-narrative is an example of a transcendent experience of childbirth that followed a first, unhappy birth.

> My mother had five babies and had a horrendous time with every one of them and she brought my sister and me up to believe

that having children was a curse and that you didn't want to go through that. I was determined that it wasn't going to be like that. Yes, it is a major life event, isn't it? It's something that you do two, maybe three or four times in your life and it's the most important thing. It's also natural; it needn't be a conflict and surrounded by technologies . . . I felt clever, very self-satisfied and special. Somehow after that I respected my body so much more. The half stone overweight didn't seem to matter very much after that.

The mother put this progressive self-narrative down to continuity of care with the midwife. As she said, 'Because you've got a relationship with someone then you're not just a patient'.

Conclusion

I have argued that midwifery represents a social model of healthcare, one that recognises the social bases of health and illness. I critiqued structuralist theories of health that explain disease or other events by recourse to a single point of reference. I argued that interpretive theories explain health as the outcome of individual negotiation of complex and contradictory discourses. Foucauldian theory inserts the importance of power relations in understanding the greater influence of some discourses over others. Foucault was less explicit about how to conceptualise individual agency. Yet this is important because partnership is pivotal in definitions of good midwifery practice. Partnership assumes an egalitarian relationship between rational equals. In order to act as an autonomous entity, individuals need to have a sense of self or self-reflexivity. I have argued that we can use the idea of self-narratives to clarify the processes whereby women harvest events from the past to explain the present and direct their actions in the future. Self-reflexivity through the construction of a self-narrative explains how resistance against powerful discourses of the body is possible, especially medical discourses relating to birth. Although discourses do not determine self-narrative, they do shape it. I have suggested 'professional generativity' as an umbrella term that imparts a vision of collaborative practice within continuity of care models to enable women to construct a progressive (that is, healthy and assertive) self-narrative.

Review questions

1 What is meant by medicalisation?

2 What is meant by a social model of health, illness and the body?

3 How does the social context affect the physical body?

4 How could you explain your choice to do midwifery by using 'the sociological imagination'?

5 What is the one characteristic shared by all structuralist theories of health?

6 What is the difference between biological foundationalism and social foundationalism?

7 What is meant by 'partnership' between the woman and her carers?

8 What is the difference between 'top-down' (structuralist) theories of power and 'bottom-up' (social constructionist or constitutive) theories of power?

9 What is a discourse?

10 How are discourses related to self-narrative?

11 Is generativity a useful concept for thinking about midwifery practice?

Notes

1 This term is derived from Nancy Fraser's (1997) essay on a viable political culture and future direction for political groups. She argues that some groups need economic redistribution and some need cultural recognition but most political groups, including women, need both. Political remedies such as 'affirmative recognition' solidify group identities and cast them into the rejected side of the accepted 'other' (e.g. marginal homosexuality against a dominant heterosexuality) but the effect is to polarise them around fixed sexualities and identities. Political remedies such as 'transformative recognition', by contrast, as in queer politics, aim to destabilise all sexual identities to make sexual preference 'a sexual field of multiple, debinarized fluid, ever-shifting differences' (p 24). That is, it accepts a diversity of experiences and orientations.

2 There is not the space here to interrogate Lacan's theory further but interested readers may go to Fraser (1997, pp 154–157) for a more sustained critique.

Online resources

Economic and Social Research Council (UK), http://www. esrcsocietytoday.ac.uk/ESRCInfoCentre/

Health Sociology Review, http://hsr.e-contentmanagement.com/

Sociology of Health and Illness A Journal of Medical Sociology, http://www.blackwellpublishing.com/journal.asp?ref=0141-9889&site=1

Sociosite: Social Science Information System based at the University of Amsterdam, http://www.sociosite.net/index.php. Australian and New Zealand References on Sociosite, http://www.sociosite.net/journals.php

References

Australian Institute of Health and Welfare 2001 Australian health trends. AIHW Cat. No. PHE 24, AIHW, Canberra

Bilton T, Bonnett K, Jones P et al 2002 Introductory sociology (4th edn). Palgrave Macmillan, New York

Bittman M, Pixley J 1997 The double life of the family. Allen & Unwin, Sydney

Brown C 1996 Body work. In: C Brbich (Ed) Health in Australia. Prentice Hall, Sydney

Darcy M, Brown S, Bruinsma F 2001 Victorian survey of recent mothers. Continuity of care: does it make a difference to women's views and experiences of continuity of care? Report No 2. Centre for the Study of Mothers' and Children's Health, School of Public Health, La Trobe University, Melbourne

Davis-Floyd R 1992 Birth as an American rite of passage. University of California Press, Berkeley

Dollahite DC, Slife BD, Hawkins AJ 1998 Family generativity and generative counselling: helping families keep faith with the next generation. In: D McAdams, E de St Aubin (Eds) Generativity and adult development: how and why we care for the next generation. American Psychological Association, Washington

Eckerman E 2000 Introduction to sociology. A study guide. Faculty of Arts, Deakin University, Geelong, Vic

Elliott A 2001 Concepts of the self. Polity Press, Cambridge

Erikson EH 1963 Childhood and Society. Norton, New York (original work published 1950)

Foucault M 1973 The birth of the clinic. Tavistock, London

Foucault M 1981 The history of sexuality, Vol. 1. An introduction. Pelican, Harmondsworth

Foucault M 1985 The use of pleasure. Penguin, Harmondsworth

Fraser N 1997 Justice interruptus: critical reflections on the 'postsocialist' condition. London, Routledge

George J, Davis A 1998 States of health: health and illness in Australia (3rd edn). Longman, Melbourne

Gergen K 1994 Realities and relationships: soundings in social construction. Harvard University Press, Cambridge, Mass.

Germov J 1998 Second opinion: an introduction to health sociology. Oxford University Press, Melbourne

Giddens A 1987 Sociology: a brief but critical introduction (2nd edn). Macmillan Press, London

Giddens A 1991 Modernity and self-identity: self and society in the late modern age. Stanford University Press, Stanford, Ca

Giddens A 1995 The transformation of intimacy: sexuality, love and eroticism in modern societies. Polity Press, Cambridge

Grosz E 1994 Volatile bodies. Toward a corporeal feminism. Indiana University Press, Bloomington and Allen & Unwin, Sydney

Gubrium JF, Holstein JA 1994 Grounding the postmodern self. Sociological Quarterly 35(4):685–703

Guilliland K, Pairman S 1995 The midwifery partnership: a model for practice. Department of Nursing and Midwifery, Monograph Series 95/1, Victoria University of Wellington, Wellington

Kent J 2000 Social perspectives on pregnancy and childbirth for midwives, nurses and the caring professions. Open University Press, Buckingham

Lane K 2000 Consumers as arbiters of professional practice? What does this mean for users of maternity services? Sociological Sites/Sights, TASA 2000 Conference, Flinders University, Adelaide

Leeder S 1999 Healthy medicine: challenges facing Australia's Health Services. Allen & Unwin, Sydney

Lupton D 1995 Medicine as culture: illness, disease and the body in western societies. Sage, London

Mills CW 1970 The sociological imagination. Penguin, Harmondsworth

Nicholson L 1999 The play of reason: from the modern to the postmodern. Cornell University Press, New York

Nurses Board of Victoria 1999 Victorian midwifery code of practice

Parsons T 1951 The social system. Routledge and Kegan Paul, London

Plummer K 1995 Telling sexual stories: power, change and social worlds. Routledge, London

Rothfield P 1995 Bodies and subjects: medical ethics and feminism. In: PA Komesaroff (Ed), Troubled bodies: critical perspectives on postmodernism, medical ethics and the body. Duke University Press, London

Synnott A 1992 Tomb, temple, machine and self: the social construction of the body. British Journal of Sociology 43(1):79–110

Taylor C 1989 Sources of the self: the making of the modern identity. Cambridge University Press, Cambridge

Turner BS 1990 Medical power and social knowledge. Sage, London

Wagner M 1994 Pursuing the birth machine: the search for appropriate birth technology. ACE Graphics, Sydney

Wearing B 1996 Gender: the pain and pleasure of difference. Longman, Melbourne

Weedon C 1992 Feminist practice and poststructuralist theory. Blackwell, Oxford

Willis E 1983 Medical dominance, division of labour in Australian healthcare. Allen & Unwin, Sydney

World Health Organization 1946 World Health Organization Constitution. WHO, Geneva

Wrong D 1998 The oversocialised conception of man. Transaction, New Brunswick, NJ

Yeatman A 1990 A feminist theory of social differentiation. In: LJ Nicholson (Ed) Feminism/postmodernism. Routledge, New York

CHAPTER 4

Risk and safety

Joan Skinner

Key terms

accountability, normality, referral, risk, safety, techno-rational discourse, values

Chapter overview

This chapter aids in the understanding of why risk is such an important concept. It begins by presenting the techno-rational or scientific approach and goes on to provide interpretations from social and cultural perspectives. What becomes clear is that the understanding and management of risk and the promotion of safety are not simple matters. However, the concerns related to risk and safety need not always engender fear and anxiety. The second part of this chapter provides a framework that the midwife can use to support safe, effective and life-affirming care within this risk environment. The framework acknowledges the complex and often paradoxical nature of midwifery practice and provides a way for the midwife to put the management of risk and safety into practice and into perspective.

Learning outcomes

Learning outcomes for this chapter are:

1 To explain the concepts of risk and safety
2 To discuss the scientific and sociocultural contexts in which risk is manifest
3 To highlight the centrality of the relationship with the woman in the provision of safe care
4 To discuss the importance of skilled midwifery care
5 To discuss the place of accountability for the use or misuse of midwifery skills
6 To discuss the place of referral and the importance of collaborative relationships
7 To acknowledge the complexity of the environment in which safe midwifery care is provided.

Introduction

The assessment of risk and the promotion and protection of safe childbirth are key elements of the provision of maternity care. Risk and safety are strongly related concepts that the midwife must come to terms with as she works alongside women as they become mothers. Safe practice minimises and 'manages' risk; risks are assessed, avoided or managed in order to provide a safe environment in which to give birth. Risk affects the lives of midwives, both in the assessment of risk in the childbearing woman, and in the management of their own risk within the medico-legal context. Yet there is something about how risk is currently constructed, not only in maternity care but also throughout the Western world, that reflects rising levels of anxiety. This increased anxiety about risk and safety is reflected in maternity care and is occurring despite a growing understanding of the causes, incidence and prevention of negative outcomes. This has been accompanied by increasing levels of intervention, accountability and surveillance, with significant implications for the way midwifery is practised (Skinner 2003). It challenges the model of birth as a normal part of human life and thus presents challenges for midwives attempting to enact in practice this model of normality. Midwives are faced with a significant paradox in attempting to work a 'birth is normal' perspective within a 'birth is risky' context. Working in this context requires the midwife to have a sophisticated understanding of the meanings of risk aversion and of safe practice.

In a sense, risk and safety have become opposing positions. There is little acceptance that taking risks is not only a normal part of life but is also essential. Without it humans do not develop. We can miss valuable and life-changing opportunities. In order to achieve safety we might sometimes put ourselves at risk of unforeseen and unknown risks. Sometimes you have to take risks to be safe, yet safe action may have unforeseen negative outcomes. Complete safety cannot be assured and there is no such thing as a risk-free birth. Risk in the current environment has become associated with the possibility of negative outcome rather than with the possibility of positive experience (Tulloch & Lupton 2003). It is the fear of negative outcome that is most often expressed. One rarely (if ever) reads reports of the risks of a positive outcome of a planned action. For example, how often is it expressed that if you plan a home birth you risk having a birth with no intervention? It is important then for the midwife practising in this environment to have an understanding of how and why risk has become so prominent and to have some tools to deal with the reality of how this affects safe practice.

Science: sourcing the evidence

The first place to investigate, and the one that holds the dominant position in current risk discourse, is the techno-rational or scientific approach. It is here that we see research dominated by epidemiology and by the randomised controlled trial and the use of this research in informing practice. These approaches to risk are focused on the mathematical calculations of risk associated with the probability of events occurring. Their main concerns are in the measurement of risks and effects. These approaches provide valuable information for the midwife in the provision of safe care and are an essential part of her knowledge base. For example, the meta-analysis of the randomised controlled trials on continuous fetal monitoring (CFM) indicates that for low-risk women, CFM increases the risk of unnecessary intervention (Thacker et al 2004). However, the application of the scientific evidence in the management of risk and the promotion of safety are seldom simple. There are several challenges that midwives face in assessing and managing risk from a science or evidence-based framework.

For the individual health practitioner there is a fundamental difficulty in extrapolating knowledge from large studies and applying it to individual situations. For example, the early identification of risk is notoriously imprecise in predicting adverse outcome for the individual (Enkin et al 2000). Once the complexity of the individual situation is identified, the ability to know what the quantified risks of an adverse event occurring are may be further eroded. The quantification of risk must take into account not only the rate of adverse outcome but also the possible benefits, and must ensure that there is some consistency in how the risks are framed (Guise 2004). The identification of risk is also tied up with control. Heyman (1998) contends that where health practitioners claim to predict the probability of an outcome for individuals, there is a tendency to attempt to make decisions on their behalf. He states: 'The health professionals' crystal ball, although providing only cloudy, probabilistic glimpses of possible futures, through the methodology of epidemiology, leads them into attempting to manage risks on behalf of their clients' (p 22). Skilled, clinical assessment and effective communication therefore remain core competencies for the midwife in assisting the client in decision-making around safe care. The scientific evidence is one important tool to inform this practice.

The techno-rational model of maternity care also has particular implications for the understanding of what is normal and so has a special importance for midwifery, which claims expertise in 'normal' birth. Understandings of what is risky and what is normal both dominate and delineate midwifery practice and yet are often seen as juxtaposed positions. Normality has changed from being a social to a scientific concept, as we have come to accept the idea that one can't know something unless it can be measured (Hacking 1990). Being normal therefore has come to mean both having no measurable risk factors and also being 'average'. This search for measurable regularity and thus quantifiable normality has given rise to rules about childbirth that have not undergone in-depth analysis (Murphy-Lawless 1998). An example of this is the decision about what constitutes a normal labour. This needed to be measurable, so statistical data of the length of labour has been applied to individual women's progress.

Deviations from the measurable, statistically assessed norm are then seen as needing to be managed and controlled. In essence, then, science in the guise of medicine has re-created and redefined 'normal' and has seen pregnancy as normal only in retrospect (Cartwright & Thomas 2001; Symon 1998; Wagner 1994).

It is within this dominant techno-rational discourse that midwifery stays firm in its claim to expertise in normal childbearing. It is a precarious position to take, given who is defining normality and who is defining risk. The challenge for midwifery is to look beyond the techno-rational definitions of normal and to claim its own. Midwifery sees birth as a normal process, not only physiologically but also socially, culturally and spiritually (NZCOM 2005). This is reflected in the commitment that midwifery has to partnership and to women-centred care. One of the risks of this perspective, however, is the possibility of decreased emphasis on the physical aspects of what we currently call normal birth—that is, birth with no intervention.

The techno-rational approach has also tended to make safety into a commodity, one that professionals are meant to be able to provide. Symon (1998), in his study of midwives' and obstetricians' attitudes to litigation, found that both midwives and obstetricians agreed that women had been given the impression that science (in the form of obstetric intervention) can achieve more than it actually can. The techno-rational model focuses on making danger visible (technology) and measurable (epidemiology) (Cartwright & Thomas 2001). But as Smythe (1998) points out, this is not always possible. There is, she says, unsafeness that is unknown. Some things can appear unannounced, suddenly and without warning. The normal and the abnormal can 'mimic' each other. She also comments that being safe or being unsafe (being at risk) is, in a sense, already there. Some women could give birth safely with no professional input and others will not give birth safely even with all the help that professionals can provide. So the midwife is there not to 'sell' a safe birth as some sort of objective measurable commodity but to support safety and to uncover, as much as she can, the risks that might threaten this safety. This unknowable nature of risk and safety means that the midwife must be skilled and vigilant.

The techno-rational approach also implies that decision-making should be made by rational experts rather than by the 'insignificant others' (Stapleton 1997). Davis-Floyd (2002) describes this approach as technocratic. Based on the pre-eminence of technology and of mind–body separation, the technocratic approach, she says, treats the 'patient' as object and sees responsibility and authority as being held by the practitioner. This approach also presupposes that both the assessment of risk and the experts themselves are objective and rational and that people will make rational decisions about what is risky and what is safe (Lupton 1999). It is based on assumptions that the evidence provides clear answers so that choices will be also be clear and self-evident. However, this is not often the case. Take, for example, clinical practice guidelines that recommend induction of labour for pregnancies that go past 41 weeks gestation. Menticoglou

and Hall (2002), on close examination of the research on which these guidelines are based, estimated that it would take 1000 inductions of uncomplicated pregnancies at 41 weeks gestation to possibly save the life of one baby. The decision about whether this is a justifiable intervention will inevitably be based on what is valued or what is feared and is therefore not a rational process. Menticoglou and Hall also highlight the possible harm caused to women and their babies by the 999 unnecessary inductions, and also to other labouring women being cared for in a maternity unit busy doing these unnecessary inductions. The use of such clinical practice guidelines, they state, also has considerable implications for litigation when they are not strictly adhered to. How midwives assist mothers to make such decisions can therefore be fraught. Who has the power to decide whether these risks are worth taking? Decisions about risk and safety are therefore not as simple as one might think.

Heyman (1998) summarises the difficulties related to the application of science and technology by saying that although the techno-rational approach has made a huge contribution to human development, it:

> cannot accurately predict most biographical outcomes, answer questions about values, or provide convincing solutions to the mind–body problem. Many of these issues come to a head in the management of health risks. [The] notion of probability, which underpins the idea of risk, does not provide a rigorous scientific tool, but only a heuristic, rule-of-thumb device which had both utility and limitations; and that the assessment of 'adversity' entails weighing up values in ways which sometimes are contested (p 2).

Heyman points out that however helpful epidemiology may be, risk decisions are not made rationally and must be understood within their social and cultural context.

Society, culture and the role of values

The management of the risks associated with childbirth then are not only understood in physical terms but must be understood within their societal and cultural contexts. As stated earlier, the current social context has highlighted risk as a central concern. This is not peculiar to maternity care. Beck (1999), a foremost sociologist in risk theory, has proposed that we now live in a 'risk society'. Modern life, he asserts, has been based on the idea that technology and science can provide the answers to our problems. Progress and controllability have been fundamental beliefs in the search for safety and security. The success of modernity, as represented by science and technology, has led to globalisation and thus to a growing understanding of the multiple ways of living and viewing the world. Modernity has also led to individualisation and a sense of self-determination. This in turn has challenged traditional social understandings including the role of women and the place of the family, leading to increasing uncertainty. This uncertainty is also reflected in the undermining of faith in science and technology, by the growing understanding that not only does technology not solve all our problems, it actually creates some of them. This uncertainly about societal roles and loss of faith in technology have led to a generalised insecurity and anxiety, along with a loss of faith in professionals and in technology. We are in a state on being 'in between', where we have not yet created social and cultural forms that replace the tenets of modernity. We are, according to Beck, not yet postmodern but are living in what he calls 'late modern' society, where we live with, among other things, the paradox of losing faith in experts while at the same time still expecting that their work will be free of negative outcomes. The levels of anxiety that are produced become counterproductive. In terms of maternity care this reflexive culture means that maternity practitioners can be constantly questioned, challenged and increasingly restricted in their practice. The accountability that results causes fear and stress not only in the practitioners but also in the consumers of maternity care, as they themselves are required to make choices with risks attached that are difficult or impossible to quantify.

Ironically this desire to avoid or control all risk in itself creates its own problems. Annandale (1996) comments that the consumerism and managerialism that have emerged as part of the risk society have tended to further increase the levels of anxiety and, paradoxically, to have undermined the quality of care that is provided. It is this combination of managerialism in the form of protocols and guidelines, and consumerism in the form of informed choice and consent, that provides the current background for midwifery practice. One needs only to reflect on the increase in caesarean section rates in light of the 'risk society' to see how this can be applied to maternity care and to midwifery. In the effort to control for all risk, both for the mother and baby and for the maternity practitioner, caesarean sections are an increasingly used intervention. Yet this intervention comes with its own risks. The dilemma for the midwife is to work in this increasingly constrained environment while providing care that is flexible and truly women-centred. And all this in an environment focused on risk aversion. The risk society as manifest in maternity care reflects the tension between both the acceptance and the rejection of modern biomedicine. Davis-Floyd (2002) accepts the valuable knowledge that biomedicine has provided but also contests its dominance. The anxiety associated with risk and safety can be seen then as having its origins in the movement beyond an uncritical acceptance of biomedicine. The resurgence of midwifery and the increase in the valuing of humanistic or holistic care could be seen as part of the movement towards a new, more postmodern way of viewing the world. We certainly seem to be in a state of transition.

Another way to view risk and safety is to take a cultural view. Cultural perspectives attend not so much to the way in which current social forms are reflective of risk (as in Beck's 'risk society') but to the way in which societal forms themselves affect the way decisions about risk are made. One of the most influential thinkers in this field is the anthropologist Mary Douglas (Douglas 1992; Douglas & Wildavsky 1982). Douglas points to the lack of uniformity in opinions about what makes something risky, how risky it might be and what should be done about it. She rejects both the scientific, objectivist approach and an individual rational choice approach to risk decision-making. Instead, she proposes that risks are decided upon according to the cultural meaning associated with them, and is critical of experts' attempts to get to the objective truth of risk by protecting it from the 'dirty' side of politics and morals. People, she proposes, do not make decisions about risk according to individualised circumstances and beliefs, but are culturally conditioned to prefer some types of decisions over others. Their beliefs and actions therefore are culturally constructed. Within any culture there will be subgroups and communities who have varied value bases and ethical systems. These ethical systems too are culturally constructed and may vary. This variety is not related to any misguided perception, as objectivists would propose, but to different political, moral and aesthetic positions (Lupton 1999).

Values and uncertainties are an integral part of these choices and Douglas proposes that the choices between risky alternatives are not value-free. Choice in the end, therefore, is essentially based on social rather than scientific knowledge. This decision-making process can also been seen as political. Who should make decisions, who and what should matter, are related to whose knowledge is regarded as authoritative. Douglas's position does acknowledge that dangers and risks are real but proposes that it is impossible to rank them in any rational sense. There are simply too many of them (Douglas & Wildavsky 1982). A cultural approach therefore helps us see risk decision-making as a result of community consensus, rather than rational individual choice. It is this community consensus that gives preference to some risks over others. We see this clearly in the decision-making processes around birth. Take, for example, a woman's decision to deliver her breech baby without intervention, compared with an obstetrician's wish to deliver her baby by caesarean section, or a woman's choice to have an epidural anaesthetic despite her midwife's commitment to normal birth. How do the women's decisions reflect their cultural and community perspectives? Whose knowledge is authoritative? How is fear being expressed? And of course, who is at risk?

Both the social and cultural interpretations of the current risk discourse speak to how blame is apportioned. Both see blame as a reflection of societal and cultural forms that have some basis in controllability. Where adverse outcomes eventuate, someone must be held accountable for the mis-management of risk. Blame then is a deflection onto someone else. Accountability for adverse outcome is required and is usually punitive. This is reflected in the 'name, blame and shame' approach that is manifest not just in maternity care or even just in healthcare but increasingly in every sphere of life. This has significant implications for health practitioners in the risk of litigation. Health practitioners, including those in maternity care, express considerable anxiety related to this risk of litigation (Aslam 1999; Cunningham 2004; Keaney 1996; Ruston 2004; Skinner 2005; Symon 1998).

Risk and safety then can be seen not only as core business for the midwife but have been made even more dominant in current maternity care by the 'risk society' in which we now live and work. The techno-rational approach to maternity care still dominates despite a growing understanding of the place of values and cultural understandings of risk and safety. The midwife must provide care that incorporates these different ways of knowing and acknowledges and deals with the complex and often conflicting perspectives inherent in these approaches. The following model offers the midwife a framework to support and assist her in this work.

Working with risk and safety: a birth stool for the midwife

This model has been developed from my research into how caseloading midwives in New Zealand manage risk in practice. The research was a mixed method study conducted in 2001 and examined the referral for obstetric consultation as a place where the expression of risk was most evident. The first part of the study was a national, total population survey of caseloading midwives and described the referral for obstetric consultation patterns. It also included an assessment of the midwives' attitudes to risk management, to referral and to the medico-legal environment. The second part of the study consisted of a series of six focus groups with midwives in a variety of New Zealand settings. The settings were selected to provide a range of perspectives and included regions across the country, both rural and urban, and small and large cities. The midwives discussed the challenges and opportunities they faced in the management of risk. The survey data were analysed with descriptive statistics and the focus group data were analysed thematically. The two data sets were then interpreted together in the development of the model. It is a model for practice focused on how midwives deal with risk.

Models can be very useful as they provide a framework for understanding the complexity of the real world and can guide our actions by defining what is important (Stewart et al 2003). What became evident during the development of this model was that dealing with risk and safety is no simple matter. It is not just about identifying risk factors and referring, or about good documentation, nor can it be compartmentalised into one aspect of midwifery practice. What also became apparent is that there is no quick fix for risk. Being a safe practitioner comes from being an effective midwife in every area of practice. The model therefore is a representation of the midwife's work. Its origins come from studying how risk is expressed in practice and it is placed within current understandings of the 'risk society'. It can also therefore be interpreted as a model for practice as a whole. The framework represents midwifery practice as a simple three-legged stool (Fig 4.1). It is a birth stool, not this time for the woman, but for the midwife. It is a tool that she can take with her and use wherever she practices. Many aspects of this 'stool' are covered in detail later in this text. The following section describes the stool and provides a

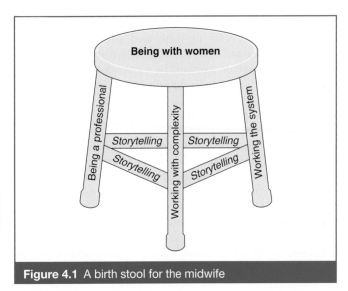

Figure 4.1 A birth stool for the midwife

framework for putting the whole of practice together in order to become a safe and effective midwife.

Being 'with women'

The most important part of a stool is of course the seat. The seat of this stool I have called 'being with women'. It represents the centrality of the midwife–woman relationship and the importance of being alongside the woman in her journey to motherhood. It is the quality both of the relationship and of the communication that is the critical factor in the maintenance of safe and appropriate care (Edwards 2000; Symon & Wilson 2002; Wilkins 2000). Relationships matter. It is within this relationship that trust is formed, information is shared, options are offered and decisions are made. Continuity of carer is important for these relationships to be formed. Being 'with women' provides the space and time for the midwife to know the woman, to understand her perspectives and to anticipate her needs. Smythe (1998), in her study of maternity practitioners' and women's understandings of the meaning of safety, comments that the relationships the midwife forms with the women are embedded in a particular social and cultural milieu that the midwife enters and uncovers. These relationships the woman has are with family, friends, other practitioners, medicine and even the media. Smythe describes the relationship as one of 'concernfulness' (Smythe 1998, p 188). It is within this concernfulness that the midwife can most effectively discern what is safe and what is not. In my research, this relationship was manifest as a sense of protection, as the midwives assisted and supported the women to make decisions and to negotiate both different forms of knowledge and the expectations of the institution. The woman's autonomy was not acknowledged in a distanced way but was protected and encouraged. Smythe describes the climate of trust and knowing that is generated in the relationship. She says that it can free the midwife to 'leap ahead, discerning what she perceives lies in the darkness' (Smythe 1998, p 188).

Pairman (2000) describes the relationship as one of professional friendship, where notions of 'being equal', 'sharing common interests', 'involving the family', building trust', 'reciprocity', 'taking time' and 'sharing power and control' are all valued (p 210). Being with women also means being with the *whole* woman. In a risk and safety context this means that the midwife doesn't separate out the physical aspects of risk from the social and cultural realities of the woman and her family. It also means that the midwife stays in connection with the woman who becomes 'at risk'. She continues to provide midwifery care and support where possible. Her care is holistic. The idea of partnership with the women can be seen as embedded within the seat of the birth stool. Central to partnership are the concepts of negotiation, equality, shared responsibility, empowerment and informed choice and consent (Guilliland & Pairman 1995). In 'being with' the woman, the midwife works towards this partnership with her. Where the relationship is new and developing, or where it is challenging and difficult, being and staying with the woman sensitively and respectfully are key factors of being a midwife. It is within this relationship that the midwife must learn to balance trust and anxiety,

Being with the woman then is a central and critical aspect of managing risk and promoting safety, yet as Smythe (1998) says, these relationships are necessary but not sufficient. Partnership is incorporated into the seat, yet this on its own is not sufficient in helping to understand the complex and challenging work of midwifery. It is, in a sense, a seat without legs. It doesn't lift the midwife off the ground. The legs of the stool provide the other aspects of practice that are vital in the provision of safe care in the current sociocultural context. Being a professional, knowing how to work the system and understanding and working with complexity, provide the stability required to stay 'with women' and to work towards partnership with them. It the legs of the midwife's birth stool that give support; the legs help to lift the midwife above the 'messy swamp' of practice (Schon 1983).

Being a professional

The first leg of the stool I have called 'being a professional'. It includes being both a skilled and an accountable practitioner. For the midwives in my study, having the skills needed to assess risk was important. The skills required are diverse and rely on a sound knowledge base. Midwifery incorporates knowledge from many different sources. It comes from within its own discipline and from other fields such as physiology, pharmacology, epidemiology and medicine. It also sources knowledge from the humanities, such as sociology and psychology. This knowledge then informs practice in the provision of safe care. A safe midwife is attentive to sound research and seeks answers to problems. However, in Smythe's (2000) study the midwives acknowledged that not all risk is assessable. Much of it is unknown and hidden. It is the midwife's task to uncover risk as much as she can, but always to remain alert and attentive, anticipating what might be lying underneath.

A skilled midwife is also a skilled communicator and listener, attentive not only to the physical factors of the woman but also to her social and cultural milieu. She seeks to understand what the woman and her family value and thus to understand how they themselves see risk and safety. She communicates her own understanding of risk and safety in a way that promotes the woman's autonomous decision-making and minimises unnecessary fear and anxiety. She is reflective of her own position and attempts to provide care that is not dominated by it. Communication with the woman and her family is based in the quality of the relationship that she develops. It is fundamental to her 'being with' the woman.

Current constructions of professional practice are also very attentive to accountability. Accountability does not necessarily mean always accepting responsibility for adverse outcome but it does mean that the midwife must be accountable for her decisions and her actions. This accountability is primarily to the woman, but also to the profession and to the public (NZCOM 2005). Accountability is a valuable tool for the midwife and she should not be afraid of it. Accountability facilitates an honest, reflective relationship. It helps to keep the midwife attentive and motivates her to maintain her knowledge and skills. It helps to keep the woman at the centre of practice.

However, it does sometimes mean that the midwife must be accountable to the public and to the profession within the medico-legal context and it is this aspect of practice that is most feared. As discussed earlier, the current state of the 'risk society' means that professionals can be blamed when an adverse outcome has eventuated. It is here that we see the midwife as being 'at risk'. She is at risk of litigation. What must be pointed out, however, is that just as the general public seem to be becoming increasingly anxious about very small probabilities of risk, so too do health professionals themselves. The risk of being held accountable within the medico-legal processes are very small and must be kept in perspective lest practice be paralysed.

There are several ways in which the midwife can protect her own safety in this context. Accurate and complete documentation will provide evidence of the care that was provided. This should include documentation of the decision-making processes, including noting the information that was provided. The midwife needs to understand and implement her professional code of ethics and the standards for care (ACMI 2006; NZCOM 2005). Safety for the midwife includes attending to the whole of practice, to all the parts of this midwife's birth stool. It remains based in the sound development of the relationship with the woman, in providing skilled care, and also in an understanding of and connection with the systems that are in place. It is supported by an understanding of, and negotiation between, the complex and often contradictory environment in which she works.

Working the system

The next leg of the stool has been called 'working the system' and is an important part of providing safe care, care that continues to be based on staying connected with the woman and her experience. I have called it 'working the system' as it is a reminder that the focus remains on being 'with women'. Midwives work the system in order to meet the needs of the woman. This leg reminds us that we do not provide care in isolation. We provide care within a system, and it is important not only to understand how the system works but also to participate in it. Three aspects of knowing the system are important. The first, and possibly the most crucial, is the development and maintenance of successful collaborative relationships with others in the system. Within my research, not only was the quality of the relationship with the woman important but the quality of the relationships with obstetricians and other midwives was also seen as crucial. The midwives felt that both they and the women were much safer where respectful, trusting relationships had been developed with those with whom they needed to collaborate. These relationships cannot be assumed but must be actively sought and maintained. They also include relationships with work partners and other midwives in the local community. It includes those who provide the secondary maternity services, the obstetricians and the midwives in the hospital. It includes forming collaborative relationships with those in the community whose services the women may also require: the GPs, the childbirth educators, the practice nurses and the local pharmacists, to name just a few. Smythe (2000) also found this in her study. She commented that trusting, collaborative relationships facilitated the sharing of what she described as concernfulness. This trust is developed within the relationship. One cannot assume or presume trust either with the woman or with other professionals. It is not automatic and must be earned. In order to do this, personal knowing is important.

The second aspect of 'working the system' relates to understanding and working with the processes that the system puts in place. The most obvious processes are guidelines and policies, but can also be extended to an understanding of the funding and contractual arrangements, of professional standards and of the required competencies. Risk management systems most clearly related to risk are the referral guidelines (Australian College of Midwives 2004; Ministry of Health 2002). These guidelines provide a framework for the midwife to use in the decision-making related to complex or 'at risk' pregnancies. No research has been undertaken as to the efficacy of these guidelines. However, there has been a wealth of evidence that risk screening processes in general suffer from low sensitivity and low specificity (Alexander & Keirse 1989; Rohde 1995; Rooney 1992). The referral guidelines could be seen as a risk-screening process and therefore can be critiqued as lacking validity as a useful tool to improve safety. However, they are also about delineating the boundaries of professional practice and attempt to facilitate inter-professional collaboration by establishing a process for the interaction. These referral guidelines (ACMI 2004; Ministry of Health 2002) can be seen as an indication of the scope of practice of a midwife, and can be used as a guide to indicate the appropriate level of care. Within my research (Skinner 2005), although some midwives found that the guidelines restricted their practice, most found that they were a useful tool in indicating when to seek obstetric assistance.

There was also a statistically significant relationship between the midwives' positive attitudes to the referral guidelines, and whether they worked in a supportive and collaborative environment.

As most midwives realise, guidelines are not always appropriate in individual circumstances and there will always be some women who do not want to follow them. Sixty-four per cent of the midwives in Symon's (1998) study of midwives and obstetricians in the United Kingdom said that they had cared for women who did not want to follow guidelines for practice. The midwives in my study also discussed this as a frequent and normal part of practice. Risk may or may not be increased when this happens. What is important, though, is that the midwife understands that this is happening and so can assess whether measures need to be put in place for added protection either for the woman or for herself. This may be as simple as keeping careful documentation.

Working the system also involves participating in organisational risk management and clinical governance processes (Cooper 2000; Wilson 2002). It is important not only to know what the organisational expectations are but also to be involved in developing them. For the midwife, managing risk and promoting safety are also about being part of the local community and being aware of the range of resources available to help. It is about knowing what is going on and participating in change processes such as research and policy development, and about taking a leadership role where needed.

This leads to the third part of working the system. It would be naive to talk about the midwife's relationship with the system without acknowledging the existence of power relationships and the need to managing the power disparities. There is a considerable play of power in the ability to define who and what is risky and what should matter (DeVries 1996; Stapleton 1997). For the midwife, the power of the institutions and the power of obstetrics are real and challenging (Freeman et al 2004). There exists a hierarchy of authoritative knowledge within maternity care in which the technical expertise of medicine is dominant (Jordan 1997). The risk discourse as it is currently constructed, principally by medicine, can be viewed and used as a tool of control and surveillance of both midwives and mothers. Power can be hidden within this risk discourse but may also be open to challenge. The midwife needs to know, however, that confronting this medical power is in itself a risky strategy and must be approached with caution (Fahy 2002).

The midwife is not only a subject of power in terms of obstetrics but can act as an agent of power. The discourse of equality central to the notion of partnership can obscure the power relations inherent in the midwife–mother relationship (Freeman et al 2004; Leap 2000; Skinner 1999; Smythe 2000). The research by Freeman and colleagues looked at how power is expressed within this relationship and investigated where expertise, experience, knowledge and legal requirements fit into a partnership model of care. Their research found that in 85% of instances where decision-making involved high-risk situations, it was the midwife who primarily made the care decisions. As a result of this finding they developed a model of decision-making in which, as risk increased, so too did the dominance of the decision-making by the midwife. The midwife, then, needs to understand the power relations that exist and work to claim her own power in the context both of providing safe care and of protecting and enhancing the power of the women. She needs to be mindful of the rhetoric of equality within what is called 'collaborative relationships' with doctors and within 'partnership relationships' with women. (See also Pairman 2005, pp 66–68, for a critique of Freeman et al 2004.)

In order to manage risk and safety, then, the midwife must learn to 'work the system'. She should keep connected and keep involved, actively participating in building collaborative relationships and in the planning of guidelines and policy. Safe practice is connected practice. Midwives need to build solid and collaborative relationships and to be involved in policy making and in research. They need to be active members of their professional organisation and develop a system for their own practice that is safe and sustainable. They need to both claim and share their power, and challenge power systems that are unjust. When midwives work in isolation they put themselves and the women for whom they care at risk.

Working with complexity

Complexity is such an integral part of midwifery care that it deserves a leg of the birth stool of its own. In being alongside women, things are often complex and unclear. The midwives in my study, in reflecting on how they managed risk, frequently talked about working in the 'grey areas', not only in the physical processes of birthing but also in the relationships that they developed with women, with medicine and with the system. There was a good deal of unknowing and uncertainty. The more experienced midwives described how these grey areas of practice became even bigger the more experienced they became. Yet as they became more experienced they also became more comfortable. Uncertainty and complexity became less disturbing. They accepted that risk and uncertainty were normal parts of practice. They accepted the need to understand and accommodate many different perspectives reflecting the differing underlying cultural and value systems in which both they and the women lived.

Midwifery practice is not simple. Developing relationships with women is not simple, being a professional is not simple, maintaining collaborative relationships is not simple, and managing risk is not simple. As Heyman (1998, p 9) states:

> Difficult decisions about risks entail weighing-up and trading-off qualitatively different values, for example autonomy versus safety, or quality of life against longevity. Such trade-offs of finely balanced but incompatible ends require value judgements which individuals and social groups make differently, and which cannot be meaningfully aggregated or anticipated. The persons most directly concerned in a health decision may have difficulty in deciding or even predicting what they would do. Health professionals who wish to help clients to manage risk need to grasp the complexities involved in such reasoning.

Dealing with risk, then, is complex and challenging work, done in the context of the primacy of 'being with the woman' and alongside astute, professional care. If it is so complex, how might the midwife go about it? Understanding some of the theory about how complex systems work might be of assistance. Complexity theory tells us that tension and paradox are natural phenomena. Problems are often not resolvable through simple cause-and-effect processes. Instead they occur in ways that are non-linear. Unpredictability is inherent in complex systems, although patterns emerge through inherent self-organisation. There always remain things that are unknowable (Plsek & Greenhalgh 2001). Paradox and uncertainty, however, are not necessarily negative. They can be used as sources of change and improvement. Complexity theory rejects the machine model of the human body and of health systems, where the whole is broken down into smaller and smaller parts for treatment or intervention. Action, then, requires a holistic approach, accepting unpredictability yet building on the emergent forces and processes that become evident. It requires careful observation and the application of astute, involved, creative and intuitive care.

The birth stool provides a framework for dealing with risk and safety, complex concepts embedded within and between complex systems. It provides a holistic approach and challenges the midwife to attend to each aspect of her practice in ways that acknowledge this. It is clear that there is no one truth about what is risky and what is safe, that truth is viewed through multiple lenses. It is the task of the midwife to understand these multiple lenses. To some extent, she can be seen as a 'paradigm broker', mediating between different ways of knowing and understanding (Skinner 1999).

Story-telling

The last part of the birth stool is the struts. Struts connect the legs with each other and with the seat, and help to hold the stool together firmly. I have called the struts of this midwife's birth stool 'story-telling'. Midwives are great story-tellers. We tell stories to share and connect with each other. The stories can be both healing and sense-making. Stories express and create the norms of practice. We tell stories in our documentation and in our formal practice review. We tell stories to the women we care for and sometimes we have to tell the story to the disciplinary bodies and to our professional organisation. Story-telling is probably the most valuable tool in the teaching and development of midwifery, as it is in story-telling that the messy and real complexity of practice is revealed and understood. Sharing stories keeps us connected with each other, helps us to understand the complexities of practice and provides a way of understanding what is expected. Stories can both challenge us and affirm us. Story-telling keeps us mindful and reflective. It brings to our attention that which we may have let go, and offers us other possibilities for action. It helps to keep our practice connected and safe.

Reflective exercise

Take some time to reflect on your own perspective on risk and safety. What is the level of tolerance for risk in your own life? How do you think this affects the way you practise, especially the way you communicate risk and safety to the woman? What are your tactics when risk becomes evident? How do you balance the evidence of risk with the woman's values? What does your birth stool look like? How would you like it to look?

Using the birth stool: putting theory into practice

Although I have described the parts of the stool separately, they are not separate at all. You will find that the themes are interconnected and are found embedded in the whole stool. In this way the stool embraces the complex and messy world of practice. The realities of real-world midwifery mean that we seldom if ever have a perfect stool. However, the good thing about a three-legged stool is that it remains stable even if it is a bit 'out of kilter'. The legs do not have to be exactly the same shape and size to be secure and sturdy. For example, where the relationship with the woman is challenging and difficult, strong, well-connected legs will support it. Where the new practitioner is still developing her skills and expertise, her relationship with the woman and the connections and involvement she develops with the system will ensure that she is supported. Where deficiencies in the system challenge the ability of the midwife in her work, an astute midwife who understands the power dynamics and the variety of apparent worldviews, and who is skilled and accountable in the context of a strong relationship with the women, can still provide safe care.

The birth stool is easily transportable and sturdy. The midwife can take it with her wherever she practises. She does, however, have to sit on the whole stool and be attentive to all its parts. If any of the parts give way, it will not provide support. It is also sometimes important to get off it to give it a polish or even just to give your legs a bit of a stretch (doing some more study or just having a holiday). It is also useful to have others looking on to warn of cracks appearing or to ensure that it is placed in the right position (professional standards or practice review). If any of the legs get too out of kilter or the glue comes unstuck, the midwife will fall off her seat—being with women will not be an option. Some of the midwives in my research were about to give up practice. For one, being with the women had become intolerable, as she found the demands too overwhelming and was unable to work the system to meet her own needs. For another, the pressure of the medico-legal environment had spoiled practice and she wished to be free of it. She no longer had trust in either her

Reflective exercise

Use each part of the birth stool to reflect on the following stories.

▸ Suzy is 34 and is expecting her first baby, conceived by IVF. She works as a program manager for a computer company and her husband is a lawyer. On her first visit with you she asks you whether she could have a home birth and how safe it would be. How would you approach this question?

▸ Karen is expecting her second baby and is now a week past her due date. She had a long labour with her first baby and had an epidural and a forceps delivery. Although this pregnancy is normal she has become increasingly anxious about the birth, and when you visit her she states that she wants an induction and another epidural, as she has heard that babies sometimes die when they are overdue. How do you manage these concerns and how do you negotiate and support Karen's final decision?

▸ Marg is expecting her fourth baby. She has had three normal births before and is relaxed and confident about this birth, although the baby is currently a breech presentation. She was shocked to be told by the obstetrician that she should have a caesarean section and is determined to have a vaginal birth with no intervention. She says she will just have you and not the doctors. How do you manage this?

▸ Beth is in labour with her first baby. She is now at the birthing unit and has been actively pushing for two hours. Although progress has been slow, Beth is coping well and the baby's heart rate has been stable. You can just see the baby's head appearing but the fetal heart rate is beginning to drop during contractions. What do you do and what do you say to Beth and her family?

medical colleagues or the women for whom she cared. She herself felt unsafe. The demands of being a professional had become overwhelming and isolating. Another was a very new midwife who had found that 'working the system' as a new practitioner was just too difficult and too scary. She lacked the support of others around her. Yet for most of the midwives there was a great deal of satisfaction, sustained by the quality of the relationships they had with the women giving birth. They were confident and safe practitioners, challenged but not overwhelmed by the complexity of their work.

Being a safe practitioner is about connectedness. It is about sitting on the birth stool: being connected with up-to-date knowledge and skills, being connected to the complex systems and processes that guide practice, being connected to co-workers, and above all, being connected with the women.

Review questions

1 How are the concepts of risk and safety related?

2 How has the techno-rational or scientific approach to birth affected the way risk is perceived?

3 How can one consider normality when risk is identified?

4 How does the 'risk' society affect the provision of maternity care?

5 What role do cultural values play in risk decisions?

6 How does the quality of the relationship that the midwife has with the woman support safe practice?

7 What else in the midwife's practice supports safe care?

8 What role does accountability play?

9 How does the midwife ensure her own safety?

10 Why is it important to have good collaborative relationships with other health providers?

11 What place do clinical guidelines play in decision making?

12 How can the 'birth stool' model of midwifery support the midwife in dealing with risk and safety?

Online resources

Australian College of Midwives 2004 National Midwifery Guidelines for Consultation and Referral, http://www.acmi.org.au/test/corporate_documents/ref_guidelines.pdf

New Zealand Ministry of Health 2002, Notice pursuant to Section 88 of the New Zealand Public Health and Disability Act 2000, http://www.moh.govt.nz/moh.nsf/7004be0c19a98f8a4c25692e007bf833/b5feb26417807a2fcc256b9f00814666/$FILE/Final%20Section%2088%20Maternity%20Notice%20April%202002.pdf. Contains New Zealand referral guidelines.

New Zealand College of Midwives Standards for Practice, http//www.midwife.org.nz/index.cfm/Standards

References

Alexander S, Keirse M (Eds) 1989 Effective care in pregnancy and childbirth. Buckingham, Open University Press

Annandale E 1996 Working on the front-line: risk culture and nursing in the new NHS. The Sociological Review 44(3): 416–436

Aslam R 1999 Risk management in midwifery practice. British Journal of Midwifery 7(1):41–44.

Australian College of Midwives 2004 National midwifery guidelines for consultation and referral. Online: http://www.acmi.org.au/test/corporate_documents/ref_guidelines.pdf

Beck U 1999 World risk society. Polity Press, Malden

Cartwright E, Thomas J 2001 Constructing risk. Maternity care, law and malpractice. In: R DeVries, C Benoit, ER Teijlingen (Eds) Birth by design. Pregnancy, maternity care, and midwifery in North America and Europe. Routledge, New York

Cooper IG 2000 Clinical risk management. In: D Fraser (Ed) Professional studies for midwifery practice. Churchill Livingstone, Edinburgh

Cunningham W 2004 New Zealand doctors' attitudes towards the complaints and disciplinary process. New Zealand Medical Journal 117(1198). Online: www.nzma.org.nz/journal/117-1198/973

Davis-Floyd R 2002 The technocratic, humanistic and holistic paradigms of childbirth. International Confederation of Midwives Conference, Vienna

DeVries R 1996 The midwife's place: an international comparison of the status of midwives. In: SF Murray (Ed) Midwives and safer motherhood. Mosby, London

Douglas M 1992 Risk and blame: essays in cultural theory. Routledge, London

Douglas M, Wildavsky A 1982 Risk and culture: an essay on the selection of technical and environmental dangers. University of California Press, Berkeley

Edwards NP 2000 Women planning homebirths: their own views on their relationships with midwives. In: M Kirkham (Ed) The midwife–mother relationship. Macmillan, London

Enkin M, Keirse M, Neilson J et al 2000 A guide to effective care in pregnancy and childbirth. Oxford University Press, Oxford

Fahy K 2002 Reflecting on practice to theorise empowerment for women: using Foucault's concepts. Australian Journal of Midwifery 15(1):5–13

Freeman LM, Timperley H, Adair V et al 2004 Partnership in midwifery care in New Zealand. Midwifery 20:2–14

Guilliland K, Pairman S 1995 The midwifery partnership: a model for practice. Wellington, Victoria University of Wellington. Monograph Series: 95/1, Department of Nursing and Midwifery

Guise J-M 2004 Vaginal birth after caesarean section. British Medical Journal 329(7462):359–360

Hacking I 1990 The taming of chance. Cambridge University Press, Cambridge

Heyman B (Ed) 1998 Risk, health and healthcare. Arnold, London

Jordan B 1997 Authoritative knowledge and its construction. In: RE Davis-Floyd, CF Sargent (Eds) Childbirth and authoritative knowledge. Cross-cultural perspectives. University of California Press, Berkeley

Keaney MA 1996 Is there a medical litigation crisis? Individual viewpoints on the perceived medical litigation crisis. Is litigation increasing? Medical Journal of Australia 164:178–179

Leap N 2000 The less we do, the more we give. In: M Kirkham (Ed) The midwife–mother relationship. Macmillan, London

Lupton D (1999) Risk. Routledge, London

Menticoglou SM, Hall PH 2002 Routine induction of labour at 41 weeks gestation: nonsensus consensus. British Journal of Obstetrics and Gynaecology 109(5):485–491

Ministry of Health 2002 Maternity services. Notice pursuant to Section 88 of the New Zealand Public Health and Disability Act 2000. Ministry of Health, Wellington

Murphy-Lawless J 1998 Reading birth and death: a history of obstetric thinking. Indiana University Press, Bloomington Ill.

New Zealand College of Midwives Inc (NZCOM) 2005 Midwives handbook for practice. New Zealand College of Midwives

Pairman S 2000 Women-centred midwifery: partnerships or professional friendships? In: M Kirkham (Ed) The midwife–mother relationship. Macmillan, London

Pairman S 2005 Workforce to profession: an exploration of New Zealand midwifery's professionalising strategies from 1986 to 2005. Unpublished Doctoral thesis. University of Technology, Sydney

Plsek PE, Greenhalgh T 2001 The challenge of complexity in healthcare. British Medical Journal 323(7313):625

Rohde JE 1995 Removing risk from safe motherhood. International Journal of Gynecology and Obstetrics 50(2):S3–S10

Rooney C 1992 Antenatal care and maternal health: how effective is it? A review of the evidence. World Health Organization, Geneva

Ruston A 2004 Risk, anxiety and defensive action: general practitioner's referral decisions for women presenting with breast problems. Health, Risk and Society 6(1):25–38

Schon DA 1983 The reflective practitioner. Basic Books, New York

Skinner J 1999 Midwifery partnership: individualism, contractualism or feminist praxis? New Zealand College of Midwives Journal (21):14–17

Skinner J 2003 The midwife in the 'risk' society. New Zealand College of Midwives Journal 28(1):4–7

Skinner J 2005 Risk and the midwife: a descriptive and interpretive study of the referral for obstetric consultation practices and attitudes of New Zealand midwives. Unpublished PhD thesis. Graduate School of Nursing and Midwifery, Victoria University of Wellington, Wellington

Smythe E 1998 'Being safe' in childbirth: a hermeneutic interpretation of the narratives of women and practitioners. Unpublished PhD thesis. School of Health Sciences, Massey University, New Zealand

Smythe L 2000 Being safe in childbirth; what does it mean? New Zealand College of Midwives Journal (22):18–21

Stapleton H 1997 Choice in the face of uncertainty. In: MJ Kirkham, ER Perkins (Eds) Reflections on midwifery. Baillière Tindall, London

Stewart M, Brown JB, Weston W et al 2003 Patient-centred medicine. Transforming the clinical method. Radcliffe Medical Press, Oxon

Symon A 1998 Litigation; the views of midwives and obstetricians. Hochland & Hochland, Cheshire

Symon A, Wilson J 2002 The way forward: clinical competence, co-operation and communication. In: J Wilson, A Symon (Eds) Clinical risk management in midwifery. The right to a perfect baby. Books for Midwives, Oxford

Thacker SB, Stroup D, Chang et al 2004 Continuous electronic heart rate monitoring for fetal assessment during labor. Cochrane Library (3). John Wiley & Sons, Oxford

Tulloch J, Lupton D 2003 Risk and everyday life. Sage, London

Wagner M 1994 Pursuing the birth machine. ACE Graphics, Sydney

Wilkins R 2000 Poor relations; the paucity of the professional paradigm. In: M Kirkham (Ed) The midwife–mother relationship. Macmillan, London

Wilson J (2002) Principles of clinical governance. In: JH Wilson, A Symon (Eds) Clinical risk management in midwifery. The right to a perfect baby. Books for Midwives, Oxford

CHAPTER 5

Ways of looking at evidence and measurement

Sally K Tracy

Key terms

case control study, cohort study, contextual scan, critical appraisal, cross-sectional study, epidemiology, ethics committee, ethnography, evidence-based midwifery, grounded theory, historical method, intervention study, levels of evidence, measurement, narrative, phenomenology, randomised controlled trial, research methodology, systematic review

Chapter overview

Measurement is crucial to the way we practise. It provides us with the basics for learning about and improving our understanding of what we do. It helps us to assess the safety and effectiveness of our practice. The purpose of this chapter is to provide an introduction to the use of measurement and seeking truth in midwifery practice and decision-making. Much of our current practice rests on both the evidence of epidemiological research and the findings of qualitative studies. You will be introduced to some of the most common epidemiological methods of research as well as some of the methods used to understand the quality and meaning of the practice of midwifery and the quality and meaning of childbirth for women. These examples of the way we measure our experiences appear, on the surface, to contradict each other. On the one hand, quantitative research such as epidemiology provides the story of populations or groups of people in the language of averages and statistically derived measures. Qualitative research, on the other hand, provides us with the story of the individual who is inextricably connected to the influences of their own context, and is only one individual in the population sample of the epidemiologist. In midwifery, both quantitative and qualitative exploration enriches our understanding of what we do. This chapter provides a summary of and an introduction to the many ways of measuring experience. It is intended to be used as an introductory tool for understanding the basics of evidence-based practice. In measuring anything, it is always important to be aware that simply through quantifying something we are in danger of disregarding, devaluing or even denying the very thing we are trying to measure.

Learning outcomes

Learning outcomes for this chapter are:

1 To explore the dimensions of evidence and measurement in midwifery

2 To introduce some of the common terms used in research, in both qualitative and quantitative methods

3 To outline the use of epidemiology in gathering evidence

4 To identify some of the pitfalls in the evidence-based movement.

Introduction

Some ways of knowing have traditionally occupied spaces at the edge of the dominant vision, the same kinds of spaces as are filled by the lives and experiences of the socially marginalised, including women. Thus, neither methods nor methodology can be understood except in the context of gendered social relations. Understanding this involves a mapping of how gender, women, nature and knowledge have been constructed both inside and outside all forms of science (Oakley 2000, p 4).

Inquiry is based on the recognition of certain connections. It is important always to be mindful that separating the knower from what is known implies a separation of one's self from another person and also implies the separation of the researcher from the subject of research (Reason 1988). The connection between understanding in the scientific and biological domain, and the experience we bring from our family, our practice, our social and political contexts, together with our use of language, is the reason we can expect to have different and multiple understandings of the world. We make sense of facts and select and organise all our observations based on the influences of previous learning and practice. Drawing stories from our reservoir of experiences and social contexts connects us through language and metaphor to understand the science behind midwifery. Understanding biological systems depends on a multiplicity of understandings, explanations and connections (Fox Keller 2002).

Seeking truth

Although there are several methods of seeking truth that may conflict or coexist with each other at various times, it is generally accepted that, in midwifery as well as medicine, some ways of arriving at the truth are more acceptable than others. The following examples will help provide you with an understanding of how many of the interventions and actions in practice have been arrived at. After reaching the end of this chapter, I hope you will return to this section and be able to discern whether or not the following methods are entirely acceptable.

Let's look at the safety of believing in something or having faith in an authoritative expert opinion. For example, many women and midwives believe that having an epidural during labour is both safe and effective. They believe that if the departments of anaesthesia and obstetrics so wholly endorse the procedure, then it is unlikely that having an epidural will have any adverse side-effects. Similarly, having a continuous CTG monitor running and recording the baby's heartbeat for the whole of labour will surely be seen as the safest way to detect anything going wrong as soon as it happens. Both these procedures were introduced as routine interventions without prior scientific validation, and are still supported by the fact that because so many women like them and they are so comforting, there seems little reason to question their routine use and safety.

Then there is the *feeling* that something is right. For years, midwives have done certain rituals because they had a gut feeling it was the right thing to do. How does this come about? For many it is the wisdom gained through the experience of looking after many women in childbirth. It may be something as simple as recommending a salt bath for the relief of the perineum, or wanting to give a baby extra fluid to complement the mother's milk supply when it seems that neither can settle happily. These are interventions that for some just feel like the right thing to suggest, even though the midwife may have no knowledge of the benefits or safety of such measures.

Very close to the feeling that something is right is the knowing through personal experience that this is the way to do something. We have seen something or heard it so often that our personal experience of the event leads us to believe it must be true. In both midwifery and obstetrics, much of what is practised is based on personal experience and learning from past mistakes. Personal experience is often characterised as being anecdotal, ungeneralisable, and a poor basis for making scientific decisions. However, it is often a more powerful persuader than scientific publications in changing clinical practice. In fact, midwives constantly use their personal judgement to affirm what they believe to be true in certain situations—the non-scientific 'rule of thumb'. This is also one of the most contentious areas in which to change attitudes and practice because it challenges one of the most strongly held methods for seeking truth—the knowledge gained through the personal experience of doing things a certain way.

Legal methods of arriving at the truth need little explanation. Here something is deemed to be true because it can be substantiated through authoritative testimony. The expert witness is seen as an authority and an expert in the subject under examination. Up until the past 15 years we were familiar with the use of the word evidence in relation to legal method. However, with the widely accepted move in medicine to evidence-based medicine, the word 'evidence' has taken a much more prominent position in the scheme of things. Box 5.1 walks you through an ethical argument in addressing the question: 'Is evidence the same as research?'

One of the most widely accepted methods of searching for truth in midwifery is through scientific method or research. Searching for truth using scientific research methods involves the systematic study of phenomena and the relations between and among phenomena using agreed rules or accepted methodologies. The systematic collection, analysis and interpretation of data minimises the contamination of results from external factors (known as bias) (Kirkevold 1997).

There are several schools of thought on how scientific method should proceed. On the one hand, it is believed that the theory and hypothesis should be developed before the research is undertaken. This is known as deductive method. It follows the thinking of Karl Popper (1972) that scientific knowledge is gained through the development of ideas and the attempt to refute them with empirical research. The dominant philosophy underlying quantitative scientific method is positivism. Positivism assumes that phenomena are measurable using the deductive principles of the scientific method. That is, the investigator starts with a theory and a hypothesis that is tested by the data (deduction).

BOX 5.1 Is evidence research?

Is evidence the same as research?

▶ In order for something (e.g. data) to be construed as 'evidence' it must be judged to be relevant and have a strong conclusion. This requires subjective interpretation, from the viewpoints of several individuals.

▶ Evidence itself does not constitute truth; rather, evidence plays a role in determining what is believed to be true. For example, in legal terms the evidence used to support various theories of what actually happened at the time of a crime is compared until one of the theories begins to hold more weight than the others, and, on the basis of the available evidence, is considered the most likely to be true.

▶ Consider how the selection of evidence to support conclusions is negotiated and debated. It is affected by social and other forces such as power, coercion and self-interest of one negotiator, or group of negotiators, vis-à-vis another. These forces then may have an impact on which conclusions or theories are ultimately selected as most likely to be true.

▶ Now consider the common practice of applying research data from studies conducted exclusively on male research participants, to female patients. The idea that data from men can be applied directly to women reflects a reductionist view of human physiology and a previously held social bias that took women's health to be an offshoot of men's health.

▶ Hence, *evidence* is a status conferred upon a fact, reflecting, at least in part, a subjective and social judgement that the fact increases the likelihood of a given conclusion being true. For any given set of phenomena, there may be many available facts that could count as evidence for more than one conclusion or theory. However, only some facts will be deemed as evidence for one successful conclusion or theory, which itself is chosen from among several options.

▶ Thus, evidence is not, as EBM implies, simply research data or facts but a series of interpretations that serve a variety of social and philosophical agendas.

(Based on an argument proposed by Gupta M 2003.)

---

experimental designs, the observations are recorded without having first manipulated the variables. In contrast to this, in experimental method there is a systematic manipulation of and control of variables. Evidence-based healthcare, or the practice of basing clinical decisions on the best available scientific evidence, is predominantly derived from experimental method. All research, whether inductive or deductive, follows the broad pattern of the research cycle.

Regardless of the method of research, this basic formula sets out the cycle of events that occur in a research process (Fig 5.1).

Qualitative research methods

Qualitative research contributes to the understanding of social aspects of health issues, through direct observation of the nuances of social behaviour (Green & Britten 1998; Pope & Mayes 2000). Qualitative research can investigate practitioners' and patients' attitudes, beliefs and preferences, and the whole question of how evidence is turned into practice. The value of qualitative methods lies in their ability to pursue systematically the kinds of research questions that are not easily answerable by experimental methods. Rigorously conducted qualitative research is based on explicit sampling strategies, systematic analysis of data, and a commitment to examining counter-explanations. Ideally, methods should be transparent, allowing the reader to assess the validity and the extent to which the results might be applicable to their own clinical practice. Qualitative research does not usually produce numerical rates and measures (Green & Britten 1998). Researchers who use qualitative methods seek a deeper truth (Greenhalgh & Taylor 1997). They aim to make sense of, or interpret, phenomena using a holistic perspective that preserves the complexities of human behaviour (Black 1994). The research often provides

The other school of thought is that research should precede theory and not be limited to a passive role of verifying and testing theory; rather, it should help to shape the development of theory (Bowling 2002) by the process of induction.

Both these strategies are used to develop the knowledge of midwifery.

Whichever method we use to try and find answers to a certain problem or situation, there are certain things that help us measure how successful the research is in answering our question. Research is measured in terms of its rigour of scientific inquiry by concepts known as reliability (the repeatability of the research) and validity (the extent to which the instruments measure what they set out to measure).

Seeking truth through empirical research involves both experimental and non-experimental research. In non-

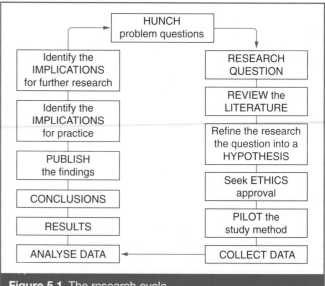

Figure 5.1 The research cycle

us with a picture of 'behind the scenes', how people are feeling, or what other forces are at work that may not be discovered in a quantitative investigation of facts.

An example of the 'behind the scenes' behaviour that affected the introduction of evidence-based leaflets into maternity hospitals in the United Kingdom was recorded by Stapleton et al (2002) when they undertook a qualitative study beside a randomised controlled trial (RCT) by O'Cathain et al (2002). In the experimental study, the researchers concluded that in everyday practice, evidence-based leaflets were not effective in promoting informed choice for women using maternity services (O'Cathain et al 2002). The qualitative study (Stapleton et al 2002) mounted alongside this RCT provided a rich insight into what was happening with the information leaflets, and found that the way in which the leaflets were disseminated affected promotion of informed choice in maternity care. The qualitative study provided the evidence for 'behind the scenes' and the bullying and coercive behaviours that had become a normal way of doing things in these maternity units. The culture into which the leaflets were introduced supported existing normative patterns of care and this ensured informed compliance rather than informed choice (Stapleton et al 2002).

Overview of qualitative methods

As a midwife you will be intimately involved in finding the answers to many questions through research evidence. However, the scope of this textbook permits only a very brief overview of some of the terms and methods you will encounter. The following summary of some of the qualitative research methods used in scientific research will give you a very brief introduction to the terminology and concepts used in qualitative research.

Phenomenology

Phenomenology is a method of constructing the meaning of (a phenomenon from) someone's experience—for example, the 'lived experience'.
- Data are gathered though interviews.
- The sample is taken from those who have experienced the phenomenon.
- The analysis follows a path of information from the research question; that is, the participant's significant phrases illustrate the researcher's interpretation.

Ethnography

Ethnography is used by the researcher to construct the meaning of culture; that is, the researcher tries to understand the insider's 'emic' view of the world. The researcher enters an unknown world and tries to make sense of it from the insider's point of view.
- Data are gathered through participant observation and interviews, and the researcher interprets the cultural patterns observed.
- The sample is taken from a cultural group living in the phenomenon. These are known as the key informants

and the general informants. The key informants are those with special knowledge who are prepared to teach the researcher.
- The analysis is undertaken on field notes and observations, and meaning is sought from cultural symbols in the informants' language.

Narrative

Narrative is a linguistic form. The narrative provides information that does not pertain simply or directly to the unfolding events. The same sequence of events told by another person to another audience might be presented differently without being any less 'true'. First, it has a finite and longitudinal time sequence—that is, it has a beginning, a series of unfolding events, and (we anticipate) an ending. Secondly, it presupposes both a narrator and a listener, whose different viewpoints affect how the story is told. Thirdly, the narrative is concerned with individuals—rather than simply reporting what they do or what is done to them, it concerns how those individuals feel and how people feel about them.

Narratives help to set a person-centred agenda and challenge received wisdom, and they may generate new hypotheses. Narratives offer a method for addressing existential qualities such as inner hurt, despair, hope, grief and moral pain, which frequently accompany, and may even constitute, people's illnesses (Greenhalgh & Hurwitz 1999).
- Data-gathering involves collecting the story the respondent has to tell.
- The sample is a convenience sample.
- The analysis of the narrative is an interpretive act; that is, interpretation (the discernment of meaning) is central to the analysis of narratives. Actual transcripts are presented in the results of narrative research.

Historical research

Historical research is mainly narrative rather than numerical. Much conventional scholarship continues to focus on the search for a single, knowable, verifiable past.
- The data consist of a systematic compilation of data regarding people, events and occurrences in the past.
- The sample tries to identify all data sources.
- The analysis involves the validity of external criticism; reliability delineates data sources by internal criticism. The reader 'hears' the narrator's 'voice' and 'sees' the actions in the story with the eyes of an 'internal' or 'external' focaliser, who may or may not be identical to the narrator (Norku 2004).

Grounded theory

Grounded theory aims to find underlying social forces that shape human behaviour. The theory emerges or is generated from the data in a manner that means most hypotheses and concepts not only come from the data, but are systematically worked out in relation to the data during the course of research (Strauss & Corbin 1998).
- Data consist of interviews and skilled observations of individuals interacting in a social setting.

- The sample is purposive—the researcher deliberately samples a particular group or setting of people who are experiencing the circumstance.
- During analysis, the researcher's task is to sift and decode the data to make sense of the situation, events and interactions observed. Often this analytical process starts during the data-collection phase. Variants of content analysis involve an iterative process of developing categories from the transcripts or field notes, testing them against hypotheses, and refining them (Mays & Pope 1995; Strauss & Corbin 1998).

Other methods

Other qualitative research methods include:

- *documents*—study of documentary accounts of events, such as meetings
- *passive observation*—systematic watching of behaviour and talk in naturally occurring settings
- *participant observation*—observation in which the researcher also occupies a role or part in the setting, in addition to observing
- *in-depth interviews*—face-to-face conversation for the purpose of exploring issues or topics in detail. Does not use preset questions, but is shaped by a defined set of topics.
- *focus groups*—method of group interview that explicitly includes and uses the group interaction to generate data (Greenhalgh & Taylor 1997).

Questions to ask

Mays and Pope (1995) suggest the following questions to ask of qualitative studies:

- Has the study contributed to our knowledge?
- Was the research question clear?
- Would a different method have been more appropriate? Was the design appropriate for the question?
- Is the context adequately described?
- Was the sampling strategy clearly described and justified?
- How was the fieldwork undertaken? Was it described in detail? Could the evidence (fieldwork notes, interview transcripts, recordings, documentary analysis, etc) be inspected independently by others; if relevant, could the process of transcription be independently inspected?
- Were the procedures for data analysis clearly described and theoretically justified? Did they relate to the original research questions? How were themes and concepts identified from the data? Was the analysis repeated by more than one researcher to ensure reliability?
- Was there an audit trail, so that another researcher could repeat each stage of the research?
- Was enough of the original evidence presented systematically in the written account to satisfy the sceptical reader of the relation between the interpretation and the evidence? (For example, were quotations numbered and sources given?)

Critical thinking exercise

Search the literature for a study that uses each of the above methodologies, and compare the written studies to see what questions are asked and how these are answered. Could the same question be answered by each of the different methodologies?

BOX 5.2 How to search

How to search for a paper on Medline or the Cochrane library:

1 To look for an article you know exists, search by text words (in title, abstract, or both) or use filed suffixes for author, title, institution, journal and publication year.
2 For a maximally sensitive search on a subject, search under both MESH headings (exploded) and text words (title and abstract), then combine the two by using the Boolean operator 'or'.
3 For a focused (specific) search on a clear-cut topic, perform two or more sensitive searches as in step 2, and combine them by using the Boolean operator 'and'.
4 To find articles that are likely to be of high methodological quality, insert an evidence-based quality filter for therapeutic interventions, aetiology, diagnostic procedures or epidemiology, and/or use maximally sensitive search strategies for randomised trials, systematic reviews, and meta-analyses.
5 Refine your search as you go—for example, to exclude irrelevant material, use the Boolean operator 'not'.
6 Use subheadings only when this is the only practicable way of limiting your search, as manual indexers are fallible and misclassifications are common.
7 When limiting a large set, browse through the last 50 or so abstracts yourself rather than expecting the software to pick the best half dozen.

(Source: Greenhalgh 1996)

Evidence-based practice

The aim of evidence-based practice, to quote from Professor David Sackett, is 'the conscientious, explicit and judicious use of current best evidence in making decisions about the care of individual patients ... the integration of individual clinical expertise with the best available external clinical evidence from systematic research' (Sackett & Cooke 1996, p 535). In other words, it is the combination of clinical judgement and clinical practical experience with information we gather to help us learn.

The following five steps in putting evidence into practice are based on the work of Sackett et al (1996):

BOX 5.3   Definitions

Some common terms used in research:

▶ *case studies*—focus on one or a limited number of settings; used to explore contemporary phenomena, especially where complex interrelated issues are involved. Can be exploratory, explanatory or descriptive, or a combination of these.

▶ *consensus methods*—include Delphi and nominal group techniques and consensus development conferences. They provide a way of synthesising information and dealing with conflicting evidence, with the aim of determining the extent of agreement within a selected group.

▶ *constant comparison*—iterative method of content analysis where each category is searched for in the entire data set and all instances are compared until no new categories can be identified.

▶ *content analysis*—systematic examination of text (field notes) by identifying and grouping themes and coding, classifying, and developing categories.

▶ *epistemology*—theory of knowledge; scientific study which deals with the nature and validity of knowledge.

▶ *field notes*—collective term for records of observation, talk, interview transcripts, or documentary sources. Typically includes a field diary which provides a record of the chronological events and development of research as well as the researcher's own reactions to, feelings about, and opinions of the research process.

▶ *Hawthorne effect*—impact of the researcher on the research subjects or setting, notably in changing their behaviour.

▶ *naturalistic research*—non-experimental research in naturally occurring settings.

▶ *purposive or systematic sampling*—deliberate choice of respondents, subjects or settings, as opposed to statistical sampling, concerned with the representativeness of a sample in relation to a total population. Theoretical sampling links this to previously developed hypotheses or theories.

▶ *reliability*—extent to which a measurement yields the same answer each time it is used.

▶ *social anthropology*—social scientific study of peoples, cultures, and societies; particularly associated with the study of traditional cultures.

▶ *triangulation*—use of three or more different research methods in combination; principally used as a check of validity.

▶ *validity*—extent to which a measurement truly reflects the phenomenon under scrutiny.

(Source: Pope & Mayes 1995)

BOX 5.4   Page's five steps

1 Find out what is important to the woman and her family.
2 Use information from the clinical examination.
3 Seek and assess evidence to inform decisions.
4 Talk it through.
5 Reflect on outcomes, feelings and consequences (Page 2002).

In *The New Midwifery*, Professor Lesley Page describes evidence in terms of 'a process of involving women in making decisions about their care and of finding and weighing up information to help make those decisions' (Page 2002, p 9). The five steps to evidence-based midwifery (Box 5.4) were adapted by Professor Page from the original work in this area undertaken by Sackett and colleagues in 1996 (Sackett et al 1996).

In step 3, seeking and assessing evidence, the original authors added that it is important to decide how *valid* something is. In other words, how close to the truth is it? It is also important to find out how *useful* it is—that is, how applicable to practice is the evidence? One thing to remember is that evidence-based midwifery should never be a 'cookbook' approach to what we do. The evidence that we bring to practice from the literature or from research should only ever inform our practice, not replace it; and it should always be taken along with a woman's individual preference for a clinical decision (Page 2002; Sackett & Cooke 1996). One of the ways of checking whether a research paper addresses the area of inquiry you are interested in is to see whether the question the research seeks to answer applies to the area of interest. To do this, we divide the question into its components to make sure it is relevant. For example:

● Does it involve a population of interest, or does the population closely resemble the one you want to understand?
● Is the intervention or treatment relevant for your area of interest?
● Is the comparison group appropriate?
● Is the outcome one that you are interested in?

This is known as the PICO method (see Box 5.5).

The appendix at the end of this chapter lists questions to ask in evaluating a clinical guideline.

Evidence-based everything

Evidence-based obstetric care is a relatively new concept, which had its origins in the early 1970s . . . this was a shift away from

---

1 Fit what you want to know into a question that can be answered.
2 Go looking for the best research to answer it.
3 Critically estimate the research for how close it is to the truth and whether it could be clinically useful.
4 Try to use the suggestions in practice.
5 Reflect on, or evaluate, what happens.

BOX 5.5   The PICO method

PICO is a way of breaking a question into its components.

P	Population or patients
I	Intervention or indication
C	Comparison group or Control
O	Outcome

opinion-based obstetrics, which up until then had been the dominant paradigm (King 2005).

The 'evidence-based' (EB) prefix moved with discreet political correctness over the years and attached itself not only to medicine, but more inclusively to EB practice, EB decision-making and EB healthcare. As the originators of the evidence-based movements concede, 'it engenders enthusiasm, anger, ridicule and indifference amongst people' (Sackett & Cooke 1996). Some have even suggested that evidence-based medicine (EBM) demonstrates the 'scientific chauvinism of the English' (Halliday 2000).

There are many claims for and against EBM. It is important for students of midwifery to spend some time reflecting on its pros and cons. Evidence-based care features very strongly in our search for evidence and measurement in practice (Chalmers 1989).

Those who question the authority of EBM believe that only studies with positive results get published, or that the *art* of patient care is threatened. Some critics say that systematic reviews may be 'pooling ignorance as much as distilling wisdom'(Naylor 1995), that 'medical muddling' is a profitable business and that the proliferation of new tests, devices and drugs continues at an unprecedented pace (Naylor 1995). Others concede that life would be very much simpler if new technologies could be appraised in rigorous studies with clinically relevant endpoints and data to guide practice (Chalmers 1989). Imagine if the question of the safety of hospital over home birth had been tested with relevant, well-designed studies of safety and satisfaction before women were expected to move from home to hospital for birth.

Many midwives claim that EBM has been used to increase the subordination and powerlessness of those practising in the hospital system—in the form of extravagant claims for the basis of interventions. Or, as Mary Stewart found in her research into 'Whose evidence counts?', the 'definitions of evidence vary widely among health practitioners . . . and are affected by the individual's own beliefs and give rise to a hierarchy in which some types of evidence are valued above others' (Stewart 2000). Many midwives would agree with the statement that 'The power of authoritative knowledge is not that it is correct but that it counts' (Jordan 1993, p 58).

BOX 5.6 EBM

One opinion on the EBM movement is that:

Evidence-based medicine (EBM) became the buzzword of the 1990s. Proponents of the method often recommend it with the zealousness of those who have received religious enlightenment (Traynor 2000).

Some followers of EBM have even stated that:

medicine has continued on a very dark and ill-informed path over the centuries, in fact, when the teachings of Galen superseded Hippocrates' first aphorism, 'life is short', sixteen centuries of dogma followed, and scientific rigour was not applied to medicine again until the appearance of Archie Cochrane and his contemporaries in the 1950's! (Halliday 2000).

Epidemiological method

The foundation and primary focus of evidence-based care is within the specialty of medical epidemiology, 'to ensure the practice of effective medicine, in which the benefits to an individual patient or population outweigh any associated harm to that same patient or population' (Muir Gray 1997, p 3). The underlying belief is that meaning can be discerned from population patterns and that a relation exists between mathematics and material reality. The epidemiologist's focus of study is the whole population, in which outcomes are described in averages and percentages, rates and risks. Then the science of chance is applied in the form of a statistical framework that gives the reader an indication of the measurement error or the uncertainty with which the result is believed to be true. This is better known as the 'confidence interval' (Jolley 1993). Epidemiology seeks to provide answers though the analysis of accumulated results of hundreds or thousands of comparable cases in population samples. The language of mathematics is used to describe the findings in terms of 'probability' and 'risk'. Such answers, arrived at through studying population samples in randomised trials and cohort studies, cannot be mechanistically applied to the individual. 'In large research trials the individual participant's unique and multidimensional experience is expressed as (say) a single dot on a scatter plot to which we apply mathematical tools to produce a story about the sample as a whole' (Greenhalgh 1999, p 324).

In other words, the answers that we gain from doing research at a population level tell us about the general population in averages and frequency measures. They do not tell us the story of the individuals who took part. In asking 'What works?', we are suggesting that research will show us how to do things the best way. The danger here is that we may unwittingly focus on very narrow 'evaluative' studies—that is, studies that demonstrate the effectiveness of an intervention, such as the randomised controlled trial (RCT), when in fact information from a whole range of types of studies, answering a variety of questions, may be more useful. (See the story of the information leaflets earlier.) In reality we practise within a complex and mostly unpredictable reality in which learning from trial and error may be an important way to make progress.

At the turn of the twentieth century, epidemiological research began to explicitly incorporate social science perspectives related to health data that could inform public policy. One of the first substantial prospective epidemiological analyses to be undertaken was a study of the socio-economic and nutritional determinants of infant mortality in the United States in 1912, by Julia Lathrop (Kreiger 2000). As sociologist Ann Oakley pointed out, the history of experimentation and social interventions is 'conveniently overlooked by those who contend that randomised controlled trials have no place in evaluating social interventions. It shows clearly that prospective experimental studies with random allocation to generate one or more control groups is perfectly possible in social settings' (Oakley 1998a, p 1240). The usefulness of the population-based results of an RCT depends on the translation of the concepts and measures used to describe groups of people into a language that can inform the decisions of an individual (Steiner 1999). The RCT is currently considered to be the orthodox and 'gold standard' scientific experimental method for evaluating new treatments. The ethical basis for entering patients in RCTs, however, is under debate. Some doctors espouse the uncertainty principle whereby randomisation to treatment is acceptable when an individual doctor is genuinely unsure which treatment is best for a patient. Others believe that clinical equipoise, reflecting collective professional uncertainty over treatment, is the most sound ethical criterion (Weijer et al 2000). The scientific principles that are applied to the design and conduct of primary research, such as the RCT, are also applied to secondary research, such as the systematic review (Chalmers et al 1992). Many regard epidemiology as 'an arcane quantitative science penetrable only by mathematicians' (Grimes & Schulz 2002). However, it must be pointed out that 'statistics is at most complementary to the breadth and judgement' of the knowledge gained from epidemiological research (Jolley 1993, p 28).

Figure 5.2 outlines the kinds of studies you will encounter in the scientific literature, both medical and midwifery, that are based on epidemiological method.

In order to find where the 'best evidence' is to support our practice we are encouraged to give research studies a ranking from the highest level, or the 'gold standard', to the lowest level of research evidence. These rankings are made explicitly on the ranking of research methods from the most reliable to the least reliable. This 'evidence hierarchy' provides an initial screening test as to whether data from research studies are derived from methods that are more or less likely to guide readers towards truthful conclusions (Gupta 2003). (Further discussion on this topic, and current debates, definitions and controversies, can be found on the Centre for Evidence-based Medicine website at http://www.cebm.net/.)

Experimental trials are limited when the study size is too small to detect rare or infrequent adverse outcomes, or when the outcome of interest is long-term and the trial would need to continue for an improbable length of time. In all these cases, observational studies may be considered more practical (Black 1996). Observational studies may be most valuable where randomising people to an intervention is inappropriate (Black 1996)—for example, randomising women to having water for birth or to having an elective caesarean section is

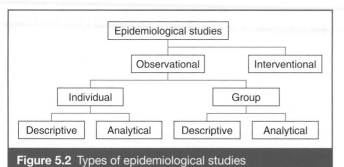

Figure 5.2 Types of epidemiological studies

BOX 5.7 Research ethics

The ethical principle governing research is that respondents should not be harmed as a result of participating in research, and they should always be asked for their informed consent to participate.

This principle is widely agreed amongst researchers. Participants should be asked to give their consent in writing after they have had written information about the aims, risks, discomforts, benefits, procedures, questionnaires and the way confidentiality and anonymity will be preserved. Hospitals and universities have ethics committees to oversee the operations of research projects from an ethical and scientific standpoint.

Before you undertake any research you must undertake to satisfy the ethics committee at the hospital or university where you work by submitting an ethics application for approval before any research begins.

---

inappropriate and also disregards the 'effect that choice itself has on therapeutic outcome' (McPherson 1994).

There is no doubt that there are limitations of empiricism as a value-neutral truth, and as the only structure for analysing our decision-making. As one physician put it, 'Evidence-based decision models may be very powerful, but are like computer generated symphonies in the style of Mozart—correct but lifeless' (Saunders 2000, p 22). From the sociologist's viewpoint, the implementation of RCTs in real-life settings causes some hazards, such as low participation and high attrition rates, problems with informed consent, unanticipated side-effects of the intervention, and possible problematic relations between research and policy. Ann Oakley, a very well-known sociologist, asks, 'What may a society obsessed with quantification have lost in terms of the value of more intimate knowledge, intuition, emotions and all the other qualities that (we) soft social scientists are renowned for going on about?' (Oakley 1998, p 1242).

Experimental method allows the investigator to have control over the population group she or he is studying, by deciding which groups will be exposed to a factor under study and which groups will become the control group. A feature of the experimental method is that the investigator can randomly allocate a subject to the experimental or the control group (Lilienfeld & Lilienfeld 1980).

- Data may consist of questionnaires, biophysical measures, structured observations and clinical trials.
- In the sample, the subjects may be randomly allocated to the experimental or the control group.
- Analysis includes inferential statistics provided in tables, which give the significance of findings in terms of a p value, or the confidence intervals.

Quasi-experimental method is similar to the above but there may be no control or randomisation. Non-experimental methods are used to gather data to describe events as they occur. These may consist of surveys, for example. The data are analysed and presented using descriptive statistics such as frequency distributions and histograms. Relationships and associations may be inferred, but not cause and effect. These methods will be covered in more detail later in this chapter.

The randomised controlled trial

Randomised controlled trials (RCTs) are often referred to as clinical trials. The difference is that each person in the trial is randomised to either receive or not receive the intervention. The clinical trial is defined as: 'any research project that prospectively assigns human subjects to intervention and comparison groups to study the cause-and-effect relationship between a medical intervention and a health outcome' (CONSORT group 2005). By 'medical intervention' we mean any intervention used to modify a health outcome. This definition includes drugs, surgical procedures, devices, behavioural treatments and process-of-care changes. A trial must have at least one prospectively assigned *concurrent* control or comparison group (International Committee of Medical Journal Editors, *JAMA* 2005; CONSORT group 2005). The rationale for conducting an RCT is to compare the outcomes of treatment given to different groups of people, while at the same time preventing the effect of systematic 'bias' on the results. The application of randomisation is the logical way to control bias in assessing the effects of certain treatments (Chalmers 1989).

> The idea is not to worry about the characteristics of the patients, but to be sure that the division of the patients into two groups is done by some method independent of human choice . . . i.e. by the use of random numbers (Cochrane 1971, p 10).

In controlling the selection bias, the aim is to be able to distinguish the effect of a certain treatment on a group of people that is separate from and not affected by the individual characteristics of that group of people. In the RCT, the logical application of controlling bias is to allocate the people who will be part of the trial by randomising them to either the treatment or the control group.

> The term random does not mean the same as haphazard but has a precise technical meaning. By random allocation we mean that each person has a known chance, usually an equal chance, of being given each treatment, but the treatment to be given cannot be predicted. If there are two treatments the simplest method of random allocation gives each patient an equal chance of getting either treatment; it is equivalent to tossing a coin. In practice most people use either a table of random numbers or a random number generator on a computer. This is simple randomisation. Possible modifications include block randomisation, to ensure closely similar numbers of patients in each group, and stratified randomisation, to keep the groups balanced for certain prognostic patient characteristics (Altman & Bland 1999, p 1209).

There are points to consider here in midwifery, however. When data are derived exclusively from randomised trials or meta-analysis, the results give us a clear idea of the efficacy of the intervention for an 'average' randomised patient. We

Definition

CONSORT
Have you seen this word when reading about randomised controlled trials? It stands for: Consolidated Standards of Reporting Trials.

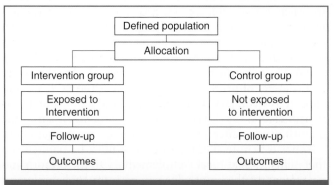

Figure 5.3 Allocation of a treatment group and a control group in an intervention study (including the randomised controlled trial)

BOX 5.8 The 'average' patient

One immediate problem in using the results of RCTs is that the conclusions refer to an 'average patient' who fulfilled the criteria for admission. When transferred to clinical medicine from an origin in agricultural research, randomised trials were not intended to answer questions about the treatment of individual patients. The trials have almost always been used to offer an average value for efficacy in groups of patients receiving the compared therapies.

(Source: Feinstein & Horwitz 1997, p 534)

will not be able to deduce, from the data we receive, any information on 'psychosocial factors and support, personal preferences of patients, and strategies for giving comfort and reassurance' (Feinstein & Horwitz 1997).

Randomised controls offer 'the protection of the public from potentially damaging uncontrolled experimentation and a more rational knowledge about the benefits to be derived from professional interventions' (Oakley 1998a, p 1242).

The systematic review

A systematic review is a concise summary of the best available evidence that addresses a sharply defined clinical question (Sackett et al 2000). In a world where more and more research findings are being published, there is a dizzying array of information for the practitioner to wade through in deciding what is best. Systematic reviews of the effects of healthcare attempt to bring together the relevant evidence on a particular intervention or treatment, so that people choosing between different interventions are more informed and can make better decisions. Regardless of whether a review is broad or narrow, the reviewer tries to identify as many of the eligible studies as possible, so that these can be included as fully as possible in the review. If appropriate, the reviewer might conduct a meta-analysis, in which the results of different trials are combined to provide a more precise estimate of the average difference between the effects of the interventions being compared. In all systematic reviews, the evidence being brought together for a particular intervention needs to be as free from bias and as reliable as possible. This is why most reviews of the effects of interventions rely exclusively on randomised trials. The process of bringing together the evidence also needs to minimise bias, and be rigorous and robust. The ultimate aim of any systematic review of randomised trials should be to ensure that relevant data on all randomised participants from all relevant trials are included (Clarke 2005).

The value of systematic reviews depends greatly on the availability and quality of the results of primary research. 'Knowledge development must be cumulative in the sense that related knowledge generated from separate research studies is integrated into a more comprehensive understanding of the topic at hand' (Kirkevold 1997, p 977).

One of the key parts of any review is to consider how similar or different the available primary studies are and what impact any differences have on the studies' results. Between-study differences or heterogeneity in results can result from chance, from errors in calculating accuracy indices, or from true heterogeneity—that is, differences in design, conduct, participants, tests and reference tests.

The steps required to undertake a systematic review are as follows:

1 The problems to be addressed are specified in the form of well-structured questions.
2 Literature searches are conducted to identify potentially relevant studies that shed light on the questions.
3 The quality of the selected studies is assessed.
4 The evidence concerning study characteristics and results is summarised, and differences between studies are explored and, when feasible and appropriate, meta-analysis helps in collating results.
5 Inferences and recommendations for practice are generated from interpretation and exploration of clinical relevance of the findings (Khan 2005).

A systematic review of the literature allows for estimations of the effects of healthcare interventions by identifying the individual, clinical and contextual factors that influence the effectiveness of that care. Overall conclusions are drawn from many studies that are believed to address the same or similar research hypotheses. An overview provides a broader look at the subject in question, as it is based on a number of studies in different settings and includes a variety of participants. Overviews are also useful in identifying the uncertainties and gaps in the research. The specific purpose of meta-analysis is to: increase statistical power for primary endpoints and for subgroups; resolve uncertainty where reports disagree; improve on estimates of effect size; and answer questions not

---

BOX 5.9 Reading a Cochrane table

▸ See Fig 5.4 for an example of a Cochrane table.
▸ The 'forest plot' is the diamond at the bottom. It depicts the pooled odds ratios.
▸ The horizontal line corresponds with each trial included and shows the difference between groups—best single—and the width of the line demonstrates the 95% confidence interval of this estimate.
▸ The black line down the middle of the picture is known as the 'line of no effect'.
▸ If the confidence interval (the horizontal line) crosses the line of no effect (the vertical line), this means either that there is no significant difference between the interventions or that the sample size was too small for us to be confident of where the true result lies.
▸ The various individual studies give point estimates of the relative risks, and the confidence intervals are so wide on some studies that they go off the page. This is depicted as an arrow.
▸ The tiny diamond below all the horizontal lines represents the pooled data from the trials, with a new, much narrower confidence interval.
▸ If the diamond overlaps the line of no effect, we can say there is probably little difference between the two interventions in terms of the primary endpoint (defined at the top of the graph).
▸ Heterogeneity can involve some serious statistics. However, the question to ask is whether there is greater variation between the results of the trials than would be conceivable through chance.

You need to think how you would interpret these results in practice.

---

posed at the start of individual trials (Sacks et al 1987). The systematic review differs from meta-analysis in that it does not necessarily statistically combine the results of studies that are critically reviewed.

Specific characteristics of a systematic review include:

● formal criteria on which studies are eligible for inclusion—this is done in order to avoid selection bias regarding inclusion or exclusion of studies
● expression of the statistical uncertainties inherent in each study by appropriate use of the confidence interval
● recognition that studies have adopted different design strategies
● in the interpretation of results, taking into account the limitation of some studies in inferring causality (Pocock et al 1994).

The systematic review is an important tool, for a number of reasons. Progress in midwifery care is achieved through research that refines, extends or refutes prior theoretical concepts to build onto that system of scientific knowledge. Knowledge that is cumulative can then be integrated into one systematic review to achieve a more comprehensive understanding (Chalmers et al 1992; Kirkevold 1997). Research must be accessible to clinicians if research-based practice is to become a reality. The value of systematic review has been demonstrated by the success of such commercial systematic review providers as the Cochrane Database.

Meta-analysis

The *Cochrane Handbook for Systematic Reviews of Interventions* lists the following reasons for considering a meta-analysis:

1 To increase power. Power is the chance of detecting a real, statistically significant effect, if it exists. Many individual studies are too small to detect small effects, but when several are combined there is a higher chance of detecting an effect.
2 To improve precision. The estimation of a treatment effect can be improved when it is based on more information.
3 To answer questions not posed by the individual studies. Primary studies often involve a specific type of patient and explicitly defined interventions. A selection of studies in which these characteristics differ can allow investigation of the consistency of effect and, if relevant, allow reasons for differences in effect estimates to be investigated.
4 To settle controversies arising from apparently conflicting studies or to generate new hypotheses. Statistical analysis of findings allows the degree of conflict to be formally assessed, and reasons for different results to be explored and quantified.

Warning: Of course, the use of statistical methods does not guarantee that the results of a review are valid, any more than it does for a primary study. Moreover, like any tool, statistical methods can be misused ... Meta-analyses of poor-quality studies may be seriously misleading. If bias is present in each (or some) of the individual studies, meta-analysis will simply compound the errors, and produce a 'wrong' result that may be interpreted as having more credibility (Deeks et al 2005, p 78).

The methods used for meta-analysis generally follow these basic principles:

(1) Meta-analysis is typically a two-stage process. In the first stage, a summary statistic is calculated for each study. For controlled trials, these values describe the treatment effects observed in each individual trial. For example, the summary statistic may be a risk ratio if the data are dichotomous or a difference between means if the data are continuous.
(2) In the second stage, a summary (pooled) treatment effect estimate is calculated as a weighted average of the treatment effects estimated in the individual studies (Cochrane Handbook 2005, p 158).

You will no doubt be familiar with the Cochrane Library graphs illustrating the probability of an outcome between two groups who have been treated differently (the treatment group and the control group). When deciding what this shows—that is, the treatment effects—the questions to ask are:
1 What is the direction of effect?
2 What is the size of effect?
3 Is the effect consistent across studies?
4 What is the strength of evidence for the effect?
See if you can work out the answers to these questions when looking at Figure 5.4.

Figure 5.4 demonstrates the outcome in terms of having to manually remove the placenta between a group of women (treatment group) who were given IM Syntometrine as the oxytocic of choice and comparing this outcome with the group of women (control group) who had been randomly allocated *not* to receive this treatment. Remember: the line that passes down the middle of the graph is called the 'line of no effect'. (This will be explained more fully later in the chapter.) To go back to our four questions:
1 *Answer*: The effect is very minimally on the positive side (the right hand side) of 1. This tells us that the treatment had a mildly positive effect—that is, having an active management of the third stage of labour was associated with having to have a manual removal of the placenta.

Review: Active versus expectant management in the third stage of labour
Comparison: Active vs expectant management (all women)
Outcome: Manual removal of placenta

Study	Treatment n/N	Control n/N	Relative Risk (Fixed) 95% CI	Weight %	Relative Risk (Fixed) 95% CI
Abu Dhabi 1997	3/827	9/821		19.9	0.33 [0.09, 1.22]
Brighton 1993	1/103	0/90		1.2	2.63 [0.11, 63.64]
Bristol 1988	16/846	22/849		48.4	0.73 [0.39, 1.38]
Dublin 1990	19/705	1/724		2.2	19.51 [2.62, 145.36]
Hinchingbrooke 1998	15/748	13/764		28.3	1.18 [0.56, 2.46]
Total	3229	3248		100.0	1.21 [0.82, 1.78]

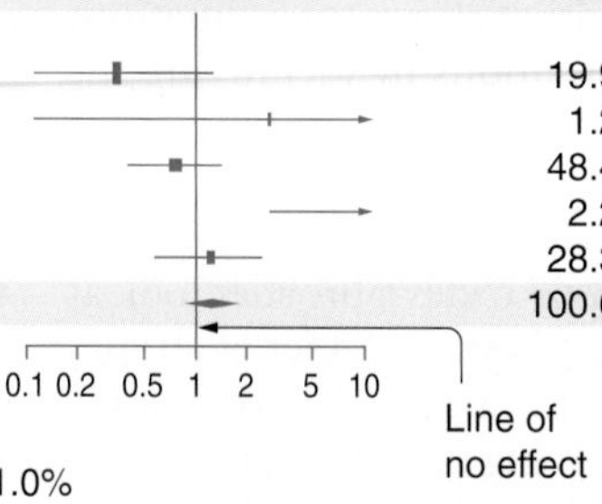

0.1 0.2 0.5 1 2   5 10

Line of no effect

Total events: 54 (Treatment), 45 (Control)
Test for heterogeneity chi-square = 13.80 df = 4 p = 0.008 I^2 = 71.0%
Test for overall effect z = 0.95 p = 0.3

Figure 5.4 Example of a systematic review and meta-analysis (based on Prendiville et al 2000)

This is called the *direction* of the effect.

2 *Answer*: The size of the effect is very small as well, because we can see that the confidence intervals of four of the studies and the pooled result all cross the line of no effect.

3 *Answer*: No, the effect is not consistent across all studies.

4 *Answer*: The confidence interval crosses 1, or the line of no effect, and therefore the strength of the evidence is not strong. The outcome may have occurred due to *chance*.

The hierarchy of evidence

According to the Oxford Centre for Evidence-based Medicine (2005):

a systematic review documenting homogeneity in the results of a large number of high-quality RCTs (randomised with concealment, double-blinded, complete follow-up, intention-to-treat analysis) provides the least-biased estimate of the effect of an intervention. This becomes Level 1 evidence, and recommendations based on it are designated Grade A. Then, because we can document progressively increasing distortions of Level 1 results as we move to systematic reviews with heterogeneity, then to individual high-quality RCTs, then to less rigorous RCTs, then to cohort studies, then to case-control studies, then to case-series, and then to expert opinion, we formed a hierarchy of levels based on this progression (CEBM Oxford 2005).

The levels of evidence in the hierarchy are listed in Table 5.1.

To recap, the results of RCTs are considered to be evidence of the highest grade, whereas observational studies are viewed as having less validity because they reportedly overestimate treatment effects (Concato et al 2000).

[Studies are] classified according to grades of evidence on the basis of the research design, using internal validity (that is, the correctness of the results) as the criterion for hierarchical ranking. The highest grade is reserved for research involving properly randomised controlled trials, and the lowest grade is applied to descriptive studies (such as case series) and expert opinion. Observational studies, both cohort studies and case-control studies, fall at intermediate levels. Although the quality of studies is sometimes evaluated within each grade, each category is considered methodologically superior to those below it. This hierarchical approach to study design has been promoted widely in individual reports, meta-analyses, consensus statements, and educational materials for clinicians (Concato et al 2000, p 1887).

Critical thinking exercise

What are the differences between the following?
▸ bad science based on poor evidence
▸ inadequate science based on insufficient evidence
▸ no science based purely on dogma.
(Source: Sharpe 2000, p 29.)

TABLE 5.1 The hierarchy of evidence

Level	Treatment/prevention
1a	Systematic review (with homogeneity) of randomised controlled trials (RCTs)
1b	Individual RCT (with narrow confidence interval)
1c	All or none of the above
2a	Systematic review (with homogeneity) of cohort studies
2b	Individual cohort study (including low quality RCT, e.g. < 80% follow-up)
2c	'Outcomes' research; ecological studies
3a	Systematic review (with homogeneity) of case-control studies
3b	Individual case-control study
4	Case-series (and poor-quality cohort and case-control studies)
5	Expert opinion without explicit critical appraisal, or based on physiology, bench research or 'first principles'

(Source: Phillips et al 2005)

Reflective exercise

What do you think of the hierarchical system for ranking evidence?

Culpepper and Gilbert (1999) point out that because the evidence hierarchy privileges certain types of data and certain types of research methodologies, phenomena not easily amenable to investigation by these privileged methods may be neglected or presumed less worthy of inquiry than those interventions best suited to the preferred methods.

Intervention studies

The RCT is an example of an intervention study. In such a study, we do not just observe exposures and outcomes in a population. We actively allocate an exposure (or intervention) to one of the study groups. The group that does not receive the intervention acts as a control group. We then follow the groups over a period of time. We compare the frequency of the outcome in the experimental group—those receiving the intervention—with the frequency of the outcome in the group not allocated the intervention. See, for example, the RCTs into continuity of midwifery care (Flint & Poulengeris 1989; Homer et al 2001; Rowley et al 1995).

The story of Semmelweis is well known. In 1848 he published his findings that the rate of fatal postpartum sepsis was 12% for obstetricians attending women in childbirth after having performed an autopsy and not washing their hands, compared to 3% for those attended by midwives who did not perform autopsies. The medical fraternity totally and unequivocally rejected his probability-based evidence. He was denounced and driven from his job, his country, and perhaps his mind, dying in a mental institution at the age of 47 (Goodman 1999).

Before accountability was determined by 'best evidence', the collective medical tradition in these years was to leave the job of clinical evaluation to the individual. The American Medical Association (AMA) code of ethics (1847) contended that character was as important a qualification as knowledge:

> . . . character must be the foundation upon which ethical action is to be built. Proper conduct among men and affairs must be left to the man, his tact, his judgement, his education and his experience.

The AMA at the turn of the century further counselled discretion and silence with regard to the practice of colleagues. No ethical alarm bells rang, then, when Charles Meigs, chairman of midwifery at Jefferson Medical College in Philadelphia, in 1859 (eleven years following the disclosure by Semmelweis) stated:

> I have practiced midwifery for many long years; I have attended some thousands of women in labour . . . passed through repeated epidemics of childbed fever, both in town and in hospital . . . After all this experience however, I do not, upon careful reflection and self-examination, find the least reason to suppose I have ever conveyed the disease from place to place in any single instance . . . a gentleman's hands are clean (Sharpe 2000, p 30).

Cohort studies

In a cohort study, we:

1 Select a study population or cohort of people who do not initially have the outcome of interest.

2 Classify the members of the cohort according to whether they have been *exposed* to the potential risk factor or not.

3 Follow the entire cohort over time and compare the incidence of the *outcome(s)* in the exposed individuals with the incidence in those not exposed.

Cohort studies are particularly useful for rare exposures and in situations where we are interested in studying more than one outcome. However, they are generally slow and expensive to carry out. They are also inefficient in investigating rare outcomes—that is why we do case control studies where we select all cases with a rare outcome and match them for variables of interest.

Case control studies

In a case control study, we:

1 Identify individual cases of the *outcome* of interest.

2 Identify a representative group of individuals who do not have the outcome. These individuals act as controls.

3 Compare cases and controls to assess whether there were any differences in their past exposure to one or more possible risk factors.

Cross-sectional studies

In a cross-sectional study, we measure the frequency of a particular exposure(s) and/or outcome(s) in a defined population *at a particular time*. Cross-sectional studies can be either descriptive or analytical.

- In a descriptive cross-sectional study, we simply describe the frequency of the exposure(s) or outcome(s) in a defined population.
- In an analytical cross-sectional study:

  1 We simultaneously collect information on both the *outcome* of interest and the *exposure* to the potential risk factor(s).

  2 We then *compare* the frequency of the outcome in the people exposed to each risk factor with the frequency in those not exposed.

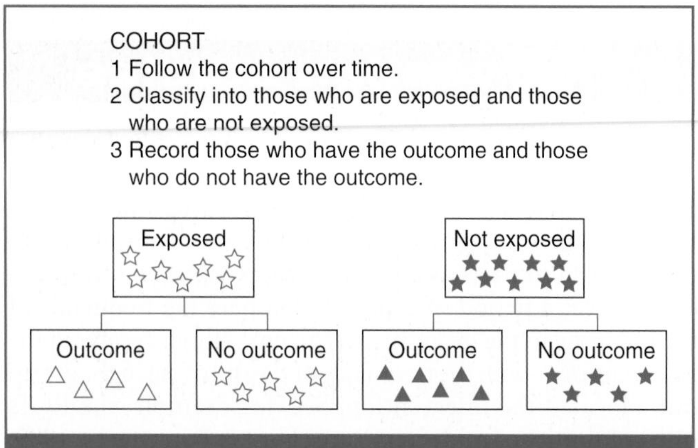

COHORT
1 Follow the cohort over time.
2 Classify into those who are exposed and those who are not exposed.
3 Record those who have the outcome and those who do not have the outcome.

Exposed   Not exposed

Outcome   No outcome   Outcome   No outcome

Figure 5.5 Cohort studies

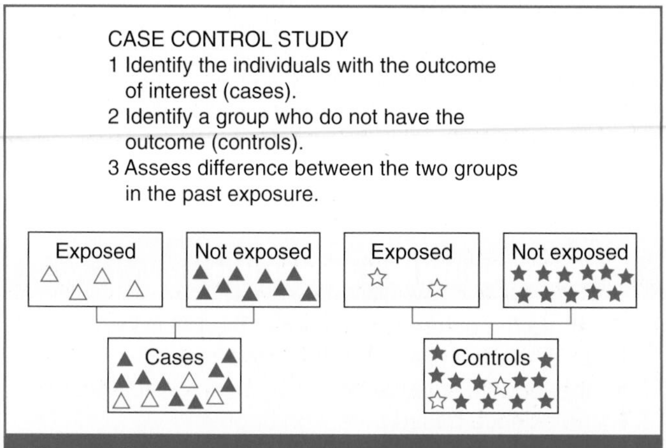

CASE CONTROL STUDY
1 Identify the individuals with the outcome of interest (cases).
2 Identify a group who do not have the outcome (controls).
3 Assess difference between the two groups in the past exposure.

Exposed   Not exposed   Exposed   Not exposed

Cases   Controls

Figure 5.6 Case control studies

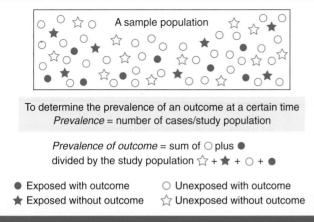

To determine the prevalence of an outcome at a certain time
Prevalence = number of cases/study population

Prevalence of outcome = sum of ○ plus ●
divided by the study population ☆ + ★ + ○ + ●

● Exposed with outcome   ○ Unexposed with outcome
★ Exposed without outcome   ☆ Unexposed without outcome

Figure 5.7 Analytical cross-sectional study design

The *prevalence* is the proportion of persons in a defined population that have the outcome under study at a specific point in time. Prevalence = the number of cases divided by the total number of people in the study population at a given time. The *incidence* of an outcome refers to the number of new cases with the outcome in a population in a defined time period.

Ecological studies

Ecological studies compare the exposure status and outcome status of *groups* rather than individuals. An ecological study thus looks for an association between an exposure and an outcome at the group level. In other words, we look to see whether the outcome is more frequent in groups where the exposure is more frequent. For each group, the exposures and outcomes are measured for the group as a whole. So, it is not possible to link the exposure of any particular individual to his or her outcome.

Bias in research studies

Bias refers to any errors in the design or conduct of a study that result in a conclusion that is different from the truth. It is particularly important that potential sources of bias are identified at the stage of study design, because you cannot usually adjust or make allowance for bias at the analysis stage. To put it very simply, if you study the wrong people, or get the wrong data from them, no amount of analysis will put it right. So, bias can ruin a study irretrievably.

The subject of bias is hotly debated in the evidence-based movement. Technical bias, publication bias and source-of-funding bias are all potential sources of systematic bias that affect the total pool of evidence and skew it in favour of experimental and commercially profitable interventions (Song et al 2000).

● *Technical bias* favours research that we know how to do, and therefore is towards phenomena that we know how

to investigate. Technical bias creates a systematic bias that influences what kinds of data are created.

● *Publication bias* refers to the differential publication by medical journals of positive and/or statistically significant results (Song et al 2000). The purpose of this practice is to make the medical literature more interesting by publishing studies where new interventions are shown to be effective. However, through publication bias, clinicians may be exposed to a group of studies that misleadingly suggests the superiority of new interventions. Furthermore, publication bias, like technical bias, can ultimately lead to the neglect of certain types of phenomena. Because getting published counts significantly in researchers' career advancement (Miettinen 1998), the researchers may choose to study a restricted group of topics that are most likely to yield publishable results, that is, topics that do not fall in the 'grey zones' of clinical practice (practices whose usefulness is uncertain or for which older research data have been equivocal) (Naylor 1995). Together, these scientific and social constructionist arguments undermine the assumption in EBM that EBM-preferred data are a representative body of data most likely to lead to truthful conclusions about the medical interventions they represent (Gupta 2003).

● *Source-of-funding bias*:

Another area for ethical concern is the effect that EBM has on the authority and power of doctors vis-à-vis other groups. EBM prioritizes certain types of clinical research and thus increases the pressure for this research to be *conducted and funded*. This results in several particular outcomes. Research funding decisions are made in the context of competing priorities so that decisions to fund clinical research are also decisions not to fund other things. As the majority of evidence-based research is conducted by physicians, EBM becomes a way of entrenching medical

---

BOX 5.11   Types of bias

Definitions of *interpretation biases*:

▶ *confirmation bias*—evaluating evidence that supports one's preconceptions differently from evidence that challenges these convictions

▶ *rescue bias*—discounting data by finding selective faults in the experiment

▶ *auxiliary hypothesis bias*—introducing ad hoc modifications to imply that an unanticipated finding would have been otherwise had the experimental conditions been different

▶ *mechanism bias*—being less sceptical when underlying science furnishes credibility for the data

▶ *'time will tell' bias*—when different scientists need different amounts of confirmatory evidence

▶ *orientation bias*—the possibility that the hypothesis itself introduces prejudices and errors and becomes a determinant of experimental outcomes.

(Source: Kaptchuk 2003)

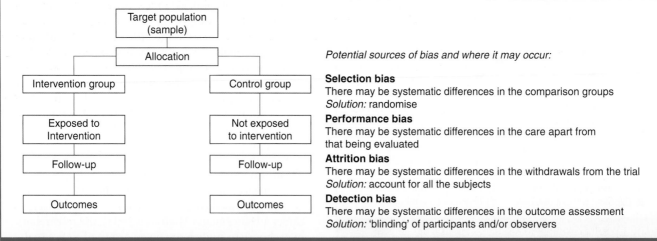

Figure 5.8 Potential sources of bias (based on sources of bias in trials of healthcare interventions in the Cochrane Handbook 2005, p 58)

authority in determining to what degree research will be funded, what questions will be researched, by whom, and thus, which results will be given priority in clinical decision-making. This occurs at the expense of those who might wish to contribute to setting the research agenda and to determining what research should be funded (Gupta 2003, p 118).

Confidence intervals

The confidence interval does as the name suggests—it allows us to feel confident (or not!) that we can apply the results we have found in our sample to the whole population. Another way of saying this is that we can *infer* the results from research to the population at large if certain situations exist (such as when we are dealing with a 'normal distribution' and are able to take a 'random sample' from the same population we are studying). Let's say we calculate from a sample of 100 healthy pregnant women that the mean weight gain (the average number of kilograms) they will gain during pregnancy will be 12 kilograms. Let's say this will be a close approximation to the average weight gained. If we were then to repeat this experiment 100 times over, with randomly selected women from the same population, we would be able to say with more certainty that the result we got (say it is 12 kilograms) is the average weight we would expect healthy pregnant women to gain in pregnancy. Of course you can see that this is a large undertaking—this is where the confidence interval comes in. Using fairly complicated statistics, we can calculate the 95% confidence interval for the average weight gain in healthy women in pregnancy. Then we can say (without having to physically repeat the experiment 100 times) that if we repeated the experiment 100 times we could be sure that 95% of the time, the mean weight gain would be somewhere around 12 kilograms. The two numbers on either side of the confidence interval tell us where the true value lies in the population. Going back to our example, we might record our finding in the following way:

Average weight gained in pregnancy = 12.0 kg (95% CI 10.5–14.2) (Our sample was randomly selected from a population of healthy pregnant women in Sydney in 2005.)

This tells us that in our study the average was 12 kg, and we can infer that 95 out of 100 times, the true value in the population will be somewhere between 10.5 and 14.2 kg. (The statistics have saved us from having to do the study 100 times and record all the weights!) Another way of saying this is that once we construct a confidence interval, we have a range of values that we can be confident includes the true value of the mean. You will meet confidence intervals when you read any quality research papers. This is an introductory guide to help you understand the very basics about confidence intervals. I have recommended further reading at the end of this chapter.

Odds ratios

One of the ways in which we can understand how an exposure or an intervention is associated with the outcome we are interested in observing, is to calculate the odds ratio. The odds ratio could be loosely described as the probability of an event happening in two groups. If the odds of an event are greater than one, then the event is said to be more likely to occur. Conversely, if the odds ratio is less than one, then the event is less likely to occur. This is a very simplistic description of a very complex statistical measure.

You are most likely to come across odds ratios in reading the Cochrane graphs in systematic reviews, so I will illustrate how to read the odds ratio using a Cochrane graph.

The graph in Fig 5.9 illustrates the odds of continuity of care during pregnancy and childbirth on the likelihood of not feeling well prepared for child care. As you can see, the odds ratio is 0.57, which is less than 1, and therefore we can deduce that continuity of care is less likely to be associated with *not* feeling well prepared for child care.

Another example of the odds (in this case the risk ratio) being less than 1 is shown in Fig 5.10. (A slightly confusing issue arises here, where the authors have used the measure 'relative risk' rather than an odds ratio. For our purposes at this stage of critical analysis they are interchangeable. At an advanced level of statistics, the meanings are slightly different.

Let's turn to Figure 5.11. Can you say in your own words what Figure 5.11 is telling us?

Now for an example of the odds being greater than 1. Figure 5.12 tells us that when comparing active versus expectant management of the third stage of labour when women in the treatment group were given IM Syntometrine as the oxytocic of choice, and comparing this outcome with the group of women (control group) who had been randomly allocated *not* to receive this treatment, there is a greater likelihood of vomiting between delivery of the baby and discharge from the labour ward. The pooled risk ratio is 2.19 with a 95%

Review: Continuity of caregivers for care during pregnancy and childbirth
Comparison: Continuity of caregivers during pregnancy and childbirth
Outcome: Not feeling well-prepared for child care

Study	Treatment n/N	Control n/N	Peto Odds Ratio 95% CI	Weight %	Peto Odds Ratio 95% CI
Flint 1989	399/503	434/498		100.0	0.57 [0.41, 0.80]
Total (95% CI)	399/503	434/498		100.0	0.57 [0.41, 0.80]

0.1 0.2   1   5 10

Test for heterogeneity chi-square = 0.00 df = 0
Test for overall effect = −3.31 p = 0.0009

Figure 5.9 Odds ratio for association between continuity of care during pregnancy and not feeling well prepared for child care (based on Hodnett 2004)

Review: Active versus expectant management in the third stage of labour
Comparison: Active vs expectant management (all women)
Outcome: Maternal dissatisfaction with third stage management

Study	Treatment n/N	Control n/N	Relative Risk (Fixed) 95% CI	Weight %	Relative Risk (Fixed) 95% CI
Hinchingbrooke 1998	27/748	46/718		100.0	0.56 [0.35,0.90]
Total	748	718		100.0	0.56 [0.35,0.90]

0.1 0.2 0.5 1   2   5 10

Total events: 27 (Treatment), 46 (Control)
Test for heterogeneity: not applicable
Test for overall effect. Z = 242 p = 0.02

Figure 5.10 Relative risk for association between active versus expectant management and maternal dissatisfaction (based on Prendiville et al 2000)

Review: Continuity of caregivers for care during pregnancy and childbirth
Comparison: Continuity of caregivers during pregnancy and childbirth
Outcome: Not feeling well prepared for labour

Study	Treatment n/N	Control n/N	Peto Odds Ratio 95% CI	Weight %	Peto Odds Ratio 95% CI
Flint 1989	359/503	396/498		100.0	0.64 [0.48, 0.86]
Total (95% CI)	359/503	396/498		100.0	0.64 [0.48, 0.86]

0.1 0.2   1   5 10

Test for heterogeneity chi-square = 0.00 df = 0
Test for overall effect = −2.99 p = 0.003

Figure 5.11 Odds ratio for association between continuity of care during pregnancy and not feeling well prepared for labour (based on Hodnett 2004)

Review: Active versus expectant management in the third stage of labour
Comparison: Active vs expectant management (all women)
Outcome: Vomiting between delivery of baby and discharge from labour ward

Study	Treatment n/N	Control n/N	Relative Risk (Fixed) 95% CI	Weight %	Relative Risk (Fixed) 95% CI
Bristol 1988	102/846	55/849		74.8	1.86 [1.36, 2.55]
Dublin 1990	10/86	2/114		2.3	6.63 [1.49, 29.47]
Hinchingbrooke 1998	47/748	17/764		22.9	2.82 [1.64, 4.87]
Total	1680	1727		100.0	2.19 [1.68, 2.86]

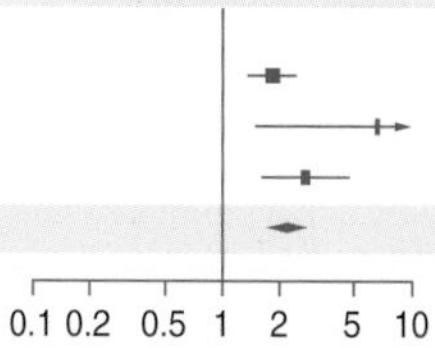

0.1 0.2 0.5 1 2 5 10

Total events: 159 (Treatment), 74 (Control)
Test for heterogeneity chi-square = 3.99 df = 2 p = 0.14 I^2 = 49.8%
Test for overall effect z = 5.80 p < 0.00001

Figure 5.12 Odds ratio for association between active or expectant management, and vomiting (based on Prendiville et al 2000)

BOX 5.12 Optimality

The concept of 'optimality' offers an alternative approach to evaluating the outcomes of clinical care. Optimality looks for the desired best possible outcome, rather than the occurrence of undesired adverse (and rare) events. In essence, it replaces the focus on risk and adverse outcomes with a focus on measuring the frequency of 'optimal' (good, desired) outcomes.

Optimality is different from the concept of 'normality'. 'Normal' is frequently defined in healthcare as the absence of abnormalities or adverse events. However, definitions of what is normal must be based on decisions about what constitutes the broad range of normal. The Dutch authors (Wiegers et al 1996) who originally used the 'optimality' approach for measuring patient care stressed that the index is not a static one, but requires close evaluation of its internal validity as it applies to different practice situations. The tool must be adapted to accommodate different or changed insights into maternity care.

(Sources: Murphy & Fullerton 2001; Wiegers et al 1996)

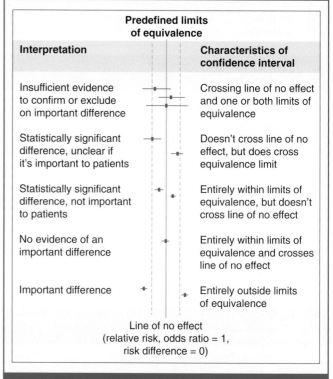

Figure 5.13 Relation between confidence interval, line of no effect, and thresholds for important differences (based on Alderson 2004)

confidence interval of 1.68–2.86. This tells us that the women who were given an oxytocic in the third stage had a greater likelihood of vomiting after birth than those who did not receive the treatment.

In summary, this has been a whistle-stop introduction to odds and risk ratios. You are advised to look at the reading list at the end of the chapter for more information.

One of the ways in which we can discern whether the results of research are going to be useful to us in clinical practice is to consider the relationship between the odds ratios, the line of no effect and another measure called the line of equivalence (which will not be explained here).

Likelihood ratios

A likelihood ratio is the percentage of ill people with a given test result divided by the percentage of well individuals with the same result. Ideally, abnormal test results should be much more typical in ill individuals than in those who are well (high likelihood ratio) and normal test results should be more frequent in well people than in sick people (low likelihood ratio). Likelihood ratios near unity have little effect on decision-making; by contrast, high or low ratios can greatly shift the clinician's estimate of the probability of disease (Grimes & Schultz 2005).

Conclusion

Turning the phrase 'evidence-based' into 'evidence-informed' was the subject of a debate in the *Midwifery Digest* (MIDIRS 2000). The author claimed that by using the word 'informed' we are more likely to be mindful of the process of midwifery knowledge that midwives understand to originate from the way women themselves understand their bodies and the process of giving birth. Lesley Page in her paper 'The backlash against evidence-based care', contends that 'evidence-based' does not necessarily mean practice based on a positivist, reductionist knowledge generated solely from within the scientific medical paradigm (Page, 1996). Others such as Mavis Kirkham claim that through research we can question the status quo, that research is also the means with which we can move from being 'expert, professional and oppressed' to an alliance with women giving birth (Kirkham 2000).

A strategic relationship between women and midwives can challenge both the economically driven imperative for research, and the legislation and control of accepted practice, and in doing so it may promote the care of previously excluded groups of women. Midwives have the opportunity to show leadership in undertaking research that is relevant to women and makes judicious use of precious research funds. To quote from Mary Stewart's research, 'the technocratic paradigm has become authoritative and highly valued, whereas a more holistic model, incorporating concepts of intuition and shared knowledge, has less credence' (Stewart 2000).

There is no doubt that evidence-based healthcare in its broadest meaning has the potential to better the lives of all women in childbirth, simply because it claims to be based in 'science' as opposed to 'authority'. It is a powerful tool with which to question the authority of obstetric practice and intervention. It is also the means with which we offer accountable and responsible care to women through informed decision-making. The RCT is currently regarded as a highly effective methodology for investigating the introduction of new technologies and treatments before they become introduced routinely. What a pity, then, that the introduction of epidurals and other highly interventionist technology was never evaluated by any rigorous, or for that matter even second-rate, scientific investigation before wholesale introduction into routine practice. In the arena of 'evidence-based everything' the RCT is an immensely valuable tool. But there is room for other methodologies and there is also room for improvement. The RCT is a relatively new and evolving method of seeking truth in maternity care that has helped to change the lives of midwives and women so far. As Chalmers noted recently, 'the greatest potential for improving research may lie in greater public involvement. Partly because of perverse incentives to pursue particular research projects researchers often seem to design trials to address questions that are of no interest to patients' (Chalmers 1989, p 1168).

BOX 5.13 Let's have SECs

As well as being vigilant in ensuring that research is ethical and meaningful to those who are researched, the use of appropriate language is something that cannot be underestimated. Ann Oakley wrote:

> Over a few commiserative drinks one evening a clinical colleague and I decided that if randomised controlled trials were renamed socially equitable comparison tests social scientists might like them better. It does not exactly run off the tongue, I know, but then neither does randomised controlled trial. Are there any takers out there? (Oakley 1998).

Count me in. Renaming the things 'socially equitable comparisons' (SECs) would locate the research language in a place much closer to the language of birth if we were to suggest having SECs rather than undertaking an RCT!

Review questions

1 What are the essential elements of a well-designed epidemiological study?

2 Name one intervention used in midwifery care that has not been researched. How would you research its effectiveness?

3 List five interventions you routinely use in your practice. Is there any published evidence to support these interventions? Is so, what level of evidence are they?

4 Using an example from practice, describe the steps you would take in applying the five steps of evidence-based practice.

5 Find an example of two areas of practice where the research underlying the practice is based on trials with a large crossover rate. How can you justify using this evidence?

6 If a study is analysed using an 'intention to treat' methodology, would you be more likely to believe the results of this trial than a population-based descriptive study? Why? What bias is likely to be evident?

7 Are randomised controlled trials meant to answer questions about the care of an individual woman? Why or why not?

8 Name some 'grey zones' of clinical practice where there is no evidence or very little evidence to support your actions.

9	What is the goal of qualitative research? Is it useful? Give an example of qualitative research that has influenced your practice.	**10**	How can qualitative methods complement quantitative ones?

Online resources

AGREE (Appraisal of Guidelines, Research and Evaluation for Europe), http://www.agreecollaboration.org

Campbell Collaboration, http://campbell.gse.upenn.edu

Canadian Health Services Research Foundation 2005 Conceptualizing and combining evidence for health system guidance, http://chsrf.ca/other_documents/pdf/evidence_e.pdf

Centre for Evidence-Based Medicine, http://www.cebm.net/levels_of_evidence.asp. (also http://cebm.jr2.ox.ac.uk/)

Centre for Reviews and Dissemination, http://www.york.ac.uk/inst/crd/wph.htm. Evidence from systematic reviews of research relevant to implementing the 'wider public health' agenda.

Cochrane Handbook for Systematic Reviews of Interventions (formerly the Reviewers' Handbook) http://www.cochrane.org/resources/handbook/index.htm. A printable version can be downloaded from www.cochrane.org/resources/handbook/.

Cochrane Library, http://www.cochrane.org

Economic and Social Research Council (ESRC), http://www.esrc.ac.uk/index.asp

Enkin M, Keirse MJNC, Neilson J et al 2000 A guide to effective care in pregnancy and childbirth, http://www.maternitywise.org/guide/ch7.html

Evidence for Policy and Practice Information and Coordinating Centre (EPPI Centre), Social Science Research Unit, Institute of Education, London EPPI Centre, http://eppi.ioe.ac.uk

National Guideline Clearinghouse, http://www.guideline.gov

Netting the Evidence, http://www.shef.ac.uk/~scharr/ir/netting/

New Zealand Guidelines Group, http://www.nzgg.org.nz

Unit for Evidence-Based Practice and Policy, http://www.ucl.ac.uk/primcare-popsci/uebpp/uebpp.htm#How

References

Alderson P 2004 Absence of evidence is not evidence of absence. British Medical Journal 328: 476–477

Altman DG, Bland JM 1999 Treatment allocation in controlled trials: why randomise? British Medical Journal 318:1209

Black N 1994 Why we need qualitative research. Journal of Epidemiology and Community Health 48:425–426

Black N 1996 Why we need observational studies to evaluate the effectiveness of healthcare. British Medical Journal 312:1215–1218

Bowling A 2002 Research methods in health: investigating health and health services. Open University Press, Buckingham, UK

Centre for Reviews and Dissemination. Evidence from systematic reviews of research relevant to implementing the 'wider public health' agenda. Online: http://www.york.ac.uk/inst/crd/wph.htm

Chalmers I 1989 Evaluating the effects of care during pregnancy and childbirth. In: I Chalmers, M Enkin, M Kierse (Eds) Effective care in pregnancy and childbirth, Oxford University Press, Oxford

Chalmers I, Dickersin K, Chalmers TC 1992 Getting to grips with Archie Cochrane's agenda. British Medical Journal 305(6857):786–788

Clarke M 2005 Individual patient data meta-analyses. Best Practice and Research in Clinical Obstetrics and Gynaecology 19(1):47–55

Cochrane AL 1971 Effectiveness and efficacy: random reflections on health services. Nuffield Provincial Hospital Trust, London

Cochrane handbook for systematic reviews of interventions (formerly the Reviewers' Handbook) 2005 Online: http://www.cochrane.org/resources/handbook/index.htm

Concato J, Nirav S, Horowitz R 2000 Randomized controlled trials, observational studies, and the hierarchy of research designs. New England Journal of Medicine 342:1887–1892

CONSORT group 2005 CONSORT statement. Checklist of items to include when reporting a randomized trial. Online: http://www.consort-statement.org/Downloads/checklist.pdf

Culpepper L, Gilbert TT 1999 Evidence and ethics. Lancet 353:829–831

Deeks JJ, Dinnes J, D'Amico R et al 2003 Evaluating non-randomised intervention studies. Health and Technology Assessessment 7(27). Online: http://www.ncchta.org/fullmono/mon727.pdf

Deeks JJ, Higgins JPT, Altman DG (Eds) 2005 Analysing and presenting results. In: JPT Higgins, S Green (Eds) Cochrane handbook for systematic reviews of interventions 4.2.5 [updated May 2005]; Section 8. In: The Cochrane Library, Issue 3, 2005. John Wiley & Sons Ltd, Chichester

Feinstein AR, Horwitz RI 1997 Problems in the 'evidence' of 'evidence-based medicine' American Journal of Medicine 103:529–535

Flint C, Poulengeris P 1989 The 'Know Your Midwife' scheme—a randomised trial of continuity of care by a team of midwives. Midwifery 5:11–16

Fox Keller E 2002 Making sense of life. Harvard University Press,

Goodman SN 1999 Probability at the bedside: the knowing of chances or the chances of knowing? Annals of Internal Medicine 130(7):604–606

Green J, Britten N 1998 Qualitative research and evidence-based medicine. British Medical Journal 316:1230–1232

Greenhalgh T 1996 How to read a paper—the basics of evidence-based medicine. Is my practice evidence-based? A context-sensitive checklist for individual clinical encounters. BMJ Publishing, London

Greenhalgh T 1999 Narrative-based medicine: narrative-based medicine in an evidence-based world British Medical Journal 318:323–325

Greenhalgh T, Hurwitz B 1999 Narrative based medicine Why study narrative? British Medical Journal 318:48–50

Greenhalgh T, Taylor R 1997 How to read a paper: papers that go beyond numbers (qualitative research). British Medical Journal 315:740–743

Grimes D, Learman LA 1996 Theory into practice: within a department. Ballières Clinical Obstetrics and Gynecology 10(4):697–714

Grimes DA, Schultz KF 2002 Descriptive studies: what they can and cannot do. Lancet 359:145–149

Grimes DA, Schultz KF 2005 Refining clinical diagnosis with likelihood ratios. Lancet 365(9469):1500–1505

Gupta M 2003 A critical appraisal of evidence-based medicine: some ethical considerations. Journal of Evaluation in Clinical Practice 9(2):111–121

Halliday 2000 Keynote address: XVII European Congress of Perinatal Medicine. Oporto, Portugal, 25–28 June 2000

Hodnett ED 2004 Continuity of caregivers for care during pregnancy and childbirth (Cochrane Review) In: The Cochrane Library (3). John Wiley & Sons, Chichester

Homer CSE, Davis GK, Brodie P et al 2001 Collaboration in maternity care: a randomised controlled trial comparing community-based continuity of care with standard hospital care. British Journal of Obstetrics and Gynaecology 108:16–22

Jolley D (1993) The glitter of the t table. The Lancet 342:27–29

Jordan B 1993 Birth in four cultures: A cross-cultural investigation of childbirth in Yucatan, Holland, Sweden and the United States (4th edn). Revised and updated by Robbie Davis-Floyd. Waveland Press, Prospect Heights, Ill.

Kaptchuk TJ 2003 Effect of interpretive bias on research evidence. British Medical Journal 326:1453–1455

Khan K 2005 Systematic reviews of diagnostic tests: a guide to methods and application. Best Practice and Research in Clinical Obstetrics and Gynaecology 19(1):37–46

King JF 2005 A short history of evidence-based obstetric care. Best Practice and Research in Clinical Obstetrics and Gynaecology 19(1):3–14

Kirkevold M 1997 Integrative nursing research—an important strategy to further the development of nursing science and nursing practice. Journal of Advanced Nursing 25:977–984

Kirkham M (Ed) 2000 The midwife–mother relationship. Macmillan, Basingstoke

Kreiger N 2000 Epidemiology and social sciences: towards a critical reengagement in the 21st century. Epidemiologic Reviews 22(1):155–163

Laws & Sullivan 2004 Australia's mothers and babies 2002. AIHW NPSU

Lilienfeld AM, Lilienfeld DE (1980) Foundations of Epidemiology. Oxford University Press, Oxford

Mays N, Pope C 1995 Qualitative research: observational methods in healthcare settings. British Medical Journal 311:182–184

Mays N, Pope C 2000 Qualitative research in healthcare: assessing quality in qualitative research. British Medical Journal 320: 50–52.

McPherson K (1994) The Cochrane Lecture 1993. The best and the enemy of the good: randomised controlled trials, uncertainty, and assessing the role of patient choice in medical decision making. Journal of Epidemiology and Community Health 48:6–15

MIDIRS 2000 What is evidence-informed midwifery? MIDIRS 10(2):149–150

Miettinen OS 1998 Evidence in medicine: invited commentary. Canadian Medical Association Journal 158:215–221

Muir Gray JA 1997 Evidence-based healthcare. Churchill Livingstone, New York

Murphy PA & Fullerton JT 2001 Measuring outcomes of midwifery care: development of an instrument to assess optimality. Journal of Midwifery and Women's Health 46:274–284

Naylor CD 1995 Grey zones of clinical practice: some limits to evidence-based medicine. Lancet 345:840–842

Norku Z 2004 Historical narratives as pictures: on elective affinities between verbal and pictorial representations. Journal of Narrative Theory 34(2):173–206

O'Cathain A, Walters SJ, Nicholl JP et al 2002 Use of evidence-based leaflets to promote informed choice in maternity care: randomised controlled trial in everyday practice. British Medical Journal 324:643–646

Oakley A 1990 Who's afraid of the randomised controlled trial? Some dilemmas of the scientific method and good research practice. In: H Roberts (Ed) Women's Health Counts. Routledge, London

Oakley A 1998 Experimentation and social interventions: a forgotten but important history. British Medical Journal 317:1239–1242

Oakley A 1998 Living in two worlds. British Medical Journal 316:482–483

Oakley A 2000 Experiments in knowing: gender and method in the social sciences. Polity Press, Cambridge

Oxford Centre for Evidence Based Medicine 2005 Levels of evidence and grades of recommendation. Online: http://www.cebm.net/levels_of_evidence.asp

Page L 1996 The backlash against evidence-based care. Birth 23(4):191–192

Page L 2002 The new midwifery: science and sensitivity in practice. Churchill Livingstone, London

Phillips B, Ball C, Sackett D et al 2005 Centre for Evidence-Based Medicine, Institute of Health Sciences Old Road Campus, Headington, Oxford, OX3 7LF, United Kingdom. Online: http://www.cebm.net/levels_of_evidence.asp

Pocock SJ, Smith M, Baghurst P 1994 Environmental lead and children's intelligence: a systematic review of the epidemiological evidence. British Medical Journal 309:1189–1197

Pope C, Mayes N 1995 Qualitative research: reaching the parts other methods cannot reach. An introduction to qualitative methods in health and health services research. British Medical Journal 311:42–45

Pope C, Mayes N 2000 Qualitative research in healthcare (2nd edn). BMJ Publishing, London

Popper KR 1972 Objective knowledge: an evolutionary approach. Oxford University Press, London

Prendiville WJ, Elbourne D, McDonald S 2000 Active versus expectant management in the third stage of labour. Cochrane Review (3). John Wiley & Sons Ltd

Reason P (1988) Human inquiry in action: developments in new paradigm research. Sage, London

Rowley MJ, Hensley MJ, Brimsmead MW et al 1995 Continuity of care by a midwife team versus routine care during pregnancy and birth: a randomized controlled trial. Medical Journal of Australia 163:289–293

Sackett DL, Cooke IE 1996 Evidence-based obstetrics and gynaecology. Ballières Clinical Obstetrics and Gynaecology 10(4):535–551

Sackett DL, Rosenberg WMC, Muir Gray JA et al 1996 Evidence-based medicine: what it is and what it isn't. British Medical Journal 312:171–172

Sackett DL, Straus SE, Richardson WS 2000 Evidence-based medicine: how to practice and teach EBM (2nd edn). Churchill Livingstone, Edinburgh

Sacks HS, Berrier J, Reitman D et al 1987 Meta-analyses of randomized controlled trials. New England Journal of Medicine 316(8):450–455

Saunders J 2000 The practice of clinical medicine as an art and as a science. Journal of Medical Ethics: Medical Humanities 26: 18–22

Sharpe VA 2000 Behind closed doors: accountability and responsibility in patient care. Journal of Medicine and Philosophy 25(1):28–47

Sleep J, Grant AM, Garcia J et al (1984) West Berkshire perineal management trial. British Medical Journal 289:587–590

Song F, Eastwood AJ, Gilbody S et al 2000) Publication and related biases. Health and Technology Assessment 4(10). Online: http://www.ncchta.org/fullmono/mon410.pdf

Stapleton H, Kirkham M, Thomas G 2002 Qualitative study of evidence-based leaflets in maternity care. British Medical Journal 324:639–643

Steiner JF 1999 Talking about treatment: the language of populations and the language of individuals. Annals of Internal Medicine 130:618–622

Stewart M 2000 Whose evidence counts? An exploration of health professionals' perceptions of evidence-based practice, focusing on the maternity services. Midwifery 17(4):279–288

Strauss A, Corbin J 1998 Basics of qualitative research: techniques and procedures for developing grounded theory. Sage, London

Traynor M 2000 Purity, conversion and the evidence-based movements. Health 4(2):139–158

Wiegers RA, Keirse M, Berghs G et al 1996 An approach to measuring quality of midwifery care. Journal of Clinical Epidemiology 49:319–325

Weijer C, Shapiro SH, Cranley Glass K 2000 For and against: clinical equipoise and not the uncertainty principle is the moral underpinning of the randomised controlled trial. British Medical Journal 321(7263):756–758

Further reading

Altman DG 1991 Practical statistics for medical research. Chapman Hall, London

Altman DG, Chalmers I, Egger M et al 2001 Systematic reviews in healthcare: meta-analysis in context. BMJ Publishing, London

Berkman L, Kawachi I 2000 Social epidemiology. Oxford University Press, Oxford

Bowling A 2002 Research methods in health: investigating health and health services. Open University Press, Buckingham, UK

Cochrane Handbook for Systematic Reviews of Interventions (formerly the Reviewers' Handbook) http://www.cochrane.org/resources/handbook/index.htm. A printable version can be downloaded from www.cochrane.org/resources/handbook/

Coggon D, Rose G, Barker DJP 2003 Epidemiology for the uninitiated. British Medical Journal Publishing, London

Darlington Y, Scott D 2002 Qualitative research in practice: stories from the field. Open University Press, UK

Deeks JJ, Dinnes J, D'Amico R et al 2003 Evaluating non-randomised intervention studies. Health and Technology Assessment 7(27). Online: http://www.ncchta.org/fullmono/mon727.pdf

Douglas E, Liamputtong Pranee 2005 Qualitative research nethods. Oxford University Press, Melbourne.

Doyle L 2003 Sex and gender: the challenge for epidemiologists. International Journal of Health Sciences 33(3):569–579

Duckitt K, Harrington D 2005 Risk factors for pre-eclampsia at antenatal booking: systematic review of controlled studies. British Medical Journal 330(7491):565

Duley L 2005 Evidence and practice: the magnesium sulphate story. Best Practice and Research in Clinical Obstetrics and Gynaecology 19(1):57–74

Economic and Social Research Council (ESRC). Online: http://www.esrc.ac.uk/index.asp

Enkin M 2000 For and against: clinical equipoise and not the uncertainty principle is the moral underpinning of the randomised controlled trial. British Medical Journal 321: 756–758

Enkin M, Keirse JNC, Neilson J et al 2000 A guide to effective care in pregnancy and childbirth (3rd edn). Oxford University Press, Oxford. Online: http://maternitywise.org/guide/about.html

Evidence for Policy and Practice Information and Coordinating Centre (EPPI Centre), Social Science Research Unit, Institute of Education, London. Online: http://eppi.ioe.ac.uk

Gordis L 1996 Epidemiology. WB Saunders, Philadelphia

Greenhalgh T 2004 How to read a paper: the basics of evidence-based medicine (2nd edn). BMJ Publishing, London

Greenhalgh T, Hurwitz B 1998 Narrative-based medicine: dialogue and discourse in clinical practice. BMJ Publishing, London

Grimes DA, Shultz KF 2005 Refining clinical diagnosis with likelihood ratios. Lancet 365(9469):1500–1505

Higgins JPT, Green S (Eds) 2005 Cochrane handbook for systematic reviews of interventions 4.2.4 (updated March 2005). Cochrane Library (2). John Wiley & Sons, Chichester. Online: http://www.cochrane.org/resources/handbook/hbook.htm

Holloway I (Ed) 2005 Qualitative research in health care. Maidenhead, UK: Open University Press.

Kranzler G, Moursund J 1999 Statistics for the terrified (2nd edn). Prentice Hall, New Jersey

Lomas J 1997 Research and evidence-based decision making. Australian and New Zealand Journal of Public Health 21(5): 439–440

Mays N, Pope C 1999 Qualitative research in healthcare (2nd edn). BMJ Publishing, London

Morse JM 1993 Critical issues in qualitative research methods. Sage, USA

Oakley A 2000 Experiments in knowing: gender and method in the social sciences. Polity Press, Cambridge

Page L 2005 The new midwifery: science and sensitivity in practice (2nd edn). Churchill Livingstone, London

Sackett DL, Straus SE, Richardson WS 2000 Evidence-based medicine: how to practice and teach EBM (2nd edn). Churchill Livingstone, Edinburgh

Silman AJ, Macfarlane GJ 2002 Epidemiological studies: a practical guide. Cambridge University Press, Cambridge

Sullivan EA, Ford JB, Chambers G et al 2004 Maternal mortality in Australia, 1973–1996. Australian and New Zealand Journal of Obstetrics and Gynaecology 44:452–457

Thacker SB, Banta HD 1983 Benefits and risks of episiotomy: an interpretive review of the English language literature, 1860–1980. Obstetric and Gynecological Survey 38(6):322–338

Vernon B, Tracy S, Reibel T 2002 Compliance, coercion and power have huge effect in maternity services. British Medical Journal 325:43

APPENDIX: Evaluating a guideline

Who developed the guidelines?
▶ Are the members of the guideline development team identified?
▶ Are all clinical perspectives represented?
▶ Are all cultural perspectives represented (e.g. African-American, Pacific Islander)?
▶ Is patient input or participation documented?
▶ Are the sponsors of the guideline identified?
▶ Are there potential conflicts of interest?

Why did they develop the guideline?
▶ Is there a clear statement of the guideline objective?
▶ Is the gap between current practice and outcomes and the recommended practice and outcomes clearly stated?
▶ Is the guideline development process described? (If so, what process was used?)
 — explicit evidence-based (includes projections of healthcare outcomes for a defined population)
 — evidence-based
 — consensus process
 — process of development not described.
▶ What is the strength of the evidence?

▶ Is there a description of the strategy used to obtain information from the medical literature?
▶ Is there a description of the strategy used to critically appraise and synthesise the evidence?
▶ Is the evidence presented in terms of absolute differences in outcome (as compared to relative differences)?
▶ Are the major recommendations of the guideline based on high-quality evidence?

Does the guideline possess the attributes of a good guideline?
▶ Are the patients that the guideline applies to clearly described and are exceptions stated?
▶ Is the guideline clear and brief?
▶ Does it provide genuine clinical guidance?
▶ Is it flexible (does it allow for clinical judgement)?
▶ Can the change in care be measured?
▶ Can it be implemented in your care delivery system?
▶ Is the information the guideline is based on current?
▶ Has the guideline been successfully piloted or implemented?

(Source: New Zealand Guidelines Group and Group Health Cooperative of Puget Sound, http://www.nzgg.org.nz)

CHAPTER 6

The place of birth

Maralyn Foureur and Marion Hunter

Key terms

birth centre, maternity unit, primary birth unit[1]

Chapter overview

This chapter focuses on the power of the place of birth to influence the behaviour of women and their midwives during childbirth. We propose that neither the type of care provider nor the model of care delivery *alone* is able to affect outcomes without sufficient attention paid to the physical and psychological environment for birth. Through exploring the complex nature of modern maternity care, with its focus on hospital birth and the use of technology to guarantee 'safety', we discover that the influence of 'environment' may be so pervasive that the full, potential benefits of 'new' systems or models, such as continuity of midwifery care, fail to be easily realised in hospital settings. Important insights into why this might occur are provided through the lens of one New Zealand study comparing the practices of midwives who move between small and large birthing units. The midwives' own words will be used to clearly illustrate what they have come to know as 'real midwifery'. The chapter begins with a brief historical account of childbirth history in Australia and New Zealand, to explore the reasons why women moved from their homes to hospitals for birth at the turn of the twentieth century and why they continue to go to hospital to give birth over a hundred years later. This will provide a context for considering what has been lost in the process and how the modern birth environment affects outcomes for women and babies, as well as midwives. This chapter aims to reveal what midwives can do to ensure that the potential benefits of midwifery-led care are optimised, no matter where the place of birth.

Learning outcomes

Learning outcomes for this chapter are:

1 To explore the impact of the place of birth on women and midwives

2 To explore different perspectives on why women moved from home to hospital for birth at the turn of the twentieth century, and to discuss what was lost in the process

3 To explore the risks and benefits of the three locations for place of birth: home, birth centre or hospital

4 To discuss the 'fear cascade', a plausible theoretical model that explains why the birth environment may affect birth outcomes

5 To describe some of the physiological consequences of birth in an unfamiliar or fearful environment

6 To describe the key competencies required for practising 'real midwifery' no matter where the place of birth.

Introduction

In the twenty-first century, birth takes place in the intimate spaces provided in women's homes, in small birth centres or primary birth units which aim to provide a home-like atmosphere, and in large hospitals surrounded by an array of technology and personnel. This chapter argues that each location exerts a powerful influence on how the woman's labour unfolds and how she will give birth and greet her baby. Importantly, each location also exerts a powerful influence on, and is influenced by, the midwife who accompanies the woman. Therefore, a comprehensive understanding of the influence of 'environment' on the physiological processes controlling labour and birth is essential for all midwives. We will endeavour to provide a point of entry into that knowledge by exploring the answers to two important questions: why did women move from home to hospital for birth, and what was lost in the process? In addition, some of the many studies that have explored the complex relationships between environment and physiology of birth will be examined in order to offer support for the proposal that this is essential knowledge for midwives. Finally, the chapter provides an in-depth discussion of the way in which one group of midwives discovered this knowledge in what they described as doing 'real midwifery'.

Birth moves from home to hospital

The turn of the nineteenth century marked the beginning of the move of childbirth into institutions throughout Britain, Europe, North America, and Australia and New Zealand. Therefore an examination of the past two hundred years of the history of childbirth in any of those countries will reveal the complex interplay of human and social forces which ultimately dislocated childbearing women from their homes and families, and moved apparent responsibility for childbirth to the medical profession based in hospitals (Graham 1997). Far from being the rational sequential scientific development that one might expect, such an examination reveals that the systems have been shaped and moulded by class and gender, fashion and fallacy, and professional and economic competition (Rowley 1998).

This chapter begins with a very brief glimpse into that history in Australia and New Zealand. While there are parallels between the development of maternity care and midwifery in Britain and Europe and among the non-Indigenous populations of Australia and New Zealand, there are also important differences emerging from Australia's initial role as a penal colony and the later development of both Australia and New Zealand as nations with booming economies where a vigorous medical profession was seeking to establish itself (Tew 1995). Mein Smith claims that in these two colonies, the revolution in the organisation of childbirth began earlier and progressed faster than in either Britain or Europe (Mein Smith 1986).

However, it should first be acknowledged that most historical accounts in both Australia and New Zealand have largely ignored the childbirth experiences and expertise of the original occupants of the land. Since we must rely on secondary sources of information, this account will do the same, in order not to misrepresent the birth traditions of either the Maori of New Zealand or the Aboriginal peoples of Australia.

The origins of midwifery in Australia

The ships of the First Fleet, which landed in Sydney in 1788, carried several women who were free settlers as well as numbers of convict women. The ships' logs record that during the long voyage to Australia, several women gave birth, allowing others to gain midwifery experience (Adcock et al 1984). The military and ship's surgeons accompanying the colonising forces probably had little or no midwifery expertise, and there were no midwives listed among either the free settlers or the convict women. Therefore it appears that midwifery in Australia began with women helping each other as best they could, accessing medical help where it was available and when it was required. Some of the women who found themselves in the role of midwife continued to assist women in childbirth and became well known, loved and respected for their abilities.

Female convicts were transported to Australia for the next fifty years in an attempt to empty English prisons of 'hardened cases' but covertly to provide sexual services for men (who outnumbered the women six to one) and ultimately to stabilise the economy of the new colony (Rowley 1998). Early census records reveal that by 1806, two per cent of women were in skilled trades, which included two women who listed their occupation as midwife, although with every woman under the age of forty-two producing a baby each year, there were clearly more than two 'midwives' in the colony (Adcock et al 1984). No 'learned' midwives were recorded among those early settlers until forty years later, when Mrs McTavish, identified as the first 'trained' midwife to settle in Australia, advertised her services in a Hobart newspaper (Barclay 1993, cited in Rowley 1998). Therefore it is reasonable to propose that the midwifery traditions of Australia were established by community-based, 'lay' midwives, without access to any theoretical knowledge or teaching other than what they had gleaned from observation and experience. These were the 'accidental' or empirical midwives of the convict era assisting women to give birth in whatever place constituted 'home'.

The first maternity hospitals in Australia

In 1820, a midwife or 'fingersmith' was appointed to the Female Factory at Parramatta, which was built to house female convicts. Some midwives chose to work in the Female Factory for short periods to gain experience before moving out into the community and private practice. Convicts in domestic service who became pregnant were sent to Parramatta for punishment and confinement. Once delivered, the women returned to their employer, often leaving the baby behind, where their infants were wet-nursed by thirty convict 'nurses' who resided there.

The Female Factory became the first maternity hospital, as the pregnancy rate among convicts was high. Soon, poor and destitute women also sought to be confined there, since the authorities were reluctant to build hospitals for the general populace. The Female Factory was eventually closed due to an epidemic of puerperal sepsis. Following the closure, convict women continued to give birth at home, as did the free settlers, attended by relatives, neighbours, or a midwife if they could afford one or find one, but rarely by a doctor.

The transportation of convicts ended in 1848 just before the discovery of gold near Bathurst in 1851. The new colony prospered. The government of the day encouraged the immigration of young single women to redress the imbalance in the sexes and to populate the country. As settlers moved out into rural areas, even neighbours were sparse, and there are numerous accounts of women being attended by Aboriginal women during childbirth (Willis 1989). Learned midwives who had received midwifery training in England and Scotland were also among the new immigrants. As the settlements grew into towns, some midwives began taking women into their own homes for 'confinement', and thus began the first private maternity homes, which were eventually to become community or primary hospitals (Shephard 1989, 1991). Later, concern over the deplorable conditions under which poor and destitute women were 'confined' in their homes led to the establishment of (initially) charitable and (ultimately) State-funded women's hospitals in the cities of Melbourne (1886) and Sydney (1893) just prior to the turn of the twentieth century (Forster 1965).

The origins of midwifery in New Zealand

Childbirth for Pakeha[2] women in New Zealand prior to the 1904 *Midwives Act* was described by Donley (1986) as a neighbourhood affair conducted in homes. Women were attended by either (English or Scottish) trained or lay midwives, who took charge of domestic responsibilities as well as supporting the woman in labour, delivering the baby and getting breastfeeding established. As in Australia, these early midwives were loved and respected for their competence and care, and there are several accounts of the good records of the pioneering midwives in terms of maternal and perinatal mortality (Donley 1986). As the towns grew and cities evolved, many midwives set up their own small, private maternity homes. It is estimated that by the turn of the twentieth century, there were over two hundred one- or two-bed maternity homes run by midwives or by doctors, located throughout the towns and cities of New Zealand (Mein Smith 1986).

The first maternity hospitals in New Zealand

Several events coalesced just after the turn of the century that initiated major changes in the way childbirth was managed, and changed it forever from a relatively private family affair into a concern of the State. Reports to Parliament had for some time recorded the fluctuating maternal and infant mortality rates in the new colony and, in particular, the rate of maternal deaths from puerperal sepsis. In 1903, a peak in the maternal mortality rate caused alarm in government circles. At the same time a Royal Commission set up in New South Wales in 1904 to investigate falling birth rates in both Australia and New Zealand found that the decline was highest among the 'better classes' and that 'while the "unfit" were having many children … [they] had a higher rate of infant mortality' (Donley 1986, p 32). The Premier, Richard Seddon, demanded action and a champion emerged in the person of Grace Neill,[3] who was easily able to persuade him that the way to increase the birth rate and improve the appalling rates of maternal and infant mortality was to register all midwives and establish State-subsidised hospitals, where the wives of working-class men (the deserving poor) could give birth in comfort and safety. This saw the setting up of St Helens Hospitals in the major centres of New Zealand, with the first established in a rented cottage in Rintoul Street, Wellington, in 1905 (Donley 1986). The hospitals provided midwifery training for both nurses and women without a nursing qualification, and offered either hospital or domiciliary care (without prejudice).

Why did women move from home to hospital?

Over the next twenty years, simultaneously in both countries, women started to move from home to hospital in increasing numbers. Why this happened is an intriguing question. A simple answer would be to find that mothers and babies died in large numbers at home in the care of midwives, and that women chose to move into hospital, where medically managed birth was safe. This is not the case, however. Different authors quote a variety of maternal and infant mortality rates, all purporting to provide evidence of either a dramatic improvement in, or worsening of, mortality as a consequence of the move (Ehrenreich & English 1973; Shorter 1983). Gaining a clear picture of what was happening at the time is difficult, and this allows different interpretations of the

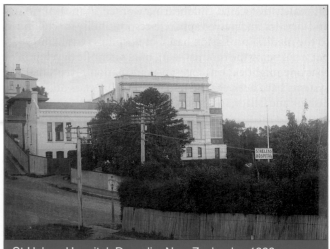

St Helens Hospital, Dunedin, New Zealand c. 1923. Reproduced with the permission of Alexander Turnbull Library, Wellington, New Zealand. Photo from the S C Smith Collection

significant events to emerge. What motivated women to move from birth at home to hospital can never be known for certain, but the parallel movement in Australia and New Zealand suggests that the motivators for the change may have been similar, and several issues can be identified which may have played a part.

The first is the issue of falling birth rates at the turn of the twentieth century and the intervention of both colonial governments in childbirth, with the aim of increasing the size of their respective populations and ensuring their health and vigour (Donley 1986). The Health Departments in both countries promoted the hospitalisation of birth in order to decrease the rate of maternal deaths particularly from puerperal sepsis, and to ensure women accessed antenatal care that would lead to the birth of a healthy baby. Both governments were disturbed by the parlous physical state of many of the men recruited into the armed forces during World War I, and saw the birth of a healthy baby as essential to the health of the nation in the event of another war (Mein Smith 1986).

Other themes relate to the views of women themselves and what they may have been seeking. Some may have sought increased material comfort around the time of the birth, because many homes in both New Zealand and Australia were described as lacking in all but the barest of necessities (Mein Smith 1986; Rowley 1998; Tew 1995). Other women may have found the promise of a temporary release from domestic burdens attractive (Tew 1995). Still others may have been seeking the support and company of other women, which had been dislocated by the Industrial Revolution (Wilson 1995), or greater access to doctors and their forceps (Loudon 1992; Rowley 1998; Tew 1995), or greater access to midwives since the lay midwife had largely disappeared from the community following the setting up of registration and hospital-based training. Added to these issues were the promises of a pain-free labour (Loudon 1992) and increased safety for themselves and their infants, largely and falsely promoted by the medical profession (Tew 1995). In New Zealand, the medical profession actively encouraged women's groups in political activity to persuade the government to build more maternity hospitals, which then became a focus for the growing power of the emerging medical specialty of obstetrics (Mein Smith 1986). All these issues have been debated in the literature cited, and the student of history is encouraged to pursue particular lines of inquiry using the references and further reading lists at the end of this chapter as a guide. It is interesting to note, for instance, that both forceps and the pain relief offered by twilight sleep were liberally administered by doctors attending women in childbirth at home, so these two reasons alone do not seem to be convincing arguments for the move to hospital (Forster 1965; Mein Smith 1986).

Far from increasing safety as promised, deaths from puerperal sepsis increased with hospital birth, in all but the St Helens Hospitals (Wood & Foureur 2005; Mein Smith 1986), but this appeared to go unnoticed by women as they started to move into hospitals in increasing numbers. Mein Smith (1986) asserts that by 1920, most New Zealand women continued to give birth at home, while approximately 35% of deliveries occurred in hospitals. In Australia, 'births in public institutions . . . increased from 3% in 1907 to 7% in 1920 but then leapt ahead to 55% in 1929' (Tew 1995, p 65), with one account quoting a rate as high as 67% for hospital deliveries in 1925 in the State of Victoria (Loudon 1992).

By 1935, deaths from puerperal sepsis were rarely seen, due to the advent of the drugs Prontosil and, later, sulphanilamide (Tew 1990). Perinatal mortality also began to decline between the world wars, due to dramatic improvements in the general health of women and raised living standards (Johanson et al 2002). However, in the minds of many, moving to hospital for birth had improved safety for women and babies, and it was not until 1990 that a critical history of maternity care undertaken by Marjorie Tew (1990) was able to convincingly demonstrate the fallacy of this belief. Today the vast majority of women in either country will give birth in hospital, be it a birth centre, primary birth unit or secondary/tertiary hospital. Home birth occurs in less than one per cent of the population of childbearing women in Australia, and although the estimated rate may be higher in New Zealand, at approximately six per cent (Pairman & Guilliland 2003), birth at home is the choice of few women. Or, paradoxically, is it that there is no choice?

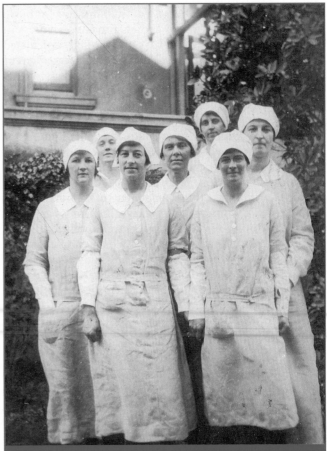

Trainee midwives, St Helens Wellington 1927. Reproduced with the permission of Archives New Zealand

What was lost in the move?

Several important things were lost in the move from home to hospital. The first was the opportunity to labour in a familiar environment. The second was the close personal and trusting relationship between the woman and her midwife and the continuous support in labour that the midwife provided. The third was the belief in the concept of birth as a normal physiological event. These were and are still universal aspects of home birth provision, and the whole package of care provides clear benefits for women (Walsh 2004). Let us explore these ideas a little more.

The concept of 'environment' is multifaceted and encompasses much more than the geographical or physical bricks and mortar of the location for birth. It is important to consider that 'environment' also includes the spiritual and emotional space and place in the mind and heart of the woman (Simkin & Ancheta 2001). We must also acknowledge that the environment too exerts a powerful influence on the midwife and that, in the future, new areas of research in what some have termed 'neuroarchitecture' (or 'psycho-geography') will improve our understanding of this concept (Foureur 2002; Lepori 1994; Newburn 2003; Page 2002; Walsh et al 2004).

In their calls for more home-like environments for birth, more continuity and more choice and involvement in decision-making, women may have unknowingly articulated their longing to replicate the idealised birth environment of home. Policy makers have attempted to put back components of the package, and researchers have undertaken numerous studies to explore the safety and impact of differences in location for birth (home, birth centre, primary unit, hospital), type of care provider (medical, midwife, doula), models of care (fragmented versus continuity of care and carer) and philosophies of care (belief in birth as a normal physiological event or only normal in retrospect; risk-embracing or risk-averse). However, if the three components of birth at home are an integrated and inseparable package, it becomes apparent that most studies to date have focused on either one or another part of the package. As a consequence, most studies are limited in what they can contribute to our understanding of this complex event. Hodnett realised the synergistic nature of caregiver and location for birth when she wrote that the environment may favourably influence caregivers' attitudes towards the care of labouring women, and that therefore it may be the influence of the caregiver *more* than just the location for birth that leads to good obstetric outcomes (Hodnett 2004). We will return to this idea later in the chapter.

Birth at home or in hospital: which is safer?

The debate concerning the safety of the home as the place of birth has been in progress for over one hundred years and no doubt will continue into the future, unless it becomes possible to conduct an extremely large trial where women are randomly allocated to either a home or a hospital birth. One such study involving only eleven women was identified during the process of systematic review published by the Cochrane Collaboration (Olsen & Jewell 1998). Because of the small size of the study, the reviewers were forced to conclude that there is no strong evidence to favour either planned hospital birth or planned home birth for low-risk women. Many other studies using less robust designs (such as observational, case control or cohort studies and audit of maternity services) have been conducted internationally, but few of these have been within Australia or New Zealand (for example, Chamberlain et al 1997; Rooks et al 1989; Young & Hey 2000). Most studies of this nature suffer from a lack of 'denominator data', meaning that the researcher cannot be certain that all women giving birth at home in their particular data set have been accounted for. Therefore, studies may under- or over-estimate the risks. However, the most recent and largest prospective cohort study of homebirth published in 2005 accurately identified all births and concluded that outcomes for homebirth women were substantially better than for low-risk American women having hospital births (Johnson & Daviss 2005). Among the 5418 women who planned to give birth at home when labour began, there was a 12.1% transfer rate at the beginning of labour. Intervention rates were significantly reduced, with epidural (4.7%), episiotomy (2.1%), instrumental delivery (1.06%) and caesarean section (3.7%). The intrapartum and neonatal mortality was 1.7 deaths per 1000 planned homebirths when congenital anomalies were excluded. This is the largest study so far to confirm the safety of homebirth.

But for mothers with a twin, breech or post-term pregnancy, the current state of evidence asserts that there is an increased risk of perinatal death at home (Bastian & Keirse 1998; Young & Hey 2000). The Johnson and Daviss (2005) paper supports the findings of the comprehensive UK study *Where to be born?*, which concluded that, given the current state of knowledge, 'there is no evidence to support the claim that the safest policy is for all women to give birth in hospital' (Macfarlane et al 2000, p 798).

However, the rhetoric that began over one hundred years ago persists, and society still views birth at home as a poor choice. Indeed, Tew (1995) identified that data had been deliberately misinterpreted in UK studies between 1958 and 1970 to support the claim that 'the family home is the most dangerous place for birth' (p 29). Tew stated that an impartial observer could clearly see that the perinatal mortality rate was higher in hospitals, yet this fact was distorted in reports of the time. Obstetricians throughout the world used the false interpretation of these statistics to influence the future development of maternity services. Midwives may also be influenced by the rhetoric and either refuse to provide a home birth option for women or unconsciously bias the way it is discussed, leading women to 'choose' a hospital birth (Walsh 2004).

The birth centre: a halfway house?

Moves to address the loss of the familiar home environment for birth appeared in the late 1970s with the call for more humanised or home-like birth spaces, culminating in the development of the birth centre in many locations throughout Australia and New Zealand (as elsewhere). Birth centres may be free-standing or located within hospitals, either adjacent to or within high-technology and medically staffed labour wards, thus enabling immediate consultation or rapid transfer if the need arises. Primary birth units may be located in urban or rural settings and share many of the attributes of birth centres. Although birth centres may differ in their structure, location, furnishings and staffing, all share a strong philosophical orientation towards assisting women to achieve normal physiological birth (Coyle et al 2001; Kirkham 2003). They are intended only for women classified as 'low risk', the very women who would fulfil criteria for birth at home. However, even in this low-risk population, numbers of women are transferred out for medical assistance or pain-relieving drugs before, during or after labour. Transfer rates vary from as low as 12% (Rooks et al 1989) to more commonly around 20% but even up to 63% in some settings (Hodnett 2004). In Australia, around 5% of women give birth in primary birth units (Griew 2003)—this includes 5379 births in birth centres in 2003, 'representing 2.1% of all confinements' (Laws & Sullivan 2005). In New Zealand the combined birth centre/primary birth unit rate in 2001 was 1% (Pairman & Guilliland 2003) and in 2003 was 15% (NZHIS 2005).

Numerous randomised controlled trials and observational studies examining the effectiveness and safety of birth centres/ primary birth units have been conducted worldwide, and have demonstrated that birth for low-risk women is at least as safe in small low-risk maternity units as it is in hospitals (Kirkham 2003; Walsh & Downe 2004). In addition, a recent consumer satisfaction survey conducted in New Zealand has revealed that women 'are more likely to be satisfied with maternity services if they birth at a primary maternity facility' (Ministry of Health 2002, p 4). In a Cochrane Systematic Review, Hodnett (2004) included evidence from six trials involving almost 9000 women, and concluded that there appear to be some benefits from home-like settings for birth. However, one recent study has raised concerns about the safety of out-of-hospital births, and it needs to be considered here (Gottvall et al 2004).

A ten-year retrospective review of the Stockholm Birth Centre undertaken by Gottvall et al (2004) revealed a trend to higher perinatal mortality in primigravid women.[4] Following scrutiny of each perinatal death by an obstetrician, Gottvall and colleagues (2004) claimed that a potential risk of birth centre care is the 'philosophy that emphasises a strong belief in the natural process' (p 77). Hodnett (2004) echoed concerns regarding the emphasis on normal birth and stated that this belief might delay recognition of imminent complications or the ability of the midwife to take averting action. However, concluding comments from Gottvall et al (2004) indicate a potential bias in the study introduced through an underlying concern with intrapartum care that does not include technology and medical assistance. Many of the perinatal deaths in the original Stockholm trial (Waldenstrom et al 1997) occurred after transfer and were associated with clearly documented suboptimal care in the receiving hospital. Gottvall and colleagues did not comment on this. On the other hand, Walsh (2004) refuted any suggestion that birth centre midwives are over-orientated to normal birth and therefore may delay recognition of complications. Walsh asserts that birth centre midwives are highly skilled practitioners with an astute awareness of normal labour and that these midwives are particularly diligent in updating their skills in emergency care. Walsh acknowledged that it might very well be the midwife's belief in physiological labour, especially for primigravid women, that enables such women to achieve normal birth in birth centres. In his most recent ethnographic study, Walsh

(2006) asserts that very little attention has been paid to organisational dimensions of childbirth care until recently. He claims that free-standing birth centres 'subvert' the processing mentality of modernist organisations such as large maternity hospitals. Birth centres demonstrate greater flexibility in labour care so as to accommodate women's preferences and enhance the autonomy of midwives and women, such that a self-managing and self-regulating ethos flourishes (Walsh 2006).

Sociologists who have paid particular attention to childbirth also show concern regarding interpretations of safety. Annandale (1988) used both quantitative and qualitative methods to study the structure of birth in a North American birthing centre. Her study included eighteen months of observation, repeated focus group interviews and content analysis of 900 women's records over a five-year period. Obstetricians did not see women unless a risk factor arose; however, Annandale commented that midwives and obstetricians disagreed about what constituted a risk factor. Midwives tended to disagree with the assertion that a post-term induction was high risk, and that intervention was required after twelve hours of rupture of membranes. Annandale found that birth centre midwives adopted strategies to maintain the 'normal', such as encouraging women to stay at home until active labour was well established. This strategy reduced the likelihood of transfer to a large hospital for perceived prolonged labour. However, Hodnett (2004) cautioned that 'just as an over emphasis on risk and intervention can lead to unnecessary interventions and avoidable complications for healthy childbearing women and their families, an over-emphasis on normality may lead to delayed recognition of or action regarding complications' (p 5).

The return of a familiar caregiver

The second component of the care package to be lost in the move was the familiar caregiver and the continuous

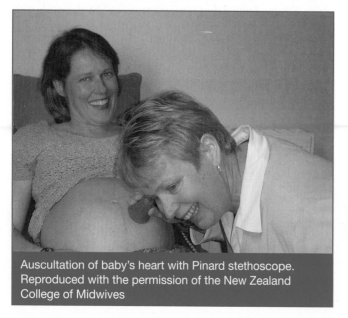

Auscultation of baby's heart with Pinard stethoscope. Reproduced with the permission of the New Zealand College of Midwives

support she provided. This has been addressed through calls for increased continuity of care, which midwives have provided, first in experimental models tested in numerous randomised controlled trials, and more latterly in New Zealand following the changes to the *Nurses Act* in 1990 leading to midwifery autonomy.

There now exists overwhelming evidence, from nearly twenty randomised controlled trials conducted in Australia, Canada, Sweden, Hong Kong, the United Kingdom, Scotland and the United States of America, that continuous labour support for women during childbirth should be the norm, rather than the exception (Biro et al 2003; National Institute for Clinical Excellence 2004; Rowley 1998; Rowley et al 1995; Waldenstrom & Turnbull 1998). It is clear that any maternity care system that is not founded on this model of care places women at increased risk of interventions such as epidural analgesia and operative birth by forceps, vacuum extraction or caesarean section. Although the short-term effects of such procedures are well documented, it is becoming increasingly apparent that these are all major interventions with potential for unanticipated, adverse, long-term physical and behavioural effects on both mothers and babies (Bahl et al 2004; Beech 1998; Carter et al 2001; DiMatteo et al 1996; Gottvall & Waldenstrom 2002; Jacobsen & Bygdeman 1998; Jacobsen et al 1990; Mayberry et al 2002). Some effects may be permanent.

The financial costs of the long-term consequences of intervention in childbirth have received less scrutiny, but even the increased costs of the procedures themselves must lead health care planners to consider more carefully the models of care to which women are subjected (Roberts et al 2000; Tracy & Tracy 2003). These findings cannot be ignored, and many maternity care systems have focused attention on ways and means of increasing opportunities for women to experience continuous labour support, with varying degrees of success.

However, while continuous labour support is a form of maternity care that should be available for all women, it is clearly not sufficient, in and of itself, to enable normal birth. Three issues will be explored here. First we will examine the New Zealand maternity care system, which has successfully embraced a model of care that provides continuous labour support for all women, but still sees women experience high and rising rates of intervention, although the rise is notably less than in other Western countries (NZHIS 2004). Second, we will consider what it is about continuity of care and continuous labour support that influences outcomes, by exploring the concept of the fear cascade (Rowley 1998). Finally, we will consider whether a better understanding of the physiology of birth contributes to keeping birth normal.

What is a 'normal birth'?

Continuous labour support aims to decrease intervention in childbirth and thereby increase the numbers of women who experience 'normal' birth. Much debate has arisen around the concept of 'normal' birth, and for the purposes of this chapter it is defined as follows: labour occurs at term, is spontaneous in onset, and there is no requirement for augmentation or analgesia; the birth occurs spontaneously, vaginally, and the mother and baby are healthy. Some authors have estimated that in the twenty-first century, fewer than one-third of women in 'developed' countries will be enabled to give birth as nature intended (Conference Reports 2001; Sandall 2004). Many women are fearful of the process and shocked by their experiences. Rates of intervention vary between and within countries, between different locations for birth (hospital, birth centre and home birth), and between different models of maternity care in the same settings (public and private, fragmented care and continuity of care). Even the rates of intervention found in randomised controlled trials of continuous labour support and continuity of care reveal differences depending on the location of the trial—whether in a labour ward or a birth centre. However, very few trials and even fewer national data collection systems report birth outcomes in terms of the numbers of women who experience normal birth. Therefore the extent (or disappearance) of normal birth has been unintentionally hidden from our gaze until very recently.

'Continuity of care' versus 'continuous labour support'

Continuity of care describes the actual provision of care by the same caregiver or small group of caregivers throughout pregnancy, during labour and birth, and in the postnatal period. This model usually implies, but may not always include, continuous one-to-one support throughout labour. Continuous labour support describes the process of one-to-one supportive care from a companion throughout labour. It is apparent from at least one systematic review that continuous labour support provided by a non-hospital caregiver is more effective at reducing interventions than support provided by members of the hospital staff (Hodnett 2004). This raises interesting questions as to why the impact of continuous labour support differs depending on the type of caregiver. Hodnett (2004) proposes that the difference results from the ability of non-hospital caregivers to give greater attention to the mother's needs, since such companions are not distracted by the diverse responsibilities of hospital employees and organisational issues such as shift changes and staff shortages. We propose that this explanation is too simplistic. If Hodnett's proposal was valid, we could expect to find low rates of intervention in maternity care systems where both continuity of care and continuous one-to-one support throughout labour from non-hospital caregivers was the norm. Arguably this is the situation that has emerged in New Zealand over the past ten years. However, while it is apparent that New Zealand women are overwhelmingly satisfied with their experiences of midwifery-led continuity of care since their emotional/social needs are well met (Ministry of Health 2002), there exists some disquiet about decreasing rates of birth without intervention (Strid 2000). Let us examine this more closely.

The New Zealand experience

Around 57,000 women give birth annually in New Zealand at tertiary and primary care hospitals, in birth centres and at home. There are approximately 2500 qualified midwives currently practising in New Zealand and they are almost evenly divided between those who work as hospital (or core) midwives and those who work as independent (or caseloading) midwives. While core midwives are employed and generally work on shifts in maternity facilities, caseloading midwives may be employed or self-employed and provide continuity of care to an identified caseload of women. All women are required to have a known caregiver or 'Lead Maternity Carer' (LMC) throughout their childbirth experience. Although a general practitioner or specialist obstetrician can be chosen by the woman as her LMC, over 78% of women choose a midwife (NZHIS 2005). If the LMC is a midwife, she will usually provide continuity of care throughout pregnancy, one-to-one continuous labour and birth support and postnatal care. The research evidence suggests that this model of care will result in low rates of intervention. However, no conclusions can be drawn at present from the emerging (and as yet incomplete) population data collections published by the New Zealand Ministry of Health (NZHIS 2003, 2004, 2005). It appears that the rates of some interventions in childbirth are continuing to climb, with the national rate of caesarean section rising from 20.8% in 2000 to 23.1% in 2003 (NZHIS 2003, 2004, 2005). However, these rates compare favourably to Australia's caesarean section rate, which increased from 20.6% in 2000 to 28.5% in 2003 (Laws & Sullivan 2002, 2005). Additionally, if LMC midwife care is compared with LMC medical care for a similar cohort of women, the intervention rates are lower (MMPO, in press). In New Zealand, the rate of unassisted vaginal birth or non-operative vaginal birth fell from 68.4% in 2000 to 67.4% in 2003, while in Australia the rate of unassisted vaginal birth fell from 68.4% in 2000 to 60.3% in 2003 (Laws & Sullivan 2005, 2002; NZHIS 2005).

What outcome statistics do not yet address is the question of whether midwifery may make a much more subtle difference to maternity outcomes than is apparent through annual statistics and trend data. While 15 years of a midwife-led and women-centred maternity service in New Zealand has not shown a dramatic change in outcome measures such as caesarean section and 'normal' birth, there is emerging evidence that New Zealand's intervention rates are slowing and appear to be reaching a plateau compared with other Western countries (Laws & Sullivan 2004; NZHIS 2005). Midwifery care may have a greater impact on primary and public health measures than has been appreciated and therefore may be more significant in bringing about social change. This means that its effects are long-term and difficult, but not impossible, to quantify in the future (Guilliland 2005). Recognised public health measures in New Zealand include outcome measures for Maori, breastfeeding rates and immunisation rates.

A recent New Zealand study into the outcomes of a million births between 1980 and 2001 showed a marked decrease in numbers of low birthweight babies born to Maori women, Pacific Island women and women from low socio-economic groups, and decreasing numbers of premature babies (Mantell et al 2004)). These groups of women are all more likely to have midwifery care and less likely to have obstetric caregivers. Over 85% of Maori women chose a midwife in 2003, versus 76% of Pakeha, and 40% chose to give birth in a primary unit, which is twice the national average (NZHIS 2005). The latest breastfeeding data also shows a very encouraging trend upwards, with an overall 4% increase in exclusive breastfeeding over three years and in some areas increases of up to 30% (NZHIS 2005). Some 95% of babies received their six-week vaccination, the highest cover for all vaccination contacts, indicating a successful midwifery transfer to the well child service that is not sustained within the next service. These measures indicate the need for a more comprehensive approach to research into outcomes in relation to type of caregiver, place of birth and trends over time.

Until then it is useful to consider a plausible explanation provided by Kitson and colleagues (Kitson et al 1998). In exploring the problems encountered in implementing research evidence in practice, Kitson et al developed a useful model described as $SI = f(E,C,F)$. In essence this means that the successful implementation of research (SI) is a function (f) of the type of evidence (E), the context (C) in which the research was produced and to which it will be applied, and the facilitation (F) that occurs to enable research implementation. It is important to consider the contexts within which the evidence of effectiveness for both continuity of care and continuous labour support was produced. The evidence in both cases is a product of numerous randomised controlled trials. Such trials usually occur in settings that are openly supportive of innovation and exploration, because they are required to invest resources to carry out such studies. They are potentially more likely to have a high awareness of evidence of effectiveness for many aspects of maternity care which may influence processes and outcomes not measured in trials. They are special places and attract staff interested in exploring the evidence base for practice.

Arguably this is not the situation in the messy everyday world of real-life maternity care. In reality, midwifery care in New Zealand is mainstream rather than experimental, as in most other countries, but midwives still work mostly in highly medicalised environments, which can clearly override the potential benefits of continuity of care and continuous labour support. They also provide care to women with a full range of risk factors, not only those considered to be 'low risk'. This in itself may be a contributing factor to the way in which midwives consider the role of intervention, given that their clients are almost never 'risk' free. The model itself may not be powerful enough to provide benefits no matter what the setting, since the setting is imbued with the power of a risk-averse belief system. We propose that increasing our understanding of how the 'package of care' actually influences the physiology of birth will provide a means to address the

environmental constraints. If midwives (and others) had a greater understanding of the physiology of birth, fearful belief systems would be overcome.

What do we know about birth physiology?

During birth, 'a range of physiological adaptations' (Ginesi & Niescierowicz 1998a) are coordinated by a delicately balanced cascade of interrelated hormones such as oxytocin, endorphins, prolactin, ACTH and more, which flood the body and brain (Ginesi & Niescierowicz 1998b; Vose 2003). This is a largely unconscious process controlled by the part of our brain that initiates and responds to emotions—the hypothalamus or primal brain. Although the process has evolved over millennia to ensure the survival of the human species and is therefore relatively robust and successful, it is clearly possible to disrupt it by stimulating the neocortex of our brain into counter-active mode. Bright lights, harsh noises, foreign smells, strange and unfamiliar surroundings, loneliness, lack of trust in companions, loss of control, invasive procedures, pain and fear are just some of the phenomena that will stimulate the neocortex. This can be more fully appreciated by examining a process named the 'fear cascade' (Figure 6.1) explored by one of the authors (MF, nee Rowley) as part of a randomised controlled trial of team midwifery in Australia (Naaktgeboren 1989; Rowley 1998; Rowley et al 1995). The fear cascade provides one plausible theoretical explanation of why the two main reasons for all interventions in childbirth—uterine inertia (failure to progress) and fetal distress—occur. This is what it suggests: A healthy increase in maternal anxiety (eustress) can be expected as labour commences and the birth approaches. Nature has intended this as a signal to find a safe place to give birth so that a helpless newborn infant can be hidden from dangerous predators. However, the fear cascade may be initiated if the level of maternal anxiety increases to the extent that high levels of the catecholamine, adrenaline, are produced. This is a component of the well-described 'fight or flight' response. Adrenaline has an impact on the continued release of oxytocin, which has a major role to play

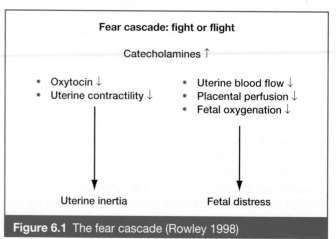

Figure 6.1 The fear cascade (Rowley 1998)

in uterine contractions (as well as many others). Disrupting the rhythmical release of oxytocin can result in incoordinate or absent contractions. This can both slow the progress of labour and increase the amount of pain experienced by the woman. The result is uterine inertia or failure to progress. On the other side of the fear cascade, the effect of adrenaline on uterine blood flow and placental perfusion can be seen. During the 'fight or flight' response, blood is diverted away from non-essential organs to the brain and limbs, and in this case the uterus is considered a non-essential organ. This may result in shifts in the amount of blood to the uterus. Even a small decrease in the volume of blood passing through the placenta can have an impact on fetal wellbeing and, thus, fetal distress may become apparent.

Finding supporting evidence for the fear cascade requires an eclectic approach to searching the literature, because the research has largely been conducted in animals and has occurred across a thirty-year span. Although results from animal research are not directly transferable to women, they do need to be given due attention. As Naaktgeboren says:

> Extrapolation from studies of parturient animals to human reproduction is inherently unwise since we assume human behaviour is much more complex than that of animals . . . but comparative obstetrics has demonstrated that . . . different species have made specific adaptations to the ecology of which they form a part; however common mechanisms which have a fundamental value, are observed in all mammals. This is just as true for the behavioural as for the physiological, endocrinological, anatomical (and many other aspects) of parturition (Naaktgeboren 1989).

Labouring undisturbed

In a classic work in 1978, perinatal psychologist Niles Newton noted the neuro-hormonal similarities between human sexual response, un-drugged birth and the let-down reflex in breastfeeding (Newton 1978). Newton suggested that all three processes were mediated by oxytocin, and that the pleasurable feelings they promoted had evolved to ensure the continuation of the species. Newton also observed that each could be inhibited by environmental disturbances, which she explored in a series of elegant experiments on mice (Newton et al 1966).

Newton randomly selected labouring mice from a laboratory mouse population and moved them from their secure nest into the hostile environment of a nest containing bedding contaminated with cat urine. She then compared the length of labour for each group of mice and found that the disturbed mice had longer labours, to the point where many did not give birth until moved back into their safe nest. Significantly fewer mice gave birth in the hostile environment. What was even more disturbing was that the newborn pups of the disturbed mice were more likely to be found dead soon after birth, suggesting that fetal damage had occurred in utero. Newton hypothesised that fear generated by the hostile environment had disturbed the production of oxytocin, slowed labour and interfered with the supply of blood to the uterus. She questioned whether the same mechanism might operate in labouring women subjected to the variations between home and hospital environments.

Newton's work offers much support for the fear cascade, at least in mice. Other research conducted with rhesus monkeys also adds some weight to the case for a fear cascade (Adamsons et al, cited in Rowley 1998). Adamsons and colleagues were also interested in the role of catecholamines and uterine blood flow. They discovered that catecholamines such as adrenaline injected directly into the fetus of a pregnant rhesus monkey had no effect on the fetus other than raising its heart rate. However, when catecholamines were injected into the mother, fetal asphyxia and acidosis could be induced, and it was postulated that this was due to the vasoconstrictor effect of catecholamines leading to impaired uterine blood flow.

There is now much more evidence concerning the impact of fear on the physiology of pregnancy in human studies, including those using ultrasound to examine uterine artery resistance in response to maternal anxiety (Teixeira et al 1999). It is now possible to demonstrate that maternal anxiety increases the uterine artery resistance index, and reduces blood flow to the baby, affecting fetal development and leading to small-for-gestational-age infants and the possibility of premature birth. All of these studies offer support for the fear cascade and suggest a role for reducing maternal anxiety through ensuring undisturbed labour as an essential

---

Reflective exercise

Take a careful look at the birth spaces in your local unit and ask yourself the following questions.

1. Can women labour *undisturbed* in this environment?
2. How can I ensure that no one disturbs the woman unnecessarily?
3. Am I disturbing her by talking too much?
4. Is there a sign on the door asking people to knock and wait for a reply if they want to come in?
5. Do unknown staff walk in unannounced?
6. Are there locks on the door?
7. Can we hear the woman next door giving birth?
8. How private is the space?
9. Who 'owns' the space when a woman is in labour and giving birth here?
10. Is the woman free to move around—to sit, stand, walk, squat, lean, lie down?
11. Are there en suite facilities for her to shower or use a bath during labour or birth?
12. Where is the bed located and what kind of bed is it?
13. Is there a space for her family/support people?
14. How welcoming is it for them?
15. Are food and drink available?
    - Is there a need to change anything?
    - How can I do that?
    - Who will help me?

aspect of keeping birth normal. Continuity of care that also includes one-to-one support throughout labour provides one way of achieving this. What 'support' should entail is well described in *The Labor Progress Handbook* by Simkin and Ancheta (2001), which provides midwives with a myriad of practical and seemingly simple ways to apply this theoretical understanding to clinical practice. The reader is urged to find a copy of this valuable publication and to share it with women and colleagues alike.

Continuity of care provides opportunities for a close and trusting relationship to develop between the woman and her midwife. Continuous one-to-one support in labour provides an opportunity to ensure that labour is undisturbed and the fear cascade is not initiated (Buckley 2003). Adding this component to the package that already includes a familiar or home-like place for birth increases the likelihood that birth will be normal. However, there is one other component of the package that appears to be essential—the belief in birth as a normal physiological process.

Belief in birth as a normal physiological process

A recent study conducted by one of the authors (MH) in New Zealand provides important insights into the power of the place of birth to influence the midwife's belief in birth as a normal physiological process (Hunter 2000, 2003). In a series of in-depth interviews conducted with caseloading midwives who cared for women in both large (secondary/tertiary) and small (primary) maternity facilities, Hunter discovered that the midwives overwhelmingly preferred to provide labour care in small maternity units, where they felt they were more able to attend to women, as opposed to attending to machines, and where they had developed additional midwifery skills. This they named as practising 'real midwifery'. In the small unit, the midwives felt truly autonomous, able to take time to let labour unfold rather than rush women along as if on a conveyor belt, able to give the woman time to settle into her labour before intruding with a vaginal examination to assess progress, and more able to tolerate the woman making noise without fear that they would be regarded as a less than competent midwife. Importantly, the midwives revealed how the additional responsibility of being alone in the small unit caused them to reflect carefully on their skills and ability to manage any challenge, keeping them alert and watchful. Despite the additional responsibility and feeling that they would 'carry the can' if anything went wrong, they were unshaken in their belief in the normal process of birth and had the confidence to enable the process to occur with minimal intervention. Hunter (2003) proposed that the following skills are necessary for midwives who practise in primary maternity units:

- the confidence to provide intrapartum care in a low-technology setting
- being comfortable with using embodied knowledge and

skills to assess a woman and her baby, as opposed to using technology
- being able to let labour 'be' and not interfere unnecessarily
- the confidence to avert or manage problems that might arise
- the confidence to trust the process of labour and be flexible with respect to time
- being willing to employ other options to manage pain, without access to epidurals
- being solely responsible for outcomes without access to on-site specialist assistance
- being a midwife who enjoys practising 'real midwifery'.

'Real midwifery' was articulated by one of the participants, named Elizabeth, as follows:

> At [the small maternity unit] it's like real midwifery in a way, because you're not interfering . . . When you are using the synto and the epidural, a lot of it's taken away from the woman and, in a lot of respects, probably taken away from you a little bit as well.
>
> . . . I think with real midwifery, a lot of it is not doing, in a way letting it happen, being there, but you're still there and you still want to make sure that things are happening as they should . . . And I think real midwifery can be not being that overpowering person there.

Midwives in primary maternity units need to have a belief in normal birth and the skills to be unobtrusive while still ensuring that labour is progressing normally. Women also need to believe that they are able to labour and give birth in a primary facility (Coyle et al 2001). Antenatal visits and childbirth education classes held at primary units generally foster women's confidence and enhance their commitment to labouring in a primary facility. In this study the midwives endeavoured to influence women with regard to place of birth, as evidenced by the following words from one of the participants:

> With first-time mums when they come to me, we talk about who has actually influenced them into thinking they need to be at a large hospital. We talk about the statistics that show women are actually safer in a smaller hospital, and a good percentage of them will end up coming to the smaller hospital (Rosemary).

Rosemary could be referring to a number of studies, including a landmark study undertaken by Rosenblatt and colleagues (1985), which showed that New Zealand women had good outcomes in primary facilities and that such facilities had an important place within a population that is dispersed throughout urban and remote rural areas.

Being confident to provide intrapartum care in a low-technology setting

Most of the participants interviewed stated that they were proficient with the technology in the large hospital. Yet they preferred practising in primary units, where there is low use of technology. Participant Elizabeth emphasises this point:

> The technology has got its place. I can go from having a woman on a syntocinon infusion and an epidural pump, to the next day,

at the small unit, and the woman is squatting in the corner, or whatever, and it is totally different.

For the midwife, being hands-off and just being there for the woman is often more challenging than being constantly busy attending to equipment and machines.

Being comfortable to use embodied knowledge and skills to assess a woman and her baby, as opposed to using technology

The ability to be attuned to embodied knowledge grows with midwifery experience, and includes the ability to listen to one's gut feelings. Using embodied knowledge does not preclude the use of technology. For example, the woman might elect to have the fetal heart monitored by Doppler to enable flexibility with positions during labour. The use of the Pinard stethoscope might require her to change position to enable the baby's heart sounds to be heard. A waterproof Doppler is a useful tool when the woman elects to have a water birth, as this enables her to remain in the water as long as she chooses.

There are times during a woman's labour when the midwife needs to step back and acknowledge the feelings and signals that arise from her own body. Embodied knowledge recognises that the mind and body are inextricably linked. Guiver (2004) undertook a grounded theory study about midwifery knowledge in relation to normal birth. Participants talked about their gut instinct, which assisted them as midwives to know whether the labour was normal. Participants in Hunter's (2000) study stated that over-use of equipment and machines meant less use of the midwife's internal senses. One participant said that switching on the cardiotocograph machine was almost simultaneous with switching off her own assessment skills related to fetal wellbeing. Another spoke of how mild tachycardia may indicate that something could be astray.

The following examples show midwives using their own assessment skills and knowledge:

> You need your eyes and your hands more than any equipment. That will tell you more than any monitors. In the large hospital you're actually thinking more in the high risk, using all the instrumentation you have, or all the technology, rather than using your own ideas or what you are seeing yourself (Cluain Meala).

> When the woman's lying there with her epidural, you're watching machines. Whereas, at the small unit, it's sort of like watching and waiting . . . and you have to have confidence in women's bodies just to let it flow (Bronnie).

The midwives talk of using their hands, eyes and own ideas through observation with the woman, as opposed to a total reliance upon equipment. Observations might entail watching and waiting. The midwife needs to have confidence that the labour will flow and progress normally. Experienced midwives know that the art of palpating contractions provides a vast amount of information, including the strength and characteristics of contractions. This is in contrast with the limited diagrammatic representation of contractions on cardiotocograph machines, which really only show the frequency of contractions.

Being able to let labour 'be' and not interfere unnecessarily

Midwives described 'real midwifery' as 'being there and letting it happen'. Sometimes it consists of 'not doing' and just letting the labour unfold. But the midwife is always watching to make sure things are progressing, without being obtrusive. Working in primary units and attending home births fosters learning about real midwifery and fosters confidence in one's own practice. High-technology settings might hinder the development of low-technology midwifery skills. Other participants echo Bronnie's words of being able to 'go with the flow' of labour in small units:

> Looking after women in the small units, there is this expectation of going with the flow. I think you have to believe that birth is normal and that women's bodies are built for the job and the majority of births are normal (Kirsty).

> You need confidence in birth as being normal and I think it's something that grows. When you leave someone alone and don't interfere, then the risk of a problem is even less (Joyce).

Being able to let labour 'be' requires a belief in normal birth and the ability to care for women without intervening unnecessarily. Guiver (2004) criticised the rhetoric that birth is only normal in hindsight and stated that birth without interventions is eminently possible with midwife-led care and a faith in normal birth.

Being confident to trust the process of labour and be flexible with respect to time

Midwives opposed the discourse of a fixed time frame for women in labour. One way in which midwives showed flexibility regarding time was through limited use of vaginal assessments. Midwives commented that an immediate vaginal assessment might not be necessary (at a primary unit) if you were very sure of presentation and engagement, if the woman was obviously contracting well and had not been in labour for too long, and if the fetal heart was normal and the woman did not want to know her dilatation:

> Sometimes women will request to have a VE just to reassure them that they are actually in established labour. I'll probably do a VE then, but if they don't request one, I'll just sit and watch for a couple of hours (Rosemary).

Coyle et al (2001) showed that women appreciated a non-interventionist approach, such as midwives keeping vaginal examinations to a minimum. In order to do this, midwives need to be adept at palpation of the presenting part, and descent and flexion of the head (Sookho & Biott 2002). Midwives also need to be willing to silently pose the question: Is it a head or could it be a breech? The presentation of the baby assumes more importance in free-standing primary units, where it might take several hours to transfer a woman with a breech presentation diagnosed in labour.

Midwives also stressed the importance of continuity of care and mutual trust where women stayed at home until labour was well established. When a woman telephoned the midwife in early labour, the midwife might offer to attend the woman at home and undertake an initial assessment that might or might not include a vaginal examination. This process reassured the woman and the midwife that labour had started, and progress was likely as the hours unfolded. The midwives placed great importance on education antenatally about the latent stage of labour and the time needed for the cervix to efface:

> This first-time mum that I am thinking of, she did have a long labour in the small unit—20 hours. It's a balance between the woman feeling relaxed in the small unit and maybe using the bath and knowing that she is coping, to going to the large hospital where we have got to use active management of labour (Kirsty).

Kirsty shows the art of midwifery in allowing the woman time, and the sense of not rushing or interfering. She also gave the woman the choice of remaining in the primary unit, as the woman and the baby were coping with the process of labour.

Most of the midwives who offered intrapartum care in small maternity units also offered women the option of having a home birth. There seemed to be similarities when the midwives described practising in small units and attending women for home birth:

> I just feel a little bit freer at the small maternity unit. It's like being at a home birth in a way really—not quite, but in a way it can be (Elizabeth).

Although all the midwives were autonomous lead maternity carers, they still felt compelled to 'do' when in a large obstetric hospital:

> The difference between a small and large hospital is that once you get into the large obstetric hospital, you feel like you've got a time frame to get out of there. Whereas, at the small unit, you don't want to interfere, you don't want to rush things (Bronnie).

The sense of a time frame appears to pervade the ambience of large obstetric hospitals and, in turn, even autonomous midwives are affected by the busyness of large hospitals and become acutely aware of time.

Being willing to employ other options to manage pain without access to epidurals

Managing pain during labour is a major challenge to women and midwives, and Leap (2000) has contributed her expertise to assist midwives. In primary maternity units, midwives have no access to epidural analgesia, and the midwives in the study preferred not to use pethidine analgesia. The key to managing pain was multifaceted, but one aspect was that the midwives tolerated noise from women during labour, as opposed to silencing them with analgesia. It is important that women are allowed to make noise during labour and to express their pain if this assists them to cope through each contraction.

Not having access to epidural analgesia taught participant Elizabeth how to work with women in labour. If epidural analgesia is on site, it is too easy to resort to this to relieve pain.

Midwives in primary facilities employed all the usual things like mobilisation, a hot pack on the woman's back, massage, homeopathy, shower, bath, pool, different positions, sitting on the toilet, rocking, squeezing the top of the hipbones and other manoeuvres. Being with the woman, going through every contraction with her, talking her through, were all viewed as methods of pain relief.

Practising as an independent midwife also changed how some of the midwives worked with women and their pain. A big difference in continuity of care is that the woman and the midwife know each other and therefore there is a sense of trust. The midwife is generally working on a one-to-one basis with that particular woman and is totally focused on her, as compared with being focused on the needs of a busy delivery unit. The 'education factor' that occurs antenatally enables a platform for working with women and their pain:

> I think that the support that you give women at one of these smaller units is more intensive. You know that if the woman has that support all the way through her labour, she is going to cope a little bit better (Rosemary).

As discussed earlier in this chapter, intensive support seems to be critical in assisting women to cope with their pain, along with trying a variety of strategies to meet the woman's needs. A calm environment creates the ambience for birth to proceed. Appropriate background music and the woman's family or supporters help to (re)create an atmosphere of normality and enable the woman to proceed with the birth process. Understanding the physiological impact of an epidural on the physiology of labour, and the potential long-term consequences of in utero exposure to narcotics for the baby may inspire both the woman and her midwife to work with the pain productively (Robinson 2001).

Being confident to avert or manage problems that might arise, and being solely responsible for outcomes without access to on-site specialist assistance

Situations arise in the course of midwifery practice where the midwife must promptly avert or manage problems. As practising midwives, we all carry memories of emergency occasions that we have been involved in and those that we have managed. It is important that practice is not coloured by a problem focus. However, our memory tends to occlude the numerous occasions when we have driven our car without incident, yet we vividly recall the one time that we had an accident. Midwives admitted that the responsibility for outcomes was greater when they practised intrapartum care in free-standing primary maternity units. Sometimes it would take hours before the woman was transferred via ambulance to the large hospital and assessed by a specialist obstetrician. In the interlude, it is the midwife who assesses the emergency situation, provides interim care and organises the urgent transfer to the large hospital.

In order to provide intrapartum care in primary units, midwives stressed the need for acute senses, awareness, alertness and the skills to react in a timely manner. A midwife in a primary unit has to know what to do immediately—there are no doctors to respond to an emergency bell.

The following participant gives an example of responding to an emergency situation:

> I had a postpartum haemorrhage the other night of 1000 ml in the small unit. I gave intramuscular syntometrine and intravenous syntocinon and I ended up putting up a drip. I knew the placenta was complete and knew the uterus wasn't contracting well. Her pulse didn't accelerate, her blood pressure never wavered, the blood had clotted; so she was able to stay there. So you just do what you would do. You don't wait and see (Mary).

Mary's assessment skills are evident in vocalising her actions. She had checked the placenta thoroughly and thus ruled out retained products. The woman had been administered two oxytocic drugs—intravenous syntocinon ensures rapid uterine contractility and intramuscular syntometrine is used to obtain a longer-acting contraction of the uterus. Mary then inserted an intravenous line to administer fluids and to provide access for an ongoing syntocinon infusion. She did not waste precious minutes trying to insert the intravenous line initially. A tourniquet can be applied to give rapid intravenous access for syntocinon administration. The woman's pulse did not accelerate and, hence, Mary was reassured that the woman was not becoming hypovolaemic and potentially shocked.

Are all midwives practising real midwifery?

In a survey administered to midwives who were not already working in a midwifery-run unit in the United Kingdom, Symon (1998) asked midwives if they would be happy to do so, taking full responsibility for a woman's care. Replies were received from 1522 midwives. The majority of midwives (76%) stated that they would happily do so, and 24% said they would not. Midwives with more than twenty years of experience, and those working in units with 2000 to 2999 deliveries per year were least likely to say 'yes'. Reasons for not wanting to work in a midwifery-run unit included: preference for consultant cover and full facilities; not having enough experience (although most of these midwives had twenty or more years' experience!); not having enough confidence; fear of complications; and fear of litigation. Symon (1998) reported the following comments from a midwife participant:

> I strongly believe that these units are an excellent means by which midwives (particularly junior ones) can develop their true midwifery skills and practice—working in an obstetric or consultant unit should be seen as a different type of practice altogether. Many of today's midwives do not seem to know the difference or care for that matter (p 45).

Graham (1997) indicated that it might be a certain type of midwife who prefers to work in settings away from the dominance of obstetricians:

> It is intuitively obvious that systems of care which give the practitioner more independence in decision making, a homely environment in which to work, continuity of involvement with women, and a focus on normality and natural childbirth will attract particular individuals (p 396).

These statements suggest that 'true' midwifery skills develop best when a midwife practises in small maternity units, whereas a different type of practice is apparent in a consultant obstetric unit. Graham concluded that more independence and a focus on normality might be more enjoyable for some midwives. It seems likely that the midwives' personal beliefs and length of time practising in a large hospital influence their choice of venue for provision of intrapartum care. There was an inverse relationship between the desire to practise in a small maternity unit and the number of years of experience the midwife had in practising in a large hospital.

Is it possible to practise real midwifery in a large hospital?

Kirkham (2003) argues that the birth centre is the place where 'the complex skills underpinning normal birth can be developed, nurtured and learned' (p 12). Whether the birth centre needs to be free-standing or whether these same skills can be nurtured in a birth centre that is part of a hospital remains to be seen (Johanson & Newburn 2001). As a space between home and hospital, birth centres may offer the greatest opportunity for both women and midwives

---

Reflective exercise

Think about the hospital labour ward with which you are most familiar and imagine that you are greeting a woman in early labour who has never been here before. Ask yourself the following questions.

1. What makes this place familiar to me—is it the smell when I walk in the door? Do I even notice it any more? I wonder what it smells like to this woman—safe and comforting, or antiseptic and scary?

2. I wonder what it sounds like to her. Is it noisy right now? What kinds of noises are there— clanking sounds of metal on metal and harsh surfaces, lots of voices, telephones and beeping machinery?

3. What does it look like—bright lights, bright, busy people, paperwork on the desk, equipment lining the corridor, signs on the wall, businesslike, efficient? Is this comforting to her? I wonder how her family (who are with her) feel right now.

4. What do I see when we walk into her room together? I wonder what she sees first and what impression it has on her and how she feels.

Remember, 'environment' encompasses all five senses—sight, hearing, touch, taste and smell—and each of these senses has an impact on the mind and heart, and therefore the physiology of childbirth.

- Is there a need to change anything?
- How can I do that?
- Who will help me?

to rediscover a profound belief in the inherently normal physiological process of birth. As with birth at home, birth centres are founded on a belief in the normality of birth, which appears to be the most influential aspect of the birth environment to consider.

Global strategies to centralise childbirth into large tertiary centres on the grounds of safety pose a serious threat not only to homebirth and birth centres but also to rural communities, who are faced with the loss of primary maternity units as locations for birth. The challenge facing maternity services today in countries like Australia and New Zealand is how to balance the need for safety with the preservation of primary-level birth facilities. A recent population-based Australian study of all women who gave birth from 1999 to 2001 showed that for low-risk women, small maternity units were not associated with higher rates of perinatal mortality, regardless of parity (Tracy et al 2006).

Conclusion

The three components of women's care that were lost when the place of birth changed from home to hospital were the familiar environment, the close personal and trusting relationship with a midwife who provided continuous care throughout labour, and a strong belief in the normal physiology of birth. All three components of the care 'package' function together, to keep birth normal. The environment for birth not only includes the geographical space where the event will unfold, but is influenced by less visible but no less powerful forces that include relationships with midwives and the beliefs, knowledge and skills they bring to practising real midwifery. The challenge for all midwives is to consider these three elements in their own practice location.

Review questions

1   What does the theoretical model known as the fear cascade contribute to our understanding of how the place of birth affects birth outcomes?

2   What role(s) does oxytocin play in birth outcomes?

3   What were the reasons for women moving from home to hospital at the turn of the twentieth century?

4   Why do different accounts of childbirth explain these events differently?

5   How similar are the childbirth histories of women and midwives in New Zealand and Australia?

6   What three things were lost when women moved from home to hospital for birth?

7   What are the potential consequences of intervention in childbirth?

8   How many women choose home birth in Australia or New Zealand?

9   Do midwives and other providers enable 'choice' for women regarding place of birth?

10 What midwifery skills are needed in order to provide care to women either at home or in primary maternity settings?

Notes

1 These terms are used interchangeably, and mean a low-technology maternity facility that does not have available epidural analgesia, operating theatres for caesarean section or on-site obstetricians, anaesthetists or paediatricians.

2 Pakeha refers to the non-Maori population of New Zealand.

3 Grace Neill was a Scottish-trained nurse and midwife who was the Chief Inspector of Hospitals in New Zealand at the turn of the twentieth century.

4 This trend was not statistically significant but has been used to discredit birth centre care and has since been critiqued by Fahy and Colyvas (2005) as having several methodological flaws.

Online resources

Website addresses are subject to change. We recommend that you try the following addresses, which were current at the time of writing. Use a search engine for locating additional sites. Search with terms including 'normal birth', 'physiological birth' and 'home birth' to gain further reading.

Active Birth Centre, http://www.activebirthcentre.com

Australian College of Midwives, http://www.acmi.org.au

Birth Works/Primal Health Research, http://www.birthworks.org/primalhealth

Friends of the Birth Centre, http://www.fbc.org.au

Home Birth Reference Site, http://www.homebirth.org.uk

Lactation Education Resources (LER), http://www.leron-line.com

LER article on pacifiers, http://www.leron-line.com/updates/Pacifiers.htm

List of references on the safety of home birth, http://www.changesurfer.com/Hlth/homebirth.html

New Zealand College of Midwives, http://www.midwife.org.nz

Penny Simkin website, http://www.pennysimkin.com

Royal College of Midwives, http://www.rcm.org.uk

Waterford Birth Centre, http://www.riverridge.co.nz

References

Adcock W, Bayliss U, Butler M et al 1984 With courage and devotion. A history of midwifery in New South Wales. Sydney: New South Wales Midwives Association

Annandale E 1988 How midwives accomplish natural birth: managing risk and balancing expectations. Social Problems 32(2):95–110

Archives New Zealand: Health—Nursing Division—Mary Lambie Collection, Series 11, Accession W2615. Archives New Zealand/Te Rua Mahara o te Kawanatanga. Wellington Office

Bahl R, Strachan B, Murphy D 2004 Outcome of subsequent pregnancy three years after previous operative delivery in the second stage of labour: Cohort study. British Medical Journal 328(311):doi:10.1136/bmj.37942.546076.546044

Bastian H, Keirse MJ 1998 Perinatal death associated with planned home birth in Australia: population based study. British Medical Journal 317(7155):384–388

Beech BL 1998 Drugs in pregnancy and labour—what effects will they have twenty years hence? AIMS UK Occasional Paper

Biro MA, Waldenstrom U, Brown S 2003 Satisfaction with team midwifery care for low- and high-risk women: a randomized controlled trial. Birth 30(1):1–10

Buckley S 2003 Undisturbed birth: nature's blueprint for ease and ecstasy. Journal of Perinatal Psychology and Health 17(4): 261–288

Carter J, Johanson R, Heycock E et al 2001 Long-term health after childbirth. British Journal of Midwifery 9(12):748–753

Chamberlain G 2000 Choosing between home and hospital delivery. British Medical Journal 320(March):798

Chamberlain G, Wraight A, Crowley P 1997 Home births: the report of the 1994 confidential enquiry by the National Birthday Trust Fund. Parthenon, London

Conference Reports 2001 Keeping birth normal: the art and the science. The Practising Midwife (4)11:38–39

Coyle K, Hauck Y, Percival P et al 2001 Normality and collaboration: mother's perceptions of birth centre versus hospital care. Midwifery 17:182–193

DiMatteo MR, Morton SC, Lepper HS et al 1996 Cesarean childbirth and psychosocial outcomes: a meta-analysis. Health Psychology 15(4):303–314

Donley J 1986 Save the midwife. New Women's Press, Auckland

Ehrenreich B, English D 1973 Witches, midwives, and nurses: a history of women healers. Old Westbury, Feminist Press, New York

Fahy K, Colyvas K 2005 Safety of the Stockholm Birth Centre Study: a critical review. Birth32(2):145–150

Fisher K, Foureur M, Hawley J 2004 Maternity services and gynaecology report 2003. Capital and Coast District Health Board, Wellington, New Zealand

Forster F 1965 Mrs Howlett and Dr Jenkins: Listerism and early midwifery practice in Australia. Medical Journal of Australia, 11(26):1047–1054

Foureur M 2002 The midwife as ontological architect. Paper presented at the 26th ICM Triennial Conference, Vienna, Austria

Ginesi L, Niescierowicz R 1998a Neuroendocrinology and birth 1: Stress. British Journal of Midwifery 6(10):659–663

Ginesi L, Niescierowicz R 1998b Neuroendocrinology and birth 2: The role of oxytocin. British Journal of Midwifery 6(12):791–796

Gottvall K, Grunewald C, Waldenstrom U 2004 Safety of birth centre care:perinatal mortality over a 10 year period. British Journal of Obstetrics and Gynaecology 111:71–78

Gottvall K, Waldenstrom U 2002 Does a traumatic birth experience have an impact on future reproduction? British Journal of Obstetrics and Gynaecology 109:254–260

Graham I 1997 Episiotomy: challenging obstetric intervention. Blackwell Science, London

Griew K 2003 Birth centre midwifery down under. In M Kirkham (ed) Birth centres: a social model for maternity care. Elsevier Science, London

Guilliland K 2005 Do women want midwives? Midwives and the New Zealand Maternity system in 2005. Proceedings, International Confederation of Midwives Conference, Brisbane. CD-ROM

Guiver D 2004 Epistemological foundation of midwife-led care that facilitates normal birth. Evidence-based Midwifery 2(1):28–34

Hodnett E 2004, 13 July 2001 Home-like versus conventional institutional settings for birth. Cochrane Review

Hunter M 2000 Autonomy, clinical freedom and responsibility: the paradoxes of providing intrapartum midwifery care in a small maternity unit as compared with a large obstetric hospital. Unpublished MA thesis, Massey University, Palmerston North, New Zealand

Hunter M 2003 Autonomy, clinical freedom and responsibility. In M Kirkham (ed) Birth centres: a social model for maternity care. Elsevier Science, London

Jacobsen B, Bygdeman M 1998 Obstetric care and proneness of offspring to suicide as adults: Case-control study. British Journal of Medicine 317:1346–1349

Jacobsen B, Nyberg K, Grondbladh L et al 1990 Opiate addiction in adult offspring through possible imprinting after obstetric treatment. British Journal of Medicine 301(76):364–371

Johanson R, Newburn M 2001 Promoting normality in childbirth. British Medical Journal 323:1142–1143

Johanson R, Newburn M, Macfarlane A 2002 Has the medicalisation of childbirth gone too far? British Medical Journal 324:892–895

Johnson KC, Daviss BA 2005 Outcomes of planned homebirths with certified professional midwives: large prospective study in North America. British Medical Journal 330:1416–1423

Kirkham M 2003 Birth centres: a social model for maternity care. Elsevier Science, London

Kitson A, Harvey G, McCormack B 1998 Enabling the implementation of evidence based practice: a conceptual framework. Quality in Health Care 7:149–158

Laws P, Sullivan E 2004 Australia's mothers and babies 2002. AIHW Cat. No. PER 28. AIHW National Perinatal Statistics Unit, Sydney

Laws P, Sullivan E 2005 Australia's mothers and babies 2003. AIHW Cat. No. PER 29. Australian Institute of Health and Welfare, Maternal Perinatal Statistics Unit, Sydney

Leap N 2000 The less we do, the more we give. In M Kirkham (Ed) The midwife–mother relationship. McMillan Press, London pp. 1–18

Lepori B 1994 Freedom of movement in birth places. Children's Environments 11(2):81–87

Loudon I 1992 Death in childbirth. An international study of maternal care and maternal mortality 1800–1950. Clarendon Press, Oxford

Macfarlane A, McClandish R, Campbell R 2000 There is no evidence that hospital is the safest place to give birth. British Medical Journal 320:798

Mantell CD, Craig ED, Stewart AW et al 2004 Ethnicity and birth outcome: New Zealand trends 1980–2001. Part 2, Pregnancy outcomes for Maori women. Australian and New Zealand Journal of Obstetrics and Gynaecology 44:537–540

Mayberry L, Clemmens D, De A 2002 Epidural analgesia side

effects, co-interventions, and care of women during childbirth: a systematic review. American Journal of Obstetrics and Gynecology 186(5):S81–S93

Mein Smith P 1986 Maternity in dispute. Government Printer, Wellington, New Zealand

Ministry of Health 2002 Maternity services consumer satisfaction survey 2002. Ministry of Health, New Zealand

Naaktgeboren C 1989 The biology of childbirth. In I Chalmers, M Enkin, MJ Keirse (Eds) Effective care in pregnancy and childbirth. (Vol. 1) Oxford University Press, Oxford

National Institute for Clinical Excellence 2004 Caesarean section clinical guideline. NICE UK

Newburn M 2003 Culture, control and the birth environment. The Practising Midwife 6(8):20–25

Newton N 1978 The role of oxytocin reflexes in three interpersonal reproductive acts: coitus, birth and breastfeeding. Paper presented at the Clinical Psychoneuroendocrinology in Reproduction: Proceedings of the Serono Symposia

Newton N, Foshee D, Newton M 1966 Parturient mice: effects of environment on labor. Science 151:1560–1561.

New Zealand Health Information Service (NZHIS) 2003 Report on maternity 2000 & 2001. Ministry of Health, Wellington

New Zealand Health Information Service (NZHIS) 2004 Report on maternity 2002. Ministry of Health, Wellington

New Zealand Health Information Service (NZHIS) 2005 Draft report on maternity 2003. Ministry of Health, Wellington

Olsen O, Jewell MD 1998 Home versus hospital birth. The Cochrane Database of Systematic Reviews 1998 Issue 3. Art. No.:CD000352. DOI:10.1002/14651858.CD000352

Page L 2002 Building for a better birth. British Journal of Midwifery 10(9):536, 538

Pairman S, Guilliland K 2003 Developing a midwife-led maternity service: the New Zealand experience. In M Kirkham (ed) birth centres: a social model for maternity care. Books for Midwives: Elsevier Science, London

Roberts CL, Tracy S, Peat B 2000 Rates for obstetric intervention among private and public patients in Australia: population based descriptive study. British Journal of Medicine 321:137–141

Robinson J 2001 Drugged babies are still becoming addicted adults. British Journal of Midwifery 9(2):90

Rooks J, Weatherby N, Ernst E et al 1989 Outcomes of care in birth centres: the national birth centre study. The New England Journal of Medicine 321(26):1804–1811

Rosenblatt RA, Reinken J, Shoemack P 1985 Regionalisation of obstetric and perinatal care in New Zealand: a health service analysis. Unpublished report for the New Zealand Government

Rowley MJ 1998 Evaluation of team midwifery care in pregnancy and childbirth: a randomised controlled trial. Unpublished PhD Thesis, University of Newcastle, Newcastle NSW

Rowley MJ, Hensley MJ, Brinsmead MW et al 1995 Continuity of care by a midwife team versus routine care during pregnancy and birth: a randomised trial. The Medical Journal of Australia 163(September):289–293

Sandall J 2004 Normal birth: a public health issue. The Practising Midwife 7(1):4–5

Shephard E 1989 The midwives of Rosewood. Wagga Wagga, Pioneer Women's Hut, NSW

Shephard E 1991 The midwives of Tumbarumba. Wagga Wagga, Pioneer Women's Hut, NSW

Shorter E 1983 A history of women's bodies. A Lane, London

Simkin P, Ancheta R 2001 The labor progress handbook. Blackwell Science, Oxford

Sookho ML, Biott C 2002 Learning at work: midwives judging progress in labour. Learning in Health and Social Care 1(2):75–85

Strid J 2000 Revitalising partnership. A consumer perspective. NZCOM Conference, Waikato, 2000

Symon A 1998 Litigation. The views of midwives and obstetricians. Hochland, Hochland, Hale, England

Teixeira JMA, Fisk N, Glover V 1999 Association between maternal anxiety in pregnancy and increased uterine artery resistance index: Cohort-based study. British Journal of Medicine 318:153–157

Tew M 1990 Safer childbirth? A critical history of maternity care (1st edn). Chapman & Hall, London

Tew M 1995 Safer childbirth? A critical history of maternity care (2nd edn). Chapman & Hall, London

Tracy SK, Tracy MB 2003 Costing the cascade: estimating the cost of increased obstetric intervention in childbirth using population data. British Journal of Obstetrics and Gynaecology 110(8): 295–300

Tracy SK, Dahlen H, Wang A et al 2006 Does size matter? A population-based study of birth in lower volume maternity hospitals for low risk women. British Journal of Gynaecology113(1):86–97

Vose C 2003 The nature of natural birthing. The Chemical Symphony of Birth. Byronchild 4(Dec–Feb)

Waldenstrom U, Nilsson C, Winbladh B 1997 The Stockholm birth centre trial: maternal and infant outcomes. British Journal of Obstetrics and Gynaecology 104:410–418

Waldenstrom U, Turnbull D 1998 A systematic review comparing continuity of midwifery care with standard maternity services. British Journal of Obstetrics and Gynaecology 105(11):1160–1170

Walsh D 2004 Birth centres unsafe for primigravidae. British Journal of Midwifery 12(4):206

Walsh D 2006 Subverting the assembly line: childbirth in a freestanding birth centre. Social Science and Medicine 62:1330–1340

Walsh D, Downe S 2004 Outcomes of free-standing, midwife-led birth centers: a structured review. Birth 31(3):222

Walsh D, El-Nemer A, Downe S 2004 Risk, safety and the study of physiological birth. In S Downe (Ed) Normal childbirth: evidence and debate. Churchill Livingstone, London

Willis E 1989 Medical dominance. Allen and Unwin Australia, Sydney

Wilson A 1995 The making of man—midwifery. UCL Press, London

Wood PJ, Foureur M 2005 Integrating research perspectives: a New Zealand maternity archive, 1907–1922. In B Mortimer, S McGann (Eds) New directions in the history of nursing. Routledge Research, Studies in the Social History of Medicine Series, Routledge, London

Young G, Hey E 2000 Choosing between home and hospital delivery. British Medical Journal 320(798):7237

Further reading

Angier N 1999 Women: an intimate geography. Virago Press, New York

Beech BL 1998 Drugs in pregnancy and labour—what effects will they have in twenty years hence? Paper presented at the AIMS UK, UK

Bistoletti P, Nylund L, Lagercrantz H et al 1983 Fetal scalp catecholamines during labour. American Journal of Obstetrics and Gynecology 147(7):785–788

Brudenell I 1996 A grounded theory of balancing alcohol recovery and pregnancy. Western Journal of Nursing Research 18(4):429

Buckley S 2001 Giving birth. The endocrinology of ecstasy. Byronchild 11–20

Calhoun BC, Jennings BM, Peniston J et al 2000 Focused obstetrical clinic for active duty junior enlisted service women: model for improved outcomes. Military Medicine 165(1):45

Campbell ND 1998 States of secrecy: Women's crimes and the practices of everyday life. Journal of Women's History 10(3): 204

Capogna G, Celleno D, Tommasetti M 1989 Maternal analgesia and neonatal effects of epidural sufentanil for cesarean section. Regional Anesthesia 14(6):282–287

D'Alessio JG, Ramanathan J 1998 Effects of maternal anesthesia in the neonate. Seminars in Perinatology 22(5):350–362

Eberle RL, Norris MC 1996 Labour analgesia. A risk–benefit analysis. Drug Safety 14(4):239–251

Fisler RE, Cohen A, Ringer SA, Lieberman E 2003 Neonatal outcomes after trial of labor compared with elective repeat caesarean section. Birth 30(2):83–88

Gimpl G, Fahenholz F 2001 The oxytocin receptor system: structure, function and regulation. Physiological Review 81(2):629–683

Greenfield S 2000 Brain story. BBC Worldwide, London

Guze BH, Guze PA 1989 Psychotropic medication use during pregnancy. Western Journal of Medicine 151(3):296–298

Haire D 1980 Birth trauma and birth injury as contributing factors to subsequent criminal behaviour and violence. Commission on Crime Control and Prevention, San Francisco

Horosita M 2001 Women's account of emergency caesarean section. Hong Kong Journal of Gynaecology, Obstetrics and Midwifery 2(1):15

Jackson DJ, Lang JM, Swartz WH et al 2003 Outcomes, safety, and resource utilization in a collaborative care birth center program compared with traditional physician-based perinatal care. American Journal of Public Health 93(6):999

Jacobsen B, Bygdeman M 1998 Obstetric care and proneness of offspring to suicide as adults: case-controlled study. British Medical Journal (317):1346–1349

Jacobsen B, Eklund K, Hamberger L et al 1987 Perinatal origin of adult self-destructive behaviour. Acta Psychiatric Scandinavia (76):364–371

Jacobsen B, Nyberg K, Grondbladh L et al 1990 Opiate addiction in adult offspring through possible imprinting after obstetrical treatment. British Medical Journal (301):1067–1070

Le Doux J 1999 The emotional brain. Simon & Schuster, New York

Marchini G et al 1989 Physiological reactions during birth. Acta Paediatrica 89(9):1082–1086

Matthiesen AS, Ransjo-Arvidson AB, Nissen E et al 2001 Postpartum maternal oxytocin release by newborns: effects of infant hand massage and sucking. [comment] Birth 28(1):13–19

Miles MS, Holditch-Davis D 1995 Compensatory parenting: how mothers describe parenting their 3-year-old, prematurely born children. Journal of Paediatric Nursing 10(4):243–253

Nathanielsz PW 1992 Life before birth and a time to be born. Promethean Press, New York

Nikkola EM, Jahnukainen TJ, Ekblad UU et al 2000 Neonatal monitoring after maternal fentanyl analgesia in labor. Journal of Clinical Monitoring and Computing 16(8):597–608

Nyberg K, Allebeck P, Eklund G et al 1992 Socio-economic versus obstetric risk factors for drug addiction in offspring. British Journal of Addiction 87:1669–1676

Odent M 1999 The scientification of love. Free Association Press, London

Pajulo M, Savonlahti E, Piha J 1999 Maternal substance abuse: infant psychiatric interest. A review and hypothetical model of interaction. American Journal of Drug and Alcohol Abuse 25(4):761

Patient C, Davison JM, Charlton L et al 1999 The effect of labour and maternal oxytocin infusion on fetal plasma oxytocin concentration. British Journal of Obstetrics and Gynaecology 106(12):1311–1313

Pert CB 1997 Molecules of emotion. Scribner, New York

Pinilla L, Gonzalez L, Tena-Sempere M et al 2001 Cross-talk between excitatory and inhibitory amino acids in the regulation of growth hormone secretion in neonatal rats. Neuroendocrinology [NLM – MEDLINE] 73(1):62

Raine A, Brennan P, Mednick S 1994 Birth complications combined with early maternal rejection at age 1 predisposes to violent crime at 18 years. Archives of General Psychiatry 51(12):984–988

Ransjo-Arvidson AB, Matthiesen AS, Lilja G et al 2001 Maternal analgesia during labor disturbs newborn behavior: effects on breastfeeding, temperature, and crying. [Comment] Birth 28(1):5–12

Raphael-Leff J 1991 Psychological processes of childbearing. Chapman & Hall, Kent

Rosenblatt DB, Belsey EM, Lieberman BA et al 1981 The influence of maternal analgesia on neonatal behaviour: II. Epidural bupivacaine. British Journal of Obstetrics and Gynaecology 88(4):407–413

Skolnick AA 1997 Lessons from US history of drug use. Journal of the American Medical Association 277(24):1919

Taylor G, Klein L, Lewis B et al 2000 Female responses to stress: tend and befriend, not flight or fight. Psychological Review 107(3):411–429

Uvas-Moberg K 1997 Physiological and endocrine effects of social contact. Annals of the New York Academy of Sciences 807(1): 146–163

Uvas-Moberg K 1998 Oxytocin may mediate the benefits of positive social interaction and emotions. Psychoneuroendocrinology 23(8):819–835

Waterstone M, Bewley S, Wolfe C 2001 Incidence and predictors of severe obstetric morbidity: case-control study. British Medical Journal 322:1089–1094

Welles B, Belfrage P, de Chateau P 1984 Effects of naloxone on newborn infant behavior after maternal analgesia with pethidine during labor. Acta Obstetricia et Gynecologica Scandinavica 63(7):617–619

Wiegers TA, Keirse MJNC, van der Zee J et al 1996 Outcome of planned home and planned hospital births in low risk women: a prospective study in midwifery practices in the Netherlands. British Medical Journal 313:1309–1313

Wittels B, Scott DT, Sinatra RS 1990 Exogenous opioids in human breast milk and acute neonatal neurobehavior: a preliminary study. Anesthesiology 73(5): 864–869

CHAPTER 7

Challenges to women's health

Caroline Homer

Key terms

alcohol, anxiety, bipolar disorder, blood-borne viruses, cannabis, chlamydia, depression, domestic violence, environmental tobacco smoke, family violence, female genital mutilation, fetal alcohol syndrome, genital herpes, gonorrhoea, hepatitis B, hepatitis C, heroin, HIV/AIDS, infibulation, legislation, mental health, methadone, schizophrenia, screening, smoking, smoking cessation programs, standard drink, STI, syphilis, universal precautions

Chapter overview

This chapter covers some of the main challenges for women during pregnancy. The following topics are discussed in detail as they are of particular relevance to midwives: mental health illnesses; smoking; alcohol and drug use; sexually transmitted diseases; blood-borne viruses; domestic violence; female genital mutilation. At the end of each topic is a critical thinking exercise and a reflective exercise. You are encouraged to undertake these as they will enhance your learning.

There are many other challenges to women's health that are of relevance to midwives. Some of these are addressed in other chapters. Others may not be directly addressed in this textbook; however, it is part of the responsibility of all midwives to learn how to seek information. Public libraries, the internet, hospital or university library databases and journals are all excellent sources of information.

Learning outcomes

Learning outcomes for this chapter are:

1 To describe the main mental health conditions and outline their effect on pregnancy

2 To describe the adverse effects related to smoking cigarettes in pregnancy

3 To describe the adverse effects related to environmental tobacco smoke on a newborn baby

4 To describe the adverse effects related to alcohol and drug use in pregnancy

5 To explain why it is advisable for women to be on methadone rather than heroin during pregnancy

6 To describe four main sexually transmitted infections, including signs and symptoms, diagnosis and management

7 To explain the risks, prevalence, effects and management of women with blood-borne viruses (HIV, hepatitis B, hepatitis C) during pregnancy

8 To compare the epidemiology and transmission rates of HIV and hepatitis C

9 To explain the prevalence of domestic violence and the specific adverse effects for women, babies and families

10 To assess some of the issues related to routine screening for domestic violence, and make suggestions for the practice setting

11 To discuss female genital mutilation (FGM) and the implications for women

12 To outline the main types of FGM and the implications for practice.

Mental health and pregnancy

Mental health disorders are common in women of childbearing age. This section discusses some of the effects of existing mental health disorders on pregnancy. Postnatal depression and psychosis are specific topics that are covered in detail in Chapter 37.

Anxiety disorders

Anxiety disorders include generalised anxiety disorder, obsessive compulsive disorder, social anxiety disorder, panic disorder, and phobias. In all of these there is an anxiety that is so overwhelming that it can interfere with a person's ability to function from day to day. A person may experience more than one anxiety disorder. Some may also experience depression with the anxiety, or have problems with alcohol or drug use (SANE Australia 2004a).

Anxiety disorders can emerge or re-emerge during pregnancy and there is an increased risk of susceptibility in the postnatal period (Altshuler et al 1998).

Initial management should include assessment, reassurance, support, cognitive behavioural therapy and social changes (Rampono 2004). Medications may be necessary if these strategies are ineffective.

Schizophrenia

Schizophrenia is a condition that affects the normal functioning of the brain, interfering with a person's ability to think, feel and act. Some people recover completely, and, with time, most find that their symptoms improve. For many, though, it is a prolonged illness that can involve years of distressing symptoms and disability (SANE Australia 2004b).

Women with schizophrenia do not have an increased risk of relapse during pregnancy if they are well before the pregnancy (Rampono 2004).

Bipolar mood disorder

Bipolar disorder is sometimes called 'manic-depression'. It affects the normal functioning of the brain, so that the person experiences extreme moods—very high and over-excited or very low and depressed. The person may be affected so much that he or she experiences the symptoms of psychosis, and is unable to distinguish what is real (SANE Australia 2004c).

Hormonal changes result in an increased risk of relapse of bipolar mood disorder during pregnancy and in the postpartum period (Rampono 2004). Little is known of the effects of bipolar disorder on pregnancy; however, the postnatal period is a time of highest risk. Postpartum relapse rates in women not treated with prophylactic mood stabilisers are 30% to 50%. Initiation of treatment with a mood stabiliser during pregnancy or immediately postpartum reduces this risk (Ward & Zamorski 2002).

The medications used to treat this disorder are complex, particularly in the first trimester. Lithium, the most commonly used medication, increases the risk of cardiovascular abnormalities in the baby. Other drugs used, such as sodium valproate and carbamazepine, are associated with spina bifida (Rampono 2004).

Women who are prescribed mood-stabilising medications should also be offered folate supplementation and prenatal screening for cardiac and neural tube defects, as indicated (Ward & Zamorski 2002).

Issues for midwives

Management of these complex mental health disorders falls beyond the scope of usual practice for midwives. Collaboration with mental health specialists, including psychiatrists, psychologists, mental health nurses and social workers, is essential to ensure that these women receive appropriate care and support. Decisions around the most appropriate management and medications need to be made with the woman and her family. Case conferences, where the woman and all those involved in her care help plan the management, are useful.

Achieving a balance between the usefulness and effectiveness of medications and the effects on the growing baby is sometimes very challenging for midwives and other clinicians. These decisions need to be made carefully in partnership with the woman and her family and the people involved in providing her care. A management plan is a useful way of disseminating this information to all concerned.

Midwives also need to ensure that women have appropriate support, especially in the postnatal period. Planning for this should occur during pregnancy and involve health and non-government organisations in partnership with the woman.

Critical thinking exercise

You are caring for a woman who tells you that she has anxiety about many issues in her life and was once labelled as having an anxiety disorder. She has never received any treatment for this; however, she seems very anxious during her pregnancy.

1 What other information should you try to obtain about this condition?
2 What resources might be useful?
3 What should be your management now?
4 What should you be putting in place for after the baby is born?

Reflective exercise

Take some time to reflect on your own experiences with mental health conditions, whether in a personal or professional capacity. How do you think your experiences might affect the way you practise and how you work in partnership with women?

Smoking and pregnancy

The relationship between smoking and pregnancy has been widely studied. Smoking during pregnancy and exposure to environmental tobacco smoke have serious health consequences for both mother and baby (English et al 1995; US Department of Health and Human Services 1990; Walsh et al 2001). Smoking in the second half of pregnancy poses the greatest risk to the health of both mother and baby. A summary of some of the negative outcomes is given in Table 7.1.

Fortunately, many of these outcomes are reasonably uncommon (e.g. placenta previa, SIDS), but the increased risks due to smoking remain a concern and are therefore important for midwives to consider carefully.

Rates of smoking in pregnancy

In one Australian state, the proportion of women smoking during pregnancy has decreased over the past five years. In 1998, almost 20% of women reported smoking in pregnancy. By 2002, the rate had decreased to 16%. Over the five-year period, among those who smoked in the second half of pregnancy, there was a trend towards smoking fewer cigarettes per day (NSW Health 2003). It is likely that these rates are similar to those reported in other Australian states and territories.

In Australia, Indigenous women have particularly high rates of smoking in pregnancy. In New South Wales in 2002, 58% of Aboriginal and Torres Strait Islander women reported smoking at some time during pregnancy, compared with 15% of non-Indigenous women (NSW Health 2003).

In New Zealand, the rates of smoking in pregnancy have also been higher in Indigenous than non-Indigenous women (Pakeha). For example, in 1999, one in two Maori women smoked during pregnancy, compared with one in four Pakeha (National Health Committee 1999).

TABLE 7.1 Estimated relative risk of negative outcomes associated with smoking in pregnancy

Negative outcomes	Relative risk (95% CI)
Spontaneous abortion	1.36 (1.32–1.40)
Ectopic pregnancy	1.46 (1.23–1.72)
Placental abruption	1.62 (1.46–1.77)
Placenta previa	1.58 (1.04–2.21)
Antepartum haemorrhage	1.62 (1.56–1.69)
Premature rupture of membranes	1.93 (1.79–2.08)
Low birthweight	2.04 (2.03–2.05)
Perinatal mortality	1.27 (1.21–1.32)
Sudden infant death syndrome	2.76 (2.66–2.86)
(Source: Walsh et al 2001)	

Environmental tobacco smoke

Exposure to environmental tobacco smoke (ETS), or passive smoking, also poses risks for pregnant woman and their babies. Children are especially vulnerable to passive smoking and it is a risk factor for SIDS (NHMRC 1997).

Women often receive advice during the antenatal period about smoking cessation, but their partners or others who live in their home are often not targeted for education. Research conducted in south-west Sydney indicated that almost none of the men attending antenatal classes had received quit smoking suggestions or advice (Mabbutt et al 2002).

Reducing smoking in pregnancy

Reducing smoking during pregnancy and exposure to ETS are important aims of antenatal care. Women are known to be more motivated to stop smoking during pregnancy and are usually in regular contact with health services and midwives (Moore et al 2002). Midwives are ideally placed to provide information and support around smoking cessation or reduction to women and their partners.

Smoking cessation programs

The most recent review in the Cochrane Library suggests that smoking cessation programs in pregnancy appear to reduce smoking, low birthweight and preterm birth, but no effect was detected for perinatal mortality (Lumley et al 2004).

'Social support is known to be an important determinant of success in smoking cessation efforts therefore … an intervention designed to increase support from a partner might lead to greater rates of successful smoking cessation' (Park et al 2004). Unfortunately, the systematic review of partner support interventions did not show an increase in quit rates and does not allow conclusions about the impact of partner support on smoking cessation (Park et al 2004).

Smoking cessation is much more complicated than merely presenting women or their partners with information, even at a time when they are probably most motivated to quit. As there is an association between social inequality and continued smoking (Oliver et al 2001), the social and cultural circumstances of women need to be considered when discussing smoking cessation in pregnancy.

Despite the challenges, the evidence in favour of routine discussions with pregnant women about smoking cessation is strong. The *Three Centres Consensus Guidelines on Antenatal Care* from Victoria in Australia recommend that smoking cessation interventions should be offered to all pregnant women who smoke or who have recently quit (Victorian Health 2001). The guidelines recommend that midwives and doctors ask women about their smoking at every antenatal visit and document this on the antenatal records. Women should be asked this question in an open-ended way, such as 'Can you tell me about your smoking?' rather than 'Do you smoke?', which will give a yes or no response.

A number of interventions have been shown to be effective once smoking is identified. These are outlined in the next section.

What works?

The review in the Cochrane Library suggests that multifaceted approaches—that is, more than one intervention—are the most effective (Lumley et al 2004). Table 7.2 summarises what is known about effective and ineffective quit smoking interventions for pregnant women (Walsh et al 2001).

Four main components of smoking cessation interventions are recommended (Walsh et al 2001): assessment, advice, assistance with quitting, and follow-up. These are outlined in Table 7.3. In New Zealand, the NZCOM provides training for midwives to assist pregnant women to change their smoking habits.

Nicotine replacement therapy, using gum and patches, is widely used in many non-pregnant populations. Some pregnant women will be using this as you can buy it over the counter in Australia and New Zealand. Its use in pregnancy, however, remains controversial as its safety is still under question. One trial of nicotine replacement therapy in pregnancy showed an overall reduction in quit rate that was the same for both intervention and placebo groups. The group who had the intervention, however, had a higher mean birthweight of 186 grams (Wisborg et al 2000).

TABLE 7.2 Effective and ineffective quit-smoking interventions for pregnant women	
	Intervention
Effective	Medical, midwifery, nursing or other counselling Self-help materials developed for the target population
Ineffective	Risk information alone Group behaviour therapy—very low attendance Self-help materials developed for different population
Insufficient evidence	Hypnosis Nicotine replacement therapy
Untested	Acupuncture Antidepressants Aversive smoking therapy
(Source: Walsh et al 2001)	

Clinical scenario

You are a midwife seeing a woman, Evelyn, for her first antenatal appointment. Evelyn is having her third baby. During the visit you find out that she smokes 10 to 20 cigarettes per day. She tells you that she did this with her other babies and there were no problems.

1 How would you discuss smoking in pregnancy with Evelyn?
2 What strategies would you use through her pregnancy in relation to her smoking?
3 How would you discuss the issue of smoking around a new baby?

TABLE 7.3 Four main components of smoking cessation interventions	
Component	**Suggested interventions**
Assessment	Avoiding questions about smoking that have simple 'yes/no' responses increases smoking disclosure.
Advice	Specific risk information tailored to the woman's current knowledge should be provided. Record in the clinical notes that advice to quit smoking has been provided.
Assistance	Check whether the woman has attempted to quit or is contemplating quitting. If she is not thinking about quitting, an attempt should be made to identify why and to respond and discuss this response. It may be necessary to dispel myths such as 'It will be easier to give birth to a smaller baby'. It is valuable to negotiate a target quit date as this seems to help people make a serious attempt to quit. Subsequent discussions should involve some behavioural tips. These need to be tailored to individual women. The five D's may be useful to use: • Delay—even for a short while • Drink water • Deep breathing • Do something different • Discuss your craving with another person. Involve the woman's partner and other members of her household in these discussions.
Follow-up	Ongoing discussions with women, reinforcing these behavioural tips, may be useful. Postnatal follow-up and discussion is also important to reduce ETS exposure for the baby.
(Source: Walsh et al 2001)	

Alcohol and pregnancy

Concerns about alcohol use in pregnancy and its effects on the baby have existed since Biblical times (O'Leary 2002). In the 1800s there were documented concerns that the children of alcoholic mothers were more likely to die prior to their second birthday than those of non-alcoholic women (Overholser 1990).

The first reported association between maternal alcoholism and a characteristic pattern of cranio-facial, limb and cardiovascular defects in the baby, which came to be known as fetal alcohol syndrome (FAS), was published in 1973 (Jones et al 1973). Since then there have been thousands of papers published that have raised concerns about the link between excessive alcohol consumption in pregnancy and FAS.

However, controversy surrounds the debate about what is considered 'excessive' alcohol intake and what quantity and frequency of consumption is required to produce adverse effects in babies (O'Leary 2002). This controversy comes from difficulties associated with measuring alcohol intake in pregnancy and making an accurate diagnosis.

Measuring and monitoring alcohol intake

Alcohol is measured in standard drinks and grams. A standard drink contains 10 grams of alcohol. One small glass of beer, wine, spirits or mixed drinks equals approximately one standard drink. Alcoholic cider and cans of premixed spirits equal at least one-and-a-half standard drinks (Alcohol Advisory Council of New Zealand 2004; National Alcohol Campaign 2002).

The *Australian Alcohol Guidelines* state that to minimise health risks, in both the short and the long term, and to gain any longer-term health benefits, the recommended alcohol intake for women (who are not pregnant or breastfeeding) is:

- no more than two standard drinks a day on average and
- no more than four standard drinks on any one day, and
- one or two alcohol-free days per week.

These guidelines are similar in New Zealand (Alcohol Advisory Council of New Zealand 2004).

Alcohol and adverse effects in pregnancy

The Royal College of Obstetricians and Gynaecologists in the United Kingdom has developed guidelines relating to the consumption of alcohol during pregnancy (Table 7.4).

Despite the lack of evidence at less than 12 standard drinks per week, it is recommended that women be careful about alcohol consumption in pregnancy and limit this to no more than one standard drink per day.

Fetal alcohol syndrome

A recent literature review on FAS provides evidence supporting the biological plausibility of alcohol as a teratogen and the link between excessive consumption of alcohol and FAS (O'Leary 2002). It is probably during the first eight weeks of the pregnancy that the primary teratogenic effects occur. Exposure later in pregnancy may affect growth and be associated with behavioural and cognitive disorders. The intellectual impairment associated with FAS is permanent, and FAS is now regarded as the leading preventable cause of non-genetic intellectual handicap (O'Leary 2002).

Overall, there appears to be no sound evidence that low levels of alcohol consumption produce FAS or other adverse effects.

The diagnosis of FAS can be difficult. This is because the syndrome can be easily confused with other disorders; there is no one clinical sign that will give the diagnosis and there is no laboratory test (O'Leary 2002). A paediatrician, preferably one with experience in this area, should make the diagnosis. Support and referral to such a health professional are the most appropriate strategies for the midwife to undertake.

Recommendations for practice

Asking women about their alcohol consumption during pregnancy is important. Women who disclose excessive

TABLE 7.4 Consumption of alcohol during g pregnancy	
Consumption of alcohol per week	**Adverse effects**
Consumption of 120gms (15 units) or more per week has been associated with a reduction in birthweight (Evidence Level III)	There are inconsistent data about the effect of social alcohol consumption on many pregnancy outcomes. Alcohol consumption of more than three drinks per week during the first trimester increases the risk of spontaneous abortion7 (O.R.=2.3; 95% C.I. ±1.1-4.5) but any effect on gestational length remains controversial. There is good evidence that social alcohol consumption does have a small negative effect on intrauterine fetal growth. Mills et al8 reported an 83gm decrement of birthweight per one to two drinks per day very similar to that found by Florey et al in the Euromac Study,9 i.e. a deficit of 66gms of birthweight per 120gms of alcohol (15 units) per week.
Consumption of 160gms (20 units) or more per week has been associated with intellectual impairment in children. (Evidence Level III)	Any impairment of neurodevelopment appears to occur at higher levels of alcohol consumption. The best information in this area comes from the Seattle Pregnancy and Health Study.10 The Seattle Group reported a decrement of five IQ points in children of mothers drinking greater than 250gms of alcohol per week, whilst at seven years of age, children of mothers drinking greater than 165gms per week had a decrement of seven IQ points. Other impairments included attention and memory deficits, arithmetic and reading difficulties.
There is no conclusive evidence of adverse effects in either growth or IQ at levels of consumption below 120gms (15 units) per week. Nonetheless it is recommended that women should be careful about alcohol consumption in pregnancy and limit this to no more than one standard drink per day. In pregnancy excessive alcohol consumers will require specific counselling and possible referral for specialist treatment. Clinics should consider providing a telephone contact number for women seeking advice and support for alcohol problems.	
Source: RCOG 1999. Reproduced from Alcohol consumption in pregnancy. Guideline no. 9, December 1999, with permission of the Royal College of Obstetricians and Gynaecologists.	

Clinical scenario

A woman you are seeing in the antenatal period tells you that she is having a couple of glasses of wine each night and a beer for lunch on the weekend. You need to work out how many grams of alcohol she is consuming per week. How would you do this? Look on the internet for descriptions of the Standard Drink to help you work it out.

Reflective exercise

Providing midwifery care to women who have problems with alcohol can often challenge our own values and beliefs. How do you feel when you see a pregnant woman drinking alcohol in a social situation? Reflect on your attitudes towards pregnant women drinking alcohol. How do you see these values affecting your capacity to provide midwifery care to these women?

If you are pregnant, or are planning to become pregnant:
- you should consider not drinking at all
- most importantly, you should never become intoxicated
- if you choose to drink, you should have less than 7 standard drinks over a week, AND no more than 2 standard drinks (spread over at least two hours) on any one day
- you should note that the risk is highest in the earlier stages of pregnancy, including the time from conception to the first missed period

The Consensus Statement produced by the NZ College of Midwives (NZCOM 2001) states that:

There is no known safe level of alcohol consumption during pregnancy. Therefore parents planning a pregnancy and women who are pregnant should be advised not to drink alcohol.

Other drugs and pregnancy

Other drugs of relevance to pregnant women include cannabis, heroin and methadone. Midwives need to have an understanding of the issues related to these drugs in pregnancy, and the referral networks and support groups that exist. An important principle in the care of women who use these drugs and others that may be harmful is to develop strong networks with other services and non-government organisations that work in this area. Midwives cannot, and should not, try to be experts in this area. It is our role to identify women with these issues and provide them with support to enable them to access

consumption should be supported and referred to specific counselling for specialist treatment. Antenatal services should provide a telephone contact number for women seeking advice and support for alcohol problems (RCOG 1999).

The *Australian Alcohol Guidelines* (National Alcohol Campaign 2002) state that:

other services and agencies who may be able to help. Other services will include drugs and alcohol networks, counsellors and peer support groups.

Cannabis

Cannabis comes from the *Cannabis sativa* plant. There are three main forms of cannabis: marijuana, hashish and hash oil.

Cannabis is a depressant drug. This class of drugs affects the central nervous system by slowing down the messages going to and from the brain to the body. Cannabis can also have mild hallucinogenic effects (Australian Drug Foundation 2003).

Little is known about the effects of cannabis on the unborn child. However, the use of cannabis during pregnancy is not recommended. If cannabis is used during pregnancy the baby may be low birthweight. Again, little is known about the effects of cannabis on breastfeeding. It is believed that some of the drug will pass through the breast milk to the baby, and the baby may become unsettled (Australian Drug Foundation 2003). The decision about whether to recommend that women who are smoking cannabis breastfeed depends on a number of factors. These include access to safe alternatives and the risks of not breastfeeding.

Heroin

Heroin is an 'opiate'. Other opiates include opium, morphine, codeine, pethidine and methadone. Pregnant women who are using heroin are encouraged to enter a methadone program as early as possible in their pregnancy. There are fewer complications associated with the use of methadone than with heroin in pregnancy (Australian Drug Foundation 2003). Reasons for this include the following:

- The unexpected periods of drug withdrawal experienced using other opiates (that can be harmful to the baby) do not occur when on a daily dose of methadone.

Critical thinking exercise

One of the most important principles in the care of women with drug or alcohol addiction is appropriate referral and multidisciplinary team work. If you provide midwifery care to a woman with these challenges, where would you obtain advice from and to whom could you refer her?

Write a list of all the people/agencies or services that might be useful.

Reflective exercise

Take some time to reflect on your own attitudes on drug and alcohol use, especially in pregnancy. How do you think your attitudes affect the way you practise, especially the way you communicate the risks to women?

- The lifestyle of women is often enhanced when on methadone treatment, resulting in improved nutrition and less stress.
- Methadone supplied by a pharmacy or treatment centre has not been 'cut' or mixed with any other potentially harmful substance that may be passed on to the baby.

Heroin crosses the placenta and can cause drug dependence in the baby. This means that these babies may experience withdrawal symptoms in the first few days. These babies need careful observation in a special care nursery using a neonatal abstinence scale or a similar method to monitor withdrawal. Injecting heroin also increases the risk of the woman contracting blood-borne viral infections such as hepatitis B, C or HIV (Australian Drug Foundation 2003).

Methadone

Pregnant women who are dependent on opiates are encouraged to enter a methadone program as early as possible in their pregnancy.

As small amounts of methadone may be passed on through breast milk, women who are on a methadone program are often encouraged to breastfeed in order to help ease the baby's withdrawal from methadone. Methadone has been found to reach its maximum level in breast milk between two and four hours after a dose, and therefore feeding the baby just before a dose or taking the methadone just before the baby has a long sleep will reduce the amount available to the baby (Australian Drug Foundation 2003).

Sexually transmitted infections and pregnancy

Sexually transmitted infections (STI) are common, although often underestimated. They have been called the 'hidden epidemic' because their scope and consequences are under-recognised by the public and healthcare professionals. The rates of STIs are increasing in most countries including Australia and New Zealand (Ministry of Health 2001; NCHECR 2004).

This section reviews the common STIs, including pathophysiology, signs and symptoms, diagnosis and management. The common STIs that will be covered are genital herpes, chlamydia, gonorrhoea and syphilis (Erian et al 2004).

Consultation and/or referral to an infectious diseases physician or sexual health nurse or doctor are important if an STI is suspected or diagnosed. Midwives must work collaboratively with other healthcare providers to ensure that STIs are recognised and treated effectively. If one STI is diagnosed, it is often wise to recommend that the woman be tested for other common STIs as well as the human immunodeficiency virus (HIV). These infections often occur together, as the modes of transmission are similar.

Notification

In Australia, chlamydia, gonorrhoea and syphilis are notifiable conditions in all states and territories This means diagnoses of these infections are notified by state/territory health authorities to the National Notifiable Disease Surveillance System, maintained by the Australian Government Department of Health and Ageing (NCHECR 2004).

In Australia, the population rates of diagnosis of chlamydia, gonorrhoea and syphilis continue to be substantially higher in the Northern Territory than elsewhere in the country. Substantially higher rates of diagnosis of chlamydia, gonorrhoea and syphilis have also been recorded among Indigenous people than in non-Indigenous people (NCHECR 2004).

Information on STIs in New Zealand is difficult to obtain as national statistics on people diagnosed are not collected and some laboratories do not provide information for population-based estimates to be made. With the exception of HIV/AIDS, STIs are not notifiable infectious diseases.

Women who are diagnosed with an STI should be counselled about referring their sexual partners for testing and treatment (Centers for Disease Control and Prevention 2002). Depending on the infection, tracing partners can go back months and even years.

Genital herpes

Genital herpes is a common infection caused by the herpes simplex virus (HSV). There are two types of HSV:
● Type 1 is usually found around the lips and is commonly referred to as a 'cold sore'.
● Type 2 is usually found around the genitals or anus.

HSV is transmitted by close skin-to-skin contact with someone who has the infection. This usually occurs during vaginal, anal or oral intercourse. However, transmission can also occur if there is skin-to-skin contact without penetrative sex. Transmission of herpes may also occur through asymptomatic shedding. This is where someone infected with herpes sheds the virus from the skin without any visible signs of herpes. Similarly, transmission may occur when people are unaware they are infected with HSV because they have no symptoms, or very minor ones that are often unnoticed (NSW Health 2004a).

TABLE 7.5 Causative agent, signs and symptoms, diagnosis and management of STIs that are most important in pregnancy

	Genital herpes	Chlamydia	Gonorrhoea	Syphilis
Causative agent	Herpes simplex virus type 2	*Chlamydia trachomatis*	*Neisseria gonorrhoeae*	*Treponema pallidum*
Signs and symptoms	Blistering and ulceration of the directly affected areas (may include labia majora, labia minor, clitoris and urethra). These can be painful, tingling or itchy.	In 70–90% of women, the infection is asymptomatic. When there are symptoms, these may include dysuria, abnormal vaginal discharge, abnormal vaginal bleeding, pelvic pain or pain during sex.	In more than 60% of women the infection is asymptomatic. Where there are symptoms, these include cervicitis and a discoloured vaginal discharge.	A primary chancre (painless sore) develops at the site after an incubation period of approximately 21 days. In the secondary stage, a rash on the palms of the hands or soles of the feet, and on other parts of the body may be seen. Second stage symptoms, if they develop, usually occur from 7 to 10 weeks after infection.
Diagnosis	A laboratory test (PCR test) is undertaken from a swab of the lesion.	Detected by swabs collected from the cervix, urethra or anus or by a urine sample. PCR test or culture is undertaken.	Detected by swabs collected from the cervix, urethra or anus and cultured for the organism.	A sample of the chancre is taken for examination. Blood tests are used to diagnose primary and secondary syphilis.
Management	Acyclovir in different doses and length of time depending on whether it is the first episode or a recurrence.	Azithromycin, doxycycline or erythromycin generally for 10 days is effective treatment.	Penicillin most commonly is used but ceftriaxone may also be prescribed. Follow-up cultures are recommended one week after completing treatment to ensure cultures are negative.	Injections of penicillin is the most common treatment. Other drugs include erythromycin and doxycycline.

The risk of transmission to the baby is high (30–50%) in women who acquire genital herpes near the time of birth, but low (< 1%) among women with a history of recurrent herpes at term or who acquire genital HSV during the first half of pregnancy. Prevention of neonatal herpes depends both on preventing acquisition of genital HSV infection during late pregnancy and on avoiding exposure of the infant to herpetic lesions during birth. In some cases, this may mean avoiding a vaginal birth (Centers for Disease Control and Prevention 2002).

Women without known genital herpes should be advised to avoid intercourse during the third trimester with partners known or suspected to have genital herpes, to reduce the chance of an episode around the time of birth.

Chlamydia

In Australia, chlamydia is the most frequently reported notifiable condition in Australia (NCHECR 2004) and its incidence is likely to be high in New Zealand. Chlamydia can affect future fertility if not treated appropriately.

Chlamydia is often referred to as 'the silent STI' because the majority of people infected do not have symptoms. Chlamydia can affect the urethra, cervix, rectum, throat and eyes and is most often transmitted through unprotected vaginal and anal sex (NSW Health 2004).

Chlamydia in newborn babies occurs because of exposure to infected cervical fluids. The infection is most often recognised by conjunctivitis that develops 5–12 days after birth. Chlamydia is the most frequent identifiable infectious cause of ophthalmia neonatorum but can also be a common cause of subacute, afebrile pneumonia at 1–3 months of age (Centers for Disease Control and Prevention 2002).

Gonorrhoea

Gonorrhoea can infect the urethra, anus, cervix, throat and eyes of both men and women. It can be transmitted through oral, anal and vaginal sex without a condom. Condoms are highly effective in preventing gonorrhoea (NSW Health 2004a).

Gonococcal infections can also be present in newborns if they have been exposed to infected cervical fluids. It is usually an acute illness than presents two to five days after birth. The infection can cause ophthalmia neonatorum, rhinitis, vaginitis, urethritis, and inflammation at sites of fetal monitoring (Centers for Disease Control and Prevention 2002).

Syphilis

Syphilis is no longer very common in Australia or New Zealand. Congenital syphilis has considerable long-term effects on babies, including deafness, and so early diagnosis and treatment are important.

In Australia and New Zealand, routine antenatal tests often include a syphilis blood test. These tests are usually the venereal disease reference laboratory (VDRL) test and the rapid plasma reagin (RPR) test. The test that is specific for syphilis is called the *T. pallidum* haemagglutination assay (TPHA). Once someone has been infected with syphilis, the infection will always show up on the TPHA test even if they have been successfully and adequately treated (Erian et al 2004).

Critical thinking exercise

Contact tracing is the term used to describe the process of finding and notifying sexual partners when a person has been diagnosed with an STI. This can be a difficult and sensitive topic and confidentiality is important. Can you think of some strategies that would assist the contact tracing process? Look on the website for your health department to find out information about notifications and contact tracing.

Reflective exercise

Many people have very negative connotations and stereotypes attached to STIs. Take some time to reflect on your own attitude to STIs. How do you think your attitude might affect the way you practise?

Blood-borne viruses and childbearing

Blood-borne viruses (BBV) are increasingly important for midwives to understand. The BBVs that have particular significance for childbearing women are the human immuno-deficiency virus (HIV), hepatitis B (HBV) and hepatitis C (HCV). This section will address issues for women and midwives in relation to these three BBVs.

While each virus has distinct transmission patterns, HIV, HBV and HCV can all be transmitted parenterally through the sharing of injecting equipment, needle-stick injuries, or piercing and tattooing with contaminated equipment. The efficiency of sexual transmission is significantly different between the viruses. This has implications for midwifery practice and mother-to-child transmission (Sasadeusz et al 2004).

Midwifery and BBVs

Midwives should institute universal or standard precautions when caring for all women, not just those who are known to be living with a BBV. This will ensure that midwives are adequately protected and that discrimination does not occur. Universal precautions include wearing protective equipment (gloves, eye shields etc) when exposed to body fluids, especially blood.

When considering the most appropriate protective equipment, it is useful to remember exactly how these infections are transmitted, and avoid 'over-reacting' when the risk is either minimal or non-existent.

Vaccination for HBV is recommended to all healthcare workers as part of an occupational screening program.

HIV/AIDS

The language of HIV/AIDS is important to understand at the outset so that the correct terminology can be used. HIV refers to the actual agent, that is, the human immunodeficiency virus. AIDS is the name of the syndrome that occurs as a result of the immune problems caused by HIV. AIDS refers to acquired immunodeficiency syndrome and includes around 26 illnesses. These are called AIDS-defining conditions—for example, invasive cervical cancer, oesophageal candidiasis, tuberculosis, recurrent pneumonia and lymphoma. Therefore, it is inaccurate to talk about 'someone having the AIDS virus'. There is no such virus.

The global picture

The number of people around the world who are, or have been, affected by HIV/AIDS is staggering. Table 7.6 reports the global summary of the epidemic to December 2004 (UNAIDS 2004). The ranges around the estimates in this table define the boundaries within which the actual numbers lie, based on the best available information.

In some parts of the world, more than half of those infected are women. For example, in sub-Saharan Africa, women and girls make up almost 57% of adults living with HIV. Young women in particular are more likely to be infected than older women. For example, in South Africa, Zambia and Zimbabwe,

young women (aged 15–24 years) are three to six times more likely to be infected than young men (UNAIDS 2004).

Some of Australia's and New Zealand's closest neighbours are struggling with an increasing HIV epidemic. For example, Papua New Guinea, which shares an island with one of Indonesia's worst-affected provinces, Papua, has the highest prevalence of HIV infection in the Pacific (UNAIDS 2004). More than twice as many young women (aged 15–24 years) as men have been diagnosed with HIV. In 2003, 1.4% of pregnant women at antenatal clinics in the capital, Port Moresby, tested HIV-positive, while in Lae, in the central highlands, 2.5% of pregnant women were HIV-positive (UNAIDS 2004).

A number of other nations in our region have reported high rates of sexually transmitted infections (gonorrhoea, syphilis, chlamydia), including Vanuatu, Samoa and East Timor. High rates of STIs are often predictors of sexual behaviour that puts women at risk of HIV. These rates are a warning sign of potential HIV epidemics in the future.

HIV/AIDS in Australia and New Zealand

In Australia, an estimated 13,630 people were living with HIV/AIDS in 2003, including around 1100 adult/adolescent women (NCHECR 2004). The annual number of new HIV diagnoses declined from around 930 in 1994 to 690 in 1999 and 780 in 2003. The annual number of HIV diagnoses in women has stayed relatively stable, but more of those diagnosed infections occurred through heterosexual intercourse—either in a high-prevalence country or with a partner from a high-prevalence country (UNAIDS 2004).

In New Zealand, to the end of June 2004 a total of 819 people (754 males and 65 females) have been notified with AIDS, and 2154 (1823 males, 313 females, and 18 sex not stated) have been found to be infected with HIV (Ministry of Health 2004).

Mode of transmission

HIV is transmitted through sexual contact, blood-to-blood contact and mother-to-child transmission.

In Australia and New Zealand, transmission of HIV continues to be mainly through sexual intercourse between men (UNAIDS 2004). In developing countries, however, transmission is primarily through heterosexual intercourse.

Blood-to-blood contact can occur during sharing of needles used in injecting drug use, blood transfusion and needle-stick injuries. Transmission through injecting drug use is uncommon in Australia and New Zealand because of early strategies to reduce the incidence of needle-sharing. Transmission through injecting drug use is particularly common in parts of Europe, Asia and the United States. In Australia and New Zealand, transmission via blood transfusion occurred before blood products were universally screened (in 1985). In countries where all blood products are screened for HIV, transmission is exceedingly rare. Needle-stick injuries rarely result in transmission. It has been reported that only 0.03% of exposures from HIV-positive individuals result in HIV transmission (Sasadeusz et al 2004).

TABLE 7.6 Global summary of the HIV epidemic to December 2004

	Number*
People living with HIV	
Total	39.4 million (35.9–44.3 m)
Adults	37.2 million (33.8–41.7 m)
Women	17.6 million (16.3–19.5 m)
Children under 15 years	2.2 million (2.0–2.6 m)
People newly infected with HIV	
Total	4.9 million (4.3–6.4 m)
Adults	4.3 million (3.7–5.7 m)
AIDS deaths in 2004	
Total	3.1 million (2.8–3.5 m)
Adults	2.6 million (2.3–2.9 m)

*Range is shown in brackets
(Source: UNAIDS 2004, www.unaids.org)

Mother-to-child-transmission can occur during pregnancy, labour and birth and through breastfeeding. The rates of mother-to-child transmission range from 20% to 45%, depending on the context. Transmission rates have been shown to be reduced significantly (to around or less than 5%) with the use of antiretroviral therapy during pregnancy, labour and after birth, and other interventions such as elective caesarean sections and avoidance of breastfeeding (Sasadeusz et al 2004).

Issues for midwives

Although HIV/AIDS is uncommon in women in Australia and New Zealand, midwives need to be aware of the infection and the implications for screening and treatment.

1 Testing for HIV in pregnancy

The first issue to address is the identification of those women with HIV infection. Treatment options during pregnancy and birth significantly reduce the risk of mother-to-child transmission of HIV. Early identification is advantageous to the baby. Identification also may mean that women can access treatments that prolong the immune deficiency effects of the virus and delay the onset of an AIDS-related condition.

Screening policies for HIV vary greatly. A survey of private obstetricians, general practitioners and directors of public maternity units found great disparity in antenatal testing policies. A policy of universal offering of antenatal testing for HIV was reported from 47% of private obstetricians, 62% of general practitioners and 23% of public maternity units (Spencer et al 2003).

Routine screening for HIV is controversial, but many are now recommending routine screening with pre- and

---

BOX 7.1 Global Coalition on Women and AIDS

The Global Coalition on Women and AIDS was launched by UNAIDS in early 2004 to highlight the effects of AIDS on women and girls and to stimulate effective action to reduce that impact. The Global Coalition on Women and AIDS is not a new organisation but a movement of people, networks and organisations supported by activists, leaders, government representatives, community workers and celebrities. Its work is focused on seven areas:

▶ preventing HIV infection among adolescent girls
▶ reducing violence against women
▶ protecting the property and inheritance rights of women and girls
▶ ensuring equal access by women and girls to care and treatment
▶ supporting improved community-based care, with a special focus on women and girls
▶ promoting access to new prevention options, including female condoms and microbicides
▶ supporting ongoing efforts towards universal education for girls.

---

post-test counselling and consent. The Royal Australian and New Zealand College of Obstetricians and Gynaecologists (RANZCOG) and the NSW Health Department recommend that all pregnant women be offered HIV screening at their first antenatal visit (NSW Health 2004a; RANZCOG 2004). The NZCOM discussed the issue in 2002 and stated that:

No consensus was reached in relation to the draft statement that had been circulating prior to the July 2002 AGM. The statement issued from the AGM was: On current evidence the New Zealand College of Midwives (NZCOM) does not support the routine screening of all pregnant women for HIV (NZCOM 2002a).

The New Zealand Ministry of Health appears to support the recommendation made by the Australian National Council on AIDS and Related Diseases (ANCARD):

In general, women identified through their medical history as being at higher risk of HIV infection should be encouraged to be tested. No pregnant woman should be pressured into HIV testing or be tested without informed consent. Conversely, no pregnant woman seeking HIV testing should be discouraged from being tested (ANCARD 1998).

This recommendation was made in 1998. The document goes on to say 'in the light of rapidly changing testing and treatment, there should be a regular (two yearly) review of antenatal testing policies and practice' (ANCARD 1998). In 2006 the New Zealand Ministry of Health announced that all pregnant women will be offered routine antenatal screening for HIV.

Routine screening is a complex matter. Midwives must consider the risks and benefits associated with both HIV infection and screening in order to decide on policy and practice.

2 A multidisciplinary approach

HIV/AIDS is complex, and so a multidisciplinary approach is necessary. An approach where continuity of carers is provided is highly beneficial. The team should consist of a midwife, obstetrician, HIV physician and HIV nurse. The team may also include a social worker or counsellor.

As the baby will require ongoing testing during the first 18 months, a paediatrician and paediatric nurse with expertise in HIV infection are also important. It is useful for the woman to meet, or have contact with, the paediatric team prior to the birth of the baby to discuss the testing and monitoring process.

3 Support and confidentiality

Pregnant women who have HIV infection experience a number of additional fears and worries in addition to the normal concerns of pregnancy. This is particularly so for women who discover in pregnancy that they have HIV infection. The diagnosis is a shock, with the whole gamut of emotions including disbelief, anger, fear and concerns for the future and the baby. These women need time and support in order to make decisions about the pregnancy and their ongoing care and use of treatments.

Non-government organisations, such as the AIDS Council in each Australian state and territory and the New Zealand

AIDS Foundation, have support groups, counsellors, resources and information that may be useful for women and families to access.

Confidentiality is essential. Some women choose to tell their family about their infection; others do not. Midwives and others involved in the care of women need to be very conscious of this when providing care, especially in a hospital ward setting. For example, if a woman's family does not know about her infection they may question why she has chosen an elective caesarean section or is not breastfeeding. These decisions must be made by the woman and respected by all those involved in her care. Other simple issues should be addressed, like removing medication charts from the end of the bed or cot, as they may have antiretroviral medications ordered, indicating the infection.

Hepatitis C

In 2003, an estimated 242,000 people living in Australia had been exposed to hepatitis C virus (HCV). Of these, 25% were estimated to have cleared their infection, 59% had chronic hepatitis C infection and early liver disease, 13% had chronic hepatitis C infection and moderate liver disease, and 3% were living with hepatitis C related cirrhosis (NCHECR 2004). In 2000, it was estimated that in New Zealand the prevalence of hepatitis C was 25,200 people, with an incidence of 1300 new cases per year. Both the prevalence and incidence are lower than Australia on a per capita basis (Nesdale et al 2000).

The test for hepatitis C only became available in 1990. Currently, there is no vaccine available for hepatitis C.

While HCV and HIV are similar is some ways, in many others they are very different. Table 7.7 illustrates some of these differences. While this comparison is in Australia, the essential differences remain the same in the New Zealand population.

Mode of transmission

The transmission of HCV mainly occurs when infected blood enters the bloodstream of another person. The most common mode of transmission in Australia and New Zealand remains injecting drug use.

The role of sexual transmission, if any, is still controversial. If sexual transmission of HCV does occur, it is at a very low level, which makes it inappropriate to routinely recommend safe sex among long-term monogamous couples.

Mother-to-child transmission occurs in approximately 5% of births. This rate may be higher in women who also have HIV infection (Sasadeusz et al 2004). Mode of birth does not appear to affect the risk of transmission. As the infection is passed parenterally, care should be taken not to damage the skin integrity of the baby (e.g. avoid scalp clips).

Mother-to-child transmission is more likely to occur if women have high levels of circulating virus; that is, the more virus the more the chance of transmission. The amount of circulating virus is measured using a test called a polymerase chain reaction (PCR). The rate of mother-to-child transmission is 6% when women have positive PCR and 0% when the PCR is negative (Dore et al 2001). Therefore, a PCR test during pregnancy is very useful to women and their care providers.

Breastfeeding is not thought to be a risk factor for transmission. No cases of transmission via breast milk have been reported (ASHM 2003).

Issues for midwives

In Australia and New Zealand, HCV is far more common than HIV, although it has received considerably less interest from the popular media and health sectors in general. Midwives are far more likely to care for a woman with HCV infection than HIV.

1 Testing for HCV in pregnancy

Routine antenatal screening for HCV in pregnancy is also controversial. The Australian National Council on AIDS, Hepatitis C and Related Diseases currently does not recommend universal screening for pregnant women (ANCAHRD 2003). It recommends that testing be offered based on risk factors.

Women are considered to be at increased risk for HCV if they have:

TABLE 7.7 Comparison of the HIV and HCV epidemics in Australia	HIV	HCV
Commencement of epidemic	early 1980s	1960s
Peak of new infections	1984	1999
Estimated current infection	13,630	242,000
Male:female ratio	17:1	1.7:1
Estimated current infection p.a.	780	14,499
Cumulative attributable deaths	6,372	unknown
Predominant transmission	Male homosexual (85%)	Injecting drug use (80%)
(Source: NCHECR 2004)		

- a history of injecting drug use
- a partner (past or present) who has injected drugs
- a tattoo or piercing
- been in prison
- received blood which later tested positive for HCV
- been on long-term dialysis
- received an organ transplant prior to July 1992 (Victorian Health 2001).

RANZCOG recommends that all pregnant women be offered hepatitis C screening at the first antenatal visit.

The issues around screening are similar to those discussed earlier in this chapter around HIV and include the need for pre-test counselling and consent (Victorian Health 2001).

2 A multidisciplinary approach

As with HIV infection, a multidisciplinary approach is essential when caring for women with HCV. An infectious diseases physician or gastroenterologist with expertise in HCV will be the most appropriate physician. Longer-term follow-up of the woman and her baby, especially to monitor liver function, needs to be offered.

3 Support and confidentiality

The issues around support and confidentiality are equally similar to the ones discussed earlier in relation to HIV. There is probably less stigma attached to an HCV diagnosis, although the recognised risk factor being injecting drug use may be difficult for some women and their families. Again, the wishes of the woman must be respected and strategies put in place to ensure confidentiality.

Hepatitis B

Hepatitis B infection is the last BBV to be considered in this section. Of those infected, 5–10% become chronic carriers, and they remain infectious to others for life.

Hepatitis B is a huge health issue around the world. More than a third of the world's population have been infected with HBV, with an estimated 350 million chronic carriers worldwide. About 25% of chronic carriers develop serious liver disease (chronic hepatitis, cirrhosis, liver cancer). HBV results in 1–2 million deaths per year (Zuckerman 1999).

Mode of transmission

Hepatitis B infection is transmitted mainly by contact with an infected person's blood or sexual fluids, or from an infected woman to her baby (NSW Health 2004b).

Prevention of hepatitis B infection depends on immunisation of all children and immunisation of household contacts of infectious cases. Infectious people should avoid exposing others to their blood or sexual fluids. Hepatitis B immunoglobulin given with vaccine to babies born to infectious mothers is also effective.

Issues for midwives

1 Testing for HBV in pregnancy

It is recommended that all women be offered screening for HBV at their first antenatal visit (RANZCOG 2004; Victorian Health 2001). There is no evidence to support a repeat test later in pregnancy (Victorian Health 2001).

The results can be interpreted using the information presented in Table 7.8. It is essential to be very clear about the interpretation of the results (see Ch 32).

2 A multidisciplinary approach

As in the other BBVs, collaboration and a multidisciplinary approach is needed in hepatitis B. Consultation with an infectious diseases physician is important so that women and families receive accurate information. In addition, long-term follow-up, similar to that for hepatitis C, is recommended.

3 Support and confidentiality

The issues around support and confidentiality are equally similar to the ones discussed earlier in relation to HIV and HCV. There is probably less stigma attached to an HBV diagnosis, as it is even more common. Nevertheless, care needs to be taken to ensure that confidentiality is maintained and that women and their families receive appropriate support.

4 Prevention of neonatal infection

Neonates whose mothers are HbsAg positive are at greatest risk of hepatitis B acquisition. Of babies infected at birth, 90% will develop chronic hepatitis B infection.

Therefore, all babies born to mothers who are HbsAg positive should be offered hepatitis B immunoglobulin (HBIG) within 12 hours plus hepatitis B vaccination. Hepatitis

---

Reflective exercise

Take some time to reflect on your own attitudes on BBV, especially HIV and hepatitis C. How do you think your attitudes affect the way you practise, especially the way you discuss the infections with women?

Critical thinking exercise

1 Appropriate referral and having a multidisciplinary team approach are essential in the care for women with a BBV. Write a list of all the people/agencies or services that might be useful in your setting.

2 Review the antenatal blood tests of a woman with HBV infection and a woman who does not have the infection. What are the features of the test that are important to understand?

3 Your manager has a policy of putting women who have hepatitis B infection in a single room for postnatal care. What are the issues in relation to this policy? Name and discuss one advantage and one disadvantage of the policy.

4 Find your hospital or health setting's policy on universal precautions. Does this reflect best practice? What is the action in the case of a needle-stick injury?

TABLE 7.8   Interpretation of hepatitis serology testing

HBsAg: surface antigen	HBeAg: e antigen	Anti-HBc: core antibody	Anti-HBe: e antibody	Anti-HBs: surface antibody	Interpretation
0	0	0	0	0	Never had HBV infection or is in the early incubation period of the infection
0	0	0	0	+	Either passive temporary immunisation with HBV infection or long-term immunisation with hepatitis B vaccine. Non-infectious
+	0	0	0	0	Late incubation period or early stages of acute infection. Infectious
+	+	0	0	0	Early stage of acute infection. Infectious
0	0	+	0	+	Indicates a past resolved HBV infection. Suggests immunity to subsequent infections. Non-infectious
0	0	+	+	+	Indicates a past resolved HBV infection. Suggests immunity to subsequent infections. Non-infectious
+	+	+	0	0	Acute or chronic infection. Infectious
+	0	+	0	0	Acute or chronic infection: stage after HBeAg has disappeared but anti-HBe not yet detected. Follow-up serology indicated. Infectious
+	+	+	+	0	Mid to late stage of acute infection or chronic carrier state. Period of seroconversion from HBeAg to anti-HBe. Follow-up serology indicated. Infectious
+	0	+	+	0	Mid to late stage of acute infection or chronic carrier state. Follow-up serology indicated. Potentially infectious
0	0	+	0	0	Resolved infection with selective loss of anti-HBs. May also represent the window phase of an acute infection with HBsAg below level of detection. Remotely potentially infectious
0	0	+	+	0	This may represent resolved infection. Remotely potentially infectious
0	+	0	0	0	A rare profile that most likely represents erroneous test result. Repeat serology.
0	0	0	+	0	Probably an erroneous test result. Repeat serology.
+	0	+	+	+	A profile observed occasionally. Infectious

<table>
<tr><td>

BOX 7.2   Discussing BBVs

Language to consider when talking with women about BBVs:

Avoid the terms:
▶ addict
▶ addiction
▶ drug addict
▶ drug abuse
▶ drug abuser
▶ intravenous.

Use the terms:
▶ injecting (rather than intravenous)
▶ drug use, not abuse
▶ injecting equipment, not needles
▶ reused, not shared (e.g. Have you ever reused someone else's injecting equipment?)
▶ withdrawal symptoms and/or dependence, not addiction
▶ new, rather than clean, equipment.

(Source: ASHM 2003)

</td></tr>
</table>

B vaccine should be administered at the same time as HBIG but in a different site.

Language

The language used is very important when discussing BBV infections with women. The National Hepatitis Education Program has developed some hints to consider when talking with women about possible or real infections (see Box 7.2).

Domestic violence and pregnancy

Domestic violence (also known as intimate partner violence or family violence) is a significant issue for women whether they are pregnant or not. A number of terms are used to refer to domestic violence in government documents and in the literature. These include 'family violence', 'intimate partner violence' and 'spousal violence'. In this chapter the term 'domestic violence' is used.

Violence against women is increasing in all cultures, societies and socio-economic groups (WHO 2000). In Australia, New Zealand and elsewhere, government and health providers have developed policies on domestic violence.

Domestic violence in pregnancy is a significant issue, as there are immediate and long-term effects on both the woman and her baby. This section discusses the prevalence of violence in pregnancy, the risks and dangers to women and their babies, and issues relating to screening, support and referral.

Challenges to determining prevalence rates

Defining and measuring domestic violence in pregnancy is challenging. Definitions include 'only physical violence' and 'physical and sexual violence', or expand to take in other forms of violence, including emotional abuse and harassment (Hegarty et al 1999; Taft 2002).

One of the other challenges is related to how women are asked about violence. Whether women are asked in person, by telephone or on a self-reporting questionnaire affects the reported prevalence rates (Taft 2002). Women who speak little English may also not disclose violence, especially if the interpreter is from their community and confidentiality is not assured. Women whose partners do not leave their sides when seeking healthcare, for example in antenatal visits, often do not disclose because of lack of opportunity (Taft 2002).

Prevalence of domestic violence in pregnancy

The prevalence of domestic violence varies depending on the context, population and measurement instruments. A review of 14 studies of violence against pregnant women reported prevalence rates between 1% and 20% (Gazmarian et al 1996). More recently, a study conducted in antenatal clinics in the United Kingdom reported prevalence rates of 2% at booking, 6% at 34 weeks of pregnancy and 5% at 10 days post partum (Bacchus et al 2004). In the United States, a study in low-risk pregnant women reported that abuse during pregnancy was reported by 6% of women (Neggers et al 2004).

An early important Australian study of more than 1000 women found that almost 30% reported a history of abuse, with around 6% reporting being abused during pregnancy. The proportion of women admitting to abuse rose over the duration of pregnancy to 9% at 36 weeks (Webster et al 1994). Women who were adolescent, single, separated, divorced or in a de facto relationship, not working outside the home or with lower levels of education, were more likely to have experienced abuse.

In New Zealand, there is evidence that domestic violence also affects a significant number of women. Research suggests that between 15% and 21% of women report having experienced physical or sexual abuse, and 44% to 53% report having experienced psychological abuse in the previous 12 months (Leibrich et al 1995; Morris 1996). While these rates are not specifically for women during pregnancy, one could hypothesise that these would translate to similar levels in pregnancy as reported elsewhere.

Effects of domestic violence

Women who suffer abuse are at risk of physical injury, gynaecological problems, complications during pregnancy and childbirth, depression, anxiety, sexually transmitted infections and eating disorders (Taft 2002).

Domestic violence can also have catastrophic effects. In the most recent report of *Maternal Deaths in Australia* there were two deaths as a result of domestic violence (Slaytor et al 2004). One was an 18-year-old woman, 18 weeks pregnant with a past history of intravenous drug use. There had been noted concerns for her regarding domestic violence. The second death occurred following a domestic dispute, in a 25-year-old woman who was nine weeks pregnant.

Avoidable factors were thought to have played a role in both deaths.

The *Confidential Enquiry into Maternal Deaths* in the United Kingdom (2001) reported that 12% of the 378 women whose deaths were investigated from 1997 to 1999 had self-reported a history of domestic violence to a health worker. Of these women, eight were subsequently murdered by a partner or close relative.

Domestic violence also affects children in the family. Exposure to violence between parents has been reported to result in higher levels of physical and psychosomatic disorders, behavioural problems, post-traumatic stress and poor educational achievements in children and young people (Taft 2002).

Implications for midwives

All health professionals, including midwives, need to be aware of the significance of domestic violence. They need to adopt a non-judgemental and supportive response to women who have experienced physical, sexual or psychosocial abuse. Midwives need to provide women with basic information about where to get help and provide continuing support whatever decision she makes about her future (Confidential Enquiry into Maternal Deaths 2001).

The New Zealand College of Midwives has a Consensus Statement about the responsibility of midwives in relation to domestic violence (NZCOM 2002b). It also provides training for midwives in relation to routine screening for family violence, and referral processes for women who disclose their exposure to violence.

Screening for violence in pregnancy

Routine screening for domestic violence has been advocated in a number of countries including New Zealand, the United States and some Australian states. The aim of screening is to enable women to disclose to healthcare providers so they can receive appropriate referral and support.

Women generally do not disclose without direct questioning unless the abuse has reached a serious level (Hegarty & Taft 2001). There are a number of barriers to women's disclosure about domestic violence (Taft 2002). These include:

- shame and/or embarrassment
- fear of the abuser and retribution
- belief that the abuse is normal and common among couples
- fear of judgemental attitudes
- her partner's presence
- believing that the abuse is her responsibility and that no one else can help.

Risks and benefits of screening

There is controversy about routine screening for domestic violence in antenatal care.

Women respond differently to the screening questions, depending on their level of fear, their degree of trust in the person asking the questions and their sense that anything can be done. Therefore, screening may not detect all women who

are experiencing abuse. The screening questions are also not always acceptable to women. A study in the United States asked women about their attitudes to being screened for physical and sexual abuse (Gielen et al 2000). When asked whether healthcare providers should routinely screen women for physical and sexual abuse, only 54% of women who reported abuse, and 42% of women who did not, agreed. A study in Sweden reported high levels of acceptability in both abused and non-abused women, with 82 and 72% respectively of these groups finding screening acceptable (Stenson et al 2001). In Australia, a pilot study reported that feedback from the 159 women who were screened over a 12-week period was very positive (Jones & Bonner 2002).

Many health settings are not well equipped to provide adequate support and referral networks, and in many places acceptable services for women do not exist. There are concerns that if undue emphasis is placed on screening and disclosure in places where effective services are in place to guarantee confidentiality and safety, women may suffer harm (Taft 2002). If screening is implemented, it is essential that the maternity service staff are aware of the available resources and support networks accessible to women.

Midwives as women

The rates of domestic violence in the community are high. It is likely, therefore, that some midwives will have been subjected to domestic violence. Midwives could be past or current victims of domestic violence. This may mean that it is difficult for these midwives to undertake screening for domestic violence. This issue needs to be acknowledged in any screening program.

It is essential that midwives who undertake screening are provided with training and ongoing support and clinical

---

BOX 7.3 NZCOM Consensus Statement

The New Zealand College of Midwives Consensus Statement on family violence is as follows.
Midwives:

- require support to address the issue of violence against women within the national family violence strategy/framework
- undertake screening of all pregnant women for violence as part of a comprehensive health assessment
- understand the effect of violence against pregnant women and in particular in relation to sexual and reproductive health
- acknowledge that the woman has the right to define choice of action/referral or support
- are familiar with referral agencies that provide support, counselling and emergency services for survivors of violence
- can provide information resources to pregnant women on local emergency support services
- do not support mandatory referral when violence has been disclosed.

(Source: NZCOM 2002)

supervision. The training should discuss the implications of screening for both women and midwives and the practicalities of screening (Jones & Bonner 2002). Ongoing support and clinical supervision are necessary for staff who are undertaking screening.

Child protection issues

Child protection must be at the forefront of concerns in relation to domestic violence. In many states and territories in Australia and in New Zealand, mandatory reporting is required if there are any concerns about children at risk, including those in domestic violence situations. Midwives need to be clear about their role and responsibilities in this area and need to work with other healthcare and non-government providers to ensure that children receive appropriate protection.

Poor communication between healthcare workers is known to be a concern in cases involving the protection of children. Appropriate referral, follow-up and documentation are therefore essential to ensure that children in potentially volatile situations have quality care and access to services and support.

Screening questions

A number of different styles of screening questions have been developed and implemented. An example is presented in Box 7.4 (Jones & Bonner 2002). The screening is only undertaken when the woman is alone with the midwife. The preamble is read out before the questions are asked. The reasons for not screening and the outcome of screening are documented.

Recommendations

A number of key recommendations have been made by the Confidential Enquiries into Maternal Deaths in the United Kingdom in relation to domestic violence (Lewis 2001):

- All health professionals should be aware of the importance of domestic violence in their practice. They should adopt a non-judgemental and supportive response to women who have experienced physical, psychological or sexual abuse and must be able to give basic information to women about where to get help. They should be able to provide continuing support, whatever decision the woman makes concerning her future.
- When a woman discloses violence this must be taken seriously. Women who are poor clinic-attenders need active outreach services.
- Local health services and community teams should develop guidelines for the identification of, and provision of further support for, these women, including developing multi-agency working to enable appropriate referrals or provision of information on sources of further help.
- Information about local sources of help and emergency help lines should be displayed in suitable places in antenatal clinics, for example, in the woman's toilets or printed as a routine at the bottom on the hand-held maternity records.

- Enquiries about violence should be routinely included when taking a social history. This may be at the booking visit.
- When routine screening is introduced, this should be accompanied by the development of local strategies for referral. This should be accompanied by an educational program for health professionals in consultation with local groups.
- Where a woman is unable to speak English, an interpreter should be provided. A partner, friend or family member should not be used for interpreting.

BOX 7.4 Preamble and screening questions

Preamble:

▶ In this health service we routinely ask all women the same questions about violence at home.

▶ This is because violence in the home is very common and can be serious and we want to improve our response to women experiencing domestic violence.

▶ You don't have to answer the questions if you don't want to.

▶ All answers to the questions will remain confidential to the health service except where you give us information that indicates that you or your children are at immediate risk of serious harm. We would discuss this with you.

Screening questions:

1 Within the last year have you been hit, slapped or hurt in any way by your partner or ex-partner?

2 Are you frightened of your partner or ex-partner?

3 Are you safe to go home when you leave here?

▶ If domestic violence has been identified in any of the above questions, continue to Question 4.

4 Would you like any assistance with this?

(Source: Jones & Bonner 2002)

Reflective exercise

Take some time to reflect on your own experiences with domestic violence whether in a personal or professional capacity. How do you think your experiences might affect the way you practise and how you communicate with women?

Critical thinking exercise

1 Screening for domestic violence should never occur with the woman's partner or family members present. What are some strategies you could use to ensure that this can occur?

2 The legislation relating to child protection and mandatory reporting varies across Australia and New Zealand. Find out what it is in your area. How will this affect your practice when asking women about domestic violence?

- Every woman should be seen on her own at least once during pregnancy to enable the disclosure of such information (Lewis 2001).

Female genital mutilation and pregnancy

The World Health Organization (WHO) has defined female genital mutilation as comprising 'all procedures involving partial or total removal of the female external genitalia or other injury to the female genital organs whether for cultural or other non-therapeutic reasons' (WHO 1997). An estimated 135 million of the world's girls and women have undergone genital mutilation, and two million girls a year are at risk of mutilation—approximately 6000 per day (Amnesty International 1997).

This definition encompasses the diversity of procedures performed by different cultural groups. The classification of FGM (see Table 7.9) provides a technical description of the types of procedures that this definition covers. Within each of the types of FGM there will be variation with respect to the amount of tissue removed.

The term 'female genital mutilation' may cause offence to some who have experienced it. Although Western societies may view the practice as mutilation, within the cultures who practise FGM it is performed with the good of the child in mind. The use of the term 'female genital mutilation' in midwifery practice has the potential to be counterproductive to the establishment of effective relationships with women. Without the development of such relationships, it may not be possible to meaningfully address the difficult and sensitive issues with which a woman affected by these practices may

need assistance (RANZCOG 1997). Sometimes terms like 'traditional female surgery', 'cutting' and 'ritual female surgery' are more useful.

Classification and terminology

Midwives need to be aware that different women may refer to the extent of the FGM differently. The WHO has devised a classification system that will be useful to define the level of FGM and to assist clarity. This will also help in the planning of the woman's care, especially for the birth.

An estimated 15% of all mutilations in Africa are infibulations. The procedure consists of clitoridectomy (where all, or part of, the clitoris is removed), excision (removal of all, or part of, the labia minora), and cutting of the labia majora to create raw surfaces, which are then stitched or held together in order to form a cover over the vagina when they heal. A small hole is left to allow urine and menstrual blood to escape. In some less conventional forms of infibulation, less tissue is removed and a larger opening is left. The vast majority (85%) of genital mutilations performed in Africa consist of clitoridectomy or excision. The least radical procedure consists of removal of the clitoral hood (Amnesty International 1997).

In some traditions a ceremony is held, but no mutilation of the genitals occurs. The ritual may include holding a knife next to the genitals, pricking the clitoris, cutting some pubic hair, or light scarification in the genital or upper thigh area (Amnesty International 1997).

Complications of FGM

A wide range of complications associated with FGM are reported, including short- and long-term physical, sexual and psychosocial problems. Some women do not experience any problems that they attribute to FGM (RANZCOG 1997).

TABLE 7.9	WHO classification of female genital mutilation
Type I	Excision of the prepuce, with or without excision of part or all of the clitoris Other terms used to describe Type I procedures include circumcision, ritualistic circumcision, sunna, clitoridectomy.
Type II	Excision of the clitoris with partial or total excision of the labia minora Other terms used to describe Type II procedures include clitoridectomy, sunna, excision and circumcision.
Type III	Excision of part or all of the external genitalia and stitching/narrowing of the vaginal opening (infibulation) Other terms used to describe Type III procedures include infibulation, Pharaonic circumcision and omalian circumcision.
Type IV	Unclassified: includes • pricking, piercing or incising of the clitoris and/or labia • stretching of the clitoris and/or labia • cauterisation by burning of the clitoris and surrounding tissue • scraping of tissue surrounding the vaginal orifice (angurya cuts) or cutting of the vagina (gishiri cuts) • introduction of corrosive substances or herbs into the vagina to cause bleeding or for the purposes of tightening or narrowing it • any other procedure which falls under the definition of female genital mutilation given above.
(Source: WHO 1997)	

TABLE 7.10	Complications associated with FGM
Immediate	• pain • bleeding • infections • injuries • urinary obstruction • death
Longer term	• vulval scarring and pain • pelvic and urinary tract infection • obstructed menstrual and urinary flow • urinary and faecal fistulae • obstructed miscarriage and childbirth • vaginal and perineal damage at childbirth
Sexual	• non-consummation due to dyspareunia, obstruction, vaginismus or painful scar tissue • trauma on deinfibulation by partner • impaired sexual response and enjoyment • problematic sexual expression or relationship conflict, if vaginal intercourse is precluded
Psychological	• reactions to the trauma of FGM itself • anxiety and depressive symptoms • effects on sexuality • conflict within family and community • responses of host communities, including health professionals • inter-generational issues regarding continuity of the practice • post-immigration anxiety and regret regarding FGM

(Source: RANZCOG 1997)

Legislation surrounding FGM

Specific legislation banning FGM has been enacted in almost all Australian states and territories and in New Zealand. Where legislation has been passed, it has the following features:

● A person who intentionally performs female genital mutilation on a person is guilty of a serious offence with a maximum penalty of at least seven years imprisonment.

● A person must not take a child from a jurisdiction, or arrange for a child to be taken from it, with the intention of having female genital mutilation performed on the child. A child is defined as someone under the age of 18 years. Again there is a maximum penalty of at least seven years imprisonment.

● There are exceptions for the performance of medical procedures that have a genuine therapeutic purpose.

Child protection legislation often also exists to protect girl children who might be deemed to be at risk of FGM. Healthcare professionals are therefore required to report incidents of FGM including situations where they believe a girl to be at risk. Reports should be made to the relevant child welfare authority (RANZCOG 1997).

Midwives and FGM

Midwives and other healthcare professionals have an important role in the prevention of FGM, and the care of women who are affected by this practice.

Considerable time is required with women who are affected by FGM to discuss all the issues and to develop trust and rapport. If possible, these women should have care from a small group of midwives throughout the antenatal, labour and birth and postnatal periods. Continuity of caregiver is important, as is knowledge about FGM and the cultural and social issues related to it.

Midwifery care

Table 7.11 presents the best practice principles for the care of women through pregnancy, labour and birth and the postnatal period. These principles are developed from work undertaken by the Royal Australian and New Zealand College of Obstetricians and Gynaecologists (RANZCOG 1997), the NSW Education Program on FGM (NSW Education Program on Female Genital Mutilation 2000) and the South Eastern Sydney Area Health Service's Women's Health Unit (South East Health 2002). These resources should be used for more information when caring for these women.

Culturally sensitive care

Female genital mutilation is a significant health issue for women and girls around the world. With increased migration and movement, midwives in Australia and New Zealand will be increasingly exposed to women who have undergone this procedure. It is essential that midwives develop skills in supporting both the physical and the psychosocial needs of this group of women. Culturally sensitive care is important if women are to feel well supported.

Critical thinking exercise

1 The legislation relating to FGM varies across Australia and New Zealand. Find out the legislation in your state or country regarding FGM.
2 Are there any national or state policies about the care of women who have experienced FGM? How can you ensure that these are incorporated into practice in your setting?

Reflective exercise

Take some time to reflect on your own attitudes on the practice of FGM. How do you think your attitudes affect the way you practise?

TABLE 7.11	Best practice principles for care of women who have undergone FGM
Antenatal	• Women with FGM should be managed by a small team of midwives and doctors to ensure continuity of caregivers, information and support • The use of sensitive language is important for women affected by FGM. • Information relating to FGM should always be given in the women's language. The depth of discussion will depend on the grading of FGM and the receptiveness of the woman and her family. Diagrams can be used to help the woman understand how she will be affected during childbirth. • After gaining consent for examination, the woman needs to be examined by the medical officer or midwife to determine the type of FGM. This can occur at a visit during the pregnancy once the midwife has developed the trust of the woman. • If she is classified as Type III or when the introitus is inadequate, then she will need deinfibulation antenatally or during the intrapartum period (see below). • Decision about deinfibulation needs to be made in consultation with the woman and her partner and undertaken between 20 and 28 weeks gestation. It can be performed as a day case, preferably under spinal or local anaesthetic. • Ensure the woman and her partner understand that reinfibulation will not be undertaken. • Communication between all involved in the care of the woman needs to be ongoing and further counselling may be needed. • Encourage the woman to have her partner/support person come to the visits. • All interventions and decisions must be documented clearly and fully in the clinical records.
Labour and birth	• Each woman will have been assessed in the antenatal period. Review the clinical notes. • Vaginal examination can be difficult. Use of one finger only may make it tolerable. • Bladder management: encourage frequent urination. Insertion of a catheter can be difficult. Urethral meatus may need to be palpated digitally prior to insertion. If a urinary catheter is inserted, leave it indwelling. • Women with Type I or II normally do not require deinfibulation. Division of adhesions normally occurs as the fetal head emerges, but on occasions deinfibulation may need to be attended.

Postnatal	• Women who have Type I or II FGM should have usual postnatal care.
	• Women who have Type III or if deinfibulation has occurred: individual assessment is required.
	  – Women need to be aware that voiding will be quicker and noisier than before.
	  – Offer urine alkaliser and analgesia.
	  – Watch for urinary retention in first 24 hours.
	  – The scar should be checked prior to discharge by the practitioner who did the deinfibulation.
	• Provide information regarding ongoing genital hygiene.
	• The midwife should become aware of cultural practices surrounding the postnatal period for individual women.
	• If the baby is a girl, there should be a discussion about FGM. Ongoing education and support needs to involve the woman's GP, social worker and child and family health nurse.

(Sources: NSW Education Program on Female Genital Mutilation 2000; RANZCOG 1997; South East Health 2002)

Conclusion

This chapter has covered a number of challenges to women's health, specifically during pregnancy.

Midwives face these challenges and many others every day in their practice. While the specifics of the challenges are different, the principles of providing woman-centred, evidence-based care always remain the same. Working with women through these challenges means listening to their stories, understanding their experiences and supporting them to make choices and decisions that are right for them. This should always be done in a non-judgemental and collaborative manner, utilising other workers and non-government agencies as appropriate. In addressing these challenges, midwives should be mindful of the need to respect and support the needs of women to be self-determining in promoting their own health and wellbeing.

Some of the issues addressed in this chapter fall beyond the scope of midwifery practice. Collaboration with others therefore is essential. Women should be provided with clear information about accessing community support agencies that are available during pregnancy, in the postnatal period and after, when the midwifery relationship is concluded. An important part of the role of the midwife is to ensure that women have developed links and networks that enable them to make connections and receive appropriate support.

Review questions

1 Which strategies may be useful for women with an anxiety disorder in pregnancy?

2 What are the major risks for the baby associated with medication used to treat bipolar disorder in the first trimester?

3 Name three adverse effects related to smoking cigarettes in pregnancy for (a) the mother and (b) the baby

4 Which two strategies have been found to result in smoking cessation in pregnancy?

5 What strategies might you use in an antenatal setting to support women who want to stop or reduce smoking?

6 What is the maximum number of standard drinks recommended for (a) non-pregnant women and (b) pregnant women?

7 What are some of the adverse effects of using heroin in pregnancy?

8 What is the management of babies whose mothers have used opiates during late pregnancy?

9 What are the signs and symptoms of chlamydia infection in women?

10 What organisms cause ophthalmia neonatorum?

11 What is the risk of mother-to-child transmission of HIV infection? How can this risk be reduced?

12 What are two issues to consider when deciding on a policy of routine screening for HIV and/or hepatitis C infections?

13 What are the estimated rates of domestic violence in pregnant women in Australia and New Zealand?

14 Why are they only 'estimated'?

15 Give two benefits and two disadvantages of routine screening for domestic violence.

16 What are three ways in which midwives can support women who have experienced domestic violence?

17 Women from which cultures are most likely to be affected by female genital mutilation?

18 Outline the features of Type III FGM.

19 What are the implications for labour and birth for women affected by Type III FGM?

20 What are some of the midwifery strategies to support women who have been affected by FGM during pregnancy and birth?

Online resources

Mental health

SANE Australia organisation, http://www.sane.org

Mental Health Information Centre, http://www.mja.com.au/public/mentalhealth

NZ Schizophrenia Fellowship, http://www.sfnat.org.nz

Richmond Fellowship (NZ), http://www.richmondnz.org

Smoking in pregnancy

Three Centres Consensus Guidelines on Antenatal Care, http://www.dhs.vic.gov.au/health/maternitycare/anteguide.pdf

Alcohol and drug use in pregnancy

Alcohol Advisory Council of NZ, http://www.alcohol.org.nz/Home.aspx

Drug-Info Clearinghouse, http://www.druginfo.adf.org.au.

Sexually transmitted infections

Centres for Disease Control and Prevention STD Treatment Guidelines, http://www.cdc.gov/std/treatment/rr5106.pdf

NSW Health Department, Sexually Transmissable Diseases, http://www.health.nsw.gov.au/health-public-affairs/publications/std/contents.html

Blood-borne viruses in pregnancy

Australian National Centre for HIV Epidemiology and Clinical Research, http://www.med.unsw.edu.au/nchecr

UNAIDS, http://www.unaids.org/en/default.asp

Ministry of Health (NZ) Hepatitis C information, http://www.moh.govt.nz/cd/hepc

New Zealand AIDS Foundation, http://www.nzaf.org.nz

Australian Federation of AIDS organisations, http://www.afao.org.au

Hepatitis C Councils, http://www.hepatitisaustralia.com and http://www.hepatitisc.org.au

Hepatitis C Resource Centre, http://www.hepc.org.nz

Domestic violence

Australian Domestic and Family Violence Clearinghouse, http://www.austdvclearinghouse.unsw.edu.au

NZ Family Violence Intervention Guidelines, http://www.moh.govt.nz

NZCOM Consensus Statement on Family Violence, http://www.midwife.org.nz

Female genital mutilation

Amnesty International, http://www.amnesty.org

RANZCOG, http://www.ranzcog.edu.au

References

Alcohol Advisory Council of New Zealand 2004 Alcohol guidelines. Alcohol Advisory Council of New Zealand

Altshuler L, Hendrick V, Cohen L 1998 Course of mood and anxiety disorders during pregnancy and the postpartum period. Journal of Clinical Psychiatry 59(suppl 2):29–33

Amnesty International 1997 Female genital mutilation: a human rights information pack. Amnesty International

ANCAHRD 2003 National hepatitis C testing policy. Australian National Council on AIDS, Hepatitis C and Related Diseases, Canberra

ANCARD 1998 HIV testing policy. Online: http://www7.health.gov. au/pubhlth/ancard/pdf/hivtest.pdf. Australian National Council on AIDS and Related Diseases, Canberra

Australasian Society for HIV Medicine (ASHM) 2003 Nurses and hepatitis C. Online: www.ashm.org.au. National Hepatitis Education Program, Sydney

Australian Drug Foundation 2003 Drug facts. Drug-Info Clearinghouse

Bacchus L, Mezey G, Bewley S et al 2004 Prevalence of domestic violence when midwives routinely enquire in pregnancy. British Journal of Gynaecology 111(5):441–445

Centers for Disease Control and Prevention 2002 Sexually transmitted diseases treatment guidelines 2002. Morbidity and Mortality Weekly Report 51(rr–6)

Confidential Enquiry into Maternal Deaths 2001 Why mothers die 1997–1999. RCOG Press, London

Dore GJ, Kaldor JM, McCaughan GW 2001 Systematic review of role of polymerase chain reaction in defining infectiousness among people infected with hepatitis C virus. British Medical Journal 315(7104):333–337

English D, Holman C, Milne J 1995 The quantification of drug caused morbidity and mortality in Australia. Commonwealth Department of Health and Human Services, Canberra

Erian M, Jones I, O'Connor V 2004 Sexually transmitted infections. In: M Finn, L Bowyer, S Carr et al (Eds) Women's health: a core curriculum. Elsevier Mosby, Sydney

Gazmarian JA, Lazorick S, Spitz AM et al 1996 Prevalence of violence against pregnant women. Journal of the American Medical Association 275(24):1915–1920

Gielen AC, O'Campo PJ, Campbell JC et al 2000 Women's opinions about domestic violence and mandatory reporting. American Journal of Preventive Medicine 19(4):279–285

Hegarty K, Sheehan M, Schonfeld C 1999 A multidimensional definition of partner abuse: development and preliminary validation of the Composite Abuse Scale. Journal of Family Violence 14(4):399–415

Hegarty K, Taft A 2001 Overcoming the barriers to disclosure and inquiry of partner abuse for women attending general practice. Australian and New Zealand Journal of Public Health 25(5):433–437

Jones C, Bonner M 2002 Screening for domestic violence in an antenatal clinic. Australian Journal of Midwifery 15(1):14–19

Jones K, Smith D, Ulleland C et al (1973) Pattern of malformation in offspring of chronic alcoholic mothers. Lancet 1: 1267–1271

Leibrich J, Paulin J, Ransom R 1995 Hitting home: men speak about abuse of woman partners. Department of Justice, Wellington

Lewis G 2001 Domestic violence. Why mothers die 1997–1999. Deaths, CEiM, RCOG Press, London, pp 241–251

Lumley J, Oliver S, Waters E 2004 Interventions for promoting smoking cessation during pregnancy (Cochrane Review). John Wiley & Sons, Chichester

Mabbutt J, Bauman A, Moshin M 2002 Tobacco use of pregnant women and their male partners who attend antenatal classes: what happens to routine quit smoking advice in pregnancy? Australian and New Zealand Journal of Public Health 26(6): 571–573

Ministry of Health 2001 Sexual and reproductive health strategy—phase one. New Zealand Ministry of Health, Wellington

Ministry of Health 2004 AIDS—New Zealand: Issue 54, August. New Zealand Ministry of Health, Wellington. Online: http://www.moh. govt.nz/aids.html

Moore L, Campbell R, Whelan A, Mills N et al 2002 Self help smoking cessation in pregnancy: cluster randomised controlled trial. British Medical Journal 325:1383–1387

Morris A 1996 Women's safety survey. Victimisation Survey Committee, Wellington

National Alcohol Campaign 2002 Australian alcohol guidelines, Commonwealth of Australia

National Health Committee 1999 Review of maternity services. Ministry of Health, Wellington

NCHECR 2004 Annual surveillance report: HIV/AIDS, viral hepatitis and sexually transmissible infections in Australia. National Centre in HIV Epidemiology and Clinical Research and the Australian Institute of Health and Welfare, Canberra

Neggers Y, Goldenberg R, Cliver S et al 2004 Effects of domestic violence on preterm birth and low birthweight. Acta Obstetrica et Gynecologica Scandinavica 83(4):455–460

Nesdale A, Baker M, Gane E et al 2000 Hepatitis C infections in New Zealand: estimating the current and future prevalance and impact. Wellington, New Zealand: Institute of Environmental Science and Research Ltd

NHMRC 1997 The health effects of passive smoking—a scientific information paper. National Health and Medical Research Centre, Canberra

NSW Education Program on Female Genital Mutilation 2000 Female genital mutilation clinical management guidelines: a self-directed learning package for health professionals. WSAHS Multicultural Health Unit, Parramatta, NSW

NSW Health 2003 NSW mothers and babies 2002. NSW Health Department, Sydney

NSW Health 2004a Report of the New South Wales Chief Health Officer: Communicable diseases—hepatitis B. NSW Health Department, Sydney

NSW Health 2004b Sexually transmitted diseases. NSW Health Department, Sydney. Online: http://www.health.nsw.gov.au/ health-public-affairs/publications/std/contents.html

NZCOM 2001 Alcohol and pregnancy: consensus statement. New Zealand College of Midwives, Wellington

NZCOM 2002a Statement from NZCOM Annual General Meeting July 2002: HIV screening in Pregnancy. New Zealand College of Midwives, Wellington. Online: http://www.midwife.org.nz/ content/documents/89/hiv.2002.doc

NZCOM 2002b Consensus statement: family violence. New Zealand College of Midwives, Wellington

O'Leary C 2002 Fetal alcohol syndrome: a literature review. Commonwealth of Australia, Canberra

Oliver S, Oakley L, Lumley J et al 2001 Smoking cessation programmes in pregnancy: systemically addressing development, implementation, women's concerns and effectiveness. Health Education Journal 60:362–370

Overholser J (1990) Fetal alcohol syndrome: a review of the disorder. Journal of Contemporary Psychotherapy 20:163–176

Park E-W, Schultz J, Tudiver F et al 2004 Enhancing partner support to improve smoking cessation. (Systematic Review). Cochrane Tobacco Addiction Group. Cochrane Database of Systematic Reviews (Issue 2)

Rampono J 2004 The psychological experience of pregnancy. In: M Finn, L Bowyer, S Carr et al (eds) Women's health: a core curriculum. Elsevier Mosby, Sydney

RANZCOG 1997 Female genital mutilation: information for Australian health professionals. Royal Austalian and New Zealand College of Obstetricians and Gynaecologists, Melbourne

RANZCOG 2004 College statement: antenatal screening tests. Royal Australian and New Zealand College of Obstetricians and Gynaecologists, Melbourne. Online: http://www.ranzcog.edu.au/publications/statements/C-obs3.pdf

RCOG 1999 Alcohol consumption in pregnancy. Royal College of Obstetricians and Gynaecologists, London

SANE Australia 2004a Anxiety disorder: fact sheet. SANE Australia

SANE Australia 2004b Schizophrenia: fact sheet. SANE Australia

SANE Australia 2004c Bipolar disorder: fact sheet. SANE Australia

Sasadeusz J, Locarnini S, Kidd M 2004 HIV, HBV, HCV: similarities and differences. In: G Dore, A Grulich, M Kidd et al (Eds) HIV/viral hepatitis: a guide to primary care. Australasian Society for HIV Medicine (ASHM), Sydney. Online: http://www.ashm.org.au/uploadFile/W_mono_1.pdf

Slaytor E, Sullivan EA, King JF 2004 Maternal deaths in Australia 1997–1999. Australian Institute of Health and Welfare, Canberra

South East Health 2002 Care of women with FGM during pregnancy, labour and birth and the postnatal period. Area Women's Health, Sydney

Spencer J, Tibbits D, Tippet C et al 2003 Review of antenatal testing policies and practice for HIV and hepatitis C infection. Australian and New Zealand Journal of Public Health 27(6):614–619

Stenson K, Saarinen H, Heimer G et al 2001 Women's attitudes to being asked about exposure to violence. Midwifery 17:2–10

Taft A 2002 Violence against women in pregnancy and after childbirth: current knowledge and issues in health care responses. Australian Domestic and Family Violence Clearinghouse, Sydney

UNAIDS 2004 AIDS epidemic update 2004. UNAIDS, United Nations, Geneva, www.unaids.org

US Department of Health and Human Services (1990) The health benefits of smoking cessation. Office on smoking and health, Rockville

Victorian Health 2001 Three Centres Consensus Guidelines on Antenatal Care Project. Mercy Hospital for Women, Southern Health and Women's and Children's Health, Melbourne

Walsh RA, Lowe J, Hopkins PJ 2001 Quitting smoking in pregnancy. Medical Journal of Australia 175:320–323

Ward R, Zamorski M 2002 Benefits and risks of psychiatric medications during pregnancy. American Family Physician 66:629–639

Webster J, Sweett S, Stoltz TA 1994 Domestic violence in pregnancy: a prevalence study. Medical Journal of Australia 161:466–470

World Health Organization (WHO) 1997 Female genital mutilation. A joint WHO/UNICEF/UNFPA statement. WHO, Geneva

World Health Organization (WHO) 2000 Women's mental health: an evidence based review. WHO, Geneva

Wisborg K, Henriksen T, Jespersen L 2000 Nicotine patches for pregnant smokers: a randomised controlled trial. Obstetrics and Gynaecology 96:967–971

Zuckerman A 1999 More than a third of the world's population has been infected with hepatitis B virus. British Medical Journal 318(7192):1213–1214

CHAPTER 8

Making decisions about fertility

Sally K Tracy

Key terms

biological clock, fecundity rates, gamete intrafallopian transfer (GIFT), intracytoplasmic sperm injection (ICSI), in vitro fertilisation (IVF), infertility, luteal support, older women, protecting fertility

Chapter overview

This chapter offers a brief introduction to fertility and reproductive issues faced by women who may not achieve pregnancy without assistance. It will introduce you to some of the physical methods of assisted reproduction, and some of the ethical dilemmas associated with fertility and reproduction technology.

Learning outcomes

The aims of this chapter are:

1 To explore the meaning of fertility and infertility

2 To identify key aspects of assisted reproduction

3 To discuss the importance of age and motherhood.

Introduction

Demographic, economic, social and administrative changes have all had a role in fertility transition (Caldwell 1999). A sustained fall in fertility is a relatively recent phenomenon. In the late eighteenth century a sustained fall in fertility began in France, and fertility declines became general in western and central Europe, as well as in English-speaking settlement countries, in the last quarter of the nineteenth century (Caldwell 1999). The reasons were complex (Caldwell 1999). Fertility decline has never been an unconscious social process; advocacy and organisation have been important. From 1950 to 1965, the world population increased by 34% and that of developing countries by 39% (Caldwell 1999). In developing countries, in the 15 years from the early 1950s until the late 1960s, life expectancy at birth had risen from under 41 years to over 52 years and the annual population growth rate had climbed from 2.0 to 2.5%, while the total fertility rate (the average number of lifetime births per woman at the age-specific birth rates at a specified date) had remained at just over six. Social theorists began to proclaim that it was unique characteristics of the Western family that had allowed or ordained fertility control, and others suggested that the socio-economic gap between the late nineteenth century West and the mid-twentieth century Third World was greater than had been thought. But by 1970 it was clear that there had been a widespread fall in fertility from about 1965 in both Latin America and Asia (Caldwell 1999).

In the three decades from 1965–70 to 1995–2000, the total fertility rate of the developing world halved from 6.0 to 3.0 births per woman. What has been less frequently noted is that between the early 1960s and the late 1990s the total fertility rate of developed countries fell by 37%, from 2.7 to 1.7. Fertility in the West fell because married women were entering the labour force in larger numbers than before, but undoubtedly the change was facilitated by the same forces that assisted the Third World: there were better contraceptives and their use had become respectable. Thus the world's annual number of births in the late 1990s was only 129 million, well below the 206 million that would have been the situation if the fertility levels of the early 1960s had been maintained.

The choice of delaying pregnancy has become the norm for many women in developed countries. Among some women, however, achieving pregnancy may be difficult or impossible at a later time. Australian and New Zealand women, like women in most developed countries, are delaying childbirth until their thirties and forties. In 1971 the average age of Australian and New Zealand women at delivery was 25.4 years, but has consistently increased since then, reaching a peak of 30.5 years in 2003 (Laws & Sullivan 2004; NZHIS 2004). Since 1971, birth rates among women in their thirties have increased while decreasing for the younger age groups. Several causative factors have been identified, such as delayed partnering, higher education, increased employment opportunities for women, longer life expectancy and improved access to and availability of contraception. At the same time, advances in assisted reproductive technologies have improved pregnancy rates among infertile couples, adding to the growing group of primiparous women aged 35 years and older.

Women's ability to conceive declines with age. Data have shown that the proportion of women who tried but did not succeed in conceiving their first child within one year increased from 6% in the 15–24 years age group to more than 30% in the 35–44 years age group (te Velde et al 1998). Adverse neonatal outcomes such as preterm birth, low birthweight, stillbirth and neonatal deaths are higher among assisted-conception births (Helmerhorst et al 2004). Infertility treatment is also an independent risk factor for caesarean section among primiparous women aged 40 and above (Sheiner et al 2001). Over half (54.3%) of all assisted reproductive technique (ART) cycles in Australia in 2002 involved women aged 35 years and over (Sullivan et al 2005, unpublished work).

Fertility

The total fertility rate refers to the number of babies a woman could expect to bear, on average, during her lifetime if she experienced current age-specific fertility rates throughout her childbearing life. In Australia, since 1961, when each woman averaged 3.55 babies, the total fertility rate has declined to 1.75 births per woman in 2002 (ABS 2003). This is notably below the replacement fertility level of 2.1 babies per woman—the number of babies a woman would need to have during her lifetime to replace both herself and her partner. This trend for fertility to drop below replacement level is occurring in most developed, and some developing, countries. Aided by effective and available methods of fertility control, Australian and New Zealand women are increasingly delaying childbearing for a number of social, economic and cultural reasons.

In 2002, the highest fertility occurred in women aged 30–34 years, at a rate of 111.2 babies per 1000 women, continuing the trend of the previous two years. This group experienced slightly higher fertility than the 25–29 year age group (104.2 babies per 1000 women). The main decline in the fertility rate over the past 20 years has occurred among the 20–24 and 25–29 age groups. Meanwhile, fertility has continued to increase in women aged 40 and over (ABS 2003), and ART has played a role in this. Recent years have seen some notable trends in reproduction. Numbers of births in Australia and New Zealand have been generally decreasing, as have fertility rates and perinatal deaths. In contrast, the proportion of multiple births has been increasing (Laws & Sullivan 2004).

'Fertility' in the colloquial sense of the word denotes reproductive capacity (rather than the demographic sense of number of live births). Aside from some medically determined causes of sterility, the reproductive capacity of a couple cannot be measured directly. Rather, it has to be assessed stochastically, by whether pregnancy occurs and how long it takes the couple to conceive (Sallmen et al 2005, p 494).

The ability to preserve fertility with various methods has become a key issue for some women. Although the need is most pressing among women with cancer, the same therapeutic options may be available for many other women who are reaching an advanced reproductive age. However, in this group, the use of the available techniques is controversial and should be considered experimental (Lobo 2005, p 64).

The peak number of oocytes in the female infant occurs at about 20 weeks gestation, when there are somewhere between 6 and 7 million oocytes. Then, by the time of birth, the number has reduced to 1 to 2 million oocytes. By the time a woman is 37 years old, she reportedly has approximately 25,000. This number drops over the years until at menopause (around 50 years for most women) she will have about 1000 oocytes left in her body (Lobo 2005, p 65). The mechanism underlying this process is poorly understood and involves multiple factors encoded by genes on the X chromosome, as well as on autosomes (Simpson 2000). Although environmental factors may be important, genetic factors predict 44% to 87% of the variance in the age at menopause (de Bruin et al 2001; van Asselt 2004). In normal women, at approximately 37.5 years of age, an accelerated atresia of the oocytes begins (Gougeon et al 1994).

This accelerated loss is poorly understood and is often associated with a small monotropic rise in the level of follicle-stimulating hormone (FSH) and decreased fecundity (Scott et al 1989; Wood et al 1992), as well as an increased risk of aneuploidy. The subtle increase in the level of FSH is thought to increase atresia, which is coupled with an accelerated loss of follicles and a further increase in FSH, thus resulting in a positive-feedback loop (Erickson et al 2000).

Accordingly, women who are destined to go through menopause at the age of 45 years (10% of the population) might be expected to have accelerated atresia and reduced fecundity beginning at the age of 32 years; however, this hypothesis has not been proved. Although it is clear that women with a strong family history of early menopause would be at risk for reduced fecundity at an earlier age, no data suggest at what age fecundity decreases. As atresia continues, both the number and the quality of oocytes fall below a critical level, and the rate of aneuploidy increases—a finding that is related at least in part to problems of the meiotic spindle resulting in nondisjunction. This process leads to a greater risk of spontaneous abortion once pregnancy occurs.

Ageing is a significant factor influencing the ability to conceive. As stated earlier, in normal women, fecundity begins to decline at a more rapid pace after the age of 37.5 years.

Premature ovarian failure, which is defined as menopause before the age of 40 years or hypergonadotrophic amenorrhea, occurs in up to 0.9% of women in the general population and has multiple causes, including the involvement of several genes. Once premature ovarian failure has been established, fertility is usually lost, although spontaneous pregnancies may occur. Familial premature ovarian failure and environmental factors that may deplete ovarian follicles define this risk category. Various environmental factors and toxic exposures may also affect the age at menopause.

Pelvic diseases—such as endometriosis, neoplasms and infection—may require surgery, which by removing and destroying cortical tissue depletes the follicular or oocyte reservoir and may lead to early menopause. In addition, pelvic surgery may lead to the formation of adhesions, which may affect the ability to conceive naturally. Among the women at greatest risk for the inability to reproduce are those undergoing treatment for cancer due to the effects of multi-drug chemotherapy.

The body fat connection

That excessive exercise or under-nutrition can postpone puberty, reduce fertility or prevent menstruation was first discovered by Rose Frisch in her pioneering studies beginning in the late 1960s. Her work describing the reproductive consequences of an altered mass of fat were largely ignored or treated with scepticism. Her hypothesis—that a critical mass of body fat is the crucial trigger of gonadotrophin secretion, both in developing girls and in mature women during reproductive life—was initially based on detailed analysis of worldwide demographic data and was later supported by highly focused clinical investigation (Reichlin 2003).

In otherwise healthy young women, a critical mass of body fat is the essential trigger of cyclical pituitary–ovarian function. A successful pregnancy requires approximately 50,000 calories stored in the form of fat. A critical body-fat mass determines the onset of menses. Excessive leanness, as in people with anorexia nervosa and some competitive athletes and professional dancers, delays the onset of puberty; after menarche has been established, excessive leanness can cause impaired ovulation, infertility and amenorrhea. Oestrogen deficiency induced by excessive exercise (and decreased fat mass) is associated with premature osteoporosis, even in runners in whom bone formation has been stimulated by exercise. On the positive side, women who have been extremely active athletically have a much reduced risk of breast cancer, presumably because they have been exposed to lower levels of oestrogen over time. These insights have been invaluable for the evaluation of women with delayed puberty and amenorrhea, and they have important social and medical implications for dancers and athletes. Though less well documented, critical body-fat mass is probably also

---

BOX 8.1 Weight and onset of menarche

Rose Frisch was the scientist who discovered, during her studies on weight gain in populations around the world, that poor rural girls had their peak rate of growth at an older age than did well-nourished urban girls. Since it was known at the time that a period of rapid growth precedes the onset of menarche, she analysed several large population studies in the United States in which the rate of growth and the age of menarche had been assessed and found that the average weight at menarche was 47 kg, whether girls matured early or late. She realised that body weight was a more accurate predictor of the age at the onset of menstruation than was chronological age.
(Source: Reichlin 2003)

important in determining pituitary gonadal activity in men (Reichlin 2003, p 870).

Time to pregnancy refers to the number of menstrual cycles it takes a couple to conceive. Fecundability, in turn, is a couple-specific probability of conceiving a recognised pregnancy per menstrual cycle, given no contraception (Sallmen et al 2005, p 494). The characteristics of 'infertile' and 'infertility' refer to couples who try for more than a year to conceive. Many infertile couples will eventually conceive, but a sterile subset cannot conceive without medical intervention (Sallmen et al 2005, p 495).

Given the irreversible nature of women's emancipation and their presence in the labour workforce, there is a relationship between public policies (maternity leave, income tax regulations), workplace conditions (part-time opportunities and the flexibility of work hours) and the availability of affordable non-parental child care that enables mothers to participate in the labour force (Hank et al 2003).

A growing body of research suggests a changing, now positive, relationship between women's education or employment and fertility with the advent of social contexts that allow women to combine childrearing and employment. Access to affordable child care is essential for this to occur (Hank & Kreyenfeld 2003).

Older women and childbirth

Most women over age 35 have healthy pregnancies and healthy babies. According to US data, the number of first births per 1000 women aged 35 to 39 years increased by 36% between 1991 and 2001, and the rate among women age 40 to 44 years leapt by a remarkable 70%. In 2002, 263 births were reported in women between 50 and 54 years of age (Heffner 2004).

Very advanced maternal age, defined as maternal age of 45 years or greater at the time of delivery, has important consequences for both mother and baby. Currently, 0.1% of all Australian and New Zealand women giving birth are in this age category (ABS 2000; NZHIS 2004). Given the trend towards delayed childbearing and the increasing availability of assisted reproductive techniques, women aged 45 and over may increasingly seek advice about the risks of embarking on a pregnancy (Callaway et al 2005).

The effect of maternal age on the outcome of pregnancy may be best assessed by examining five specific factors (Heffner 2004) that can negatively affect the desired outcome of a pregnancy—a healthy mother and baby. These are:

- declining fertility
- miscarriage
- chromosomal abnormalities
- hypertensive complications
- stillbirth.

It is not unusual for a woman in her mid-thirties or older to take longer to conceive than a younger woman. Age-related decline in fertility may be due, in part, to less frequent ovulation, or to problems such as endometriosis, in which

tissue similar to that lining the uterus attaches to the ovaries or fallopian tubes and interferes with conception. While women over age 35 may have more difficulty conceiving, they also have a greater chance of bearing twins. The likelihood of naturally conceived (without fertility treatment) twins peaks between ages 35 and 39, then declines.

Miscarriage is defined as spontaneous pregnancy loss before the twentieth week of gestation. Karyotyping of the products of conception after miscarriage indicates that about two-thirds are chromosomally abnormal (Heffner 2004). There is a strong relationship between maternal age and miscarriage rates. At 20 years of age, the rate is about 10%. It increases to a high of more than 90% among women 45 years of age or older. This high miscarriage rate contributes significantly to decreasing fertility among older women (Heffner 2004, p 1927).

The success rate using donor eggs from younger women for in vitro fertilisation supports the hypothesis that deterioration occurs in the quality of the ova with advancing maternal age (Heffner 2004).

Both chronic hypertension (that antedates pregnancy) and pregnancy-induced hypertension usually occur during the second half of a pregnancy and include both hypertension without proteinuria and the many variants of the disorder pre-eclampsia. All forms of hypertension can complicate pregnancies by restricting fetal growth and may necessitate premature delivery when the health of either the mother or the fetus is in jeopardy. The risk of hypertensive complications of pregnancy increases steadily as women age; such complications are twice as likely among women 40 years of age or older as among younger women (Heffner 2004, p 1928).

How should we counsel young women when they ask about their reproductive choices? Generally speaking, the decade between 25 and 35 years of age would seem to be ideal. A woman's education is typically complete, she has usually gained some experience in her professional arena, and pregnancy is at its safest. For women between 35 and 45 years

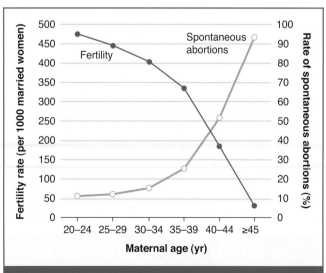

Figure 8.1 Fertility and miscarriage rates as a function of maternal age (based on Heffner 2004)

of age for whom earlier childbearing is not an option, this decade remains safe enough that maternal age alone should not be a contraindication to childbearing. However, women do face decreasing fertility and a moderate increase in the risks of miscarriage and chromosomal abnormalities as they pass 40 years of age. Perimenopausal and postmenopausal pregnancy remains an option for those women who are lucky enough to find themselves healthy and sufficiently wealthy to pursue it (Heffner 2004, p 1929).

The risk of bearing a child with certain chromosomal disorders increases as a woman ages. The most common of these disorders is Down syndrome, a combination of mental retardation and physical abnormalities caused by the presence of an extra chromosome 21 (humans have 23 pairs of chromosomes). At age 25, a woman has about a 1 in 1250 chance of having a baby with Down syndrome; at age 30, a 1 in 1000 chance; at age 35, a 1 in 400 chance; at age 40, a 1 in 100 chance; and at 45, a 1 in 30 chance. Most pregnant women who are 35 or older are offered the option of prenatal testing (with amniocentesis or chorionic villus sampling) to diagnose or, more likely, rule out Down syndrome and other chromosomal abnormalities. About 95% of women who undergo prenatal testing find that their baby does not have one of these disorders. If prenatal testing rules out chromosomal defects and the mother is healthy, the baby probably is at no greater risk of birth defects than if the mother were in her twenties.

Most miscarriages occur in the first trimester for women of all ages. The rate of miscarriage in older women is significantly greater than that in younger women. A recent Danish study found that about 9% of recognised pregnancies for women aged 20 to 24 ended in miscarriage. The risk rose to about 25% at age 35 to 39, and more than 50% by age 42 (Nyobo Anderson et al 2000).

While women in their late thirties and forties are very likely to have a healthy baby, they do face more complications along the way. Besides the increased risk of diabetes and high blood pressure, women over 35 have an increased risk of placental problems. The most common placental problem is placenta praevia, in which the placenta covers part or all of the opening of the cervix. First-time mothers over age 40 were up to eight times as likely as women in their twenties to have this complication. Some studies suggest that women having their first baby at age 35 or older are at increased risk of having either a low birthweight or preterm baby (born at less than 37 full weeks of pregnancy). These risks rise modestly but progressively with a woman's age, even if she does not have age-related chronic health problems such as diabetes and high blood pressure. The Danish study also found that women over age 35 had an increased risk of ectopic pregnancy (in which the fertilised egg implants in the fallopian tube) (Nyobo Anderson et al 2000).

Teenage pregnancies

Among teenage mothers in Australia and New Zealand the birth rate continues to decline. In Australia the birth rate for women aged 15–19 years declined from 27.4 births per 1000 women in 1982 to 17.1 in 2002. Even in the last few years, the decline has been large, down from 22.0 in 1992 to 17.7 in 2000. Compared with the 1982 rate, the 2002 rate represents an overall decline of 38% (ABS 2003).

Thirty years ago, a study of 37 developed countries including Denmark, Finland, Norway and Sweden showed a relationship between low fertility rates and openness about sexual matters, government policy for providing contraceptives to young unmarried women, well-organised teaching about contraception in schools, and a high percentage of the population living in large cities (Jones et al 1985). It is believed that the main reason for a drop in abortion rates worldwide is increased use of contraceptive methods (Henshaw 1999) and in the Netherlands a national emphasis on the importance of contraceptive methods, ongoing positive sex education in schools, and easily accessible, low-cost and friendly contraceptive services are the main reasons for low fertility and abortion rates (Ketting & Visser 1994).

In Sweden, contraceptive services for young people were introduced and are run by midwives (Bender et al 2003). The greater accessibility of contraceptive methods in Sweden was made possible through the immediate development of teenage clinics, which now comprise over 200 nationwide (Bender et al 2003). The link between fertility and use of contraception was considered important, and its preventive effect regarding abortion was recognised. Sweden also developed an effective link between sex education in schools and contraceptive services for young people (Bender et al 2003).

In industrialised countries, *Chlamydia trachomatis* is the predominant infectious agent causing pelvic inflammatory disease and, as a result of damage to the fallopian tubes, accounts for up to half of all ectopic pregnancies. The substantial financial costs of genital chlamydial infections result from hospital treatment for pelvic inflammatory disease, ectopic pregnancy and infertility, which may include in vitro fertilisation.

World population trends

Since 1968, when the UN Population Division predicted that the world population, now 6.3 billion, would grow to at least 12 billion by 2050, the agency has regularly revised its estimates downwards. It now expects world population to plateau at 9 billion. We are experiencing a profound demographic shift as a result of two forces: increasing longevity and declining fertility. The best-known example of shrinkage is in Italy, where women were once symbols of fecundity. By 2000, Italy's fertility rate was Western Europe's lowest, at 1.2 births per woman. Its population is expected to drop 20% by mid-century. Denmark was below population replacement level in 1970 at 2.0 births per woman, and slid to 1.7 by 2001 (Kurjak & Carrera 2005).

Demographics of New Zealand women

The age of mothers has changed over the past 20 years, with the number of women giving birth over 30 years of age

TABLE 8.1   Projected population growth

Location	Total population, 2004 (billions)	Projected population, 2050 (billions)	Average growth, 2000–2005 (billions)
World	6.378	8.919	1.2
More developed regions	1.206	1.220	0.2
Less developed regions	5.172	7.699	1.5
Least developed countries	0.736	1.675	2.4

Data are from the United Nations Population Fund. More developed regions comprise North America, Japan, Europe, Australia and New Zealand. Less developed regions comprise all regions of Africa, Latin America, the Caribbean, Asia (excluding Japan), Melanesia, Micronesia and Polynesia. The least developed countries are defined according to the standard United Nations designations.
(Source: Rosenfield & Schwartz 2005)

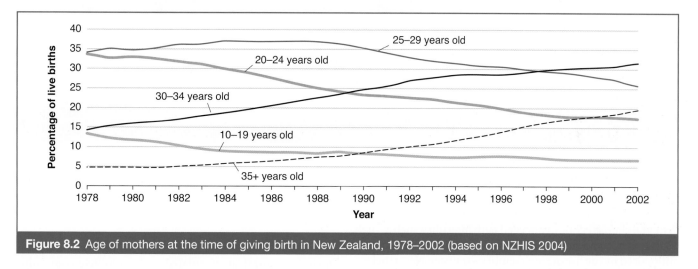

Figure 8.2 Age of mothers at the time of giving birth in New Zealand, 1978–2002 (based on NZHIS 2004)

steadily increasing, while births among younger women have decreased. The reducing rate for teenage women is a result not of a declining fertility rate but of an increasing abortion rate, and the birth rate in women under the age of 19 remains high by international standards. Young pregnant women—especially those without sufficient family support—require significant support from health and social services. In the 2002 Maternity Services Consumer Survey, women aged 15–19 years were less likely than older mothers to have been satisfied with maternity services (New Zealand Ministry of Health 2004).

Although the age distribution of mothers may have changed over time (Fig 8.2), the percentage of births by each ethnic group has changed very little.

In 2002 the average age for New Zealand women to have a baby was 29.7 years, and 56.3% of New Zealand births were to women between the ages of 25 and 34 years. Seven per cent of births were to those under 20 years (3697/53,037), 19.5% (10,338/53,037) to Maori women, 10.8% to Pacific women (5714/53,037), and 7.7% to Asian women (4082/53,037).

In 2002, Maori women tended to have children at a younger age than women in other ethnic groups (Fig 8.3). The most common age for a Maori woman to give birth was 20–24 years. Of all births to teenage mothers (under 20 years of age),

44.1% (1629/3697) were to Maori women. Asian women most commonly gave birth between 25 and 34 years of age, and accounted for 1.7% (64/3697) of the teenage births.

Methods of assisted reproduction

Conception depends on a woman releasing an egg each month. The egg enters the fallopian tube where it meets the sperm. A sperm cell penetrates the egg in the process known as fertilisation. The resulting embryo is transported down the tube to the uterus, where it implants into the uterine lining (endometrium) a few days later. In general, 75% of couples will achieve a spontaneous pregnancy within six months of exposure, 90% by a year and 95% by two years. Three major factors determine the chances of a natural conception: female age, sperm quality and duration of exposure. It is well known that the risk of an adverse outcome after in vitro fertilisation (IVF) is attributable in large part to the greatly increased rate of multiple births. The rates of multiple gestation after IVF in Europe and the United States are 26.4% and 35.4%, respectively (Thurin et al 2004), underscoring the magnitude

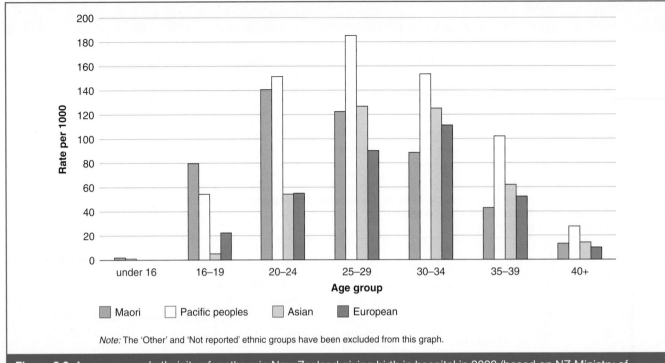

Figure 8.3 Age group and ethnicity of mothers in New Zealand giving birth in hospital in 2002 (based on NZ Ministry of Health 2004)

of the problem. However, higher risks of preterm delivery and low birthweight have also been observed for singletons conceived by IVF and have been attributed at least in part to parental characteristics associated with infertility, such as high maternal age and nulliparity; these, of course, would not be influenced by the use of single-embryo transfer. Nevertheless, a substantial reduction in multiple births after IVF would dramatically decrease the risks associated with prematurity and low birthweight for children born after IVF (Thurin et al 2004).

In vitro fertilisation

In vitro fertilisation involves four basic steps: ovarian stimulation, egg recovery, insemination and, finally, embryo replacement. Couples with less than two years exposure need only consider IVF with proven tubal disease, significant semen abnormalities and moderate to severe endometriosis. Couples with unexplained infertility of less than two years, in women aged less than 35, need only consider IVF after two or more years of trying, and after a year in women older than 35. Minimal endometriosis is unlikely to be the cause of a delay in conception. Although IVF was originally devised for women with tubal damage or dysfunction, in combination with intracytoplasmic sperm injection (ICSI) it is a very effective method to treat male factor infertility. In vitro fertilisation treatment may be used in selected instances with donated eggs, sperm or embryos.

It is important to establish the cause of infertility before proceeding to IVF. Investigations would usually include checks of ovulation, tubal patency and an ultrasound for the female partner. A semen analysis is required for the male partner.

Ovarian stimulation

During a natural unstimulated cycle, a follicle containing a single egg develops to maturity. To produce more eggs it is necessary to stimulate the ovaries with a group of drugs known as gonadotrophins. Ovarian hyperstimulation (an excessive response) is a major and potentially life-threatening complication associated with gonadotrophins.

It is safest to monitor the response of the ovaries by daily oestrogen measurements and ultrasound. Ultrasound scans are used to see the number and size of the follicles and to judge when to do the egg recovery. The oestrogens are necessary to determine the ovarian response to stimulation. By interpreting the results of ultrasound and oestrogen, the specialist will determine the best time to perform the egg collection. About 36 hours before the egg collection is due, an injection of human chorionic gonadotrophin (hCG) is given to initiate the final process of egg maturation. Precise timing is necessary, as the eggs will be suitable for recovery 34 to 36 hours after the hCG injection.

Egg collection

This is done under sedation or general anaesthetic using a vaginal ultrasound probe. A needle is guided through the top of the vagina into the ovary. Each follicle is aspirated through the needle using a suction device.

Insemination and fertilisation

The eggs are identified in the laboratory and placed in culture medium. They are then placed in dishes in an incubator. The male partner produces a semen sample by masturbation and this is prepared in the laboratory. A number of motile sperm are extracted and used to inseminate the eggs some hours later. It takes about 18 hours for fertilisation to be completed, and about 12 hours later the embryo starts to divide. Two or three days after egg collection, when the embryos have reached the 2–6 cell stage, they are ready to be replaced into the woman's uterus.

Embryo transfer

This is a most important step and is best performed under ultrasound guidance. A maximum of two embryos may be replaced. Couples should consider the replacement of a single embryo to prevent a twin pregnancy. There is no evidence that bed rest makes a difference to the outcome and most units recommend resuming normal activities.

Luteal support

Hormone supplementation in the form of hCG injections, progesterone pessaries or injections is usually recommended after embryo transfer, to support the uterine lining.

Embryo freezing

Most IVF clinics offer embryo freezing and storage for spare embryos. However, not all surplus embryos are suitable for freezing, not all survive the procedure, and the implantation rate after transfer is lower than with fresh embryo transfer.

Abandoned cycles

The abandoned cycle rate varies considerably between units. Cycles may be abandoned before egg recovery as the ovarian response is either inadequate or excessive, and before embryo replacement if no eggs are recovered, or the eggs fail to fertilise or the embryos don't divide. In many instances it will be possible to try again using alternative drugs or methods, such as intracytoplasmic sperm injection (ICSI) for failed fertilisation.

Occasionally IVF cycles are abandoned because of a high risk of ovarian hyperstimulation. (The risk of ovarian hyperstimulation is increased in women with polycystic ovaries.) In these circumstances the cycle may be cancelled during ovarian stimulation and restarted with a lower dose of drugs, or allowed to proceed but all the embryos are frozen and replaced when the ovaries have returned to normal.

The ovarian hyperstimulation syndrome is potentially life-threatening. This syndrome occurs in about 2% to 3% of cases and consists of severe nausea and vomiting, a rapid gain in weight, abdominal swelling and shortness of breath. The fluid and electrolyte imbalance needs careful management in experienced centres. It starts a week after the hCG injection and is made worse by pregnancy.

Support when undergoing treatment

It is well recognised that undergoing assisted conception treatment, particularly IVF, is stressful both emotionally and physically. It is essential that patients fully understand the proposed treatment program and the commitment in time required for monitoring the cycle. Most clinics have information sheets and some have support groups to help in times of stress. All licensed centres are obliged to offer independent counselling to patients considering IVF treatment. This may prove helpful, as it gives the opportunity for a couple to discuss their infertility and treatment confidentially with an impartial person.

Gamete intrafallopian transfer

Gamete intrafallopian transfer (GIFT) can be considered both a sophisticated form of artificial insemination and a simplified form of IVF. The management of a patient in a GIFT treatment cycle is usually exactly the same as for an IVF cycle, up until the point at which the oocytes (eggs) have been recovered. A number of drug regimens are used to stimulate the ovaries to produce multiple oocytes, and these are always discussed with the couple at the time the treatment is started.

The growth of the ovarian follicles in which the eggs are developing is always monitored with a combination of serial ultrasound scans and often blood or urine tests. When the follicles are considered to be mature enough, arrangements are made for the patient to receive an injection of hCG and the egg recovery procedure is planned some 34–36 hours later.

Most clinics now will recover the oocytes by the transvaginal ultrasound directed technique, as for IVF. Some clinics will, however, recover the eggs laparoscopically. Once the oocytes have been collected and identified, the best two or three are selected. A preparation of the husband's sperm is taken into a fine catheter, together with the eggs, the tube is gently inserted under direct vision through the laparoscope into the outer ends of one or both fallopian tubes and the egg/sperm mixture is injected into the tube(s). At the end of this procedure, the patient is returned to the ward to recover, and will go home the same day.

Most patients are given either injections or pessaries of the hormone progesterone and some 15 days later a pregnancy test is carried out to determine whether there is early evidence of a pregnancy.

GIFT is generally found to be slightly more successful than IVF in most clinics. This is probably because the fallopian tube is a more physiological environment for fertilisation to occur in than in a laboratory culture dish. However, the procedure does require a laparoscopy, and most clinics now do not generally believe that the extra inconvenience of and potential discomfort of a laparoscopy makes the slightly increased pregnancy rates worthwhile. If a clinic is achieving good results with IVF, then it will generally not do GIFT. Clinics achieving poorer success rates with IVF may find that GIFT is considerably more successful and therefore recommend it.

Pregnancy rates for IVF are commonly quoted as being in the range of 15–30% and for GIFT, 25–30%.

Intracytoplasmic sperm injection

Intracytoplasmic sperm injection (ICSI) was introduced into clinical treatment for certain types of infertility in 1992. It is a type of IVF treatment that involves the injection of a single sperm straight into each egg. The fertilised egg (embryo) can then be transferred into the womb of the woman as in a normal IVF cycle.

The live birth rates for ICSI and conventional IVF are similar—about 23% per cycle, in the most recently published Human Fertilisation and Embryology Authority (HFEA) data from the United Kingdom (2005).

What does ICSI involve?

Intracytoplasmic sperm injection is similar to conventional IVF in that gametes (eggs and sperm) are collected from each partner. To achieve fertilisation, a single sperm is taken up in a fine glass needle and is injected directly into an egg. The eggs are then incubated and examined. Usually one or two embryos may then be transferred back into the womb of the woman two or three days after fertilisation. Some eggs may not survive the injection process and not all eggs collected will be of a high-enough quality or mature enough to be suitable for injection.

When is ICSI used?

In conventional IVF the eggs and the sperm are mixed together in a dish and the sperm fertilise the eggs naturally. ICSI by-passes the natural processes involved in a sperm penetrating an egg, and is therefore used when there are problems that make it difficult to achieve fertilisation naturally or by conventional IVF. It is used when:

● the sperm count is very low
● the sperm cannot move properly or are in other ways abnormal
● the sperm have been retrieved directly from the epididy-mis (PESA) or the testicles (TESA/TESE), from the urine, or by electro ejaculation
● there are high levels of antibodies in the semen
● there have been previous fertilisation failures.

Men who have very few sperm (oligozoospermia) or no sperm (azoospermia) in their semen, or who have high numbers of abnormal sperm that are unable to fertilise an egg, would previously have had little or no chance of fathering their own genetic offspring.

Like IVF, ICSI is an invasive procedure. However, unlike IVF, ICSI involves injecting a sperm directly into an egg, therefore allowing the use of sperm that may not otherwise be able to fertilise an egg. For these reasons, concerns about the potential risks to children born as a result of ICSI have been raised, and several follow-up studies have been published.

ICSI is still a relatively new technique, and all children conceived using ICSI are still very young. Consequently, follow-up studies involve relatively small numbers of children

> **BOX 8.2** **Terms used in ART**
>
> ▶ *PESA*—percutaneous epididymal sperm aspiration, involving sperm being retrieved directly from the epididymis using a needle.
> ▶ *TESA*—testicular sperm aspiration, involving sperm being retrieved directly from the testes using a needle.
> ▶ *TESE*—testicular sperm extraction, involving sperm being retrieved from a biopsy of testicular tissue.

and do not include effects that may only be seen in older children or in the next generation. Follow-up studies are extremely important. The complexity of the process of egg and sperm production means that even if an individual possesses a normal number of chromosomes, their gametes could potentially have an abnormal number. It is not possible to detect beforehand which eggs or sperm have chromosomal abnormalities, and gametes that might not have been able to participate in natural fertilisation could therefore be used in ICSI. Babies born after ICSI have been reported to have new chromosomal abnormalities in up to 3% of cases. The rate in the general population is around 0.6% (HFEA 2005).

The procedure

The woman is stimulated for follicle (the tiny sack in the ovary that carries the egg) production, as in conventional IVF. Egg recovery is identical to that for routine IVF, but sperm treatment differs according to individual patient circumstances and, even if obtained from the ejaculate, often requires a modification of the procedures used for IVF. This modification uses a high centrifugation method to concentrate the contents of the seminal plasma into the size of a tiny fraction of a teardrop from which just a few sperm can be obtained and extracted. In certain circumstances micro-injection needles are used (approximately 12 times thinner than a strand of human hair) to isolate single sperm from the seminal plasma.

Whichever method is used—centrifugation or single sperm isolation—it is essential that the sperm be washed free of the seminal plasma. The human egg aspirated from the follicle is surrounded by thousands of spacialised cells—the cumulus cells (these perform a 'nursing' role while the egg is in the follicle). These cumulus cells are removed by treatment with hyaluronidase, a natural enzyme that is produced by the sperm during its passage through the cumulus cells while in the fallopian tube. In less than a couple of minutes the enzyme digests away the cells, leaving the egg encased in a few layers in another type of specialised cells. These are mechanically removed by the embryologist using gentle suction into a very finely pulled glass tube. The egg denuded of almost all its surrounding cells is then accessible for ICSI.

The ICSI procedure per se begins by first immobilising the sperm. This is often performed by transferring the sperm into a viscous solution, which dramatically slows down its motility. In its sluggish state the single sperm has its tail permanently immobilised—this has been shown to be an extremely important part of the process. The sperm is then aspirated into the tiny micro-needle and carefully maintained at its tip. The micro-injection needle is manipulated using a micro-manipulator, which has extremely fine control capabilities. The egg itself is held onto another micro-tool by gentle suction to keep it firmly positioned. The micro-needle containing the sperm is pushed gently up against the outer shell (zone pellucida) and carefully pushed through the shell, through the outer membrane of the egg and directly into the centre of the egg itself—in the egg's cytoplasm.

Once the needle is inside the egg, a tiny amount of cytoplasm is aspirated into the micro-needle to mix with the sperm and ensure that the egg has been properly penetrated. Despite the tiny size of the egg (approximately seven times smaller than the average full stop), the membrane is a very elastic structure and can be extensively stretched without actually being ruptured. Once the embryologist is certain that the egg has been penetrated, the sperm and cytoplasmic mixture is injected back into the egg. This procedure rarely causes residual damage to the egg, and has no lasting effects on further development. The whole procedure is performed under a high-powered microscope. In some cases, immotile but living sperm is used. It is therefore important for the embryologists to be able to distinguish between dead and living immotile sperm. In this situation a solution is used that causes the tail of a living but immotile sperm to curl. The curled tail indicates that the sperm is actually living. It is these that the embryologist selects with the micro-needle.

Once isolated, the sperm can then be transferred to the viscous solution and treated in the same way for the ICSI procedure. At the end of the injection procedure the micro-injection needle is carefully withdrawn and suction on the egg is released. The egg is washed through a few changes of normal culture medium, and left overnight in an incubator at 37°C in conditions similar to routine IVF culture. The subsequent culture procedures, checking for fertilisation, cleavage of the fertilised egg and transfer of any embryos to the womb, occur in the same routine manner as for conventional IVF.

Laws about donation

In New Zealand and parts of Australia, the identity of donors is recorded. Knowing about our genetic heritage can help us to understand who we are. This can be important:

- for the psychological and emotional wellbeing of donor-conceived people. Many of them, like people who have been adopted, are naturally curious about their genetic origins.
- for medical reasons. Inherited characteristics may predispose the offspring to certain medical conditions. Knowing the medical history may help to get an early diagnosis and effective treatment for an inherited disease.
- for family relationships. Family secrets can undermine trust and lead to conflict and stress. They can also suggest to children (and others) that their parents are ashamed of how they were conceived.
- for donor-conceived people's future relationships. There is a small but real risk that two people who are genetic

siblings could have children together without realising they were related. If parents tell their children they were donor-conceived they will be able to check this out.

- for donors. Donors are often curious about the children they may have created. Under the law they are able to find out from the clinic how many children were born as a result of their donation. They will not be able to identify them by name, however, although children will be able to find out who the donor was and may wish to contact them.

Demographics of assisted reproduction

Following the introduction of assisted reproductive technologies (ART), including intracytoplasmic sperm injection (ICSI), in vitro fertilisation (IVF) and ovulation induction (OI) with clomiphene citrate or follicle-stimulating hormone (FSH), the past 20 years have seen a steady increase in multiple pregnancy rates (Bolton et al 2003). Rates for twins are increased by approximately 20 times and higher-order multiple pregnancies by 400 times in women undergoing treatment with ART. When compared with singleton births, twins have a six-fold increased risk of mortality and for triplets the risk is 10- to 20-fold higher. The proportion of multiple births that are the result of fertility treatments is unknown in New Zealand, as a result of inadequacies in birth record information (Bolton et al 2003).

In Australia

In Australia, among babies born in 2002, 2.3% were following the use of ART. These babies had a lower average birthweight than all Australian babies, with 20.9% of pregnancies being preterm. Almost half the women with ART pregnancies gave birth via caesarean section (49.4%). Of ART pregnancies there were 3845 singletons (79.1%), 988 sets of twins (20.3%) and 26 sets of triplets (0.5%). In total, 20.9% were multiple pregnancies.

Since 1979, assisted reproductive technology (ART) has been used in Australia to help couples achieve pregnancy. The main procedures used in ART treatment cycles include IVF, ICSI and GIFT. Data on treatment cycles and outcomes of pregnancy are collected annually from all 25 ART centres in Australia and four in New Zealand and collated into an Australian and New Zealand assisted conception data collection. The data collection is funded by the Fertility Society of Australia and is maintained at the National Perinatal Statistics Unit (NPSU). Results of treatments and outcomes of pregnancies in previous years' treatments were reported annually in the past, from the Assisted Conception Data Collection (ACDC). With the implementation of the new Australian and New Zealand Assisted Reproduction Database (ANZARD) collection in 2002, the results of the treatments and their pregnancy outcomes can be reported as a single cohort in the same year in the AIHW Assisted Conception series (Laws & Sullivan 2004, p 61).

In 2002, the average age of women giving birth after ART treatment was 33.7 years, 4.3 years older than the average age of all Australian and New Zealand mothers (29.4 years). In 2002, the average duration of ART pregnancies was 37.6 weeks. Of all ART confinements, 20.9% were preterm, reflecting a much larger proportion of preterm births compared with all Australian births (7.0% preterm). The proportion of ART singleton babies that were preterm was 10.9%, compared with 58.2% for ART twins. For all Australian singletons, the proportion of preterm babies was 6.3% and for twins 52.9% (Laws & Sullivan 2004).

Mothers of ART babies had a higher incidence of caesarean section (49.4% of all ART births) compared with all Australian deliveries (27.0%). Since 1997, the caesarean section rate has been steadily increasing, from 41.9% to 49.4%. The average caesarean section rate between 1993 and 2002 was 44.4%, twice that of all Australian pregnancies during the same period (21.6%). In 2002, the average birthweight of all ART babies was 2943 grams, 415 grams lower than the average birthweight of all Australian babies (3358 grams). The proportion of ART babies of low birthweight (less than 2500 grams) was 24.1%, and of very low birthweight (less than 1500 grams), 5.3%. The proportions for all Australian babies in 2002 were 6.9% and 1.5%, respectively. The average birthweight for singleton ART babies was 3263 grams, 130 grams lower than the average birthweight of all singleton Australian babies (3393 grams) (Laws & Sullivan 2004, p 62).

Birth outcomes following ART

In vitro fertilisation was introduced into practice with little formal evaluation of its effects on the health of the children conceived with this procedure. Following the introduction of intracytoplasmic sperm injection in 1992, there was a concern that infants conceived with the use of assisted reproductive technology might have an increased risk of birth defects (Hansen et al 2002; te Velde et al 1998). A study published in the *New England Journal of Medicine* in 2002 (Hansen et al 2002) found that infants conceived with assisted reproductive technology were more than twice as likely as naturally conceived infants to have major birth anomalies diagnosed during the first year of life, and were also more likely to have multiple major anomalies. The increase in the risk of a major birth anomaly associated with assisted conception remained significant when only singleton or term singleton infants were

Scenario

Issues in assisted reproduction

The first case involved Lu and John B. who used in vitro fertilisation (IVF) with donor eggs and donor sperm. The embryos were subsequently implanted in a genetically unrelated woman (the 'surrogate' mother) for gestation and birth. The Bs intended to rear the resulting child as their own. Before the child, Jay, was born, the couple separated and John wanted to have nothing to do with the child.

In the first trial in this case the judge found that Jay was parentless [regardless of the fact that six adults had been involved in her 'production'].

This decision was reversed on appeal, and the appeals court decided that because, under California law, a husband who consents to his wife's artificial insemination becomes the legal father of the child, a husband and wife [should be] deemed the lawful parents of a child after a surrogate bears a biologically unrelated child on their behalf . . . [since] in each instance a child is procreated because a medical procedure was initiated and consented to by intended parents. Thus, the court concluded that Lu and John were Jay's legal parents. To make sure no one missed the analogy, the court expanded on it, stating that gestational surrogacy and artificial insemination are exactly analogous in this crucial respect: both contemplate the procreation of a child by the consent to a medical procedure of someone who intends to raise the child but who otherwise does not have any biological tie. The court did not like the idea of people who are responsible for the creation of a child turning around and disclaiming any responsibility after the child is born. Since the court believed that John 'caused' the birth of Jay simply by signing a contract, the court had no problem concluding that the same logic that made him the legal father made Lu (his wife at the time the contract with the surrogate mother was signed) the legal mother, since she agreed to the 'procreative project' at the start. The appeals court nonetheless concluded that 'things might work out for the best'. The court conceded that John may have agreed to the surrogate-mother arrangement simply 'as an accommodation to allow Lu to surmount a formality' but observed that 'human relationships are not static; things done merely to help one individual overcome a perceived legal obstacle sometimes become much more meaningful'.

There is no legal basis for such musings, according to George J Annas, writing in the *New England Journal of Medicine* (1998).

(Sources: Annas 1998; Buzzanca v. Buzzanca, 61 Cal. App. 4th 1410 1998)

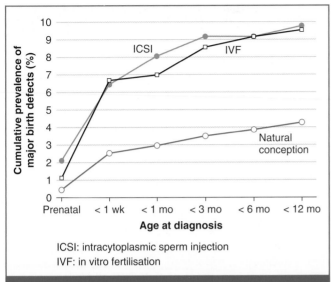

ICSI: intracytoplasmic sperm injection
IVF: in vitro fertilisation

Figure 8.4 Cumulative prevalence of diagnosed major birth anomalies in singleton infants, according to age at diagnosis (based on Hansen et al 2002)

considered, as well as after adjustment for maternal age and parity, the sex of the infant, and correlation between siblings. Furthermore, the estimates of the prevalence of anomalies reported to the registry by one year of age in the assisted-conception groups were well in excess of the 6% prevalence of major birth anomalies (Hansen et al 2002, p 729).

An excess risk of major birth anomalies in infants conceived with assisted reproductive technology is plausible due to the older age of the couple concerned as well as the underlying cause of their infertility. The risk of anomalies may be associated with medications used to induce ovulation or to maintain the pregnancy in the early stages and factors associated with the procedures themselves. These procedures may involve freezing and thawing of embryos, the potential for polyspermic fertilisation, and the delayed fertilisation of the oocyte (Hansen et al 2002).

Complication rates

Complication rates in subfertile women have been ascribed to increased maternal age, lower parity and multiple births resulting from fertility treatment. A large population cohort of women attending a fertility clinic between 1989 and 1999 who subsequently delivered singletons were more likely to develop complications of pregnancy including pre-eclampsia and antepartum haemorrhage than the general obstetric population after adjustment for confounders such as age and parity (Thomson et al 2005). While the calculated relative risks for abruption and placenta praevia are high for subfertile women, the absolute increase in risks is extremely small. Only 0.5% more subfertile women had abruption and 0.7% more had placenta praevia than control women, indicating the importance of considering both the statistical and the

clinical significance of any findings. Fertility treatment did not seem to affect the rate of maternal complications or the rates of obstetric intervention. The researchers found that subfertility did increase the risk of delivering by caesarean section, although this could be partially attributed to the anxiety surrounding these pregnancies, which may lower obstetricians' thresholds for intervention. The association between rates of complications and obstetric intervention by obstetricians has been noted before (Bell et al 2001).

Conclusion

Wide disparities exist in the availability, quality and delivery of infertility services between the resource-rich and resource-poor nations of the world. Approximately 80 million people worldwide are infertile. Most countries in the industrialised West have declining fertility rates marked by late marriage, postponed childbearing and primary infertility. In contrast, in the developing world, there is little voluntary effort to postpone childbearing, and early first marriage is common. However, a high prevalence of sexually transmitted infections and infections acquired as a result of inadequate healthcare result in increased rates of secondary infertility (Nachtigall 2006). In developing societies, childlessness is often highly stigmatised and leads to profound social suffering for infertile women in particular, yet most infertile people in the developing world have virtually no access to effective fertility treatment.

In countries such as New Zealand and Australia, however, in just over two decades, assisted reproduction techniques have evolved from a laboratory curiosity to a commercialised, industrialised technology responsible for thousands of births. Human reproduction has always been a matter of philosophical debate and social controversy. In resource-rich nations, the debate has grown more complicated through continued technical evolution. Both hopes and concerns have been raised simultaneously about the legitimacy of pre-embryo research, the slippery slope of pre-implantation embryo diagnostic testing and eugenic implications, and the fundamental and philosophical problem of the status of the embryo.

Among the resource-poor women of the world, an estimated 250 million years of productive life are lost every year as a result of reproductive health problems. The inability to determine when and how many children to have limits a woman's life choices (UN 2005). More than a decade after the 1994 Cairo International Conference on Population and Development (ICPD), and a global consensus that reproductive rights are central to human rights, sustainable development, gender equality and the empowerment of women (UN 2005), millions of women still do not have access to contraceptive services. Maternal mortality rates remain essentially unchanged and many women still die from complications of unsafe abortions. Both fertility and reproductive health problems remain the greatest burden of the world's poorest women.

Review questions

1   Name four reasons for infertility in women.

2   Name five major reasons for 'subfertility' or infertility in men.

3   What is ovulation induction (hormone treatment)? How would you describe this treatment to women?

4   What is artificial insemination (AI) using the partner's sperm and intra-uterine insemination (IUI)? How would you describe these processes?

5   What is the difference between gamete intra-fallopian transfer (GIFT), in vitro fertilisation (IVF) and intra-cytoplasmic sperm injection (ICSI)?

6   Do you think there should be a register of sperm donors? If so, what are the ethical issues associated with donor insemination?

7   Describe the issues identified in question 6 from the point of view of a male donor (father's point of view).

8   Describe the issues from the point of view of an adolescent wanting to trace her biological parents. Address the implications of the importance of genetic information.

9   What are some of the adverse outcomes of assisted reproduction for women? Have these changed over the past 10 years? If so, what has changed?

10 What are the risks of multiple births following assisted reproduction? Are these significantly different from those of multiple births following unassisted reproduction?

Online resources

Abortion services in New Zealand, http://www.abortion.gen.nz/regional/capitalcoast.html

Human Fertilisation and Embryology Authority (HFEA) website, http://www.hfea.gov.uk

Infertility Network UK (INUK), http://www.infertilitynetworkuk.com

References

Annas GJ 1998 The shadowlands—secrets and lies and assisted reproduction. New England Journal of Medicine 339(13):935–939

Australian Bureau of Statistics (ABS) 2003 Births, Australia, 2003. Cat. No. 3301.0. ABS, Canberra

Bell J, Campbell DM, Graham WJ et al 2001 Do obstetric complications explain high caesarean section rates among women over 30? A retrospective analysis. British Medical Journal 322:894–895

Bender SS, Geirsson RT, Kosunen E 2003 Trends in teenage fertility, abortion, and pregnancy rates in Iceland compared with other Nordic countries, 1976–99. Acta Obstetrica Gynecologica Scandinavica 82:38–47

Berkowitz GS, Skovron ML, Lapinski RH et al 1990 Delayed childbearing and the outcome of pregnancy. New England Journal of Medicine 322:659–664

Bolton P, Yamashita Y, Farquhar CM 2003 Role of fertility treatments in multiple pregnancy at National Women's Hospital from 1996 to 2001. Australian and New Zealand Journal of Obstetrics and Gynaecology 43:364–368

Caldwell J 1999 Paths to lower fertility. British Medical Journal 319:985–987

Callaway LK, Lust K, McIntyre HD 2005 Pregnancy outcomes in women of very advanced maternal age. Australian and New Zealand Journal of Obstetrics and Gynaecology 45:12–16

de Bruin JP, Bovenhuis PAH, van Noord PA et al 2001 The role of genetic factors in age at natural menopause. Human Reproduction 16:2014–2018

Erickson GF 2000 Ovarian anatomy and physiology. In: RA Lobo, J Kelsey, R Marcus (Eds) Menopause: biology and pathobiology. Academic Press, California, pp 13–32

Gougeon A, Ecochard R, Thalabard JC 1994 Age-related changes of the population of human ovarian follicles: increase in the disappearance rate of non-growing and early growing follicles in aging women. Biology of Reproduction 50:653–663

Hank K, Kreyenfeld M 2003 A multilevel analysis of child care and women's fertility decisions in Western Germany. Journal of Marriage and Family 65:584–596

Hansen M, Kurinczuk JJ, Bower C et al 2002 The risk of major birth defects after intracytoplasmic sperm injection and in vitro fertilization. New England Journal of Medicine 346:725–730

Heffner LJ 2004 Advanced maternal age—how old is too old? New England Journal of Medicine 351:1927–1929

Helmerhorst FM, Perquin DA, Donker D et al 2004 Perinatal outcome of singletons and twins after assisted conception: a systematic review of controlled studies. British Medical Journal 328(7434):261

Henshaw SK, Singh S, Haas T 1999 Recent trends in abortion rates worldwide. International Family Planning Perspectives 25:44–48

Human Fertilisation and Embryology Authority (HFEA) 2005 Guide to infertility. Online: http://gtiaccess.hfea.gov.uk/

Jones EF, Forrest JD, Goldman N et al 1985 Teenage pregnancy in developed countries: determinants and policy implications. International Family Planning Perspectives 17:53–63

Ketting E, Visser AP 1994 Contraception in the Netherlands: the low abortion rate explained. Patient Education and Counselling 23:161–171

Kurjak A, Carrera JM 2005 Declining fertility in the developed world and high maternal mortality in developing countries. Journal of Perinatal Medicine 33:95–99

Laws PJ, Sulllivan EA 2004 Australia's mothers and babies 2002.

AIHW Cat. No. PER 28.2004. Perinatal Statistics Series No. 15. AIHW, Canberra

Lobo RA 2005 Potential options for preservation of fertility in women. New England Journal of Medicine 353:64–73

Nachtigal RD 2006 International disparities in access to infertility services. Fertility and Sterility 85:871–875

New Zealand Health Information Service (NZHIS) 2004 Report on maternity 2002. Ministry of Health, Wellington

Nybo Andersen AM, Wohlfaht J, Christens P et al 2000 Maternal age and fetal loss: population based register linkage study. British Medical Journal 320:1708–1712

Reichlin S 2003 A review of female fertility and the body fat connection. (Women in culture and society) by Rose E. Frisch. Chicago: University of Chicago Press. New England Journal of Medicine 348:(9):869–870

Roberts CL, Tracy S, Peat B 2000 Rates for obstetric intervention among private and public patients in Australia: population based descriptive study. British Medical Journal 321:137–141

Rosenfield A, Schwartz K 2005 Population and development—shifting paradigms, setting goals. New England Journal of Medicine 352(7):647–649

Sallmen M, Weinberg CR, Baird DD et al 2005 Has human fertility declined over time? Why we may never know. Epidemiology 16(4):494–499

Scott RT, Toner J, Muasher X et al 1989 Follicle-stimulating hormone levels on cycle day 3 are predictive of in vitro fertilization outcome. Fertility and Sterility 51:651–654

Sheiner E, Shoham-Vardi I, Hershkovitz R et al 2001 Infertility treatment is an independent risk factor for cesarean section among nulliparous women aged 40 and above. American Journal of Obstetrics and Gynecology 185(4):888–892

Simpson JL 2000 Genetic programming in ovarian development and oogenesis. In: RA Lobo, J Kelsey, R Marcus (Eds) Menopause: biology and pathobiology. Academic Press, California, pp 77–94

te Velde ER, van Baar AL, van Kooij RJ 1998 Concerns about assisted reproduction. Lancet 351:1524–1525

Thomson F, Shanbhag S, Templeton A et al 2005 Obstetric outcome in women with subfertility. British Journal of Gynaecology 112:632–637

Thurin A, Hausken J, Hillensjo T et al 2004 Elective single-embryo transfer versus double-embryo transfer in in vitro fertilization. New England Journal of Medicine 351:2392–2402

UN Population Fund 2005. State of world population. Online: http://www.unfpa.org/swp/swpmain.htm

van Asselt KM, Kok HS, Pearson PL et al 2004 Heritability of menopausal age in mothers and daughters. Fertility and Sterility 82:1348–1351

Wood C, Calderon I, Crombie A 1992 Age and fertility: results of assisted reproductive technology in women over 40 years. Journal of Assisted Reproduction Genetics 9:482–484

CHAPTER 9

Transitions

Jan Pincombe

Key terms

attachment theory, bonding, family health, life transitions, transition to fatherhood, transition to motherhood, transition to parenthood

Chapter overview

Having a baby is a life-changing event, and transition to the role of mother, parent or father has been described as both exhilarating and exhausting. This chapter explores some of the main aspects of life transitions to motherhood, family health and the transition to parenthood and fatherhood.

Learning outcomes

Learning outcomes for this chapter are:

1 To discuss the main theories concerning life transitions with respect to the birth of a baby

2 To highlight the importance of maternal–infant attachment and bonding

3 To provide information for expectant women on admission to maternity units or midwifery-led models of care

4 To discuss the role of men's transition to fatherhood.

Introduction

In this section we see that life transitions, including birth, becoming a mother, a parent or father, are generally accompanied by ritual, and that the rituals vary from society to society.

In the past, the birth of a baby was recognised as a major life transition. According to Levy-Shiff (1994) and Ball (1994), researchers have theorised that this time in a woman's life represents a period of crisis and a watershed in her life. However, more recently they have conceptualised birth in terms of developmental phases with associated 'personal, familial, social and more often professional changes' (Levy-Shiff 1994, p 591).

Draper (2003) examined the history of the development of transition, or what has been referred to as ritual theory, and discusses the theory of 'rites of passage' in her paper exploring men's transition to fatherhood. The seminal work carried out by anthropologist van Gennep (1960) argues that 'rites of passage' represent a way of understanding traditional societies' rituals and rites. He describes customary behaviour in these rituals and rites that go with 'changes of place, state, social position and age' (Froggat 1997, p 124) van Gennep (1960) proposes that common life cycle events include childbirth as well as puberty, marriage and death. He suggests that these customary behaviours consist of three main groups and that 'all rites of passage have a similar tripartite form of separation, transition and incorporation' (Froggatt 1997, p 124).

van Gennep's (1960) work analyses particular ceremonies that took place around pregnancy and childbirth in different cultures from writings during the 1880s, and as a consequence his work reflects the attitudes of that time. He writes how, in some cultures, the woman during her pregnancy is separated from her society, her family and at times even members of her own gender. He describes the period of pregnancy as one of transition, and ultimately with the birth of the child, the associated 'rites' that take place, the woman being reintegrated back into her society, often with an elevated place, often depending to some extent on the gender of her baby, with the birth of a son in many communities providing additional status for the woman. According to van Gennep (1960), transitional rites and ceremonies vary according to particular cultures. He also refers to the transition period as 'limen'. The limen 'constituted a boundary in its own right and time (and place) where the people passing through the rite are cut off from the wider structure of society' and represented 'a time and a place of withdrawal from the normal mode of social action' (Froggatt 1997, p 125). van Gennep's work was extended by Turner (1969, 1977, 1987). Turner differentiated between traditional and small-scale societies and suggested that 'liminial' be reserved for 'ritual and myth telling' and the term 'liminoid' be reserved to mean 'modern symbolic inversions and expressions of disorder' (Froggatt 1997, pp 125, 127).

In current writings, the theory of transition has also been linked to structural-functionalist roots by Draper (2003, p 66), who argues that despite this, transition theory can be seen to be useful as a framework for 'illuminating contemporary transitions across the life course'. Rituals are common in all cultures and are written about extensively by anthropologists, who associate rituals with transitional periods in life. Hospital culture is well known for its rituals. Midwifery researchers and scholars suggest that hospital rituals surrounding birth often do not support birthing women and their families, but rather favour hospital rules and regulations (Hunt & Symonds 1995; Kirkham 2000).

Philpin (2002, p 144) suggests that 'ritual' has been used in a negative way to refer to 'unthinking, routinised action by nurses, which lacks any empirical foundation'. She carried out an electronic data-based literature search from 1960 to 2000 to explore the term 'ritual', which revealed two broad themes: 'First, the complex issues surrounding the definition of ritual, including the relationship between rational and irrational action; and second, the purposes served by ritual' (Philpin 2002, p 144). Any exploration of the transition to motherhood must take into account these myths and rituals surrounding birth.

Transition to motherhood

Becoming a mother is recognised as a significant transition in the life of a woman, often giving rise to ambivalent feelings and emotions (Barclay et al 1997; Mercer 2004; Percival & McCourt 2000; Rogan et al 1997), and feelings of being ill prepared for the role (Schmied & Everitt 1996). Feminist Rich (1976), writing during the 1970s, promoted the idea that motherhood had the potential to provide a source of creativity and joy, although she also raised the issue that birth in contemporary industrial societies is often dominated by men.

Rogan and colleagues (1997) propose that there are three broad theories that underpin research and practice in the transition to early motherhood and the postpartum period. They assert that role attainment and its cognitive aspects reflect one theoretical approach (Rubin 1967a,b, 1984). Rubin's work encompasses two main aspects, namely attaining the maternal role and the recognition of the baby. She articulates the importance of the changes that take place when becoming a mother, and her work has been influential for some scholars in their approach to research on the postpartum period.

Another theoretical approach according to Rogan et al (1997, p 878) involves 'behavioural and psychosocial aspects of transition' and is illustrated in the work by Burr (1972) and Rossi (1968). Their sociological frameworks have been largely adopted by nursing and midwifery researchers and is typified by the work carried out by Mercer (1981, 1985, 2004), who examined aspects of parenthood that are impeded or enhanced by behavioural and psychological conditions that affect the transition to motherhood.

The third area described by Rogan et al (1997) encompasses 'emotional ties between mother and her infant' (Ainsworth

1962; Gottlieb 1978; Klaus & Kennel 1976, 1982; Rogan et al 1997, p 878). Essentially this work concerns attachment theories and bonding between mother and child.

Attachment and bonding with the baby

What is attachment?

Attachment theories provide a theoretical understanding of the importance of the bonding between mother and newborn. Attachment has been defined as 'the tendency of the young organism to seek closeness to particular individuals and to feel more secure in their presence' (Atkinson et al 1993, p A-31). What became known as attachment theory has antecedents in animal studies. One of the first recorded studies in the psychology literature to test out attachment was an experiment to investigate whether contact comfort was more important than feeding. Harlow and Zimmerman (1959) raised baby rhesus monkeys with surrogate mothers. Each baby had two 'mothers', one a food source and made of wire, the other with no food and made of cloth. The mothers were always available to the baby monkeys. The researchers found that the baby monkeys spent decreasing time with the wire mother monkey and increasing time with the cloth-covered mother. They also found that baby monkeys showed a tendency to use the 'cloth mother' from which to explore the environment, and when they were afraid they clung to the cloth mother. These findings were in contrast to the current theories of the time, which predicted that the babies would develop a stronger bond with the wire mother because it fed them. These experiments demonstrated the importance of bonding and the importance of the mother in being able to provide comfort to their offspring.

John Bowlby's work also built on the idea of attachment. He hypothesised a control systems model of attachment and provided, for the time, a very different approach to understanding the development of the mother (caregiver) and infant relationship (Broberg 2000). The aim of the system was to enhance survival and reproduction of the species (Bowlby 1969). To achieve this, the infant needed to maintain close proximity to the caregiver for protection against real or feared danger. Bowlby (1969) suggested that all infants who receive basic care from their caregiver developed some level of attachment. However, not all infants were able to access their caregiver as a secure base from which to explore their world, and the caregiver needed to be able to respond to the infant's attachment requirements. This came to be known as the caregiving system. More recently, research on the capacity of babies and young children to adapt positively to changed circumstances has been published and consistent. It is understood that children need kind, supportive care from one or more caregivers who may or may not be the mother. Bowlby (1980) later acknowledged that an infant may form selective attachments to a number of caregivers. Moreover, once established, the security of the parent/infant bond remains stable over time.

Ainsworth and colleagues (1978) were the first to provide descriptions of the caregiving system that is essential to the development of the attachment relationship. Ainsworth's work was based on the idea that parental stimulation, especially in response to the infant's signals, was critical in developing attachment. Further, she hypothesised that in developing maternal responsiveness between infant and mother, a secure base was established that allowed the infant to explore her or his environment and create an emotionally stable attachment. These studies were carried out in the context of a 'strange situation'. Infants separated or reunited with their primary caregiver responded in a particular pattern categorised as securely attached, avoidance behaviour or anxious/ambivalent behaviours. Those infants who were securely attached to their primary caregiver confidently explored their environment and used their caregiver as a secure base. The infants who were judged to be 'avoidant' explored their environment but ignored their caregiver on reunion. Anxious/ambivalent infants became anxious when separated and were reluctant to explore their environment (Ainsworth et al 1978).

More recently, animal studies in rats have demonstrated the positive effects of maternal care on baby rats. Specifically,

> i) a causal relationship between maternal behaviour and stress reactivity in the offspring and ii) the transmission of such individual differences in maternal behaviour from one generation of females to the next (Francis et al 1999, p 1155)

has been found. An earlier study by some members of this team (Lui et al 1997, p 1659) established, from their research, that those adult rats whose mothers demonstrated more licking and grooming of their pups in the first 10 days of life showed:

> reduced plasma adrenocorticotropic hormone and corticosterone responses to acute stress, increased hippocampal glucocorticoid receptor RNA expression, enhanced glucocorticoid feedback sensitivity and decreased levels of hypothalamic corticotropin-releasing hormone messenger RNA. Each measure was significantly correlated with the frequency of maternal licking and grooming (all r's > –0.6).

Studies of non-human mammals have been important as they have allowed examination of ways of promoting secure attachment between human mothers and infants in conditions that would have made observation difficult or experimentation unethical had humans been used. One study referring to the importance of animal experiments examined the effects of home visiting after the birth of a baby (Armstrong et al 1999), specifically looking at maternal–infant bonding during work on early home-based interventions. This work was predicated on the importance of the first few years of a child's life as a 'critical period' in the child's brain development (Wynder 1998). A randomised controlled trial (RCT) was carried out to investigate the effect of a home-visiting program in 181 families classified as vulnerable (Armstrong et al 1999). Recruitment to the trial was carried out using a self-report questionnaire called the Brisbane Evaluation of Needs Questionnaire (BENQ). This tool contained questions that identified families at risk. Two levels of risk identification were used. The first level consisted of 'physical domestic violence, identified childhood abuse of parent, sole parenthood, or ambivalence to the pregnancy (sought termination, no antenatal care)' and the second level consisted of:

> maternal age of less than 18 years, unstable housing (three or more moves in the preceding 2 years), financial stress (often concerned about having adequate food, or making ends meet), less than 10 years of maternal education, low family income (< A\$16,000 per annum), social isolation, history of mental health disorder, drug, or alcohol abuse (either parent) and domestic violence other than physical abuse; the presence of three or more of these risk factors enabled selection (Armstrong et al 1999, p 238).

Those families that met the inclusion criteria and gave informed written consent were randomised to a control group ($n = 91$) or the intervention group ($n = 90$). The intervention group received weekly home visits from a child health nurse for six weeks, fortnightly up to three months and then monthly up to six months. The intervention was multifaceted and consisted of the following aims:

> i) establish a relationship of trust with the infant's family; ii) enhance parenting self-esteem and confidence by reinforcement of success; iii) provide anticipatory guidance for normal child development problems such as crying or sleep behaviour variants; iv) promote preventative child healthcare; and v) facilitate access to appropriate community services (Armstrong et al 1999, p 238).

In addition to this, the child health nurse met with a social worker and paediatrician in a weekly case conference for the planning of care for the family and child. A variety of instruments were used to measure maternal and child health outcomes in this study group at six weeks postnatally. A 30-item self-report questionnaire called the Parent Questionnaire, the Edinburgh Post Natal Depression Scale (PNDS) (Cox et al 1987), Parent Domain (PD), which is a subset of the Parenting Stress Index (Abidin 1990), The HOME Inventory (Caldwell & Bradley 1984) and the Modified Patient Satisfaction Questionnaire (Ware et al 1976) were administered to both groups at six weeks. Significant differences were found between groups for postnatal depression, with the intervention group demonstrating better (lower) levels ($F1,169 = 7.35$, $p < 0.050$) than the control group. The scores for the PSI subscale that measured perception of parent–child interaction showed a statistically significant main effect ($F1,169 = 8.72$, $p < 0.05$), showing that there were better scores in the intervention group, illustrating higher levels of confidence among this group. The HOME inventory scores were better on all but one subscale for the intervention group ($p < 0.001$ to $p < 0.003$). Also, greater satisfaction levels were statistically significant in the intervention group for all subsets of the Modified Patient Satisfaction scale. The findings for this study showed the overall good effects of this targeted home-based intervention for vulnerable families.

Armstrong and colleagues (2000) carried out a follow-up of the RCT with participants at four months. The intervention group and the control group each consisted of 80 families. There were significant differences between the intervention group infants' immunisation status and the control group, with higher levels of completed immunisation in the intervention

group ($p < 0.05$). The intervention group also self-reported fewer bruises and injuries.

The EPND scores at six weeks were better (lower) for the intervention group but were not maintained at the four months assessment interval. The total HOME score for the intervention group on all subscales showed better scores (statistically significant) than the control group. The researchers pointed out the positive effects of this intervention but argued for longer-term follow-up studies to confirm the results collected at six weeks and four months post partum.

A volunteer home-visiting program in the outer metropolitan area of Sydney using a phenomenological approach was carried out by Taggart et al (2000). The emphasis of this program was on implementing a volunteer home-visiting program to prevent child abuse and neglect. Interviews were carried out with the coordinator of the project, 10 volunteers and 15 mothers involved in the project. The descriptions of the experiences of the three groups were reported, with excerpts from the mothers' interviews. Emotional support was one of the main issues identified as being a critical issue. One example quoted in the paper consisted of the following:

> I had no family support, three children at home and was totally incapacitated after a traumatic birth, and my husband had to go interstate with work. It's really hard. I thought that I'd have to rely on friends, who have their own families. Both our Mums are old and live far away (M12) (Taggart et al 2000, p 5).

Friendship and motherhood was also one of the main themes, and it was important to these mothers that they were helped emotionally by being able to talk about their worries and having someone who would listen to them.

Involvement of midwives

Midwives have the opportunity to be intimately involved with promoting best midwifery practice in the following way. Immediately after the birth of their baby, mothers can be encouraged by midwives to hold their babies directly against their skin, thus encouraging bonding, maintaining the baby's optimum temperature and promoting the initiation of breast feeding within one hour of the baby's birth (Ashmore 2001).

Kangaroo mother care, or skin-to-skin contact, has been found to have beneficial effects for both mother and baby. It has been described in the following way: the baby is held in an upright position by the mother, with skin-to-skin and chest-to-chest contact, and held between her breasts for approximately one to two hours (Ludington-Hoe 1993). In

---

Reflective exercise

Reflect on what you can do as a midwife to promote bonding between the woman and her baby immediately after birth. This may require providing strategies to encourage the maintenance of a quiet and secure environment in what is a sometimes a noisy place for having a baby.

a RCT with low birthweight babies randomised to kangaroo mother care versus traditional care 'kangaroo care' has been found to be safe to use with low birthweight babies whose diagnosis is considered clinically stable (Charpak et al 1997; Ruiz-Pelaez et al 2004).

Maternal role attainment and adjustment

Maternal role attainment and adjustment has a history of development that is recorded in the North American literature and has also been adopted by some Australian midwifery researchers. In this section the North American background, followed by Australian studies and their relevance to midwifery, is reviewed.

According to Rubin (1975), a consistent American view of motherhood expressed during the 1960s and 1970s was that after the birth of a baby everyone lived happily ever after. Rubin (1975) argued that this attitude was responsible for shorter hospital stays for birthing women during the period from 1960 to 1986. Reviews of the effects of early discharge during this time reflected mainly the experiences of women who had had extensive prenatal education and postnatal follow-up, with little research into 'the needs and experiences of low-risk puerperal women' (Ruchala & Halstead 1994, p 83).

Ruchala and Halstead (1994) point out that a complication of reduced length of hospital stay after birth was that little time was available for mother–infant relationships to be assessed by midwifery staff. They reported that women experiencing uncomplicated births were discharged from 12 to 48 hours after the birth of their baby. They carried out interviews with 50 women in their homes two weeks after discharge from the maternity unit. The results from the coding of the interview data demonstrated that the majority of the women indicated that postnatally their experiences were 'hectic' and consisted of 'a time of adjustment' (Ruchala & Halstead 1994, p 85). Postnatal fatigue was also reported as a major part of their experiences, with 22 (44%) of the women expressing this view and how it adversely affected their relationship with their partner and other family members. Six (24%) of the primiparous women and 8 (32%) multiparous women stated that they experienced 'crying' episodes. The authors concluded that many mothers reported fatigue and still had emotional and physical concerns connected to the birth of their baby to deal with. They suggested that mothers should be supported with follow-up telephone calls and to encourage women to participate in support groups.

The relationship between maternal role attainment and postpartum depression was explored by Fowles (1997). She recruited 168 primiparous women during the last trimester of their antenatal period, with 136 of those women participating in her study and completing standardised questionnaires 9–14 weeks after the birth of their baby. Each of the women completed four questionnaires—the Edinburgh Postnatal Depression Scale (EPDN) and three questionnaires that investigated maternal role attainment, namely the 'Myself as Mother Scale'.

The 'My Baby Scale' reported re-test reliability estimates ranging from 0.64 to 0.77 and estimated each mother's evaluation of her infant. The Perceived Competence Scale, which assessed mothers' views of their competence in feeding and infant care, demonstrated a Cronbachs' Alpha ranging from 0.83 to 0.93. Fowles found that 'maternal depression had a negative relationship with women's confidence in the mothering role' (Fowles 1997, p 90).

The implications for practice were that most mothers felt confident by four months in their mothering, supporting the earlier work by Mercer (1985). However, she suggested that 2–3 months after the birth of their baby, women should be evaluated for postnatal depression. She also indicated the importance of role models for women so that they can be exposed to appropriate parenting behaviours to instill feelings of confidence in the new mother.

This section has explored the work of theorists who have supported a maternal role attainment approach. However, Mercer (2004) recently expressed the view that perhaps the term 'becoming a mother' more completely reflects the transition to motherhood theory. This is demonstrated in one of her recent articles, where she writes:

> Women's descriptions of the life-transforming experience in becoming a mother with concomitant growth, development and new self-definition are not adequately encompassed in MRA terminology. The maternal persona continues to evolve as the child's developmental challenges and life's realities lead to disruptions in the mother's feelings of competence and self-confidence. The argument is made to replace 'maternal role attainment' with 'becoming a mother' to connote the initial transformation and continuing growth of the mother identity (Mercer 2004, p 231).

The view Mercer reflects in this most recent article is more aligned with Australian midwifery researchers and scholars, such as the work by Barclay et al (1997), who support the 'becoming a mother' theoretical stance.

Studies examining mothers' readiness to assume their role

Various research studies have explored women's readiness to assume their mothering role. The functional status of first-time mothers was investigated by McVeigh (2000) in an Australian-based study. McVeigh and Charboyer (2002, p 107) defined 'functional status' in a later study as 'mothers' readiness to assume infant care responsibilities and resume self-care, household, social and community, and occupational activities'.

McVeigh (2000) explored the relationship between anxiety and functional status in first-time mothers. Her work was based on earlier research by Fawcett et al (1988), who developed a multidimensional measurement instrument they called Functional Status After Childbirth (IFSAC). The tool consisted of a 36-item scale and was found to have an inter-rater reliability estimate of 97% and a Cronbach's alpha of 0.70 (Fawcett et al 1988).

McVeigh (2000) sent the IFSAC questionnaire to 200 first-time mothers residing in a regional health area of New

South Wales, who attended maternal child health centres. The Speilberger State Anxiety Inventory (Speilberger 1983) and a short socio-demographic questionnaire were also included in the package sent to each participant. The response rate was 86% ($n = 173$) at six weeks, with 73% ($n = 146$) responding at three months and 71% ($n = 142$) at six months. At six weeks the results showed a 'significant inverse relationship between total functional status score and maternal anxiety ($p = 0.015$), social and community activities and maternal anxiety ($r = -0.234$, $p = 0.002$) and self-care and maternal anxiety ($r = -0.226$, $p = 0.003$)' (McVeigh 2000, p 16).

Although the statistical results were slightly different at three months and six months, they were also significant at these points. Also, mothers who were found to be highly anxious were also found to have babies who were more likely to be unsettled ($p < 0.001$) and babies who were more likely to sleep less at night ($p < 0.001$). These mothers were also more dissatisfied with their role ($p < 0.0001$). McVeigh (2000) suggested that the implementation of continuity midwifery-led models of care may offer midwives a better opportunity to identify women at risk of maternal anxiety. She also recommended that midwives be involved in the design and introduction of programs to identify maternal anxiety in expectant and postpartum women in order to improve satisfaction with being a mother.

Applications to midwifery practice

Midwives can support women after the birth of their baby by listening to what women have to say. Gamble and colleagues (2004) discuss counselling processes that can assist those women who experience psychological distress following childbirth. In their study they investigated strategies used by 16 midwives during counselling with women after the birth of their baby. The analysis of the interviews revealed three main themes. The first consisted of 'opportunities to talk about the birth'. Midwives indicated that although they were familiar with the term 'debriefing' they preferred to use an approach that consisted of a 'woman-led discussion' (Gamble et al 2004, p 18). This technique allowed for input from the midwife as required. Midwives also suggested that women should have the opportunity to discuss their birthing experience when they are ready to, and more than once if required. The second theme was 'developing an understanding of events', and midwives suggested that going though the 'labour record with them' was a useful approach (Gamble et al 2004, p 18). They also suggested that, in the event of an operative procedure, the medical officer should debrief the woman. The third theme was that of 'minimising feelings of guilt', and midwives strongly supported the view that women should not see themselves as 'failing' and that positive affirmations and suggestions should be given to women, such as, 'I think that was a very good decision' (Gamble et al 2004, p 18).

Transition to parenthood

Vimpani (2001) has claimed that parenting is a vital public health priority facing Western societies. The transition to parenthood, according to de Montigny and Lacharite (2003), has been a focus for study for more than 50 years, with most studies concentrating on the role of the mother.

Education for parenthood

Evidence from the literature suggests that, in preparation for parenthood, information about parenthood provided by health professionals during prenatal classes is oriented around the birth of the baby. This has resulted in postnatal issues being insufficiently covered (Nolan 1997; O'Meara 1993). Nolan (1997, p 26) recommends that pregnant women be given more information about practical baby-care skills and opportunities to discuss 'postnatal emotional issues' during antenatal classes. Collington (1998) discusses the importance of midwives being able to provide educational advice to parents about all aspects of pregnancy care, so that parents can make informed choices about care and thereby be empowered.

Coming in for the birth of the baby

Maternity hospitals provide literature for pregnant women and their partners during the antenatal period, and information about when women should contact their midwife. For example, women who book into one of the maternity hospitals in Adelaide, South Australia, are advised that:

- if more than 20 weeks pregnant, the woman should contact her midwife if in a Midwifery Group Practice (MGP) or the midwife in the delivery suite
- if less than 20 weeks pregnant she should contact the midwife in the Women's Assessment Service (WAS).

Women are provided with information about signs or feelings that they might experience which should lead them to come into the maternity unit. For example, the maternity teaching hospital in Adelaide also encourages women to contact the hospital if they experience any of the following:

- Their water breaks (even though they may not be experiencing contractions).
- The contractions are regular.
- They are experiencing increasing abdominal discomfort.
- There is any blood loss.
- The baby's movements reduce.
- They are uncertain of what is happening.
- They are concerned or anxious.

Women are also given a list of suggested requirements for their baby, which they are advised to bring in with them (see Box 9.1). They are also requested to bring their pregnancy health record with them. This 'hand held record' contains confidential information about their progress during pregnancy. In some states of Australia this data is now entered into an electronic database.

BOX 9.1   Advice given to expectant mothers

Things to bring to hospital:

▶ your Pregnancy Hand Held Record
▶ your birth plan
▶ things you might choose to use in labour (discussed in antenatal classes), e.g. a selection of music tapes or CDs
▶ casual clothes to wear during the day if desired
▶ 2 night dresses (minimum)
▶ dressing gown and slippers
▶ 2 maternity bras
▶ plenty of comfortable underpants
▶ cordial if desired
▶ pen
▶ toiletries, e.g. soap, shampoo, toothbrush and toothpaste
▶ 1 large box of tissues
▶ 1 box of nipple pads/washable nursing pads
▶ 4 packets of sanitary pads
▶ your own pillow if desired.

For your baby:

▶ 40 disposable nappies or
▶ fasteners/nappy pins if you are going to use cloth nappies (Cloth nappies are provided by the hospital if you do not wish to use disposable nappies.)
▶ 6 pilchers (not plastic) if using cloth nappies
▶ baby care products for your baby while in hospital—for example, baby wipes and gentle lotions or creams (optional)
▶ mittens (optional).

(Source: *Having your Baby at the Women's and Children's Hospital* 2003, pp 16, 17)

In New Zealand all women hold their own notes and there are moves to standardise these notes based on the New Zealand College of Midwives Maternity Notes. These documents will provide three records within the one set of notes—one for the woman, one for the midwife and one for data collection and payment purposes.

Mothers' postnatal needs not being met

Research into women's transition to motherhood has demonstrated that many women are often unprepared for the transition to parenthood, and particularly for postnatal self-care and baby care. Several studies have also found that women's postnatal needs are not being met (Cook & Stacey 2003; Henderson 2000; McKellar et al 2002). The National Health and Medical Research Council (1996) suggests that many women feel abandoned during the postpartum period.

Dissatisfaction with postnatal experiences was voiced by women in a study carried out in the United Kingdom (Ockelford et al 2004). An at-home interview conducted with 39 multiparous and primiparous 'white' and Indian women 13 weeks after the birth of their babies was carried out to investigate women's views about their postnatal experiences at two time points retrospectively. The first time point for

women's views about their experiences was their immediate postnatal stay, and the second was as they were leaving to go home. The most mentioned problem for women during their early postpartum stay was shortages of midwifery staff and the resultant lack of attention to the care of their baby and their own wellbeing. Some women indicated that that was a reason for leaving the postnatal ward earlier than they had planned. Their recorded experiences of leaving hospital and going home reflected their feelings of difficulties with the transition from postnatal stay to home with a new baby.

Teaching mothering skills

Postnatal research in Australia has shown that women experience feelings of exhaustion, often linked to shorter length of postnatal stay in traditional care situations. This trend, according to Maloni (1994), has provided fewer opportunities for teaching mothering skills. Other reasons for new mothers to be less exposed to mothering are the greater percentage of women working until the birth of their baby, and growing mobility leading to greater geographic distance from relatives.

In most states of Australia, postnatal early discharge is common after childbirth and in some states, 'mothers in the public healthcare system undergo mandatory early discharge' (Emmanuel et al 2001, p 16). Various reasons have been proposed, that have been associated with encouraging early postnatal discharge. They have included economically driven requirements (Buist 1997). In some cases it has been due to women's choice (Nolan 1997). Buist (1997) reported in an article published in the *Australian Medical Journal* that early discharge rates had increased to 32% of mothers in 1994 from 20.2% in 1991.

Some studies have found that early discharge is as safe as traditional postnatal stays (Grullon & Grimes 1997). Women's satisfaction with early postnatal stays has been investigated by Carty and Bradley (1990), who found that the group of women discharged early at 12–24 hours were more satisfied with midwifery care than those in the four-day postnatal stay group. The first group was designated to 12–24 hour early discharge with four home visits, the second group was discharged at 25–48 hours with three home visits, and the third group had a four-day stay and received one home visit. The variation in the number of home visits and the small sample size ($n = 131$) may have confounded the results, so caution needs to be exercised with these findings.

The influence of shorter length of postnatal stay on women's breastfeeding duration at six weeks post partum and maternal depression at five to eight months has been investigated by Brown et al (2004) in three population-based surveys. They studied women who birthed in Victoria, Australia, during '1 week in 1989, 2 weeks in 1993 and 2 weeks in 1999' (Brown et al 2004, p 202). The response rate for each survey point was 71.4% (790/1107) for 1989, 62.5% (1336/2138) for 1993 and 67% (1616/2412) in 1999. They found that at the end of the 1990s, the standard length of stay was two to three days for a public patient, although women with private health insurance had five days or longer postnatal stays. Only 27% of privately insured women in the survey were discharged earlier than five days postnatally. There were no significant differences between women's responses in the three surveys for shorter length of stay, depression and breastfeeding duration at six weeks.

A systematic review of the literature by Brown et al (2005) examined eight trials with 3600 women who were discharged early from maternity hospitals. Their results were inconclusive. There was no evidence to support any adverse findings with respect to early discharge, but due to limitations caused by methodological problems this could not be entirely ruled out. They also indicated that the importance of the effect of support at home by a midwife was as yet unclear. They recommended that large trials investigating the effect of early discharge be carried out (Brown et al 2005).

Early discharge from maternity services was one aspect reported in the *Review of Maternity Services in New Zealand* (National Health Committee 1999). A postal survey was completed by 11,511 women and a telephone survey was conducted with 1000 women who had recently had a baby in New Zealand. Results from the survey showed that 'nearly 10% of mothers in New Zealand are now discharged home on the day of delivery', and that 'two thirds of respondents had hospital stays of between two and five days, with 22% having a stay of one day or less' (National Health Committee 1999, p 24). Although 82% of women reported that they had a choice with respect to how long they stayed in hospital, most women indicated that there was pressure to leave quickly or the 'understaffed postnatal wards provided incentives to leave' (National Health Committee 1999, p 24). The quality of the hospital environment and postnatal hospital care left room for considerable improvement, according to women who responded to the surveys. However, those women who had a lead maternity caregiver (LMC) and rural women recorded higher satisfaction levels with their hospital care than other women who did not have an LMC or came from a non-rural area.

In 2003, the Ministry of Health published the outcomes of the Maternity Services Consumer Satisfaction Survey, a follow-up to the 1999 survey. This evaluation adopted similar methods to the 1999 survey for comparative purposes. It included some minor changes which incorporated three new questions and some improvements to several existing survey questions (Ministry of Health 2003).

The 2003 survey reported on the views of 2909 New Zealand women who gave birth between February and March 2002. The findings from the survey indicated that although the maternity services framework had not changed since the 1999 survey, responses from women confirmed that it was essential that they choose an LMC. Women also indicated the importance of having a vital role in decision-making about their care as well as opportunities for choices about their care.

The importance of parent group support has been heightened due to early discharge of women and their babies from maternity units (Hanna et al 2002). Notwithstanding the contribution of community-based midwifery services, parent groups are particularly important for first-time parents, according to these writers. In Australia, various levels of government funding are provided for formal parenting courses, through which informal groups can be formed, or for directly arranging or expediting meetings of new parents. For example, in Victoria, Australia, women are provided with eight sessions concentrating on 'parenting skills, relationship development and social support in order to increase confidence and skills in parenting' (Hanna et al 2002, p 209).

Family health

Policies to improve family health have been legislated by Australian state governments (for example, in South Australia, 'Every chance for every child. Making the early years count. A framework for early childhood services in South Australia 2003–2004', Department of Human Services 2003). The Australian federal government has also developed legislation to improve family health (see 'Participation Support for a More Equitable Society', Department of Family and Community Services 2000; and in Sydney, '"Families first" outcomes evaluation framework', Fisher et al 2002).

New Zealand also has extensive legislative reforms articulated in various reports to advocate and support New Zealand families (for example, see 'New Zealand Families Today', Ministry of Social Development 2004).

Improving family health through education

A Cochrane Review that investigated postnatal parental education for improving family health was carried out by Gagnon and Barkum (2003). They acknowledged that the transition to parenthood was both exciting and overwhelming, and suggested that parents may receive an overload of information during prenatal classes and may not assimilate postnatal information during this time. They also suggested that early discharge from maternity units may also contribute to deficits in new parents' knowledge about self-care and care for their newborns.

McKellar and colleagues (2002), using action research methods, investigated a strategy to enhance postnatal education for new mothers. Focus groups were carried out with six midwives and seven first-time mothers to find out their views about how information to improve postnatal information could be presented to new mothers. From the thematic analysis of the focus groups, a written educational resource was designed. One theme indicated that respondents believed that consistent and relevant information was important. Mothers indicated that developing knowledge and confidence in caring for their baby—that is, baby-care and self-care—were the most important aspects. The educational resource was designed from this information. Women also revealed that because midwives did not have sufficient time to spend with first-time mothers, this presented a significant factor in preventing women from being able to effectively learn to care for their baby and to learn about their own care.

A questionnaire was then developed to find out women's views about the effectiveness of the resource. Seventeen mothers were surveyed and the results indicated that they believed that the resource was easy to read and contained clear and helpful information without the need to read through an extensive amount of literature. Importantly, 81.70% of women felt that the education resource had contributed to their confidence in providing baby-care and self-care (McKellar et al 2002). It should be noted, however, that the number of women surveyed was very small and therefore caution should be exercised regarding any generalisation to other populations.

According to Brown et al (2002), after the birth of a baby, education and interventions vary considerably, with birth mainly taking place in institutional settings in Western countries. However, globally, for most women birth takes place in the home, where education is provided mainly by informal structures, which can be immediate female members of the family and extended family (Moran et al 1997).

Maternity payment

Family health has been linked to socio-economic status and historically the maternity payment provided to women in Australia for having a baby was referred to as a 'baby bonus'. It was first introduced in Australia by the federal government in 1912 at the sum of five pounds (Thompson 2004). The authorities at the time believed that:

It would increase the declining birthrate; diminish maternal and infantile mortality, and make childbearing safer for women. In the nine years following its introduction, the birth rate steadily decreased. There was no substantial reduction in the maternal or infantile death rates, and the number of women attended in childbirth by a doctor greatly increased—medical attendance was greater in the State of Victoria despite the Midwives' Act in Victoria (Kingston 1977, cited in Thompson 2004, p 17).

Maternity payment guidelines in Australia are outlined on the Australian Government, Family Assistance, website (see the list of online resources at the end of this chapter). The purpose is outlined and it is stated that maternity payment is not income-tested, can be made as a lump-sum payment and replaces the 'existing maternity allowance and the Baby Bonus'. Eligibility for maternity payment is outlined on the website as:

A parent of a baby if the parent meets all other eligibility criteria at any time within 13 weeks of the baby's birth; or

A parent of a stillborn baby if the parent would have met all the other criteria if the baby had not been stillborn; or

A claimant who is entrusted with the care of a newborn baby if the claimant meets all other eligibility criteria within 13 weeks of the baby's birth and if the claimant is likely to continue to have care of the child for no less than 12 weeks; or

A claimant who, before a baby is 26 weeks of age, has the baby entrusted to their care because the claimant will be adopting the baby, provided the claimant meets all other eligibility criteria within 13 weeks of the baby coming into the care of the claimant.
(http://www.familyassist.gov.au/Internet/fao/fao.nsf/content/publications-factsheets-m...4/12/2005, p 1)

Further eligibility criteria:

the claimant and the baby must meet Australian residency requirements

the claimant must be legally responsible, either alone or with another adult, for the day-to-day care, welfare and development of the baby; and

the claimant must satisfy tax file number requirements; and

the claimant must lodge an effective claim within 26 weeks of the baby's birth or, in the case of adopting parents, within 26 weeks of the baby coming into their care.

These eligibility criteria change from time to time and midwives should encourage women to check the website for up-to-date information. This is particularly important, as documentation is required to be submitted to government agencies in a timely manner in order to register for benefits.

Maternity care is free to all New Zealand women, although private obstetricians are entitled to charge women for care.

In New Zealand, a 'maternity payment' is not provided to parents but a variety of possible benefits are available to women and families who meet certain criteria. For example, the Domestic Purposes Benefit is available to sole parents (mothers or fathers). A sickness benefit is available for those who have had to stop working or reduce their working hours due to sickness, injury, pregnancy or disability. Low- and middle-income families can access the Childcare Subsidy program and the OSCAR Subsidy to help pay for early childcare and after-school programs. Working for Families is a package of financial support designed to assist low- and middle-income families to work and raise a family. Further details about available subsidies can be found through the New Zealand Ministry of Social Development website (see online resources at the end of this chapter).

Men's transition to parenthood

Draper (2003) writes about the importance of men's transition to fatherhood as being an integral part of their partners' transition to motherhood. She suggests that this transition needs to be viewed within the context of understanding that it is represented as a matrix and encompasses the baby, siblings and grandparents as well as the father.

Fathers' attendance at their babies' birth

According to Dellman (2004, p 20), during the early 1900s, anthropologists recorded various instances of fathers' 'bizarre behaviour' during their wives' labour, with the husbands not attending the actual birth but participating in ceremonies. For example, in one reported ceremony this behaviour involved 'building bridges for the infant's soul'.

In Western societies in the late twentieth and early twenty-first centuries, men's attendance at the birth of their baby has been shown to be high—approximately 96% of men are reported to have attended their partner giving birth (Dellman

2004). Interestingly, Odent (1996), who is well known for his early work on encouraging the presence of the father at birth, has more recently suggested that 'men should be kept away from the birth' as in his view they increase the levels of stress in their partner and slow down their partner's labour (Neile 1997, p 120). Odent has also commented that 'the labouring woman doesn't need support' (Odent 1996, p 46). Odent (cited in Walters & Kirkham 1997, p 105) also states that:

> Men sometimes find it hard to observe, accept and understand a woman's instinctive behaviour during childbirth. Instead they often try to keep her from slipping out of a rational, self controlled state … it is not mere coincidence that in all traditional societies women in labour are assisted not by men but by other women who have had children themselves.

However, Vehvilainen-Julkunen & Liukkonen (1998, pp 10–11) report in their paper on transformation from man to father that 'fathers appreciate being asked about their experiences and opinions' and that 'the presence of fathers at childbirth has been shown to be a highlight in the life of both parents'.

Walters and Kirkham (1997) also write about the father's presence at birth, and indicate that major changes have occurred since the 1950s when, they argue, it would have been a radical event if the father had been present at the birth. They suggest that by the 1980s, the father's attendance at the birth was expected. However, by the 1990s there were reports of the experience of birth being 'overwhelming' and suggestions that a doula can provide positive strategies to the partner so the partner can assist the woman and be supported as well (Walters & Kirkham 1997, p 105).

Studies examining the transition to fatherhood

Researchers claim that studies have focused more on the role of the mother, with little research addressing men's attitudes to their partner's pregnancy (Thomas & Upton 2000). However, due to changes in society, with more men attending antenatal classes with their partners and the birth, there has been a small trend towards examining the role of the father (Dellman 2004). This is reflected in the following studies.

A qualitative study was carried out by Barclay and Lupton (1999) into the experiences of 15 first-time Australian fathers in a series of semi-structured interviews carried out over four time-points. The first interview was done just prior to the birth of the baby and three interviews were carried out post birth over five to six months. Although the majority of the men interviewed looked forward to fatherhood, some men found it 'more uncomfortable than rewarding' (Barclay & Lupton 1999, p 1013). Discourse analysis was applied to the textual data and some themes were revealed in their comments about bonding. For example, one father reported that bonding with his infant did not occur immediately. The following is an extract of comments by 'Juan' (Barclay & Lupton 1999, p 1017):

> I thought as a father there would be a bond there straight away with the child. I thought it would just come naturally. I thought because he was mine I was going to be immediately attracted to

this child and love would come naturally. I was surprised I wasn't overcome with feelings for him straight away.

A change in the relationship between partners was also a theme. Positive and negative aspects from the participants' interviews were recorded by researchers. However, 'Peter's' comments demonstrated simple pleasures in being involved in his changed role. He indicated that:

> We'll go down to … a local park and take the baby and the dog with us. We try to do this every second, if not each weekend. We usually go about lunch time when there is no one else around, we just take some sandwiches and water for the dog and enjoy ourselves' (Barclay & Lupton 1999, p 1018).

Barclay and Lupton (1999, p 1019) stated how, in the future, the 'new fatherhood' might be achieved, and that structural and societal changes would be needed in Western society in order for this change to occur. In their view, 'mutually supportive and enriching early parenting is currently unachievable' (Barclay & Lupton 1999, p 1019). Further, they argued that this was not due to men not wishing to be involved in 'close, caring relationships with their infants' but more about how 'fatherhood is represented and understood' (Barclay & Lupton 1999, pp 1019–1020).

A survey carried out by Vehvilainen-Julkunen and Liukkonen (1998) with 137 fathers attending the birth of their baby in a university hospital in Finland showed a response rate of 81% ($n = 107$). Younger fathers reported feeling uncomfortable during the birth more often than others.

A grounded theory approach was used by Barclay et al (1996) to study 53 first-time fathers who attended antenatal clinics with their partners. The resultant analysis of the textual data revealed five categories—'anxiety, ambivalence, adjustment, separation and need to know'—and the core category was defined as 'development' (Barclay et al 1996, p 14). 'Development' represented one of the more positive categories, and the authors indicated that in their interviews, the men stated concepts such as 'excitement, growth of self and of relationships with partner, expected child and their family involvement and closeness' (Barclay et al 1996, p 20).

Baafi and colleagues (2001) argued that midwives should be encouraged to understand the impact that a new baby has on the father, and that men should be afforded greater recognition during this period. They suggested that during the transition to fatherhood, men should be encouraged to develop strategies to deal with their role. The authors administered a quantitative survey to 204 men residing in a regional area health service in New South Wales. Data were collected at three and six months, and a response rate of 63% ($n = 128$) was recorded. Early results showed that 94% of men who responded were satisfied most of the time with their role of fatherhood.

First-time fathers' adjustment to their role and factors affecting their transition were investigated by Buist et al (2002). Two hundred and twenty men were recruited from a large maternity teaching hospital in Melbourne, Australia. The researchers used a longitudinal repeated measures design that included questionnaires assessing 'parity history, social support, marital satisfaction, anger, anxiety and gender role stress' at a prenatal interview, followed by interviews postnatally at four months after the birth of their baby (Buist et al 2002, p 172). Prenatal and postnatal distress was measured using the EPDS. The most distressing time for men was experienced at the time of their first interview, which was held during their partners' prenatal period; this was especially so for those men who were younger, employed part-time and who had been in shorter relationships. Distress was reported to become less during the postnatal period, although it was shown to negatively affect the attachment of men to their infant. However, the transition to fatherhood for most men was dealt with effectively. The authors suggested that problems with transition to parenthood could be reduced if attention was paid to men's anxieties antenatally.

These studies suggest that the transition to fatherhood represented profound changes in men's lives. This was particularly so for first-time fathers, who experienced issues relating to changes in their relationship with their partner.

Ways in which midwives can involve fathers

Midwives can facilitate the establishment of communication between father and baby by suggesting the use of baby massage (Whitehouse 2001). Mackereth (2003) writes about teaching fathers baby massage, and although only one father took part in the study, the case study that is reported suggested that 'Mike' (the father) found good effects from the first time he used the massage technique. These good effects had benefits for all members in the family. This was demonstrated when their baby, who also had eczema, slept through the night after the massage for the first time.

With Mike, the only father, in the four case studies, his overwhelming concerns were problems with the baby waking frequently during the night and her eczema, which was being treated with a cream containing 1% hydrocortisone. Both the parents and the infant were not resting fully. Mike reported that this had left both their baby and themselves tired and irritated during the day—this was their first child. Mike reported that following the first massage session his baby slept through the night for the first time. In the group sessions he reported that she had slept every night without disturbance since massage had become part of the daily routine. Importantly, he also reported that her eczema had also improved, possibly from a combination of the massage with oil and the improved sleep. Mike said that carrying out the massage session was their quality time, doing something together, which was not centred on changing nappies or feeding, it was also a time to interact, notice developmental changes and play. Joining the baby massage classes also provided opportunities to meet other parents and see his baby start to play with others (Mackereth 2003, p 150).

Conclusion

This chapter has presented some of the main aspects of life transitions—transition to motherhood, transition to parenthood, family health and men's transition to fatherhood. The evidence suggests that this is a time of great change for women, their babies and families. The challenge for midwives is to ensure that women, their babies and families are supported and provided with information that will assist them to be competent and confident mothers.

Review questions

1 Explain the role of rites and rituals in childbirth and the transition to parenthood.

2 Describe the major attachment theories relating to maternal and infant bonding.

3 Discuss how kangaroo mother care can assist in bonding between mother and newborn.

4 Briefly list the main maternal role and attainment theories.

5 Describe actions that midwives can apply when women experience psychological distress after the birth of their baby.

6 Describe the signs and feelings that women experience that should lead them to come into the maternity unit.

7 Discuss the importance of teaching mothering skills to women in the immediate postpartum period.

8 Discuss the effects of shorter length of stays for mothers on breastfeeding outcomes.

9 Describe eligibility for maternity payments for Australian and New Zealand women.

10 Discuss strategies that midwives can use to include men in the parenting role.

Online resources

Australian Government, Family Assistance Office, http://www.familyassist.gov.au/Internet/FAO/FAOl.nsf/content/publications-factsheet 11.07.2004

Ministry of Health, New Zealand http://www.womenz.org.nz/pol%20alerts/Govt%20QandA.doc

Ministry of Social Development, New Zealand, http://www.msd.govt.nz

References

Abidin R 1990 Parenting stress index (3rd edn). Charlottesville, VA

Ainsworth MD (Ed) 1973 The development of infant-mother attachment. University of Chicago, Chicago

Ainsworth MD 1962 The effects of maternal deprivation: a review of findings and controversy in the context of research strategy. In: MD Ainsworth et al (Eds) Deprivation of maternal care. Schocken, New York, pp 287–357

Ainsworth MD, Blehar MC, Waters E et al 1978 Patterns of attachment: a psychological study of the strange situation. Erlbaum, Hillsdale, NJ

Armstrong KL, Fraser JA, Dadds MR et al 1999 A randomized controlled trial of nurse home visiting to vulnerable families with newborns. Journal of Paediatric Child Health 35:237–244

Armstrong KL, Fraser JA, Dadds MR et al 2000 Promoting secure attachment, maternal mood and child health in a vulnerable population: a randomized controlled trial. Journal of Paediatric Child Health 36:555–562

Ashmore S 2001 Implementing skin-to-skin contact in the immediate postnatal period. MIDIRS Midwifery Digest 11(2):247–250

Atkinson RL, Atkinson RC, Smith EE et al 1993 Introduction to Psychology (11th edn). Harcourt Brace, Sydney

Baafi M, McVeigh C, Williamson M 2001 Fatherhood; the changes and challenges. British Journal of Midwifery 9(9):567–570

Ball JA 1994 Reactions to motherhood: the role of postnatal care (2nd edn). Books for Midwives, Hale, Cheshire

Barclay L, Donovan J, Genovese A 1996 Men's experiences during their partner's first pregnancy: a grounded theory analysis. Australian Journal of Advanced Nursing 13(3):12–24

Barclay L, Everitt L, Rogan F et al 1997 Becoming a mother—an analysis of women's experience of early motherhood. Journal of Advanced Nursing 25:719–728

Barclay L, Lupton D 1999 The experiences of new fatherhood: a socio-cultural analysis. Journal of Advanced Nursing 29(4):1013–1020

Bowlby J 1969 Attachment and loss. Hogarth, London

Bowlby J 1980 Attachment and loss. Vol. 3. Loss: sadness and depression. Basic Books, New York

Brazier J, Harper R, Jones N et al 1992 Validating the SF-36 health survey questionnaire: new outcome measure for primary care. British Medical Journal 305:160–164

Broberg AG 2000 A review of interventions in the parent-child relationship informed by attachment theory. Acta Paediatrica 434(89):37–42

Brown S, Bruinsma F, Darcy M et al 2004 Early discharge: no evidence of adverse outcomes in three consecutive population-based Australian surveys of recent mothers, conducted in 1989, 1994 and 2000. Paediatric and Perinatal Epidemiology 18:202–213

Brown S, Davis P, Faber B et al 2002 Early postnatal discharge from hospital for healthy mothers and infants (Protocol for a Cochrane Review). Cochrane Library (1). John Wiley & Sons, Chichester

Brown S, Small R, Faber B et al 2005 Early discharge from hospital for healthy mothers and term infants. Cochrane Database of Systematic Reviews. Cochrane Library (1). John Wiley & Sons, Chichester, ID#CD002958

Buist A 1997 Counting the costs of early discharge after childbirth. Medical Journal of Australia 167:236–237

Buist A, Morse C, Durkin S 2002 Men's adjustment to fatherhood: implications for obstetric healthcare. Journal of Gynecology and Neonatal Nursing 32(2):172–180

Burr WR 1972 Role transition: 'a reformulation of theory'. Journal of Marriage and the Family 34:407–416

Caldwell B, Bradley R 1984 Home observation. Measurement of the environment. University of Arkansas at Little Rock, Little Rock

Carty E, Bradley C 1990 A randomized, controlled evaluation of early postpartum discharge. Birth 17(4):199–204

Charpak N, Ruiz-Pelaez J, Figueroa Z et al 1997 Kangaroo mother versus traditional care for newborn infants < 2000 grams: a randomized, controlled trial. Pediatrics 100(4):682–688

Collington V 1998 Do women share midwives' views of their educational role? British Journal of Midwifery 6(8):556–563

Cooke M, Stacey T 2003 Differences in the evaluation of postnatal midwifery support by multiparous and primiparous women in the first two weeks after birth. Australian Journal of Midwifery 16(3):18–24

Cox J, Holden J, Sagovsky R 1987 Detection of postnatal depression. Development of the 10-item Edinburgh Postnatal Depression Scale. British Journal of Psychiatry 150:782–786

Davis-Floyd R 1994 The ritual of hospital birth in America. In: JP Spradley, DW McCurdey (Eds) Conformity and conflict. Readings in cultural anthropology. Harper-Collins, New York

de Montigny F, Lacharite C 2003 Fathers' perceptions of the immediate postpartal period. Journal of Gynecology and Neonatal Nursing 33(3):328–339

Dellman T 2004 'The best moment of my life': a literature review of fathers' experience of childbirth. Australian Journal of Midwifery 17(3):20–26

Department of Family and Community Services 2000 Participation support for a more equitable society. Final Report of the Reference Group on Welfare Reform. DFCS, Canberra

Department of Human Services 2003 Every chance for every child. Making the early years count. A framework for early childhood services in South Australia 2003–2004. DHS, Adelaide

Draper J 2003 Men's passage to fatherhood: an analysis of the contemporary relevance of transition theory. Nursing Inquiry 10(1):66–78

Emmanuel E, Creedy D, Fraser J 2001 'What mothers want'. A postnatal survey. Australian College of Midwives Inc. 14(4):16–20

Fawcett J, Tulman L, Meyer S 1988 Development of the inventory of functional status after childbirth. Journal of Nurse-Midwifery 33(6):252–260

Fisher K, Kemp L, Tudbull J 2002 'Families first' outcomes evaluation framework. University of New South Wales, Sydney

Fowles E 1997 The relationship between maternal role and attainment and postpartum depression. Healthcare of Women International 19:83–94

Francis D, Diorio J, Lui D et al 1999 Nongenomic transmission across generations of maternal behavior and stress responses in the rat. Science 286(5):1150–1158

Froggatt K 1997 Rites of passage and the hospice culture. Mortality 2(2):123–136

Gagnon AJ, Barkum L 2004 Postnatal parental education for improving family health. Cochrane Database of Systematic Reviews 2003, Issue 1. Art. No CD004068. DOI:10.1002/14651858. CD004068. (This version first published online: 20 January 2003 in Issue 1, 2003.)

Gamble J, Creedy D, Moyle W 2004 Counselling processes to address psychological distress following childbirth: perceptions of midwives. Journal of the Australian College of Midwives 16–19

Gottlieb L 1978 Maternal attachment in primiparas. Journal of Obstetrical, Gynaecological and Neonatal Nursing 7:39–44

Grullon K, Grimes D 1997 The safety of early postpartum discharge: a review and critique. Obstetrics and Gynaecology 90(5):860–865

Hanna B, Edgecombe G, Jackson C et al 2002 The importance of first-time parent groups for new parents. Nursing and Health Sciences 4:209–214

Harlow HF, Zimmerman RR 1959 Affectional responses in the infant monkey. Science 130:421–424

Having your baby at the women's and children's hospital 2003 Women's and Children's Hospital Adelaide, January 2003

Henderson C 2000 Postnatal care needs are not being met. Midwifery 8(8):472–474

Hunt S, Symonds S 1995 The social meanings of midwifery. MacMillan, London

Kingston B (Ed) 1977 The world moves slowly: a documentary history of Australian women. Cassell Australian, Stanwell, NSW

Kirkham M 2000 How can we relate?. In: M Kirkham (Ed) The midwife–mother relationship. Palgrave MacMillan, UK

Klaus MH, Kennell JH 1976 Maternal–infant bonding. Mosby, St Louis

Klaus MH, Kennell JH 1982 Parent–infant bonding (2nd edn). Mosby, St Louis

Levy-Shiff R 1994 Individual and contextual correlates of marital change across the transition to parenthood. Developmental Psychology 30(4):591–601

Ludington-Hoe S 1993 Kangaroo care. Bantum Books, New York

Lui D, Diorio J, Tannenbaum B et al 1997 Maternal care, hippocampal glucocorticoid receptors, and hypothalamic-pituitary-adrenal responses to stress. Science 277:1659–1662

Mackereth PA 2003 A minority report: teaching fathers baby massage. Complementary Therapies in Nursing and Midwifery 9:147–154

Maloni J 1994 The content and sources of knowledge about the infant. Maternal-Child Nursing Journal 22(4):111–120

McKellar L 2002 Congratulations, you're a mother: a strategy for enhancing postnatal education for first-time mothers investigated through an action research cycle. Unpublished honours thesis, University of South Australia, Adelaide

McKellar L, Pincombe J, Henderson A 2002 Congratulations. You're a mother: a strategy for enhancing postnatal education for first-time mothers investigated through an action research cycle. Australian Midwifery 16(1):24–31

McVeigh C 2000 Anxiety and functional status after childbirth. Australian College of Midwives Inc. 13(1):14–18

McVeigh C, Charboyer W 2002 Reliability and validity of the Inventory of Functional Status after childbirth when used in an Australian population. Nursing and Health Sciences 4:107–112

Mercer R 1981 A theoretical framework for studying factors that impact on the maternal role. Nursing Research 30:73–77

Mercer R 1985 The process of maternal role attainment over the first year. Nursing Research 34:198–204

Mercer R 2004 Becoming a mother versus maternal role attainment. Journal of Nursing Scholarship, Third Quarter:226–232

Ministry of Health 2003 Maternity Services Consumer Satisfaction Survey. NOH, Wellington

Ministry of Social Development 2004 New Zealand families today. Online: http://www.familiescommission.gov.nz/-8k-28Aug 2005

Moran C, Holt V, Martin D 1997 What do women want to know after childbirth? Birth 24(1):14–18

National Health and Medical Research Council (NHMRC) 1996 Options for effective care in childbirth. Commonwealth of Australia, Canberra

National Health and Medical Research Council (NHMRC) 1998 Review of services offered by midwives. Commonwealth of Australia, Canberra

National Health Committee 1999 Review of maternity services in New Zealand. National Health Committee, Wellington

Neile E (1997) Control for black and ethnic minority women: a meaningless pursuit. In: M Kirkham, E Perkins (Eds) Reflections on midwifery. Baillière Tindall, London

Nolan M 1997 Antenatal education: failing to educate for parenthood. British Journal of Midwifery 5(1):21–29

O'Meara C 1993 A diagnostic model for the evaluation of childbirth and parenting education. Midwifery 9:28–34

Ockleford E, Berryman J, Hsu R 2004 Postnatal care: what new mothers say. British Journal of Midwifery 12(3):166–171

Odent M 1996 Why labouring women don't need support. Mothering 80:46–50

Percival P, McCourt C 2000 Becoming a parent. In: L Page (Ed) The new midwifery: science and sensitivity in practice. Churchill Livingstone, Edinburgh, pp 185–222

Philpin S 2002 Rituals and nursing: a critical commentary. Journal of Advanced Nursing 38(2):144–151

Rich A 1976 Of woman born. Bantam Books, New York

Rogan F, Schmied V, Barclay L et al 1997 'Becoming a mother'—developing a new theory of early motherhood. Journal of Advanced Nursing 25:877–885

Rossi AF 1968 Transition to parenthood. Journal of Marriage and the Family 30(1):26–39

Rubin R 1967a Attainment of a maternal role: Part I. Process. Nursing Research 16:237–245

Rubin R 1967b Attainment of a maternal role: Part II. Models and referents. Nursing Research 16:342–346

Rubin R 1975 Maternity nursing stops too soon. American Journal of Nursing 75:1680–1688

Rubin R 1984 Maternal identity and the maternal experience. Springer, New York

Ruchala P, Halstead L 1994 The postpartum experiences of low-risk women: a time of adjustment and change. Maternal-Child Nursing Journal 222:83–89

Ruiz-Pelaez JG, Charpak N, Cuervo LG 2004 Kangaroo mother care, an example to follow from developing countries. British Medical Journal 329:1179–1181

Schmied V, Everitt L 1996 Post-natal care: poor cousin or priority area? In: L Barclay, L Jones (Eds) Midwifery trends and practice in Australia. Churchill Livingstone, Melbourne

Spielberger C 1983 Manual for the state-trait anxiety inventory (Form Y). Self-evaluation questionnaire. Consulting Psychologists Press, Palo Alto

Taggart AV, Short S, Barclay L (2000) She has made me feel human again: an evaluation of a volunteer home-based visiting project for mothers. Health and Social Care in the Community 8(1):1–8

Thomas SG, Upton D 2000 Professional issues. Expectant fathers' attitudes towards pregnancy. British Journal of Midwifery 8(4):218–221

Thompson F 2004 Mother and midwives. The ethical journey. Books for Midwives, Sydney

Turner BS 1969 The ritual process. Penguin, Harmondsworth

Turner BS 1977 Transformation, hierarchy and transcendence: a reformation of van Gennep's model of the structure of rites de passage. In: SF Moore, BG Myeroff (Eds) Secular ritual. Van Gorcum, Amsterdam

Turner BS 1987 Medical power and social knowledge. Sage, London

van Gennep A 1960 The rites of passage. University of Chicago Press, Chicago

Vehvilainen-Julkunen K, Liukkonen A 1998 Fathers' experiences of childbirth. Midwifery 14:10–17

Vimpani G 2001 The role of social cohesiveness in promoting optimum child development. Youth Suicide Prevention Bulletin 5:20–24. Australian Institute of Family Studies, Melbourne

Walters D, Kirkham M 1997 Support and control in labour: doulas and midwives. In: M Kirkham, E Perkins (Eds) Reflections on midwifery. Baillière Tindall, London

Ware JE, Snyder MK, Wright WR 1976 Development and validation of scales to measure patient satisfaction with medical care services. Vol 1, Part A. Review of literature, overview of methods, and results regarding construction of scales (NTIS Publication PB 288-0329). National Technical Information Service, Springfield

Whitehouse K 2001 The touch of life. Practising Midwife 4(11): 28–32

Wynder EL 1998 Introduction to the report on the conference on the 'critical' period of brain development. Preventative Medicine 27:166–167

CHAPTER 10

Professional frameworks for practice in Australia and New Zealand

Sally Pairman and Roslyn Donnellan-Fernandez

Key terms

Australian College of Midwives, Australian Midwifery Action Project, code of ethics, code of practice, competencies, New Zealand College of Midwives, maternity services, medicalisation, midwifery regulation, professionalism, Register of Midwives, regulatory framework, standards of practice

Chapter overview

This chapter outlines current and evolving professional and regulatory frameworks guiding midwifery practice in Australia and New Zealand. While professional frameworks for midwifery arise from the profession itself, regulatory frameworks reflect societal understandings of midwifery and wider interests than those of midwifery alone. Regulatory frameworks provide the statutory boundaries for midwifery practice and define the extent of professional autonomy each state affords to midwifery. This chapter explains the relationships between regulatory and professional frameworks in both countries and how these frameworks affect midwifery practice.

Learning outcomes

Learning outcomes for this chapter are:

1 To describe current and evolving professional frameworks that guide midwifery practice in Australia and New Zealand

2 To describe the links between definition and scope of practice of a midwife, philosophy, code of ethics, and standards for practice with midwifery standards review and recertification (NZ), and continuing professional development (Australia)

3 To articulate an understanding of the term 'professionalism' and differentiate between 'old' and 'new' professions

4 To articulate differentiations in the development of the midwifery profession in New Zealand and Australia, with respect to history, role, functions and structure

5 To differentiate between midwifery regulation in New Zealand and midwifery regulation in Australia, and express an understanding of regulatory principles in common

6 To describe the role and function of the Midwifery Council of New Zealand and the various regulatory authorities for midwifery in Australia

7 To explain the relationship between regulatory and professional frameworks and their application to midwifery practice.

Introduction

As a health profession, midwifery in both Australia and New Zealand is governed by legislation that determines, to a greater or lesser extent, the scope of midwifery practice, the level of midwifery autonomy, processes for entering the profession (registration), expected standards for practice (competencies), and mechanisms for accountability and regulatory control. The purpose of this regulatory framework is to ensure the safety of the public by ensuring that midwives are appropriately qualified, competent and safe to practise midwifery. The legislation reflects society's understanding of and assumptions about midwifery at the time the legislation was enacted. The effect of such legislation is to determine how midwifery interfaces with other providers of maternity services, how midwifery fits within the structures of maternity and health services, and the extent of its professional jurisdiction. Particularly in the case of Australia, regulatory legislation does not necessarily reflect current midwifery practice or, indeed, women's views of the kinds of midwifery services they wish to receive. It may well reflect the interests of other professional groups such as medicine, or of the state, in determining the direction of maternity services. Indeed, 'as both a licensing authority and a source of funding, the state can enhance or diminish the control that an occupation or profession has at any given time over the provision of particular services' (Tully 1999, p 3).

While legislation provides a regulatory framework for midwifery practice, midwives in both Australia and New Zealand also operate under professional frameworks that guide and determine practice. The New Zealand College of Midwives (NZCOM) and the Australian College of Midwives (ACM, formerly ACMI) are the midwifery professional organisations in their respective countries. Both provide direction for midwifery practice through setting philosophy, standards for practice, and ethics and practice guidelines that midwife members are expected to follow. Both organisations also have a political role in working on behalf of midwives to strengthen and protect midwifery and in working to ensure that maternity services meet the needs of childbearing women.

These two frameworks are complementary. Regulation focuses on public safety, while professions focus primarily on midwifery and midwives. Both are concerned with ensuring a competent and safe midwifery workforce but the profession generally has wider concerns and can undertake political action, whereas regulation is constrained by the limits of the legislation.

The way in which regulatory and professional frameworks have developed in each country reflects their unique historical, social, political, cultural and economic contexts. Australia and New Zealand share a common history of colonial settlement from Britain in the early nineteenth century and both countries have Indigenous peoples who have suffered and continue to suffer the effects of colonisation. However, for all their commonalities, Australia and New Zealand have evolved

differently into the modern nations they are today. So too have their professions of midwifery. This chapter briefly traces the historical development of midwifery in both countries and then provides an overview of the regulatory and professional frameworks that determine the practice of midwifery in Australia and New Zealand.

Professions and professionalism: what do they mean?

The *Concise English Dictionary* defines a profession as 'an occupation involving high educational or technical qualifications' or 'the body of persons engaged in such a vocation'. Further, 'a professional' is defined as 'one who has skill or proficiency in an art or science, and who makes their living by the practice of this knowledge, as distinguished from one who engages in it for pleasure'.

Professionalisation can be considered 'the process by which an occupation moves toward a special form of control called a profession' (Aydelotte 1985, p 127). In addition to laying claim to a special knowledge base that is socially sanctioned, and deriving economic benefit from the application of this knowledge, there is also an active political dynamic and legal legitimation of any claim to professional status that has led to the assertion that professions are the creation of a ruling class. The sociologist Elliot Friedson, in defining the attributes and characteristics required for full professional status in relation to the medical profession, advanced this view, stating:

> A profession attains and maintains its position by virtue of the protection and patronage of some elite segment of society which has been persuaded that there is some special value in its work (Friedson, cited in Ehrenreich & English 1973, p 47).

Ehrenreich and English, building on Friedson's work, show how professional groups maintain political and economic monopolisation of their field by exercising 'control over their institutional organisations, their theory and practice, their profits and prestige' (1973, p 20). Additionally, they establish that:

> An occupational group doesn't gain a professional monopoly on the basis of technical superiority alone. A recognised profession is not just a group of self-proclaimed experts; it is a group which has authority in the law to select its own members and regulate their practice, i.e. to monopolise a certain field without outside interference (1973, p 47).

In other words, a profession uses its knowledge base as 'an ideological cover in its struggle for power and status' (Tully 1999, p 30). A profession's knowledge base is contingent on the complex interactions that take place between professions, the state and client or consumer groups and thus is highly variable (Tully 1999).

Abbot picked up on the dynamics of interactions between professions in his development of what he called the 'system' of professions (Abbott 1988). Abbott identified professionalism as a system of interprofessional competition that focuses on disputes over jurisdiction. He defined 'jurisdiction' as the link between a profession and its work and argued that it 'is the history of jurisdictional disputes that is the real, the determining history of professions' (Abbott 1988, p 20). A profession's work is the control of tasks.

> The tasks themselves are defined in the profession's cultural work. Control over them is established by competitive claims in public media, in legal discourse and in workplace negotiation. A variety of settlements, none of them permanent, but some more precarious than others, create temporary stabilities in this process of competition (Abbott 1988, p 84).

Gendered professions

Divinity, law and medicine are three longstanding and traditional professions. Each group has a long and entrenched history of patriarchal tradition in Western societies and has attained the attributes of a profession described above. It is well documented that throughout their histories each has sought to exclude women from entry or from the professional societies and organisations in which members exercise political influence, or marginalised women to non-lucrative and less prestigious areas of practice. This behaviour needs to be considered in the context of the historical control and cultural views of defined sex roles in Western industrialised societies, whereby the female sex role was considered to be incompatible with that required for professional achievement (Speedy 1987). For instance, medicine extended its social and legal legitimacy as the dominant health profession during the nineteenth and twentieth centuries, aided by the ideals and activities of Western imperialism, the rational doctrines of the Enlightenment and the principles of modern mechanisation (Grimshaw et al 1996; Willis 1983). Synchronously, midwifery was downgraded and/or made illegal in many Western societies, in the face of the new licensed professional (predominantly male), specialist medical practitioner, the obstetrician and gynaecologist (Anderson 2002; Donley 2002; Finklestein 1990).

While the improved status of women in contemporary Western society has enabled some to be admitted into the traditional professions, issues around sex differences and power dynamics remain. Men continue 'to control the means by which their particular perspectives are privileged, through their control of political, religious, and literary discourses' (Torres 1992, cited in Shachar 2001, p 4). In relation to childbearing, Lane (2002) and Reiger (2001, 2003) show that the scientific paradigm and its attendant consequences is now firmly institutionalised in law, medical recruitment and clinical practice in contemporary Australian society, including mainstream models of care sponsored by the funding mechanisms of the modern nation state. While the medical discourse of childbirth is being challenged in New Zealand by the development of a midwife-led and women-centered maternity system, it is still deeply entrenched, and the maternity service still reflects the global phenomena of medicalisation and technological intervention that characterise every Western society (Pairman & Guilliland 2003).

Tully (1999) argues that a more useful way of understanding the relations between gender and professionalising activity is to conceptualise gender as a resource rather than a relation of social domination or inequality. Her examination of midwifery in New Zealand shows how midwifery was able to use the gender of its practitioners as a resource in a context where women were demanding more 'women-centred' care and the state had given priority to this women's agenda. Tully contends that New Zealand midwifery deliberately reconstituted itself as a feminist form of professional practice. Central to this practice is the concept of a 'partnership' between midwives, as female health professionals, and women who share their understanding of birth as a normal life event.

> In positioning midwives and birthing women as 'partners' who shared responsibility for the pregnancy/birth, midwifery leaders drew on feminist understandings of the importance of women taking control over their lives and health in general, and their reproductive experiences in particular. Feminist concerns about issues of responsibility, control, empowerment and choice were put at the centre of midwifery's definition of itself as a profession with a 'moral obligation to work in partnership with women' (Tully 1999, p 49).

'Old' and 'new' styles of professionalism

The attributes that characterise a profession have been described as

- a strong level of commitment;
- long and disciplined educational process;
- unique body of knowledge and skill;
- discretionary authority and judgement;
- active and cohesive professional organization;
- acknowledged social worth and contribution (Speedy 1987, p 20).

However, a profession's social power is even more important than its expertise or knowledge, or the commitment of its members. This social power is achieved through a social mandate for practice, and the social mandate comes from political action.

> An occupation becomes a profession not because of the good work of its individual members, but because the occupation as a whole wins a state or social mandate to practise.

> When a class recognises itself as a class, it can organise itself politically . . . professionalism in this sense is quite simply not something that can be achieved by hard work or study. Professional status comes from political action (Katz Rothman 1984, p 300).

Ehrenreich and English reminded us of the contradictions inherent in professional status when they stated:

> We must never confuse professionalism with expertise. Expertise is something to work for and to share: professionalism is—by definition—elitist and exclusive, sexist, racist and classist (Ehrenreich & English 1973, p 42).

These notions of professions as 'expert' with a rational, scientific and masculinist approach to knowledge characterise 'old' style professionalism, which continues to define dominant professions in Western industrialised societies. For many midwives, the characteristics of 'old' professions are antithetical to midwifery because they are seen as separating midwives and women from each other, and midwives have asked why midwifery would want or need to be a profession (Cronk 2000; Wilkins 2000). In contrast, the New Zealand midwifery model of midwifery partnership provides an example of 'new' professionalism (Guilliland & Pairman 1995; Pairman 2005; Tully 1999). This latter model has been described as characterising the 'new midwifery' of the future, in which knowledge about the body is constructed as the outcome of relationships and interactions between people (Lane 2002; Page 2003). The characteristics of old and new professionalism can be differentiated as: mastery of knowledge versus reflective practice; unilateral decision processes (patient as dependent, colleagues as differential) versus interdependent decision processes (patient empowered, colleagues engaged as equals); autonomy and self-management versus supported practice teamwork; individual accountability versus collective learning, responsibility and accountability; and detachment versus engagement (Health Workforce Advisory Committee 2005).

We move on now to explore midwifery's approach to professionalism in both Australia and New Zealand.

Midwifery as a profession in Australia

Midwifery in Australia is in a state of transition and at this stage does not reflect the attributes of either 'old' or 'new' professions (Barclay et al 2003).

Influences of competing discourses of childbearing

Understanding the evolution of a professional framework for midwifery practice in Australia in the twenty-first century is contingent on examining and understanding the historical, political, cultural, economic and race relations of Australia's early foundation as a colonial settlement of the United Kingdom and its subsequent development into a modern nation state. These developments encompass the socio-political, professional and economic arrangements and relationships that underpin the evolution of its current health infrastructure (Anderson 2002; Duckett 2000; Grimshaw et al 1996; Reiger 2003). Additionally, understanding recent critique of contemporary economic, political and cultural forces that have influenced government policy, including competing trends towards both market-driven health services and institutionalised state-sponsored health services, consumer and professional activism, and the women's movement during the twentieth century, is also vital in understanding influences on the future framework for professional midwifery practice in Australia (Barclay et al 2003; Donnellan-Fernandez & Eastaugh 2003; Maternity Coalition 2002; Reiger 2001).

Mainstream Australian maternity services are fragmented into antenatal, intrapartum and postnatal spheres, and maternity care has been constructed within an industrial nursing framework whereby the midwife's role is confined to a set roster and specified hours. This historical structural division

of labour has created conflict among groups advocating an elitist, specialist, professionalising route for midwifery, and those that place women at the centre of the decision-making process, such as 'partnership' models of midwifery, in which care is part of the continuum of an established relationship (Reiger 2001). Within such a context, continuing questions need to be asked about how and where professionalisation as a strategy for midwifery sits in relation to current discourses of birth as a social construct. This includes consideration of the emerging ethos of relationship between women and midwives being articulated as 'partnership' models of birth in countries such as New Zealand, where midwifery autonomy has been actualised in practice and is visibly regulated (Pairman 2000; Guilliland & Pairman 1995).

In examining the Australian history of childbearing, Reiger (2003) and Lane (2002) have analysed the evolution and construction of birth as the medicalisation of the body and of social life. Both authors propose that professionalisation has been a response to the state-sanctioned medical practice monopoly in childbearing, including the historical subordination of midwifery as a branch of specialist nursing practice. This is supported by contemporary Australian midwifery researchers' claims of the practice of medical obstetrics on normal, healthy women as a form of 'occupational imperialism' to ensure ongoing medical strategic control and financial monopoly of maternity services. Twofold effects have been a national lack of access for consumers to midwifery-based services and continuing lack of midwifery autonomy and job satisfaction, resulting in deskilling and increasing attrition rates from the midwifery workforce (Brodie 2002; Tracy et al 2000).

The sites where midwives have been able to practise autonomously in Australia, such as birth centres and home birth, have been limited and marginalised by barriers that include: a lack of state-sponsored policy frameworks and funding mechanisms; interprofessional rivalry and philosophical clashes with medical and nursing groups; and, since mid-2001, national withdrawal of professional indemnification arrangements for self-employed midwives despite continuing state-subsidised arrangements for the medical profession (Donnellan-Fernandez 1996, 2000; Donnellan-Fernandez & Eastaugh 2003). Although midwifery claims to be a profession, its professionalisation strategy is still in its infancy (Lane 2002). Lane (2002, p 30) suggests that 'Midwives need to ask themselves how much autonomy they wish to exercise in their practice and how they understand the relationship between the body and society'. In common with the findings of Sandall (1997) in the United Kingdom and Lazarus (1997) in North America, her research leads her to advocate for diversity in models of midwifery practice, to suit 'both women and a range of women's needs' (Lane 2002, p 39).

Australian Midwifery Action Project (AMAP)

The most recent comprehensive report on midwifery in Australia is that of the Australian Midwifery Action Project (AMAP) (Barclay et al 2003). This project facilitated the collaboration of industry partners, researchers, relevant organisations and the wider community through an action-oriented research process. Over the life of the project, the primary outcome has been a series of publications investigating the service delivery, educational, policy and regulatory environments affecting midwifery nationally. Important secondary outcomes have been 'to analyse and facilitate collaboration and communication across all of these sectors', in addition to 'informing the development of national and state initiatives to improve maternity services' (Barclay et al 2003, p 61). The findings of AMAP are a legacy of the history of many of the forces identified above, and the report is significant in that it underlines barriers to the future of midwifery in Australia. Particularly problematic at the beginning of the twenty-first century is the national status of the midwife. In summary this includes:

the lack of a coherent approach to the role of the midwife—the invisibility of midwives in policy, planning and regulation, and problems in contemporary midwifery education offered by schools of nursing. These include lack of symmetry between various stakeholders with regard to the role of the midwife; her sphere of practice, her skills, degree of professional autonomy and legal responsibilities forms a singular and monolithic barrier to the emergence of a fully functional midwifery profession. The future potential of midwifery as a provider of primary healthcare to all women, regardless of designated medical risk status, rests on the capacity of educational, regulatory and service institutions to mobilise a unified vision of midwifery practice and the requisite skills and legal framework to achieve it (Barclay et al 2003, p 57).

Professional status

Specific challenges have recently been mounted to midwifery's capacity to fulfil its professional status in Australia, in the areas of educational process, body of knowledge, discretionary authority and judgement, and cohesive professional organisation.

Educational process

While a unique body of knowledge and skills in midwifery is asserted in the 'International Definition of a Midwife' (ICM 1990) and accepted by the Australian College of Midwives Inc., recent mapping and critique of inconsistencies and minimum practice standards in midwifery education programs in Australia have highlighted both a lack of opportunities for students to participate in midwifery models, and the fact that current assessment regulations for midwifery fall well short of those required by the regulation bodies of other industrialised countries (ANMC 2004; Leap et al 2002). These findings are hardly surprising, given Australian midwifery's history, education infrastructure, resources and industry/labour force expectations of a skill set and accompanying set of socialised relationships that are constructed as 'add-ons' to specialist nursing practice (Donnellan-Fernandez 2000).

Body of knowledge

Recent interviews by Lane (2002) with Australian midwives showed that midwifery is not a static, discrete body of knowledge, and that midwives cannot be classified into discrete obstetric assistant/medical models or professional/independent midwifery models. Rather, most could be classified as 'hybrid' and reflecting the needs of a variety of practice settings rather than a model determined by midwifery.

Discretionary authority and judgement

While the Australian College of Midwives (ACM), as the peak 'professional' body for midwives in Australia, has articulated national standards for midwifery practice and education, it currently has no statutory mandate to enforce these standards in law in all Australian states and territories. At present there are no nationally consistent midwifery educational or practice standards that are either universally endorsed or are statutorily enforceable by the Australian nursing regulatory authorities in each of the eight states and territories of the nation—that is, there is no 'discretionary authority' or professional regulatory jurisdiction that is legally sanctioned. Rather, midwives in most Australian states and territories are ambiguously licensed as nurses, a position that is not legislatively consistent with professional midwifery practice or regulation in other areas of the Western world, or consistent with the principle of regulation in the public interest (Brodie & Barclay 2001; Donnellan-Fernandez 2001).

Cohesive professional organisation

Until the late 1970s, midwives in Australia were largely subsumed within nursing organisations. In 1979 a National Midwives Association was formed concurrent with an emerging professional consciousness. Subsequent incorporation and membership of the International Confederation of Midwives (ICM) has seen the ACM develop over the past 20 years to become the accepted national organisation for midwives. In addition to shaping standards for professional midwifery practice it has developed educational programs, participated in health policy development and provided a significant information network for its members (Barclay et al 2003).

However, despite ACM articulation of comprehensive objectives (see the discussion of the role and function of the ACM later in this chapter), recent analysis indicates that the ACM has not yet achieved the same cohesion, public profile or political influence as some of its international sister organisations, such as the New Zealand College of Midwives and the Royal College of Midwives UK. Membership consists of less than a quarter of midwives estimated to be currently practising, with the majority (who are employed by state and territory governments in public sector hospitals) remaining members of the principal industrial body for nursing in Australia, the Australian Nursing Federation (Reiger 2003).

Birth culture and institutionalisation

Despite current global evidence that supports universal access for all healthy childbearing women to midwifery-led care (WHO 1996), the dominant, state-sanctioned birth culture in Australian society at the beginning of the twenty-first century remains that of institutionalised medicine (CDHAC 1999;

Maternity Coalition 2002). This culture is characterised by state sponsorship of medicine, including over-representation of techno-industrial models of 'professional' practice, which view the birthing body as a 'machine' and generate profits or health-funding outcomes that are defined in a market-driven economy (Davis-Floyd & Sarjeant 1997; De Vries et al 2001). In common with many other affluent, industrialised Western nations, in Australia this culture is entrenched at the level of government policy, funding and existing health infrastructure (AGPC 2004; Donnellan-Fernandez & Eastaugh 2003; Reiger 2003).

Despite two decades of state, territory and national inquiries into birthing services in Australia, including accompanying recommendations expressing women's repeated requests for 'choice, continuity and control', there is a vacuum in national government policy and political will to enable the funding, infrastructure and service reform recommendations of these reports to be implemented (Maternity Coalition 2002).

With three exceptions (Victoria, New South Wales and Western Australia), no state or territory government in the past decade has articulated a comprehensive policy for maternity services reform based on primary health principles that enables the midwife to work to the full scope of practice as defined in the International Definition of the Midwife. Maternity policy in Victoria, New South Wales and Western Australia envisage restoring midwifery to a primary health role in the delivery of state-based maternity services (New South Wales Health Department 2000; State of Victoria, Department of Human Services 2004; Western Australian Government 2004). Despite recent evidence that rates of obstetric intervention in labour and birth are lowest among women experiencing care from midwives in public-sector facilities, a culture of expensive medicalised childbirth is the norm for the majority of women in Australia (Homer et al 2001a; Roberts et al 2000, 2002). Maternity care options for women living in regional, rural and remote areas of Australia are limited to state-funded medical providers, and in many instances access to local services and culturally appropriate services, particularly for Indigenous women, are either non-existent or in short supply (Maternity Coalition 2002). While this is the current context for childbearing women and midwifery practice in Australia, some models of midwifery continuity of care are beginning to evolve (Homer et al 2001b).

Redefining professionalism in New Zealand

The current status of midwifery as a profession in New Zealand is somewhat different to that in Australia. New Zealand midwives are an autonomous and distinct professional group. They were granted a social mandate for autonomous practice in 1990 through the Nurses Amendment Act and over the subsequent 15 years have established midwifery as the main provider of maternity services based on a model of autonomous caseload practice and midwifery partnership. Largely through the influence of midwifery, New Zealand's maternity service has been reshaped to a women-centred and midwife-led service in which each woman can access one-to-one continuity of midwifery care from early pregnancy through to six weeks post partum, no matter what the course of her childbirth experience and which other providers need to be involved, and no matter where she chooses to give birth (Pairman & Guilliland 2003). New Zealand midwifery, perhaps more than any other, most closely meets the International Definition of the Midwife by practising within the full scope of midwifery practice (International Confederation of Midwives 1990; Midwifery Council of New Zealand 2004a).

For New Zealand midwifery, these achievements are the culmination of years of planned political and professional activity to bring about the necessary changes to legislation, to societal understandings of birth and midwifery, and to midwifery's understanding of itself as a profession that is deeply intertwined with women. The central tenet of New Zealand midwifery's professional identity is that midwifery *is* the partnership between women and midwives (Guilliland & Pairman 1995; New Zealand College of Midwives 2005). By constituting midwifery as 'midwifery partnership', New Zealand midwifery has sought to replace traditional notions of professionalism with one in which relationships between midwives and women are negotiated and where power differentials are acknowledged and actively shifted from the midwife to the childbearing woman.

This recognition that midwifery is a partnership between a woman and a midwife resulted from the combined political activity of maternity consumer groups and the New Zealand College of Midwives, which led to the *Nurses Amendment Act 1990* and the one-to-one caseload model of midwifery practice that developed subsequently.

Although New Zealand has had a regulated midwifery workforce since the *Midwives Act 1904*, the scope of midwifery practice diminished as a result of increasing hospitalisation and medicalisation of childbirth from the early 1920s onwards (Donley 1986; Mein Smith 1986; Pairman 2002, 2005; Pairman & Guilliland 2003; Papps & Olssen 1997). Women were encouraged to birth in hospitals to avoid the risks of puerperal infection in the home, to access 'pain-free' birth and because of unfounded claims that hospitals were safer than home. That hospitalisation led to fragmented maternity care, loss of control for women and their families, increased medical intervention and use of technology, loss of confidence in women's bodies, and increased fear of birth, has been well documented and is reflected throughout the Western world (Donley 1986; Donnison 1988, Kitzinger 1988; Mein Smith 1986; Papps & Olssen 1997; Tew 1990). Institutional organisation and power structures also affected midwives, who lost their one-to-one community-based practice with women to become 'doctor assistants' and 'specialists' in aspects of maternity care. By 1971, midwifery was no longer visible as a separate profession and was incorporated into nursing as 'specialist nursing practice'. Legislative changes in 1983 and 1986 further undermined the definition and scope of practice of midwifery, which reached an all-time low, where only a handful of home birth midwives remained practising in a way that bore any resemblance to the International Definition of Midwifery (Donley 1986; International Confederation of Midwives 1990).

It was this near-demise of midwifery that led to its rebirth. In reclaiming their identity as separate from nursing, midwives used their professional group, the Midwives Section of the New Zealand Nurses Association, as a vehicle for political action. Initially this activity was focused on reclaiming the International Confederation of Midwives (ICM) definition of a midwife as a 'person' rather than a 'nurse' (as the Nurses Association had redefined it) and on separating midwifery education from nursing (Pairman 2002). However, midwives soon realised that their interests were divergent from those of nursing and could never be served by the (larger) nursing professional organisation. Midwives disbanded the Midwives Sections and in 1989 formed a separate midwifery professional organisation, the New Zealand College of Midwives (Donley 1989; Guilliland 1989).

Maternity consumer groups were also active at this time, seeking to gain control over their birth experiences and to decrease the dominance of the medical model over maternity services (Strid 1987). These women had faith in midwifery and argued for a return of the autonomous midwife, who they believed would be more likely to share power with women through a more women-centered and normal-birth philosophy of practice (Dobbie 1990; Strid 1987).

Recognising that their aims were mutual, midwives and women joined together in a combined political strategy that would first reinstate midwifery autonomy, secondly enable women to have a choice of midwifery care, and thirdly enable the development of direct entry midwifery education to produce the new type of midwife that would be required for this autonomous scope of practice.

A key outcome was that midwives recognised the benefit to themselves and to women of their political partnership, and they gave meaning to this partnership by incorporating partnership constitutionally into every aspect of the New Zealand College of Midwives. Midwifery 'consciously recognises that the only real power base we have rests with the women we attend' (Guilliland 1989, p 14). The active involvement of women in the New Zealand College of Midwives has continued to strengthen midwifery. 'Women's participation in the midwifery profession has given midwives a public, legal and socially sanctioned mandate for practice' (Guilliland & Pairman 1995, p 19). This social mandate carries with it a moral obligation for the midwifery profession to provide the kind of service women want. The continued involvement of women (consumers) in the policy formation and processes of the College ensures that midwives uphold the needs and wishes of women.

It was this understanding of the link between professional autonomy and women's need to have control over their birthing experiences that was the basis of New Zealand midwifery's determination to redefine professionalism.

Although not attracted by the traditional 'power over' model of professionalism, it recognised the potential benefit of professional autonomy. As Oakley and Houd (1990, p 114) contend, 'the exclusion from childbirth of autonomous midwifery restricts the care options available to childbearing women and inevitably promotes the definition of childbearing

as a pathological medicalised event'. New Zealand midwives and women believed that if midwifery autonomy were reinstated, then midwives would have the ability to once again practise within their traditional role as a guardian of normal birth (Strid 1987). Each midwife who worked in this way would be a 'positive presence who focuses on the childbearing woman and the baby, with the knowledge and skills required, but also with a sensitivity and respect for the individuality and uniqueness of each woman and her choices for birthing' (Strid 1987, p 15). Writers such as Barbara Katz Rothman supported these beliefs when she stated:

> I have come to see that it is not that birth is managed the way it is because of what we know about birth. Rather, what we know about birth has been determined by the way it has been managed. And the way childbirth has been managed has been based on the underlying assumptions, beliefs and ideology of medicine as a profession (Katz Rothman 1984, p 304).

The determination to provide women and midwives with the opportunity to co-create new knowledge and understandings of childbirth that would lead to women regaining control and choice in childbirth and to society once again recognising childbirth as a normal life event rather than an illness was the impetus for political activity to reinstate midwifery autonomy. Through the experience of this political partnership, midwives were able to conceptualise a 'new' model of professionalism.

> By redefining the professional–client relationship as one of 'partnership' in which each partner contributes knowledge and experience, it also embraces feminist criticisms of the hierarchical power relations inherent in the doctor–patient relationship and the consequent devaluing of women's knowledge (Tully & Mortlock 1999, p 175).

In recognising the knowledge and experience of women/clients as well as midwives, Midwifery partnership does not afford midwifery expertise and knowledge the same epistemological priority it held in the 'old' model of professionalism (Tully 1999). In midwifery partnership both midwives and women have recognised authority and the midwife's role moves from 'expert' to 'reflective practitioner' whose task is to support, guide and accompany a woman within a more equitable, interdependent and empowering relationship (Tully 1999). In redefining its practice as partnership, midwifery has differentiated its services from those offered by other providers and claimed jurisdiction over 'normal' birthing services. Thus partnership with women is an effective professionalising strategy for midwives (Tully 1999).

The challenge for midwifery is to maintain its partnership relationships with women; and, as will be discussed, the professional and regulatory frameworks of New Zealand midwifery both aim to ensure that this occurs. By articulating midwifery as a partnership, New Zealand midwives have redefined traditional notions of professionalism. However, midwives need to understand this definition and midwifery needs to reinforce the implications of this 'new' style of professionalism for midwifery practice so that midwives do not abuse their power and authority.

Instead of seeking to control childbirth, midwifery seeks to control midwifery, in order that woman can control childbirth. Midwifery must maintain its women-centered philosophy to ensure that its control of midwifery never leads to control of childbirth (Guilliland & Pairman 1995, p 49).

Development of the midwifery profession in New Zealand

Structure and functions of the New Zealand College of Midwives

The New Zealand College of Midwives (NZCOM; the College) is the professional organisation for midwifery in New Zealand. Established in 1989, the College has provided a focus for midwifery's understanding of itself as a profession separate from nursing, and now represents over 80% of all practising midwives in New Zealand. Its commitment to midwifery

partnership has meant that from its inception, women consumers have been members as of right and the constitution provides for regional and national membership by individual women and consumer groups. The consumer membership votes for four representatives to the National Committee from consumer organisations such as Parents Centre New Zealand, Home Birth Aotearoa, La Leche League and The Plunket Society. As the voice for midwifery in New Zealand, the College is involved in a wide variety of activities, both professional and political, to meet the needs of individual midwives, the profession as a whole, and birthing women as its partners and the focus of its interests, by working to maintain a strong and autonomous midwifery profession. The role and functions of the College are summarised in Box 10.1.

The College structure is simple (see Fig 10.1). New Zealand is divided into 10 regions, each with its own regional committee and governance responsibility. The chairpersons (all midwives) of each of the 10 regions are members of the National Committee, along with the four consumer representatives, two midwifery student representatives and

---

BOX 10.1 NZCOM role and functions

The role and functions of the New Zealand College of Midwives are listed below.

Professional practice advice and information
- for all midwives
- for District Health Boards (DHBs)
- for Ministry of Health/government ministries
- for regulatory body/other statutory authorities
- for consumers and consumer organisations
- for other professions
- for the public

Professional development/standards
- for all midwives
- Midwives Handbook
- liaison with DHBs
- expert witness training
- professional development program
- portfolio development and support
- Section 88 negotiations/interprofessional liaison
- contractual advice and policy development

Quality assurance
- Midwifery Standards Review Process for all midwives
- complaints resolution committees for women
- training programs

Education
- NZCOM continuing education workshops/programs
- consensus statements/practice guidelines
- DHB practice workshops
- smoke change workshops
- family violence workshops
- liaison with midwifery education providers
- liaison with DHB midwifery educators

Liaison
- with consumers
- with Maori
- with government/statutory bodies/health organisations/non governmental organisations
- international midwifery organisations
- other professional groups

Research
- Secretariat for Joan Donley Midwifery Research Collaboration
- Biennial Research Forum

Communication and promotion
- journal
- midwifery news
- biennial conference
- publications
- website
- promotional material
- media

Legal advice and representation
- professional indemnity insurance
- legal representation

Financial management/membership management

two Maori midwife representatives. Two Kuia or elders (Maori and Pakeha), the President and Chief Executive lead the Committee. The National Committee meets three times a year to fulfil its governance role. It works in a non-hierarchical and women-centred model that includes extensive consultation processes and consensus decision-making. The National Committee employs the Chief Executive, who in turn employs the staff of the National Office. These staff, some of whom are midwives, carry out the day-to-day work of the College as represented in Box 10.1.

As it has evolved, the College has recognised the need for other midwifery-specific organisations to meet the business and industrial needs of midwives. Considerable thought went into the establishment of these organisations to ensure that their structure, functions and governance mechanisms did not become blurred with the College and dissipate the overall strength and unity of the midwifery voice. As shown in Fig 10.1, the College has created three separate but parallel organisations: the Midwifery and Maternity Provider Organisation (MMPO), the Midwifery Employment Representation and Advice Service (MERAS), and the Joan Donley Midwifery Research Collaboration (JDMRC). Each organisation has its own governance structure and specific role and functions, and its links to the College are maintained through College representation to its governance structure and through the requirement for midwives to first be members of the College before they can access services from any of these organisations.

The Midwifery and Maternity Provider Organisation (MMPO)

The College established the MMPO in 1997 as a separate limited-liability company with its own governance structure. Its purpose is to support the business practices of midwives who carry caseloads and are remunerated through the Maternity

Benefit Schedule. It does this through managing the claiming of fees on behalf of midwives and through provision of standardised midwifery notes that facilitate compliance with data provision and reporting.

Each page of the Maternity Notes is in triplicate: one copy remains with the woman as her birth story and personal record, one is kept by the midwife as her clinical and legal record, and the third is sent to the MMPO for fee-claiming purposes and for clinical data entry into the NZCOM midwifery database. Midwives receive their fee payment together with a report on their clinical outcomes and statistics, which they take to their annual Midwifery Standards Review.

The majority of self-employed midwives throughout New Zealand use this service, and the MMPO also manages the midwife claims for some DHB and Community Trust employers.

NZCOM contracts the MMPO to enter the clinical data from the maternity notes for its midwifery database. It then uses the database to produce a national report on midwife outcomes that analyses the aggregated and anonymous data.

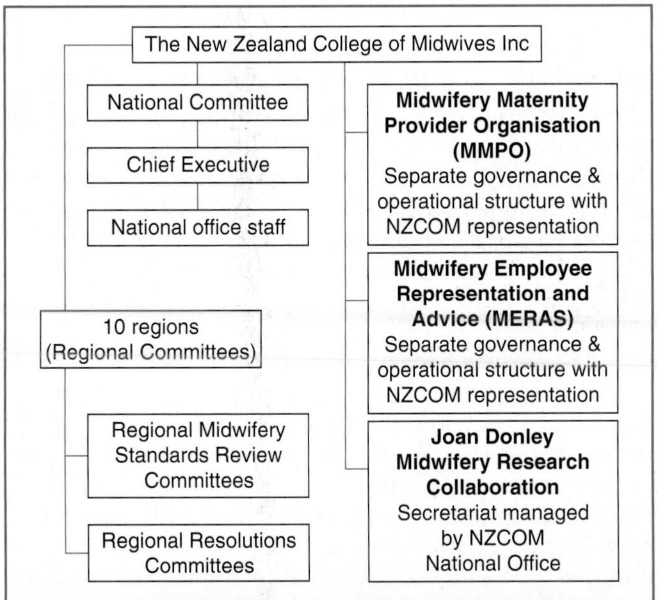

Midwifery Employee Representation and Advisory Service (MERAS)

MERAS is the union for employed midwives. Its formation arose from the wish of College members for a more midwifery-focused representation in the workplace. Until 2003, industrial representation for midwives was only available through the New Zealand Nurses Organisation (NZNO), and salaries and conditions to meet the needs of employed midwives and their various practice models could only be recognised through a variation of the nursing agreement.

In 2005, MERAS achieved a collective agreement specifically for midwives. This agreement covered midwives in all 21 District Health Boards. It not only improved conditions and pay levels for employed midwives but also framed the industrial document within a professional midwifery model and reflected the need for all midwives to focus on professional codes and practice standards. It paved the way for a new midwifery professional development model for employed midwives that is distinct from nursing.

The Joan Donley Midwifery Research Collaboration (JDMRC)

The Collaboration is housed in the College and is named after midwife Joan Donley, the founder of the NZCOM and midwife author and researcher. It is the evidence-based arm of the New Zealand College of Midwives. Its purpose is to encourage and facilitate research cooperation between all midwifery education providers. It hosts a research forum once every two years, specifically for postgraduate midwifery students and hospital midwifery educators to develop research ideas and proposals or present the results of work carried out.

Professional activities

The leadership of the NZCOM has been a major driver in the development of the midwife-led and women-centered

Figure 10.1 Structure of the New Zealand College of Midwives

maternity service that New Zealand enjoys today (Pairman 2005; Pairman & Guilliland 2003). Its leadership has also been essential in the development of midwifery as a strong and autonomous profession. There have been many processes through which the College has worked and continues to work with midwives to build their professional identity and enhance professional standards. These include:

- developing its philosophy and setting standards for practice and an ethical framework (NZCOM 2005)
- producing consensus statements about practice, an education framework and breastfeeding guidelines
- providing education for midwives on family violence and how to screen for and refer women in situations of violence (on contract from the Ministry of Health (MOH))
- providing education for midwives on smoking in pregnancy and how to assist women to change their smoking habits (on contract from MOH)
- publishing resources to guide practice and professional development (e.g. *Midwives Handbook for Practice*, Midwives Portfolio)
- convening disciplinary forums to build practice consensus
- developing mentoring frameworks
- promoting rural networks and locum support
- advising and monitoring pre-registration midwifery education programs.

Perhaps one of the College's most innovative and important professional developments is its Midwifery Standards Review (MSR) process. This, together with its Resolutions process, provides a quality assurance process for midwifery practice in New Zealand that aims to improve and maintain professional midwifery standards. Each region of the College has standing committees for its MSR process and its Resolutions process. As will be discussed later, the College's MSR process is an essential feature of the Recertification Program established in 2005 by the Midwifery Council of New Zealand for all midwives.

Midwifery Standards Review

The Domiciliary Midwives Society initially established Midwifery Review in 1988 to review the practice of home birth midwives. This was in response to moves by obstetric and hospital management to try and impose hospital practices and protocols on the home birth service. As more midwives moved into independent practice after 1990, the College realised that it needed to provide a similar quality assurance mechanism for all midwives. Consequently, in 1992, the College adopted the domiciliary review process and modified it to include the College's standards of practice. Eventually the Domiciliary Midwives Society dissolved and became part of the College, and all midwives are now reviewed under the same criteria.

Midwifery Standards Review committees comprise two midwives, nominated from the region, and two consumers, nominated from consumer organisations. The region endorses all members. All reviewers attend a College-run national training program that seeks to ensure a standardised approach to MSR throughout the country and to help reviewers develop the personal and communication skills necessary for the reviewer role.

Midwives prepare for review by examining their previous year's work, analysing their annual birth outcomes (statistics), considering feedback from women clients (collected via client evaluations by a third party and provided to the midwife for her review), and undertaking a self-assessment against the NZCOM Standards for Practice.

Midwives meet individually with the Review Committee and have the opportunity to explore and discuss their midwifery practice through a supportive and educative process. A main outcome is the joint development of a Professional Development Plan that is revisited at the next review.

It was caseloading midwives who initially undertook MSR and usually presented for review each year. In 2003, NZCOM began encouraging core midwives (hospital midwives not working in caseload models) to undertake review, and since 2005 the Midwifery Council has made MSR mandatory for these midwives every three years, while it expects caseloading midwives to continue with annual review.

Resolution Committees

While the review process is consciously midwife-centered, the College's commitment to partnership with women is reflected in the establishment of Resolution Committees. These committees focus on consumers, and any woman who has concerns about the midwifery care she has received can use this process. One midwife and one consumer make up the committee and also participate in a national training program. The committee helps a woman to resolve her issues, sometimes through facilitating a meeting with the midwife or by providing a forum in which a woman can have her concerns heard and discussed. If resolution is not possible, the committee assists the woman to access other available avenues.

Midwifery as a profession in New Zealand

The New Zealand College of Midwives displays a strong level of commitment to midwifery and to ensuring a midwife-led and women-centred maternity service. Midwifery in New Zealand claims a unique body of knowledge and skill as a guardian of normal birth that arises from its model of midwifery partnership, and it is this experiential knowledge that may be its greatest contribution to the discipline.

The contribution midwifery makes to society is recognised by the authority it has been granted over midwifery, and thus 'normal birth', through legislative changes. As a result, midwives have wide jurisdiction to make midwifery judgements and provide midwifery care on their own responsibility. Legislative authority means that midwifery as a profession is self-regulating and must therefore ensure that midwives provide appropriate standards of care and are accountable for their midwifery judgements. The control of a sphere of practice is never static, and the College must be constantly vigilant to maintain midwifery's position as the main provider of primary maternity services.

While midwifery in New Zealand can claim to have achieved a great deal, it still faces challenges in consolidating its status as a profession and in ensuring that its service really does make a positive difference to the lives of New Zealand women, particularly in a global context of increasing medicalisation and technology. An important ongoing role of the profession is to encourage and assist midwives to act on their personal and professional autonomy and use their midwifery knowledge with confidence in an endeavour to reduce the impact of these global ideologies on childbearing women and their families (Guilliland 2004).

Development of the midwifery profession in Australia

Challenges to a professional framework for midwifery practice in Australia

Australian midwifery has evolved beside and in relation to medical dominance, and the emergence of medical dominance parallels the development of the nation state (Grimshaw et al 1996). Although most births still took place at home at the beginning of the twentieth century, the first half of the century saw birth shifted to hospital and a well-established culture of medical birth (Reiger 2003). Hospitalisation for birth has led to fragmented and episodic care, confined to sites dominated by medicine and where funding, resources and labour force have been concentrated. Within many of these environments, application of complex medical technologies and procedures, implemented by multiple providers, are prioritised over human relationships and basic primary healthcare measures. This distortion is common in many Western industrialised societies and is reinforced by vested market interests in health, 'as it complements and abets continuing fragmentation and colonisation of women and babies' bodies by expensive Western science, practice, products and "health systems" across their life span' (Donley 2002; Donnellan-Fernandez & Eastaugh 2003; Shachar 2001).

Australian midwifery reflects this same history of erosion and colonisation by powerful 'others', including medicine, nursing and the nation state, and 'this has resulted in the erosion of women's birthing power, and state and statutory endorsement of the "invisible" midwife' (Donnellan-Fernandez & Eastaugh 2003).

The Australian Midwifery Action Project (Barclay et al 2003) makes 21 specific recommendations for reform in education, regulation, sphere of practice, cultural safety, maternity service funding mechanisms, industry expectations and community interest in order to achieve community-orientated maternity services and midwifery-led, women-centered care. Synchronously, the formation and replication of grassroots, state, territory and national organisations calling for implementation of reforms in maternity care have been steadily increasing their profile, strategic planning and political activity in the Australian community over the past decade, supporting a social mandate and political platform for increased midwifery autonomy (Donnellan-Fernandez & Eastaugh 2003; Johnston & Newman 2005; Reibel 2004). The ACM, in collaboration with women, is a significant stakeholder in this discourse.

Structure of the Australian College of Midwives

The Australian College of Midwives (ACM) was established from the National Midwives Association (formed in 1979), whose membership broke away from the Australian Nursing Federation, the chief federal industrial body for nurses in Australia. Membership of the ACM across all states and territories of Australia comprises approximately 3000 midwives. National midwifery workforce data suggest that this figure comprises approximately 30% of all practising midwives (Tracy et al 2002).

The ACM is governed by a constitution and by-laws that outline the aims and objectives of the College, the terms and categories of membership status, the functions and powers of the National Executive Committee, and provide for a federated structure with equal representation from each of the eight state and territory ACM Branches (New South Wales, South Australia, Tasmania, Queensland, Victoria, Western Australia, Northern Territory and Australian Capital Territory). Membership of the National Executive (NEC) comprises one delegate from each state and territory, who is elected and nominated by each branch for two years prior to each Biennial Conference. Office bearers for the positions of President, Vice-President, Secretary and Treasurer are nominated and elected by delegates comprising the NEC.

The eight state and territory branches of the ACM operate as autonomous bodies charged with the responsibility of fulfilling the aims and objectives of the College. Each is governed by its own articles of association (which must be in harmony with the national constitution), and branch executives can authorise the formation of sub-branches within their region. Although the ACM has always sought to establish alliances and effective working relationships with women and maternity consumer groups, it is only in the past five years that amendment of the inaugural national constitution and articles of association of state and territory branches have enabled women consumers as members of right.

The National Executive meets up to four times per year to fulfill its governance role, and there is a Biennial General Meeting that is usually held in conjunction with the Biennial National Midwifery Conference. The NEC employs the Chief Executive Officer, who employs the staff of the National Office. In 2003 the National Office was relocated from Melbourne to Canberra.

The cooperative federalism model of governance that dictates the current structure of the ACM has both strengths and challenges in a country as large as Australia, and replicates the Westminister model on which the Australian system of government is based—that is, an overarching national constitution with two tiers of governance that enables state and territory, in addition to federal, debate and input into decision-making.

Role and functions

College membership is through membership of a state or territory branch. The NEC carries out certain duties at the request of the International Confederation of Midwives (ICM), as a member association. The NEC acts in response to issues raised at branch level, and may delegate tasks to the various branches for research and action. See Box 10.2 for a summary of the College's vision and purpose, key strategic goals and functions.

While state sponsorship of autonomous midwifery practice in New Zealand is currently guaranteed via legislated funding (Maternity Benefit Schedule) and regulatory process (Midwifery Council of New Zealand), this is not the case in Australia. Consequently, unlike MMPO and MERAS, which represent the business and industrial interests of midwives in New Zealand, there has been no development of parallel organisations in the Australian context, apart from the Australian Society of Independent Midwives, whose membership of self-employed midwives remains small. There are currently no equivalent structures within the ACM, which to date, despite vigorous government lobbying, has been unable to secure professional indemnification arrangements for self-employed midwives since this was withdrawn nationally in mid-2001. In public health facilities in Australia, the majority of midwives, as employees of the state, have had no collective salary agreements that are independent of the eight state-based Nursing Awards under whose conditions, terms and pay structures they are employed. Recent introduction of an Annualised Salary Agreement for Midwives (as a variation to a state-based Nurses Award) took four years to negotiate in one state, and in 2005 has been expanded to all public sector sites in that state (Nurses South Australian Public Sector Enterprise Agreement: 2004, Midwifery Caseload Practice Agreement). Negotiations continue in other states individually, between Area Health Services and the Nurses Union.

Australian College of Midwives Framework for Midwifery

In March 2004, the ACM established the Australian National Education Standards Taskforce (ANEST) to undertake a national review of current ACM philosophy, codes of ethics and practice, education standards and position statements,

---

BOX 10.2 ACM role and functions

The role and functions of the Australian College of Midwives are as listed below.

Vision and purpose:

▶ To be the leading organisation shaping Australian maternity care

▶ To provide a unified political voice for the midwifery profession

▶ To support midwives to reach their full potential

▶ To ensure all childbearing women have access to continuity of care by a known midwife

▶ To set professional practice and education standards.

Key strategic goals:

▶ To be an accessible, efficient, transparent organisation providing valued services to members

▶ Consistent and timely political representation to influence policy development and decision making Australia wide

▶ To make midwifery a public health strategy

▶ To achieve National Standards for midwifery education and practice that are internationally recognised.

Functions:

▶ To act as the political voice of the midwifery profession in Australia

▶ To further the professional, educational and social interests of midwives in Australia

▶ To promote and maintain high standards of maternity care

▶ To set national professional practice and education standards that are internationally recognised. (An accreditation process for Independently Practising Midwives has been established since 1990. Current ACM negotiations with the Australian

Council of Safety and Quality are working towards a proposal for funding to support development of a Continuing Professional Development process for all midwives that is linked to the new national midwifery standards framework. It is envisaged that the CPD process will closely parallel the Standards Review system adopted by NZ Midwifery (ACMI 2005).)

▶ To provide continuing education programs for midwives

▶ To act as a consultant to government bodies in the development of health policy that makes midwifery a public health strategy

▶ To provide an information network for midwives throughout Australia and all organisations affiliated with the International Confederation of Midwives

▶ To provide a forum for professional midwifery discussion and debate

▶ To disseminate current information via the ACM journal, national newsletter, Biennial National Midwifery Conferences, and through state Branches and the media

▶ To provide scholarships for midwives to undertake research and to assist in the promotion of the education and practice of midwifery through administration of the Australian Midwifery Scholarship Foundation Biennial National Midwifery Conferences, and through state branches and the media

▶ To provide scholarships for midwives to undertake research and to assist in the promotion of the education and practice of midwifery through administration of the Australian Midwifery Scholarship Foundation.

(Source: ACM 2005)

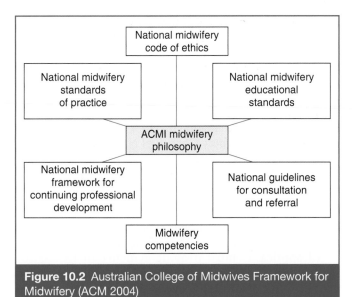

Figure 10.2 Australian College of Midwives Framework for Midwifery (ACM 2004)

and to propose a Professional Development Framework (see Fig 10.2). At the same time, the Australian Nursing and Midwifery Council (established in 1992 and changing its name to include midwifery in 2005), whose stated brief is to lead a national approach with state and territory regulatory authorities in developing statutory standards for nursing and midwifery, funded a project to research the role and scope of practice of midwives and to develop national competency standards for midwifery. This project was completed in late 2005 and ANMC National Competency Standards for the Midwife (ANMC 2005a) will replace the ACM Midwifery Competency Standards (2002).

Australian National Standards for Midwifery Practice

It is currently a time of significant change, challenge and upheaval for diverse factions and groups of midwives in Australia with regard to developing a cohesive national framework for professional standards.

Attempts to meet international standards in the education of Australian midwives have seen the introduction of three-year Bachelor of Midwifery Degree programs at several universities in two Australian states in 2002, with further states and universities commencing these courses in 2006, in alignment with the ACM National Standards for three-year Bachelor of Midwifery courses. This strategy, projected to help address current industry shortages and an ageing midwifery workforce, comprises a professional paradigm shift in midwifery education in Australia, and has undoubtedly advanced the agenda of developing a national midwifery framework that is compatible with international standards. It has also heightened tensions with industry, professional and industrial groups in nursing, and highlighted gaps in current regulatory frameworks, particularly with regard to the absence of endorsed national regulatory standards against which to measure continuing competence in midwifery.

The ACM national website currently hosts a variety of endorsed professional publications, including:
- ACM Midwifery Philosophy Statement (2004)
- National Midwifery Guidelines on Consultation and Referral (2004)
- National Position Statement on Midwifery Education (2004)
- Code of Practice for Midwives (2000)
- Code of Ethics (2001)
- Midwifery Competency Standards (2002) (www.acmi. org.au).

Newly developed National Competency Standards for the Midwife (ANMC 2005a) were released by the Australian Nursing and Midwifery Council in January 2006, following extensive consultation with midwives around Australia. Members from the Australian National Education Standards Taskforce of the ACM acted as Reference Group for the Project Management Group at the University of Technology, Sydney, which undertook development of the midwifery standards on behalf of the ANMC. The standards have been approved by each state and territory nursing and midwifery regulatory body to provide a nationally consistent framework by which the performance of midwives can be measured. The Code of Practice for Midwives (2000) and Code of Ethics (2001) are under review, with the ANMC in late 2005 tendering a joint project of a National Review of the Code of Ethics and Code of Conduct for Nurses in Australia, and the development of a National Code of Ethics and Code of Conduct for Midwives in Australia. The project, announced in January 2006, will involve collaboration between regulatory, professional and industrial bodies including the ANMC, the ACM, the ANF and the Royal College of Nursing. The project is due for completion in 2007.

Midwifery regulation in New Zealand

In December 2003, a new regulatory authority, the Midwifery Council of New Zealand, was established with the passing of the *Health Practitioners Competence Assurance Act 2003* (HPCAA). This historic event provided final recognition that midwifery is a profession in its own right, as the Midwifery Council took over all regulatory functions and responsibilities from the Nursing Council.

The Midwifery Council comprises six midwives and two lay members, and its focus is on protecting the public and ensuring that they receive safe and competent midwifery care. It does this by carrying out a number of statutory functions that came into force on 18 September 2004 (see Ch 11).

Midwifery Scope of Practice

The HPCAA required each profession to define its scope(s) of practice. The Midwifery Scope of Practice (see Box 10.3) further amended previous modifications made by NZCOM to the ICM definition of a midwife in order to ensure that the Midwifery Scope of Practice statement appropriately

---

BOX 10.3 Midwifery Scope of Practice

The midwife works in partnership with women, on her own professional responsibility, to give women the necessary support, care and advice during pregnancy, labour and the postpartum period up to six weeks*, to facilitate births and to provide care for the newborn.

The midwife understands, promotes and facilitates the physiological processes of pregnancy and childbirth, identifies complications that may arise in mother and baby, accesses appropriate medical assistance, and implements emergency measures as necessary. When women require referral midwives provide midwifery care in collaboration with other health professionals.

Midwives have an important role in health and wellness promotion and education for the woman, her family and the community. Midwifery practice involves informing and preparing the woman and her family for pregnancy, birth, breastfeeding and parenthood and includes certain aspects of women's health, family planning and infant well-being.

The midwife may practise in any setting, including the home, the community, hospitals, or in any other maternity service. In all settings, the midwife remains responsible and accountable for the care she provides.

(*In relation to a preterm baby the Midwifery Council defines the six-week postpartum period as commencing from the expected date of birth rather than the actual date of birth. That is, Council recognises that the postpartum midwifery role for preterm babies *may* extend beyond six calendar weeks.)

(Source: Midwifery Council of New Zealand 2004a)

---

reflected current midwifery practice in New Zealand (ICM 1990; NZCOM 1993, 2002).

The Midwifery Scope of Practice provides a broad statement of the boundaries of what a New Zealand midwife can do *on her own professional responsibility*. It provides a legal definition of New Zealand midwifery practice. It does not mean that every midwife must practise the full scope all the time. Rather, it is expected that all midwives can demonstrate that they are *able* to practise the full scope, even if their daily practice is more restricted. The Midwifery Scope of Practice reflects what the public expects from anyone holding the title of 'midwife' (Midwifery Council of New Zealand 2004b).

Competencies for entry to the Register of Midwives

In setting the competencies required of midwives in order to gain registration in New Zealand, Council amended competencies initially developed in 1996 by the Nursing Council in collaboration with NZCOM. The competencies for entry to the Register of Midwives (see Box 10.4) provide the detail of the skills, knowledge and attitudes expected of a midwife working within the Midwifery Scope of Practice. Where the Midwifery Scope of Practice provides the broad

boundaries of midwifery practice, the competencies provide the detail of how a registered midwife is expected to practise and what she is expected to be capable of doing. These are minimum competence standards required of all midwives who register in New Zealand. Again, not all midwives will necessarily demonstrate all competencies all the time in their everyday practice. However, the Council requires all midwives to make an annual declaration that they are *able* to meet these competencies (Midwifery Council of New Zealand 2004b).

Registration as a midwife in New Zealand

The Midwifery Council is responsible for setting policy and managing the process for registration in New Zealand of its own midwifery education graduates, overseas registered midwives, and midwives applying from Australia.

All applicants must provide evidence of fitness for registration, specified qualifications, and competence to practise in the Midwifery Scope of Practice as measured by the Competencies for Entry to the Register of Midwives. Midwives applying from Australia under the *Trans Tasman Mutual Recognition Act 1997* (see Ch 11) are deemed to be registered, but along with other overseas applicants are likely to have conditions placed on their practice.

Common conditions that apply to Australian and other overseas midwives are that they work in peer-supported contexts such as maternity hospitals or group practices, and that they cannot prescribe medications until they have completed courses that orientate them to New Zealand's maternity and midwifery services and a course in pharmacology and prescribing.

Midwives educated in New Zealand must complete an approved three-year Bachelor of Midwifery program. These programs are mainly 'direct entry' for women without a previous nursing qualification, although there is a slightly shorter route for the few nurses who still wish to change careers and become midwives. The Bachelor of Midwifery programs began in 1992 and have been the only route to midwifery registration since 1996.

Continuing competence as a midwife

A central tenet of the HPCAA (2003) is that all health practitioners must demonstrate ongoing competence to practise in order to be issued with an annual practising certificate. The Midwifery Council makes this assessment through its Recertification Program.

All midwives make a declaration of their competence each year. Over each subsequent three-year period they must: work across all aspects of the Midwifery Scope of Practice; undertake certain compulsory education to update skills in cardiopulmonary resuscitation (CPR), infant resuscitation and certain other clinical skills identified by the Midwifery Council; undertake a certain amount of elective continuing education; and complete a certain amount of professional activity (Midwifery Council of New Zealand 2004d).

A key element of the recertification program is that every midwife is required to undergo the NZCOM's Midwifery

---

BOX 10.4   Revised competencies for entry to the Register of Midwives

Competency 1

'The midwife works in partnership with the woman throughout the maternity experience.'

Explanation

The word 'midwife' has an inherent meaning of being 'with woman'. The midwife acts as a professional companion to promote each woman's right to empowerment to make informed choices about her pregnancy, birth experience and early parenthood. The midwifery relationship enhances the health and well-being of the woman, the baby and their family/whanau. The onus is on the midwife to create a functional partnership. The balance of 'power' within the partnership fluctuates but it is always understood that the woman has control over her own experience.

Competency 2

'The midwife applies comprehensive theoretical and scientific knowledge with the affective and technical skills needed to provide effective and safe midwifery care.'

Explanation

The competent midwife integrates knowledge and understanding, personal, professional and clinical skills within a legal and ethical framework. The actions of the midwife are directed towards a safe and satisfying outcome. The midwife utilises midwifery skills that facilitate the physiological processes of childbirth and balances these with the judicious use of intervention when appropriate.

Competency 3

'The midwife promotes practices that enhance the health of the woman and her family/whanau and which encourage their participation in her healthcare.'

Explanation

Midwifery is a primary health service in that it recognises childbirth as a significant and normal life event. The midwife is therefore responsible for supporting this process through health promotion, education and information sharing, across all settings.

Competency 4

'The midwife upholds professional midwifery standards and uses professional judgement as a reflective and critical practitioner when providing midwifery care.'

Explanation

As a member of the midwifery profession the midwife has responsibilities to the profession. The midwife must have the skills to recognise when midwifery practice is safe and satisfactory to the woman and her family/whanau.

Each of the above competencies has a number of criteria that provide detailed measures of how a midwife would demonstrate her competence against each competency statement. The full list of competencies and criteria can be found on the Midwifery Council of New Zealand website (www.midwiferycouncil.org.nz).
(Source: Midwifery Council of New Zealand 2004c)

Standards Review process either annually or every three years. As part of the review, the MSR committee focuses on the midwife's ability to meet the NZCOM standards for practice and the Midwifery Council Competencies and assists the midwife to identify a personal development plan for the forthcoming year(s).

Midwives are randomly audited to ensure they comply with the requirements of the Recertification Program.

Competence review

Where it has reason to be concerned about a midwife's competence to practise, the Council can carry out a competence review. It establishes a Competence Review Panel to make an assessment of a midwife's competence. If concerns are identified, the Council has various powers, such as requiring the midwife to complete a specific competence program, undertake further education or work under certain conditions. If Council believes that a midwife poses a risk of serious harm to the public, it has the power to suspend a midwife from practice.

Disciplinary functions

All complaints made by consumers about midwives are investigated by the Health and Disability Commissioner and assessed in relation to the Code of Health and Disability

Services Consumers' Rights, and findings are reported to the Midwifery Council. If the Commissioner decides the matter is a serious professional matter, he or she may refer it on to the Director of Proceedings, who may then decide to lay charges against the midwife. The HPCAA established a separate tribunal, the Health Practitioners Disciplinary Tribunal (HPDT), to hear allegations of professional misconduct. The HPDT can impose various penalties, including suspension, fines and cancellation of registration.

The Midwifery Council has established a Professional Conduct Committee (PCC) to which it can refer matters for investigation. Such matters may include notifications of practice below required standards of competence and conduct, and notification of convictions for certain offences or against certain legislation. The PCC can investigate, call for evidence and receive evidence or submissions. It can make recommendations to the Council and can lay charges before the HPDT.

Other functions

The Midwifery Council has powers to seek information about any midwife who is notified as being unable to practise appropriately because of some physical or mental condition and to apply conditions to that midwife's practice in order to protect both the public and the midwife. The Council also has

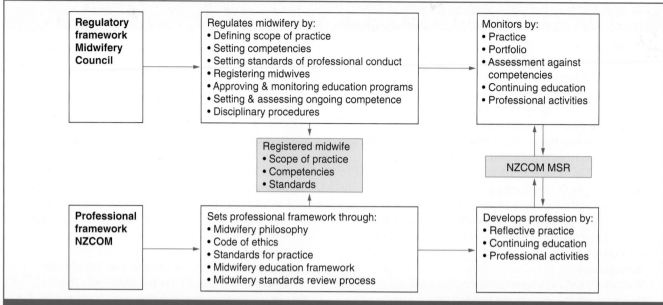

Figure 10.3 Relationship between professional and regulatory frameworks for practice in New Zealand (based on Midwifery Council of New Zealand 2004d)

an important role in approving and accrediting midwifery education providers, programs and courses.

Relationship between the New Zealand College of Midwives and the Midwifery Council

Although they are separate organisations, the roles of the Council and NZCOM are complementary. The Council provides the regulatory framework within which midwives must practise, and it sets the minimum standards required for public safety. NZCOM provides the professional framework in which midwives practise, and it aims to develop and support high standards of midwifery practice. Both organisations have an interest in ensuring that the regulatory processes for midwives are integrated in a professional framework and that appropriate standards of midwifery practice are maintained so that the public can be assured of safe and competent midwifery care. Figure 10.3 shows the interface of these professional and regulatory frameworks.

Midwifery regulation in Australia

Midwifery Scope of Practice

The International Definition of the Midwife has been recognised as the basis for the definition of the role and scope of practice in many Western industrialised countries, including Australia, where it has been used to develop various local and national standards and underpins all curriculum documents for entry to practise midwifery. The midwife's primary role and responsibility is to understand, support and facilitate the physiological processes of pregnancy, labour and the postnatal period with women, within parameters of cultural safety. Additionally, midwives are responsible for identifying deviations from normal and consulting, referring and working collaboratively with other health professionals where required (ACM 2004).

Recent consultations undertaken by the Australian Midwifery Competencies Project: Round Three (Homer 2004) on the role and scope of practice of midwives in Australia have seen the National Executive Committee of the ACM affirm its commitment to the current ICM Definition of the Midwife, including the requirement that this definition be included in any review of standards for practice in Australia (ACM National Executive 2004). Other areas for discussion have related to the timeframe surrounding the woman/midwife partnership postpartum, the inclusion of pre-pregnancy care in the midwife's scope of practice, and midwifery's relationship to sexual and reproductive health, encompassing areas such as family planning. During the course of these discussions the Technical Working Group of WHO (1999) definition of the postnatal period has been acknowledged (i.e. one hour after delivery of the placenta until the first six weeks after giving birth). In the main, debates have focused on existing tensions in maintaining international comparability and alignment while ensuring that the role and scope of practice remains broad, including the attendant consequences for regulation, education and overlap with other professional groups (ACM National Executive 2004).

National midwifery competencies

Competencies for midwives serve as the minimum requirement for licensure/registration to practise. In the Australian context, competencies 'provide details of the skills, knowledge and attitudes expected of a midwife to work within the midwifery scope of practice'(ANMC 2005b, p 6). They detail how a

---

BOX 10.5   Domains and competencies

Domains and competencies for Australian midwifery are listed below.

Domain 1: Legal and professional practice

▶ *Competency 1*—Functions in accordance with legislation and common law affecting midwifery practice

▶ *Competency 2*—Accepts accountability and responsibility for own actions within midwifery practice

Domain 2: Midwifery knowledge and practice

▶ *Competency 3*—Communicates information to facilitate decision-making by the woman

▶ *Competency 4*—Promotes safe and effective midwifery care

▶ *Competency 5*—Assesses, plans, provides and evaluates safe and effective midwifery care

▶ *Competency 6*—Assesses, plans, provides and evaluates safe and effective midwifery care for the woman and/or baby with complex needs

Domain 3: Midwifery as primary healthcare

▶ *Competency 7*—Advocates to protect the rights of women, families and communities in relation to the provision of maternity care

▶ *Competency 8*—Develops effective strategies to implement and support collaborative midwifery practice

▶ *Competency 9*—Actively supports midwifery as a public health strategy

▶ *Competency 10*—Ensures midwifery practice is culturally safe

Domain 4: Reflective and ethical practice

▶ *Competency 11*—Bases midwifery practice on ethical decision-making

▶ *Competency 12*—Identifies personal beliefs and develops these in ways that enhance midwifery practice

▶ *Competency 13*—Acts to enhance the professional development of self and others

▶ *Competency 14*—Uses research to inform midwifery practice

(Source: ANMC 2005)

---

provider is to practise and what they are expected to be capable of doing, in contrast to definition and scope of practice, which provide the 'broad boundaries' of midwifery practice (ANMC 2005b, p 6).

Domains and competencies deemed relevant for Australian midwifery are those indicated in Box 10.5. A domain is defined as 'a cluster of competency standards that characterise a central aspect of midwifery practice,' and a competency is 'a combination of attributes underlying some aspect of successful professional performance' (Homer et al 2004, pp 7–16). Within each competency are elements that contain examples of competent performance known as cues (Homer et al 2004).

States and territories: legislation

Brodie and Barclay (2001) have recently undertaken a comprehensive analysis of state and territory statutory regulation of midwifery education and practice standards as part of AMAP research. A systematic content analysis of each of the eight nursing statutes purporting to regulate midwifery in Australia was undertaken. Serious deficiencies in the current regulatory system were identified and reflected concerns about midwifery practice, regulation and education in Australia that have been expressed over the previous two decades in relation to issues of international parity, power and outcomes for childbearing women and their infants (Barclay 1985, 1986; Barclay & Haddon 1993; Bogossian 1998; Chamberlain 1998; Donnellan-Fernandez et al 2001; Hancock 1992; Summers 1995; Tracy et al 2000; Waldenstrom 1996, 1997). Midwifery continues to be regulated by nursing and is not recognised as a separate profession to nursing, a position that continues to be contested by women, midwives, the ACM and some regulatory authorities in Australia. Most recently, the Australian Nursing and Midwifery Council added midwifery to its name to indicate recognition of the separate nature of midwifery by that organisation (AMALG 2000; Barclay et al 2003; Donnellan-Fernandez & Eastaugh 2003; Phelan 2005; Reiger 2003).

Registration, continuing competence and disciplinary functions

In the Australian context, 'midwife' describes a registered/regulated health professional who has undertaken either a nursing degree with subsequent postgraduate 'midwifery' education, or, more recently, a comprehensive three-year Bachelor of Midwifery Degree (i.e. direct entry route). Midwifery in Australia continues to experience inconsistent and de facto regulation under the auspice of nursing legislation in most of the eight states and territories. This position has historically been contingent on social and professional acceptance of a legislated identity that has classified midwifery as a branch of specialist nursing practice. Lying within this regulatory misappropriation is a series of anomalies and ambiguities that vary among the states and territories and includes: varying educational requirements in midwifery curricula; declaration of competence in accordance with national nursing competencies in some states and territories; an annual declaration of continuing competence in midwifery when the practising certificate renewal is issued by the regulator, but no mandated requirement for demonstration of midwifery standards review; professional misconduct committees and disciplinary tribunal and process constituted under nursing frameworks. These anomalies call into question the credibility of assessment and regulation processes for midwives in Australia at the national level and create further difficulties and inconsistencies with respect to Mutual Recognition legislation. Urgent legislative ambiguities currently exist for students graduating from three-year Bachelor of Midwifery Degree programs who have not undertaken nursing studies or clinical competencies in nursing. Similarly, midwives arriving from overseas and seeking employment in Australia who have not been educated via nursing pathways are confronted with the same inconsistencies.

Recent developments

Beginning in 2003, and subsequent to National Competition Policy Review of professional regulation over the previous decade (COAG 1999) and intense lobbying by women and midwives, amendments to the Nurses Acts in New South Wales, the Northern Territory and the Australian Capital Territory are now naming midwifery as a discrete field alongside nursing in the titles of their Boards. Western Australia currently also has a Nurses and Midwives Bill before the WA Parliament, to replace the existing WA Nurses Act 1992 (ANF 2006). It may be naive, however, to assume that, without further direct lobbying and pressure from midwifery organisations and consumers, nationally consistent standards for statutory midwifery regulation will be prominent on the government's agenda. Much work remains to be done if a comprehensive, nationally consistent approach to regulating the midwifery profession, as has recently occurred in New Zealand, is to be achieved in all Australian states and territories. Recent recommendations in the National Productivity Report, chaired by Mike Woods, advocate the merging of Australia's 90 existing registration boards for health professionals into one national entity (AGPC 2004; Cresswell 2006).

National legislation and regulation

Regulated labour force arrangements that construct and distort midwifery as a branch of specialist nursing practice ensure a continuing division of labour to serve the interests of institutionalised medical birthing practice in Australia. Vigorous consumer activism in the second half of the twentieth century has highlighted tensions between medicalised mainstream maternity services available in the Australian context and a rising identity crisis in midwifery practice and education (NMAP 2002). This climate has implications for regulation of the midwifery workforce. Ongoing sponsorship of the medical model of childbirth by the modern nation state via health funding, infrastructure support, and maintenance of current regulatory arrangements makes the continuing relationship between nursing and the regulation of midwifery practice highly significant, and open to critique in both the social and the professional domains (Donnellan-Fernandez & Eastaugh 2003).

Friedson's assertion that 'a profession is a group that has authority *in the law* to select its own members and to regulate their practice'(cited in Ehrenreich & English 1973, p 47) requires nationally consistent education requirements for midwifery and nationally consistent practice standards that are universally endorsed by Australian nursing and midwifery regulatory authorities, including the Australian Nursing and Midwifery Council. Although the ACM is appropriately engaged in articulating national standards for midwifery practice and education, it currently has no statutory mandated authority on behalf of midwives or women, to ensure in the public interest that these standards are being met.

The first principle of professional regulation through legislation is that it should be in the public interest (COAG Committee on Regulatory Reform 1999). The public interest of

---

> **BOX 10.6 AMALG Vision Statement**
>
> ▸ Women and midwives work in partnership to ensure culturally appropriate care that is safe, affordable and accessible.
> ▸ Midwives are autonomous practitioners who provide woman-centred care.
> ▸ Midwifery legislation will protect and strengthen the woman and midwife partnership.
>
> (Source: AMALG 2000)

---

naming *what* is being regulated cannot be overstated. Reform and innovation that acknowledges a discrete legislated identity and mandate for regulation of the midwifery profession in Australia is supported by current scientific evidence and policy directives of the World Health Organization that recognise midwives as the most appropriate, cost-effective providers for women experiencing healthy pregnancy and childbirth (WHO 1996). Although national midwifery legislation is precluded by the Australian constitution and cooperative federalism model in which state and territory governments retain responsibility for legislating with respect to provision of services and regulation of trade and commerce, national consistency in midwifery regulation across state and territory borders is possible, desirable and expected under the terms of Mutual Recognition. This aim has been articulated in the Vision Statement and Terms of Reference of the Australia Midwives Act Lobby Group (AMALG) since 2000 (AMALG 2000) (see Box 10.6).

Encompassed within a mandate for national regulation is the agenda to legitimise and fund, through legislative reform, authorisation of services already undertaken by midwives, such as test ordering for normal pregnancy and childbearing, diagnostic imaging, prescribing and referral practices (NHMRC 1998). Unlike New Zealand, where midwives are reimbursed for services via the Maternity Benefit Schedule, in Australia, midwives are excluded from federal funding mechanisms provided through Medicare and HIC (Health Insurance Commission) Agreements via which medical practitioners providing midwifery services maintain their state-supported monopoly on maternity care (Australian Government Productivity Commission (AGPC) 2004; Maternity Coalition 2003). These current economic and legislative arrangements deny Australian women equity in accessing midwifery-based care.

Relationship between professional and regulatory frameworks in Australia

The national professional framework for midwifery and current regulatory jurisdictions in each state and territory demonstrate inconsistency and a lack of integration. However, political alliances between the community and midwives are beginning to drive a reform agenda that demands consistency and integration of these areas, in the interest of public safety. This includes the need for a discrete legislated identity for the midwifery profession in Australia (www.maternitycoalition. org.au; www.amalg.asn.au). Kahn articulated the notion of language as an instrument of control, describing it as 'the repository of all power relations' (cited in White 1999). That midwifery is a contested site is evident both in the discourses on childbirth in Australia and in the historical regulation of midwifery as specialist nursing practice. How midwives name themselves and their practice is significant, with the importance of naming in nursing and midwifery having been well described by White (1999), Leap (1999) and Brodie & Barclay (2001).

The process of emancipation for midwifery in Australia within a context of dominance by the nursing profession is evolving and gaining momentum through multiple paradigm shifts, including: introduction of a national professional standards framework for midwives in Australia; introduction of direct, comprehensive three-year university degree programs for midwifery education; implementation of continuity of midwifery care services in mainstream health settings across the nation; legislative amendment of state and territory Nurses Acts to recognise the discrete discipline of midwifery; increasing professional awareness of interdisciplinary practice domains; and public demand for greater accountability from providers of healthcare.

A professional framework underpinned by the International Definition of the Midwife, based on national standards for midwifery education and practice, and linked to continuing professional development and competence, is articulated by ACM (2005). Uniform endorsement and adoption of these national midwifery standards by the Australian Nursing and Midwifery Council and current regulators is essential to protect the public interest, to promote and maintain high standards of maternity care in Australia, and to underpin and further the goal of realising nationally consistent midwifery legislation in all states and territories within the next five years.

Conclusion

This chapter has provided a brief overview of the professional and regulatory frameworks for midwifery practice in Australia and New Zealand. While midwifery in both countries is claimed to be a profession, New Zealand midwifery has a legal and professional framework that supports this claim. Australian midwifery faces a number of challenges to bring about legislated change that will recognise midwifery as separate from nursing, through regulation and to change funding, insurance and other institutional processes that will support midwifery's professional framework and aspirations. Although professional frameworks are extremely important, legislated changes are essential if midwifery is truly to be self-determining as a profession.

Review questions

1. What are the main characteristics of a profession and why is it important for midwifery to be a profession?

2. What does the concept of 'professionalism' mean for midwifery?

3. How do current social/partnership models of birth affect the notion and development of midwifery as a profession in Australia and New Zealand?

4. How is the midwifery scope of practice (as defined in the WHO definition and by the NZ Midwifery Council) enabled or constrained in both the Australian and New Zealand contexts?

5. What is the relationship between scope of practice and competencies?

6. What is the purpose of regulation of midwifery and how does it work?

7. What has been the influence of history, role, functions and structure on the midwifery profession in both Australia and New Zealand, and how is this manifest currently in delivery of maternity services in each country?

8. How does the relationship between the professional and regulatory frameworks influence midwifery practice in Australia and New Zealand?

9. How does New Zealand's Midwifery Standards Review process work to improve standards of midwifery practice?

10. What might be the impact of deregulation of midwifery?

Online resources

Australian College of Midwives, http://www.acmi.org.au
Australian Institute of Health and Welfare, National Perinatal Statistics Unit, http://www.aihw.gov.au/npsu/report

Australian Nursing and Midwifery Council, http://www.anmc.org.au
Maternity Coalition Inc., http://www.maternitycoalition.org.au
Midwifery Council of New Zealand, http://www.midwiferycouncil.org.nz
New Zealand College of Midwives Inc., http://www.midwife.org.nz

New Zealand Ministry of Health, Manatu Hauora, http://www.moh. govt.nz

References

Abbott A 1988 The system of professions—an essay on the division of expert labour. University of Chicago Press, Chicago

Anderson W 2002 The cultivation of whiteness: science, health and racial destiny in Australia. Melbourne University Press, Melbourne

Australian College of Midwives Incorporated (ACMI) 2004 Midwifery News, p 14

Australian College of Midwives Inc. (ACMI) National Executive 2004 Written communication/directive provided via CEO to members of ACMI ANEST, December 2004

Australian College of Midwives Incorporated (ACMI) 2005 National website. Online: www.acmi.org.au, accessed January 2005

Australian Government Productivity Commission (AGPC) 2004 Review of national competition policy arrangements: public hearings. Maternity Coalition submission/evidence, 7 December 2004. Online: www.pc.gov.au/inquiry/ncp

Australian Midwives Act Lobby Group (AMALG) 2000 Commentary Paper. Online: www.amalg.asn.au

Australian Nursing & Midwifery Council 2004 Newsletter, November 2004

Australian Nursing and Midwifery Council (ANMC) 2005a National Competency Standards for the Midwife. ANMC, Canberra

Australian Nursing and Midwifery Council (ANMC) 2005b Midwifery Project Report: researching the role and scope of practice of Australian midwives and the development of competency standards for midwives. ANMC, Canberra

Australian Nursing Federation 2006 Australian Nursing Journal 13(7):8

Aydellote M 1985 Nursing: societal discontent and professional change. In: R Wieczorek (Ed) Power, politics and policy in nursing. Springer, New York

Barclay L 1985 Australian midwifery training and practice. Midwifery 1:86–96

Barclay L 1986 One right way: the midwife's dilemma. Canberra College of Advanced Education, Canberra

Barclay L, Haddon E 1993 The education of midwives in Australia: current trends and future directions. Conference proceedings, Eighth Biennial Conference: Midwifery: A Family Affair, 15–17 September 1993, ACMI, Adelaide, South Australia

Barclay L, Brodie P, Lane K et al 2003 Australian Midwifery Action Project (AMAP) Report, Vols 1 and 2. Centre for Midwifery and Family Health, University of Technology, Sydney

Bogossian F 1998 A Review of midwifery legislation in Australia: History, current state and future directions. Australian College of Midwives Journal 11(1):24–31

Brodie P 2002 Addressing the barriers to midwifery: Australian midwives speaking out. Australian Journal of Midwifery 15(3): 5–14

Brodie P, Barclay L 2001 Issues in the regulation of Australian midwives. Australian Health Review 24(4):113–118

Chamberlain M 1998 Midwifery and the next millennium: issues for the future. Australian College of Midwives Journal 11(1): 7–8

COAG Committee on Regulatory Reform 1999 Guidelines for the review of regulation of the professions under national competition policy. AGPS, Canberra

Commonwealth Department of Health and Aged Care 1999 Rocking the cradle. Report on the Senate Community Affairs Committee Inquiry into Childbirth Procedures. AGPS, Canberra. Online: http://www.aph.gov.au/senate/committee/history/index.htm. Community

Commonwealth Office for the Status of Women 2002 Focus on women: Indigenous women of Australia & New Zealand. AGPS, Canberra

Cresswell A 2006 Health plan calls for bypass of GPs. The Australian, 19 January. Online: http://www.theaustralian.news.com.au/ printpage/o,5942,17866415,00.html

Cronk M 2000 The midwife: a professional servant? In: M Kirkham (Ed) The midwife–mother relationship. Macmillan, London

Davis-Floyd R, Sarjeant C (Eds) 1997 Childbirth and authoritative knowledge: cross cultural perspectives. University of California Press, Berkeley

De Vries R, Benoit C, Van Teijlingen et al (Eds) 2001 Birth by design: pregnancy, maternity care, and midwifery in North America and Europe. Routledge, New York

Dobbie M 1990 The trouble with women. The story of Parents Centre New Zealand. Cape Cately, Whatamongo Bay

Donley J 1986 Save the midwife. New Woman's Press, Auckland

Donley J 1989 Professionalism. The importance of consumer control over childbirth. New Zealand College of Midwives Journal September: 6–7

Donley J 2002 Globalisation of midwifery. Celebrating diversity within unity, Conference Proceedings, New Zealand College of Midwives Seventh Biennial National Conference, pp 211–217

Donnellan-Fernandez R 1996 Personal, professional, structural and cultural challenges to autonomous practice: a midwife's perspective. Conference Proceedings, Autonomous Practice in Nursing and Midwifery, Australian Nursing Federation, Adelaide, pp 58–69

Donnellan-Fernandez R 2000 Autonomous private midwifery practice: a retrospective 1994–2000. Childbirth in Isolation Conference Proceedings, ACMI Goldfields Sub Branch, Kalgoorlie, Western Australia & Promaco Conventions

Donnellan-Fernandez R 2001 Midwifery legislation. Birth Matters, The Journal of the Maternity Coalition Inc., June 5(2):2–4

Donnellan-Fernandez R, Eastaugh M 2003 Midwifery regulation in Australia: a century of invisibility. Innovations in regulation. Conference Proceedings, Sixth International Conference on the Regulation of Nursing and Midwifery, CD-ROM, Nurses Board Victoria, Melbourne

Donnellan-Fernandez R, Eastaugh M, Glenie C 2001 Legislating midwifery in Australia: politics, action and renewal in the 21st century. Conference Proceedings of Politics, Action & Renewal in the 21st Century: Fourth Australian Women's Health Conference, Adelaide

Donnison J 1988 Midwives and medical men. A history of the struggle for the control of childbirth (2nd edn). Historical Publications, London

Duckett SJ 2000 The Australian healthcare system. Oxford University Press, Melbourne

Ehrenreich B, English D 1973 Witches, midwives and nurses. Writers & Readers Publishing, London

Finklestein J 1990 Women, pregnancy and childbirth. In: J Scutt (Ed) Baby machine: reproductive technology and the commercialisation of motherhood. Green Print Merlin Press, London

Grimshaw P, Lake M, McGrath A et al 1996 Creating a nation 1788–1990. Penguin, Melbourne

Guilliland K 1989 Maintaining the links. New Zealand College of Midwives Journal (1):14

Guilliland K 2004 A hundred years of midwifery and what have we learnt about ourselves? Centenary Oration. Midwifery News (34):4–6, 28–29

Guilliland K, Pairman S 1995 The midwifery partnership: a model for practice. Department of Nursing and Midwifery Monograph Series 95/1. Victoria University, Wellington

Hancock H 1992 Midwifery education: whither will we wander? Australian College of Midwives Journal 9: 7–10

Health Workforce Advisory Committee 2005 Fit for purpose and for practice: a review of the medical workforce in New Zealand. Ministry of Health, Wellington.

Homer C 2004 Australian Midwifery Competency Project: Draft Three. Online: www.anmc.org.au/Projects

Homer C, Brodie P, Leap N 2001b Establishing models of midwifery continuity of care: a handbook for midwives and managers. Centre for Family Health and Midwifery, UTS. ISBN 0-9579592-0-6

Homer C, Davis G, Brodie P et al 2001a Collaboration in maternity care: a randomised controlled trial comparing community-based continuity of care with standard hospital care. British Journal of Obstetrics and Gynaecology 108:16–22

Homer et al 2004, Australian Nursing and Midwifery Council Project, Round 3 consultation document, Nov 2004 – Jan 2005

International Confederation of Midwives (ICM) 1990 Definition of a midwife. Position statement 90/1. ICM, London

Johnston J, Newman L 2005 Maternity care: a human rights issue? Journal of the Maternity Coalition 9(1):3–5

Katz Rothman B 1984 Childbirth management and medical monopoly: midwifery as (almost) a profession. Journal of Nurse-Midwifery 29(5):300–306

Kitzinger S 1988 The midwife challenge. Pandora Press, London

Lane K 2002 Midwifery: a profession in transition. Australian Journal of Midwifery 15(2):26–31

Lazarus E 1997 What do women want? Issues of choice, control and class in American pregnancy and childbirth. In: R Davis-Floyd, C Sarjeant (Eds) Childbirth and authoritative knowledge: cross cultural perspectives. University of California Press, Berkeley

Leap N 1999 Defining midwifery as we develop woman-centred practice. Conference proceedings, Eleventh Biennial Conference: Hearts, Hands and Minds, Midwifery in the New Millenium, 2–4 September 1999. ACMI, Hobart, Tasmania

Leap N, Sheehan A, Barclay L et al 2002 Mapping midwifery education in Australia survey: Findings of the AMAP Education Survey. AMAP Report Vol 2

Maternity Coalition/AMALG 2003 Submissions to the Commonwealth Review of the Medicare Funding Agreement. Online: http://www.maternitycoalition.org.au, http://www.aph.gov.au/senate_medicare

Maternity Coalition, Australian Society of Independent Midwives, Community Midwifery WA Inc. 2002 The National Maternity Action Plan (NMAP). Online: www.maternitycoalition.org.au

Mein Smith P 1986 Maternity in dispute in New Zealand 1920–1939. Historical Publications Branch, Department of Internal Affairs, Wellington

Midwifery Council of New Zealand 2004a Midwifery scope of practice. www.midwiferycouncil.org.nz

Midwifery Council of New Zealand 2004b Midpoint. Newsletter of the Midwifery Council of New Zealand, September

Midwifery Council of New Zealand 2004c Competencies for entry to the Register of Midwives. Online: www.midwiferycouncil.org.nz

Midwifery Council of New Zealand 2004d Midpoint. Newsletter of the Midwifery Council of New Zealand, December

New South Wales Health Department 2000 The NSW Framework for Maternity Services 2000–01

New Zealand College of Midwives (NZCOM) 1993 Midwives handbook for practice. NZCOM, Christchurch

New Zealand College of Midwives (NZCOM) 2002 Midwives handbook for practice. NZCOM, Christchurch

New Zealand College of Midwives (NZCOM) 2005 Midwives handbook for practice. NZCOM, Christchurch.

National Health and Medical Research Council (NHMRC) 1998 Review of services offered by midwives. AGPS, Canberra

Oakley A, Houd S 1990 Helpers in childbirth. Midwifery today. Hemisphere Publishing, on behalf of the World Health Organization, London

Page L 2003 One-to-one midwifery: restoring the with woman relationship in midwifery. Journal of Midwifery and Women's Health 48(2):119–125

Pairman S 2000 Woman centred midwifery: partnerships or professional friendships. In: M Kirkham (Ed) The midwife–mother relationship. Macmillan, London, pp 28–52

Pairman S 2002 Towards self-determination: the separation of the nursing and midwifery professions in New Zealand. In: E Papps (Ed) Nursing in New Zealand. Critical issues, different perspectives. Pearson Education, Auckland

Pairman S 2005 Workforce to profession: an exploration of New Zealand midwifery's professionalising strategies from 1986 to 2005. Unpublished doctoral thesis, University of Technology, Sydney

Pairman S, Guilliland K 2003 Developing a midwife-led maternity service: the New Zealand experience. In: M Kirkham (Ed) Birth centres: a social model for maternity care. Books for Midwives, London

Papps E, Olssen M 1997 Doctoring childbirth and regulating midwifery in New Zealand. Dunmore, Palmerston North, NZ

Phelan M 2005 Australian Nursing and Midwifery Council: new council name marks an historic change in care for pregnant women. Australian Midwifery News, Autumn: 6–8

Reibel T 2004 Community midwifery—what it means for women. Birth Matters, Journal of the Maternity Coalition Inc., September 8(3):5

Reiger K 2001 Our bodies, our babies: the forgotten women's movement. Melbourne University Press, Melbourne

Reiger K 2003 Difficult labour: struggles to change Australian maternity care. The AMAP Report 2:41–58

Roberts C, Algert C, Douglas I et al 2002 Trends in labour and birth interventions among low risk women in New South Wales. Australian New Zealand Journal of Obstetrics and Gynaecology 42(2):176–181

Roberts C, Tracy S, Peat B 2000 Rates of obstetric intervention among private and public patients in Australia: a population based descriptive study. British Medical Journal 321(7254): 137–141. Online: http://bmj.com/cgi/content/abstract/321/7254/187

Sandall J 1997 Midwives: burnout and continuity of care. British Journal of Midwifery 5(2):106–111

Shachar O 2001 The invisible female patient: the new reproductive technologies. Discourse in the medical literature. Online: http://www.pantaneto.co.uk/issue2/shachar.htm

Speedy S 1987 Feminism and the professionalisation of nursing. Australian Journal of Advanced Nursing 4(2):20–28

State of Victoria, Department of Human Services 2004 Future directions for Victoria's maternity services. Online: http://www.health.vic.gov.au/maternitycare/pubs.htm

Strid J 1987 Midwifery in revolt. Broadsheet 153:14–17

Summers A 1995 For I have ever so much more faith in her ability as a nurse: the eclipse of the community midwife in South Australia 1836–1942. Unpublished PHD thesis, Flinders University, South Australia

Tew M 1990 Safer childbirth? A critical history of maternity care. Chapman and Hall, London

Thoroughgood C, Thiele B, Hyde K 2003 Community Midwifery Program WA Inc. Evaluation 1997 – Dec 2001. Community Midwifery Program WA Inc, WA. Online: http://www.communitymidwifery.iinet.net.au

Tracy S, Barclay L, Brodie P 2000 Contemporary issues in the workforce and education of Australian midwives. Australian Health Review 23(4):78–88

Tully E 1999 Doing professionalism differently: negotiating midwifery autonomy in Aotearoa/New Zealand. Unpublished doctoral thesis, University of Canterbury, New Zealand.

Tully E, Mortlock B 1999 Professionals and practices. In: P Davis, K Devo (Eds) Health and society in Aotearoa New Zealand. Oxford University Press, Auckland

Waldenstrom U 1996 Midwives in current debate and in the future. Australian College of Midwives Inc. Journal 9:3–9

Waldenstrom U 1997 Challenges and issues for midwifery. Australian College of Midwives Inc. Journal 10:11–17

Western Australian Health Department 2004 Healthy future for Western Australians. Final report of the Health Reform Committee, WA Government, March 2004

White J 1999 Midwifery practice: always a political act. Australian College of Midwives Inc. Journal 12(1):6–13

Wilkins R 2000 Poor relations: the paucity of the professional paradigm. In: M Kirkham (Ed) The midwife–mother relationship. Macmillan, London

Willis E 1983 Medical dominance: the division of labour in Australian healthcare. Allen & Unwin, Sydney

World Health Organization (WHO) 1992 International definition of the midwife. WHO, Geneva

World Health Organization (WHO) 1996 Care in normal birth: a practical guide. Maternal and Newborn Health / Safe Motherhood Unit, Family and Reproductive Health, WHO, Geneva

World Health Organization (WHO) 1999 Technical Working Group definition of the postnatal period. WHO, Geneva

Further reading

Aboriginal Women of Central Australia 1985 Congress Alukura by Grandmother's Law. Model of healthy public policy

Australian Capital Territory Health 1994 ACT Maternity Services Review. Commonwealth Department of Health and Family Services, Canberra

Australian Institute of Health and Welfare National Perinatal Statistics Unit (2002 data). Online: http://www.aihw.gov.au/npsu/report

Australian National Education Standards Taskforce (ANEST) 2004 Draft ACMI Standards for midwifery practice

Bell D 1998 Ngarrindjeri Wurruwarrin: a world that is, was, and will be. Spinifex Press, Melbourne

Chief Nursing Officer's Office 2001 Enhanced Role Midwife Project. Department of Health, Government of Western Australia

Department of Health NSW 1989 Maternity services in New South Wales. Final report of the Ministerial Taskforce on Obstetric Services in NSW (Shearman Report). Department of Health Publication No. (HSU) 89-007

Friedson E 1970 Profession of medicine. Harper & Row, New York

Health Department of Victoria 1990 Having a baby in Victoria. Final Report of the Ministerial Review of Birthing Services in Victoria, Melbourne

Jag Films Pty Ltd 2001 Birth rites. Producer: Jennifer Gheradi

James H, Willis E 2001 The professionalisation of midwifery through education or politics. Australian Journal of Midwifery 14(4): 27–30

Jellet H 1901 A short practice of midwifery for nurses. Churchill, London

Kent J 2000 Social perspectives on pregnancy and childbirth for midwives, nurses and the caring professions. Open University Press, Buckingham

Kildea S 2000 And the women said . . . reporting on birthing services for Aboriginal women from remote top end communities. Women's Health Strategy Unit, Territory Health Services, Northern Territory Government

Lane K 1999 Autonomous midwifery in Australia: the safer alternative. Birth Matters, Journal of the Maternity Coalition Inc. 3(2):6–12

McKinnon C 1987 Feminism unmodified. Harvard University Press, Cambridge

National Health and Medical Research Council (NHMRC) 1996 Options for effective care in childbirth. AGPS, Canberra

Nixon A, Byrne J, Church A 2003 Final evaluation of the Community Midwifery Program, Northern Women's Community Health Centre, Northern Metropolitan Community Health Service, Adelaide. Online: http://www.whs.sa.gov.au/pub/final_document_Evaluation_CMP.pdf

Office of the Status of Women, Department of the Prime Minister & Cabinet 1993 Women—shaping & sharing the future. The new national agenda for women 1993–2000 (2nd edn). AGPS, Canberra

Scutt J (Ed) 1999 Baby machine: reproductive technology and the commercialisation of motherhood. Green Print Merlin, London

Select Committee on Intervention in Childbirth Report 1995 Western Australian Legislative Assembly

Stewart M 2000 Ngalangangopum Jarrakpu Purrurn: mother and child. The women of Warnum as told to Margaret Stewart, Australia

Torres L 1992 Women and language: from sex differences to power dynamics. In: C Kramarae, D Spender (Eds) The knowledge explosion: generations of feminist scholarship. Teachers College Press, New York

CHAPTER 11

Legal frameworks for practice in Australia and New Zealand

Helen Newnham and Jackie Pearse

Key terms

common law, regulation, statute[1]

Chapter overview

The law regulates and controls the practice of midwifery and provides legal redress for clients who have been injured after contact with a member of the midwifery profession. This chapter provides an overview of the main statutes from Australia and New Zealand that affect midwifery practice. An understanding of the law and how it operates is essential for safe practice and so that midwives can fulfil their legal responsibilities both to clients and to the midwifery profession.

Learning objectives

Learning outcomes for this chapter are:

1 To summarise key legislation affecting midwives in Australia and New Zealand as they relate to regulation and control of the midwifery practice

2 To examine the role and function of nursing/midwifery regulatory authorities

3 To discuss the legal responsibilities of midwives when undertaking midwifery practice

4 To examine privacy issues as they pertain to midwifery practice and patient access to information

5 To discuss the legislative requirements for the notification of births and deaths in midwifery practice

6 To explain the avenues of complaint for clients following an adverse incident

7 To examine the role and the function of the Coroner's Court as it relates to midwifery practice.

Introduction to the law

The primary functions of the law are to provide protection to citizens, to administer and regulate entitlements, and to sanction those who offend against the norms and values of any society, as those norms and values are expressed within its legal system. In Australasia the generic term 'law' refers to the Acts of Parliament (statutes), regulations, and the common law, each of which govern the lives and actions of citizens within our respective societies.

Why is the law important to midwives?

All midwives must be aware of the legislative context in which they practise and they must be sufficiently cognisant of 'the law' to enable them to fulfil their legal and professional obligations to their clients, profession and society. The law confers duties on practitioners and provides for the protection of the fundamental rights of health consumers. There may be significant consequences for a midwife where harm results from an act or omission in the delivery of health care. Following an incident a midwife may face a civil action brought by the mother or parents of a newborn, or a criminal action brought by the authorities, or a disciplinary hearing brought by the regulatory authority. Ignorance of the law is no excuse. Every midwife should be aware of the law in the jurisdiction in which she practises.

Midwifery practice in both Australia and New Zealand is governed by a large number of statutes. This chapter summarises key Australian and New Zealand statutes to help midwives understand the breadth of their legal responsibilities.

Australia, unlike New Zealand, is a federation with six states and two territories, each with a legislative body making laws that affect the practice of midwives. In a chapter such as this it is impossible to cover all the laws governing the practice of midwifery in Australia; instead, it provides an overview of certain key pieces of legislation and professional issues governing midwives. Midwives are encouraged to be aware of the laws of the jurisdiction in which they practise.

The chapter is divided into sections addressing the laws that pertain to midwifery regulation, public safety, privacy and personal information, and midwifery practice. Each section provides information first for Australia and then for New Zealand. As New Zealand midwives may prescribe drugs on their own responsibility there is a section on specific legislation pertaining to this. It is understood that Australian midwives are involved in the administration of medications and need to be familiar with relevant legislation in their jurisdictions. However, specific information on that legislation is not provided in this chapter. In the final section, the role of the coroner is addressed for Australia and New Zealand together, as the function and purpose of a coronial inquest is similar in both countries.

Key statutes on regulation of midwifery practice

Midwifery regulation in Australia

Overview

In 1901 the Federation of Australia came into existence. The Commonwealth of Australia consists of six states and two territories, each with its own statutory authority to regulate the practice of nursing and midwifery. Section 51 of the Australian Constitution gives the federal or Commonwealth legislature certain powers to make laws for the 'peace, order and good government of the Commonwealth'. Therefore, the Commonwealth Government has power to pass laws in the national interest but this does not include the regulation of professions. Until such time as the states and territories concede that power to the Commonwealth, or the Constitution is changed, Australia will remain with eight jurisdictions—six states and two territories—regulating the practice of nursing and midwifery. Although similarities exist between the states and territories, there are also differences. It is not possible to provide a comprehensive review of all the legislation in the area in a chapter such as this, and midwives are encouraged to familiarise themselves with the legislation in the jurisdiction in which they practise.

Mutual recognition legislation

Prior to the introduction of mutual recognition legislation, a nurse or midwife who wished to practise in another state or territory had to apply for registration. Each case was assessed individually and required the submission of evidence of registration in the first state. Mutual recognition legislation first introduced by the Commonwealth in 1992 and subsequently adopted by the states and territories has in part facilitated the process of registration from one state to another but is well short of a national registering authority. The main principle of the legislation is that a person registered in one state is entitled to be registered in another state for the equivalent occupation (section 17 *Mutual Recognition Act 1992* (Commonwealth (Cth))). If any conditions are placed on practice, or the registration of a nurse or midwife is cancelled or suspended in one state following a disciplinary hearing, the person's registration in another state is similarly affected. However, the other state may vary or waive any conditions set in the first state if this is considered appropriate given the circumstances (section 33 *Mutual Recognition Act 1992* (Cth)).

All states and territories, with the exception of Western Australia and Tasmania, have Trans-Tasman mutual recognition legislation allowing for registration of nurses and midwives between Australia and New Zealand.

Midwifery regulation

Until the early twentieth century, midwives mostly practised independently and without regulation. Tasmania was the first state in Australia to regulate midwives with the *Midwifery Nurses Act 1901*. Victoria regulated midwives with the *Victorian Midwives Act 1915*, followed by South Australia in 1920 and New South Wales in 1923 (www.nursesreg.nsw.gov.au/). All midwives in Australia are now registered and regulated by nursing and midwifery registering authorities in their respective states or territories.

Professional regulatory authorities

Each state has a Nurses Act or Nurses and Midwives Act and accompanying Regulations. The names of the Acts and governing bodies vary from jurisdiction to jurisdiction (see Table 11.1).

The legislation sets out the role and function of the regulatory authorities including the composition of the Board or Council and the procedure for disciplinary hearings.

The ACT, NSW and the Northern Territory, in addition to Australia's peak nursing body, the Australian Nursing and Midwifery Council (ANMC), have incorporated 'midwifery/ midwives' into the title of their legislation and nursing regulatory authorities in recognition of midwifery as a separate discipline.

Generally the legislation has a common purpose, namely to maintain acceptable standards within the practice of nursing and midwifery and to ensure that clients are not misled as to whether their health carer has met the requirements of the state (Wallace 2001). By registering nurses and midwives, setting and maintaining standards, and inquiring into alleged misconduct, the public is protected. The wording of the Acts varies from jurisdiction to jurisdiction and while some specifically state in the objects that the purpose of the Act is the protection of the public, others do not. By way of example, the *Nurses and Midwives Act 1991* (NSW) states the following:

Section 2A of the Nurses and Midwives Act 1991, NSW
(1) the objects of the this Act are:

(a) to protect the health and safety of the public by providing mechanisms to ensure that nurses and midwives are fit to practise, and
(b) to provide mechanisms to enable the public and employers to readily identify nurses and midwives who are registered or enrolled under the Act.
(2) The Board must exercise its functions under the Act in a manner that is consistent with these objects.

The titles of 'nurse' and 'midwife' are protected under the legislation with penalties for unauthorised use. Generally there are two divisions of the register for nurses and midwives in the various states and territories. Comprehensive and general nurses are recorded in Division 1 and enrolled nurses in Division 2. On successful completion of an accredited course, midwives are endorsed or recorded in Division 1 of the register. Once registered, a midwife must notify the appropriate authority of her intention to practise as an independent or private midwife. The notification is usually in a prescribed form, such as the Health (Notifications By Midwives) Regulations 1994, WA.

In New South Wales, the Nurses and Midwives Board will recognise courses leading to a Bachelor of Midwifery without the previous requirement of a nursing qualification. Midwives who are nurses will remain on the register for nurses with an endorsement for midwifery.

Powers and functions of the regulatory authorities

Although the boards and council have expressed their powers and duties differently, in essence they have a common purpose. Section 16(1) of the *Nurses Act 1999* (SA) identifies the functions of the Nurses Board of SA as follows:

(a) to regulate the practice of nursing in the public interest;
(b) to determine the scope of nursing practice;
(c) to approve courses of education or training that provide qualifications for registration or enrolment as a nurse under this Act;

TABLE 11.1 Statutes regulating the practice of nursing and midwifery in Australia

State/territory	Name of the Act	Board/Council
Australian Capital Territory	*Nurses Act 1988* *Health Professionals Act 2004*	ACT Nursing and Midwifery Board
New South Wales	*Nurses and Midwives Act 1991*	Nurses and Midwives Board of NSW
Northern Territory	*Health Practitioners Act 2004*	The Nursing and Midwifery Board of the Northern Territory
Queensland	*Nursing Act 1992*	Queensland Nursing Council
South Australia	*Nurses Act 1999*	Nurses Board of SA
Tasmania	*Nurses Act 1995*	Nursing Board of Tasmania
Victoria	*Nurses Act 1993*	Nurses Board of Victoria
Western Australia	*Nurses Act 1992*	Nurses Board of WA

(d) to determine the requirements necessary for registration or enrolment under the Act;

(e) to investigate the fitness of persons to practise as nurses in this State, and to investigate the professional conduct of nurses who are registered or enrolled under this Act;

(f) to endorse codes of conduct for nurses;

(g) to endorse professional standards, including definitions and titles;

(h) to authorise areas of specialist nursing practice for inclusion on the register or roll under this Act;

(i) to determine and recognise special practice areas for the purposes of this Act;

(j) to exchange information with other registering authorities for nurses;

(k) to provide advice to the Minister as may be appropriate;

(l) to carry out other functions assigned to the Board by or under this Act, or by the Minister.

Midwives should consult the relevant legislation in their jurisdiction.

Disciplinary action

As part of its role in protecting the public, each board or council has the power to investigate professional misconduct by a nurse or midwife and recommend that a disciplinary hearing take place. The process is initiated by a complaint, which may be from a patient, a member of the public or another health professional, often a Director of Nursing. The complaint is then investigated and the matter may or may not proceed to a disciplinary hearing. If the complaint is considered frivolous or vexatious it may not be pursued.

Most states have a two-tiered system where, for instance in New South Wales, a Professional Standards Committee is set up to review complaints, and should a finding of professional misconduct be made the matter is referred to the Nurses and Midwives Tribunal. Following an enquiry, the name of the midwife may be removed from the Register or Roll. In Western Australia, an informal or formal inquiry may be held. A nurse or midwife can only be de-registered following a formal inquiry.

Section 4(1) of the *Nurses and Midwives Act 1991*, NSW defines 'professional misconduct' as 'Unsatisfactory professional conduct of a sufficiently serious nature to justify the removal of the nurse's name from the Register or Roll'. The NSW *Nurses and Midwives Act 1991* distinguishes 'unsatisfactory professional conduct' as less serious than 'professional misconduct' and defines the term in section 4(2) as:

(a) any conduct that demonstrates lack of adequate:
  (i)   knowledge,
  (ii)   experience,
  (iii) skill,
  (iv)   judgement, or
  (v)   care
  by the nurse or midwife in the practice of nursing or midwifery.

The onus of proof is on the board or council to prove the allegation against the nurse according to the civil standard of proof, which is on the balance of probabilities.

Under section 61 the Nurses Board of Western Australia has further powers to conduct a disciplinary hearing where: registration has been obtained by fraud; a nurse has been convicted of an offence, is addicted to or misuses alcohol, any deleterious drug or suffers from a mental or physical disorder that renders the person unfit to practise as a nurse.

Section 61(g) of the *Nurses Act 1992*, WA provides that the Board may take action against a person who is guilty of unethical conduct as a nurse by reason of:

(i)   carelessness
(ii)   incompetence
(iii) impropriety
(iv)   misconduct
(v)   a breach of this Act; or
(vi)   non-compliance with any condition or restriction imposed under this Act.

The purpose of a disciplinary hearing is not to punish the nurse or midwife but to protect the public. While many nurses who appear before a disciplinary hearing no doubt consider the process punitive, that is not its main purpose. While an aggrieved patient may notify the Board or Council of the alleged misconduct, the hearing does not provide for a compensation payment to be paid to the patient. Should a patient wish to be compensated for the loss incurred, a civil action must be brought through the courts. The Boards or Council have the power to set up an independent committee of enquiry, which conducts a hearing into the alleged misconduct. The names of the committees, procedure and composition of the committee hearing the disciplinary matter varies but each jurisdiction provides for a process designed to protect the public by ensuring that nurses and/or midwives are fit to practise. Some proceedings are open to the public.

In the ACT, the complaint process is controlled by the *Nurses Act 1988*, the *Health Professionals Boards (Procedures) Act 1981* and the *Community Health Services Complaints Act 1993*. It is anticipated that from 2005 in Western Australia, the state Administrative Tribunals will conduct hearings into what were previously formal hearings dealt with by the Professional Standards Committee of the Nurses Board. The Board will continue to conduct informal hearings but it will no longer have the power to suspend or de-register a nurse or midwife.

While the procedure and composition of the committees investigating the alleged misconduct varies from jurisdiction to jurisdiction, most are informal. The rules of evidence do not apply, with the exception of formal enquires in Western Australia. However, a hearing is governed by rules set out in the relevant legislation and incorporates the principles of natural justice. The main principles are that the accused must know of the allegations, and must be able to state their case, and that 'no one may sit in judgement of another who has a vested interest in the outcome' (Wallace 2001, p 16). Following a disciplinary hearing, a right of appeal exists within the respective legislation. By way of example, a breach in the rules of natural justice would give a midwife the right to appeal to another judicial body according to the specific legislation.

The penalties imposed by the Boards or Council following a finding of guilty vary but in general range from a censure to de-registration. By way of example, the Nurses Board of Victoria may, under section 41 of the *Nurses Act 1993*, impose the following penalties after an informal hearing where a nurse or midwife has been found guilty of unprofessional conduct which is not of a serious nature:

   (a)   that the nurse undergo counselling;

   (b)   that the nurse be cautioned;

   (c)   that the nurse be reprimanded;

   (d)   that the nurse undertake further education of the kind stated in the determination and complete it within the period specified in the determination.

The Nurses Board of Victoria can, under section 48 of the *Nurses Act 1993*, Vic, impose the following penalties after a formal hearing:

   (a)   require the nurse to undergo counselling;

   (b)   caution the nurse;

   (c)   reprimand the nurse;

   (d)   require the nurse to undertake further education of the kind stated in the determination and to complete it within the period specified in the determination;

   (e)   impose conditions, limitations or restrictions on the registration or endorsement of registration of the nurse;

   (f)   impose a fine on the nurse of not more than 10 penalty units;

   (g)   suspend the registration or endorsement of registration of the nurse for the period specified in the determination; or

   (h)   cancel the registration or endorsement of registration of the nurse.

The number of complaints received in 2002–03 represents a substantial increase in the number of complaints received by the Nurses Board of Western Australia from the previous year. In the same period, nine formal hearings were conducted with three pending, and 13 informal hearings with two pending (Nurses Board of Western Australia 2003, p 13).

Midwifery regulation in New Zealand

Nurses Act 1977

The *Nurses Act 1977* was the governing legislation for nurses and midwives in New Zealand until 2003 and it established the Nursing Council of New Zealand as the statutory body. It was the role of the Nursing Council, amongst other things, to regulate registration of local and overseas nurses and midwives, issue annual practising certificates, approve educational programs, and investigate and hear complaints against nurses and midwives as part of its disciplinary function.

The regulation of midwives was transferred from the Nursing Council to the Midwifery Council of New Zealand as a result of the *Health Practitioners Competence Assurance Act 2003* (HPCAA). This legislation repealed the *Nurses Act 1977*, and other health professional legislation, and established the Midwifery Council as the responsible authority to regulate the practice of midwifery.

Nurses Amendment Act 1990

Before considering the HPCAA in more detail, it is useful to briefly reflect on the enactment of the *Nurses Amendment Act 1990*, as the passing of this Act represented a major victory for midwives and women in New Zealand. Prior to this Amendment Act, the requirement for a doctor to oversee maternity care and be present at every birth meant that women were limited in the type of care they could access. Women who wanted to birth at home struggled to find a doctor willing to attend the birth. The 1990 Amendment removed the medical monopoly on maternity care and as a consequence enabled greater choice for women about who cared for them during pregnancy and birth, and where they gave birth.

For midwives, the advantages accompanying the Amendment Act were equally significant. As a profession, midwifery regained its professional autonomy and midwives were given a socially mandated right to practise independently of medical practitioners and medical oversight. In her introduction to an information booklet for providers, the Honorable Helen Clark, then Minister of Health, stated:

> Statistics reflect the benefit of a commitment to natural childbirth, of continuity of care of the client and the rejection of unnecessary intervention. The majority of women have been socialized to perceive birth as an illness. The challenge of this legislation is to change this perception (Department of Health 1990, p 1).

This was a socially and internationally unique statement. It represented an affirmation by government of the importance of natural childbirth and provided a statutory recognition that midwives were appropriate caregivers for women experiencing normal birth.

The Amendment Act also enabled midwives (through changes to other legislation) to provide a full range of maternity services, including the right to order laboratory tests and ultrasound scans, to prescribe drugs for antenatal, intrapartum and postnatal care, including the controlled drug pethidine, to refer clients to specialists, and to admit women to public hospitals under midwifery care.

The Amendment Act enabled experimental midwifery education programs to be established and paved the way for direct entry midwifery education, which is now the most common route to midwifery registration in New Zealand. The Amendment Act was also a key step in the attainment of pay equity for midwives. This equity was reinforced through a ruling of the 1993 Maternity Tribunal, which stated that general medical practitioners and midwives provided the same level of maternity care and should be paid the same amount for providing that service.

Health Practitioner's Competence Assurance Act 2003 (HPCAA)

A key aim of this omnibus Act was to bring all registered health practitioners under one regulatory framework rather than enact a separate piece of legislation for each professional group. The HPCAA was highly significant for New Zealand midwives as it established what may be the world's first solely midwifery council—a council completely separate from nursing and medicine. Its establishment has removed the final barrier to full professional autonomy for midwives.

The HPCAA (2003) sets out the functions of the various professional councils, or, as they are termed, Responsible Authorities. In summary, each authority is required to:

- maintain a public register
- authorise registration
- set standards of clinical, cultural and ethical competence
- monitor and accredit educational institutions, programs and degree courses
- review and promote the competence of practitioners
- issue annual practising certificates
- notify appropriate persons or bodies, where the practice of a health practitioner may pose a risk of harm to the public
- establish health and disability procedures for practitioners whose health or habits are affecting their practice.

Each council or authority will additionally establish a 'scope of practice' for the profession it regulates, and identify any health services that are to be termed 'restricted activities' and therefore only able to be performed by health practitioners who are competent to practise such activities.

The HPCAA (2003) gives the Midwifery Council a wide scope to establish Professional Conduct Committees and Competence Review Committees to investigate and review the conduct and/or competence of any midwife. If valid concerns are identified, the Council may require that midwife to undergo a competence program to ensure that she is practising to a safe and reasonable standard, and may impose restrictions on the midwife's practice to ensure protection of the public while improving her standard of practice.

The HPCAA (2003) also divides the disciplinary and regulatory functions of the councils and establishes a new Health Practitioner's Disciplinary Tribunal (HPDT), which will hear all professional misconduct charges against all professionals. The Tribunal has a legal chair and among its members are one lay person and three peers from the same profession as the respondent practitioner. The process of investigation and the hearing procedures are contained on the HPDT website (see list of online resources later in this chapter). If, following a hearing, there is a finding of professional misconduct against a midwife, the penalties that may be imposed include censure, suspension or restrictions on practice, such as the requirement for supervision or that the midwife work in a specific area, for up to three years, a fine of up to $30,000, or removal of the midwife's name from the register. Part of the penalty would include an award of costs against the midwife and there would normally be publication of the midwife's name and details of the HPDT decision in the media and practice journals. Any midwife who is unhappy with a decision of the tribunal may appeal to the High Court of New Zealand.

Other statutes that protect public safety

Complaint procedures and professional negligence in Australia

Unlike New Zealand, Australia does not have a no-fault liability scheme to compensate injured clients. Following an adverse event, a client may choose to seek redress in a number of ways. They may go directly to the healthcare provider, which may be an institution or midwife. Alternatively, they may sue the midwife for negligence or they may take their grievance to a health complaints authority.

Professional negligence

Negligence is part of tort law, which seeks to compensate persons injured through an act or omission of another. The purpose of this is to put the person in the position they would have been in had they not been injured (Forrester & Griffiths 2001). Damages are intended to compensate the injured party, not to punish—that is the role of criminal law (Skene 2004).

Civil liabilities legislation has been enacted in the states and territories in response to the so-called medical insurance crisis (Skene 2004). Legislation now provides for a statutory basis for the principles of negligence, which were based on common law principles. It is presumed that in interpreting the statutory provisions, the courts will apply the general principles of negligence evolved through the common law (Balkin & Davis 2004).

In negligence, the plaintiff must prove that a duty of care was owed, that there was a breach in the duty of care, that is, the standard of care fell below that of an ordinary reasonable midwife given the circumstances, and that the damage or injury was a reasonably foreseeable consequence of that breach.

There is no question that a midwife owes a client a duty of care. To successfully argue otherwise would in most cases be extremely difficult. Lord Atkin, in the now famous case of *Donoghue v Stevenson* [1932] AC 562 at 580, established to whom a duty of care is owed.

> You must take reasonable care to avoid acts or omissions which you can reasonably foresee would be likely to injure your neighbour. Who then in law is my neighbour? The answer seems to be persons who are so closely affected by my act that I ought reasonably to have them in contemplation as being so affected when I am directing my mind to the acts or omissions which are called in question.

The statutory duty of care is identified in section 5B of the *Civil Liability Act 2002*, WA Similar provisions exist in other jurisdictions within Australia.

Section 5B

(1) A person is not liable for harm caused by that person's fault in failing to take precaution against a risk of harm unless–

   (a) the risk was foreseeable (that is, it is a risk of which the person knew or ought to have known);

(b) the risk was not insignificant; and

(c) in the circumstances, a reasonable person in the person's position would have taken those precautions.

(2) In determining whether a reasonable person would have taken precautions against a risk of harm, the court is to consider the following (amongst other relevant things)–

(a) the probability that the harm would occur if care were not taken;

(b) the likely seriousness of the harm;

(c) the burden of taking precautions to avoid the risk of harm;

(d) the social utility of the activity that creates the risk of harm.

Once a duty is established, the plaintiff must prove that the midwife breached her duty of care or that it was her fault that the injury occurred. The test used to establish a breach is one of reasonableness. The standard required of a midwife is an objective test according to what a 'reasonable midwife' would or would not have done in the circumstances. In determining whether the standard has been met, the court will consider not only expert evidence but various documents such as appropriate statutes, hospital policy and the midwife's case notes.

In proving causation, the traditional test in Australia has been the 'but for' test. The 'but for' test is expressed as, but for the actions of the defendant the plaintiff would not have been injured. However, it is not an exclusive test (Skene 2004, p 230). Civil liabilities legislation now requires a factual causation, that is, whether the harm was caused by the negligence and whether 'it is appropriate to extend the scope of the tortfeasor's (defendant's) liability to the harm so caused (scope of liability)' (s 5C *Civil Liability Act 2002*, WA).

The plaintiff always bears the onus of proof, according to the civil standard of proof, namely, on the balance of probabilities (s 5D *Civil Liability Act 2002*, WA). The defendant does not have to prove that he or she was not negligent but rather raise sufficient evidence to throw doubt on the plaintiff's case (Wallace 2001).

Health complaints authorities in Australia

Each state and territory has an independent health care complaints body, set up under specific legislation to deal with complaints about health care providers and services (see Table 11.2). The health complaints authorities are in recognition of an increase in patients' rights (Wallace 2001) and acknowledgement that it may not be appropriate to take every grievance through the courts. Forrester and Grifffiths (2001) suggest that while the aim of tort law is to maintain quality health care through the threat of litigation, this is not always the case.

An aggrieved patient may choose not to purse litigation through the courts. The process is time-consuming, expensive and stressful whether or not the case proceeds to court. An alternative means of resolution is through a health complaints authority, where the patient can make a complaint about the health care provider. The legislation varies from jurisdiction to jurisdiction but in general the aim of the legislation is to

TABLE 11.2 Australian health complaints authorities	
Legislation	**Complaints body**
Community Health Services Complaints Act 1993, ACT	Community and Health Service Complaints Office
Health and Community Services Complaints Act 1998, NT	Health and Community Services Complaints Commission
Health Rights Commission Act 1991, Qld	Health Rights Commission
Health and Community Services Complaints Act 2004, SA	Health and Community Services Complaints Commion
Health Complaints Act 1995, Tas	Health Complaints Commissioner
Health Care Complaints Act 1993, NSW	Health Care Complaints Commission (HCCC)
Health Services (Conciliation and Review) Act 1987, Vic	Health Services Commissioner
Health Services (Conciliation and Review) Act 1995, WA	Office of Health Review

provide an independent body for the resolution of complaints between health consumers and providers.

In general a complaint must allege that the health service provider acted unreasonably in one or more areas, such as: not providing a health service; in the manner of providing a health service; denying or restricting the user's access to the records kept by the health provider; in disclosing or using the user's health records or confidential information or in the fee charged (s 25 *Health Services (Conciliation and Review) Act 1995* WA). There is an expectation that the patient will have attempted to resolve the issue with the health care provider before making a complaint (s 30 *Health Services (Conciliation and Review) Act 1995* WA).

The commissioner or director of the health complaints authority has the power to investigate and conciliate a matter arising from a complaint. For a matter to be conciliated requires the consent of both parties. If appropriate, the matter can be referred to the registering authority of the professional involved for investigation (s 32 *Health Services (Conciliation and Review) Act 1995*, WA).

Complaint procedures and professional negligence in New Zealand

Health and Disability Commissioner Act 1994 (HDCA)

Part of the impetus for the appointment of a Health and Disability Commissioner (HDC) was calls from consumer groups for an independent person or watchdog that could investigate complaints against health professionals. Another driver for the establishment of the office of the HDC was the abject failure of health professionals to regulate themselves and prevent the occurrences that lead to inquiries such as that which became known as the 'Cartwright Inquiry' (Cartwright 1998).

Despite initial government support for a Health Commissioner, it was almost a decade before the first Health and Disability Commissioner was appointed. The Commissioner's first task was to draft a Code of Health and Disability Services Consumers' Rights ('the Code'). This Code sets out 10 fundamental rights for any person receiving a health or disability service. These include the right to:

- respect
- fair treatment
- dignity and independence
- proper standards
- communication
- information
- make informed decisions
- support
- teaching and research protections
- complain.

The Code is a regulation under the substantive Act and is enforceable by law.

The HDCA requires all midwives to practise according to the Code, and it provides an avenue for complaint and prosecution of any midwife who is found in breach of its provisions. The HDC is now the primary complaints organisation in New Zealand and the Office filters and manages almost all complaints against all health practitioners.

A lesser-known requirement of the Code is that any midwife who personally receives a complaint must respond to the complainant within five working days. This is in keeping with the aim of the Act, which is to deal with complaints in a simple, speedy and efficient way, and its underpinning philosophy of early mediation and resolution. Where such resolution cannot be achieved, or is unrealistic given the seriousness of the complaint, the matter will be investigated, the midwife notified of the allegations against her, and statements of witnesses and evidence will be gathered. It is usual for the Commissioner to refer the complaint, and responses, to midwifery experts, who will assist the Commissioner in the consideration of the clinical issues and who will provide an opinion on the reasonableness or otherwise of the midwife's practice and decision-making during the relevant events. Eventually a decision will be made as to whether, in the Commissioner's opinion, the midwife's conduct constitutes a breach of the Code.

During this process the midwife is given at least two opportunities to respond and comment on the case against her, although unfortunately she may not be aware of much of the evidence until very late in the investigation. The first opportunity is following initial notification of the complaint, where she is requested to provide a full report on her involvement to the Commissioner. The second opportunity is upon receipt of the Commissioner's Provisional Opinion, which will set out the evidence and proposed finding. Often it is only at this point that the midwife becomes aware of the full extent of the complaint against her, and it is important that she

fully address any adverse evidence before the Commissioner's Opinion is finalised.

If the Commissioner finds the midwife in breach, she or he may make a range of recommendations including written apology, further education, and mentoring. Since the establishment of the Midwifery Council, the Commissioner has begun to recommend that the Council consider whether or not to conduct a competence review of the midwife's practice.

In serious cases the Commissioner will notify the midwife that he or she is referring the matter to the Director of Proceedings. The Director is an independent statutory officer and will determine whether the complaint reaches the threshold of seriousness to warrant laying a charge of professional misconduct before the Health Practitioner's Disciplinary Tribunal and whether, additionally, damages should be sought before the Human Rights Review Tribunal.

Once the Commissioner has finalised his or her Opinion, an anonymous version is circulated to the professional bodies, the complainant, the practitioner(s), to employers and sometimes to external bodies such as the Minister of Health or the police. It may also be placed, for educational purposes, on the Commissioner's website in the hope that similar complaints can be averted. An identifiable copy of the Final Opinion is sent to the Midwifery Council. The Council can decide to take action on the matter, if it decides that it raises professional issues that need to be addressed, even if the Commissioner is not taking the complaint further.

In some cases the Commissioner may liaise with the Midwifery Council earlier in the process. This might occur if the Commissioner had serious concerns about the safety of the midwife's ongoing practice. Alternatively, if the Commissioner came to the view that the midwife had health or disability issues and that these were affecting her ability to practise safely, then the Commissioner might refer the matter to the Health Committee of the Midwifery Council.

The most common areas of complaint against midwives under the HDC jurisdiction relate to poor communication, poor documentation, lack of informed consent, failure to recognise and act on deviations from normal, particularly with respect to fetal heart patterns and failure to progress in labour, and failure to refer women to a specialist in a timely and appropriate manner. These same themes occur in obstetric or maternity complaints across almost all international jurisdictions.

Human Rights Act 1993 / Human Rights Amendment Act 2001

This Human Rights Act is notable for midwives as it established the Human Rights Review Tribunal (HRRT) (previously known as the Complaints Review Tribunal). If a practitioner is found in breach of the *Human Rights Act 1993*, the *Privacy Act 1993* or the *Health and Disability Commissioner's Act 1994*, an 'aggrieved person' or someone acting on their behalf can seek damages of up to $200,000. The claim may cover pecuniary (monetary) loss and expenses reasonably incurred by the complainant and any loss of benefit the person might reasonably have expected to obtain, but for the breach that occurred.

Under the HDCA it was only the Director of Proceedings who could lay proceedings before this Tribunal. With the advent of the HPCAA, where there is a finding of breach of the Code, any aggrieved person may seek damages before the HRRT, irrespective of whether or not the Director of Proceedings considers that the threshold of seriousness has been met.

The usual HRRT process is that a charge is laid alleging that the breach of the Code has caused humiliation, loss of dignity and injury to the feelings of the complainant or, as the case may be, to the aggrieved person. Once this is received, the Tribunal notifies the parties and sets down a date for a formal hearing. The Human Rights Review Tribunal is made up of a minimum of three people, one of whom is legally trained. The hearings are held in public and witnesses may be summonsed to give evidence. Witnesses have the same privileges and immunities as in court proceedings. Parties may be legally represented and the procedure is similar to that of District Court hearings or disciplinary tribunals. Decisions of the Tribunal must be in writing and be properly reasoned. An Appeal may be lodged against any decision of the Tribunal to the High Court.

Injury Prevention, Rehabilitation and Compensation Act 2001

New Zealand has a comprehensive 'no fault' accident and insurance scheme whereby any person suffering personal injury by accident receives financial compensation and assistance. Part of this is that any claimant who receives cover under the scheme is then effectively barred from bringing suit against a registered health professional. While there are a few exceptions to this rule, the extent of this cover means that New Zealand midwives are largely protected from civil action or law suits against them.

The *Injury Prevention Rehabilitation and Compensation Act 2001* (IPRC) is the most recent version of the Accident Compensation legislation. This legislation was amended in 2005 to simplify the cover criteria and claims process for injuries arising from treatment and make this more consistent with the rest of the ACC scheme.

For a claimant to receive cover for personal injury by accident they must, where a registered health professional has been involved in their care or treatment, bring themselves under the medical misadventure provisions of the IPRC. This section was amended in 2005, replacing the two generic categories of Medical Mishap and Medical Error with a new category of Treatment Injury. Under this amendment, the ACC no longer has to find fault to consider a treatment injury claim for cover, or limit cover to injuries that are 'rare and severe'.

A treatment injury is a personal injury that has occurred within the context of treatment provided by, or at the direction of, one or more health professionals. There must be a direct causal link between the injury and the treatment. Treatment injury cover is for outcomes that are abnormal, unusual or exceptional having regard to the patient's particular circumstances, and such events are not expected to happen often. In the context of treatment injury, personal injury is defined as either the death of a person; physical injury; mental injury suffered by a person because of physical injury; and/or damage to dentures or prostheses that replace a human body part.

Treatment is defined as:

The giving of treatment; diagnosis; choice of treatment, including a decision not to treat; failure to provide treatment, or to provide it in a timely manner; provision of prophylaxis;

Obtaining or failing to obtain informed consent from the legally appropriate person;

Failure of any equipment, device, or tool used as part of the treatment process, including failure of any implant or prosthesis, other than by an intervening act (e.g. a fall, which would be considered under the accident provisions of the scheme) or fair wear and tear; and

The application of any relevant support systems, including policies, processes, practices and administrative systems (ACC information sheet 2005).

A key objective of the changes was to encourage health providers to make claims earlier and with more comprehensive information to facilitate the timely provision of assistance by ACC to claimants. Ideally, claims for treatment injury should be made on behalf of the patient (claimant) by the registered health professional who provided the treatment that caused the injury. With the removal of the 'fault' aspect, the health professional will be able to provide information to the ACC without fear of reprisal.

There are numerous claims for ACC cover and most New Zealand midwives will deal with a claim every three to five years. The claims are wide ranging but common examples (under the previous category of medical error) included: a failure to accurately diagnose a complication of pregnancy or labour; a tendency to normalise abnormalities, such as where the midwife does not recognise the significance of abnormal tracings, attributing reduced variability to a sleeping trace, or where she does not respond appropriately to warnings of possible fetal distress such as thick meconium, or does not recognise the signs of an obstructed labour. Another bracket of claims related to a lack of, or delays in, appropriate specialist referral. This is a frequent allegation where babies are born with severe asphyxia or are later found to have cerebral palsy.

There have also been a number of less serious claims for complications of perineal lacerations, particularly when the extent of the tear is incorrectly diagnosed by the midwife or where the laceration is left unsutured without documented evidence that the woman has consented for this to happen.

ACC claims have arisen less commonly with respect to postnatal care but may occur where a midwife fails to accurately identify haemolytic jaundice or kernicterus in a baby and the parents later make a claim for a baby's hearing loss or resultant brain damage.

Claims under the old category of medical mishap were rare and included cases where the baby was unexpectedly large or there was a malpresentation or a shoulder dystocia and Erb's palsy resulted, or where the woman sustained an injury to her coccyx or back during labour, or where there was radial nerve damage after an appropriately sited intravenous infusion.

The ACC no longer reports individual medical error decisions and trends to the HDC, registration authorities and employers unless the ACC determines that there is risk of public harm. The ACC continues to collect and make available non-identifiable trend data.

Crimes Act 1961

The Crimes Act has a number of sections, 150A–157, often dubbed the 'duty sections', which require all health professionals to meet a reasonable standard of skill and care in their practice, while operating on patients, and while doing dangerous acts such as administering surgical or medical treatment including administering complex intravenous drug therapy, epidural anaesthesia and drugs (Mellars et al 1995).

The concept of the 'reasonable standard' has been adopted from the common law and is basically linked to the question: 'What would a reasonable midwife do, or not do, in these circumstances?' Usually the adjudicating body will determine the evidence of what constitutes reasonable practice after they have heard the evidence of expert witnesses from the same professional group as the practitioner under scrutiny.

Other criminal charges

Midwives should remember that they are subject to the whole realm of law, just like any other citizens. However, unlike other citizens, a conviction for serious traffic or drug offences, assaults or dishonesty offences may have the additional result

for a midwife of a professional misconduct hearing, and a loss of her right to practise.

Statutes on privacy and access to personal information

Australian privacy legislation

Patients do not own their records. They are owned by the person or institution who made them, but patients have a right to access the information contained in them (Skene 2004, p 236). Patients in the public sector have access through state and federal freedom of information legislation. At common law there was no right of access to patient records in the private sector, although access could be gained through the process of litigation. In 2000 the Commonwealth *Privacy Act 1988* was amended to provide access for private patients to their records. It also provides patients with access to their personal information held by Commonwealth agencies. The ACT, New South Wales and Victoria have enacted legislation to provide private patients with access to their medical records.

The *Privacy Act 1988* (Cth) sets out Information Privacy Principles (IPPs) (s 14), which pertain to government agencies, and National Privacy Principles (NPP) (Sch 3), which pertain to private institutions and doctors.

The Principles provide instruction on the collection of information, use and disclosure of information, quality of information, security of information, type of information held, access to information, correction of information, use of unique identifiers, anonymity options, international transfer of information and circumstances in which information may be collected. Midwives should familiarise themselves with these principles.

The *Privacy Act 1988* (Cth) established the office of Privacy Commissioner to investigate and deal with complaints or breaches under the Act.

New Zealand statutes on privacy and information

Health (Retention of Health Information) Regulations 1996

These regulations impose an obligation on midwives to retain original health information about their clients, both mothers and babies, for a minimum of 10 years. The information may be retained in any form the midwife thinks fit. Health information for the purposes of the regulation may include midwifery diaries, travel logs and phone logs if clinical details are noted in such documents. In the event of retirement or a midwife ceasing practice, this information can be transferred to the client or, if the client is dead, to that individual's personal representative, or to another provider. Although such transfer is possible, this may have significant legal risk if a claim is later brought against the midwife and the midwife no longer has access to the notes in order to mount a defence.

Reflective exercise

1   There is a wide diversity of views about what drugs or equipment should reasonably be available for midwives to use. What equipment do you think should be available to you as a midwife to ensure the safety of the women and babies you care for? If this equipment is not available, what is your responsibility?

2   Hera is a 40-year-old woman pregnant with her fifth child. She has a history of severe postpartum haemorrhage and has experienced a previous obstructed labour. She has refused referral to a secondary care provider or a specialist, and chooses to birth at home
  ● What issues does the midwife face?
  ● What are her legal responsibilities?
  ● What steps should the midwife take in relation to the legal and ethical ramifications of any decisions?

An exception to this Regulation is that original health information may be subpoenaed in some jurisdictions, in which case the midwife is entitled to release the records to the appropriate authority.

Health Information Privacy Code 1994 / Privacy Act 1993

Although the *Privacy Act 1993* establishes certain privacy principles regarding the collection, correction, use, disclosure, storage and access to personal information, the rules with respect to the health information of identifiable individuals comes under the Health Information Privacy (HIP) Code. This Code applies to all 'agencies' providing healthcare, such as hospitals and individual practitioners. The following is summarised from the Privacy Commissioner's document 'Health Information Privacy Code 1994'. The Code consists of 12 privacy rules covering the collection (in most cases this will be from the individual concerned), storage, access to, retention and correction of any health information obtained by health professionals. The Code also sets certain limits on the use and disclosure of an individual's health information. If any information is to be shared with other agencies such as a well child provider or medical practitioner, this should be discussed with the woman.

Most midwives who practise in partnership with women will either provide a copy of any health information collected, such as clinical notes, or give the woman a summary of what has been documented at each visit. The woman should be informed of her rights in relation to provision of information and to access or correct any information gathered. Midwives must ensure that the woman comprehends the information being given. If she is unfamiliar with English or is having trouble understanding what is being said, then an appropriate family member, friend or interpreter may need to be used or the midwife may need to provide a written summary of the woman's rights under the HIP Code. Care must be made not to make unfounded assumptions regarding the ethnicity and language ability of any person.

Health information, including diaries, lab results, scan reports and phone logs, must be stored to prevent loss, unlawful access by others, or misuse of the information. All files should be safely stored, in a locked cupboard or cabinet, and not in the boots of cars, as is the practice of some community midwives. Access to the notes, including any faxed information, should be strictly limited. When a woman requests access to her information, the Code outlines the time frame in which a midwife by law must respond to the request.

The Privacy Commissioner reminds us that while health information is created to provide care and treatment, it may also be used for other purposes such as clinical or financial audit, for administration purposes and for training and education. If such additional purposes are envisaged, they should be disclosed when the information is collected, although generally if the information is to be used for collateral purposes it will be transferred to a non-identifying form. Where disclosures are made without the consent of the individual, they must be made only to the extent necessary to meet the particular purpose or permitted request.

> ### Reflective exercise
>
> John is the partner of Sue, a woman you cared for two years ago. He phones and says that he is in a custody and paternity dispute and wants a copy of Sue's midwifery notes to show that he was actively involved in the birth of their son.
> 1. Who do the notes belong to?
> 2. Is John entitled to a copy?
> 3. Is there any circumstance in which you would release the notes?

> ### Clinical point
>
> There may be times when a midwife will observe evidence of violence or neglect of a baby and this will lead to concern about the baby's life or safety. If the matter is not urgent then the midwife should document her concerns and involve social workers, Family Start program support, general practitioners or family or whanau to help the parents and prevent future harm. On rare occasions, however, the midwife may consider that immediate intervention should take place and she will need to urgently report the mother, father or partner to the appropriate agency. Technically this may constitute a breach of confidentiality, but the midwife who acts in good faith and has reasonable grounds to believe that her actions are necessary to prevent serious or imminent harm to a child is likely to have a defence.

Complaints

Any complaints alleging a breach of privacy may be made to the Privacy Commissioner—Te Mana Matapono Matatapu. If complaints cannot be resolved with the assistance of the Commissioner, then the complainant may seek orders, declarations or damages from the Human Rights Review Tribunal.

Legislation on midwifery practice

Australian legislation

Notification of birth

Each state and territory has legislation that requires the notification and registration of births, deaths and marriages. Under the Births, Deaths and Marriages Acts in the respective states and territories, the definitions of birth, child and whether a stillborn is registered as a birth and/or a death vary, but all agree on the gestation and weight parameters of a stillborn.

A 'stillborn' is a child that exhibits no sign of respiration or heartbeat, or other sign of life, after birth and that:

(a) is of at least 20 weeks' gestation, or

(b) if it cannot be reliably established whether the period of gestation is more or less than 20 weeks, has a body mass of at least 400 grams at birth (s4 *Births, Deaths and Marriages Registration Act 1995*, NSW).

The South Australian legislation goes further and states that a birth 'does not include the product of a procedure for the termination of pregnancy (s 4 *Births, Death and Marriages Registration Act 1996*, SA).

In the ACT, New South Wales, South Australia, Victoria and Tasmania, a stillborn or stillbirth is registered as a birth but not a death. In Western Australia and Queensland, a stillborn is registered as a birth and a death.

In Queensland, South Australia, Tasmania and Western Australia, a birth is defined as the expulsion or extraction of a child from its mother. A child is further defined as including a stillborn. In the ACT, New South Wales, the Northern Territory and Victoria, a birth includes a stillbirth.

Failure to provide the details to the appropriate authority is an offence. The purpose of the notification is so the particulars of the birth can be entered into the Births, Death and Marriages Register of the state or territory in which the child was born. Health legislation provides for the requirement of notification of a birth whether stillborn or a live birth. Under the respective legislation, a midwife who attends a birth is required to notify the appropriate authority. A specific form for the purpose is provided in the respective legislation. The time frame for notification varies from jurisdiction to jurisdiction but ranges from 24 hours in Victoria to one month in Western Australia.

In Western Australia a neonatal death is defined as 'the death of a live-born child within 28 days after the birth'.

In Victoria a perinatal death means:

(a) the death of a live-born child within 28 days after the birth; or

(b) a stillbirth.

In Western Australia, for the purposes of burial under the *Cremation Act 1929*, WA and the *Cemeteries Act 1986*, WA, a dead body 'means the body of a deceased person (who was born alive) and includes the body of an infant of not less than 7 months gestation that was still-born'. Unless the parents wish to conduct a funeral there is no requirement in law in Western Australia to do so for a stillborn of less than 28 weeks.

Abortion laws in Australia

Each state and territory has provisions in their respective criminal legislation that make abortion unlawful. A breach of the legislation generally carries severe criminal penalties. 'An abortion can be defined as the untimely expulsion of the fetus from the uterus either spontaneously or by artificial means' (Forrester & Griffiths 2001, p 196). However, provisions do exist for a termination of pregnancy to take place in specific circumstances. Case law in Victoria and other states such as R v Davidson [1969] VR 667 allows for an abortion to be lawful in circumstances where the medical practitioners are of the view that the procedure is necessary to preserve the woman's physical and mental health. However, as Rankin (2001, pp

233–4) points out, at no stage are the views of the woman taken into account.

In South Australia, Section 82A of the *Criminal Law Consolidation Act 1835*, SA further provides that a medical practitioner must perform the abortion in a prescribed hospital. Additionally, the woman must have been a resident of South Australia for at least two months prior to the termination, and again it is a medical decision to perform the abortion.

Following an incident in Western Australia where two doctors were charged under the Criminal Code for performing an abortion in 1998, the abortion laws were changed and are now one of the most liberal in Australia. An unlawful abortion is still a crime as per section 199 of the Criminal Code 1913, WA. Previously an unlawful abortion attracted a term of 14 years' imprisonment. Under the amendments to the Criminal Code 1913, WA and the *Health Act 1911*, WA, an unlawful abortion by a medical practitioner attracts a fine of $50,000. An abortion performed by a person other than a medical practitioner is still a crime and attracts a penalty of five years' imprisonment. Provided the requirements of Section 334 of the *Health Act 1911*, WA are met, no offence has been committed. The provisions require that a woman must give 'informed consent' to the procedure. The requirements for 'informed consent' are met when the woman is advised of 'the medical risk of termination of pregnancy and of carrying a pregnancy to term' and a medical practitioner has offered to refer the woman for appropriate counselling (s 334 *Health Act 1911*, WA). Alternatively, if the pregnancy is more than 20 weeks, the matter is referred to a committee of two medical practitioners from a panel of six, who agree that the mother or unborn child has a severe medical condition that in their clinical judgement justifies the termination. The legislation changes in Western Australia do to some extent take the focus away from the criminal law. The doctor can make the decision based on a reasonable belief that if the abortion were not performed the woman would suffer serious mental or physical harm. However, it is still not abortion on demand.

New Zealand legislation

New Zealand Public Health and Disability Act 2000

Under Section 88 of the *New Zealand Public Health and Disability Act 2000* the Crown, or a District Health Board, may issue a notice of the terms and conditions on which payment will be made to those providing a public health service. One example is the Notice Pursuant to Section 88 of the *New Zealand Public Health and Disability Act 2000* for Maternity Services, which sets out the terms and conditions for the provision of maternity services. Key appendices to the Notice include the Guidelines for Consultation with Obstetric and Related Specialist Medical Services; the Standard Terms and Conditions of Access to a Maternity Facility or a Birthing Unit, and the Indications for Ultrasound Scanning. These appendices require the practitioner to consult and refer women according to the guidelines and set up the expectation that midwives will practise according to the standards set down by their professional bodies.

The national Access Agreement is also included in the Section 88 Notice and this requires the midwife, subject to the woman's informed consent, to comply with the protocols and policies set out by the hospitals to which she admits her clients. Often midwives are unaware that as soon as they have accepted any payment under the Notice, they are deemed to have agreed to comply with all the terms and conditions and appendices of the Notice and that they are then bound to follow these protocols and policies.

A further issue for midwives claiming payment under Section 88 is that their claims may be subjected to an extensive random audit. If the midwife is audited she must be able to demonstrate that she has provided the services that she has been paid for, and be able to prove this provision through documentation. Generally the auditors take random copies of the midwife's notes and check these against what was claimed. Any failure of the midwife to substantiate claims during the investigation may lead to money being recovered from her, or, in the worst-case scenario, prosecution of the midwife for fraud in the District Court.

Births, Deaths and Marriages Registration Act 1995

The midwife has several legal responsibilities with respect to the birth of a baby. The first is to determine whether the baby is born alive or is stillborn. While this may seem an obvious distinction to make, there are times in practice where a midwife may confuse the two states, and this can lead to significant legal difficulties.

Live birth is the complete expulsion or extraction from the mother of a product of conception, irrespective of the duration of pregnancy which, after such separation, breathes or shows any other evidence of life, such as beating of the heart, pulsation of the umbilical cord, or definite movement of the voluntary muscles, whether or not the umbilical cord has been cut or the placenta is attached.

Stillbirth means the issue from its mother of a stillborn child. A stillborn child is a dead fetus which, whether or not the umbilical cord had been severed or the placenta has detached, at no time after issuing completely from its mother breathed or showed any other sign of life (such as beating of the heart, pulsation of the umbilical cord, or definite movement of the voluntary muscles), and weighed 400 grams or more when it issued from its mother or issued from its mother after the 20th week of pregnancy.

When a baby is born alive or stillborn, a Notice of birth must be completed and sent to the Registrar of Births, Deaths, and Marriages within five working days of the birth. Generally this notification is the responsibility of the occupier of the hospital where the birth took place, and a person attending the birth, such as a midwife, endorses it. Where the birth takes place at home, the midwife will usually complete the Notice.

The parents or guardians or any baby born alive or stillborn must also be registered with the Registrar of Births, Deaths and Marriages within two months of the birth. Every death must also be notified to the Registrar of Births, Deaths and Marriages within three working days after the disposal of the body. This notification is made by the person who carries out this disposal. Where an inquest has occurred, the coroner must make the notification to the registrar within three working days after the completion of the Inquest.

In most cases the coroner only becomes involved where the cause of death is unclear, or there are concerns about the circumstances surrounding the death. It is then up to the coroner to decide whether a post mortem is required to ascertain the cause of death. If a coroner does commence an investigation, a medical certificate stating the cause of death cannot be signed until after the coroner has completed his or her inquiries. This means that no one, including a funeral director or family member, can take charge of the baby's body without first obtaining the appropriate certificate, burial order or the coroner's order authorising its release. It is only once these formalities are completed that the family can bury or cremate their baby. This can be a stressful and difficult time for families, particularly Indigenous families such as New Zealand Maori, where whanau members would normally stay with the baby from the time of death to the burial or cremation.

In some stillbirth situations a doctor need not sign a certificate of stillbirth. Midwives should note that Section 46A of the *Burial and Cremation Act 1964* states that where a baby is stillborn, either a medical practitioner who was present at the birth or examined the baby after the birth, or if no doctor was present, a registered midwife who was present at the birth, may certify that the baby was born dead. The midwife must have been present at the birth and therefore in the situation of a precipitate birth where the midwife arrives just after the birth and finds a baby dead, she should not sign the certificate.

Adoption Act 1955

From time to time midwives become involved in adoptions, particularly where adoptions take place within an extended family grouping or whanau. Midwives should be aware that the New Zealand Adoption Acts set out a statutory procedure that must be followed before an adoption can legally take place. A midwife cannot act as an agent, and nor can she broker an adoption arrangement between parties. If a midwife is caring for any woman considering an adoption of her baby, the midwife should ensure that the woman is referred to the appropriate state agencies. This will usually require the early involvement of a social worker.

Contraception, Sterilisation and Abortion Act 1977

The key responsibility of midwives under this Act is to be aware of the referral requirements for any woman seeking abortion. Often it is the midwife to whom a woman will come for diagnosis or confirmation of pregnancy. It is illegal for any midwife to help a woman procure an abortion. If any woman does not want to continue a pregnancy then the role of the midwife is to refer her to a doctor for further counselling and assessment.

Legislation on drug administration and prescribing (New Zealand)

Medicines Act and Regulations

There is a plethora of Acts and Regulations relating to the prescription and administration of drugs, and this section attempts to pull together the key points of the law as it relates to midwives.

New Zealand midwives have been able to prescribe a range of drugs and medications related to antenatal, intrapartum and postnatal care since 1990. The Medicines Regulations 1984 as amended by the Medicines Regulations 1984, Amendment No 3, gave a statutory mandate for midwives to prescribe a range of medications and brought midwives under the Medicines Regulations 1984. Section 39 of the Regulations (1984/143) states that:

> (6) No registered midwife shall
> (a) Prescribe for any patient a quantity of any prescription medicine that exceeds 3 months supply; or
> (b) Prescribe any prescription medicine otherwise than for antenatal, intrapartum or postpartum care.

Although the law is a bit convoluted, this basically legislates that a midwife may prescribe for the normal conditions of pregnancy—that is, within the Scope of Midwifery Practice. Midwives should not prescribe for pre-existing medical conditions or complex pregnancy conditions.

Section 41 of the Medicines Regulations 1984 prescribes the form of any prescription, which must include:

- that it shall be legibly and indelibly printed
- the date, address and personal signature of the prescriber
- the title, surname, initial and address of the person for whom the prescription is given
- the name, strength, dose, frequency of dose, and method of administration of the medicine
- the number of occasions on which the medicine may be supplied
- the interval between dates of supply
- the period in which the medicine is to be used.

Whenever a midwife prescribes a medication, there must be a discussion about the reason for the prescription, the effects, side-effects and contraindications to that medication, an identification of any allergy or previous problems with the medication, and a clinical assessment of the appropriateness of the medication for that person, in the presenting circumstances. Ultimately where the drug is given, the practitioner must demonstrate that this was done with the informed consent of the client. An exception to this is an emergency, such as where there is a seriously depressed neonate who might be given naloxone, or where a woman is experiencing an overwhelming postpartum haemorrhage and becomes unconscious and is administered intravenous fluids and possibly blood products. In most cases, however, such scenarios will have been discussed antenatally and the woman's views ascertained prior to this occurring.

Clinical point

Requirements for prescriptions for controlled drugs. Medicines Act Amendment No 11 (1995/75)
Prescriptions should be legibly and indelibly written, signed and dated, include the midwife's address, the name of the drug, the amount of the drug, the dose and frequency of the drug, the surname, initials and address of the person for whom the drug is intended and bear the words 'for midwifery use only'.

Urgent prescriptions

Section 40A of the Medicines Amendment Regulations 2001 enables a registered midwife to request an urgent prescription orally (in person or by phone) to a pharmacist to whom he or she is known personally. She must then forward a written script of the oral communication within seven days. The schedule of this Amendment also discusses standing orders with respect to controlled drugs, although in practice it would be unusual for a midwife to use this mechanism, because if a controlled drug is required, the midwife or her back-up should either already be in attendance or should immediately attend to assess the woman.

Controlled drugs

Section 8 (2) of the *Misuse of Drugs Act 1975* as amended by the *Nurses Amendment Act 1990* enables any registered midwife to prescribe, supply and administer the controlled drug pethidine to a patient under her care but the frequency of administration is strictly regulated. The Misuse of Drugs Regulations 1977, Amendment No. 9 (1990/222) states that pethidine may be supplied to the patient of a midwife on not more than two occasions, and should be supplied at an interval specified by the midwife, the first being not more than four days after the prescription and the second being not more than four days after the termination of that interval.

Any prescription must be written on a Controlled Drug prescription form, and in hospital must be written on the drug sheet. Amendment No. 10 (1993/157) updates the requirement to keep a Controlled Drug Register in hospital wards. Midwives cannot prescribe benzodiazepines such as clonazepam, diazepam and temazepam, as they are class C Part V controlled drugs.

Coroner's Court legislation and process

The office of coroner is an ancient one and each state and territory in Australia and New Zealand has a Coroner's Act. The coroners legislation requires certain deaths to be reported and provides for penalties for failure to inform the coroner of a 'suspicious death'. If the death has been reported to the coroner then the midwife is no longer under an obligation to do so. Home birth midwives in particular should be cognisant of the requirements for reporting a death in the jurisdiction in which they operate.

The coroner investigates those deaths where certain facts need to be established to determine how the person died. 'The office of the coroner is established to provide a means of investigation of certain situations where death results, to identify impropriety or negligent activity' (Forrester & Griffiths 2001, p 242). The wording and the requirements for an inquest vary. However, the purpose is to investigate sudden or unexplained deaths and to establish whether the death resulted from natural causes or from unlawful homicide. The coroner generally has the power to order a post mortem, investigate deaths where a person has died in custody, in a mental health facility or under the care and control of a member of the police force, while in prison or under child welfare legislation (s3 *Coroner's Act 1996*, WA).

The number of deaths referred to coroners in New Zealand and Australia is growing and it is increasingly likely that a midwife, at some time in her career, will be involved in a coronial investigation or that she will be called to give evidence at an inquest. This can be a difficult and stressful experience and it is therefore important for midwives to be aware of the procedures set out in the coroners legislation governing her practice.

When the coroner's office is notified of a death, the body should be left until such time as the coroner's office instructs the hospital that the body can be moved to the morgue. All intravenous lines, catheters and drains are left in situ or capped as necessary. The midwife or midwives involved in the care should make notes regarding the case, as these can then be used to assist in a statement given to the police.

Not all deaths fit into the category of 'suspicious circumstances' and the coroner may dispense with the inquest once satisfied that the death was from natural causes. The legislation varies—in some cases the coroner has a discretionary power to hold an inquest and in others it is mandatory to hold an inquest. For completeness and accuracy it is suggested that the relevant legislation be consulted.

In Australia and New Zealand, uniformed police officers assist the coroner in these inquiries. They gather evidence and interview or request reports from those involved. Sometimes the police will ask midwives to disclose information or the clinical records. Poor records may indicate that the care given to the patient prior to death was also inadequate. If asked for an interview or a written statement, or for originals or copies of the notes, a midwife would be well advised to seek independent legal advice. The hospital may offer legal advice from their lawyers. However, a situation may arise where the interests of the midwife and those of the institution are in conflict.

Midwives who are involved in these inquiries are witnesses, not parties, and there are fundamental protections to which they are entitled. A midwife is entitled to give a written report at a later time and she can refuse to be questioned at all by the police until she has spoken to a lawyer or taken professional advice. It is important that midwives do not give evidence when they are distressed, exhausted or worried about the woman and her family, or when they have not had access to the clinical records, as any unwitting errors that they make may later adversely affect their credibility. When she does speak with police the midwife should always retain a copy of any evidence or statement that she provides, and she should keep the contact details of any officer that she speaks to or who phones her. She should also carefully read through any statement or answers to questions that she makes before signing this as correct. If the matter goes to an inquest, the midwife's evidence may either be accepted 'on the papers', in which case she may not have to actually attend the hearing, or she may be summonsed as a witness and will then be required to be sworn in and to read her statement in open court.

In Australia, magistrates appointed as coroners do not conduct trials; they merely establish the facts as to the identity of the deceased, the cause of death and the circumstances surrounding the death, so the death can be recorded under the births, deaths and marriages legislation.

The coroner is concerned with causation, not fault. A Coroner's Court is generally more informal than an ordinary court and the rules of evidence do not apply. Nevertheless, the Coroner's Court has many of the trappings of an ordinary court. It is a public hearing, where witnesses give sworn evidence and are questioned by the coroner and may be cross-examined by lawyers representing the various parties. Witnesses can be summonsed to give evidence and the coroner can impose penalties should a witness fail to appear. Often media are present and report on what takes place.

It is not the role of the coroner to find a person or persons liable in negligence or guilty of a crime, but rather to establish how the person died. The coroner cannot frame his or her findings in a way that indicates either the guilt or negligence of a person involved with the person prior to the death. In New Zealand, if a coroner makes an 'adverse comment' about the acts or omissions of any provider, then he or she is required to give that person—or in the case of adverse comment about a dead person, to give the family—at least seven days' notice of the proposed comments. This enables the person or their representative to make submissions to the coroner in order to answer and defend the comments before the finding is released. If the coroner believes that an indictable offence has been committed, the appropriate authority, in most cases the Director of Public Prosecutions, is notified. The findings at inquest may provide relatives of the deceased with information indicative of negligence. It is then up to the relatives to pursue the matter through the civil courts.

At the conclusion of an inquest, a coroner may comment on any matter in relation to a death, including public safety or the administration of justice, and make recommendations. For instance, in New South Wales, an elderly patient died after suffering severe burns from a hot water tap in a shower. She was shocked by the rush of water and was unable to turn the tap off. By the time help arrived, she had been severely scalded and subsequently died. The coroner recommended that the temperature of water in hospitals and nursing homes be thermostatically controlled to avoid a similar occurrence in the future. While it is a recommendation, the appropriate departments have a responsibility to act on such a recommendation (Staunton & Chiarella 2003). Under New Zealand legislation, the coroner is also charged with making recommendations to try to bring to the attention of the public the circumstances of the death, in the hope of avoiding future similar deaths.

In Western Australia, a coroner may refer the matter to the registering authority/disciplinary body if the coroner believes that they may wish to inquire into the conduct of a member of that profession (s 50 *Coroner's Act 1996*, WA). Although other legislation may not have that express provision for informing a regulatory authority, the findings of a coroner may form part of a disciplinary hearing against a midwife.

Summary

It may be surprising to find that so much law applies to midwifery practice, but midwives can be reassured that they are rarely the subject of criminal or civil proceedings. It is hoped that this chapter has provided a helpful guide to the key statutes that relate to midwifery practice in Australia and New Zealand.

Review questions

1   What is the legislation that governs the regulation of midwifery in your state/country and what are the main functions of this legislation?

2   What is the definition of 'professional misconduct' in the state/country where you practise?

3   What would you do if someone made a complaint against your practice?

4   In New Zealand, what are your responsibilities under the Code of Health and Disability Services Consumers' Rights?

5   What is the process for consumers/clients to make a complaint about their care in your state/country?

6   What privacy requirements govern your practice?

7   Where and how should health information be stored (in your state/country)?

8   Can a midwife broker an adoption in New Zealand?

9   What documentation must be completed when a baby is born (in your state or country)?

10 What is the role of the coroner?

Note

1   (Where definitions differ between Australia and New Zealand they are provided in the text.) *Statute*: a law made by an Act of Parliament passed by a majority of elected representatives. (Orsman & Wattie 2001). *Regulation*: (for the purposes of this chapter) a rule or other order issued by a ministry or (government) department under authority delegated by parliament. A regulation has the force of law in Australia and New Zealand. *Common law*: originally defined as the ancient unwritten law of England, but it has come to mean the system of law based on old customs or court decisions, as distinct from statute law or the laws enacted by parliament (Orsman & Wattie 2001).

Online resources

Accident Compensation Corporation, www.acc.co.nz
Australasian Legal Information Institute, www.austlii.edu.au
Australian Government, Office of the Privacy Commissioner, www.privacy.gov.au
Health and Disability Commissioner, www.hdc.org.nz
Midwifery Council of New Zealand, www.midwiferycouncil.org.nz
Nurses and Midwives Board NSW, www.nmb.nsw.gov.au
Pharmaceutical Management Agency of New Zealand, www.pharmac.govt.nz

Privacy Commissioner, Te Mana Matapono Matatapu, www.privacy.org.nz
Public Access to Legislation Project, www.legislation.govt.nz

References

Balkin R, Davis J 2004 Law of torts (3rd edn). Lexis Nexis Butterworths, Sydney

Cartwright SR 1998 The report of the Commission of Inquiry into allegations concerning the treatment of cervical cancer at National Women's Hospital and into other related matters. Government Printing Office, Auckland

Department of Health 1990 Nurses Amendment Act 1990: Information for health providers. Department of Health, Wellington

Forrester K, Griffiths D 1991 Essentials of law for health professionals. Harcourt, Sydney

New Zealand Register of Births 1995 How to register the birth of your child. Register of Births, Wellington, September 2005

Nurses Board of Western Australia 2003 Annual report 2002–2003

Nurses Board of Western Australia 2004 Annual report 2003–2004

Orsman HW, Wattie N (Eds) 2001 The Reed dictionary of New Zealand English (3rd edn). Reed, Auckland

Rankin M 2001 Contemporary abortion law: the description of a crime and the negation of a woman's rights to abortion. Monash Law Review 27(2):229–252

Skene L 2004 Law and medical practice: rights, duties, claims and defences (2nd edn). Lexis Nexis Butterworths, Sydney

Staunton P, Chiarella M 2003 Nursing and the law (5th edn). Saunders: Baillière Tindall, Sydney

Wallace M 2001 Health care and the law (3rd edn). Law Book Company, Sydney

Statutes

Adoption Act 1955 [NZ]

Birth Deaths and Marriages Registration Act 1995, [NZ]

Birth Deaths and Marriages Registration Act 1995, NSW

Birth Deaths and Marriages Registration Act 1996, NT

Birth Deaths and Marriages Registration Act 1996, SA

Birth Deaths and Marriages Registration Act 1996, Vic

Birth Deaths and Marriages Registration Act 1997, ACT

Birth Deaths and Marriages Registration Act 1998, WA

Birth Deaths and Marriages Registration Act 1999, Tas

Birth Deaths and Marriages Registration Act 2003, Qld

Burial and Cremation Act 1964 [NZ]

Cemeteries Act 1986, WA

Children, Young Persons and their Families Act, 1989 [NZ]

Civil Liability Act 2002, WA

Community Health Services Complaints Act 1993, ACT

Contraception, Sterilisation and Abortion Act 1977 [NZ]

Coroners Act 1988 [NZ]

Coroner's Act 1996, WA

Cremation Act 1929, WA

Crimes Act 1958, Vic

Crimes Act 1961 [NZ]

Criminal Code 1913, WA

Criminal Law Consolidation Act 1835, SA

Donoghue v Stevenson [1932] AC562

Health (Notifications by Midwives) Regulations 1994, WA

Health Act 1911, WA

Health Act 1937, Qld

Health and Community Services Complaints Act 1988, NT

Health and Disability Commissioner Act 1994 [NZ]

Health Care Complaints Act 1993, ACT

Health Care Complaints Act 1993, NSW

Health Care Complaints Act 1995, Tas

Health Information Privacy Code 1994 [NZ]

Health Practitioners Act 2004, NT

Health Practitioner's Competence Assurance Act 2003 [NZ]

Health Professionals Boards (Procedures) Act 1981, ACT

Health Professionals Act 2004, ACT

Health (Retention of Health Information) Regulations 1996 [NZ]

Health Rights Commission Act 1991, Qld

Health Services (Conciliation and Review) Act 1987, Vic

Health Services (Conciliation and Review) Act 1995, WA

Hospital Regulations 1993 [NZ]

Human Rights Act 1993 [NZ]

Human Rights Amendment Act 2001 [NZ]

Injury Prevention Rehabilitation and Compensation Act 2001 [NZ]

Medicines Amendment Act 1999 [NZ]

Medicines Amendment Regulations 1995 [NZ]

Medicines Amendment Regulations 2001 [NZ]

Medicines Regulations 1984 [NZ]

Misuse of Drugs Act 1975 [NZ]

Misuse of Drugs Regulations 1977 [NZ]

Mutual Recognition Act 1992 (Cth)

New Zealand Bill of Rights Act 1990

New Zealand Public Health and Disability Act 2000

Nurses Act 1977, [NZ]

Nurses Act 1988, ACT

Nurses Act 1992, WA

Nurses Act 1993, Vic

Nurses Act 1995, Tas

Nurses Act 1999, SA

Nurses Amendment Act 1990 [NZ]

Nurses Amendment Act 2003, NSW

Nurses and Midwives Act 1991, NSW

Nursing Act 1992, Qld

Nursing Act 1999, NT

Ombudsman Act 1972, SA

Privacy Act 1988, Cth

Privacy Act 1993 [NZ]

Protected Disclosures Act 2000 [NZ]

R v Davidson [1969] VR 667

Regulations Act 1936 [NZ]

The Constitution of the Commonwealth of Australia

Further reading

Johnson S (Ed) 2004 Health care and the law (3rd NZ edn). Thomson, Brookers, Wellington

Mellars C, Cronin L, Merry A 1995 Is nursing a crime? Kai Tiaki: Nursing New Zealand, p 26

Newnham H 2003 Fetus v mother: who wins? Australian Journal of Midwifery 16(1):23–26

Pearse J 1998 Informed consent—issues for midwives. Presentation to the 5th National Midwifery Conference. Journal of NZ College of Midwives, p 22

Seymour J 2000 Childbirth and the law. Oxford University Press, Oxford

Slane B 2002 Guthrie tests: a report by the Privacy Commissioner. Office of the Privacy Commissioner, Auckland

Slane B 1999 On the record: a practical guide to health information privacy. Office of the Privacy Commissioner, Auckland

CHAPTER 12

Ethical frameworks for practice

Lynley Anderson and Bronwen Pelvin

Key terms

autonomy, beneficence, bioethics, code of ethics, ethics, informed consent, justice, non-maleficence

Chapter overview

This chapter outlines the philosophical underpinnings of midwifery and the history of the development of bioethics. The principles adopted in order to understand moral ethical approaches and informed consent are explored. The codes of ethics of the International Confederation of Midwives (ICM), the Australian College of Midwives (ACM) and the New Zealand College of Midwives (NZCOM) are also presented and discussed.

Learning outcomes

Learning outcomes for this chapter are:

1 To explore the philosophical framework of midwifery from a bioethical perspective

2 To describe moral concepts associated with midwifery professional practice

3 To outline the development of bioethics

4 To describe the four-principle approach to ethics

5 To provide a history of the development of the international codes of ethics

6 To examine the current midwifery codes of ethics in Australia and New Zealand.

The world of the midwife

Throughout history, midwives have assisted the birthing woman with companionship, guidance, knowledge and support. Midwifery has developed out of a particular human need and to respond to women as they experience a common and universal biological and physiological process.

However, midwifery is also created and affected by the social context in which it exists. Shifts in the way society is structured and functions affect how midwifery is practised. Some of those shifts have been discussed in earlier chapters, and have had a major impact on the place of midwifery in society. Other social reforms will affect how midwives respond to women in their care. There have been a number of interesting changes in society since the Second World War. Improvements have occurred in health, education and general levels of wealth. Such improvements, along with developments in levels of information and communication, have seen a move from attention to basic concerns of life to the challenging of authority and hierarchy within our society. The civil rights movement and the women's movement were two such changes that gathered force at around this time. These created a climate of growing social awareness of the need for widening the scope of activity to groups in society that had previously been denied. There has also been an increase in inclusiveness of all members of society, and an increased focus on individuals having a say in matters that affect them. This has led to a focus on what individuals want for their own life, with much emphasis on achieving goals and outcomes for the education, work, lifestyle, material possessions and so on that the individual decides upon. Individuals also began to challenge medical authority, wanting to have more say in their own treatment and care. The move to individuals having a greater say and involvement in their care has changed the way midwives and women interact.

In the West, we have to some extent distanced ourselves from our two biological endpoints, birth and death. Medicalisation and specialisation of both of these elemental human processes have removed them from the communities in which the birthing woman or the dying person lives. Healthcare is now most often delivered to individuals away from their homes, in institutions developed specifically for the purpose of delivering complex health services, with trained health professionals or specialists providing the care. Maternity care provision has also commonly been drawn into modern styles of health service delivery, with the development of large hospital-based services providing midwifery and medical services to women at the time of birth rather than through the continuum of the woman's maternity experience.

Some midwives and women in the West may look enviously at other cultures whose day-to-day existence is closer to the reality of birth and dying, and its impact. While there might be some appeal in this, there are also harsh realities faced by these communities, including the very real risks of dying, disability and loss associated with giving birth, to which the West is able to provide many solutions. At the same time, proximity to pregnancy, giving birth and breastfeeding ensures that young women in these cultures have absorbed knowledge of the process. They learn from a young age that birth is a normal physiological process that occurs as part of the nature of life despite the individual risks and outcomes that they observe.

We have also professionalised the people who provide care to those who are birthing or dying, so the knowledge is contained within the professional person. We now live in an age of 'expert-ism', with the public expecting that the 'expert' will have the answers to their life issues and the experiences and problems they encounter in living.

The sharing of the 'expert's' knowledge with a person and their family/whanau is dependent on the professional person's desire to share knowledge and power, and that is dependent on their plan and desire for their own life—are they an ambitious person, for example, wanting to succeed in their own professional realm? Do they wish to have 'power over' others to build up their sense of their own power? Do they have a social conscience, desiring to assist others by sharing knowledge and resources with others in their immediate community?

Philosophical underpinnings of midwifery

Over the course of a midwife's working life, whether she is aware of it or not, she will be using a framework for understanding and making sense of the way in which she practises midwifery and the style of care she provides to women and babies. For example, how much the midwife shares her knowledge and the degree to which she works alongside the woman and her family will be determined by the midwife's own particular philosophy about the manner in which care should be provided. This philosophy will have come from a number of sources, including her own belief system incorporating her cultural understandings, from the society in which she lives, as well as those from the midwifery profession. This framework could be thought of as being constructed from her values or those things she considers morally important.

Ethical reasoning informs a midwife's everyday clinical practice. The way a midwife relates to and interacts with a woman and her family, and the styles of care she chooses, all have an underlying ethical basis. Recognising the ethical dimensions of clinical practice is important in meeting the needs of the woman and her family and also in meeting the professional standards laid down by midwifery bodies.

A midwife will also encounter a number of complex ethical issues during the course of her professional life. Some of these might cause her to stop and think about what is the right course of action to take in the particular situation; in others, she might be very clear about the correct course of action. How she responds to these issues will depend on the ethical factors she believes most relevant to the issue.

Applying these values is not necessarily a simple task. For example, there might be problems if her ethical values conflict with those of the woman she is caring for, or the institution she may be working in. What if the ethical values she was raised with conflict with those of her profession? These questions raise some interesting issues for midwives, particularly with regard to the process of thinking through ethical issues arising in clinical practice.

Some examples of ethical issues that can arise in practice might include those where:

- the midwife perceives that the woman is making a decision that is not in the woman's best interests or her baby's best interests—for example, the woman may drink heavily or be taking non-prescription drugs during pregnancy
- the best interests of the baby compete with those of the mother—for example, the woman develops a life-threatening illness in pregnancy and refuses treatment to ensure her baby's survival; or the woman develops a complication of pregnancy and refuses treatment despite the fact that her baby will be severely affected or may die as a result
- a woman is limited in her ability to make decisions—this might be due to an oppressive partner, or mental disability or traumatic brain injury.

New reproductive and birthing technologies can also pose ethical issues for midwives. The rise of genetics and particularly prenatal genetic screening may stir ethical unease in many midwives, especially if abortion is involved. Because women now have fewer children, the pressure exists for each child to be the 'perfect' child, and the idea that there are now ways of ensuring that each child is 'perfect' can be enormously attractive to some people. Involving women in research also raises ethical concerns.

There is little doubt that these and many other contentious issues make midwifery an ethically interesting and sometimes challenging occupation. On reading a list of potential ethical concerns such as those listed above, many people will have a 'gut' response to some issues. And while this kind of response might be a good indicator that there is indeed an issue involved, gut instincts may be based more on our distaste for or level of discomfort with a situation. Being able to recognise an ethical issue in clinical practice is a good start, but getting to the heart of why these might be troubling, and beginning to unravel the issues requires a more systematic response. For that we begin by turning to the academic discipline of bioethics.

Bioethics is commonly described as a branch of applied moral philosophy.[1] In the midwifery context, bioethical approaches can be used to provide reasoned analysis of the array of ethical concerns. Ethical analysis can assist a midwife to untangle the issues involved in a particular situation, helping to identify and clarify the moral concerns and at times help her to find a resolution to the problem. We can explore an ethical problem using a variety of approaches. Each approach acts to highlight a different aspect of the particular problem.

Moral ideas from everyday life

All of us are familiar with moral concepts (although they might not have been identified as such) from our upbringing.

As young children we are taught a range of important moral ideas. We learn, for example, the importance of telling the truth and of not hurting others, the significance of keeping our promises and respecting the views of others, and about sharing, to name a few. These concepts are reinforced by our own experiences of what it feels like to be caught telling lies or to be hurt by others.

Much of the time these ideas work well—we keep our promises and others keep their promises to us, or we are kind to others, and so on. However, problems soon arise when we discover that in order to follow one concept, we can no longer comply with another. For example, if we are asked by a friend who is trying on clothes, 'Do I look fat in this?' we might begin to question whether honesty is indeed the best policy. So while honesty is an important concept for a young child to learn, later we might learn that complete honesty might cause harm to the feelings of others and that it may be better to say nothing or modify our statements than to tell the complete truth. However, as an individual moves into professional practice it is important to know when to apply which moral idea. For example, honesty may not be best when giving clothing advice to overweight friends, but for a woman in labour who has decisions to make, honesty will be required from her caregivers in order for her to make an informed decision.

Moral concepts in professional practice

As a student trains to become a midwife, moral ideas become increasingly important. Many of these are written into professional codes of practice that establish particular ethical standards of behaviour that midwives are expected to meet. These will be discussed later in the chapter.

Law and ethics

Expectations about the quality and standards of all health professionals in their dealings with those in their care may also be expressed in legislation. For example, getting informed consent from a woman prior to undertaking any treatment or care is now an expectation under New Zealand law. For a woman to be able to make a decision about her care, she must receive information about why something is being suggested and what it might mean to make each choice, as well as the risks and benefits, and so on. And so honesty is an example of a moral idea from early life that develops new meaning and legal expectations in professional midwifery care.

However, ethical reasoning is not simply an application of legal expectations in professional life. Law and ethics have much common ground, and yet they are distinct disciplines. What is ethically acceptable might differ significantly from what is legally acceptable. For example, some laws might be ethically unacceptable. There may also be times when an activity is not illegal but could certainly be considered ethically dubious. For example, imagine a woman who says she will take her lonely friend out to the movies, but later gets invited to a party with some people she has been trying for some time to impress. The woman then calls her friend to say she is sick, in order to break their arrangement so she can go to the party. Although she hasn't done anything illegal, we could question her standard of ethics.

A reason sometimes given by health professionals for complying with legislation put in place to protect those they care for is fear of legal reprisals for failure to do so. An example of this might be when getting informed consent from a woman. It is often heard that this is only done to avoid getting into trouble with the law. However, such a motivation—fear of legal punishment—fails to comprehend the ethical value in informing women, including acknowledging and respecting a woman's right to make decisions for herself.

The history and development of bioethics

Bioethics emerged during the last half of the twentieth century, partly in response to the revelation of unethical and unchecked action by doctors and scientists, but also in response to the exceptional clinical developments in healthcare at around that time, as well as the social changes already outlined at the beginning of this chapter. At the end of the Second World War, Nazi doctors being tried at Nuremberg revealed that horrific experiments had been carried out on prisoners of war and others. While many attributed these actions to the horrors of war and the monstrous Nazi regime, that doctors could be involved in such atrocities in the name of research was of major concern. Protection of research participants from unethical research was an important development resulting from the Nuremberg Trials.

Unethical research was found not to be limited to war when, in 1966, Henry Beecher wrote his famous article entitled, 'Ethics and clinical research'. This article uncovered 22 research studies he claimed were unethical, being carried out in US hospitals. The desire to improve clinical care had led many researchers to disregard the health and wellbeing of the research subject, many of who were vulnerable or considered to be of lower social class.[2] The Beecher article demonstrated that all was not well with medicine and science, particularly in the world of research. The need to protect the participants in research became paramount.

Developments in clinical medicine were burgeoning around this time and these also contributed to the development of ethical reflection on their use. One such clinical example of this kind of development was that of regular kidney dialysis in 1961—this provided an opportunity for lives to be extended where they previously would have ended. However, a shortage of dialysis machines meant that decisions had to be made about who should get this precious resource.

In New Zealand, the growth of bioethics can, in part, be attributed to the revelation of our own unethical research at National Women's Hospital in Auckland. In 1987, two journalists published an article in an Auckland magazine. This article detailed the research of Associate Professor Herbert Green into carcinoma in situ of the cervix (cervical cancer). A small number of doctors at the hospital collaborated with the authors after their own earlier attempts to call a halt to the

study had failed. The authors claimed that Professor Green (a consultant obstetrician and gynaecologist at National Women's Hospital in Auckland) had conducted a medical experiment in which conventional treatment was withheld without the women's knowledge and consent over a period of nearly 20 years. Professor Green believed that carcinoma in situ did not lead to invasive cancer, despite this being recognised internationally at the time. The intense public interest generated by the article led to the Minister of Health appointing Judge Silvia Cartwright to head an inquiry. The Inquiry validated the allegations of the article, concluding that 'for a minority of women, their management resulted in persisting disease, the development of invasive cancer and, in some cases, death' (Cartwright 1988). The Inquiry did not limit itself solely to the research project but also explored other related issues, such as patients' rights, medical power and hierarchy, and the problems of effective problem solving in medical institutions. The Cartwright Inquiry can be understood as the first public scrutiny of medical practice, research, education and institutions in New Zealand. One of the most significant outcomes in New Zealand has been the development of the Code of Health and Disability Services Consumers' Rights, which enshrines a code of patients' rights under legislation. Another important outcome has been the development of ethical review of research through a system of ethics committees.

The Cartwright Inquiry and the subsequent developments in patient rights and ethical review of research could not simply have occurred at any time; it needed the right socio-political conditions in which to emerge. The second wave of feminism and the rise of women's health issues surrounding women's reproductive choices was one of the significant issues of this time, creating a climate ripe for the examination of the practices of those in authority. Bioethics therefore has, to some degree, developed out of a social movement that challenges traditionally held authority and has been involved in empowerment of those who are socially marginalised.

Approaches to ethics

The four-principle approach to healthcare ethics

The framework most commonly seen within the bioethics literature is that of the four principles developed by Beauchamp and Childress (2001). These include: autonomy, beneficence, non-maleficence and justice. Although originally developed with medicine in mind, many of these concepts are valuable in other health professional contexts and will be discussed here. This framework also has some shortcomings, which will be discussed later in the chapter.

Autonomy

The term 'autonomy' literally means self-rule or self-determination. It means having the freedom to make decisions in line with how we want our life to be. Autonomy is based on the idea that we all have our own experiences, identities and significant features in our life; therefore it is thought that we will have the ability to judge what is best for us.

Autonomy means self-determination. In any individual case, autonomy may be influenced by the cultural values and beliefs of the individual.

The principle of autonomy requires that the right of each person to individual beliefs, desires, values and goals be respected and safeguarded.

Healthcare involves an agreed transaction between providers and user of services. Since the relationship behind the transaction is often one of unequal value, special care is required to ensure respect for the autonomy of users.

Respect for autonomy involves seven key points:

· effective communication
· adequate information
· comprehension
· competence
· absence of coercion
· the right to refuse proposed treatments and/or procedures
· advocacy (Ministry of Health, New Zealand 1991, p 9).

In healthcare, the concept of autonomy involves respecting the ability of a person to make choices about their treatment and for those choices to be respected. It implies that the individual has the competence to make decisions for themselves and also that they should not be coerced or forced into making decisions.

Autonomy in healthcare is a relatively recent development in line with the social changes outlined earlier. It has come about due to a rise in individualism and a growing desire for people to have increasing involvement in their own care. It is also a direct challenge to medical paternalism, where the doctor has traditionally been held to know what is best. The rise in autonomy has meant a shift in the locus of decision-making in healthcare from the healthcare professional to the person himself or herself.

Informed consent

One of the most important ways in which we can commonly see the principle of autonomy in action is through the process of informed consent. In the midwifery context, informed consent involves providing information to the woman and allowing her to either consent or refuse the suggested course of action.

Informed consent has two main components—the providing of information, and the giving of consent. These two components can be broken down further to:

● information
● comprehension
● competence
● voluntariness.

Take the example of a woman being presented with the option of a vitamin K injection for the baby following delivery. The midwife would need to provide *information* to the woman, telling her what vitamin K is and what it does, what the procedure entailed, what risks and benefits are associated with the injection (including short- and long-term benefits and risks), how much pain the baby would be expected to experience due to the injection, any possible effective alternatives, and what if any costs the woman might be expected to incur, and so on. The information needs to be provided in a way that the woman can understand. This does not mean that the woman should to be spoken down to, but that the information should be given at a level that is comprehensible to the woman, and is jargon-free. Midwives sometimes wonder how much information to give about a particular topic. Should they give out information about very rare complications related to some procedures? There are common concerns that this kind of information could frighten some people and put them off a procedure that might otherwise be helpful. In order to answer this we need to return to the concept of autonomy. To be truly respectful of autonomy, midwives are required to give the information. The extent of the information that needs to be given has been a topic under scrutiny in recent times, particularly in the courts.

The 'consent' part of informed consent involves considering the competence of the woman to give informed consent and the voluntariness of that decision. Under New Zealand law, every person is presumed competent to consent unless proved otherwise. For some, it may take more explanation, and the use of diagrams and other methods, but the presumption should be that nearly all women are able to give consent. Questioning the competence of a woman simply because she is making a choice that the midwife doesn't agree with is not acceptable and not in line with a respect for autonomy.

Consent should also be *voluntary*, meaning that it should not be coerced. An example of coercion would be if a midwife carrying out research tells a woman that she will withdraw some element of care if the women does not agree to take part in the research. The woman who consents under these circumstances could be said to have been coerced.

Informed consent should be viewed as an ongoing conversation between the midwife and the woman, not a one-off event. In this way the midwife is always checking with the woman that care is proceeding along lines that she is comfortable with.

We all are aware that some people will not be able to be autonomous, including a person with a severe and acute psychiatric illness, or severe brain injury. In these situations we might rightly question the competency of this person. There may be times, for example when people who are normally competent temporarily lose such ability, due, for example, to the administration of an anaesthetic or due to unconsciousness. Under these circumstances care can be provided that is perceived to be in that person's best interests, until such time as they recover their competency.

Beneficence

Acting in the way described above, in a way that promotes the best interests of others, involves the principle of beneficence. The principle of beneficence determines that we act in such a way as to provide benefit to or improve the wellbeing of those we provide care for. This is one of the fundamental principles underlying the provision of healthcare. The very purpose of healthcare in all its many forms is to improve the health and wellbeing of its recipients.

However, there are many accounts of what might constitute a benefit or an improvement in wellbeing. We know that people are different from each other—some like a life full of challenge and risk, while others prefer life to be more sedentary. Because we all differ, deciding on what a benefit is for others is a particularly difficult and dangerous task, and is best left to the individual to decide for themselves, unless they are unable to do so.

When dealing with pregnant women, the issue is compounded because caregivers might want to take into consideration the interests of the baby. How far should we go to safeguard the wellbeing of the baby? For most of the time, the best interests of both coincide: good nutrition for the mother will mean good nourishment for the dependent fetus. However, the interests of the two will diverge when a woman acts in a way that threatens the future of the unborn baby—by consuming excessive alcohol, for example, or using drugs. Should we override the wishes of the mother to defend the interests of the baby? This idea has been carried out with some pregnant women detained due to substance abuse, or forced to undergo a Caesarean section against their wishes. Some might point out that the woman has an interest not to be harmed by such detention or forced surgery, while others might claim that the interests of the baby outweigh the interests of the mother in both bodily integrity and freedom.

Non-maleficence

Non-maleficence can be understood simply as 'do no harm'. This principle requires that we do nothing that will harm or injure a person in our care. But what one person thinks as a harm may not be a harm for someone else. For example, a woman may consider that experiencing a birth without pain relief would be to suffer a great harm, whereas another woman might feel that to miss out on the birth process by taking pain relief would be harm. Given that we all differ in our preferences, the difficulty lies in how to determine what a harm is.

Justice

Within healthcare, the principle of justice dictates that healthcare services should be distributed fairly. There are two important ways in which this can be understood in healthcare. The first is with regard to providing care to people without discrimination. We need to take care that we are not discriminating against people because of their race, religion, sexual orientation, marital status and so on. Imagine two women needing midwifery care: one woman is married, has a mild heart condition and is having her third baby; the other is living in a lesbian relationship and is having her first baby. Do we provide different levels of care for each person? According to the principle of justice, both are given good quality care. However, that does not mean that we have to give out exactly the *same* care to each woman. Each will have different requirements: the woman having her first baby may require more time than the woman having her third. She may

require more detailed explanation about certain tests and procedures than the other woman, who has been through it all before. The woman having her third may require a little more attention in other areas, such as support with the two other children, and care with regard to how her heart condition might be responding to pregnancy and birth. So while each woman may require different care and more of the midwife's time at certain times during pregnancy and birth, this is due to the individual needs of each of the women, and not because of their marital status or sexual orientation.

The principle of justice may also have us pay attention to the allocation of resources on a much wider scale than that facing an individual midwife. In our society, for example, many people do not have equal access to a number of social benefits and appear to carry greater social burdens than the rest of us. Some of these inequalities can be expressed in poorer health statistics related to morbidity and mortality. Most caring societies wishing to promote at least some egalitarian principles would wish to ensure a basic quality of life for its most vulnerable and disadvantaged members. Policies will therefore need careful consideration to ensure that the distribution of health services does not exacerbate any existing inequalities in health, but attempts to mitigate them.

Some criticisms of a principles approach
No solution

Many authors have identified problems associated with a principles approach to ethical issues in healthcare. One of the most commonly identified problems is that the principles do not solve our problems for us. They might highlight particular issues and supply a framework for thinking about the issues, but provide no instruction on how to balance or rank the principles when they conflict.

No single unifying theory

Another criticism in the literature is that the principles do not represent a single theory, but result from taking a bit from one theory and a bit from another. For example, autonomy is said to be a concept borrowed from a Kantian idea of respect for persons and beneficence from John Stuart Mill (a utilitarian). Because each of these concepts comes from conflicting moral theories, criticisms are made that the principles lack internal consistency and should therefore be rejected.

Feminist objections

Feminist bioethicists have also objected to a principles approach to bioethics. Their objections centre on the failure of the principles to fit the moral experiences of women, and the lack of regard to the particularities of a given situation. They also claim that there is a lack of attention to the political and social dimensions of a situation, and therefore a lack of attention to issues of power and dominance in our society. Some feminist authors also object to the principles approach, saying that because they have emerged from a Western philosophic tradition, they are therefore male-dominated and male-orientated, and at times have been misogynistic.

Having emerged from a desire to protect vulnerable research participants, it appears odd that bioethics hasn't readily taken on some of the concerns of feminism, especially as many of the concerns appear to be paralleled. However, despite this, early bioethical writing has largely neglected the views of women, even when the topic has been of central concern to women. There has also been scant understanding of the hierarchical nature of medical institutions and its exclusion of women's voices and experiences. Many feminists have identified the gender blindness that exists in standard ethical theory and analysis, and have sought to remedy this by developing and promoting a feminist approach to bioethics.

Feminist approaches to ethics in healthcare

Feminist approaches to bioethics do not speak in one voice. Just as there are different approaches to feminist thought, so too there are multiple voices in bioethics. These might include liberal, cultural, radical, Marxist and psychoanalytical approaches, each highlighting a different aspect of oppression and possible solutions that might be appropriate.[3]

Feminist approaches to bioethics have focused on the 'concern to understand and eliminate the oppression of women in all its guises'(Crosthwaite 2001, p 32). However, although feminists are primarily interested in removing oppression based on gender, their moral opposition would expand to all forms of oppression. There are a number of areas in which a feminist approach to ethics would challenge traditional approaches to bioethics. A prominent writer in feminist bioethics, Susan Sherwin, has proposed that a feminist approach to bioethics might include not only re-examining existing areas of discussion using a lens of feminism, but also widening the debate to hear from other perspectives and turning to issues that concern these groups. She also suggests that feminist approaches would also use alternative methods for analysis and reflection (Sherwin 1998).

So how would this approach differ practically from a principles approach? An example might be that of a woman undergoing cosmetic surgery to enlarge her breasts. While a principles approach might consider factors such as her competence to consent and a discussion of her autonomous right to choose, a feminist approach might raise concerns about the subordination of women to oppressive ideas of beauty and youth and how women might be forced to conform to these in order to get work or please a partner.

Objections to a feminist approach

One of the most common criticisms of a feminist approach is that it does not offer an alternative moral guide. While a feminist approach might help to open the debate to wider issues than those presented under the four principles, those advocating other approaches might argue that feminism doesn't help to resolve the issue. Feminist approaches also vary widely, and so there are vastly different ways in which to respond.

Ethic of care

The ethic of care arose from women's experiences of caring for others. This theory is commonly used in nursing and specifically values the caring work that is done predominantly by women. The ethic of care originated from the work of Carol Gilligan (1982) who, in response to claims that women were morally less developed than men, theorised that women and men reasoned differently. When she asked a group of 11-year-old boys and girls how they would respond to an ethical problem, she discovered that males used principles more frequently, relying on the principle of justice in response to the case. Girls, on the other hand, made decisions based on which response provided the best outcome for maintaining the different relationships in the case. On the basis of this, and her work on women making abortion decisions, Gilligan created her theory. She argued that because women are involved in caring relationships due to their capacity to get pregnant, give birth and mother children, they are more attuned to the nurturing role and therefore would place greater emphasis on the quality of relationships. Caring 'involves responding to the particular, concrete, physical, spiritual, intellectual, psychic, and emotional needs of others' (Tronto 1989, p 174). An ethic of care values and fosters the web of relationships that exist between people. In many ways the ethic of care provides a challenge to what is sometimes referred to as the 'masculine' way of thinking that values abstract principles over the detail and particulars of caring. It takes account of the moral dimensions of care and what it means to care for others.

Some problems with an ethic of care

One of the problems with an ethic of care most commonly identified within the literature relates to the limits it places on women and men. If caring and relationships are indeed something that women do best, then how are they to escape it? Should we therefore expect women to take on the caring role in our society? Not surprisingly, many feminists object to an ethic of care because it appears to trap women in a biologically determined role. Understanding men as less able to care could be understood as freeing them from any expectation of caring. Men may also want to be involved in caring work, but may be limited because they are not thought to have such abilities under this theory.

Midwifery codes of ethics

As a way of explaining the nature of midwifery, professional organisations and regulatory bodies produce statements reflecting what the profession believes about itself. This is usually represented by a statement of philosophy—the values and belief system that underpin the working of the profession—or a mission statement that clearly identifies the purpose for which the organisation exists. Codes of ethics are written as guides to the correct or proper way for members of the profession to conduct themselves.

Codes of ethics act as a distillation of centuries of knowledge and wisdom that guides members of a profession in the 'right' way to maintain their relationships with the client group to whom they provide services. They guide the behaviour of members of the profession in a way that ensures that individual practitioners reflect the values on which the profession is based. Codes of ethics often reflect the highest human values as identified by religious, humanitarian and philosophical systems that have developed over centuries.

The frameworks created by the midwifery Codes describe and encapsulate the world and culture of midwifery. They provide the midwife with a reference point for making decisions about appropriate midwifery conduct in everyday practice as well as in situations that require complex examination and decision-making. Codes of ethics enable the midwife to examine her own values and beliefs and her professional conduct to see whether it fits within the midwifery values and belief system. Most importantly, these Codes assist each midwife to experience herself as part of a larger world—the world of midwifery, a world within the bigger world that consistently expresses certain values and beliefs about the best way for the world to work in the interests of women and the midwives that care for them.

The midwife has a role to play in guiding and supporting women and their families through the experience of childbearing in a way that assists them to make sense of the experience and derive maximum benefit from it for their ongoing life. It is critical that the midwife has a good grasp of the values and beliefs that the profession espouses so that she can display these in her everyday interactions with all the women she has contact with. This is irrespective of the role she may be in. She may be providing one-to-one continuity of care; she may be working shifts in a maternity facility—a birthing centre, a primary unit, a secondary or tertiary facility; she may be a manager of midwifery services or a facility; she may be an educator or professional advisor. The onus is on each individual midwife to ensure that she is grounded within the ethical framework of the profession so that she expresses its values and beliefs in her everyday work.

Codes of conduct and standards of midwifery practice are a further development and expression of ethical frameworks and provide guidance to the midwife and others about the standard of care women can expect from a member of the profession. Standards of Practice assist the midwife to apply the ethical framework in her daily practice and her relationships with the woman and her family. They assist her with her relationships with other midwives and colleagues of other professions with whom she works, as well as those who determine the shape of maternity service provision. Codes of conduct and standards of midwifery practice require ongoing application so that the midwife internalises the values and beliefs they express and, in that way, the midwife herself becomes the expression of those values and beliefs in the world.

Midwifery philosophies, codes of ethics, codes of conduct and Standards of Midwifery Practice give the midwife a valuable tool to use when she is reflecting on practice and developing herself into a critically reflective midwifery practitioner by giving her a framework for the expected behaviour of the professional midwife.

Three different midwifery organisations' codes of ethics are presented here in full to give a sense of what these guiding documents say about the way in which professional midwives are expected to behave.

International Confederation of Midwives Code of Ethics

The International Confederation of Midwives (ICM) represents the world's midwives. It has 85 Member Associations in 75 countries throughout the world. It exists to 'advance worldwide the aims and aspirations of the midwives in the attainment of improved outcomes for women, their newborns and families during the childbearing cycle using the ICM midwifery philosophy and model of care' (ICM 2005).

The goals of the ICM are to:

- work to improve women's health globally
- promote and strengthen the midwifery profession
- promote the aims of the organisation internationally.

To guide the profession of midwifery worldwide, the ICM has developed its Code of Ethics (Box 12.1) through a consultative process with its member associations.

Australian College of Midwives code of ethics

The Australian College of Midwives (ACM) is the professional organisation for midwives in Australia. It has a national office in Canberra and branches in the capital cities of each state or territory. Its purpose is:

- to provide a unified political voice for the midwifery profession
- to support midwives to reach their full potential
- to set professional practice and education standards
- to ensure that all childbearing women have access to continuity of care by a known midwife.

The ACM has developed a code of ethics (Box 12.2) to guide and support the midwifery profession in Australia.

New Zealand College of Midwives philosophy and code of ethics

The New Zealand College of Midwives (NZCOM) is the professional organisation and recognised 'voice' of midwives in New Zealand. NZCOM works in partnership with maternity consumer groups such as Parents Centre New Zealand, the Home Birth Association, La Leche League and individual women to ensure high-quality maternity services in New Zealand. The organisational structure of NZCOM reflects and supports this partnership between women and midwives by ensuring a place for women as well as midwives at every level of the College and in every College process. Through working in partnership with women the College aims to ensure that midwives remain professionally autonomous and that women have the opportunity to be in control of their childbearing experiences. The College has a national office based in Christchurch.

BOX 12.1 ICM Code of Ethics

PREAMBLE

The aim of the International Confederation of Midwives (ICM) is to improve the standard of care provided to women, babies and families throughout the world through the development, education, and appropriate utilization of the professional midwife. In keeping with its aim of women's health and focus on the midwife, the ICM sets forth the following code to guide the education, practice and research of the midwife. This code acknowledges women as persons with human rights, seeks justice for all people and equity in access to healthcare, and is based on mutual relationships of respect, trust, and the dignity of all members of society.

THE CODE

I. Midwifery relationships

a. Midwives respect a woman's informed right of choice and promote the woman's acceptance of responsibility for the outcomes of her choices.

b. Midwives work with women, supporting their right to participate actively in decisions about their care, and empowering women to speak for themselves on issues affecting the health of women and their families in their culture/society.

c. Midwives, together with women, work with policy and funding agencies to define women's needs for health services and to ensure that resources are fairly allocated considering priorities and availability.

d. Midwives support and sustain each other in their professional roles, and actively nurture their own and others' sense of self-worth.

e. Midwives work with other health professionals, consulting and referring as necessary when the woman's need for care exceeds the competencies of the midwife.

f. Midwives recognize the human interdependence within their field of practice and actively seek to resolve inherent conflicts.

g. The midwife has responsibilities to her or himself as a person of moral worth, including duties of moral self-respect and the preservation of integrity.

II. Practice of midwifery

a. Midwives provide care for women and childbearing families with respect for cultural diversity while also working to eliminate harmful practices within those same cultures.

b. Midwives encourage realistic expectations of childbirth by women within their own society, with the minimum expectation that no women should be harmed by conception or childbearing.

c. Midwives use their professional knowledge to ensure safe birthing practices in all environments and cultures.

d. Midwives respond to the psychological, physical, emotional and spiritual needs of women seeking healthcare, whatever their circumstances.

e. Midwives act as effective role models in health promotion for women throughout their life cycle, for families and for other health professionals.

f. Midwives actively seek personal, intellectual and professional growth throughout their midwifery career, integrating this growth into their practice.

III. The professional responsibilities of midwives

a. Midwives hold in confidence client information in order to protect the right to privacy, and use judgement in sharing this information.

b. Midwives are responsible for their decisions and actions, and are accountable for the related outcomes in their care of women.

c. Midwives may refuse to participate in activities for which they hold deep moral opposition; however, the emphasis on individual conscience should not deprive women of essential health services.

d. Midwives understand the adverse consequences that ethical and human rights violations have on the health of women and infants, and will work to eliminate these violations.

e. Midwives participate in the development and implementation of health policies that promote the health of all women and childbearing families. Revised May 1999

IV. Advancement of midwifery knowledge and practice

a. Midwives ensure that the advancement of midwifery knowledge is based on activities that protect the rights of women as persons.

b. Midwives develop and share midwifery knowledge through a variety of processes, such as peer review and research.

c. Midwives participate in the formal education of midwifery students and midwives.

(Source: International Confederation of Midwives 1993 Code of Ethics)

The College has developed both a philosophy and a code of ethics (Box 12.3) to guide the practice of midwifery in New Zealand. The philosophy of NZCOM is as follows:

Midwifery care takes place in partnership with women. Continuity of midwifery care enhances and helps protect the normal process of childbirth.

Midwifery is holistic by nature: combining an understanding of the social, emotional, cultural, spiritual, psychological and physical ramifications of women's reproductive health experience; actively promoting and protecting women's wellness; promoting health awareness in women's significant others; enhancing the health status of the baby when the pregnancy is ongoing.

Midwifery is: dynamic in its approach; based upon an integration of knowledge that is derived from the arts and sciences; tempered by experience and research; collaborative with other health professionals.

BOX 12.2 ACM Code of Ethics

I. The professional responsibilities of midwives

A Midwives in their professional capacity should at all times maintain standards of personal conduct, which reflect credit upon the profession.

B Midwives respect and maintain confidentiality of client information in order to protect the client's right to privacy, and use professional judgement when sharing information necessary to achieve healthcare goals.

C Midwives are accountable for their decisions and actions related to outcomes of their care of women.

D Midwives may refuse to participate in activities for which they hold deep moral opposition: however the emphasis on individual conscience should not deprive women of essential health services or respect for her culture.

E Midwives participate in the development and implementation of health policies that promote the health of women and childbearing families.

F Midwives are accountable for the dissemination of unbiased, current information to promote informed choice by women.

II Practice of midwifery

A Midwives provide care in partnership for women and childbearing families with respect for cultural diversity.

B Midwives encourage realistic expectations of childbirth by women within their own society.

C Midwives use their professional knowledge in collaboration with women ensuring that women are not harmed by conception, childbearing or birthing practices in all environments and cultures.

D Midwives respond to the psychological, physical, emotional and spiritual needs of women seeking healthcare whatever their circumstances.

E Midwives actively seek spiritual, intellectual and professional growth throughout their midwifery career, integrating this growth into their practice.

III Midwifery relationships

A Midwives respect a woman's right to make an informed choice and acknowledge her choice and support her in that choice.

B Midwives encourage and support women in their right to participate actively in decisions about their care. Midwives empower women to speak for themselves on issues affecting the health and welfare of women and their families in their culture/society.

C Midwives support and sustain each other in their professional roles, and actively nurture their own and others' sense of self-worth.

D Midwives liaise with other health professionals as necessary to ensure that women's needs for care are met.

E Midwives recognise the human interdependence within their field of practice and actively promote co-operation and mutual understanding.

IV Advancement of midwifery knowledge and practice

A Professional development encompasses a range of activities related to the advancement of midwifery knowledge, is based on skills, evidence based practice and inquiry that protects the rights of women.

B Midwives are responsible for maintaining a core of professional knowledge, through reflection on current practices and the initiation of new research.

C Midwives implement quality standards of practice through processes such as peer review, continuous quality improvement and research.

D Midwives support and actively participate in the education of midwifery students and each other.

(Revised 2001)

(Source: ACM, Code of Ethics)

(Currently under review)

Midwifery is a profession concerned with the promotion of women's health. It is centred upon sexuality and reproduction and an understanding of women as healthy individuals progressing through the life cycle.

Midwifery care is given in a manner that is flexible, creative, empowering and supportive (NZCOM 2005, p 3).

Despite the three Codes originating in three different midwifery organisations, there are consistent themes expressed in the statements. Broadly, there are three areas of midwifery ethical responsibility:

● the midwife's responsibility to the women she cares for
● the midwife's professional responsibilities
● the midwife's role in the wider community.

Underpinning the relationship the midwife has with the woman are respect for the woman's autonomy and culture. This is demonstrated by the need for the midwife to follow a process of giving unbiased and current information so that the woman makes informed choices and gives her consent for the care the midwife provides. The midwife has a responsibility to treat the woman's information as private and confidential. The midwife is responsible for meeting the woman's needs whatever circumstances the woman finds herself in. The word 'partnership' is used to describe the nature of the relationship between the midwife and the woman in the codes of ethics developed in Australia and New Zealand, and there is a clear expectation that the midwife will work in this way with the women for whom she cares.

Professionally, the midwife carries the responsibility and accountability for the care that she provides. This includes the necessity to recognise the limitations of her knowledge, experience and expertise and to make the necessary referrals to others. The midwife is responsible for her own ongoing education and professional development throughout her

BOX 12.3 NZCOM Code of Ethics

Responsibilities to the woman

a] Midwives work in partnership with the woman.

b] Midwives accept the right of each woman to control her pregnancy and birthing experience.

c] Midwives accept that the woman is responsible for decisions that affect herself, her baby and her family/whanau.

d] Midwives uphold each woman's right to free, informed choice and consent throughout her childbirth experience.

e] Midwives respond to the social, psychological, physical, emotional, spiritual and cultural needs of women seeking midwifery care whatever their circumstances, and facilitate opportunities for their expression.

f] Midwives respect the importance of others in the woman's life.

g] Midwives hold information in confidence in order to protect the right to privacy. Confidential information should be shared with others only with the informed consent of the woman unless there is a danger to her or her baby's life.

h] Midwives are accountable to women for their Midwifery practice.

i] Midwives have a responsibility not to interfere with the normal process of pregnancy and childbirth.

j] Midwives have a responsibility to ensure that no action or omission on their part places the woman at risk.

k] Midwives have a professional responsibility to refer to others when they have reached the limit of their expertise.

l] Midwives have a responsibility to be true to their own value system and professional judgements. However, Midwives' personal beliefs should not deprive any woman of essential healthcare.

Responsibilities to the wider community

a] Midwives recognise the Maori people as Tangata Whenua of Aotearoa and honour the principles of partnership, protection and participation as an affirmation of the Treaty of Waitangi.

b] Midwives encourage public participation in the shaping of social policies and institutions.

c] Midwives advocate policies and legislation that promote social justice, improved social conditions and a fairer sharing of the community's resources

d] Midwives acknowledge the role and expertise of community groups in providing care and support for childbearing women.

e] Midwives act as effective role models in health promotion for women throughout the life cycle, for families and for other health professionals.

Responsibilities to colleagues and the profession

a] Midwives support and sustain each other in their professional roles and actively nurture their own and others' sense of self-worth.

b] Midwives actively seek personal, intellectual and professional growth throughout their career, integrating this into their practice.

c] Midwives are responsible for sharing their Midwifery knowledge with others.

d] Midwives are autonomous practitioners regardless of the setting and are accountable to the woman and the Midwifery profession for their Midwifery practice.

e] Midwives have a responsibility to uphold their professional standards and avoid compromise just for reasons of personal or institutional expedience.

f] Midwives acknowledge the role and expertise of other health professionals providing care and support for childbearing women.

g] Midwives take appropriate action if an act by colleagues infringes accepted standards of care.

h] Midwives ensure that the advancement of Midwifery knowledge is based on activities that protect the rights of women.

i] Midwives develop and share Midwifery knowledge through a variety of processes such as peer review and research.

j] Midwives participate in education of Midwifery students and other Midwives.

k] Midwives adhere to professional rather than commercial standards in making known the availability of their services.

(Source: NZCOM 2005)

career. She has a responsibility to herself and her own moral code; she can refuse to participate in activities but she is not ethically able to deprive women of midwifery care. As a member of the midwifery profession, the midwife has a responsibility to support, sustain and nurture other midwives and to educate midwifery students and her colleagues. She also has responsibility for the advancement of midwifery knowledge while protecting the rights of women.

Within society, midwives act as role models for other women in the communities in which they live. They carry responsibility for ensuring that women and midwives have a say in the development of health policies that promote and protect the health of women and childbearing families, particularly working with women to set policy for the provision of maternity services.

The role of the midwife carries many responsibilities and these are specified in the codes of ethics for the profession. Clearly, these are not to be taken lightly. At the same time, the work of midwives is involved with the most joyous and life-affirming moments in the lives of women and their families. The ethical responsibilities that they carry need to be balanced with the satisfying role of assisting women to become mothers.

Ethics in practice

We have now explored some ethical theories and have looked at the codes of ethics for midwives; it is time to examine how the ethical frameworks work in practice. The following are real-life scenarios that midwives deal with in their everyday work. Read through the scenarios and use the following information to work out how you will deal with such matters when they arise in your practice.

Scenario 1

Mary and Phil are expecting their first baby and have engaged Trudy as their midwife. They have decided to have their baby at home and are very keen to have no intervention in the birth process. Mary goes into labour in the early hours of one morning and contacts Trudy after about four hours. Trudy visits and, during a palpation of Mary's abdomen, determines that the baby is lying in a breech position. Trudy explains the extra risks of a breech birth to Mary and Phil, and advises them that current practice recommends that they transfer to hospital for the birth and consult with an obstetrician. Mary and Phil decide that they do not want to change their plans, and they let Trudy know that they still want to go ahead with a home birth.

The midwife involved with this couple will need to be aware that Mary and Phil are making decisions from a position of little knowledge of the experience of birth but a great deal of knowledge of themselves, their capabilities and the type of birth they want to experience. One of the ethical responsibilities of the midwife is to provide Mary and Phil with the necessary and appropriate information to ensure that they are making an informed choice and understand what they are choosing. There is also the ethical issue of building up Mary's belief in herself as a birthing woman and there is a fine line between giving a woman the facts of this situation and not scaring her about the physiological process she is already embarked upon. The experience of the midwife in breech birth and the length of time she has been a practitioner are likely to have an impact on her ability to 'be with' Mary and Phil as they make this decision. It will influence the way in which she guides them through the decision-making process.

This case raises some interesting questions, such as: Are the risks to the baby from being born breech outweighed by Mary's claim to autonomy and her ability to determine the matter for herself? Irrespective of Mary and Phil's decision on where to have their baby, what is the midwife's responsibility to them? How does the midwife deal with the fact that there can be competing ethical responsibilities in dealing with an issue? Is there any overriding responsibility the midwife has in relation to Mary? Who might the midwife consult with if she is unsure of her responsibilities in this scenario? What is she entitled to do if she totally disagrees with Mary

and Phil's decision to stay at home? What support mechanisms might be put in place so that additional assistance and specialist expertise is immediately available should any complications arise during the birth or should the baby need resuscitation? Would consent need to be sought from Mary and Phil in anticipation of calling for specialist assistance if required?

Scenario 2

Sheralyn is expecting her first baby. She is 36 and has a career as a partner in a law firm. She makes it clear at her booking visit with the midwife that she plans to have a caesarean section at 39 weeks and will go back to work full time when the baby is eight weeks old, employing a nanny to take care of her child. She asks the midwife to refer her to an obstetrician who will provide this care.

In responding to this case, a midwife might want to begin by examining the choice Sheralyn is making. As pointed out earlier, there are good reasons why we might wish to support a woman in her choice and not override her views—after all, Sheralyn will probably be the best judge of what might be appropriate for her. The potential harms that may result from Sheralyn's choice might also need to be clarified and discussed with her. However, she may claim that such harms may be less significant for her than those associated with vaginal delivery. Turning now to feminism to explore this case, we would find that different branches of feminism would take differing views. For example cultural feminism may highlight the gendered nature of healthcare and how women are being influenced by beliefs that women's bodies are out of control and should be taken under the care of medicine. They might argue that such beliefs detach a woman from the capabilities and power of her body to give birth naturally. However, radical feminists might argue that women can only free themselves from oppression by removing the ties to reproduction. This group would want women to have a wide variety of choices that suit a variety of women and perhaps not to be subject to traditional ideas of childbirth.

For the midwife in clinical practice, Sheralyn's decision may not fit well with her philosophical position, and she may have to make a decision about whether she will continue care or pass her on to an obstetrician and midwife who specialise in this kind of care.

Scenario 3

Jenna is 16 years old and is pregnant with her first child. She first found out she was pregnant when she was already at 22 weeks gestation. Jenna was unhappy to discover she was pregnant but was too far advanced to meet the criteria for an abortion.

(continued)

Scenario 3—cont'd

She is now 25 weeks pregnant and has been heavily involved in binge drinking and sniffing solvents. Jenna was recently picked up in the street by police for disorderly behaviour while intoxicated. Sophie is Jenna's midwife, but they have had little contact because Jenna doesn't often make it to appointments. Jenna's mother says she is at her wits end with Jenna, as Jenna won't listen to her

Using the four principles to explore this case might instruct the reader to think about how we can benefit Jenna and her baby. Getting her away from solvents and alcohol would certainly benefit both her and her baby, but does this justify detaining her? This could risk alienating her from her caregivers and her baby when she realises that this is not happening to her friends who aren't pregnant. This raises another issue: should women be subject to a loss of freedom because they are pregnant? Another way of looking at this case might be to use an ethic of care. Jenna, her baby and her mother will still have some sort of a relationship long after the involvement of health professionals. How could a midwife foster such relationships? Planning appointments to suit Jenna might be a start. However, this may require some creative work from the midwife. Involving Jenna and her mother in her own care as much as possible will also help both of them feel more connected to the process.

Scenario 4

Cherry has been a midwife for five years and has recently taken on a position as a case-loading midwife in a hospital team. She has taken over the case-load of another midwife who has gone on maternity leave. Cherry has been in the position for three months and there is one woman, Marlene, who she is finding it difficult to get along with. Marlene is very critical of Cherry and keeps referring back to the things that her previous midwife said and did. Marlene is expecting her third baby and is now 35 weeks pregnant. Cherry is feeling increasingly uncomfortable in providing care to Marlene and is thinking about what her next step needs to be to resolve the situation.

In considering this scenario, the midwife has to weigh up her ability to develop a positive relationship with the woman to whom she is providing care. The midwife has the responsibility to provide a professional standard of care to the women for whom she provides midwifery care, and at the same time there is an expectation that there will be a working partnership between the two individuals involved. There are a number of approaches that can be taken when considering this scenario.

What is the nature of the partnership when one or other of the participants does not get on with the other? How is it possible to provide effective and professional midwifery care in this circumstance? Whose role is it to make the partnership work? What steps need to be taken when the relationship is not working for the midwife? In the absence of other care being available to the woman, what are the responsibilities of the midwife who is already involved with her? One aspect of this situation to consider is the developmental challenge provided to the midwife in terms of her ability to provide care to a wide range of women.

Research ethics and midwifery

The midwifery encounter does not just begin and end with maternity services as we commonly understand them to be. There is also potential for midwives to be involved in research. Having due regard for the research participant in research is also of ethical concern.s

Many midwives have a desire to understand more about pregnancy, childbirth and the social context in which these occur. This may be partly driven by aspirations to understand more or improve their own practice and the experience for women and their families. There is also a move within healthcare to base practice on firm foundations of knowledge rather than on an unsupported belief, theory or anecdote. All these factors have meant that many healthcare providers, such as midwives, are involved in research. However, whenever people are part of a research study there is always the potential for harm.

Ethical review of research involving human participants

We know from earlier in the chapter that research participants have not always fared well, and concern for their welfare has, at times, been lacking. There has been recognition worldwide that safeguards are required to ensure that the welfare of research participants is protected. In New Zealand and Australia, a formal process of ethical review for any research involving human participants is carried out by research ethics committees.

It may be thought that the review process is sometimes an unnecessary step in research. It could be claimed that midwives have the best interests of their clients at heart and so it is not necessary for anyone other than the midwife herself to decide about the ethical status of her research. However, midwives also undertake research because of their own interests—to publish, obtain degrees and advance their own profession. But the real issue here is not so much mixed motivation as the fullest possible protection of potential and actual research participants. It is widely agreed that this requires all proposed studies to be assessed by research ethics committees who have no vested interests in the research.

Ensuring the wellbeing of research participants

Consent

The primary means by which the wellbeing of participants is ensured is through participant consent. Ethical review aims to ensure that as far as possible no research participant will ever be the subject of research without his or her full, informed and continuing agreement. Ways of achieving consent include information sheets describing the intended research written in such a way as to be readily understood by someone new to the area of study. Participants need time to think about participation, and the option to withdraw without penalty, which means that there will be no reduction in the level or quality of care provided if they decide not to take part.

But even with all this in place, consent can be subtly compromised, for example in the actual circumstances in which it may be sought. A particular problem in midwifery-based research might be the occasions where the prospective participants are the clients of the researcher. The enthusiasm of the researcher-midwife for the research or the gratitude of a woman for what the midwife has done or is doing for her may make it difficult for the woman to refuse a request to participate in research. Overcoming these problems requires careful consideration of *how* women are approached and *who* makes that approach.

Calculating harms and benefits

Ethical review of healthcare research is commonly concerned not only with whether or not the risks of taking part in research are acceptable. This issue precedes the concern with consent and places some onus on the researcher to make sure that the planned research is minimally harmful *before* consent is requested.

Here it may be argued that midwifery research is unlikely to be harmful because midwifery research is likely to involve the woman as an informant, where she is asked to take part in an interview or questionnaire. The levels of risk of such research must be low compared to being in the trial of a new drug. But harm can come from all kinds of sources, including questioning and interviewing. *What* is asked, and *how* it is asked, are of ethical interest.

In addition, some research, while not actually producing harm, is incapable of producing benefits—because the design of the study is inadequate, for example. Research that cannot meet its own aims is pointless, and in such a case if the research proceeded then any risk or even inconvenience to the participants would be unacceptable.

Confidentiality

It is common for ethics committees to demand that those who participate in research have their identities protected in any published (that is, publicly available) form of the research, unless they have agreed to being identified. Research undertaken by midwives commonly involves women telling their experiences, and care must be taken to ensure that confidentiality is maintained.

Innovative practice

In any clinical practice, such as midwifery, there is constant innovation. Midwives will become aware of new techniques and may see situations where they can try these, believing that they may be just what the woman needs. This kind of evolving innovative practice is common but raises some ethical questions, such as: Is this practice effective in the situation where I am using it? Can it cause harm? These questions cannot be addressed without proper research. Midwives, as with all healthcare professionals, need to be alert to when a developing practice requires research to validate its use before it becomes a new and accepted practice.

Research involving people automatically raises ethical issues, and there is international agreement that a process of ethical review centred on certain key issues is essential. These include consent, confidentiality and an evaluation of harms and benefits. In the midwifery context there are some specific subtle issues that arise in relation to these and to the question of what counts as, and/or needs, research.

Conclusion

This chapter has introduced the ethical constructs of the midwifery profession. It has presented codes of ethics for the midwifery profession and examined how these create the midwifery world. It has also presented the development of bioethics and critiques of the bioethical approach as an introduction to ethical thinking in the provision of healthcare. Finally, it has looked at ethical dilemmas that midwives may confront in their everyday practice and the guidance that professional codes of ethics may provide the individual midwife in exploring the dilemmas that arise.

Review questions

1　Briefly describe the philosophical underpinnings of midwifery.

2　Discuss the way in which ethical reasoning can affect the everyday clinical practice of midwives, and provide a case scenario.

3　What strategies can midwives employ in applying moral concepts to their professional midwifery practice?

4　Discuss the importance of gaining informed consent from women undergoing treatment or care.

5 Briefly discuss the history and development of international codes of bioethics.

6 List the components of the four-principle approach to healthcare ethics.

7 Discuss, in a paragraph, the idea of 'do no harm' and its application to midwifery care.

8 Describe the history of the development of international midwifery codes of ethics.

9 Briefly discuss the current code of ethics of the Australian College of Midwives Incorporated (ACMI).

10 Name three elements from the philosophy and code of ethics of the New Zealand College of Midwives.

Notes

1 Strictly speaking the term 'bioethics' is used to refer to the moral concerns in all areas of life, including human, animal, plant and environmental areas. However in this chapter we will limit this term to refer to ethical analysis of midwifery practice only.

2 Examples of such research can be seen in the Tuskegee experiments uncovered in 1972. For further discussion see McNeill, *The Ethics and Politics of Human Experimentation* (in Further reading).

3 For further detail on the different varieties of feminism see Rosemary Tong, *Feminine and Feminist Ethics* (in Further reading).

Online resources

Australian College of Midwives, http://www.acmi.org.au

Childbirth Connection, http://www.chilcbirthconnection.org/home. asp?Visitor=Professional. Note the report on a recent study of women's choice of caesarean section.

International Confederation of Midwives, http://www.international midwives.org

Midwifery Council of New Zealand, http://www.midwiferycouncil.org. nz

New Zealand College of Midwives, http://www.midwife.org.nz

Nursing Midwifery Council, http://www.nmc-uk.org. See in particular circular 8/2006

References

Beauchamp T, Childress J 2001 Principles of biomedical ethics (5th edn). Oxford University Press, New York

Brenner J, Gillies J, Pickering N 2004 The ethics of health infomatics. Mediflex, Auckland

Crosthwaite J 2001 Gender and bioethics. In: H Juhse, P Singer (Eds) A companion to bioethics. Blackwell, Oxford

Gilligan C 1982 In a different voice. Harvard University Press, Cambridge

International Confederation of Midwives (ICM) 1993 International code of ethics for midwives

International Confederation of Midwives (ICM) 2005 Mission statement

Ministry of Health New Zealand 1991 Principles and guidelines for informed choice and consent. Ministry of Health, Wellington

New Zealand College of Midwives (NZCOM) 2005 Midwives handbook for practice. NZCOM, Christchurch

Sherwin S 1998 Health care. In: A Jaggar, IM Young (Eds) A companion to feminist philosophy. Blackwell, Mass., pp 420–428

Tronto J 1989 Women and caring: what can feminists learn about morality from caring? In: AM Jaggar, S Bordo (Eds) Gender/ body/knowledge: feminist reconstructions of being and knowing. Rutgers University Press, New Brunswick, NJ, pp 172–187

Further reading

Charlesworth M 1993 Bioethics in a liberal society. Cambridge University Press, Cambridge

Gillett G, Campbell A, Jones G 2001 Medical ethics (3rd edn). Oxford University Press, Melbourne

International Confederation of Midwives 1993 International code of ethics for midwives

Jecker N, Jonsen A, Pearlman R 1998 Bioethics: an introduction to the history, methods and practice. Jones and Bartlett, Sudbury

Johnstone M 1994 Bioethics: a nursing perspective (2nd edn). WB Saunders, Sydney

Mappes T, DeGrazia D 1996 Biomedical ethics (4th edn). McGraw-Hill, New York

McNeill P 1993 The ethics and politics of human experimentation. Cambridge University Press, Cambridge

New Zealand College of Midwives 2005 Midwives handbook for practice. NZCOM, Christchurch

Nie J-B, Anderson L 2003 In: J Peppin, M Cherry (Eds) Bioethics in New Zealand: A historical and Sociological Review. Swets Zeitlinger Lisse

Pickering N, Anderson L 2004 The importance of ethical review in midwifery research. Journal of the New Zealand College of Midwives 30:15–16

Taylor R 2004 Midwifery, professional misconduct and codes of ethics: an analysis of findings by the Accident Corporation, the Health and Disabilities Commission and the New Zealand Nursing Council 1996–2003. New Zealand College of Midwives 8th Biennial National Conference Proceedings

Tong R 1993 Feminine and feminist ethics. Wadsworth, Belmont, CA

Tronto J 1989 Women and caring: what can feminists learn about morality from caring? In: AM Jaggar, S Bordo (Eds) Gender/ body/knowledge: feminist reconstructions of being and knowing. Rutgers University Press, New Brunswick, NJ, pp 172–187

Wolf S 1996 Feminism and bioethics. Oxford University Press, New York

Acknowledgements

The authors would like to acknowledge Claire Gallop for her valuable comments on an earlier draft. The authors would also like to thank Neil Pickering and the *Journal of the New Zealand College of Midwives* for permission to use sections regarding research ethics. The original article was co-authored with the first author of this chapter.

CHAPTER 13

Life skills for midwifery practice

Bronwen Pelvin

Key terms

autonomy, boldness, commitment, companionship, curiosity, decisiveness, empathy, friendliness, generosity, honesty, integrity, life skills, negotiating, organisational skills, positivity, practicality, reflectiveness, relationships, robustness, self-care, self-knowledge, self-responsibility, work–life balance

Chapter overview

This chapter identifies a number of 'life skills' that are required for midwives to fulfil their role in working 'with' women through the life experiences of pregnancy, birth and new mothering. These life skills include the development of personal attributes needed to be in relationships with women and of skills that assist midwives to sustain and maintain their midwifery practice.

This chapter is experiential, as it provides the personal perspective of one midwife with a long involvement in midwifery practice across all settings and draws on knowledge derived from practice rather than theory. Unlike other chapters in this book, this chapter is not based on research or other evidence from current literature. Instead, the author offers guidance to midwives based on her knowledge and understandings and derived from reflective midwifery practice.

Learning objectives

Learning outcomes for this chapter are:

1 To explore the role of a midwife and the nature of midwifery practice

2 To identify and explore the essential qualities of a midwife

3 To identify and explore the life skills necessary to undertake the work of a midwife

4 To identify and explore concepts of 'self-care' and 'work–life balance' in relation to sustaining midwifery practice.

Introduction

Women rarely go through their childbearing experiences totally on their own. Each woman comes with not only her own personal context but also her social context. Each woman's personal context is made up of her life stage, stage of personal development, educational background, spiritual beliefs, personal values that she holds and the nature of her relationships with those in her immediate social circle. Her social context consists of the wider community, social group, ethnic or religious community that she lives within and the values and beliefs that those groups hold and how these influence the woman's life.

Consequently, a midwife has to develop the ability to make an analysis of the total context of each woman and her family/whanau as well as the ability to develop a meaningful and purposeful working relationship with each woman as together they travel the journey of pregnancy, birth and the postnatal period. The way these working relationships develop will depend to a large extent on each individual midwife and where she is on her own professional and personal development journey. The learning she does as a midwifery student and the knowledge she gains through her practice experiences unite into her journey of development as a professional midwife.

The nature of midwifery practice requires the development of skills and abilities within each midwife to support the work that she is required to do in her working relationships with each woman and her family. It is useful for a midwife to understand the skills and abilities that will continue to develop along with her midwifery practice as she builds practice wisdom through her experiences as a midwife.

Midwifery, centered as it is in human relationships and assisting an individual through a universal, yet highly personal and intimate life experience, requires practitioners who are able to bring sensitivity, support, compassion and generosity to those for whom they are providing care. The position of midwife is one of privilege—the intimate nature of the work places a midwife in a position of close proximity, learning, noticing and observing how a woman functions at a fundamental level and in her relationships with those nearest and dearest to her, as she experiences one of life's pivotal events. Midwifery relationships, at their best, facilitate not only the physiological process of pregnancy, giving birth and the early mother–baby relationship but also the growth and development of each woman and a deepening of her relationships with those in her family/whanau.

This chapter discusses the personal qualities and skills a midwife needs in order to be able to meet the demands of her profession. Midwifery education programs can assist individuals to prepare for the role of midwife by helping students begin to develop the necessary skills and abilities. This chapter will focus on identifying some of the life skills required to carry out, support and sustain the work of a practitioner of the art and science of midwifery.

The nature of midwifery and the role of the midwife

Midwifery is concerned with the making of mothers. At the core of midwifery is the relationship between each mother and her baby. Midwives know that this relationship is critical for the baby's physical, mental, emotional and spiritual survival. Midwives know that this relationship has a profound effect on the mother's sense of her own power, her ability to give and nurture life and her core sense of herself as a woman and as a human being. Midwives understand the intensity of the feelings attached to this experience and the need for the mother to allow herself the deepest sense of love that she may yet have experienced. Midwives know that it is critical for the baby to grow and develop in a world of love, understanding, generosity and abundance, in order to lay the foundations for its ongoing development for the rest of its life.

There is also the nature of each woman's relationships with the others in her immediate family/whanau/social network to consider. Midwives facilitate the development of the necessary support systems so that family and friends will support the mother in her primary role in ensuring the wellbeing of the baby. The midwife acts as a source of information and guidance; she acts as an educator of the wider family group and the community. As life has become more technologically advanced and complex, the midwife acts as holder of some fundamental truths of human existence, the things we can and must do to ensure that our lives have depth and meaning and that we are connected with each other. This is expressed around the universal act of giving birth; the truths evident here are applicable to the rest of our lives.

The role of the midwife is a large one in whichever society the midwife lives and works. It is a role that the individuals who take up midwifery grow into. Each midwife does not emerge from her educational program 'fully formed'. As a new practitioner, each midwife cannot be expected to have the wisdom of the ages in her bones. It can be expected that she will have the competencies of a registered midwife and a willingness to go on learning through her experience.

Developing the role of the midwife

The ability to enact a particular role within a society requires development that occurs in a certain way. First it requires integration of the individual's own context and personal development with the requisite knowledge, skills and abilities of the role. Second, it requires acknowledgement that maturity and wisdom both develop over time and that therefore an individual who pursues midwifery will mature over time into a 'self-actualised' midwife, able to meet the obligations that the role and society demand.

Consequently, the focus is on developing each midwife's ability to know herself as a person and as a professional practitioner. Midwifery will make certain demands on those who practice, demands that, in the main, will be a pleasure and a joy for the midwife to meet. However, some demands will challenge the midwife to the foundations of her own sense of herself and her belief in the purpose of life and the nature of meaningful work. Fortunately, a midwife's experience takes place over many periods of time, as midwives take on different roles within the profession and move in and out of full- and part-time work depending on their personal life circumstances. There is an interesting synergy to an individual's development as a midwife. To be a midwife requires a certain degree of personal development and maturity; but the practice of midwifery itself provides important opportunities for individuals to develop maturity and wisdom. Each midwife's professional life can be viewed as a continuous stream of learning opportunities and challenges. In so doing it is useful to identify some of the qualities that will sustain each midwife in her ongoing midwifery life and keep her open to learning from the deep and rich experiences that midwifery practice offers.

Qualities for midwives

Robustness

Being robust means being able to withstand what life presents to you, able to pick yourself up after being knocked over and carry on. The word 'robust' means strong and healthy, sturdily built, requiring and displaying physical strength. In the case of the midwife, this is translated into the mental, emotional and spiritual characteristics necessary to assist women and their families through the experience of childbearing and the number of challenges that can occur in any life experience.

Midwives deal with life 'in the raw', life as it is lived by women who rely on them for information, support and guidance. This means each midwife has to develop the ability to deal with what is happening in the 'here and now' and continue to work with each woman and her family to support them through their experiences. This requires stamina, fortitude and physical and emotional strength as well as the ability to keep thinking, assessing and planning.

Empathy

Empathy is the ability to sense and understand someone else's feelings as if they were one's own. It is necessary for midwives to develop this ability to a high degree in order that they can put themselves in each woman's position and have a sense of what it is like for her. There is a potential danger in a midwife over-identifying with a woman, and this may lead to a desire to have the woman's experience for her or to protect her from the experience that she is having. Empathy has to be tempered by the ability to set clear boundaries and have respect for each woman and her autonomy. The ability to empathise leads to acceptance of another and understanding of what their life is like for them.

Empathy is derived from communicating with each woman to discover what her feelings are about any given situation that arises in her experience. There is no room here for making assumptions about what a woman may or may not be experiencing. Whatever a midwife thinks a woman is experiencing needs to be checked out to ensure that the midwife is not projecting her own thoughts and feelings into the situation.

Companionship

The word 'midwife' is derived from the Old English *mid*, meaning 'with' and *wif*, meaning 'woman'. At the core of the word is the concept of being a companion to a person, being alongside them, journeying together. Thus a midwife takes on the role of a companion and the nature of the work requires her to be able to assist a woman to make sense of her experience bit by bit and as a whole. But it is not just being a companion; it is being a companion in a certain way.

Midwifery companionship is based on midwifery knowledge, knowledge derived and distilled from centuries of attending women in childbirth. This includes knowledge of: the anatomy and physiology underlying the physical process of reproduction; human psychology, developmental psychology and the nature of human relationships; social, cultural and spiritual contexts of each woman; and women's wellness, place in society and networks of support. Midwifery companionship is grounded in the belief of each woman's ability to give birth—to grow and nurture a baby through pregnancy; to initiate, go through labour and give birth; and to nurture and care for a newborn infant and sustain its life in the first weeks after birth. Midwifery companionship is also grounded in respect for each woman, her life experience so far, and both the woman's and the midwife's own capacities to learn from experience.

Honesty

Honesty is the quality of being truthful and trustworthy. It can be applied to relationships where openness and sincerity characterise the interactions between the participants, who present themselves as they are.

In midwifery, honesty pertains to the ability of a midwife to present herself, her way of working, her knowledge, beliefs, assessments, opinions and the available evidence about her choices for care to each woman truthfully so that meaningful discussions can occur about the care needed by each woman and her family/whanau. There is an art to presenting the midwifery 'truth' while still leaving room for a woman and her family/whanau to express the truth of the matter from their perspective. There is an art to being able to contain more truths than just one's own and to work for a way forward if the truths are different or in conflict.

Commitment

Commitment is about honouring the intended purpose of each midwife/woman relationship, and a midwife is involved in providing services that meet the maternity needs of women and their families. A midwife has to develop the ability to be committed to the work and to each woman for whom she cares. She will do this in different ways, depending on the midwifery role she is in. One of the most binding commitments a midwife can make is to provide continuity of care to a woman throughout her childbearing experience. A midwife makes herself available to respond to a woman and the unpredictable nature of her experience, whenever and however it occurs.

Midwives working in other midwifery roles—shift work within a maternity facility, as a midwifery educator or advisor—also express commitment to their work by being available for the work at regular times and being available to others during the times of work and often outside those times of work as well. When at work, these midwives express their commitment to the profession by engaging with the women for whom they care, the students they teach and the midwives and others they advise.

The law requires commitment from registered midwives. There are regulatory requirements that midwives have to meet and, depending on how maternity services are managed, contractual obligations for service to fulfil. The midwifery profession requires commitment from midwives. The profession expects them to provide midwifery care to a professional standard, and articulates what the professional standard of care is and what midwives need to do to provide it.

Integrity

Integrity implies consistency between the spoken word and the actions of an individual. It can be defined simply as honesty, the capacity for truthfulness, but there is an extra dimension connected to being united or whole. The word can be applied to a person's functioning to describe the way in which their behaviour reflects their expressed belief system and their intentions. As a professional person, a midwife has an ethical responsibility to be consistent in what she says and does. This also applies to her words and actions being consistent with the professional expectations of her as reflected by professional regulatory requirements, codes of ethics and philosophical statements.

Decisiveness

The role of the midwife requires the ability to make decisions. Decision-making requires the midwife to take in all the information about a certain issue, practice or course of action, weigh up the information and determine what aspects of the issue are more critical or pressing, examine her own thoughts and beliefs about the information, and come to a decision about what is required or what advice to give the woman and her family. In most situations, this process can be leisurely and thoughtful, but there are also circumstances that require decisions to be made quickly because the life or wellbeing of the woman or her baby is at stake.

Curiosity

Pregnancy, labour, birth and the postnatal period are biological, physiological, mental, emotional and spiritual processes that a woman experiences. This means they are as dynamic and varied as each woman who experiences them. A midwife is involving herself in a life event and it is being lived forward, without the benefit of hindsight, until it is completed. A midwife will benefit from curiosity in her work—the eagerness to know or find out.

Despite her basic knowledge of the process of childbearing, each time a midwife encounters the experience it is with a different woman. Each time she encounters the childbearing experience with the same woman, the woman is in a different place on her developmental journey and the process is another singular event in her life—it is 'this time', not the last time or the next time. Nothing can be assumed or taken for granted.

Curiosity will enable a midwife to sustain her interest in the childbearing process. It will open her up to being responsive to what is in front of her, continuing to learn, assess and report on the event for the woman and her family/whanau.

Practicality

Midwives are often known and respected for their sense and practicality. Practicality is derived from experiences and actual use rather than from theory. The involvement of midwives with women in their everyday lives affords them a wonderful opportunity to see women coming up with practical solutions to the management of pregnancy, labour and the care of the newborn. As women, midwives have often had these experiences themselves and can report on what they have found helpful. They can also report what they have noticed in other women's childbearing experiences and contribute to the dissemination of knowledge. In this way midwives act as conduits of sensible, useful and effective responses to the situations women encounter as they journey through their childbirth experience.

Boldness

Courage, confidence and fearlessness typify the midwife's functioning in the world. This is not a profession for retiring, 'shrinking violets'! When a midwife deals with all the possibilities and variations of a physiological life event and the potential for disappointment, grief, shock and trauma as well as enormous joy, elation, love and compassion, she must develop the capacity to be bold—to go where no one else has gone, to risk uncertainty and to respond to changing and unknown situations.

Women and their families/whanau can face their deepest fears as they approach childbirth in today's risk-averse society. There is a strong drive for guarantees and perfect outcomes, not least because women have fewer babies than they have ever had before in the history of the human race. They want every baby, particularly their baby, to be perfect. The opportunity to learn about the nature of life from many different experiences is reduced and maximum learning has to be derived from the experiences that each person has. Medical dominance of the reproductive process and the reflection of that dominant view in the media has created a degree of fear in the community that the midwifery profession, coming as it does from a belief in a woman's ability to grow, nurture, give birth to and feed her own baby, has to withstand.

It is work in itself to present a different view of childbirth to women informed by magazines, newspapers, radio and television that seem intent on sensationalising only the most dramatic and often negative stories about birth. It requires effort to sustain a belief in the physiological process and to defend women's ability to achieve their biological purpose with a minimum of intervention from any quarter. From a midwifery perspective, there is a need to support this approach to ensure that women are built up in their sense of their own competence. This is essential for the wellbeing of women, babies, families and society; and midwives, individually and collectively, have a great responsibility to contribute.

Reflectiveness

Introspection is an essential ability for a midwife in order to process and make sense of her professional experiences. She needs the ability to reflect on her practice in order to grow and develop in experience and practice wisdom. She needs to reflect on her own functioning with women and their families to learn more about ways in which she can make a positive contribution to their lives.

A midwife must be able to both reflect internally and express that reflection in the company of others, to ensure that she is maintaining practice in the way in which the profession expects. A midwife also has to be able to place her own personal, professional experience within the context and frameworks that create the midwifery world.

Friendliness

The nature of midwifery work requires midwives to move in and out of women's lives and the lives of their family/whanau members. A midwife needs to develop an open and welcoming demeanour that demonstrates goodwill towards others, a quality reflected in the word 'friendliness'. Being friendly carries the suggestion of being on the same side, disposed towards being helpful and supportive. It is this concept that is reflected in the slogan 'Midwives help people out' used in the New Zealand College of Midwives' promotional material.

Generosity

Generosity is a quality that women value highly from their midwife or the midwives who attend them while they are in hospital. Generosity means a willingness to give time, attention, knowledge; freedom from pettiness and meanness; the sense of abundance and plenty. Women appreciate midwives giving them the necessary time to deal with their concerns, to assist them through the decision-making process, attending them throughout their labour and birth, providing support and knowledge as they respond and develop as mothers in the postnatal period—all in an unhurried, stress-free and easy manner.

There will be times in every midwife's life when she finds herself unable to continue to be generous. At this time she needs to resource herself adequately through taking a break, talking with family, friends and colleagues, seeking professional guidance or assistance and other means, in order to restore her faith in herself and human nature, to enable her to again approach her work in the spirit of generosity.

Positivity

Positivity in the midwifery profession is the quality that assists women to believe in their ability to grow and develop a baby during pregnancy, to experience labour and give birth and to become a mother. This quality is grounded in a midwife's belief, knowledge, understanding and experience of a woman's physiological process and her body's ability to do what, from a biological and evolutionary point of view, she is designed and equipped to do. Positivity is characterised by affirmation of each woman and the biological process she is undergoing, as well as expressing certainty in that process and in a woman's ability to learn throughout her experience.

Midwives are fortunate that they are in touch with a life-giving process on a regular basis, and with new life as they greet each new baby along with its mother, her family and her friends. There is magic in birth and in seeing a woman in all her power and glory. There is magic in the resolution of difficult obstetrical problems to a safe outcome and a happy meeting of mother, baby and family. It is this magic that nurtures positivity in individual midwives and the profession. It can be used to replenish and restore midwives so they can support and nurture other women and families through the same process.

In summary

Naturally, these are not the only qualities that midwives will have or continue to develop. The qualities described above are some of those that a midwife will find useful for sustaining herself as a practitioner. The ongoing development of all of these qualities in a midwife will ensure that the women and the families with whom a midwife comes into contact, will benefit from her involvement with them.

The qualities described above give some indication of the expansive nature of midwifery work. As one person within a network of women, families and communities, a midwife, by the nature of her involvement in an individual's intimate life experiences, has a wide sphere of influence. Think of a pebble being dropped into a pond—the initial impact may be small but ripples spread in ever-widening circles—a midwife in her working life touches many lives.

Reflective exercise

1. Get together with one other student from your class. Discuss the preceding qualities and identify which ones you have developed well in your functioning; which ones you have but need to develop further; and which ones are absent from your functioning.
2. Identify three ways in which you can strengthen each quality that is under-developed and one way in which you can begin to develop the qualities that are absent from your functioning.
3. Write down your findings and your plan, for future reference.

Sustaining midwifery practice

Let us now move on to explore the way in which a midwife can sustain herself to be able to express these qualities within her working life and fulfil her role as a midwife.

Self-knowledge

How does a midwife come to know herself as both a person and a midwife? Every midwife needs to gain a sense of herself as a 'work in progress', on her own unique professional and personal journey. Inherent in the nature of professional practice is the concept of ongoing and continual learning from experience. Central to the professional midwifery practitioner is the idea that the learning and knowledge gained from all she experiences will be integrated into her functioning, and that her clients will benefit from the practice wisdom she develops over time.

The nature of midwifery work will assist a midwife to develop the sense of being a 'work in progress' as she accompanies the women she cares for through the dynamic life process we call 'having a baby'. The contact with many, many women, some of them other midwives, in various stages of personal and professional development, provides opportunities for a midwife to reflect on her own life stage and her own development simply through exposure to other people's lives. Throughout the span of her midwifery career, in the various roles she enacts in the midwifery world, a midwife is exposed to many ideas, personal stories, personal visions, ways of being and doing things, lifestyles and life choices that will inform and guide her when making decisions for herself.

During the process of learning about midwifery, many students are introduced to the concept of journaling as a powerful, reflective tool for their own learning. Journaling, or simply writing about what she experiences, enables a midwife to discriminate between her personal responses to what happens within her midwifery practice and her professional responses informed by what she knows and believes about midwifery along with professional midwifery knowledge and perspectives, professional ethics and standards.

Midwives also involve themselves in many opportunities to reflect on their own functioning as midwives. This can occur in informal discussions and dialogue with women and other midwifery practitioners; conversations with colleagues in passing in corridors and ward offices in hospitals; midwifery practice meetings; involvement with midwifery students; and picking up information from newspapers, magazines, television, the movies, the internet and many other sources. A midwife will also involve herself in more formal learning opportunities such as Midwifery Standards Review; peer review; formal sessions with a midwifery mentor or supervisor; formal courses and involvement in postgraduate study; preparing and giving teaching sessions; subscriptions to midwifery journals and magazines; internet searches and literature reviews on particular topics. A midwife can connect to her professional group and is likely to involve herself to a greater or lesser degree with the professional activities that occur.

Many midwives will also make use of their own life experiences to inform their practice. They may do this informally and as part of their journaling exercises. They may also participate in personal development sessions or workshops. Examining the effect of personal experience both past and present may form part of the exploration of practice behaviour undertaken with mentors, supervisors or as part of midwifery conversations with peers and colleagues. Midwives may participate in professional development processes and find that these also have personal development outcomes for them.

As her practice progresses and develops in this way, a midwife will become much clearer about herself as a practitioner. If she is involved in marketing herself or the practice she belongs to, or presenting herself to reviewers or her peers, she will need a clear sense of herself as a midwife in order to present herself well. The idealism with which she is likely to present herself at the beginning of her career will be replaced with practice knowledge and wisdom developed from her own experience, as this is integrated into the way she is as a practitioner and the way in which she works. She will develop objectivity about herself and her own behaviour as a midwife and this will assist her in assessing her own performance, as well as creating new ideas about the best way in which she can fulfil her role.

As part of her developing consciousness, a midwife also becomes aware of her capabilities and her limitations as a practitioner. As a new practitioner, a midwife is conscious of her limitations and inexperience; at the same time she is aware of the amount she has to learn and is eager to develop herself as a practitioner. Through the experience she has in providing care for women, a midwife will begin to add her own experience to the knowledge and competence she has gained as a student midwife.

Once a midwife begins to integrate her experience into her functioning, and through reflection on practice both formally and informally, she becomes more conscious of her capabilities. Developing awareness of capabilities brings awareness of limitations. A midwife then needs to discern whether her personal and professional limitations will affect her development as a practising midwife. She is also able to discriminate more easily between the effect she can have on the women to whom she provides midwifery care and the other influences on those women from their own lives, their own experience and their own value systems.

As this learning takes place within individual midwives over time, they become more able to recognise that they cannot be all things to all women. They are likely to develop a wide range of referral options for women to assist them to support their physiological processes instead of being restricted to the medical, obstetric paradigm. Midwives also become more aware of community-based support networks for women and their families/whanau. This will include local maternity consumer organisations, support groups and counselling services as well as social and government agencies that have a role in supporting women at this time in their lives. This knowledge enables midwives to direct women to appropriate sources of information and support. Midwives learn how to use referral judiciously to benefit each woman and her individual circumstances.

There is no doubt that the development of a midwife's consciousness of her functioning is a critical factor in her ability to sustain herself as a practitioner and within the profession. Midwifery is a large role to take on and there are many demands made on a midwife, particularly when she provides continuity of care to women. Different practitioners will respond differently to the demands of midwifery and may choose to be involved in different areas of practice because, for them, that is the best way for them to manage the demands of the professional role. It is important that as midwives we are just as sensitive, understanding and appreciative of our colleagues' ways of being midwives as we are of our own.

Autonomy

Autonomy means self-determination, the ability to be self-governing. It can be applied to individuals, groups, communities, societies and states. Autonomy will be influenced by many and varied factors, including values and belief systems, cultural and ethnic origins as well as personal and professional desires and goals.

Midwifery is often described as an autonomous profession. This concept is used to declare its independent functioning, distinct from the medical profession and the nursing profession. The concept is also used to demonstrate that midwifery has its own distinct body of knowledge, its own view of the world derived from that knowledge, and that it is self-determining in its educational pathways, philosophy, ethics and standards.

There is a point at which the notion of autonomy applies to each individual midwife, bestowing on her the freedom to determine her own actions and behaviour within the midwifery context. There is also a point at which the notion of autonomy applies to the midwife's personal life. Obviously, there is integration between the personal and the professional life of any midwife, and the degree of integration will influence

---

Reflective exercise

1. Think about your own degree of autonomy in your life. Are you completely self-determining and in charge of the course your life takes?
2. What influences the decisions you make about your own path in life?
3. What are the thoughts and beliefs you have that prevent you from doing what you want to?
4. Write a summary of what you have discovered and a paragraph on any steps you will take to develop the sense you have of yourself as completely autonomous.

---

and inform both her professional and personal functioning and decision-making processes.

Autonomy implies that actions are the result of deliberate and informed decisions rather than reactivity and unconscious behaviour. It is in a midwife's best interests for her to develop the ability to function as an autonomous individual, clear about what she is deciding and why, both personally and professionally. Her perception of herself as autonomous will depend on her personal development as an autonomous person in her own life. If the midwife has not developed as an individual who is free to make decisions in her own best interests, knowledgeable about her own personal circumstances and possible consequences of her actions, she *may* be able to function autonomously as a midwife but it will be much more difficult for her to do so.

Self-responsibility

Responsibility refers to the ability or authority to act or decide on one's own, without supervision. It also refers to the person who is answerable for an action. Responsibility comes from the same root as the verb 'to respond'. To every action or event, a midwife has a response and her response will be both personal and professional. Her response(s) will then influence, inform and direct the actions she takes in relation to what she encounters. Self-responsibility refers to the ability to be responsible and account for one's own thoughts, feelings, actions and decisions. It requires the individual to develop the ability to state, 'Yes, I did that, I made that decision, I gave that information, I thought that, I felt that' and, if necessary, to explain further.

Self-responsibility is closely aligned with autonomy. It adds an extra dimension to the concept of self-determination by indicating that the people who decide carry the full weight of the decision on their own shoulders. It is nicely summarised in the phrase: 'The buck stops here!'.

For a midwife, self-responsibility begins with the way in which she engages with the profession, initially as a student and then as a practitioner, whether providing hands-on midwifery care, educating midwifery students and other midwives, managing midwifery services or advising the profession. The ability to carry responsibility for one's own

---

Reflective exercise

1. Consider the person you were five years ago. Write a paragraph on what sort of person you were at that point in your life—identify your character traits, the things you thought about, your dreams, goals, plans, what you thought and felt about things.
2. Now write a paragraph on yourself as you are now, describing the same things.
3. Write another paragraph identifying what is the same about you and what has changed in that period of time.

actions and behaviour grows exponentially with the midwife as a practitioner. From the moment of registration, each midwife is responsible in law for her professional actions. She carries that responsibility as an adjunct to all her activities, including some of her personal decisions. It will benefit her greatly to develop and practise the ability to be accountable for her actions and decisions.

A midwife is also responsible for the way in which she organises and conducts herself in the profession and for carrying out her professional activities in a professional manner—that is, as determined by the profession through its regulations, standards and ethical codes. If a midwife is employed to provide women with midwifery care, it is likely that her employer will have expectations of her professional functioning. Within her employed role, whatever it may be, there is a professional expectation that an individual midwife will be responsible for her actions and decisions.

As part of her responsibility, a midwife will also need to be able to determine and negotiate responsibilities within each midwifery partnership she forms with the women for whom she provides care. There is no need for a midwife to assume responsibility over a woman and her actions and decisions. However, there is a need to be able to negotiate who is responsible for what and to tread the fine, and sometimes difficult, line of shared responsibility and shared decision-making.

Occasionally, in a midwifery partnership, a midwife is required by professional imperatives to assert her midwifery authority. This will be a rare event, given the collaborative nature of midwifery partnerships, occurring only when a midwife believes that life is in danger. A midwife must be sure of her position and clear with the woman about why this needs to occur and discuss with her in what situations she may need to assert her professional authority.

As each midwife grows professionally throughout her career, she will learn to carry her various responsibilities with ease and lightness. When she works in true partnership with women, each midwife will have a clear understanding of what is her responsibility and what responsibilities the woman retains.

Developing and negotiating relationships

Midwifery is itself a relationship—a negotiated partnership between a woman and the midwife caring for her. This means that a midwife has to develop a way of establishing, continuing and finishing the relationships she has with women and their families; midwifery colleagues and practice partners; other professional colleagues; employers; consumer and other community groups; and members of the public and so on. Women come to the midwifery partnership in varying stages of their ability to develop working relationships with a midwife. Therefore it falls to the midwife to develop a functional partnership with each woman for whom she provides care. The midwife takes a leadership role in establishing the partnership, sustaining it throughout the life of the partnership and negotiating its completion.

Over a practice lifetime, a midwife will have contact with thousands of women and their families. She will engage with women in a variety of settings and will be working in a variety of midwifery roles. She may be 'their' midwife—providing continuity of midwifery care throughout a woman's childbearing experience and possibly over several experiences for the same woman and her family. She may be working in a hospital and meeting women briefly as they progress through the institution during an aspect of their childbearing experience. Or she may have a longer involvement with women who are in hospital several times in a pregnancy or for a long period of time. She may have fleeting involvement with women as part of a secondary care 'team' providing care in an urgent or emergency situation. She may be an educator or a manager and have involvement with women at a distance as she works with students or the midwives who are providing care.

In all these situations, a midwife has to use her ability to develop a relationship easily and sometimes quickly, as this enables her to work with a woman and her family/whanau, being alongside her to achieve the most satisfying birthing experience that she can have, given her personal circumstances, whatever they may be.

Each midwife will have her own way of developing this relationship according to the ethical principles and frameworks expressed in chapters 12 and 14. Each midwife needs to consider her own ability to do this and develop whatever skills she requires to make the process of building the relationships with women and their significant others pleasurable, effective and able to rise to the challenges that will eventuate. For the vast majority of midwives, this is learned on the job, by having successes, making mistakes, having another go and learning the most effective way to keep working together to benefit the woman and her experience of having a baby.

Organisational skills

Every midwife must develop the ability to organise her own workload. This applies whether she is managing a caseload of women for whom she provides continuity of care or whether she is employed to work 8–12 hour shifts in a maternity facility. It applies if she is self-employed, employed, in an educator role or a managerial one, or working in a professional advisory capacity.

A midwife organises and manages the things she must do to meet the obligations she has to women and their families, her employer, the profession and within the law. She must have good organisational skills, whether she is responsible for providing all the care for women through the continuum of childbearing or only part of the care as a shift worker in a maternity facility.

A major component of the ability to organise work is the ability to plan. A midwife has to plan how she will achieve whatever she has to achieve within the time available. Because of the nature of midwifery work—it is involved with a life process that does not always follow a straightforward path—a midwife also needs the ability to change the plan and to make alternative arrangements for the work that she planned. Fortunately for midwives, they work with women who are in the main going through a healthy life event without any extra requirement for care. This often means that whatever they had planned for providing care to women can quite safely be postponed while the midwife attends to the more urgent matter. This can range from attending a birth, to an emergency situation, an urgent need or, indeed, the midwife's own illness or family situation.

Time management is a critical factor in the ability to organise. Unfortunately, lateness can become habitual, as many midwives fail to take into account the human element of midwifery work when planning their time and do not factor in the extra time needed to deal with the concerns of individual women they are scheduled to see. Obviously, part of a midwife's work is unpredictable but much of what midwives do can be planned methodically, as long as enough time is allocated to each midwifery exchange. One way to demonstrate the importance with which a midwife views an individual woman and her experience is to behave in a way that recognises that her time is as valuable as the midwife's time and to give plenty of notice when existing arrangements have to be altered.

Because midwives are, in the main, women who work with other women, there is an acceptance of how women's lives work. Consequently, there is an acceptance by women receiving care from midwives of the nature of the midwives' work and a tolerance of the situations that arise. This does not lessen the need for midwives to explain how they work and the alternative arrangements they plan for women in their own absence. Midwives should not take the goodwill of

---

Reflective exercise

1   Write a description of your organisational style and how you think it will contribute to your work as a midwife. How will it assist you? How will it hinder you?
2   What do you need to change about the way you organise and plan your life and work in order to become a successfully functioning midwife?

---

their clients for granted or use it as an excuse for poor time management and disorganisation.

For midwives providing continuity-of-care to women, one of the most important considerations in organising their practice is ensuring clear back-up arrangements. Midwives often make mutually beneficial arrangements for back-up and 'cover' with one or more midwives, depending on whether they practise as a sole practitioner, in a midwifery partnership with one other midwife or in a group practice. It is common within group practices for the midwives involved to work in pairs for back-up to ensure that women do not have to meet a stream of midwives who 'might' provide their care.

Midwives working shifts in a maternity facility often care for a number of women at any one time, providing antenatal and postnatal care. This also requires organisation and planning to deliver the necessary care in a defined time period without feeling stretched or stressed.

Many of the decisions involved in organising an individual midwife's life and work come down to a matter of personal choice. As long as women understand clearly how the service is provided and who provides it, and feel that they are getting the individual attention that they need, they are usually satisfied with the way in which midwives work.

Self-care

Midwifery is an important role in any society. Midwives form part of the grass-roots systems in the community that carry information and wisdom about how people function in groups and communities over time. They also hold important knowledge about the nature of life, death, the meaning of human experiences and in particular the role of giving birth and the nature of the parenting relationship. Midwives carry a great deal of responsibility to the women they care for, to the profession through regulation and professional expectations, and to society in general for the nature of the work they do with families in their community and the contribution they make to the wellbeing of the communities in which they live.

Consequently, midwives also carry responsibility for ensuring that they are able to continue to do their work, in whichever setting they choose to work, in a way that is sustainable for them. Individual midwives have to make their own assessment of what they personally require to sustain them in the role they have chosen. What she requires may not be totally clear to a midwife when she begins practising in the profession, and the first few years of practice will be a time for coming to understand the nature of the work, the demands it makes on her and of her, as well as working out the things she needs to sustain and develop in order to withstand the demands of working with women and their families at a profoundly intense period in their lives.

There are several areas for the midwife to consider as she determines the best way in which she can look after herself so that she can continue to work in a fresh and thoughtful way.

Work–life balance

For a midwife to be able to bring her best professional functioning to her work, she needs to ensure that she has the appropriate balance between work and other aspects of her life.

Each midwife has to find out what that appropriate balance is, and this will depend on the phase of her life. Is she a single woman with no dependants starting out in the profession? Or is she a mother with children whose needs she has to consider when planning how she will contribute to the workforce? Does she have elderly parents she needs to care for? Have her children left home now, leaving her free to work more in a job she loves? Has she worked for many years and does she now want to have more time to pursue other interests?

The answers to any or all of the above questions will depend on each midwife as she considers her own life path and the personal and professional goals she has for herself at any given time. Whatever answers each midwife comes up with will determine the way in which she becomes involved with the profession and will influence the way in which she chooses to work: case-loading midwifery and how many women she will take on in a year; working with one or two other midwives or being part of a bigger practice; working core shifts in a maternity unit; or working in some other area of practice in a different way.

There is also the matter of holidays and leisure activities. Midwives who are employed to work in maternity units on 8- or 12-hour shifts perhaps have a more ordered life, and of course some midwives choose to work this way so that they *can* have a more ordered life with scheduled time off and regular holidays from work.

Midwives who attach themselves to women and provide continuity of midwifery care have a more unpredictable life. They are responsive to the women they care for, who are caught up in a reproductive life experience that has its own timetable that often does not fit with the way in which we try to order our world. Consequently it is both more important and more difficult for midwives working in this way to ensure that they schedule regular time off and take enough holidays each year to rest and recover from the demands made on them.

Sleep is also a factor for caseloading midwives, as they can become sleep-deprived when attending long labours or many women in the same time period. The work of a midwife does not finish when the baby is born—it begins in earnest as the midwife supports and guides the women in the first days of her baby's life so that she and her baby get off to a good start with each other. It becomes critical that the midwife paces herself to cope with these demands and calls for help from her back-up colleagues when necessary, so that she gets the essential rest she needs to be able to keep going with her work.

Having fun and enjoyment

All midwives have to consider how they can work in a way that allows them to derive maximum enjoyment and satisfaction from their experience as a midwife. Without enjoyment, the work of the midwife becomes unsustainable at a personal level. The work of a midwife is sufficiently important that the individuals who work in the profession have to feel a sense of purpose and satisfaction for them to be able to continue to provide women and their families with the support, guidance and care that they require.

Fortunately, being with women when they go through pregnancy, labour and birth and as they achieve motherhood is a very positive experience that is often reward in itself, and a midwife does get a sense of her work being important to the wellbeing of the world. As midwives progress in the profession, they get a sense that they are responsible, not for what happens to women, but for their own professional functioning and the contribution that they make. A midwife begins to understand that she is part of something greater than herself and can carry the work lightly even though she is dealing with serious matters that can sometimes be life-threatening. Developing her acceptance of what is happening and her ability to respond to what is happening will free a midwife to enjoy the unpredictable nature of the work and her involvement with the women and their families, whatever role and relationship she has with them and other midwives.

Fun can be derived in many ways in the work of a midwife. Many midwives have cheerful working relationships with their midwifery colleagues and make the most of opportunities to share midwifery experiences and stories with each other. The ability to do this both at work and socially lightens the load of responsibility that many midwives feel through their involvement with women as they go through the birthing process. Midwifery conferences are particularly renowned for midwives letting their hair down and having a good time with each other. It is important for individual midwives to have colleagues with whom they can share stories of the humorous, satisfying, problematic and sometimes tragic experiences they encounter. Each midwife needs to ensure that she is connected with a group of colleagues with whom she meets regularly, as a release valve for all the responsibility she holds in relation to her work.

Obviously, there is also fun outside of midwifery and it is critical for every midwife to have other activities in which she is pursuing something she enjoys. This can be as simple as regularly organised family activities, gardening, going to the movies, tramping or bushwalking, singing, sports such as cycling, running, canoeing, karate and so on, or any other hobby or leisure pursuit. By participating in activities she enjoys completely outside of midwifery, the midwife replenishes her resources so that she can continue to provide good-quality midwifery care to women. She can bring a more rounded and balanced life perspective to her work and this will benefit those with whom she works, both women and midwives.

Setting boundaries

The concept of boundaries comes from the self-assertiveness movement of the 1970s and 1980s, as women developed themselves to take on a fuller role in society after the second wave of feminist thinking. Boundary setting is a particularly important aspect of freeing oneself from the dependency models of human functioning and creating a strong sense of self and self-determination.

For midwives working in maternity units, this may never become an issue, or they may find it useful to consider the matter of boundaries when dealing with particularly demanding women and their families. Caseloading midwives may find that boundary issues can and do arise with some women for whom they care.

It is the role of a midwife to know the purpose of the work she does with women and to support women to become autonomous in their own lives. Midwives are also autonomous as health professionals, and tensions can arise in the relationship between a midwife and a woman if what the woman wants from the midwife and what the midwife is prepared to offer do not match up. The midwife has to have ability to make an assessment of what the woman is requesting and to determine whether it is in the best interests of the woman for the midwife to meet the request. She then needs to have a discussion with the woman and resolve the matter to the point where the relationship continues or finishes in an amicable way. This can include the midwife ensuring that the woman receives care from another midwife or maternity service.

While midwives can be a source of information and support to women, it is not the role of the midwife to provide everything a woman requires or to fix her life up for her. A midwife has a role in assisting the woman to determine what she needs, and a role in helping her find the appropriate information and develop the necessary support networks to ensure that her needs are met. Midwifery is very specific in its role—the role of the midwife is to provide maternity services to women. There are other agencies in society and other community groups to meet some of the non-maternity needs of women for whom a midwife is caring. Having a good knowledge of those agencies and groups is one way for midwives to ensure that they are not taken advantage of and can fulfil their own role in an appropriate way. Midwives need not be all things to all the women they care for and in that way protect themselves from being overburdened by the role of the midwife.

Standing strong, being in control

Midwifery teaches all of us that we are not in control of the processes of life. We are also not in control of what other people choose to do—they make their own decisions and have their own successes and mistakes. Although we have more understanding of the processes involved than ever before, having a baby remains predictably unpredictable.

> ### Reflective exercise
>
> 1   List seven ways in which you plan to take care of yourself in the first two years of your midwifery practice.
> 2   Beside each item, plan the steps you will take to achieve that goal.

Midwifery, however, does hold some things to be true and it is this that contributes and informs midwifery knowledge: working in partnership with women; informed choice and consent; assessing health and wellbeing; recording and documentation; planning care with women; practising safely; accountability to women and the profession; and reflection on practice.

A midwife grounded in midwifery knowledge, tempered by her own experience that she has reflected on and made sense of within the framework of midwifery's philosophy, ethics and professional standards, will develop her own authority. This will enable her to stand strongly in the face of the challenges that will come her way. These challenges will come from women she attends and their families, as well as members of other professional groups who do not understand the nature of midwifery, and other groups in society who have different agendas than the one midwifery espouses.

The one thing a midwife does have control over is her self: the way in which she gets involved and engages with women and their families; her midwifery colleagues; her employers; the profession; members of the community and the public; and members of allied health professions. All this is in her control and will reflect how well she has internalised the midwifery philosophy. Her own functioning as a midwife will give her much material on which to reflect when she engages in the informal and formal processes that contribute to her ongoing development as a midwifery practitioner.

Conclusion

This chapter has focused on the development of some of the abilities and attributes that will assist a midwife to derive the maximum personal and professional benefit from the work she does. It has identified a wide range of qualities for midwives to consider when thinking about their work and what they need to develop to sustain them. It has provided a general and broad look at life skills needed by midwives for their work to be satisfying and educational.

As all midwives are individuals who bring their own personal life qualities, learning styles and personal/professional goals to their work, this chapter cannot provide specific advice to individuals about their career path or development required to meet particular challenges. Ideas are presented here for the reader to consider as they reflect on their own development in the profession of midwifery.

Recommended reading

Davis E 1987 Heart and hands. A midwife's guide to pregnancy and birth (2nd edn). Celestial Arts, Berkeley

Flint C 1986 Sensitive midwifery. Heinemann Midwifery, London

Gaskin IM 1980 Spiritual midwifery. The Book Publishing Company, Summertown

New Zealand College of Midwives 2005 Midwives handbook for practice. NZCOM, Christchurch

PART B
Practice

PARTNERSHIP

SECTION ONE

CHAPTER 14

Theoretical frameworks for midwifery practice

Sally Pairman and Judith McAra-Couper

Key terms

active participation, assimilation, being equal, being with, continuity of caregiver, control, cultural awareness, cultural safety, cultural sensitivity, culturally safe practice, culturally unsafe practice, emancipation, empowerment, equality, independent profession, individual negotiation, informed choice, informed consent, midwifery partnership, practice wisdom, professional friendship, reciprocity, 'self' in practice, self-responsibility, shared power, shared responsibility, support, theoretical frameworks, Treaty of Waitangi, trust, with woman, women-centred

Chapter overview

This chapter discusses two theoretical frameworks—cultural safety and midwifery partnership—that can be used by midwives to guide their practice. Both frameworks were developed in New Zealand and arose out of that country's unique historical, social and cultural context. However, both can be applied to midwifery practice in Australia and other countries, as the principles articulated in each theory describe values, beliefs, understandings and behaviours that any midwife can embrace.

Both theories focus on relationships. Cultural safety enables a health practitioner to examine her or his beliefs, values and culture, and to understand how these might affect the person who is the recipient of care, with their different cultural understandings. Culturally safe care is provided when the recipient of that care determines that it is safe for them. Midwifery partnership provides a model for a midwife/woman relationship. Involving trust, shared control and responsibility and shared meaning, it is a reciprocal relationship negotiated and understood by the partners—a childbearing woman and a midwife. Like cultural safety, midwifery partnership aims to shift power from the midwife to the childbearing woman and seeks to redefine accepted definitions of the midwife as 'expert'. Ultimately, cultural safety and midwifery partnership are about self-determination, whereby the childbearing woman is recognised as 'expert', able to define her own needs, to control her own experiences, and to determine the appropriateness of the midwifery care she has received.

Learning outcomes

Learning outcomes for this chapter are:

1 To explain the origin of the term 'cultural safety' and the development of this theory

2 To describe the principles of cultural safety

3 To describe the difference between caring for a woman as the midwifery 'expert' and working with a woman as an equal partner

4 To explain the principles of midwifery partnership

5 To discuss the implications of midwifery partnership and cultural safety for professionalism

Midwifery and relationships

Midwifery is about *relationships*—between women and midwives, between women's families and midwives, between midwives, and between other health professionals and midwives. These relationships are the medium through which midwifery is practised and they take place in varying contexts and over varying periods of time.

Midwifery involves working with women and their families through the significant and universal life event of childbirth. Childbirth is a physiological process in which healthy women are able to birth healthy babies with the minimum of interference or assistance. This physiological process is also mediated by cultural and social norms and practices that strongly influence how women feel about their ability to birth, where they feel safe to birth, who they want with them during birth and what cultural practices are important to them during birth and new motherhood.

Universally, midwives understand that their role is to support and enhance this physiological and cultural process by being alongside a woman and her family as a companion or guardian (Kaitiaki), using specific expertise and knowledge to ensure a safe transition to new motherhood that meets the individual needs of each woman and family (Donley 1986). This midwifery expertise is as much about knowing when not to interfere in the physiological process of pregnancy and birth as it is about recognising when and how to intervene in a way that will facilitate and enhance the woman's ability to give birth or to confidently mother her new baby.

While midwives in Australia, New Zealand and elsewhere lost this role during the twentieth century through the hospitalisation and medicalisation of childbirth, they are now reclaiming it. In New Zealand, and increasingly in Australia, midwives work in contexts that enable them to provide continuity of midwifery care throughout the entire childbirth process from pregnancy, through labour and birth, to the completion of the postnatal period at six weeks. Working with women over this nine- to ten-month period enables women and midwives to really get to know each other in a way that is much more intimate and personal than was the case when women arrived in the maternity unit to be cared for by midwives with whom they had no prior relationship. Internationally, midwives are now exploring and claiming a more personal relationship with each childbearing woman that is based on mutual respect, shared understanding and trust, and which breaks down power inequalities previously inherent in health professional/patient relationships in favour of one that is negotiated and equitable (Kirkham 2000a; Page 2000).

To work in equal and negotiated professional relationships requires self-knowledge, personal security, integrity and maturity. The midwife can no longer rely on her professional role as 'expert' to guide her practice. Instead she must open herself as a person to each woman she works with and be willing to recognise and embrace the woman as an equal partner, as together they explore the physical, emotional, social and spiritual ramifications of childbirth for that woman. The midwife brings her midwifery knowledge and understandings to the relationship, as the woman brings her knowledge and experiences. But rather than directing care, the midwife works 'with' the woman to support her to take up her power as a woman and as a mother so that she can direct and control her own birthing experience.

Theoretical frameworks for practice

Two theoretical frameworks have been developed in New Zealand that can provide some guidance for midwives engaging in these types of relationships with women. Midwifery partnership describes and explores how midwives can work in partnership with women. Cultural safety supports partnership relationships through focusing on invisible structures of power that exist between any two partners and in wider contexts within health service institutions and society. Cultural safety, like midwifery partnership, seeks to make these power differentials visible so that both partners can negotiate how they work together and ensure that the woman, as the recipient of care, receives care that meets her needs and leaves her individuality intact and strengthened.

Cultural safety and midwifery partnership both also have a political imperative. Cultural safety challenges any personal, professional, institutional and social issues and structure that 'diminishes, demeans or disempowers the cultural identity and wellbeing of an individual' (NCNZ 2002, p 7). Midwifery partnership challenges professional power structures and medical dominance over childbirth, through recognising childbearing women as active partners of equal status in the shared experience of maternity care (Guilliland & Pairman 1995).

What is a theoretical framework?

Rosamund Bryar (1995) contends that the essence of the art of midwifery is intuition and empathy that is informed by theory, knowledge and reflective thinking. Exercising the art of midwifery requires combining the personal qualities of the midwife with reflective thinking about how theory and knowledge can best be used in the care of individual women. 'Theory provides a structure within which midwives can compare the present experiences of the woman they are caring for with the responses identified in the theory' (Bryar 1995, p 5).

Theory arises from midwifery practice and from a range of other disciplines. The thinking of midwives about this theory in relation to their daily practice with women will lead to further development of practice theories. Theory is an integrated set of defined concepts and statements that present a view of a phenomenon and can be used to describe, explain, predict and/or control that phenomenon (Burns & Grove 1995).

The relationship between concepts can sometimes be presented diagrammatically to illustrate how the author visualises the links between the concepts. It can also be presented through language that explains the relationship between concepts. Models and theories are 'mental constructs or images developed to provide greater understanding of events in the physical, psychological or social worlds ... and are intended to be tested, modified or abandoned in the light of new evidence' (Bryar 1995, p 40). Theoretical frameworks are tools for making sense of and explaining reality, and for thinking about practice. They provide ways in which midwifery care may be examined, understood, tested and developed.

The two theoretical frameworks presented in this chapter, midwifery partnership and cultural safety, arose from practice, and describe and explain living processes (relationships) that are always engaging, challenging and changing. 'Partnership' and 'cultural safety' exist only in encounters between individuals, groups or cultures, and have a moral and ethical imperative as well as a theoretical one. Both theoretical frameworks identify a number of concepts and values, and these are described below as tools for helping midwives to think about themselves and explore how they engage with others in their professional roles as midwives.

The origins of cultural safety and midwifery partnership

Cultural safety and midwifery partnership were both developed in New Zealand and both arose out of its unique historical, cultural and social context. New Zealand's constitutional and legislative structure is founded on the Treaty of Waitangi, signed in 1840 between Maori (New Zealand's Indigenous peoples) and the British Crown. The Treaty of Waitangi articulates a particular relationship between Maori and generations of settlers who have come to New Zealand since the early 1800s. This relationship is a bicultural partnership between Maori and the Crown that recognises the unique place and status of the Indigenous people and assures the place of both Maori and the colonists in New Zealand (Ramsden 1990, 2002).

Rapid British colonial expansion in the nineteenth century meant that immigrants from Britain and the four continents as well as the Pacific rapidly outnumbered Maori. There has been ongoing debate and dispute about the meaning of the Treaty and biculturalism in a society made up of a variety of ethnicities, languages and religions. These debates have been compounded by a long-standing struggle by Maori to have the Crown recognise and meet its partnership obligations under the Treaty. The 1980s and 1990s saw increased efforts by Maori and government to address Treaty claims and construct a bicultural relationship based on the principles of partnership, protection, participation and equity. One result of this work has been that the notion of 'partnership' is culturally embedded in New Zealand society.

New Zealand women drew on this cultural understanding of partnership when they actively sought changes to the way in which maternity services were delivered, and in particular demanded the choice of a midwife as their caregiver for childbirth (Dobbie 1990; Strid 1987). In the mid-1980s, maternity consumer organisations joined with midwifery's professional organisation (at that time the Midwives Section of the New Zealand Nurses Association, now the New Zealand College of Midwives) in an organised political campaign to reinstate midwifery autonomy and enable women to have a choice of caregiver for childbirth (Donley 1989; Guilliland 1989). The campaign took place in a context in which women's issues were high on the political agenda and the Cartwright Inquiry had raised awareness of patients' rights and issues of informed consent (Guilliland & Pairman 1995). Together, women and midwives succeeded in bringing about change, and the resulting 1990 Amendment to the *Nurses Act 1977* reinstated midwives as practitioners in their own right and gave women the choice of a doctor or a midwife or both as their lead caregiver for childbirth.

Another result of this political campaign was midwifery's recognition of its political partnership with women and its determination to enact this partnership by establishing representation for women (as maternity service consumers) at every level of midwifery's professional structure, the New Zealand College of Midwives. It was then only a short step for midwives to understand that their individual relationships with women were also partnerships, or could be. Exploration of the political and professional relationships between midwives and women has led the New Zealand College of Midwives (NZCOM) to identify partnership as a philosophical stance, a standard for practice and an ethical principle (NZCOM 2005).

New Zealand midwifery is redefining midwifery professionalism to mean midwifery partnership as it seeks to replace traditional hierarchical professional relationships with relationships that are negotiated and in which power differentials are acknowledged and actively shifted from the midwife to the childbearing woman so that she can control her own birthing experience (Guilliland & Pairman 1995). New Zealand midwifery has also embraced cultural safety as developed by Irihapeti Ramsden and required of all New Zealand nurses and midwives by the Nursing Council of New Zealand (since 2003 replaced for midwives by the Midwifery Council of New Zealand) in its competencies for entry to the registers of nurses and midwives (NCNZ 2002; Ramsden 2002). The NZCOM Standards for Midwifery Practice require midwives to be 'culturally safe' and the Midwifery Council of New Zealand's (MCNZ) Competencies for Entry to the Register of Midwives require that the midwife 'apply the principles of cultural safety to the midwifery partnership' (NZCOM 2005, p 13; MCNZ 2004a).

Cultural safety and midwifery partnership in other contexts

The theoretical frameworks of cultural safety and midwifery partnership both explore relationships and therefore, although both arose out of the New Zealand context, are applicable in other countries, cultures or contexts. Indeed, the Australian Midwifery Competency Project identified that a role of the midwife is to work in partnership with women and to ensure that midwifery practice is provided in a culturally safe environment (Homer 2004).

In any context, midwifery must be concerned with relationships because, unlike any other health profession, midwifery is privileged to have the opportunity to be 'with' women throughout the life experiences of pregnancy, birth and new motherhood. In their professional roles, midwives are able to develop relationships with women that last up to 10 months (sometimes longer) and they have the opportunity to work with women in their own homes and communities, away from the influence and control of institutions. In such settings the traditional practitioner/patient relationship, where the practitioner is the 'expert' and has the authority to make decisions, is clearly inappropriate. Midwives who work within continuity-of-care models work in contexts in which relationships are valued and where midwifery care such as support, caring and enabling is recognised as skilled midwifery practice. Midwives and childbearing women in these settings need to develop relationships of equity, trust and mutual understanding. So too do midwives and women working within the constraints of hospital services with fragmented care, insufficient staffing numbers, hierarchies and organisational control. Such settings can undermine midwifery knowledge and midwifery confidence and trust, making it difficult for midwives to support women in taking control of their own birthing experiences (Kirkham 2000a). Both midwives and women need to take hold of their power in order to begin to change the culture of these institutions. The political partnership of women and midwives experienced in New Zealand offers some guidance (Guilliland & Pairman 1995; Kirkham 2000b).

No matter what the context, midwives should examine their relationships with childbearing women because these relationships are at the heart of midwifery practice. When New Zealand women fought for midwifery autonomy they did so because they believed that midwives would provide an alternative model to medicine—a model of care in which women would be in control as the decision-makers (Strid 1987). These same arguments are being made by Australian women and midwives seeking to strengthen midwifery autonomy through legislative and practice changes (Maternity Coalition 2002).

Midwifery autonomy in New Zealand brought with it a social mandate for midwives to practise independently of other health professions so that they could provide the kind of care that women wanted. This social mandate carries with it a moral obligation for midwifery to provide the service that women have called for. There is also a moral obligation to recognise and respect individual differences in those we work with as midwives, no matter what other structures encourage us to do so. For New Zealand midwives, 'there would still be a moral imperative to engage in the difficult and complex quest to achieve meaningful partnership with Maori, even if there were no Treaty of Waitangi' (Hinchcliff 1997, p 300). The same is true in Australia, where Australian midwives have a moral obligation to engage meaningfully with Aboriginal peoples in order to create maternity services that will meet their needs.

Midwives in any country and from any cultural context will work with childbearing women who are different from them. Midwives need to examine their relationships with the women they care for if women are to become active agents in their own care (Kirkham 2000b). Cultural safety and midwifery partnership provide frameworks for achieving meaningful relationships between midwives and childbearing women.

Cultural safety

Cultural safety is defined as:

> The effective nursing[1] or midwifery practice of a person or family from another culture, and is determined by that person or family. Culture includes, but is not restricted to, age or generation; gender; sexual orientation; occupation and socio-economic status; ethnic origin or migrant experience; religious or spiritual belief; and disability.
>
> The nurse or midwife delivering the nursing or midwifery service will have undertaken a process of reflection on his or her own cultural identity and will recognise the impact that his or her personal culture has on his or her professional practice. Unsafe cultural practice comprises any action which diminishes, demeans or disempowers the cultural identity and well-being of an individual (NCNZ 2002, p 7).

Intrinsic to the concept and practice of cultural safety is the notion of 'right relationship'. Whether that relationship is between two persons, two groups, two cultures or two countries, right relationship recognises and honours the rights and responsibilities of each (McAra-Couper 2005). Cultural safety seeks to establish the practice of right relationship at a personal, professional and institutional level.

What is meant by 'culture'?

> . . . we learn from the experiences of the past to correct the understanding of the present and create a future which can be justly shared (Ramsden 2002, p 182).

The understandings of culture expressed in nursing and midwifery in New Zealand today have evolved over a long period. It is important to be familiar with this evolution of understandings in order to appreciate the significance and place of cultural safety.

Historically, in New Zealand and elsewhere, culture was invisible in nursing and midwifery curricula. In part this reflected a context in which assimilation was prevalent. Despite the existence of the Treaty of Waitangi, assimilation policy influenced the social thinking of the nineteenth and early twentieth centuries, and led to the establishment of structures and processes that denied differences between Maori and Pakeha in an attempt to make Maori like Pakeha and absorb them into Pakeha-dominated culture and society (Walker 1987).

In this context, nurses and midwives were encouraged to give care to patients 'irrespective of differences such as nationality, culture, creed, colour, age, sex, political or religious belief or social status' (Ramsden 1990, p 79). This understanding of culture informed the practice of nurses in New Zealand until the early 1970s. It was well intentioned but served only to reinforce assimilation (Spence 2001). The long-term consequences of assimilation are suppression and destruction of the culture of Indigenous people, which results in mental, physical and spiritual stress (NCNZ 1992). This stress is seen only too readily in the present-day health statistics of Indigenous peoples in New Zealand and Australia and throughout the world.

In the 1970s a new understanding of culture developed. In New Zealand, as elsewhere, anthropological understandings of culture emerged which led to greater cultural awareness and cultural sensitivity. Transcultural nursing theory, developed by nurse theorist Madeline Leininger in the early 1970s, influenced nursing education. Transcultural nursing was based on nurses having knowledge about a range of different cultures from which they could respond therapeutically to their client's needs (Papps 2005). Nurses and midwives were taught to gather information about the beliefs, patterns and behaviours of other cultures, so that they would be able to identify 'specific cultural patterns that occurred' and provide culturally sensitive care (Richardson 2000, p 32; Spence 1999). Nurses and midwives were taught about the concepts of cultural awareness (becoming aware of difference) and cultural sensitivity (sensitivity to the legitimacy of difference and the impact the midwife's own culture may have on others) (NCNZ 2002). Nursing and midwifery knowledge considered culture and race from the perspective of the nurse or midwife, as an observer, exploring and understanding what makes the other person different from themselves (Ramsden 2000; Richardson 2000). Such approaches allowed the nurse or midwife to be patronising and powerful as they identified the needs of people from other ethnic groups, and did not require any self-knowledge or change in attitude (Ramsden 2000). In New Zealand, the dominance of transcultural nursing in nursing education and practice was challenged by the alternative theory of cultural safety.

Developed in the 1980s by Maori nurse educator, Irihapeti Ramsden, cultural safety or Kawa Whakaruruhau, provided another theoretical framework for understanding culture. This socio-political definition of culture had the Treaty of Waitangi as its starting point, and involved recognition that power needed to be shared and racism de-institutionalised (Spence 1999). Cultural safety focused on the socio-political factors that affected health care (Richardson 2000).

By contrast, notions of cultural sensitivity and cultural awareness avoided the more difficult recognition of power relationships that existed in the delivery of health care and led to cultural stereotypes and simplistic notions such as cultural checklists (Ramsden 2000). Cultural safety focused not on the 'other' but on the nurse and midwife. The process of cultural safety began with self-reflection and attitude change (see Fig 14.1). This process required the nurse or midwife to recognise themselves as 'powerful bearers of their own life experience and realities and the impact this may have on others' (Ramsden 2000, p 117).

The notion of power is inherent in the concept of and processes associated with cultural safety. The nurse or midwife is challenged to recognise her or his personal power and the power of the institutions and society in which they work and live (Richardson 2000). Cultural safety is primarily about establishing trust, gaining a shared meaning of vulnerability and power, and carefully working through the legitimacy of difference (Ramsden 2000). Cultural safety makes visible the invisible structures of power (including our own) and attempts to transform anything that creates inequality and inequities in the health services. In the New Zealand context this also includes actions that do not uphold the Treaty of Waitangi in the delivery of health services.

Figure 14.1 describes the progression of students towards understanding cultural safety and the difference in meaning of the commonly used terms 'cultural safety', 'cultural sensitivity' and 'cultural awareness'.

Thus cultural safety and transcultural nursing present different theoretical understandings of culture. Transcultural nursing exists in a multicultural context and focuses primarily on defining culture as race and ethnicity (Ramsden 2002). Transcultural nursing places the nurse or midwife in the position of 'external observer' for the purpose of providing culture-specific care. On the other hand, cultural safety addresses the issue of power between the client (woman) and the nurse (midwife) and interprets 'culture' in the broadest possible sense (Ramsden 2002).

Cultural safety
Is an outcome of nursing and midwifery education that enables safe service to be defined by those who receive the service.

Cultural sensitivity
Alerts students to the legitimacy of differences and begins a process of self-exploration as the powerful bearers of their own life experience and realities and the impact these may have on others.

Cultural awareness
Is a beginning step towards understanding that there is a difference. Many people undergo courses designed to sensitise them to formal ritual and practice rather than to emotional, social, economic and political context in which people exist.

Figure 14.1 Developing understanding of cultural safety (based on Ramsden 2002)

Leininger's culturally congruent care model is different from Cultural Safety in that nurses and midwives need to move from treating people *regardless* of colour or creed towards a model of treatment that was *regardful* of all those things that make them unique (Ramsden 1993, p 5 (our emphasis)).

This movement from 'regardless to regardful' is one of the most important contributions cultural safety makes in ensuring the safety of the care that midwives give.

The development of cultural safety

Irihapeti Ramsden's theory of cultural safety arose from her experiences in the late 1980s in teaching student nurses, and her attempts to include Maori health issues and the Treaty of Waitangi in her teaching (Ramsden 2005). Her frustrations in trying to teach about difference and racism in a context of assimilation, where culture was seen only as ethnicity, led her to develop strategies for teaching about Maori health issues in nursing. These strategies were articulated in her framework, 'A Model for Negotiated and Equal Partnership', which was adopted by all schools of nursing soon after (Ramsden 1989).

In 1988, Irihapeti Ramsden was commissioned to run a national hui (meeting), the Hui Waimanawa, which involved over 100 participants including Maori nursing students. According to Irihapeti, it was a first-year nursing student at that hui who first coined the term 'cultural safety' and permitted Irihapeti to use the term in her subsequent work. The student stood at the hui and spoke about the expectation of legal safety, ethical safety, safe clinical practice and safe knowledge bases for nurses and asked, 'What about cultural safety?' (Ramsden 2005, p 17). Irihapeti Ramsden published her document, Kawa Whakaruruhau: Cultural Safety in Nursing Education in Aotearoa' in 1990. The Nursing Council of New Zealand accepted it, along with 'A Model for Equal and Negotiated Partnership', thus legitimising the term 'cultural safety' in nursing and midwifery language (Ramsden 2005).

At several hui held in the late 1980s and early 1990s, a variety of definitions for cultural safety were debated. The hui of the Whanau Kawa Whakaruruhau defined culturally safe practice as 'actions which recognise, respect and nurture the unique cultural identity of tangata whenua and safely meet their needs, expectations and rights' (Hill, cited in Whanau Kawa Whakaruruhau 1991, p 7). This hui also defined 'culturally unsafe practice' as 'any actions which diminish, demean, or disempower the cultural identity and well being of the individual' (ibid).

Cultural safety required appropriate health services to be provided for all New Zealanders. However, the need to address Maori health as a result of the enduring effects of colonisation had become urgent (Spence 2004). Therefore, much of the early work around cultural safety was concerned first and foremost with trying to identify ways in which health services could address the poor health status of Maori (Ramsden 2002). While colonisation was primarily the reason for the poor health status of Maori, it was also the reason for the development of cultural safety, and the initial processes of teaching cultural

safety needed to deal with colonial history. Therefore cultural safety teaching included analysis of the historical, political, social and economic realities that were affecting Maori Health (Ramsden 2002). Nursing and midwifery students needed a 'profound understanding of the history and social function of racism and the process of colonization' to become culturally safe practitioners (Ramsden 2002, p 180).

In 1991, the Nursing Council commissioned Irihapeti Ramsden to write guidelines that would assist schools of nursing (and midwifery) to incorporate cultural safety (Kawa Whakaruruhau) into the education curricula (Papps 2002). In the council's view it was important that such guidelines would provide a process through which students would understand difference and dominance and so 'demonstrate flexibility in their relationships with people who are different from themselves' (NCNZ 2002, p 12).

These guidelines became council policy in 1992 and required student nurses and midwives to be educated:

- to examine their own realities and the attitudes they bring to each new person they encounter in their practice;
- to be open-minded and flexible in their attitudes toward people who are different to them and to whom they offer or deliver service;
- not to blame the victims of historical and social processes for their current plight (NCNZ 1992, p 1).

In these guidelines the Nursing Council's definition of cultural safety more clearly articulated a shift in power to the client (Papps 2005). Cultural safety was now defined as:

The effective nursing of a person/family from another culture by a nurse who has undertaken a process of reflection on [her] own cultural identity and recognises the impact of the nurse's culture on [her] own nursing practice. Unsafe cultural practice is any action which diminishes, demeans or disempowers the cultural identity and well-being of an individual (NCNZ 1992, p 1, glossary).

The incorporation of cultural safety into nursing and midwifery curricula from 1992 meant that education required:

- the nurse and midwife to acquire insight and analysis of themselves as cultural safety shifted the focus from other to self (Ramsden 2000)
- attitudinal change through reflection on self (Ramsden 2000)
- that clients be cared for regardful, not regardless, of all that makes them unique (Ramsden 2002)
- that the nurse and midwife understand that the care they provide is defined as safe by those who use their service (Ramsden 2002)
- that at the end of the educational process the 'most vulnerable in our society' can say that the nurse/midwife was safe (Ramsden 2000, p 5).

Unfortunately, few nurse educators had the educational preparation to teach cultural safety or to understand that culture was an important influence on people's health, and students were not provided with clear definitions of culture. Where culture was equated with ethnicity, students were often taught Maori language, songs and dance instead of learning about their own cultural identity and its impact on their nursing or midwifery practice (Papps 2005).

The confusion continued in media reports that condemned the teaching of cultural safety in nursing, claiming that attention to this aspect of the curriculum was to the detriment of other more important areas such as 'medical' knowledge. Papps suggests that opposition to and confusion about cultural safety arose because it aims to do two separate but interrelated things. First it aims to address nurses' and midwives' conscious or unconscious attitudes towards any cultural differences, and second, it aims to raise awareness about imbalances in the health status of Maori (Papps 2002). Because it teaches about the effects of colonisation on the health of Maori, cultural safety has been misunderstood as being about only one culture (Papps 2002). What was not understood was that cultural safety is about addressing power relationships between nurses or midwives and the recipients of their care. Where historically nurses were taught to provide care *irrespective* of colour or creed and to treat everyone the same, cultural safety requires nurses and midwives to be '*respective* of the nationality of human beings, the culture of human beings, the age, the sex, the political and the religious beliefs of other members of the human race' (Ramsden 2005, p 7). Rather than the nurse or midwife deciding what is culturally safe, it is the patients or clients who determine whether they feel safe with the care they have received (Ramsden 1995, cited in Papps 2002).

Intense political and media scrutiny of cultural safety eventually led to an investigation by a Parliamentary Select Committee in 1995. Cultural safety was 'depicted as politically inspired while the curriculum of clinical nursing practice was apolitical and neutral' (Papps 2005, p 26). Several recommendations from this enquiry were actioned by the Nursing Council but it remained firm that the name 'cultural safety' would not change and that the Treaty of Waitangi would remain as the basis for nursing and midwifery education (Papps 2005).

In 1996, the Nursing Council published new guidelines in which the definition of cultural safety was broadened and focused less on Maori issues such as structural, political or social causes of the poor health status of Maori (Ramsden 2002). It emphasised relationships between nurses and midwives and clients who differ from them by age, gender, sexual orientation, socio-economic status, ethnicity, religious or spiritual belief and disability (NCNZ 1996). Council recognised that while cultural safety originated from the experience of Maori, its principles needed to be broad-based and apply to all people. 'Culture, in the cultural safety sense, includes all people who differ from the cultures of nursing and midwifery' (NCNZ 1996, p 8).

By 1996, the Nursing Council definition of cultural safety had evolved to include the consumer in determining 'effective nursing or midwifery care' (NCNZ 1996, p 9). The council said:

> Cultural safety is the experience of the recipient of care. Cultural safety is well beyond cultural awareness and cultural sensitivity.

MIDWIFE'S STORY 1

It was obvious from the moment we walked in that there was a lot of tension in the room, and the night staff looked relieved to be going home. The young woman, who was a Pakeha and aged about 17, was looking straight ahead and not really acknowledging us at all. The boyfriend was sitting in the corner with his Walkman plugged in and his eyes closed, and the mother of the young woman looked as if she was about to pounce on us. You could feel the hostility and anger. The first thing the mother said was, 'I suppose you are going to tell us she is not in labour either'. The midwife pulled up a stool and sat next to the woman and reassured the mother that she was not about to say such a thing after being in the room only a short time. The midwife then did nothing except sit there with her hand on the woman's abdomen feeling for the contractions—she did this for 30 minutes. The young woman gradually looked at her and then talked to her and the mother sat down and touched her daughter and a conversation took place. I could not believe the difference in the room and in the bodies of the mother and the pregnant young woman. The boyfriend even had a peek to see if it was safe to come out. The midwife listened to the baby's heart and then sat there for another 30 minutes just feeling the contractions and talking to the woman and her mother. Eventually, after an hour, when it was clear that the contractions were not establishing the young woman into labour, the midwife talked to the family about what was happening in terms of the contractions, early labour, first babies and so on. They eventually went home and she did come back four hours later in established labour and had her baby five hours after that. I asked the midwife why she had handled it this way. She replied that when she walked into the room it was clear that everyone was upset, angry and anxious, and until she had established trust and had gained a rapport with them it was a waste of time doing anything. It was important for them to feel safe, supported and listened to before any other options were offered.

Questions
1 Describe the 'culturally unsafe' issue presented in this story.
2 Describe what the midwife did to ensure that the woman and her family were safe.
3 Identify the principle/s of cultural safety that the midwife adhered to, which ensured that her practice was culturally safe.
4 Describe ways in which midwives can ensure that their practice is culturally safe (e.g. 'listening' to what is unspoken).
5 Describe how you would have handled this situation, in order to ensure the cultural safety of the woman and her family.

It gives people the power to comment on care leading to reinforcement of positive experiences. It also enables them to be involved in changes in any service experienced as negative (NCNZ 1996, p 10).

Ramsden (2000) argued that this all-inclusive definition of cultural safety meant that there was a need for a new curriculum design. She believed it was time for a stand-alone course in Maori health, so that the integration of cultural safety in its broadest sense could occur without threat to the issues of Maori health and the Treaty of Waitangi (Ramsden 2000).

Guidelines released by the Nursing Council in 2002 made this distinction. Cultural safety teaching was separated from teaching of the Treaty of Waitangi and Maori health in order to avoid confusion about the nature of cultural safety (NCNZ 2002). Nursing and midwifery education is now expected to prepare nurses and midwives to face and deal with personal, professional, institutional and social issues that affect the provision of safe midwifery care to women and their families.

It was Irihapeti's view that the future evolution and direction of cultural safety will not focus on the customs, habits and cultural practices of any group, but rather will continue to be about an analysis of power and relationships of power (Ramsden 2002). Cultural safety is simply an instrument that allows the woman and her family to judge whether the health service and delivery of health care is safe for them (Ramsden 2002). Therefore, the next step in this journey of cultural safety will need to be centred on the facilitation of a process whereby women and their families can tell midwives about the safety of the care they receive (Ramsden 2002).

Principles of cultural safety

The Nursing Council of New Zealand believes that cultural safety is facilitated by communication, understanding the diversity in worldviews, and the impact of colonisation (NCNZ 2002).

It identifies four principles of cultural safety:

● Cultural safety seeks to improve the health status of all New Zealanders.
● Cultural safety seeks to enhance the delivery of health and
● disability services through a culturally safe workforce.
● Cultural safety is broad-based and broad in its application.
● Cultural safety focuses closely on 'understanding of self, the rights of others and the legitimacy of difference' (Ramsden 2002, p 200; NCNZ 2002).

Nursing and midwifery education is based on these principles and the Nursing Council expects that it will lead to a nursing and midwifery workforce that will practise in a culturally safe way as defined by recipients of the care. The learning outcomes they identify are that nursing and midwifery students will have:

● examined their own realties and attitudes that they bring to practice
● assessed how historical, political and social processes have affected people's health
● demonstrated and continue to 'demonstrate flexibility in their relationship with people who are different from themselves' (NCNZ 2002, p 12).

In her doctoral thesis, titled 'Cultural safety and nursing education in Aotearoa and Te Waipounamu', Irihapeti

---

MIDWIFE'S STORY 2

I was a student midwife working on the delivery unit with a hospital midwife when at handover we were sent to Room 9. There was a woman aged 42 having her fifth baby. Her pregnancy had been uneventful and everything was progressing normally in labour and it was thought that she was close to birthing. The midwife we took over from was very anxious, as she said it was impossible to get near the woman to 'do' anything to her. I looked over and saw that the woman was surrounded by her four grown-up daughters in a semi-circle around the bed, and it was true that there was not a spare inch for any midwife to get into the birthing space. The midwife introduced herself and me to the woman and her daughters, who acknowledged us—just. The midwife then stood back and watched, and said to me, 'This baby will be born soon'. I whispered to her, 'How are you going to be part of this baby's birth?' and she said, 'I don't think I am and I don't need to be'. It soon became clear that the baby was about to be born—the daughters formed a tight circle around their mother as she birthed their new brother into the world. The midwife had a towel ready and as one of the daughters lifted the baby up and welcomed the baby with song and prayer, the midwife dried the baby and we were allowed in to 'do'. This experience has stayed with me and reminded me time and time again about to whom birth belongs and just what the role of the midwife is in the birthing process.

Questions

1 Describe the culturally safe and culturally unsafe issue in this story.

2 The night midwife felt anxious because she could 'not do anything' to the woman, while the other midwife was more relaxed because she knew the mother and baby were safe. Describe the skills that would have been needed to keep the situation culturally safe if something had had to be 'done' for the baby or the woman.

3 Identify the principle/s of cultural safety that the midwife adhered to, which ensured that her practice was culturally safe.

4 Describe the questions you would ask a woman to find out what was important to her and what would ensure a culturally safe experience for and her family.

Ramsden (2002) makes a number of statements that may also be interpreted as principles of cultural safety:

● Care is provided within a framework of recognising and respecting the difference of every person.
● Professional trust is established between the midwife and the woman and her family or whanau.
● The differences between the woman and her family or whanau are 'identified and negotiated' (Ramsden 2002, p 118).
● The woman and her family or whanau decide the definition of safe care.

- The power relationships between the providers and recipients of care are addressed, including the transfer of power from those who provide the service to those who receive the service (Kearns 1997).

Implications for midwifery practice

Learning about cultural safety and thinking about its implications for practice can be challenging. Students who are part of the dominant culture (such as being a white New Zealander with a European background) can be challenged by issues such as history, the Treaty of Waitangi, biculturalism and cultural safety, and may perceive these as irrelevant or unimportant. McIntosh (1988) claims that members of the dominant culture are socialised in such a way that they do not recognise their privilege in society and instead 'think of their lives as morally neutral, normative and average' (p 16). In other words, when people are part of a dominant culture, they believe that the ways in which they experience the world are natural and normal, and are the same for everyone. Understanding that this is not the case can be disturbing, challenging and alienating for students if the process of coming to awareness is not facilitated with sensitivity and care. It is important that a framework that is working towards the transformation of everything that diminishes, demeans and disempowers, does not do precisely this in working towards awareness.

Spence (2004) suggests that the process of engaging with people who differ from the nurse and midwife is unlikely to ever be free of tension. She argues that nurses (and midwives) need to learn to live with the uncertainty and paradox that difference constantly presents to them. The process of becoming culturally safe and learning to live with uncertainty and paradox takes courage, patience and kindness: courage to enter into the process, patience to stay with the process, and kindness towards self and others in the struggle with what the process requires. As Ramsden reminds us, the process of cultural safety calls for 'excellence in the service to other human beings' (Ramsden 2000, p 12).

We finish this section by acknowledging that cultural safety was 'designed as an educational process by Maori and it is given as koha [gift] to all people who are different from the service providers, whether by gender, sexual orientation, economic or educational status, age or ethnicity' (Ramsden 2002, p 181).

Midwifery partnership

As described earlier, New Zealand midwifery has developed a model for practice within its unique historical, social and cultural context. The notion of midwifery as a partnership between the woman and the midwife arose from midwifery's reflection on its successful political partnership with maternity consumer groups, which had brought about the Nurses Amendment Act in 1990 and reinstated midwifery autonomy. The New Zealand College of Midwives gave primacy to this partnership relationship by ensuring that women (consumers) had a rightful place at every level in the structure of the

Critical thinking exercise

Cultural safety is not about extraordinary events but about the everyday situations midwives find themselves in. It is the handling of these ordinary situations that requires a midwife to be culturally safe.

College and in the development of all policy and decisions. Midwifery recognised that its only power base came from the women it worked with and that together they could bring about further changes to the maternity services that would benefit both (Guilliland 1989). Thus the philosophy, standards for practice and ethical statements of the College all recognised the importance of partnership to midwifery practice (NZCOM 2005).

However, it was not until 1994 that this partnership relationship was examined in depth and an attempt was made to explain what partnership meant for midwives and how it could be practised (Guilliland & Pairman 1994).

Evolving understandings of midwifery partnership

By 1994, four years after midwifery autonomy had been reinstated, many midwives were discussing and reflecting on their new understandings of childbirth and of their role as midwives, which were arising as a result of the longer-term relationships they could now have with women throughout pregnancy, labour, birth and through the postnatal period to six weeks, and in which they were now the sole or main caregiver.

In 1994, Karen Guilliland and one of us (SP) wrote *The Midwifery Partnership: a model for practice* in an attempt to explore the relationships that were developing between midwives and their clients in the new context of midwifery autonomy and continuity of care (Guilliland & Pairman 1995). In this exploration, the authors attempted to identify the common characteristics and components of these relationships, and developed a set of principles and a model to guide midwives in their practice of partnership.

The model of midwifery partnership was published in 1995 and appeared to strike a chord with many midwives in New Zealand and overseas, because it has added to the profession's understanding of the relationships between midwives and women. It has become a required text in all schools of midwifery and has been used as a framework for midwifery curricula and models of midwifery practice in both New Zealand and overseas, including Australia.

As more midwives have been able to work in continuity of care models with women, their understanding of midwifery partnership has deepened, and midwives have become more aware of the personal attributes they need to develop in order to work in partnership relationships. In 1998, one of us (SP) completed Master's research that sought to further examine the relationship between midwives and childbearing women (Pairman 1998). In this study, six independent (caseloading

MIDWIFE'S STORY 3

I was with my independent midwife at home, discharging one of the women I had followed through as part of my student midwifery case-load. Sue was 42 and had just had her sixth baby, and in the presence of all the family I was doing the discharge examination. I asked Sue what type of contraception she would use, noting that she had used contraception for the last three years. She looked away from me and even looked embarrassed. I realised that this was an embarrassing topic for her, so to make it easier I said, 'Will you take the same contraception as last time?'. The midwife who had been talking to one of the relatives looked over at me and changed the subject and went onto another part of the discharge form. We never went back to the question of contraception and when I questioned the midwife about it later, she said, 'Sue took the contraception in secret so no one knew about it because of her family's values and beliefs'. Sue had told the midwife that in taking the contraception she felt she was betraying her family, culture and religion but that she did not want to have another child and so had done it in secret. Sue had said that children were seen as a blessing from God and so the more children, the more blessed. It appeared that contraception was not something that was discussed in the way I had assumed and in fact was a taboo subject. I felt so bad about this mistake on my part—it never fails to amaze me the assumptions I have when it comes to caring for and working with women.

Questions

1. Describe the culturally unsafe issue in this story.
2. Identify and explore the principle/s of culture safety that would have ensured culturally safe practice in this instance.
3. Describe how this situation could have been handled to ensure that it was a culturally safe experience for this woman.
4. Describe your own culture and identify five things that are really important to you.
5. Describe how the assumptions, beliefs and values that you hold may affect your practice as a midwife.
6. Identify three ways in which you can ensure that your practice as a midwife will be culturally safe.
7. Explore how you might feel and what you might do if a woman or her family told you that they felt unsafe with you.

documented. However, as the context for midwifery practice has evolved it has become necessary to revisit the model and explore its application for midwives who do not work in continuity of care and independent practice models. This work is under way and is expected to be published in 2006 (Pairman 2005).

Overview of midwifery partnership: a model for practice

Midwifery partnership is defined as:

> A relationship of 'sharing' between the woman and the midwife, involving trust, shared control and responsibility and shared meaning through mutual understanding (Guilliland & Pairman 1995, p 7).

This relationship constitutes midwifery because it is the medium through which a midwife works with a woman through the shared experience of pregnancy, labour and birth and the postnatal period to six weeks that makes up the Midwifery Scope of Practice (MCNZ 2004b).

Although a single diagrammatic representation is presented here, it is important to recognise that each relationship a midwife has with each woman she works with will be different. The key to midwifery partnership is that both partners are recognised as individuals who make equally important contributions to the relationship. Both partners negotiate the relationship and how it unfolds over time to take account of and respect their differences, needs and wishes. This negotiation is overt and requires active participation by both partners, as well as clear communication. Each woman's childbirth experience is unique and the respective roles of each midwife and each woman will vary to reflect these individual experiences and needs. The negotiated outcomes of each partnership will be different for each midwife/woman pair and therefore few partnership relationships will look the same. Because it is a professional relationship, the midwife is responsible for initiating the partnership and working with the woman to achieve this. The principles outlined below provide guidance for a midwife to achieve this.

The partners

The two partners in a midwifery partnership are a midwife and a woman. They enter into a relationship for the purposes of receiving and giving midwifery care and together they share the woman's life experiences of pregnancy, labour and birth and the postnatal period. As mentioned previously, this nine- to ten-month time frame sets the boundaries of midwifery care and enables a midwife and a woman to get to know each other in a way that makes their relationship distinctly different from usual health professional/client relationships.

Each partner will bring a unique contribution to the relationship. The woman brings her beliefs, values, knowledge, expectations, experiences and fears. She is the expert on herself and knows what she wants for this birth experience. In the model, the woman's partner, children and family/whanau surround her. The woman defines who these people are and

and self-employed) midwives and six of their clients were individually interviewed and also participated in two focus group meetings. The participants were actively involved in analysis of the data and identification of the emerging themes. At the final stage, participants compared the findings of the study with the model of midwifery partnership as developed by Karen and one of us (SP). Refinements were suggested and the participants 'teased out' midwifery partnership to also mean 'professional friendship' (Pairman 1998, 1999, 2000).

Subsequently, no further formal developments to the theoretical framework of midwifery partnership have been

the role they play in her life and through this birth experience. She will be influenced by the beliefs, values and culture of this group. The midwife, too, comes from her own social context and personal culture. However, because she is in this relationship in a professional role, the midwife is depicted in the model surrounded by midwifery's professional framework of standards and ethics that guide her practice. Both partners will also be shaped by the wider cultural and social context of the society in which they live. This will include the impact of socio-economic structures and environment, including health and maternity services. Both partners will also be influenced by dominant societal ideologies and historical determinants such as gender and class.

As the examination of cultural safety has shown us, the midwife needs to have worked through and reflected on her cultural identity, what it is that she brings with her to any midwifery relationship and how these beliefs and values could affect the woman with whom she is working. The midwife needs to recognise each woman as an individual, and respect and acknowledge her differences, working with the woman to ensure that she provides care in a way that the woman determines will meet her needs.

The model shown in Figure 14.2 depicts midwifery partnership as two equal and intertwined circles. The equal size of the circles represents the equality of both partners. The intertwined segment depicts the shared experience of pregnancy and childbirth, which provides the immediate context for each midwife–woman relationship, and the woman symbol in this section indicates the woman-centered nature of the partnership.

In Pairman's (1998) study, additional concepts were added to both the woman circle and the midwife circle to make more explicit the contributions that both make to the relationship and also to make more overt the qualities that women seek from midwives and that midwives can bring to their relationships with women (see Fig 14.3). These concepts arose from the data and were verified by the participants.

To the 'woman' circle were added the concepts of 'seeking professional care', 'seeking active participation, self-responsibility and control', 'seeking trust, respect, equality and openness' and 'being female'.

As Bizz, one woman in the study, said:

I wanted someone that I could initially build a trust in and get to know leading right up to the birth. Just that more personal and

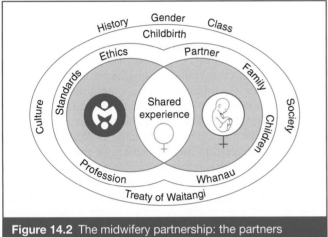

Figure 14.2 The midwifery partnership: the partners (based on Guilliland & Pairman 1995)

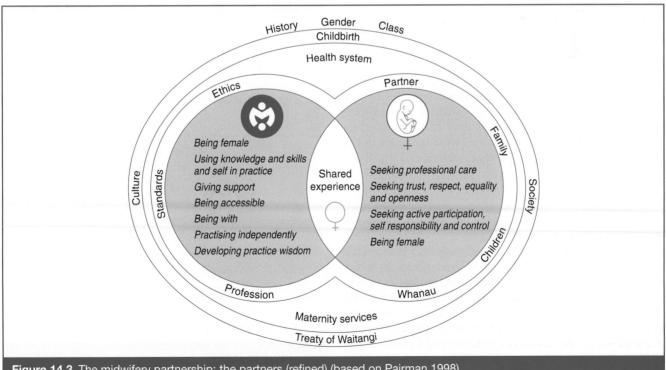

Figure 14.3 The midwifery partnership: the partners (refined) (based on Pairman 1998)

trusting relationship. And hearing the same things from the same person . . . it was important that it was someone I could talk to quite confidently, someone approachable . . . it was important too that she was a woman . . . to have an equal relationship (BF, in Pairman 1998, p 75).

Bizz's expectations were not unusual, according to Chris, one of the midwives, although she does raise the question of whether these aspects will be so clearly articulated by women once continuity of midwifery care is easily accessible to all.

Some people are very keen right from the beginning to be responsible for their own care and make their own decisions and they want information and can pretty much handle it themselves, making their decisions. You tend not to have women coming to you who want to be told what to do. I think the women that choose to come to midwifery care, and it's probably changing, but a lot of them come because they are already prepared to stand up and be counted and make their own choices because it's still going against the consensus, I think of society as a whole. Their mothers, aunts, husbands, society, which says, 'You must have a doctor, you know you've got to be safe', and the feeling is that a midwife isn't . . . I guess for a lot of women they are already in a place where they are wanting to and do make their own choices (CS, in Pairman 1998, p 82).

Exploration of the way in which midwives worked with women identified that midwives contributed more than just their midwifery knowledge and experiences to the relationship (Pairman 1998). Midwives also exhibited other attributes. Broadly, these were described as being 'with woman' and involved: the way a midwife used knowledge, skill and 'self' in practice; her accessibility to women; the way in which she provided emotional support to women and her specific skill in supporting women in labour; and the way she brought herself as a woman to each relationship. Thus within the midwife circle, the concepts of 'being female', 'giving support', 'being accessible', 'using knowledge, skill and "self" in practice' and 'being with' were added. In addition to her ability to be 'with woman', the midwife also brought her ability to reflect on her practice and to develop and trust her practice wisdom. Midwives recognised that practising midwifery independently was both conscious and active and extended beyond their work as midwives into their daily lives and affected their personal identities. These attributes were included in the midwife circle as 'developing practice wisdom' and 'practising independently'.

Philosophical underpinnings

Midwifery partnership relies on the midwife, and often also the woman, holding certain philosophical beliefs. These beliefs provide the supporting structure for midwifery partnership because they direct the practice of midwifery. In many ways these beliefs are what distinguish midwifery from other disciplines involved in the provision of maternity care. Midwives around the world share these philosophical positions and they are inherent in the international definition of a midwife articulated by the International Confederation of Midwives (ICM) (Association of Radical Midwives 1986; Australian Nursing and Midwifery Council 2005; Davis

1987; Flint 1986, 1993; Gaskin 1980; Houd 1993; ICM 1990; Page 1988, 1993; Midwifery Council of New Zealand 2004; Midwives Alliance of North America 1991). These philosophical beliefs are that: pregnancy and birth are normal life events; midwifery provides continuity of caregiver; midwifery is an independent profession; and midwifery is women-centered (see Fig 14.4).

Pregnancy and childbirth are normal life events

The belief that pregnancy and childbirth are normal life events is one of the fundamental differences between the midwifery and medical models of childbirth. While a myriad of definitions of 'normal' exist, in this context it is generally understood to mean that pregnancy and childbirth are unique physiological processes and critical events in women's lives that mark transitions to motherhood and create families (Beech & Phipps 2004).

In Western societies, the rise of faith in science and technology has led to the development of maternity services that tend to trust machines and technology more than physiology. Rather than seeking ways to support and enhance physiology, research has looked for ways to control childbirth in order to guarantee a healthy baby (and mother) at the end. As a result, the culture of childbirth that is constructed in Western societies is deeply entrenched in medicalisation, so that most births take place in hospitals, most women experience some form of surgical, technological or pharmacological intervention and many midwives are actively involved in implementing these interventions (Crabtree 2004). Medical management of childbirth has become the norm. In this context, both women and midwives have lost confidence in women's bodies and their belief in physiology is undermined. As Downe and others have identified, midwifery's claim to be the guardian of normal birth while apparently actively implementing a variety of interventions during pregnancy and birth is paradoxical (Downe 2004; Kirkham 2000b). Even where models of midwifery support one-to-one care from a midwife, such as in New Zealand, intervention rates in childbirth continue to rise, although they may be beginning to plateau.

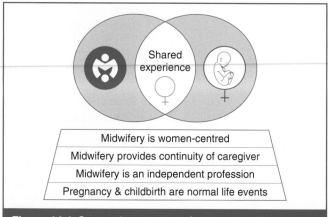

Figure 14.4 Supporting structure for the midwifery partnership (based on Guilliland & Pairman 1995)

Clearly the belief that pregnancy and childbirth are normal life events is not enough on its own, although it must be the first place to start. Downe and McCourt (2004) argue that childbirth must be understood as unique to each woman and her baby, and recognise

> the interaction and connectivity between her personal and familial history, the environment in which she labours, the attitude and response of the caregiver(s), and a multitude of other factors (Downe & McCourt 2004, p 20).

The challenge for midwives in recognising the complexity and uncertainty of childbirth is to explore personal and contextual influences on the way they practise and the way they protect and facilitate normal birth.

> By being more acutely aware of the overt and subtle ways in which medical ideology frames our practice and continues to operate, we can seek ways in which to challenge, resist and reframe this practice (Crabtree 2004, p 98).

In Chapter 6, Foureur and Hunter propose that the 'package' required to keep childbirth normal comprises three strands: a close personal and trusting relationship with a midwife who provides continuity of care throughout the childbirth experience; a strong belief in the normal physiology of childbirth; and a familiar environment for birth that enhances and supports the belief that childbirth is normal. This is supported by Pairman and Guilliland (2003), who suggest that midwives and women need locations for birth that are not dominated by the medical-model philosophy of birth, in order to strengthen their understandings of birth as a physiological process and reduce their reliance on technological interventions for routine screening and pain relief. To this end, midwives and maternity service managers need to actively promote both home and primary facilities/birthing centres as the most appropriate places for the majority of women to give birth (Pairman & Guilliland 2003). Downe and McCourt (2004) suggest that systems of care need to be reframed before any other interventions to promote normal birth can work. Instead of framing childbirth on the basis of 'simplicity, certainty and pathology', as is the case in the medical model, childbirth needs to be reframed as 'unique normality'. A maternity system that responds to women's unique normality is 'most likely to engage with complexity and uncertainty, and to maximise holistic well-being, while ensuring appropriate responses to pathology when it arises' (Downe 2004, p 174).

Midwifery partnership is about recognising each woman as uniquely normal. This belief is internalised for both women and midwives as they experience childbirth as a continuum and as women birth 'in their own way, unfettered by imposed belief systems' (Guilliland & Pairman 1995 p 35). When midwives and women work together throughout the childbirth experience and in women's own environments, midwives begin to understand the range of 'normal', which can only be defined individually for each woman (Katz Rothman 1984). The challenge for midwifery is to promote practice from these understandings so that in midwife-led care at least, childbirth really is reframed as 'uniquely normal'. Perhaps then midwifery's challenge to the medicalisation of childbirth can be truly effective.

Midwifery is an independent profession

Independent midwifery practice exists when the midwife works in partnership with the woman to provide the complete service throughout pregnancy, labour, birth and the postnatal period on her own responsibility (Guilliland & Pairman 1995, p 37). Independence relates to the way the midwife practises, not to where the woman gives birth or the employment status of the midwife.

The key aspect of independent practice is autonomy—that is, a specific philosophy and body of knowledge, together with the ability to practise without reference to another discipline. For midwifery this means being able to provide care across the scope of midwifery practice and the freedom to make decisions with the woman about care. Autonomy also requires accountability and responsibility for these midwifery judgments and actions. Autonomy does not mean practising alone. In midwifery partnership, decisions are always discussed and negotiated with each woman, and the midwife is firstly accountable to her. Midwives also work with other midwives and often discuss their midwifery judgments and uncertainties with their midwifery colleagues. When additional care is required, these judgments will include deciding when to involve an obstetrician or other specialist in a woman's care. Midwives who practise independently will take responsibility for ensuring that roles and expectations are clarified when others become involved in a woman's care, that communication is good and that the woman remains the primary decision-maker.

That midwives can practise independently is important to both midwives and to women. As will be discussed later, it is this recognition of professional autonomy that provides the foundation for the development of new understandings and knowledge that places the control of childbirth with women instead of doctors or midwives.

Midwifery provides continuity of caregiver

Continuity of caregiver means 'one midwife (and her back-up colleague) providing midwifery care throughout the entire childbirth experience' (Guilliland & Pairman 1995, p 39). Continuity of caregiver in a one-to-one relationship is fundamental to midwifery because it enables midwives to work in their full scope of practice in a way that other disciplines do not. It is what distinguishes midwifery as a profession. It gives midwives the ability to build partnerships with women because it provides them with time to get to know each other and to develop trust. In relationships that span pregnancy and beyond, there is time to work with each woman to discuss her wishes and her fears for birth and motherhood, and to build her confidence in herself. There is time to work with families to build their confidence and to uncover their fears and misconceptions. Decision-making becomes much easier because there is time for each woman to explore information and to think through options to come to decisions that are right for her. Midwives and women have time to talk about labour, pain, the impact of the environment, uncertainty and complexity, so that, ideally, by the time a woman goes into labour she is willing and confident to 'let go' and to trust her body to give birth.

Midwives working outside the continuity model (core midwives) provide the essential link for the caseloading midwife and the woman when they require extra or supportive care. Core midwives' partnership relationship with the woman's chosen midwife ensures that the continuum of care is possible for most women regardless of their need for obstetric intervention.

There is now a significant amount of evidence that care provided by teams of midwives in continuity-of-care models is associated with a reduction in the use of some technological and pharmacological interventions, and that women prefer this type of care (Sandall 2004). Although there are no randomised controlled trials of caseloading (one-to-one) midwifery, the evidence of the importance of supportive relationships during pregnancy and continuous one-to-one support during labour is clear (Hodnett et al 2003; MIDIRS 1996; Oakley et al 1996). Despite this research knowledge, it is often not acted upon and outside New Zealand many maternity services do not enable and support midwives to develop and maintain one-to-one models of practice (Kirkham 2000b).

Midwifery is women-centred

In midwifery partnership, 'women-centredness' is important in three main ways. First, midwifery only exists 'to facilitate the optimal experience of birth for pregnant women and their babies' (Guilliland & Pairman 1995, p 41). Secondly, midwifery recognises the centrality of women's experiences by ensuring that its focus is on the woman, who defines her needs. The midwifery relationship is with the woman, who has the primary relationship with her baby. A woman-centred philosophy does not separate the needs of the mother and baby, viewing them rather as an integrated whole, where the needs of one will be the needs of the other. Women-centredness is not a denial of the important part the family plays in the woman's life, but rather acknowledges that it is she who has the primary relationship with her family, not the midwife, and it is she who decides how her family will be involved.

Finally, a women-centred philosophy ensures that women are seen as individuals, each with different needs and different cultural identities. As Bizz described, a women-centred approach takes account of each woman's particular context.

> The midwife spoke about my pregnancy as a whole thing with me, Eric and the baby, rather than just my body and my baby inside it (BF, in Pairman 1998, p 183).

And Kate explained:

> It's the whole family dynamics; it's the people who are close to her. It's not just the woman; it's everyone that affects her and everything that affects her (KS, in Pairman 1998, p 183).

Women-centredness just means working with a woman in whatever way she wants. For the women in Pairman's study

(1998), the involvement of their families was crucial and their expectations were that the midwife would facilitate the involvement of their families in these shared experiences of pregnancy and childbirth.

Theoretical concepts

The philosophical beliefs outlined above provide the conditions within which midwifery partnerships can form. However, the successful establishment and maintenance of a midwifery partnership relies on the integration of certain principles in how the partners relate to each other. These principles are: individual negotiation, equality, shared responsibility and empowerment, and informed choice and consent (see Fig 14.5).

It is on this aspect of midwifery partnership that the findings from Pairman's (1998) study had the most impact, and refinements were made in order to make more explicit the way in which midwives and women 'work together' in

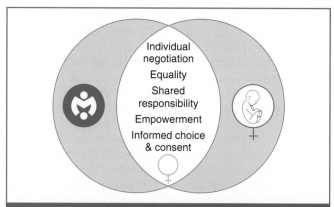

Figure 14.5 Principles inherent in the partnership (based on Guilliland & Pairman 1995)

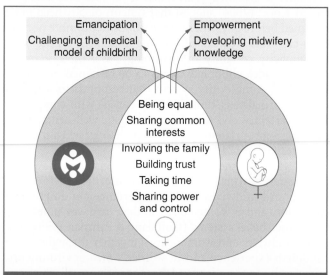

Figure 14.6 Principles inherent in the partnership model and outcomes of midwifery partnership (based on Pairman 1998)

a midwifery partnership. The refined model identified the following concepts as describing how midwives and women worked together: 'being equal', 'sharing common interests', 'involving the family', 'building trust', 'reciprocity', 'taking time' and 'sharing power and control' (see Fig 14.6).

These concepts incorporated most of the original concepts identified in the midwifery partnership model (see Fig 14.5), but were more specific and focused to a greater extent on how a midwife and a woman actually worked together.

The refined model also made the outcomes of midwifery partnership more explicit. Empowerment was identified as an outcome for both women and midwives, as was emancipation. The developments of new knowledge about midwifery and about birth and the challenge this midwifery model of care poses to the medical model of childbirth were identified as two specific outcomes that resulted from empowerment and emancipation of the midwife and woman within midwifery partnership. The refined model is presented in Figure 14.7.

The concepts discussed below are key principles from both models that exemplify the way in which midwifery partnership is enacted. In many ways these concepts overlap in their meaning, and it is their integration that characterises midwifery partnerships.

Negotiation

The underlying premise of the partnership is that it is individually negotiated, recognising the essential contribution of each (Guilliland & Pairman 1995, p 44). Each partner brings different things to the partnership, but both partners must participate and contribute if the partnership is to work. Negotiation is a process by which a midwife and a woman work though issues such as power-sharing, decision-making, and mutual rights and responsibilities, and make their expectations of each other explicit. Negotiation relies on open and effective communication and a positive sense of self. It is a process for working things out and coming to mutual understandings and agreements. It is a mutating, changing, synchronous pattern of give and take that facilitates movement towards a shared purpose (Henson 1997, p 79).

Each partnership will be different because of the unique characteristics of each partner and the way they negotiate the relationship.

Equality and reciprocity

In a partnership, both partners have equal status and must feel equal. This does not mean that a midwife and a woman are the same or that they bring the same things to their relationship

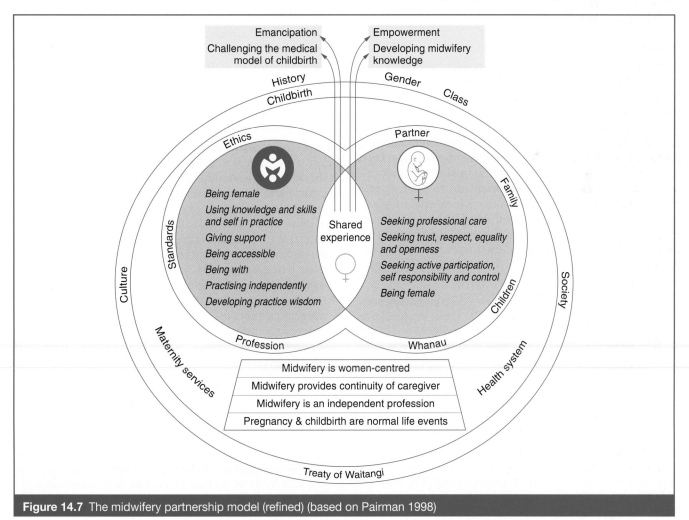

Figure 14.7 The midwifery partnership model (refined) (based on Pairman 1998)

or that they have the same roles. They are different and this difference is recognised and respected. As Amy, a woman in the study, commented: 'She was there to do her job and not be bossy and I was there to do a job and not push her around' (AA, in Pairman 1998, p 122). And Bizz said:

> I trusted her professionalism and all her knowledge, but I felt very equal with her. I needed her expertise and I was very confident in it, but I suppose her confidence built my confidence. So I didn't feel at any stage that she was in any way above me, looking down on me or anything like that (BF, in Pairman 1998, p 117).

The contributions that both make to their relationship are equally valued and the process of getting to know each other and working together is reciprocal. Reciprocity means a two-way sharing or mutual exchange that creates shared meaning and is beneficial to both. Mutual involvement of both partners strengthens and deepens their relationship and has positive effects on both partners. As Chris, one of the midwives in the study, explained:

> It's two way . . . that the woman feels relaxed and comfortable, supported . . . if she feels she can trust you with herself and particularly the vulnerability in labour . . . I think that's a real privilege for us to have that trust, and it works the other way, that you trust the woman to tell you what her needs are and if she's not happy or wants something else (CS, in Pairman 1998, p 122).

Trust and time

As women and midwives get to know each other, they learn to trust each other. Trust is essential in any healthy human relationship and in midwifery partnership trust underpins information sharing, decision-making, power sharing and empowerment. When two people trust each other they feel safe with each other and willing to expose their vulnerabilities because they know the other person will respect these. Faced with the uncertainty of childbirth, it is important for women to trust their midwives and for midwives to trust women. No amount of talking or preparation can predict how each unique birth experience will unfold and there is always a time when women and midwives have to 'let go' and trust the process—trust physiology, trust women's bodies, and trust themselves. As Linda, one of the women in the study, explained:

> I felt that if something was going wrong she'd give me plenty of advance warning and I wouldn't have to yell at her to take me . . . like she knew that I was scared, she knew how I was feeling. Because we discussed Lauren's birth quite in detail, and so she knew where I was coming from and so I felt very comfortable with her . . . after Brianna was born, the way she lifted her up . . . I felt very safe with her having Brianna as well . . . I trusted her totally . . . I trusted her to show it (the placenta) to me and it was alright. It was alright because I felt safe with her (LF, in Pairman 1998, p 121).

Trust develops over time and therefore continuity of caregiver enhances the development of trust. Midwives who visit women in their own homes during pregnancy are able to get to know each woman in her own context and in surroundings where she is comfortable and in control. Often

family will be involved. In these more relaxed settings both partners have the opportunity to really get to know each other. Dianne said:

> Just the development of the relationship. It does take a while to get to know someone. And you're inviting them to partake in something that's going to happen only once or twice in your lifetime. So you want to be sure that the person who's attending you is going to respect your wishes and is going to be on the same wavelength as you (DMcD, in Pairman 1998, p 127).

There are several dimensions to time: the time that midwives give to each visit that enables full discussion; being accessible to women at other times when necessary; the length of the relationship from early pregnancy through to about six weeks after birth; and for some midwives and women, the opportunity to work with each other again in subsequent pregnancies so that their relationships can continue to develop over years. This ability to spend time is valued by both women and midwives. As Dianne said:

> She'd come and spend an hour with us . . . I was really appreciative of all the time she did spend with us, so that the experience that we had was really amazing . . . it wasn't just a five minute 'Are you OK?'. Because sometimes I think that you need longer . . . you really need that time to go through and talk about what was going on (DMcD, in Pairman 1998, p 126).

As mentioned already, the capacity of a midwife to develop a personal and trusting relationship with a woman over nine to ten months is one of the unique differences between midwifery and other health professions involved in the provision of maternity care.

Sharing power and responsibility

In midwifery partnership, both partners exercise power. The balance of power is negotiated and mutually agreed. Power is shared through sharing information, by the way decisions are made and by recognising and enhancing each woman's sense of control. Feeling in control during childbirth leads to a sense of satisfaction, fulfilment and positive wellbeing (Green et al 1990). The exercise of power and personal control is dependent on having the resources and options that allow choice, being adequately informed about choices, being involved in decision-making and being able to implement those decisions once they are made (Walker et al 1995). Midwifery partnership provides a framework within which a woman can achieve a sense of personal control. In an equal and negotiated relationship, where both partners trust each other and feel safe, midwives can actively support women to take hold of their power and make decisions without imposing their own beliefs. As Kay explained:

> I present women with all the information that's available and then they make the choices of what they want to do . . . I give them information, usually research based, about things they want to know . . . I think there is a danger that some midwives put their experiences onto women . . . sometimes that's okay and sometimes it's not, because it's not actually your experience, it's their experience so it should be totally theirs, it should be unique (KF, in Pairman 1998, p 135).

Dianne also described this kind of decision-making:

> It was at the back of my mind that she must have her own feelings about what should be done but it never came through. That's what I found really amazing about her, that I never felt in any way that whatever she carried with her (because I believe that anyone who makes a decision—there's a whole lot of other things as to why they make that decision), and I never felt she brought any of that into the situation . . . she was there but she never moved in (DMcD, in Pairman 1998, p 134).

Along with the power to make decisions and be in control comes responsibility for those decisions. While midwives are always professionally accountable for their midwifery judgements and actions, in midwifery partnership women also take responsibility for the outcomes of decisions jointly made. As Dianne described, taking responsibility and making decisions can be an empowering process:

> You've got to take responsibility and I think once you take responsibility for your life you can do so much more. It's tied up in a circle—you can evolve much beyond that. It's like taking hold of your life. If you take responsibility then if you get a bad thing out of it then you learn from your mistake. If you get a good thing out of it then you get a real buzz. It's not anyone else's—they might have contributed to it, but it's like 'yeah, I did that and I can take the credit for it' . . . even today I look at Jessica and I find it really amazing that she grew up in me. I ate really healthy and I felt whatever I did would be reflected in Jessica, and I wanted a really good healthy baby . . . then at the end we got this fantastic little baby who was really alert from day one. Even now she's raring to go. I take a wee credit for that (DMcD, in Pairman 1998, p 168).

Empowerment and emancipation

Midwives are privileged in that their professional role enables them to be alongside women and families through the important and life-changing processes of pregnancy, childbirth and early motherhood. The midwifery role is mainly to support and assist women in a way that 'recognises that the physical, emotional, and spiritual aspects of pregnancy and birth are equally important' (Page & Hutton 2000, p 1). Midwifery aims to enable women to recognise their personal power and strengths and increase women's sense of autonomy and confidence as mothers and as women. These are lofty aims but because pregnancy and birth are such life-changing events they often cause women to ask questions about themselves and their lives and seek to make changes. As Nicky Leap (2000, p 5) said, 'The question marks of pregnancy are the beginning of a process of grappling with the uncertainty and decision-making that will persist throughout the experience of raising a child'. For some women, having a midwife ask them what they want for their birth may be the first time they have had the opportunity to make any choices in their lives. Kate commented:

> It's a nice feeling to see a woman go from thinking that everyone else owns, or has a right to dictate, to deciding—and to see it spill over into other areas is really neat . . . and start questioning other areas and other things in her life . . . that's a major plus I think to work with a woman over a longer time (KS, in Pairman 1998, p 166).

Midwives can work with women in ways that facilitate empowerment for women and this in turn can be empowering for midwives. Key facilitation skills for midwives are believing in women and inspiring confidence, and knowing when to intervene and when to withdraw (Leap 2000). As Julie described:

> Every message they get is about self-responsibility . . . asking information at the beginning, saying, 'How is your baby moving? What do you notice about yourself? How have you felt?' and actually listening . . . what we're doing is checking that she's observing and aware of herself and her baby, and I believe women take that on (JR, in Pairman 1998, p 143).

Although midwives share significant life events with women, they are involved in women's lives for only short periods. Their involvement with women can be empowering if they work to facilitate independence and self-determination rather than dependence. One way to do this is to encourage women to build their own networks of support rather than relying on midwives, who will not be there for the long-term. As Chris explained:

> I like to think that the focus is that they're developing their own independence and their own networks to support them, because when you move towards leaving them at six weeks postpartum or whenever, I usually find, not quite that you're rejected, but that you're not needed anymore. By the time you finish they're competent, confident and managing and have set up networks to keep going (CS, in Pairman 1998, p 150).

Midwifery partnership can be empowering for both women and midwives. As midwives work with women in this way, their beliefs about birth and about midwifery are reinforced and strengthened. Observing the uniqueness of each woman's birth experience builds midwives' confidence about the ranges of 'normal' that are possible and builds trust in women's bodies. Sharing and negotiating power and decision-making and being able to see the outcomes of these decisions strengthens midwives' trust and confidence in women, and in themselves as autonomous practitioners.

Midwifery partnership also has emancipatory potential. Women who experience midwifery partnership often encourage other women to seek this type of care. 'Emancipation is a dynamic state of being in which self-knowledge (enlightenment) and self-advocacy (empowerment) are connected to knowledge and advocacy for others' (Henderson 1995, p 66). As most systems of maternity care in Western societies are still entrenched in the medical model, there is huge scope for women to persuade other women through the telling of their stories about the normalcy of birth and the benefits of one-to-one midwifery care. New Zealand and Canada are two examples of where political action by women has led to significant structural and philosophical changes in the way maternity services are delivered and the development of more women-centred models of care.

Professional friendship

The women in Pairman's (1998) study believed that the term 'professional friend' encompassed what they felt about the midwife/woman relationship and their experience of midwifery partnership. This term describes the relationship between midwives and women as friendship but also recognises the professional focus of the relationship and its time-limited nature (Pairman 2000). As Bizz explained:

> I think we had a really good relationship, actually. It was more of a friend relationship, but a friend you could trust in—a professional friend you could rely on (BF, in Pairman 1998, p 163).

Pairman's study teased out midwifery partnership to mean 'professional friendship'. As described, the refinements made to the partnership model in this study provided further depth and understanding of the concepts by exploring how women and midwives experienced midwifery partnerships. Further exploration of the notion of professional friendship will contribute to midwifery's understanding of the practice of partnership.

Potentials and possibilities for partnership

Midwifery partnership, then, is a relationship of sharing based on mutual respect and trust that has the potential to enrich the lives of both women and midwives. Although the partnership model arose from New Zealand's unique historical, social and cultural context, it can be applied in other settings. New Zealand midwives have claimed that 'midwifery *is* the partnership between the woman and the midwife' (Guilliland & Pairman 1995, p 33). This is because midwives work always in relationships with women (Guilliland & Pairman 1995. These relationships are the medium through which midwives provide care and have a powerful impact on how women receive this care. Midwifery partnership identifies a set of principles that enable midwives to develop relationships with women that are intrinsically different from the usual health professional/client relationships. In midwifery partnerships, women are recognised as autonomous individuals undergoing a significant and transformative but 'normal' life process. Women need midwives' specialised expertise, knowledge and wisdom to support and guide them through this process but must also contribute their own expertise, knowledge and wisdom if the experience is to meet their needs. In midwifery partnerships, midwives and women both have recognised expertise and they collaborate to ensure that the childbirth experience is safe and fulfilling for the woman. The processes of collaboration, sharing and negotiation required in midwifery partnerships strengthen and empower both midwives and women. New Zealand midwifery has redefined professionalism to mean midwifery partnership and claimed a new professional role as 'partner' rather than 'expert'.

Working in partnership is demanding. It requires self-knowledge on the part of midwives, strong and effective communication skills and a secure sense of self. It also takes time and the ability to be reflective. Like any human relationship it will not be possible to get it 'right' every time,

and each new relationship with a woman can add to a midwife's understanding of herself and how she works with women, if she is willing to examine these. The model of midwifery partnership provides guidance to midwives wanting to develop partnerships with women, and the concepts discussed above are a starting place for reflective practice and learning about partnership.

Midwifery partnership is definitely enhanced when midwives work in one-to-one continuity of care models as autonomous practitioners. Even when this is not possible, midwives can incorporate some of the principles of partnership into their care of women in more fragmented settings where the midwife and the woman do not know each other. Acknowledging our professional power and finding ways to shift that power to women is challenging but still possible even in the most fleeting of encounters with women. The way midwives write in women's maternity notes and the language they use can empower or disempower women.

Midwifery partnership also provides a model for the development of political partnerships between maternity consumer groups and midwifery professional organisations. There is always the opportunity for midwives to get to know their local community and to establish relationships with maternity consumer groups. As seen in New Zealand, these women can be a force for social change. Change can happen in small steps. The successful implementation of one-to-one care in a single maternity unit can lead to further developments as more women demand this type of care and more midwives demand to work in this way.

As midwife-led maternity services are developed they need to be supported, ideally by the wider health organisations. However, even if support is not forthcoming from managers and employers, midwives can do a great deal to support each other and empower themselves as a group. Pairs of midwives working together to provide care to a caseload of women should join other pairs to create larger groups. These larger groups can provide support, friendship, mentoring and safe places to debrief and problem solve. They can also provide political strength when necessary.

Where midwives and women experience continuity-of-care relationships based on partnership, they begin to understand childbirth differently. If each woman's experience is different, then it follows that protocols, timeframes and routinised midwifery care will not enhance women's diverse childbirth processes. In such settings a midwife has to 'question many of the taken-for-granted assumptions of the medical setting and the medical model. And she finds herself constructing a new model, a new way of explaining what she sees' (Katz Rothman 1984, p 304). Midwifery partnership creates the opportunity for new knowledge (midwifery knowledge) to develop for both

Critical thinking exercise

Are midwifery partnership and cultural safety the same? If so, explain their similarities. If not, explain their differences.

midwives and women that can begin to challenge the medical model as the dominant paradigm for childbirth.

Conclusion

Midwifery partnership provides a framework for a negotiated and reciprocal relationship of equity and power sharing. Cultural safety provides a framework for recognising cultural 'difference' between a midwife and a woman, the power inherent in the professional role of a midwife and the impact that the culture of the midwife may have on her professional practice. A key aspect of cultural safety in relation to midwifery practice is that it is the childbearing woman and her family, not the midwife, who determine that the midwifery care is effective and 'safe'. Together these frameworks identify and explain the unique nature of New Zealand's midwifery and maternity practices.

Review questions

1 Describe 'culture' as defined by the New Zealand Nursing Council.

2 Describe 'cultural safety' as defined by the New Zealand Nursing Council.

3 Describe culturally safe practice.

4 Describe culturally unsafe practice.

5 Who determines whether a midwife's practice is culturally safe?

6 Describe the difference between transcultural nursing and cultural safety.

7 Describe the relationship between colonisation and cultural safety.

8 Describe the difference between cultural awareness, cultural sensitivity and cultural safety.

9 Describe the movement from 'regardless' to 'regardful' of what makes a person unique and how this relates to cultural safety.

10 Describe how power and structures of power are related to cultural safety.

11 List the principles of cultural safety.

12 Describe midwifery partnership as defined by Guilliland and Pairman (1995).

13 What are the supporting philosophical positions of midwifery partnership?

14 Identify five important concepts that describe how a midwife and a woman work together in partnership

15 How is empowerment achieved in midwifery partnership?

Note

1 This section talks of nurses and midwives because cultural safety was developed in an era when nursing and midwifery were still closely intertwined educationally and were both regulated by the Nursing Council of New Zealand, which defined cultural safety as a competency for practice for both nurses and midwives.

Online resource

Irihapeti Ramsden's 2002 doctoral thesis on cultural safety, http://culturalsafety.massey.ac.nz/thesis.htm

References

Australian Nursing and Midwifery Council 2005 Role, scope of practice and development of national competency standards for midwives. Online: https://www.anmc.org.au/, accessed 31 March 2005

Association of Radical Midwives 1986 The vision: proposals for the future of the maternity services. ARM, London

Beech BL, Phipps B 2004 Normal birth: women's stories. In: S Downe (Ed) Normal childbirth: evidence and debate. Churchill Livingstone, London

Burn N, Grove SK 1995 Understanding nursing research. WB Saunders, Philadelphia

Bryar R 1995 Theory for midwifery practice. MacMillan, London

Crabtree S 2004 Midwives constructing normal birth. In: S Downe (Ed) Normal childbirth: evidence and debate. Churchill Livingstone, London

Davis E 1987 Heart and hands. A midwife's guide to pregnancy and birth (2nd edn). Celestial Arts, Berkeley, California

Dobbie M 1990 The trouble with women. The story of Parents Centre New Zealand. Cape Catley, Whatamongo Bay

Donley J 1986 Save the midwife. New Women's Press, Auckland

Donley J 1989 Professionalism. The importance of consumer control over childbirth. New Zealand College of Midwives Journal, September:6–7

Downe S 2004 Aspects of a controversy: summary and debate. In: S Downe (Ed) Normal childbirth: evidence and debate. Churchill Livingstone, London

Downe S, McCourt C 2004 From being to becoming: reconstructing childbirth knowledges. In: S Downe (Ed) Normal childbirth: evidence and debate. Churchill Livingstone, London

Flint C 1986 Sensitive midwifery. Heinemann Midwifery, London

Flint C 1993 Midwifery teams and caseloads. Butterworth-Heinemann, Oxford

Gaskin IM 1980 Spiritual midwifery. The Book Publishing Company, Summertown, TN

Green J, Coupland V, Kitzinger J 1990 Expectations, experiences and psychological outcomes of childbirth: a prospective study of 825 women. Birth (17):15–24

Guilliland K 1989 Maintaining the links—a history of the formation of the NZCOM. New Zealand College of Midwives Journal, September:14–15

Guilliland K, Pairman S 1994 The midwifery partnership: a model for practice. New Zealand College of Midwives Journal, October:5–9

Guilliland K, Pairman S 1995 The midwifery partnership: a model for practice. Monograph series: 95/1. Department of Nursing and Midwifery, Victoria University of Wellington, New Zealand

Henderson D 1995 Consciousness raising in participatory research: method and methodology for emancipatory inquiry. Advanced Nursing Science 17(30):58–69

Henson RH 1997 Analysis of the concept of mutuality. Image: Journal of Nursing Scholarship 29(10):77–81

Hinchcliff J 1997 Values integrating education: an exploration of learning in New Zealand. Mirilea Press, Pukekohe

Hodnett ED, Gates S, Hofmeyer GJ et al 2003 Continuous support for women during childbirth. Cochrane Library (4). John Wiley & Sons, Chichester

Homer C 2004 Australian Midwifery Competency Project. Draft Three. Online: www.anmc.org.au/projects

Houd S 1993 The spirit of midwifery. Keynote address, proceedings of the International Confederation of Midwives, 23rd International Congress, Vancouver, May, pp 75–86

International Confederation of Midwives 1990 Definition of a midwife. Position Statement 90/1, ICM, London

Katz Rothman B 1984 Childbirth management and medical monopoly: midwifery as (almost) a profession. Journal of Nurse-Midwifery 29(5):300–306

Kearns RA 1997 A place for cultural safety beyond nursing education? New Zealand Medical Journal 110:23–24

Kirkham M (Ed) 2000a The midwife–mother relationship. Macmillan, London

Kirkham M 2000b How can we relate? In: M Kirkham (Ed) The midwife–mother relationship, Macmillan, London

Leap N 2005 The less we do the more we give. In: M Kirkham (Ed) The midwife–mother relationship. Macmillan, London

Maternity Coalition, AIMS (Australia), Australian Society of Independent Midwives, Community Midwifery WA Inc. 2002 National maternity action plan for the introduction of community midwifery services in urban and regional Australia. Author

McAra-Couper J 2005 Right relationship and cultural safety. Unpublished paper. Auckland University of Technology, Auckland

McIntosh P 1988 White privilege: unpacking the invisible knapsack. Online: http://www.utoronto.ca/acc/events/peggy1, accessed 8 August 2004

MIDIRS 1996 Support in labour. Informed Choice Leaflet No 1. MIDIRS/NHS Centre for Reviews and Dissemination, Bristol/York

Midwives Alliance of North America 1991 MANA Core Competencies for basic midwifery practice, MANA, Bristol, VA

Midwifery Council of New Zealand (MCNZ) 2004a Competencies for entry to the register of midwives. Online: http://midwiferycouncil.org.nz/main/Competencies/, accessed 31 March 2005

Midwifery Council of New Zealand (MCNZ) 2004b Midwifery Scope of Practice. Online: http://www.midwiferycouncil.org.nz/main/Scope/, accessed 31 March 2005

New Zealand College of Midwives (NZCOM) 2005 Midwives handbook for practice. NZCOM, Christchurch

Nursing Council of New Zealand (NCNZ) 1992 Guidelines for the cultural safety component in nursing and midwifery education. NCNZ, Wellington

Nursing Council of New Zealand (NCNZ) 1996 Guidelines for the cultural safety component in nursing and midwifery education. NCNZ, Wellington

Nursing Council of New Zealand (NCNZ) 2002 Guidelines for cultural safety, the Treaty of Waitangi, and Maori health in nursing and midwifery education and practice. NCNZ, Wellington

Nursing Council of New Zealand (NCNZ) 2005 Guidelines for cultural safety, the Treaty of Waitangi and Maori health in nursing education and practice. NCNZ, Wellington

Oakley A, Hickey D, Rajan L et al 1996 Social support in pregnancy: does it have long-term effects? Journal of Reproductive and Infant Psychology 14:7–22

Page LA 1998 The midwife's role in modern healthcare. In: S Kitzinger (Ed) The midwife challenge. Pandora Press, London

Page LA 1993 Midwives hear the heartbeat of the future. Keynote address, proceedings of the International Confederation of Midwives, 23rd International Congress. Vancouver, May

Page LA (Ed) 2000 The new midwifery. Science and sensitivity in practice. Churchill Livingstone, London

Page LA, Hutton E 2000 Introduction: setting the scene. In: LA Page (Ed) The new midwifery. Science and sensitivity in practice. Churchill Livingstone, London

Pairman S 1998 The midwifery partnership: an exploration of the midwife/woman relationship. Unpublished masters thesis, Victoria University of Wellington

Pairman S 1999 Partnership revisited: towards midwifery theory. New Zealand College of Midwives Journal 21(October):6–12

Pairman S 2000 Women-centred midwifery: partnerships or professional friendships? In: M Kirkham (Ed) The midwife–mother relationship, Macmillan, London, pp 207–226

Pairman S 2005 Workforce to profession: an exploration of New Zealand Midwifery's professionalisation strategies from 1986 to 2005. Unpublished doctoral thesis. University of Technology, Sydney

Pairman S, Guilliland K 2003 Developing a midwife-led maternity service: the New Zealand experience. In: M Kirkham (Ed) Birth centres: a social model for maternity care. Books for Midwives, London

Papps E 2002 Cultural safety: what is the question? In: E Papps (Ed) Nursing in New Zealand. Critical issues, different perspectives. Pearson Education, Auckland

Papps E 2005 Cultural safety: daring to be different. In: D Wepa (Ed) Cultural safety in Aotearoa New Zealand. Pearson Education, Auckland

Ramsden I 1989 A model for negotiated and equal partnership. Author, Wellington

Ramsden I 1990 Kawa whakaruruhau: cultural safety in nursing education in Aotearoa. Ministry of Education, Wellington

Ramsden I 2000 Cultural safety / Kawa whakaruruhau ten years on: a personal overview. Nursing Praxis in New Zealand 15(1):4–12

Ramsden I 2002 Cultural safety and nursing education in Aotearoa and Te Waipounamu. Unpublished PhD thesis, Victoria University of Wellington

Ramsden I 2005 Towards cultural safety. In: D Wepa (Ed) Cultural safety in Aotearoa New Zealand. Pearson Education, Auckland

Richardson F 2000 What is it like to teach cultural safety in a New Zealand nursing education programme? Unpublished Masters thesis, Massey University, Palmerston North

Sandall J 2004 Promoting normal birth: weighing the evidence. In: S Downe (Ed) Normal childbirth: evidence and debate. Churchill Livingstone, London

Spence DG 1999 Prejudice, paradox and possibility: Nursing people from cultures other than one's own. Unpublished PhD thesis, Massey University, Palmerston North

Spence D 2001 The evolving meaning of 'culture' in New Zealand Nursing. Nursing Praxis in New Zealand 17(3):51–61

Spence D 2004 Prejudice, paradox and possibility: the experience of nursing people from cultures other than one's own. In: K Kavanagh, V Knowlden (Eds) Many voices, toward caring culture in healthcare and healing. Wisconsin: University of Wisconsin Press, pp 140–180

Strid J 1987 Maternity in revolt. Broadsheet 153:14–17

Walker R 1987 Nga Tau Tohetohe, years of anger. Penguin, Auckland

Walker J, Hall S, Thomas M 1995 The experience of labour: a perspective from those receiving care in a midwife-led unit. Midwifery 11:120–129

Further reading

(Readers are also advised to peruse the reference list above.)

Cronk M 2000 The midwife: a professional servant? In: M Kirkham (Ed) The midwife–mother relationship. Macmillan, London

Ehrenreich, B, English D 1973 Witches, midwives and nurses: a history of women healers. The Feminist Press, Glass Mountain Pamphlet, New York

Wepa D 2001 An exploration of the experiences of cultural safety educators. Unpublished Masters thesis, Massey University, Palmerston North

Whanau Kawa Whakaruruhau 1991 Cultural safety. Hui of the whanau kawa whakaruruhau. Apumoana Marae, Rotorua

Wilkins R 2000 Poor relations: the paucity of the professional paradigm. In: M Kirkham (Ed) The midwife–mother relationship, Macmillan, London

CHAPTER 15

Working in partnership

Nicky Leap and Sally Pairman

Key terms

continuity of care, core midwife, decision-making, partnership, persuasion, professional friend, professional judgement, midwifery role, professionalism, relationship, self-determination, women-centred care

Chapter overview

This chapter provides an overview of how midwives can work in partnerships with women and with other midwives through an exploration of key aspects of partnership practice.

Working in partnership takes maturity, self-knowledge, honesty, commitment and professionalism. It is demanding and challenging but ultimately rewarding and satisfying. It can benefit both partners. To work in partnership requires a midwife to move beyond her professional role and expose and share herself as a person with the women for whom she provides care. This chapter identifies some important aspects of partnership practice and explores how midwives can integrate these aspects into their own midwifery practice.

Learning outcomes

Learning outcomes for this chapter are:

1 To explore the meaning of 'partnership' between women and midwives

2 To identify key aspects of partnership practice

3 To understand the importance of midwifery partnership to midwifery practice and women's experiences of childbirth

4 To develop strategies for the integration of partnership into midwifery practice.

Introduction

The central tenet of midwifery is that it is a relationship between a midwife and a woman and that this relationship is one of partnership (Guilliland & Pairman 1995; Kirkham 2000). The development of this partnership relationship relies on midwives being able to work in continuity-of-care models so that mutual trust and understanding between midwives and women can evolve over time. Partnership relationships provide a context from which there is potential for both women and midwives to be enriched by exploring the inherent possibilities within the self (Guilliland & Pairman 1995; Siddiqui 1991).

Promoting normal (physiological) birth is only one aim of midwifery care. Equally important is the aim of supporting women to be confident in their roles as mothers, with the consequent positive impact on families and communities. A one-to-one relationship between a midwife and a woman over nine to ten months of the childbirth process provides a unique opportunity for midwives to reinforce and support women's abilities as decision-makers and their sense of self-determination. Confidence in her body and in her self will stand a woman in good stead as she takes on the complex role of mother that is central to the healthy functioning of a family.

While personally demanding, working in partnership with women is also extremely rewarding and empowering for midwives. One-to-one continuity of care provides a context in which midwives can truly embrace their full role and scope of practice and explore what it means to 'be with' women during childbirth. This meaning will differ for each midwife, who will identify and develop her[1] own practice strategies to enhance her partnership relationships with women.

This chapter looks at some of the practicalities and issues relating to practising in partnership with women and with the aim of promoting women's confidence and sense of self-determination. The chapter also examines the partnerships that midwives form with midwifery colleagues. The philosophy and particular nature of midwifery partnership is explored, with practical references to an approach that:
- minimises disturbance, direction, authority and intervention
- maximises the potential for physiology, common sense and instinctive behaviour to prevail
- places trust in the expertise of the childbearing woman
- shifts power towards the woman (Leap 2000, p 2).

Partnership: overview of some evidence

There is a growing awareness of the benefits to women of being able to access one-to-one continuity of midwifery care (or midwifery caseload practice), which is the foundation of partnership (Benjamin et al 2001; Hodnett 2004; Homer et al 2001; Homer et al 2002a; Page et al 2001; Sandall et al 2001). Although most studies are of continuity of care from a small group of caregivers rather than one-to-one care, the benefits for women include increased satisfaction with their care and a reduced likelihood of: being admitted to hospital antenatally; having drugs for pain relief in labour; having an episiotomy; and their baby requiring resuscitation (Sandall 2004). These benefits extend to women who experience complications and need to also have care provided by obstetricians, paediatricians and other medical specialists (Farrell et al 2002; Homer et al 2002b).

A central component of midwifery caseload practice is continuous support in labour, which has a positive impact on both women's experiences and birth outcomes (Hodnett 2004). Women who have continuous support are more likely to have a spontaneous vaginal birth, less likely to use analgesia in labour, less likely to have an operative birth or caesarean section and are more likely to be satisfied with the birth experience (Hodnett 2004).

In New Zealand, where over 78% of women receive continuity of care through caseload midwifery models, the impact of this care in improving outcomes for women and babies is beginning to be recognised (NZHIS 2005). Rather than a dramatic decrease in intervention rates, it appears more likely that continuity of midwifery care may make a positive impact on outcomes and health over a longer timeframe (Guilliland 2005). For example, since the commencement of this one-to-one partnership model of midwifery care in 1996[2], perinatal mortality rates have continued to decline, antenatal admission rates for women with serious complications have declined, 95% of babies receive their six-week immunisation (a rate higher than at any other time in the immunisation schedule), rates of exclusive breastfeeding at six weeks and three months are increasing, and women's satisfaction with their maternity service is high and continues to increase (Guilliland 2005; Ministry of Health 1999, 2001, 2003; NZHIS 2003, 2004, 2005).

The picture for Maori and Pacific Island women as well as women from lower socio-economic groups is also positive. Maori and young women from lower socio-economic groups are more likely to choose midwives as their lead care providers, and Maori women are more likely to birth in primary maternity facilities than any other ethnic group (NZHIS 2005). A study of over a million births from 1980 to 2001 shows that while preterm birth rates for Maori women are still higher than for non-Maori women, there has been a slight decline in the rates for Maori and Pacific Island women, in contrast to a marked increase for European women (Craig et al 2004). While rates for small for gestational age (SGA) babies have decreased for Maori, Pacific Island and European women over this period, the rate of decline for Pacific Island and Maori women has been greater (Craig et al 2004). Despite the high rates of preterm birth and SGA among Maori women, perinatal mortality rates for Maori communities are equal to or lower than those of other ethnic groups (NZHIS 2000).

Intervention rates in childbirth continue to increase in New Zealand as elsewhere in developed countries. However, while New Zealand's caesarean section rate has slowly increased to 23.1% in 2003, the increase appears slower and lower than in Australia, where the rate was 28.3% in 2003 (Laws & Sullivan 2005; NZHIS 2005; Ministry of Health 2001). Other measures such as instrumental births and induction of labour have declined in recent years, and epidural rates have barely increased (23.3% in 1997 to 24.4% in 2003). Midwifery care is linked to better outcomes than care with general practitioners and obstetricians, with higher normal birth rates and lower rates of caesarean section, instrumental births, episiotomies and epidural use (NZHIS 2004).

The context for childbirth in Western societies is characterised by the increasing use of intervention and technology, and the reasons for this are complex. Reducing unnecessary intervention in childbirth and reframing birth as a physiological life process is no simple matter, but providing midwifery care through one-to-one continuity of care in partnerships with women is one place to start (Page 1995). The relationship between a woman and a known midwife can ameliorate the impact of institutionalisation (Berg et al 1996; Halldorsdottir & Karlsdottir 1996; Kirkham 2000) and repeated studies demonstrate that women's feelings about this relationship and the related interactions override all other factors when women reflect on their experiences of labour (Hodnett 2002, 2004).

Partnership and the role of the midwife

The International Confederation of Midwives definition and scope of practice of a midwife (accepted in Australia and adapted in New Zealand) identifies that midwives work with women during pregnancy, labour and birth and the postnatal period—identified by the World Health Organization[3] as six weeks following birth—in the provision of 'woman-centred' midwifery care (ACMI 2005; Midwifery Council of New Zealand 2004; NZCOM 2005). The childbirth experience is a discrete period of profound significance to women and their families/whanau. Unlike any other episode where people seek healthcare, pregnancy, birth and breastfeeding are physiological processes. 'Woman-centred care' is articulated as different from the care given by other practitioners in that, throughout centuries and across cultures, women have asked midwives to be alongside them in their journey to motherhood in a relationship of mutual trust and respect embodying feminist principles and focusing on the individual needs of each childbearing woman (Guilliland & Pairman 1995; Thompson 2004).

In maternity services in New Zealand, and to a lesser extent in Australia, women can access models of care where midwives are alongside them throughout this period as primary carers. What women seek from midwives is support and skills in addressing the physical, emotional, social and spiritual aspects of a rite of passage that has far-reaching consequences for all involved and for the wellbeing of societies (Kirkham 2000; Kitzinger 1988; Thompson 2004).

Many of the currently compartmentalised components of woman-centred care are linked through relationship. The midwife becomes a 'professional friend' (Pairman 1998, 2000a; Wilkins 2000), supporting a woman to give birth in a way that she believes to be right for her and her baby. This relationship includes an emotional engagement, each party placing the other within a personal and biographical context (Wilkins 2000). Women have articulated the concept of the midwife as 'professional friend' where the following factors apply:

> The midwife and the woman work together in a particular way that integrates the notions of 'being equal', 'sharing common interests', 'involving the family', 'building trust', 'reciprocity', 'taking time' and 'sharing power and control' (Pairman 2000a, p 210).

The concept of 'professional friend' embodies characteristics of friendship within a professional relationship formed for the purpose of providing professional midwifery care and ending at completion of the childbirth process (Pairman 1998). Working with women in partnership as a 'professional friend' involves the integration of knowledge, skills and attitudes as reflected in the philosophies, competencies and other standards of the midwifery professions in both New Zealand and Australia. The midwifery role of 'being with woman' (the meaning of the Anglo-Saxon word *mid-wyf*) underpins these professional frameworks and is recognised by midwives internationally.

As identified in Chapter 14, the midwife–woman relationship was first articulated as a feminist concept involving partnership by New Zealanders Sally Pairman and Karen Guilliland in their 1995 monograph, *The Midwifery Partnership: A Model for Practice* (Guilliland & Pairman 1995). The notion of 'being with' as opposed to 'doing to' is associated with rites of passage such as birth and death (Powell Kennedy et al 2003). Fundamental to this understanding is recognition of the autonomy of the individuals involved in these significant events. The midwife's role is to 'be with' each woman and support her independence and growth through pregnancy and birth so that she feels strong and confident in her abilities as a woman and as a new mother (Katz Rothman 1991).

> At every stage of our interactions with childbearing women, as midwives, we should be adopting behaviours that will ensure that women can take up the power that will enable them to lead fulfilling lives as individuals and as mothers. This process of empowerment may have far reaching consequences in terms of women's feelings of self worth and confidence (Leap 2000, p 4).

In order to promote confidence in women, the midwife needs to be secure and confident in herself, both as a woman and as a midwife (Kirkham 2000). This often entails a mature approach to resisting the temptation to 'make things better', 'sort everything out' and take control as the 'expert'. It also means understanding how to avoid creating dependencies. There is a danger that 'needy' midwives can create 'needy' women' and inadvertently create dependencies that interfere with a woman's sense of her own expertise and ability to be self-determining.

Instead of seeing themselves as the 'experts' who need to 'instruct' and 'educate' women, midwives need to conceptualise the relationship as one based on mutual learning and

Critical thinking exercise

1   Continuity of midwifery care is common in New Zealand, but not in Australia. Think about the implications for women who cannot access continuity of midwifery care. How might this affect their relationships with midwives? What impact could this have on their experiences of maternity care?

2   If you work in a setting where continuity of care is not available to women or midwives, how can you incorporate some of the principles of partnership into your midwifery practice? Think of six changes you can make to your practice that will help you to develop a more equal relationship with the women you work with and to give them a stronger sense of power and control.

reciprocity (Guilliland & Pairman 1995; Pairman 1998). This begins with the midwife asking open-ended questions and having good listening skills.

> If a relationship is such that the practitioner does not listen, does not come to know the hopes and fears of the woman, does not respond to her anxieties, then the mode of care can only ... be based on the semblance of what the practitioner thinks should be happening. It lacks attention to the things that are 'mattering'. It traps the woman into a passive role of accepting inappropriate, unsafe care, rather than freeing her to involve herself in the accomplishment of personalised care that promotes all that is safe (Smythe 1998, p 202).

If midwifery is about promoting self-determination for women, then the notion of 'advocacy'—often seen as an important part of the nursing role—needs to be questioned. Arguably women should be advocating for themselves if they are to feel powerful. In most situations this is possible, particularly where the relationship with a midwife has enabled the woman to access information and articulate her needs. Where pain in labour or severe illness interferes with this process, the midwife may have a role in presenting the woman's wishes but this is done from a position of knowledge and trust that has been established and negotiated. This is all part of being clear about expectations at the initial visit and subsequently as the relationship develops.

Valuing women's expertise

Valuing a woman's expertise in monitoring her baby's well-being throughout pregnancy and in the early weeks of motherhood is often about stepping back and sending a message of trust. The balance between 'trusting the process' and being alert to signs that there is a need to intervene—either by making suggestions or by taking action—is a core midwifery skill that is often invisible and is hard to articulate

in its complexity. The individuality and unpredictability of each woman's experience means that often both women and midwives find themselves in situations where they feel they are outside their comfort zones and where they need to draw on courage as well as knowledge and experience.

Thus 'being with' encompasses the ability of midwives to trust the process of birth while using practice wisdom to guide and intervene as necessary. Because midwives cannot always be certain about their decisions or women's decisions, the balance between trusting and facilitating a process, and intervening through action, is finely balanced and individual to each woman's experience. It takes a degree of maturity on the part of the a midwife, and characteristics and skills such as honesty, integrity, decisiveness, practicality, reflectiveness, generosity, positivity and autonomy.

Working in partnership with women

The beginning of the relationship

The fundamental starting point for partnership is the recognition that women and midwives both have expertise that will contribute to an optimal experience for each woman and her family. The way in which both a midwife and a woman will contribute to the relationship needs to be individually negotiated. Each will bring different expectations and skills.

> The woman, with her knowledge of self and family...brings a willingness to participate actively in her care, sharing responsibility for her decisions and assuming control over her experience. The midwife, from her foundation of professional standards and ethics, brings her ability to be 'with woman'. In this, she utilises her knowledge, skills and self in practice and is accessible and supportive to the woman (Pairman 2000a, p 210).

Women seek midwifery care because of the knowledge and skills that midwives bring to the relationship. Indeed, the only reason for midwives to be involved with women is to bring this expertise. Safety is a priority for women and they expect midwives to act on their professional judgements.[4] At the same time, making professional judgements does not give midwives licence to deny women choices or to make decisions on their behalf under the guise of 'professional judgement'. Partnership requires each midwife and each woman to clarify their expectations of each other, to understand the philosophical base from which each works and to work out together the limits and extent of decision-making processes.

Partnership is linked to continuity of care because it takes time for midwives and women to get to know each other, to trust each other, to clarify and negotiate expectations. The best place for these discussions to occur, at least initially, is in the woman's home, where she is comfortable and the midwife is a guest. Working in partnership means working in a relationship where the power balance between the partners is equalised and negotiated. When midwives visit women in their homes for the booking visit, there is a subtle shift of power to the woman, and midwives and women can get to know each other on a more personal level in an environment that is familiar to the woman. Generally, women feel more confident in sharing information and thus the midwife is able to get a sense of what matters to the woman as well as her social context.

During pregnancy

Subsequent visits can be negotiated according to both the woman's and the midwife's situations. There may be value in most of these being at the midwife's practice premises if this means that the woman will be able to meet other pregnant women and attend antenatal groups; however, there may be reasons why it suits both for all antenatal care to take place in the woman's home. Either way, as identified in Chapter 17, there are many benefits when the midwife carries out a visit in late pregnancy to bring together the woman's supporters and plan for labour and the early postnatal period (Kemp 2003). The woman identifies the people in her family/whanau and community who will play a role in her experience of labour, birth and mothering and, where appropriate, the midwife can facilitate situations that ensure these support structures thrive. She can talk through likely events and how the woman might react to them, and enable time to discuss everyone's roles and expectations.

The value of midwives facilitating groups as opposed to running classes is also discussed in Chapter 17. This approach is about a social model of midwifery care, one that sees bringing women together in groups as a crucial strategy to develop a forum where they can learn from each other and develop friendships and support networks (Leap 1991). As suggested by Mavis Kirkham, 'linking women with others makes them stronger' (Kirkham 1986, p 47). Where the focus of antenatal groups is on antenatal care as well as education and support, significant improvements in outcomes have been identified in disadvantaged communities in the United States (Ickovics et al 2003; Schindler Rising 1998).

Telling the story

Where midwives work in partnership with women, they tend to develop a different attitude towards how maternity records are developed and kept. This includes encouraging the woman to write in her notes, using woman-friendly, descriptive language, avoiding alienating abbreviations and enabling the woman to keep a copy of the record when the midwifery partnership ends approximately six weeks after the baby's birth. Anecdotal evidence suggests that women cherish the record of their pregnancy, labour and the early weeks following birth, particularly where a story has been told using language that does not shy away from emotions.

During pregnancy, women can record how they felt at each stage of their pregnancy where the record stays with the woman rather than with the caregiver or institution. The concept of 'woman-held' maternity records is increasingly being seen as an important principle in maternity care and is a fundamental component of the midwifery partnership model. However, there is still resistance to their use in some quarters where midwives are employed and therefore an overview of the evidence relating to this subject may prove useful.

Woman-held maternity records are popular with women and are widely used in New Zealand (Hendry 2003) and the United Kingdom (Hart et al 2003). In Australia, although their use has been encouraged by government policy (NHMRC 1996; NSW Health Department 2000), widespread introduction has been relatively slow. Freedom of information, access to and ownership of medical records are current and controversial issues in Australia, and the debate provokes emotional responses (Phipps 2001). However, it can be argued that where midwives work in partnership with women, the maternity record reflects the relationship and is one of the contributory factors in sharing power and shifting the dominant culture of professionalism that potentially disempowers women.

The advantages of women carrying their own maternity care notes were first argued in the 1980s in the United Kingdom (Draper et al 1986; Lovell & Elbourne 1987; Lovell et al 1986). Since then, numerous authors have identified that this initiative encourages women's active participation in their care, improves communication between practitioners, and enhances communication between caregivers and women. Furthermore, women who carry their own notes have an increased sense of control and are unlikely to lose their records (Brown & Smith 2004; Elbourne et al 1987; Fawdry 1994a,b; Holmes et al 2005; Homer et al 1999; Lovell et al 1987; Phipps 2001; Young 1991).

A WHO collaborative study in eight developing countries identified that a woman-held maternity record plays an important role in primary healthcare and health promotion. The WHO concluded that the concept should be widely adapted for local use due to its effectiveness in the promotion of continuity of care, the early recognition of 'at-risk' women, the promotion of self-referral and self-care, and the generation of local health information (Shah et al 1993). On the basis of this research, the argument has been made for the widespread use of woman-held maternity records as a tool to promote women's active partnership in their care (Fallon 1994).

The language of partnership

Consideration of how midwives engage with women around the maternity record raises issues concerning the language midwives use and how this both reflects and constructs the culture in which midwifery practice is enacted (Leap 1992). Working in partnership with women involves finding opportunities to counteract the 'official' language of midwifery, namely the language of obstetrics, with its emphasis on measuring and setting norms (Kirkham 1986, 1993, 1997). This often begins with midwives getting together to explore how language reinforces the status quo of institutions and the technocratic model of birth (Davis-Floyd 1994), but also how language can challenge power dynamics.

The next step is for midwives to engage in an ongoing process of analysing how the unfolding of this awareness is played out in practice, in particular how we avoid the tendency to be trapped in dichotomous thinking. However, it has been suggested that in identifying the difference between woman-friendly language and the language of obstetrics, we are at risk of creating a new set of dynamics that mirror those that potentially disempower women. Fielder and colleagues (2004) have explored how the language of midwifery has a tendency to both force and reflect dichotomous thinking. They suggest that midwives have learned to think in binary opposites and that there is merit in addressing dualism in language use and the effect it has on both thinking and practice. The authors explore the types of opposites used by midwives and identify how this way of thinking has been learned from society, medicine and the culture of midwifery itself.

> Midwifery thinking and writing is full of opposites: normality-abnormality, safe-unsafe, health-illness, life-death, safety-danger (or in more contemporary jargon, risk), pathology-salutology, professional-lay, autonomy-dependency. There are also dichotomous, although less literally opposite pairs of concepts, such as breast-bottle, home-hospital, physiology-pharmacology, midwifery model-medical model, and midwife-obstetric nurse (Fielder et al 2004, p 6).

Fielder et al (2004) suggest that our expressions of opposites often imply value judgements that separate off what is unacceptable within social, medical and midwifery norms. If one side of an opposite is seen as 'good' there is the potential to demonise the other side as 'bad'. This polarisation can become a habit, manifesting in bullying behaviour and underpinning much of the horizontal violence that is endemic in midwifery practice (Leap 1997).

Dichotomous thinking also has the potential to force people and ideas into rigid standpoints that reduce richness and complexity (Sherwin 1989). According to Fielder et al (2004, p 7), the challenge is to make sure that dualistic thinking does not hamper our acknowledgement of different stages in colleagues' careers or thinking, that we continue to explore all the 'invisible between the extremes', and that we analyse and resist the effects of binary thinking on midwifery practice. This includes engaging with women around the complexities of uncertainty and questioning how our hierarchical rhetorical positioning of 'normal' affects women whose experiences fall outside such constructs.

Critical thinking exercise

1. Examine the maternity notes used in your local maternity facility. How is information recorded in these notes? Do these notes tell the story of women's experiences in pregnancy and birth? How could they be changed?

2. Midwives often resist writing stories in women's notes because they perceive that this takes too much time. What factors in your local maternity facility support story telling in the maternity notes? What factors inhibit this practice? How can these be changed?

The notion of binary opposites was initially developed by Jacques Derrida (Caputo 1997), who identified that language cannot escape the built-in biases of the cultural history that produced it. Hidden mechanisms are always at work, subtly influencing meaning in language. Identifying these underlying assumptions can be the first step in demonstrating the concealed power of symbols to shape thinking. According to Derrida (Caputo 1997), no one escapes these elusive qualities of language and being caught up in the subconscious networks of meaning that affect how we communicate ideas and experiences. As midwives, it is important to remain acutely sensitive to the conscious and subconscious historical, social and linguistic 'constructedness' of our beliefs and practices, and how, within processes of social negotiation, meanings are ever-shifting (Herrick 2001, p 52).

During labour and birth

In the current context of intervention and technology that characterises Western maternity services, it can be difficult for midwives to hold on to their belief in birth as a physiological process and to trust women's bodies to give birth. Indeed, several generations of midwives in Australia and New Zealand have had their confidence in physiological birth challenged through the twentieth century as childbirth was removed from the family and community and became instead a fragmented and hospital-based event in which midwives were unable to fully enact their 'with women' role (Davis-Floyd 1994; Guilliland & Pairman 1995). However, despite these challenges, many midwives and women have retained their belief in childbirth as a normal life event and in midwifery's expertise in facilitating this process. Latterly, the professional frameworks developed by midwifery's professional organisations in New Zealand and Australia have clearly articulated midwifery's role in promoting and protecting normal birth.

Midwives must have confidence in themselves as women and understanding of their role as facilitators and companions on a life journey if they are to instil confidence in women (Thompson 2004). Trusting the childbirth process and trusting women and their bodies is arguably one of the most important contributions midwives can make to women's sense of their ability to give birth and breastfeed their babies. Midwives have the benefit of working with many women through their childbirth experiences, and through these experiences they build up a store of knowledge of and expertise in the range of 'normal' and the varied manifestations of physiology.

When midwives see normal birth happening time and again, they develop trust in the process and confidence in women's bodies. They need to call on this belief when working with women who may only experience childbirth once or twice and who often do not have the same embedded belief and understanding of their ability to give birth. Midwives need to believe in women when women do not believe in themselves, when they are overwhelmed with the intensity of labour and have reached a point where they feel they cannot go on. This is the time for a midwife to step forward and, with certainty, encourage and express belief in the woman so that she can move forward with support.

A key skill for midwives is in knowing when to intervene during labour and when to stand back. A balance needs to be achieved in providing support and guidance or 'hands-on' care when necessary and promoting each woman's sense of self-achievement by drawing on her own strengths and those of her family and support people.

However, staying in the background while the woman and her family take centre stage does not mean that the midwife is a spectator of an event that will inevitably unfold in a certain way no matter what is done. There are a myriad of contextual factors that can interrupt the flow of labour or challenge a woman's self-confidence. A midwife needs to be alert to these factors and work to facilitate an environment in which the woman is supported to give birth or to mother her baby in her own way. The midwife's role is one of watchful anticipation, constantly assessing what is happening with the woman and comparing it to her store of experience and knowledge (Powell Kennedy 2004). An experienced midwife will begin to recognise patterns and be able to identify when the woman's experience is no longer within the realm of 'normal' for her and when it is necessary to intervene to prevent further complications. Being able to make professional judgements and act when required is essential for the provision of safe midwifery care.

Partnership and decision-making

If we acknowledge the importance of engagement in relationships, the process of decision-making becomes less about presenting a range of options as if they were all equal and much more about listening to women and helping them to mesh decisions with their lifestyles, beliefs and backgrounds (Thompson 2004).

Involving women in decision-making can have far-reaching implications for women as new mothers. For many women there may also be consequences in terms of learning about the life-long process of weighing up factors in order to make decisions. Within the partnership model, the midwife can enable situations in which women have a chance to develop their confidence in this area, with acknowledgement that the midwife also grapples with the uncertainty and complexity that surrounds much decision-making (Downe & McCourt 2004).

Women have identified that the amount of control and involvement they have during pregnancy, labour and the early weeks of new motherhood affects how they feel as new mothers (Green et al 1988, 2000). This sense of control is related to autonomy, which in turn is related to identity and a sense of personhood (Griffiths 1995). This notion may well be linked to the discovery that, where midwives can facilitate situations in which women are able to make decisions that are relevant to their lives, there is the potential for short- and long-term improvements to health and social outcomes (Ickovics et al 2003; Oakley et al 1996; Sandall et al 2001). However, the idea that individuals are free to make decisions that enable a sense of control needs to be addressed with caution. Often there is a denial of the role that social inequalities, particularly poverty, play in restricting the ability of women to make changes in their lives, or even to engage in a process of making choices.

The three 'C's in midwifery—choice, control and continuity of care (Page 1993)—are allied to the contemporary notion of 'informed choice' (Department of Health 1993; NHMRC 1996, 1998; Page 2000). Often there is little recognition of the complex nature of 'informed choice' and the fact that the person who does the 'informing' will play a major role in determining the 'choice' that is made (Leap 2000). Choices are limited by intersections of ideology, resources, class, race and other factors, such as obstetric regimens and value systems, over which women have little control (Leap & Edwards 2006). Recognition of these complexities is important if midwives are to engage with women in ways that recognise the pitfalls of the notion of 'informed choice' and prioritise mutual discussion and information sharing:

The technocratic culture of childbirth (Davis-Floyd 1994) maintains that decision-making in any situation should be based on the assessment of 'safety' and 'risk'. For women, safety is undoubtedly a key issue but the interpretation and meanings associated with risk and safety may be at odds with those identified by professionals. Where midwives work in partnership with women, there is the opportunity for both to explore how their individual social considerations and cultural values might affect the woman's decision-making process. This may well be more about safeguarding and promoting emotional wellbeing and personal integrity than about avoiding physical damage to their bodies and babies (Edwards 2005). Examples might include a woman who has been traumatised by a previous birth deciding to take control in a subsequent pregnancy by planning an elective caesarean section or home birth in situations where obstetric advice suggests other courses of action in the name of 'safety'.

Other examples of women making decisions that prioritise social and emotional safety occur in remote Australian communities, where women often feel that it is more dangerous to be removed from their families at 38 weeks to await birth in far-away tertiary referral hospitals than to give birth in their local communities (Kildea 2003). Some women decide not to leave their local community even though they know that there are no immediate caesarean section facilities. In many societies, particularly in rural areas, where women are expected to leave home to wait to give birth in distant maternity units, 'safety' is about protecting their other children and their homes from potential harm during their absence.

In the Northern Territory of Australia, up to 20% of Indigenous women who are flown out of their remote communities in late pregnancy to await birth in a tertiary referral hospital manage to hitch a lift back home (Kildea 1999). For these women, issues of 'safety' may include having their babies in their communities, according to customary law, surrounded by women they know, who speak their language and uphold customs that are seen to make babies strong (Kildea 2003).

In any situation where women are needing to make difficult decisions that are not necessarily straightforward in terms of recognised notions of 'safety' and 'risk', the attitudes of midwives play an important role in how women feel about the process, including how they reflect on the impact of the decisions they have made. This is especially important when midwives are challenged by the decisions that women make and find it hard to support their choices. Clear messages to women that the midwife trusts their ability to weigh up all the factors and make appropriate decisions, particularly in difficult circumstances, may go a long way to building up women's confidence in their ability to cope with the challenges of new motherhood (Edwards 2005).

Challenging the paradigm of professionalism

Working in partnership, women and midwives are truly exposed and open with each other. Each midwife is known as both a woman and a midwife to each woman she works with; it is therefore not possible for midwives to hide themselves behind their professional persona of 'midwife'.

In her research into what women want from community midwives, Ruth Wilkins (1993) discusses the emotional engagement necessary for such relationships to work well. Wilkins defines how the traditional notions of professionalism situate midwives and the women they attend in different social dimensions. She suggests that where midwives engage with women according to the ideals of professional distance, their biographical, social and psychological self is excluded from practice, leading to a distancing from women. Clinical assessment, monitoring and the giving of advice take precedence over building partnerships based on mutuality and subjectivity. In a similar vein, Mary Cronk (2000) suggests that the enacting of professional status reinforces the public perception that 'the expert knows best'. Cronk draws on transactional analysis theory to identify how this power imbalance directly reinforces a parent–child relationship that disempowers and patronises women.

In order to challenge the ideology of professional distance, midwives need to have an awareness of the potential for power imbalance within the midwife–woman relationship (Flemming 1998, 2000; Guilliland & Pairman 1995; Pairman 2000a, 2005). Applying this within each individual partnership relationship requires midwives to develop finely tuned skills in self-awareness. This includes an understanding of the potential effect of the use of self during interactions, and an awareness of the significance of informal interactions and the impact of environment on relationships. It also means resisting the pressure to give women certainty, and instead engaging with women in a dialogic process that embraces complexity and uncertainty (Downe & McCourt 2004).

Grappling with uncertainty is an ongoing process in life that is central to the challenges of becoming and being a mother (Leap 2000). The confidence to approach parenting in this way can develop when women and midwives have connection based on reciprocity, mutuality, personal disclosure and the removing of the anonymity and stereotyping that tends to dominate institutionalised care (Halldorsdottir & Karlsdottir 1996). These dynamics can most easily be encompassed within relationships involving continuity of care (Edwards 2005). Women have identified that such relationships provide the engagement, trust and nurturing needed for women to feel safe enough to move through birth to motherhood in an exciting process of discovery that is led by the woman (Edwards 2005).

As well as being a central issue for women as mothers, grappling with uncertainty is a core feature of midwifery. As midwives, we purport to engage in 'evidence-based' practice while often not recognising that there is no evidence for at least 80% of the situations we find ourselves in when it comes to 'informed decision-making' (Sackett et al 1997). Lesley Page's (2000) framework, the 'Five Steps to Evidence Based Midwifery', enables midwives to address this uncertainty around evidence. Use of this framework in practice ensures a woman-centred approach to making and reflecting on decisions in partnership.

Partnership and 'persuasion'

Interactions between midwives and women that involve mutual trust will inevitably address the conditioning that women and their families have been exposed to about birth and mothering. Sometimes this means exploring how these influences might obscure a woman's ability to make choices in her or her baby's best interest (Leap 1996b). Decisions are heavily influenced by the persuasive elements of the birth culture the woman happens to be in (Davis-Floyd & Sargent 1997). Rather than concentrating on an approach dominated by the ethos of 'informed choice', it may be a legitimate part of a midwife's role to counteract the conditioning that a woman has had that might inhibit the choices she makes. This might mean persuading the woman of the safety of home birth, for example, or convincing her to breastfeed her baby.

Many people will feel uncomfortable with this idea, given the awareness of how women are coerced within the technocratic model of birth and how easy it is to influence the decisions women make. However, it is worth considering how elements of persuasion underpin all our day-to-day interactions (Herrick 2001, 2004). To imagine that we can give information in an unbiased way without an element of persuasion is naive. It can be argued that persuasion plays a role in resistance to the highly persuasive dominant birth culture in suggesting alternative philosophies and actions. As Young (1998) discusses, positive action is needed to counteract the conditioning to which childbearing women are exposed in Western society. Women approach midwives in order to access their knowledge and experience; persuasion may therefore play an important role in how midwives respond to the investment and trust that women place in midwives as together they explore uncertainty, potential and possibilities.

Partnerships with other midwives

Midwives do not work in isolation. In midwifery caseload practice models, midwives generally work in partnership with another midwife in order to provide a 24-hour-a-day service to women. Often a midwife-pair will be part of a larger group practice and a third midwife from this practice may also be involved to provide cover for holidays and other leave including sickness.

However, the relationships that midwives have with each other offer more than a practical 'back-up' (Leap 1996a). These relationships also have the potential to provide:

- friendship, support, laughter and fun
- reflection in and on practice (Schon 1983)
- debriefing
- the sharing of ideas, information and evidence
- a safe place to express uncertainty and fear
- mentoring and peer review
- support for students and new graduates
- opportunities to locate individual experiences in the wider political context
- strategising and action to enable political and policy change
- the breaking down of hierarchical barriers
- a sense of 'belonging' and professional identity.

It is important that midwives choose their midwife partners, as it is essential to share a similar philosophy and approach to work when sharing a caseload. Like midwife–woman relationships, relationships between midwives rely on time to get to know each other and to develop trust. According to Sandall (1997), there is an imperative for midwives to meet regularly and to decide themselves how to manage their workloads and their time off, as these factors are linked to work satisfaction and the avoidance of burnout. Midwives need to like and trust their midwife partners so they can be assured that women will receive consistent midwifery care to similar professional standards.

Midwives work in partnership not only with their midwife partner but also with midwives employed in maternity units on 'shifts'. In New Zealand, the role of these midwives has changed in response to the development of midwifery caseload practice. Currently, most women still birth in a maternity facility and the majority come into the unit under the care of their own midwife, known as their lead maternity carer (LMC). Employed midwives find themselves involved directly in the care of women with serious complications who have been admitted under the care of the hospital obstetric team, or for the few women who choose a doctor for their LMC or who arrive without a named caregiver. Therefore, a new role has been articulated for the 'core' midwife, one that is based on supporting the primary midwife–woman partnership

(Campbell 2000; Pairman 2000b). The core midwife is recognised as the 'wise woman' of the maternity unit; her skills in facilitating and negotiating the interface between primary services and secondary/tertiary services have a major impact on each woman's experience of birth and each midwife's ability to continue to provide the woman's midwifery care, even when obstetric interventions may be required. In order for this to happen, both LMC midwives and core midwives have to develop clear understandings of each other's roles and the need to work in partnership in the interests of woman-centred care. These relationships are enhanced where midwives have had the chance to work in both roles.

Other partnerships: the midwife in the community

As primary health practitioners who cross the interface between hospital and community services, the majority of a midwife's work takes place in the community. This means that midwives need to have a sophisticated understanding of the importance of networking and establishing partnerships with other agencies and practitioners in their local communities in initiatives that employ the principles of primary healthcare[5] and community development.

Effective partnerships underpin the role of midwifery as a woman-centred, public health strategy (Kaufmann 2000, 2002). Midwives who are community based, providing continuity of care that 'follows the woman' across the interface of community and hospital services, are ideally placed to engage with women around strategies for health promotion, including addressing social exclusion and isolation (Leap 2004). They therefore need to understand the social determinants of health and the complex politics of how inequalities affect women's lives.

In particular, there are opportunities for midwives to 'dovetail' their services and liaise with child health nurses, well child services and community-based organisations. Because the midwife is alongside the woman on her journey through pregnancy, birth and the initial weeks of new motherhood, she is ideally placed to keep an overview of all the interacting needs of the woman in terms of accessing appropriate services and support structures. This is about physical, emotional and cultural safety. Midwives can engage with women in ways that avoid dependency and maximise the potential for women to learn from each other and build supportive networks in the community:

> The midwife maintains the 'midwifery overview' ensuring that all the interwoven elements of a woman's life are kept in relief, whatever the events that unfold. The midwife works with the woman and her community, collaborating with other health professionals if necessary, to ensure that everything is done to ensure a safe and supported transition to new motherhood, taking into consideration the woman's individual circumstances and wishes (Leap 2000, p 4).

Moving on

Giving birth is a powerful and transformative process. Women who are partners in their care with midwives and who are involved in making decisions about that care are more likely to find childbirth positive, even when they have experienced unplanned intervention. Women who have felt in control of their experiences are more likely to feel strong and independent in their roles as new mothers (Kitzinger 1991).

As the end of the midwifery relationship approaches at four to six weeks following birth, it is useful for both the woman and the midwife to reflect on the experience, including the midwifery input. Even when formal feedback is sought from women, as in New Zealand's Midwifery Standards Review Process, it is always useful to talk with women to find out which aspects of the midwife's care were useful and which were not. This enhances each midwife's opportunity to learn from each partnership relationship in terms of her personal and professional development and practice wisdom.

Ideally, at the end of the professional relationship, each woman should move on in her life with her sense of self intact, with pride in her achievements and with confidence in her mothering role. The partnership she and the woman have engaged with will have opened doors for both in terms of potential possibilities, joy and learning.

Conclusion

This chapter has explored the importance of partnership to women and midwives and has examined how midwives can work in partnerships, not only with women for whom they provide midwifery care, but also with other midwives with whom they work. A key feature of midwifery partnership is that it recognises the autonomy of both partners and therefore requires midwives to move beyond their professional persona to engage instead with women in a mutual relationship that recognises and supports women's expertise and self-determination. Partnership requires midwives to develop a key midwifery skill—achieving a balance between trusting and facilitating a process midwives know to be physiological for most women, and intervening through action when the process is no longer physiological. Keeping women and babies safe through making and acting on appropriate professional judgement is at the heart of the midwife's contribution to partnership.

Review questions

1 What is meant by the term 'midwifery partnership'?

2 Identify six essential characteristics of a partnership relationship between a midwife and a woman.

3 How might working in partnership be of benefit to women and to midwives?

4 How would you go about establishing a partnership relationship with a woman?

5 What skills might be necessary to work in partnership relationships with women?

6 How might you develop the skills necessary to work in partnership relationships?

7 What are the benefits of working in partnership with other midwives?

8 What are important considerations when thinking about entering a partnership with a midwifery colleague?

9 What role do midwives play in the interface between maternity and midwifery services and other community agencies?

10 Distinguishing between 'normality' and complications is a key midwifery role. What attributes does a midwife require to fulfill this role?

Online resources

Australian College of Midwives, http://www.acmi.org.au
Midwifery Council of New Zealand, http://www.midwiferycouncil.org.nz
New Zealand College of Midwives Inc., http://www.midwife.org.nz

Notes

1 The word 'woman' is used here in recognition that over 99% of midwives are women. It does not mean to exclude men who are midwives, who will have other dynamics to explore within the relationship, based on the politics of gender and power relationships in society.

2 While midwifery autonomy was reinstated in 1990, the LMC model of one-to-one continuity of care did not commence until 1996. From 1990 to 1996 women could choose both a midwife and a doctor as caregivers and many did so. The LMC model requires women to choose one primary caregiver and by 2004 some 78% of women chose a midwife as their LMC.

3 WHO Technical Working Group 1999 Postpartum care of the mother and newborn: A practical guide. Birth 26(4):255–258.

4 For example, a woman who is bleeding heavily immediately following birth does not want to engage in a long conversation about her 'choices' regarding the administration of an oxytocic. She trusts the midwife's expertise in acting swiftly and appropriately in the interest of safety.

5   Equity and access, services based on need, community participation, collaboration, community based care, affordable care and sustainability.

References

Australian College of Midwives Inc. 2005 National website: www.acmi.org.au, accessed January 2005

Benjamin Y, Walsh D, Taub N 2001 A comparison of partnership caseload practice with conventional team midwifery care: labour and birth outcomes. Midwifery 17:234–240.

Berg M, Lundgren I, Hermansson E et al 1996 Women's experience of the encounter with the midwife during childbirth. Midwifery 12:11–15

Brown H, Smith H 2004 Giving women their own case notes to carry during pregnancy. Cochrane Database of Systematic Reviews (2), amended 20 January 2004

Campbell N 2000 Core midwives—the challenge. Proceedings of the New Zealand College of Midwives Sixth National Conference, Cambridge, 28–30 September, pp 187–193

Caputo JD (Ed) 1997 Deconstruction in a nutshell: a conversation with Jacques Derrida. New York: Fordham University Press

Craig E, Mantell C, Ekeroma A et al 2004 Ethnicity and birth outcome: New Zealand trends 1980–2001. Part 1. Introduction, methods, results, overview. Australian and New Zealand Journal of Obstetrics and Gynaecology 44:530–536

Cronk M 2000 The midwife: a professional servant? In: M Kirkham (Ed) The midwife–mother relationship. Macmillan, London

Davis-Floyd R 1994 The technocratic body: American childbirth as cultural expression. Social Science and Medicine 38:1125–1140

Davis-Floyd R, Sargent C 1997 Childbirth and authoritative knowledge: cross cultural perspectives. University of California Press, Berkeley, CA

Department of Health 1993 Changing childbirth (Cumberledge Report). Department of Health, HMSO, London

Downe S, McCourt C 2004 From being to becoming: reconstructing childbirth knowledges. In: S Downe (Ed) Normal childbirth: evidence and debate. Churchill Livingstone, Edinburgh

Draper J, Field S, Thomas H et al 1986 Should women carry their antenatal records? British Medical Journal 292(6520):603

Edwards NP 2005 Birthing autonomy: women's experiences of planning home birth. Routledge, London

Elbourne D, Richardson M, Chalmers I et al 1987 The Newbury maternity care study: a randomised controlled trial to assess a policy of women holding their own obstetric records. British Journal of Obstetrics and Gynaecology 94(7):612–619

Fallon PD 1994 An argument for home-based maternal records in the United States. Family and Community Health 17(2):52–59

Farrell TJ, Homer C, Davis GK et al 2002 The risk associated pregnancy team: an Australian approach to collaborative care. Proceedings of the 26th Triennial Congress of the International Confederation of Midwives (ICM), Vienna

Fawdry R 1994a Antenatal casenotes 1: comments on design. British Journal of Midwifery 2(7):320–327

Fawdry R 1994b Antenatal casenotes 2: general comments. British Journal of Midwifery 2(8):373–374

Fielder A, Kirkham M, Baker K et al 2004 Trapped by thinking in opposites. Midwifery Matters: Journal of the Association of Radical Midwives 102:6–9

Flemming V 1998 Autonomous or automatons: an exploration through history of the concept of autonomy in midwifery in Scotland and New Zealand. Nursing Ethics 5(1):43–51

Flemming V 2000 The midwifery partnership in New Zealand: past history or a new way forward? In: M Kirkham (Ed) The midwife–mother relationship. Macmillan, Basingstoke

Green JM, Coupland VA, Kitzinger JV 1988 Great expectations: a prospective study of women's expectations and experiences. Child Care and Development Group, University of Cambridge, Cambridge

Green JM, Renfrew MJ, Curtis PA 2000 Continuity of carer: what matters to women? A review of the evidence. Midwifery 16:186–196

Griffiths M 1995 Feminisms and the self: the web of identity. Routledge, London

Guilliland K 2005 Do women want midwives? Midwives and the New Zealand maternity system in 2005. Unpublished paper presented at the 27th Congress of International Confederation of Midwives, Brisbane, 24–28 July 2005

Guilliland K, Pairman S 1995 The midwifery partnership: a model for practice. Victoria University, Department of Nursing and Midwifery Monograph Series, Wellington

Halldorsdottir S, Karlsdottir SI 1996 Journeying through labour and delivery: perceptions of women who have given birth. Midwifery 12(2):48–61

Hart A, Jones A, Henwood F et al 2003 Use of client held records in the maternity services. British Journal of Midwifery 11(11):668–669, 672–674

Hendry C 2003 MMPO update: development of woman-held notes by the MMPO. Midwifery News 31:26

Herrick J 2001 The History and theory of rhetoric: an introduction (2nd edn). Allyn & Bacon, Needham Heights, MA

Herrick J 2004 Argumentation: understanding and shaping arguments. Strata Publishing, State College, PA

Hodnett ED 2002 Pain and women's satisfaction with the experience of childbirth: a systematic review. American Journal of Obstetrics and Gynaecology 186(5):S160–S172

Hodnett ED 2004 Continuity of care givers during pregnancy and childbirth. Cochrane Review, Oxford

Holmes A, Cheyne H, Ginley M et al 2005 Trialling and implementing a client-held record system. British Journal of Midwifery 13(2):112–117

Homer C, Davis G, Everitt L 1999 The introduction of a woman-held record into a hospital antenatal clinic: the bring your own records study. Australian and New Zealand Journal of Obstetrics and Gynaecology 39(1):54–57

Homer C, Davis G, Brodie P et al 2001 Collaboration in maternity care: a randomised controlled trial comparing community-based continuity of care with standard hospital care. British Journal of Obstetrics and Gynaecology 108:16–22

Homer C, Davis G, Cooke M 2002a Women's experiences of continuity of midwifery care in a randomised controlled trial in Australia. Midwifery 18(2):102–112

Homer C, Farrell T, Brown M et al 2002b Women's worry and the risk-associated pregnancy team. British Journal of Midwifery 10:256–259

Ickovics JR, Kershaw TS, Westdahl C et al 2003 Group prenatal care and preterm birthweight: Results from a two-site matched cohort study. Obstetrics and Gynecology 102:1051–1057

Katz-Rothman B 1991. In labour: women and power in the birth place. WW Norton, London

Kaufmann T 2000 Public health: the next step in woman-centred care. RCM Midwives Journal 3(1):26–28

Kaufmann T 2002 Midwifery and public health. MIDIRS Midwifery Digest 12(suppl 1):S23–S26

Kemp J 2003 Midwives', women's and their birth partners' experiences of the 36 week birth talk: a qualitative study. Unpublished thesis. Florence Nightingale School of Nursing and Midwifery, Kings College, London

Kildea S 1999 And the women said … report on birthing services for Aboriginal women from remote Top End communities. Territory Health Service, Darwin

Kildea S 2003 Risk and childbirth in rural and remote Australia. Paper presented at the Seventh National Rural Health Conference, The art and science of healthy community-sharing country know how, Hobart

Kirkham M 1986 A feminist perspective in midwifery. In: C Webb (Ed), Feminist practice in women's health. John Wiley, Chichester, pp 35–49

Kirkham M 1993 Communication in midwifery. In: J Alexander, V Levy, S Roch (Eds) Midwifery practice: a research-based approach. Macmillan, Basingstoke

Kirkham M 1997 Stories and childbirth. In: MJ Kirkham, ER Perkins (Eds) Reflections on midwifery. Baillière Tindall, London, pp 183–204

Kirkham M 2000 The midwife/mother relationship. Macmillan, London

Kitzinger S (Ed) 1988 The midwife challenge. Pandora, London

Kitzinger S 1991 Childbirth and society. In: I Chalmers, M Enkin, M Keirse (Eds) Effective care in pregnancy and childbirth. Oxford University Press, pp 99–109

Laws PJ, Sullivan EA 2005 Australian mothers and babies 2003. Cat. No. PER 29. Australian Institute of Health and Welfare, Sydney

Leap N 1991 Helping you to make your own decisions—antenatal and postnatal groups in Deptford SE London. VHS video. Available from Birth International, www.birthinternational.com.au

Leap N 1992 The power of words and the confinement of women: how language affects midwives' practice. Nursing Times 88(12):60–61

Leap N 1996a Caseload practice: a recipe for burnout? British Journal of Midwifery 4(6):329

Leap N 1996b Persuading women to give birth at home—or offering real choice? British Journal of Midwifery 4(10):536

Leap N 1997b Making sense of horizontal violence in midwifery. British Journal of Midwifery 5(11):689

Leap N 2000 The less we do, the more we give. In: M Kirkham (Ed) The midwife–mother relationship. Macmillan, Basingstoke

Leap N 2004 Journey to midwifery through feminism: a personal account. In: M Stewart (Ed) Pregnancy, birth and maternity care: feminist perspectives. Books for Midwives, London, pp 185–200

Leap N, Edwards N 2006 The politics of involving women in decision making. In: L Page, R Campbell (Eds) The new midwifery: science and sensitivity in practice (2nd edn). Churchill Livingstone, London

Lovell A, Elbourne D 1987 Holding the baby—and your notes. Health Service Journal 19 March:335

Lovell A, Zander LI, James CE et al 1986 St Thomas' maternity case notes study. Why not give mothers their own case notes? Cicely Northcote Trust, London

Lovell A, Zander LI, James CE et al 1987 The St. Thomas's Hospital maternity case notes study: a randomised controlled trial to assess the effects of giving expectant mothers their own maternity case notes. Paediatric and Perinatal Epidemiology 1(1):57–66

Midwifery Council of New Zealand 2004 Midwifery Scope of Practice. Online: http://www.midwiferycouncil.org.nz.

Ministry of Health 1999 Obstetric procedures 1988/89 – 1997/98. MOH, Wellington

Ministry of Health 2001 Report on maternity 1999. Ministry of Health, Wellington

Ministry of Health 2003 Maternity services consumer satisfaction survey 2002. MOH, Wellington

National Health & Medical Research Council (NHMRC) 1996 Options for effective care in childbirth. AGPS, Canberra

National Health & Medical Research Council (NHMRC) 1998 Review of services offered by midwives. Commonwealth of Australia, Canberra

NSW Health Department 2000 The NSW Framework for Maternity Services (No. (NB) 000044). NSW Health Department, Sydney

New Zealand Health Information Service (NZHIS) 2000 Fetal and infant deaths. Ministry of Health, Wellington

New Zealand Collge of Midwives (NZCOM) 2005 Midwives handbook for practice. NZCOM, Christchurch

New Zealand Health Information Service (NZHIS) 2003 Report on maternity 2000 and 2001. Ministry of Health, Wellington

New Zealand Health Information Service (NZHIS) 2004 Report on maternity 2002. Ministry of Health, Wellington

New Zealand Health Information Service (NZHIS) 2005 Draft report on maternity: maternal and newborn information 2003 (unpublished)

Oakley A, Hickey D, Rajan L et al 1996 Social support in pregnancy: does it have long term effects? Journal of Reproductive Health and Infant Psychology 14:7–22

Page L 1993 Redefining the midwife's role: changes needed in practice. British Journal of Midwifery 1(1):21–24

Page L 1995 Effective group practice in midwifery: working with women. Blackwell Science, Oxford

Page L 2000 The new midwifery: science and sensitivity in practice. Churchill Livingstone, London

Page L, Beake S, Vail A et al 2001. Clinical outcomes of one-to-one practice. British Journal of Medicine 9:700–706

Pairman S 1998 The midwifery partnership: an exploration of the midwife/woman relationship. Unpublished masters thesis. Victoria University of Wellington

Pairman S 2000a Woman-centred midwifery: partnerships or professional friendships? In: M Kirkham (Ed) The midwife–mother relationship. Macmillan, Basingstoke, pp 207–226

Pairman S 2000b Revitalising partnership. Panel presentation. New Zealand College of Midwives Sixth National Conference, Cambridge, September (unpublished)

Pairman S 2005 Workforce to profession: an exploration of New Zealand midwifery's professionalising strategies from 1986–2005. Unpublished professional doctorate thesis, University of Technology, Sydney

Phipps H 2001 Carrying their own medical records: the perspective of pregnant women. Australian and New Zealand Journal of Obstetrics and Gynaecology 41(4):398–401

Powell Kennedy H 2004 Orchestrating normal: the art and conduct of midwifery practice. Paper presented at the Second International Conference on Normal Labour and Birth, Grange-over-Sands

Powell Kennedy H, Rousseau A, Kane Low L 2003. An exploratory metasynthesis of midwifery practice in the United States. Midwifery 19:2003–2214

Sackett D, Richardson W, Rosenberg W et al 1997 Evidence-based medicine: how to practise and teach. Churchill Livingstone, Sydney

Sandall J 1997 Midwives' burnout and continuity of care. British Journal of Midwifery 5(2):106–111

Sandall J 2004 Promoting normal birth: weighing the evidence. In: S Downe (Ed) Normal childbirth: evidence and debate. Churchill Livingstone, Edinburgh

Sandall J, Davies J, Warwick C 2001 Evaluation of the Albany Midwifery Practice: final report. Nightingale School of Midwifery, Kings College, London

Schindler Rising S 1998 Centering pregnancy: an interdisciplinary model of empowerment. Journal of Nurse-Midwifery 43(1): 46–54

Schon D 1983 The reflective practitioner: Basic Books, New York

Shah PM, Selwyn BJ, Shah K et al 1993 Evaluation of the home-based maternal record: a WHO collaborative study. Bulletin of the World Health Organization 71(5):535–548

Sherwin S 1989 Philosophical methodology and feminist

methodology: are they compatible? In: A Garry, M Persall (Eds) Women, knowledge and reality. Unwin & Hyman, Boston

Siddiqui J 1991 The therapeutic relationship in midwifery. British Journal of Midwifery 7(2):111–114

Smythe 1998 'Being safe' in childbirth. A hermeneutic interpretation of the narratives of women and practitioners. Unpublished doctoral thesis. Massey University, Palmerston North

Thompson F 2004 Mothers and midwives: the ethical journey. Books for Midwives, Edinburgh

Wilkins R 1993 Sociological aspects of the mother-community midwife relationship. Unpublished PhD thesis, University of Surrey.

Wilkins R 2000 Poor relations: the paucity of the professional paradigm. In: M Kirkham (Ed), The midwife–mother relationship. Macmillan, London

WHO Technical Working Group 1999 Postpartum care of the mother and newborn: A practical guide. Birth 26(4):255–258

Young D 1991 Who should hold the medical record—provider, parents, or both? Birth 18(1):2–4

Young D 1998 First class delivery: the importance of asking women what they think about their maternity care. Birth 25(2):71–72

CHAPTER 16

Working in collaboration

Sally K Tracy and Suzanne Miller

Key terms

collaboration, competency, consultation, referral

Chapter overview

Collaborative practice is integral to the safety of midwifery practice. Midwives, as primary caregivers, need to make evidence-based decisions regarding when an individual woman in their care may need a referral or consultation with another caregiver during pregnancy, labour, birth or the postnatal period. This chapter outlines the means of collaboration between midwives, the women they care for and the other health professionals with whom they may need to collaborate.

Learning outcomes

Learning outcomes for this chapter are:

1 To describe the frameworks within which midwives practise

2 To explore the nature of collaboration, consultation and referral.

Introduction

Engagement in collaborative effort is the midwife's *raison d'être*. 'Working together' is the thread that runs through every aspect of midwifery practice. The most fundamental understandings of the midwifery partnership model involve women and midwives working together to achieve positive experiences for all. Collaboration between women and midwives has undergone widespread political change throughout the late 1980s and 1990s, and has brought about the establishment of a truly women-centred maternity service in New Zealand, and a movement towards this in Australia. At every level, from the individual woman and midwife, through the professional and regulatory bodies, it is women and midwives working collaboratively who determine the vision and direction for the future of maternity services (DOH 1993; NMAP 2002; NZCOM 2005).

Midwifery care is centred on promoting and protecting birth as a normal physiological process. For most birthing women, the totality of their care falls within the scope of midwifery practice. There are occasions, however, when the complexity of a woman's experience may require that she also have some input from other health professionals. Midwives are skilled at assessing whether referral for consultation or transfer of clinical responsibility is necessary. To assist midwives with their decision-making, in both New Zealand and Australia referral guidelines have been developed that outline a range of circumstances where referral may be warranted.

Collaborative practice is integral to the safety of midwifery practice and enshrined in midwifery policy. The New Zealand College of Midwives Code of Ethics states that: 'Midwives have a professional responsibility to refer to others when they have reached the limit of their expertise' (NZCOM 2005, p 5). Similarly, the Midwifery Scope of Practice, which legally defines midwifery in New Zealand, requires that: 'When women require referral, midwives provide midwifery care in collaboration with other health professionals' (MCNZ 2004b).

The competencies for entry to the Register of Midwives provide further clarification of what generally and specifically constitutes midwifery practice, in terms of the profession's and the public's expectation of woman-centred care. The Definition and Scope of Practice provides the broad boundaries of midwifery practice, whereas competencies provide the detail of how a midwife is expected to practise and what she is expected to be capable of doing (MCNZ 2004 a,b). There are a set of minimum competencies required of all midwives who register in New Zealand and Australia. It is expected that all midwives will demonstrate that they are able to meet the competencies relevant to the position they hold (Homer et al 2005, p 5). These two competencies are reproduced in Box 16.1.

BOX 16.1 Competencies for entry to the Register of Midwives

New Zealand Competency 2

The midwife applies comprehensive theoretical and scientific knowledge with the affective and technical skills needed to provide effective and safe midwifery care.

Performance criteria:

▶ Assesses the health and well-being of the woman and her baby throughout pregnancy, recognising any condition which necessitates consultation with or referral to another midwife, medical practitioner or other health professional.

▶ Identifies factors in the woman or her baby during the labour and birth which indicate the necessity for consultation with, or referral to, another midwife or a specialist medical practitioner.

▶ Provides and is responsible for midwifery care when a woman's pregnancy, labour, birth or postnatal care necessitates clinical management by a medical practitioner.

▶ Regularly and appropriately assesses the health and well-being of the baby and initiates necessary screening, consultation and/or referral throughout the postnatal period.

▶ Assesses the health and well-being of the woman and baby throughout the postnatal period and identifies factors which indicate the necessity for consultation with or referral to another midwife, medical practitioner, or other health practitioner.

▶ Collaborates and co-operates with other health professionals, community groups and agencies where necessary.

Australian Competency 8

Develops effective strategies to implement and support collaborative midwifery practice.

Demonstrates effective communication with midwives, healthcare providers and other professionals.

▶ Adapts styles and methods of communication to maximise effectiveness.

▶ Uses a range of communication methods including written and oral.

▶ Liaises and negotiates with colleagues at all levels to build systems and processes to optimise outcomes for the woman.

▶ Discusses and clarifies with relevant healthcare providers interventions that appear inappropriate or unnecessary and negotiates a collaborative plan.

▶ Demonstrates effective communication during consultation, referral and handover.

Establishes, maintains and evaluates professional relationships with other healthcare providers.

▶ Recognises the role of other members of the healthcare team in the provision of maternity care.

▶ Identifies and responds to factors that facilitate or hinder professional relationships.

▶ Invites, acts upon, and offers, constructive feedback on midwifery practice from peers and colleagues.

(Sources: ANMC 2005; MCNZ 2004a)

Systems that enable midwives to work collaboratively are valued. The components of supportive systems include effective communication, consultation and referral between professionals. A collaborative relationship with medical colleagues is an important aspect of midwifery practice.

Collaboration also includes working with others when the care of women falls outside the midwives' scope of practice. For example, the care of women with mental health conditions is seen as one area where collaboration is particularly needed (Homer et al 2005).

The nature of collaboration

Successful collaborative practice requires several conditions. First, and most importantly, the woman must remain at the centre of the process. In order that she may participate in informed decision-making, information-sharing must occur in a context where her values and philosophical beliefs are respected and upheld. Midwives can assist women to critically examine the evidence presented to them, and help them make sense of those aspects that appear conflicting or inconclusive. When the woman is central to the collaborative process, her ability to tease out the important elements (to her) of both midwifery and obstetric practice will mean that she can formulate a plan of care that will best meet her needs. Edwards (2000, p 81) uses the phrase 'a potentially radicalising effect on the maternity system' to describe what can happen when the relationships between caregivers and women become the organising principle around which care is structured.

Many scholars have added depth to the discussion of preconditions for successful collaborative practice. Dorne has drawn together a number of these in what she describes as the Ten Major Tenets of Collaboration (Dorne 2002, p 17). They are as follows:

- provision of a non-competitive/non-hierarchical environment
- partnership between parties based on shared power and authority
- the ability to jointly define work processes, relationships, mutual objectives and goals
- joint responsibility/accountability for decision-making
- secure self-identity enabling clearly defined roles, with an emphasis on the function of each party
- power based on knowledge/expertise as opposed to power based on role and role function
- mutual trust, respect, cooperation and commitment
- time and space for open and effective communication and conflict resolution
- recognition/valuing of how differing perspectives inform decision-making
- interdependence of work with dependent/independent functions within the collaborative practice.

It is easy to see how these theoretical aspects could fit within the context of midwifery/obstetric collaborations. In practice it must be acknowledged that a maternity service that contains all these elements is rare, but certainly an admirable goal. It must be remembered also that midwives are accountable for their midwifery actions, regardless of who accepts 'clinical responsibility'.

Stapleton (1998) builds on the idea of mutual trust and respect as essential attributes of collaboration, and explores the notion of professional maturity. She believes that 'individuals who feel secure and competent professionally can communicate their discipline's strengths, value, limitations and contributions to colleagues from other disciplines' and adds that this requires 'a high level of professional maturity and confidence in one's professional knowledge and clinical skills' (Stapleton 1998, p 14). Effective communication is another crucial prerequisite for working together. It requires that 'members listen to each other's perspective yet are assertive in presenting their point of view' (Henneman et al 1995, p 106).

Midwives participating in a reflective midwifery partnership are in a position to have a positive impact on women's experiences in situations where referral is required. In addition to honouring the woman's own knowing about herself and her body, she can assist the woman to educate herself well, so that the consultation is not one in which the 'specialist' is the only 'expert'. Thus a woman will ask the questions that will *meaningfully* aid her decision-making, rather than following a predetermined protocol that may not reflect her values or beliefs. Whilst it is true that some obstetricians find this challenging, it can only serve to expand their horizons and increase their understanding of childbirth not just being about the removal of a baby from a woman's uterus.

Midwives need to remain mindful of the fact that *within* midwifery there is an enormous resource and body of knowledge, and that sometimes it is to our colleagues that we should turn for discussion and advice. Experienced midwives know well how judicious one needs to be about some indications for referral—the 'large-for-dates' baby, for example. We need to be clear that the experience of consultation will not negatively affect the woman's confidence in her ability to birth normally when the obstetrician has told her she has a high likelihood of needing a caesarean section. We are of course obliged to discuss the recommendation for referral with the woman, and support her decision to consult or not, as the case may be. But we need to balance the content of her consultation with midwifery knowledge about moulding, pelvic mapping, optimal baby positioning, working with labour pain, and mobility in labour to enhance her likelihood of normal birth.

Sometimes the woman may request referral, or may self-refer to health professionals other than obstetricians/paediatricians/anaesthetists. It might be an acupuncturist, osteopath, homoeopath or naturopath who can best assist with the particular issue the woman faces. A respectful collaborative process can be achieved here also. Indeed, because of a greater appreciation for holism displayed by complementary therapists, many midwives find working alongside these practitioners very fruitful and mutually satisfying for all involved.

Professional collaborations

The midwifery profession is becoming increasingly involved in building relationships with the professional bodies of other health disciplines. This is to ensure that those involved in the production of clinical guidelines for practice, and policy discussions are aware of the full scope of midwifery practice. This 'top down' approach also ensures that the voice of pregnant women is heard at the highest levels, as an expectation of consumer involvement operates at this level also.

Two recent examples of this in New Zealand have been the participation by midwives in the GBS New Zealand Consensus Working Party, which has produced guidelines for risk assessment and treatment approaches for Group B Streptococcus infection (MOH 2005), and the New Zealand Guidelines Group, a collaboration between midwives, obstetricians, consumers, paediatricians, GPs, maternity managers and midwifery and medical educators, which has produced best practice guidelines in relation to the care of women with breech presentation or previous caesarean birth (New Zealand Guidelines Group 2004). These documents contribute much to our understanding of evidence-based care and will lead to increased consistency of advice to pregnant women faced with making decisions about aspects of their care.

The New Zealand Referral Guidelines

In New Zealand, the Referral Guidelines are contained in Appendix 1 of the Notice Pursuant to Section 88 of the New Zealand *Public Health and Disability Act 2000*.

The stated purpose of the Guidelines is that they be 'used to facilitate consultation and integration of care, giving confidence to providers, women and their families' (Ministry of Health 2000, p 31). Circumstances in which the Guidelines may be varied are outlined, acknowledging the fact that midwives and others providing maternity services have a wide range of skills, and that where one's level of expertise allows, departures from the Guidelines may occur. In this instance, the midwife should be able to justify her course of action, and documentation reflecting the process of information sharing and decision-making with the woman should appear in the clinical record.

The process of referral can take many forms. In general, the booking interview is often the time when the woman will disclose a situation that may require referral. If this is because of something in her medical or maternity history, the midwife can discuss the recommendation for referral and, with the woman's informed consent, initiate the process immediately. Other indications for referral may arise later in the pregnancy—for example, the discovery of a twin pregnancy, or breech presentation that persists near term. Referral will occur in such instances as the particular issue arises.

If after discussion of the recommendation for referral the woman consents to consult, the midwife is responsible for writing a letter to request a consultant review. This letter should provide enough pertinent information to enable the obstetrician to adequately assess the woman's situation. At the very least, the letter will contain:

- the woman's name, address, date of birth, National Health Index number, gravidity/parity and contact details
- the reason that referral is sought
- a brief statement outlining her medical and/or maternity history
- any relevant supporting documentation (e.g. blood test or ultrasound reports)
- her lead maternity carer's name and contact details.

Whether or not the midwife accompanies the woman to the appointment is negotiated between the midwife and the woman. Some advantages of having the midwife present are that it can facilitate the process of 'three-way discussion' more easily, and some women find that the presence and support of the midwife can make the encounter less stressful. The midwife will be able to interpret the content of the discussion after the appointment if any issues need clarification. On the other hand, some women feel that the presence of the midwife might cause the obstetrician to withhold certain information or to consider the woman incapable of understanding complex information or needing her 'hand held' in some way.

The main outcome of the consultant review will be the formation of an ongoing plan of care that reflects the woman's informed choices regarding who will have clinical responsibility, who will provide her primary care if transfer occurs, and if not, then whether and when further consultation should occur. All these decisions should be clearly documented in the clinical record so that there is no confusion as to roles and responsibilities. Referral for consultation does not imply that the clinical responsibility for the woman's care will be assumed by the secondary service.

The Guidelines define three categories or 'levels of referral' and consequent action.

Level 1

The lead maternity carer (LMC) *may recommend* to the woman (or parents in the case of a baby) *that a consultation with a specialist is warranted* given that her pregnancy, labour, birth or puerperium (or the baby) is or may be affected by the condition. *Where a consultation occurs, the decision regarding ongoing clinical roles/responsibilities must involve a three-way discussion between the specialist, the LMC and the woman concerned. This should include discussion on any need for and timing of specialist review.* The specialist will not automatically assume responsibility for ongoing care. This will depend on the clinical situation and the wishes of the individual woman.

Level 2

The LMC *must recommend* to the woman (or parents in the case of a baby) *that a consultation with a specialist is warranted* given that her pregnancy, labour, birth or puerperium (or the baby) is or may be affected by the condition. *Where a consultation occurs, the decision regarding ongoing clinical roles/responsibilities must involve a three-way discussion between the specialist, the LMC and the woman concerned. This should include discussion on any need for and timing of specialist review.* The specialist will not automatically assume responsibility for ongoing care. This will depend on the clinical situation and the wishes of the individual woman.

Level 3

The LMC **must** recommend to the woman (or parents in the case of a baby) **that the responsibility for her care be transferred** to a specialist given that her pregnancy, labour, birth or puerperium (or the baby) is or may be affected by the condition. *The decision regarding ongoing clinical roles/responsibilities must involve a three-way discussion between the specialist, the LMC and the woman concerned.* In most circumstances the specialist will assume ongoing responsibility and the role of the primary practitioner will be agreed between those involved. This should include discussion about timing of transfer back to the primary practitioner.

The Australian Midwifery Consultation and Referral Guidelines

The aim of the *National Midwifery Guidelines for Consultation and Referral* (2004) is to provide an evidence-based, national framework for consultation and transfer of care between midwives, doctors and other professionals, and to promote a system of care based on the principal of close cooperation between primary-, secondary- or tertiary-level maternity caregivers and the woman involved:

- at booking
- during pregnancy and the antenatal period
- during labour and birth
- during the postnatal period.

Primary maternity care is where the responsibility for maternity care rests with the primary-level maternity care provider—in this case, the midwife. Secondary maternity care is where the responsibility for maternity care rests with the medical practitioner, such as a GP or specialist obstetrician, or the medical staff on duty in the referral hospital. Tertiary-level maternity care is when responsibility for maternity care rests with a team of providers in a tertiary-level hospital. This may include an obstetrician and/or physician who specialises in fetal–maternal medicine, neonatology or other highly specialised services.

The Guidelines (2004) reflect the following guiding principles:

- As a primary caregiver, the midwife, together with the woman, is responsible for decision-making.
- An informed-choice agreement between the midwife and the woman at booking should outline the extent of midwifery care, in order to make women aware of the scope and limitations of midwifery care. This will include an explanation of these Guidelines with the woman.
- If problems occur during pregnancy or birth, the midwife may consult with her peers in the first instance, or consult directly with a secondary- or tertiary-level caregiver and refer when appropriate.
- The midwife discusses care of a woman, consults, or transfers primary care responsibility according to the Guidelines.
- The secondary- or tertiary-level care provider may also refer the woman back to primary care at any time if the condition that prompted referral is no longer a risk factor.
- The severity of the condition will influence these decisions.

Three main steps in consultation and referral

(The information in this section is from the Australian College of Midwives (2004) *National Midwifery Guidelines for Consultation and Referral.*)

When an abnormality or complication presents during a woman's care, it is recommended that the midwife undertake one or more of three main steps:

A Discuss the issue/condition with another midwife and/or with a medical colleague.

B Consult with a medical practitioner.

C Transfer responsibility for the woman's care to a medical specialist.

A. Discussion with another midwife and/or with a medical colleague

a The midwife may recommend to the woman (or parents in the case of the baby) that consultation with a medical practitioner is warranted, given that her pregnancy, labour, birth or postnatal time (or the baby) may be affected by the condition.

b It is the midwife's responsibility to initiate a discussion with, or provide information to, another midwife or medical practitioner, with whom the care is shared, in order to plan and provide care appropriately.

c Where a consultation occurs, the decision regarding ongoing clinical roles/responsibilities must involve a three-way discussion between the medical practitioner, the midwife and the woman.

d This should include discussion of the need for (if any), and timing of, medical practitioner review.

e The medical practitioner will not routinely assume responsibility for ongoing care. This will depend on the clinical situation and the wishes of the individual woman.

f Areas of discussion and involvement must be clearly agreed upon and clearly documented.

B. Consultation situation

a A consultation refers to the situation where a midwife recommends the woman consult a medical practitioner, or where the woman requests another opinion of a medical practitioner.

b The individual situation of the pregnant woman is evaluated and agreements are made about the responsibility for maternity care based on the Guidelines.

c It is the midwife's responsibility to initiate a consultation and to clearly communicate to the medical practitioner that she is seeking a consultation.

d The consultation involves addressing the issue that led to the referral, a 'face-to-face' assessment, and the prompt communication of the findings and recommendations to the woman and the referring professional.

e Where a consultation occurs, the decision regarding ongoing clinical roles/responsibilities must involve a three-way discussion between the medical practitioner, the midwife and the woman concerned. This should include discussion on any need for, and timing of, medical practitioner review.

f The medical practitioner or midwife will not automatically assume responsibility for ongoing care. This will depend on the clinical situation and the wishes and needs of the individual woman.

g After consultation with a medical practitioner, it should be clear whether primary care and responsibility:
   1 continues with the midwife, or
   2 is transferred to the medical practitioner.

h The medical practitioner may be involved in, and responsible for, a discrete area of the woman's care, with the midwife maintaining overall responsibility within her scope of practice.

i Where urgency, distance or climatic conditions make a 'face-to-face' consultation between a woman and a medical practitioner impossible, the midwife should seek advice from the medical practitioner by phone. The midwife should document this request for advice in her records, and discuss with the woman the advice received.

j Areas of discussion and involvement must be clearly agreed upon and clearly documented.

C. Transfer to secondary or tertiary care

a When primary care is transferred, permanently or temporarily, from the midwife to a medical practitioner, the medical practitioner assumes full responsibility for subsequent decision-making in consultation with the woman.

b When primary care is transferred to a medical practitioner, the midwife may continue to provide midwifery care and support within her scope of practice, in collaboration with the medical practitioner.

c Areas of discussion and involvement must be agreed upon and clearly documented (ACMI 2004, pp 11–13).

The Guidelines include a summary of these responsibilities (Table 16.1) and a decision diagram for use by midwives (Fig 16.1).

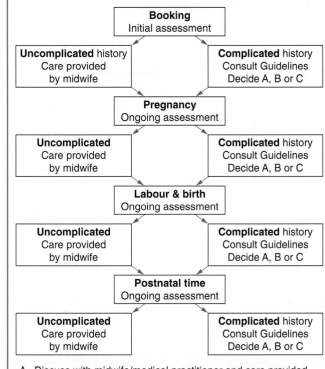

A Discuss with midwife/medical practitioner and care provided by midwife
B Consultation with medical practitioner and care continues with midwife or is transferred to medical practitioner
C Transfer care to medical practitioner

When there is any doubt, consultation is recommended.

Figure 16.1 A decision diagram for use by midwives in daily practice (based on ACMI 2004)

Conclusion

Collaboration in maternity care involves the incorporation of the woman as partner in all decision-making processes in addition to working with others to implement the most appropriate and effective care. The challenge of collaborative practice is always to find a balance between midwifery skills, the notion of intensive 'presence' and minimal intervention, and the practice of medicine, in particular obstetrics, with its emphasis on technological expediency. Achieving collaboration and cooperation between the professional groups involved in maternity care involves recognising and acknowledging each other's particular expertise. Birth is a disorderly business. The multiple strategies of midwifery practice are negotiated through the intensity and immediacy of each birth experience, rather than defined in advance (Maher & Souter 2002). The way midwives work with each other, with women and with their professional colleagues shapes the experience of birth for both women and their families.

TABLE 16.1 Summary of responsibilities

Code	Description	Care provider
A. Primary maternity care	The responsibility for maternity care in the situation described is with the midwife.	Midwife
B. Consultation and possible transfer of care to medical practitioner	Evaluation involving both primary and secondary care needs. Under the item concerned, the individual situation of the woman will be evaluated and agreements will be made about the responsibility for maternity care.	Medical practitioner and/or midwife, depending on agreements
C. Transfer of care to medical practitioner	This is a situation requiring medical care at a secondary or tertiary level for as long as the situation exists.	Medical practitioner (Where appropriate the midwife continues to provide midwifery care or support.)

(Source: ACMI 2004)

Clinical scenario

'Megan' (35 years old) came to me to discuss the provision of midwifery care for her fourth pregnancy. Her maternity history was as follows:

1988 SRM at 32/40. Syntocinon induction leading to spontaneous vaginal birth of 1900 g daughter
1990 40/40 Normal birth of 3090 g daughter
2001 40/40 Normal birth at home of 3250 g daughter.

Megan's third pregnancy had been complicated by a diagnosis of pulmonary embolus at 32/40 gestation. For the remainder of that pregnancy, Megan had injected herself daily with the anticoagulant medication Clexane. Postnatally she medicated with warfarin for four months, which involved daily blood tests for the first couple of weeks to monitor her INR ratio. Megan gave birth to this baby at home 'against medical advice', with the support of two experienced midwives. She had now moved cities and wanted to plan a similar experience for this baby's birth. Megan had made many dietary and lifestyle changes since the birth of her third child. She had stopped smoking, and was taking flaxseed oil and vitamin E supplements.

I discussed the Referral Guidelines with Megan, with particular reference to the fact that a history of PE was a 'Level 3' indication for referral, i.e. that I must recommend that her care be transferred to a specialist. At this stage Megan was happy to be referred to a haematologist, but not to an obstetrician. Her perception was that this wasn't about birthing her baby, it was about avoiding the recurrence of clot formation, and that for her a haematologist was the more appropriate person to see. Megan also had a consultation with a local GP who specialises in nutritional medicine, in order to confirm that the supplements she was taking were the most

appropriate dosages, and were safe to continue taking during pregnancy.

Megan saw the haematologist, who recommended that she wear TED stockings, and begin taking Clexane at once. Megan was very reluctant to begin medicating in the absence of symptoms. Together we explored the evidence for thromboprophylaxis in terms of its effectiveness in reducing the incidence of recurrent clot formation, and its safety profile both in pregnancy and during lactation. Megan found the Royal College of Obstetricians and Gynaecologists Guideline 'Thromboprophylaxis during pregnancy, labour and after vaginal delivery' (Nelson-Piercy 2004) very useful in assisting her decision-making about whether or not to anticoagulate this pregnancy, because it described a number of clinical scenarios and what to do for each. Megan was able to identify her own particular risk profile, which included having four persisting risk factors (her age, her past history of PE, her prothrombin gene mutation, and her protein S deficiency). This enabled her to make an informed choice, which ultimately led to her beginning Clexane at 23/40 into her pregnancy. Megan was thrilled to have made it to this gestation without taking medication.

Further discussion took place between Megan and myself about the advisability of also consulting an obstetrician. I was clear with Megan that I needed to be able to demonstrate that she had made an informed decision regarding place of birth, and that even though we had discussed at length the pros and cons of home birth in this situation, I needed to be sure that she had had the opportunity to discuss it from an obstetric point of view too. We talked about how the decisions she made could affect me

Clinical scenario—cont'd

professionally in the event of an adverse outcome. Even though she accepted full responsibility for her decisions, the process that could ensue in this circumstance could involve her and her family in a lengthy process if a complaint was laid by a third party. Megan agreed to see an obstetrician, and by now her clinical record was becoming fairly full, with the content and outcomes of every discussion being carefully documented!

Megan's visit to the obstetrician was disappointing. We were hoping to achieve a respectful collaborative process, but instead the consultation resulted in Megan's even stronger resolve to avoid the secondary service at the hospital. The first question that was asked of her was whether or not she intended to 'hand over care'. Megan replied that she needed to know what care was being offered by the hospital in order to make that choice. Megan outlined that for her the critically important thing was that her midwife would be able to remain involved in her care. In this institution, if a woman's reason for referral is a '3' and care is transferred, the midwife can no longer provide the primary midwifery care. At this point the obstetrician stated that there wasn't much point in continuing the conversation, except to suggest to Megan that she ought to think about how it would feel for her husband if she died and he was left to raise four children alone.

The remainder of Megan's pregnancy was straightforward. She remained in my care and had two more appointments with the haematologist, who assisted us in formulating a plan of care regarding how to manage the Clexane/warfarin transfer at the time of labour. Her GP worked with us to order blood tests that were outside the scope of what a midwife can normally prescribe. Megan went into spontaneous labour at 38/40, and birthed her beautiful first son at home in three hours. She had a physiological third stage and her blood loss was minimal. She took warfarin for six weeks postnatally.

I think Megan's story serves us well in illustrating how collaboration can occur in an environment where mutual respect and trust are present. There was clear role definition between myself, the GP and the haematologist. Where professional trust and respect were absent, collaboration could not happen effectively. Because there was a perceived 'overstepping' of my midwifery scope of practice, and because of policy constraints that precluded my ongoing involvement, the obstetrician was unable to accommodate Megan's informed choice to have me remain involved in her care.

It should be remembered that the 'outcomes of maternity care that are of concern to midwives are broader than just measures of mortality' (Page 2000, p 69). When women are making assessments about risk, they may weigh up risk and safety in ways that differ from ours. It may be their view that 'hospital birth itself poses physical and emotional risks because of the greater likelihood of invasive and damaging interventions' and that their 'attempts to decrease risk, by avoiding technology, unfamiliar surroundings and strangers, could be interpreted from the standpoint of medical ideology as increasing risk' (Edwards 2000, p 65).

In Megan's case, as well as determining her 'risk factors', we endeavoured also to look at those factors that could reasonably lead us to expect a good outcome, 'salutary factors' in the new jargon (Downe 2004, p 18). Megan had already given birth at home whilst on anticoagulant medication, without adverse events occurring, and had 'normal' postnatal progress. I believe that it is important to balance what we know from research, with what else we know from experience, wise clinical judgement and what the woman brings to the equation too. This fits neatly with White's assertion that 'reflective practice is a legitimate way of generating . . . knowledge' and that '"clinical artistry" is as essential as scientific or empirical evidence' (White 1997, p 175).

Review questions

1 Describe the central tenets of collaborative practice.

2 Is *cooperation* different from *collaboration*? If so, in what way?

3 How would you describe national competency standards to a new intake of midwifery students?

4 What are the 'domains' of midwifery competency?

5 Describe, in your own words, what you understand as the competencies that relate to legal and professional responsibilities.

6 What do you understand by the statement: 'Midwifery is a public heath strategy'? How would you describe the need for collaboration in this strategy?

Review questions—cont'd

7   Describe the competencies that relate to the performance of midwifery practice, including assessment, planning, implementation and evaluation.

8   How legally binding are the consultation and referral guidelines that guide your practice?

9   How would you describe the complementary roles of midwives and obstetricians?

10 What do you understand by the notion of 'turf war'? How can this be addressed in practice?

Online resources

Australian Nursing and Midwifery Council, http://www.anmc.org.au

Australian Midwives Code of Practice, http://www.acmi.org.au/text/corporate_documents/practice.pdf

Midwifery Council of New Zealand, http://www.midwiferycouncil.org.nz

New Zealand College of Midwives, http://www.midwife.org.nz

References

Australian College of Midwives Inc. (ACMI) 2004 National Midwifery Guidelines for Consultation and Referral. Online: http://www.acmi.org.au/text/publications/publications.html

Australian Nursing and Midwifery Council (ANMC) 2005 National competencies for the midwife. Online: http://www.anmc.org.au

Department of Health (DOH) 1993 The Cumberledge Report: changing childbirth: the report of the expert maternity group. HMSO, London

Dorne A 2002 Collaboration between Healthcare Professionals, what does it mean? The rhetoric and the reality. Research paper. Victoria University of Wellington, Wellington.

Downe S 2004 From being to becoming: reconstructing childbirth knowledges. In: S Downe (Ed) Normal childbirth, evidence and debate. Elsevier, Churchill Livingstone, Philadelphia

Edwards N 2000 Women planning homebirths: their own views on their relationships with midwives. In: M Kirkham (Ed) The midwife-mother relationship. MacMillan, Hampshire, pp 55–91

Henneman E, Lee J, Cohen J 1995 Collaboration: a concept analysis. Journal of Advanced Nursing 21:103–109

Homer C, Pincombe J, Thorogood C et al 2005 An examination of the role and scope of practice of Australian midwives and the development of competency standards for midwifery. Final report. UTS and Australian Nursing and Midwifery Council

Maher JM, Souter KT 2002 Midwifery work and the making of narrative. Nursing Inquiry 9:37–42

Midwifery Council of New Zealand (MCNZ) 2004a Competencies for entry to the Register of Midwives. Online: http://www.midwiferycouncil.org.nz/content/library/Competencies_for_Entry_to_the_Register1.pdf, accessed 1 January 2004

Midwifery Council of New Zealand (MCNZ) 2004b Midwifery scope of practice. Online: http://www.midwiferycouncil.org.nz/main/Scope/, accessed 1 January 2004

Ministry of Health (MOH) 2000 Public Health and Disability Act 2000

Ministry of Health (MOH) 2005 New Zealand Technical Working Group. Online: http://www.nzma.org.nz/journal/117-1200/1023/

Ministry of Health Maternity Services 2002 Notice Pursuant to Section 88 of the New Zealand Public Health & Disability Act 2000

National Maternity Action Plan (NMAP) Maternity Coalition 2002. Online: www.maternitycoalition.org.au/nmap/html

Nelson-Piercy C 2004 Thromboprophylaxis during pregnancy, labour and after vaginal delivery. Royal College of Obstetricians and Gynaecologists Guideline No. 37

New Zealand College of Midwives (NZCOM) 2004a Code of ethics. Online: http://www.midwife.org.nz/index.cfm/Ethics, accessed 1 January 2004

New Zealand College of Midwives (NZCOM) 2004b NZCOM consensus statement. Group B Streptococcus (GBS). Online: http://www.midwife.org.nz/content/documents/127/GBS-_NZCOM.pdf, accessed 21 February 2005

New Zealand College of Midwives (NZCOM) 2005 Midwives handbook for practice. New Zealand College of Midwives, Christchurch.

New Zealand Guidelines Group 2004 Care of women with breech presentation or previous caesarean birth. NZGG, Wellington

Page LA 2000 Using evidence to inform practice. In: LA Page (Ed) The new midwifery. Churchill Livingstone, London

Stapleton S 1998 Team building. Making collaborative practice work. Journal of Nurse-Midwifery 43(1):12–18

White S 1997 Evidence-based practice and nursing: the new panacea? British Journal of Nursing 6:175–178

CHAPTER 17

Promoting physiological birth

Nicky Leap

Key terms

antenatal groups, community midwifery, empowerment, home birth, interdisciplinary learning, interdisciplinary rivalry, midwifery caseload practice, midwifery continuity of care, normal birth, pain in labour, physiological birth, social support, 36-week home visit

Chapter overview

The focus of this chapter is the promotion of physiological birth by midwives. Strategies are suggested, including the need to develop systems and an organisational culture that nurtures the potential of birth to transform lives and strengthen women, their families and societies.

The imaginary story of the birth of Jason Smith, presented in this chapter as a scenario, can be used for discussion and analysis in small groups. As a similar group exercise, practitioners and students can present 'real life' stories from practice in order to analyse the factors that can promote or inhibit physiological birth in any given situation. Such an exercise can be incorporated in continuing professional development exercises such as peer review, interdisciplinary learning, case review and workshops.

Learning outcomes

Learning outcomes for this chapter are:

1 To explore the practicalities, sensitivities and systems that promote physiological birth

2 To highlight the factors and organisational culture that can inhibit this approach in midwifery practice.

3 To explore the evidence concerning continuity of midwifery care

4 To provide information about midwifery practices that enhance physiological birth.

Introduction

In this chapter, the phrase 'promoting physiological birth' is used deliberately as an alternative to the commonly heard phrase 'the midwifery art of keeping birth normal'. As Holly Powell Kennedy (2004) has suggested, the notion of 'normal' is hardly in keeping with the midwifery philosophy of embracing the concept of each woman's birth being viewed by her as essentially 'special'. However, women and most maternity care providers are unlikely to use the term 'physiological', and the word 'normal' is embedded in the documentation and discourses that shape and reflect contemporary maternity service provision. Importantly, the term 'normal' is used to identify the primary domain of the midwife, a sphere of practice that is clearly defined as separate from the technological or medical interventions associated with complications, identified here by the World Health Organization (WHO):

> The midwife appears to be the most appropriate and cost effective type of care provider to be assigned to the care of normal pregnancy and birth, including risk assessment and the recognition of complications (WHO 1996, p 6).

Fulfilling this role is not as straightforward as it might seem. Midwives in Western countries often work in hospitals where computerised summaries identifying 'normal birth' do not necessarily reflect physiological processes or the efforts of practitioners to promote physiological birth. This was identified in an important epidemiological study of 1464 births in five consultant maternity units in the United Kingdom (Downe et al 2001). Once women who had artificial rupture of membranes, induction and acceleration of labour, epidural anaesthesia or episiotomy were removed from the equation, only 16.9% of women having their first baby and 30.1% of women having a second or subsequent baby could be classified as having a 'normal' birth. This study shrinks the domain of midwives as 'guardians of the normal' and raises questions as to whether we are 'failing' in this role (Beech 1997). Furthermore, there are mounting concerns about the limited learning opportunities for practitioners where the promotion of physiological birth is limited by 'technocratic' approaches in institutions (Davis-Floyd 2001; Kitzinger 2000; Leap 2002).

In suggesting strategies to promote physiological birth, this author is mindful of the fact that the majority of midwives are working in institutions where 'normal' birth is not the most common experience for women. The underlying power dynamics in these situations can subvert the efforts of midwives to promote physiological birth and practise according to their full role and scope of practice. Addressing these issues starts with an understanding of how these dynamics have evolved over recent centuries.

The midwife as 'guardian of the normal'

A long history of interprofessional rivalry lies behind the 1996 WHO statement and the contemporary rhetorical notion of the midwife as 'guardian of the normal'. Before men entered the birthing arena, most women in European countries were attended at home by women they knew, one of whom might well be referred to as 'the midwife' due to her acknowledged role and expertise (Wilson 1995). If problems occurred, it was not unusual for a more experienced midwife to be called to help out. As described in the diaries of Catherine Schrader, a seventeenth-century midwife who was called to complicated births in Holland, this often involved internal podalic version and bringing the baby out by its feet (Marland 1987).

A core professionalising strategy used by midwives in Western countries in the eighteenth and nineteenth centuries was the relinquishing of complicated (and lucrative) birth practice to the medical profession in return for the domain of 'normal childbirth' (Donnison 1977; Leap & Hunter 1993). This strategy responded to, and set up, a dynamic that has had far-reaching consequences in terms of gender and class inequalities and the collective psychological effects of subordination (Witz 1992). Pathology was the pivotal factor for role division, and doctors were presented as the superior professionals, educated at a higher level than midwives in order to carry out rescuing manoeuvres associated with the complications of childbirth. In comparison, the midwife's role was shrunk to that of 'caring' for women who did not need interventions, and to recognising problems and calling for a doctor to 'correct' the situation and intervene in a timely fashion.

The fraught negotiations that led to the role delineation between midwives and doctors have given way to a situation with its own set of interprofessional tensions. While fulfilling the imperative to adopt good collaborative relationships with obstetricians in the interests of women and safe practice, the midwife often defines the boundaries of 'normal' in situations that are intricate and unclear. She[1] engages with women and makes decisions in a culture dominated by the ideologies of authoritative medical science and its quest for certainty. Evidence-based protocols and policies often do not 'fit' with the complexity of individual women's psychosocial situations and the impact of the environment. This has led to a childbirth culture in which it is increasingly difficult to find consensus on what constitutes 'normal birth' other than an absence of technical intervention (Downe & McCourt 2004).

The rationale for promoting physiological birth

The boundaries of what is considered 'normal' are at the heart of the passionate discussions that happen whenever midwives get together. In recent years, midwives have been addressing these issues by identifying the complexity of their role in being 'with woman' and promoting physiological birth. This is often explained in terms of the potentially self-transformative nature of birth and the profound long-term consequences of empowerment for women, their families and society (Leap 2004; Leap & Anderson 2004). The promotion of physiology begins in early pregnancy and is about far more than aiming for an uncomplicated birth. It is concerned with a journey to motherhood that will have profound consequences for each individual woman in terms of how she feels about herself, her body and her capabilities (Thompson 2004). Whether or not she eventually gives birth without intervention, a woman who feels powerful is in a good situation to take on becoming a new mother.

> Birth is not only about making babies. Birth is also about making mothers—strong, competent, capable mothers who trust themselves and know their inner strength (Katz Rothman 1996, pp 253–4).

Sadly, the opposite is also true—women can end up feeling disempowered and emotionally fragile as a result of an experience of childbirth that rendered them passive in the face of intervention (Kitzinger 2000). This chapter explores some of these issues, relating them to the practicalities of midwifery practice and initiatives that optimise women's potential to feel good about their experiences of pregnancy, giving birth and nurturing a new baby. Some strategies are suggested that might help to promote physiology, even in situations where midwives are 'swimming against the tide' of interventionist thinking. The word 'interventionist' rather than 'medicalised' is used in an attempt to acknowledge that it is not only doctors who can hinder physiological birth.

The imaginary story below will be used to tease out some of these issues. Within the culture of maternity care in industrialised countries, where health professionals who are strangers to the woman often provide fragmented care in busy, under-staffed maternity units, this is a familiar story.

This story describes well-meaning midwives and doctors struggling to provide a safe, kind service under conditions

Scenario

The birth of Jason Smith at St Average Hospital

This is an everyday story about the birth of a baby at St Average hospital. It's the story of the birth of Jason Smith, first child of Mary and Wayne Smith. Mary is a receptionist in a hotel and has continued working up until she was 34 weeks pregnant. She has not had any problems in her pregnancy and has been coming to the antenatal clinic regularly, where, after waiting for over an hour, she has seen a different person at each visit for a 15-minute check-up. She attended antenatal classes at the hospital but could not persuade Wayne to come with her to these. Wayne is a motor mechanic. He's a shy man who doesn't like hospitals. Secretly he's very worried about being with Mary when she's in labour. He's scared that he'll faint, and is worried about seeing Mary in pain. He didn't want to go to the classes in case they showed a video that might make him pass out or want to vomit. He has heard stories from his mates at work that make him shudder. Mary found the classes useful. They reinforced her idea that she would 'try for a normal birth', but it is comforting to know that the epidural is there if she can't cope.

One Sunday evening, a week past her due date, Mary starts having some low, period-type pains. She thinks her waters may have broken. She is very scared, and so is Wayne, who rings the hospital. The midwife on the phone asks him a lot of questions: 'How often are the contractions?', 'How long do they last?', 'What colour is the water?', ' Is the baby moving?'. The midwife suggests that it may be early days yet but to come in if they're worried. They are worried. They go in to St Average.

When Mary and Wayne get to the 'delivery suite' at St Average, they are assigned to the care of midwife Sally, in Room 11. Sally is friendly and efficient, asks Mary lots of questions, including whether she has been to classes and what her choices are for pain relief. Mary says she's not sure how she'll cope, as she has a low pain threshold and already these pains are severe. The midwife says, 'We'll take it one step at a time, shall we? You're coping well at the moment.' She talks Mary and Wayne through all the 'natural' methods of pain relief, and then explains that if Mary can't cope with the pain, there are other things to help—she explains the pros and cons of gas, pethidine and epidurals.

Sally the midwife gives Mary a hospital gown and carries out a series of tests—takes Mary's temperature, pulse and blood pressure, tests her urine, and palpates her abdomen. She places Mary on the monitor and explains the trace to Wayne, who is fascinated and remains glued to every variation in the lines. Sally reassures Mary that the baby's heartbeat looks really good. She explains that she is looking after someone in the room next door, that she'll come back in ten minutes. She gives them a bell to ring if they need her.

It will be a while before Sally can get back to Mary. Next door, Sophie's contractions are suddenly very strong. She is having her second baby, and in order to have continuity of care with someone she trusts, Sophie has booked with a private obstetrician, Edward Richman. Sally helps her get down onto all fours on a mattress on the floor. Sophie is bellowing. Sally asks someone to phone Dr Richman to come.

Scenario—cont'd

He arrives ten minutes later as the baby's head is crowning. Edward insists that Sophie get up onto the bed, cuts an episiotomy and hands her a healthy baby girl, who will be called Anna. Sophie and her partner thank Edward profusely. There is much jubilation all round.

Meanwhile, back in Room 11, Mary and Wayne are still anxiously watching their baby's heartbeat on the monitor. Eventually Sally asks Rita, another midwife, to go and check on Mary. They all look at the trace and admire its reassuring variations. According to the machine, Mary is having what Rita interprets as 'irregular tightenings'. Mary says that they are quite painful and Rita responds gently by telling Mary that she's doing really well and that 'Bub's happy' but it looks as though it's early days yet. She asks Mary what she has decided she'd like for pain relief if she needs it later. She reiterates what is on offer and tells Mary that, as her waters may have broken, the doctor will come and examine her and have a look at her cervix using a sterile speculum.

Alexandria, the new resident, examines Mary. She is kind and gentle but Mary finds the examination painful. Alexandria asks Mary what choices she has made for pain relief. She reassures her by saying, 'It's great if you can manage the pain but you don't have to be a martyr. If you're going to have an epidural don't wait until it's really bad before getting it inserted'.

It seems that Mary's waters have broken but her cervix is still long and firm. She is offered the choice of going home and waiting for the contractions to establish, with daily review at the hospital, or having a 'bit of help to get things going'. She is too scared to contemplate going home and the thought of 'getting things going' is appealing. Mary has some prostaglandins to help soften her cervix. She is given some sedatives to help her get some sleep, and

Wayne goes home to get some rest.

The ensuing chain of events over the next day is familiar to all who have worked in large maternity units. For Mary these events will remain embedded in her memory until the day she dies. She was very grateful to have an epidural to help her cope with the fierce contractions induced by a Syntocinon infusion. The pethidine she had had earlier hadn't touched the pain. She had a kind midwife called Sandra with her for most of the labour. Sandra was a mature woman whom Wayne would later describe as 'really knowing her stuff'.

Little Jason Smith is pulled into the world with the aid of a Ventouse after the monitor showed signs that he really would be 'better off out than in'. He is a fine, healthy baby, albeit a little confused about how to find his way around Mary's breast. He is taken to the nursery for a few hours to be observed because he is 'breathing up a bit'.

Wayne didn't faint. He is in awe of Mary and thanks God for the 'life saving wonders of modern medicine'. Mary and Wayne are very grateful to the staff of St Average and give them a huge box of chocolates when they go home with Jason four days after his birth.

Mary is given the name of a child health clinic she can go to get Jason weighed and where she can access advice about breastfeeding. She is pleased about this because Jason still seems a bit confused about how to latch on and her nipples are very sore. Her Mum, Jenny, is coming to stay for a couple of weeks, but Jenny is very unsure about how to support Mary in breastfeeding Jason. Jenny's own experience left her thinking she was 'unable to make enough milk' and that formula was the only option in these circumstances.

Thus begins the new life of Mary and Wayne as proud parents of little Jason Smith . . .

hampered by fragmented care, staff shortages, public expectations, medical dominance and all the other components of the stresses associated with maternity service provision in large tertiary maternity units. At every stage of the story, these well-meaning members of staff reinforce Mary and Wayne's belief that Mary will need some form of pain relief. In the spiralling cascade of intervention, Mary is rendered passive and dependent on the expertise of strangers.

As this is not a 'real' story, there is the opportunity to wind back the clock and explore how the experience might have been different for Mary, Wayne and their baby, Jason, had circumstances been otherwise. The re-telling of this story enables scrutiny of a range of changes to practice, some of which are within the grasp of the practitioner and others that

would require significant changes to systems. The evidence for these strategies will be woven throughout the process of looking at how we might reconstruct the 'everyday story' of the birth of Jason Smith.

Promoting physiological birth

Access to midwifery care

From the scenario, some might question the usefulness of midwifery care, given that Mary and Wayne appear grateful and happy about the birth of their son, Jason. Although the members of staff at St Average were all strangers to Mary and Wayne, they were friendly, kind and competent, which is what women say is important to them (Green et al 1998; Lee 1997).

Such challenges raise complex questions about how to evaluate women's experiences of birth in terms of their 'satisfaction' and how midwifery and the promotion of physiological birth might be implicated. It can be argued that women have a vested interest in evaluating their experience positively in the postnatal period and that, in many situations, it is impossible for women to know how their experience might have been otherwise. For example, research in South Australia has shown that women like Sophie chose private obstetric care because they had no knowledge of midwifery. However, once such women were exposed to midwifery care, they identified that they would choose it in subsequent pregnancies (Zadoroznyj 2000).

Had Mary lived in New Zealand, she would have had considerably more chance of finding and getting to know a midwife who would be present during her labour. Legislative processes have enabled the majority of women in New Zealand to choose a publicly funded lead maternity carer to provide them with continuity of care.

This is an important consideration because midwives can play a crucial role in promoting psychosocial wellbeing. This was identified by Anne Oakley and colleagues (Oakley et al 1990, 1996) in a randomised controlled trial, which showed that the effect of midwives making themselves available, in a 'listening ear' capacity throughout pregnancy, had profound long-term consequences for the relationships and social lives of women, their children and their families.

Midwifery continuity of care

The anxiety of pregnant women who do not know which midwife will be there in labour for them, and whether this makes a difference to outcomes, has not been well captured by researchers on the whole. Confusion about the term 'midwifery continuity of care' and what it actually means in practice has added to the difficulty of making comparisons in research studies, particularly in exploring how women feel about their care (Sandall 2004). Furthermore, the notion of randomising women in studies does not lend itself to enquiry into choices, processes and relationships. However, a Cochrane Review (Hodnett 2004) identified that continuity of care from midwives has the potential to make a significant difference to the promotion of physiological birth when comparisons are made with standard care from physicians and midwives, as identified in Box 17.1.

Midwifery caseload practice

An increasing body of literature identifies the need for studies to look specifically at the midwifery continuity of care provided in a caseload practice model. Non-randomised studies of this form of care suggest that there are improved outcomes for women where they are able to establish relationships with midwives during pregnancy (Benjamin et al 2001; Page et al 2001; Sandall et al 2001).

BOX 17.1 Continuity vs standard care
Cochrane Review of caregivers during pregnancy and childbirth
Women experiencing continuity of care from a team of midwives were:
▶ less likely to be admitted to hospital antenatally
▶ less likely to have pharmacological pain relief
▶ less likely to have babies needing resuscitation
▶ less likely to have an episiotomy
▶ more likely to attend antenatal education programs
▶ more likely to be pleased with their antenatal, intrapartum and postnatal care.
(Source: Hodnett 2004)

The Albany Midwifery Group Practice in the United Kingdom is held up as an example of a community-based midwifery group practice that operates a caseload practice model and makes a difference to outcomes in a disadvantaged community (Reed 2002a,b). An evaluation of this group practice identified the fact that the midwives were very successful at facilitating normality in pregnancy and birth (Sandall et al 2001). Significant differences in outcomes were reported in terms of: increased satisfaction and rates of normal vaginal birth; home birth and breastfeeding rates; and reduced rates of induction, caesarean section, use of pharmacological pain relief, and perineal trauma (Sandall et al 2001).

Preliminary evaluations of the Northern Women's Community Midwifery Project (NWCMP) in the northern suburbs of Adelaide suggest that similar positive outcomes for women can be achieved through replicating the model in other contexts (Nixon et al 2003). The NWCMP has similar features to the Albany Midwifery Group Practice, in that the midwives:

- are community-based in a publicly funded model
- cover a geographical area of extreme socio-economic deprivation
- offer booking visits and a 36-week visit in the woman's home
- run antenatal and postnatal groups
- offer home birth as an option.

Offering home birth

In light of such evidence it might be a good starting point for the reconstruction of the story of the birth of Jason Smith to provide Mary with a midwifery continuity-of-care model in her pregnancy, one that gives her options about the place of birth. Given that the birth of Jason Smith could be reconstructed in any way, it would be possible to tell a story that starts with Mary booking with independent midwives for birth at home. There are good reasons to suggest that such services should be publicly funded. Internationally, home birth has been shown to be a safe option for a carefully selected group of women (Ackermann-Leibrich et al 1996; Anderson

& Murphy 1995; Campbell & Macfarlane 1994; Chamberlain et al 1997; Davies 1996; Murphy & Fullerton 1998; Olsen 1997; Olsen & Jewell 1998; Tyson 1991; Wiegers et al 1996). Similar findings have been demonstrated in Australia and New Zealand (Crotty et al 1990; Gulbransen et al 1997; Woodcock et al 1990), although poor outcomes have been associated with women with risk-associated pregnancies, such as twins and breeches, opting for birth at home in Australia (Bastian et al 1998).

While women in New Zealand can choose to give birth within publicly funded maternity services, in Australia the development of such options is in its infancy. Publicly funded, community-based midwifery programs that incorporate home birth options in a publicly funded healthcare system have been successfully implemented in both Western Australia (Thiele & Thorogood 1997; Thorogood et al 2002) and South Australia (Nixon et al 2003), with safe outcomes for both mothers and babies and high levels of satisfaction for women and midwives.[2]

Given the evidence that planned home birth is just as safe as birth in hospital for the majority of women, like Mary, who have uncomplicated pregnancies (Olsen & Jewell 1998), the promotion and support of home birth as a mainstream option for women has to be a major tactic in promoting physiological birth. Resistance to such a proposal is enshrined in the discourse of contemporary maternity services. With this in mind, the House of Commons Select Committee on Maternity Services (2003) proposed that all midwives, GPs or obstetricians should be enabled to attend a home birth during their training in order to challenge their prejudices and familiarise them with the promotion of normal birth (House of Commons 2003). Anecdotal evidence suggests that attending a birth at home has a significant effect on the practice of both midwives and doctors by giving them an insight into the profound nature of birth and the power of physiology.

Public awareness of the safety of home birth also needs to be addressed. As identified by the Albany Midwifery Practice, where over 50% of women give birth at home, it is possible to convince people that home birth is a safe option, even where they would never have considered it before. This practice has been able to show that where known midwives engage with women and their supporters throughout pregnancy, in particular during a home visit in late pregnancy and where decision-making about the place of birth is reserved for labour, home birth can be seen as a safe option for the majority of women, with a significant decrease in operative birth and medical interventions (Reed 2002a,b).

Reconstructing Jason's story

In order to make full use of reconstructing the birth of Jason Smith, we will not simplify the story by turning it into one about home birth. However, we will enable Mary to book with a group of midwives who have a woman-centred approach to providing continuity of care. The reconstructed story speaks of the difference this makes to how the story unfolds.

Scenario

Reconstructing Jason's birth: Mary's booking

When Mary suspects that she is pregnant, she goes to her local community centre, where she knows there are midwives who advertise a free pregnancy testing service twice a week at set times. The midwives are in a group practice and have their own premises in the community centre where women can access advice and information and attend a variety of support groups. The midwifery group practice is linked to the publicly funded maternity service provided at St Average Hospital.

The midwife who confirms that Mary is pregnant sets out the various options for maternity care and gives Mary some written information so that she can go home and discuss these options with Wayne. It does not take Mary and Wayne long to decide that they will book with the midwifery group practice. Fiona is the midwife assigned to be Mary's primary midwife. She phones Mary and arranges to come to her home to carry out the booking visit at a time when Wayne can be present. By the end of this leisurely visit, Mary and Wayne feel excited and very relieved. Fiona has made them feel that they are very special. She leaves the pregnancy record with Mary and encourages her to fill in any parts that she wants to and to make a note of any questions she has for subsequent visits.

Fiona encourages Mary and Wayne to attend the antenatal groups that the midwives run in their practice. Instead of classes where the midwives instruct the women, these antenatal groups are organised so that each week someone comes back to the group to tell their story. Mary can go to the group as often as she likes, starting in early pregnancy, so she will hear many different stories. She will learn from other women and will make friends who will be her support network when she is at home with a new baby. Wayne decides he might go with Mary to some of the evening groups now that he has met Fiona and likes her.

Mary's confidence about giving birth starts to grow.

Antenatal groups

Mary has booked with a midwifery group practice that sees bringing women together in groups as a crucial strategy to develop a forum where they can learn from each other and develop friendships and support networks (Leap 2000). As suggested by Mavis Kirkham, 'linking women with others makes them stronger' (Kirkham 1986, p 47).

This model of antenatal support and information sharing has been explained by women who have benefited from such groups, in a video: *Helping You to Make Your Own Decisions* (Leap 1991). The concept of running groups instead of classes is based in a women-centred philosophy. Women set the agenda in the groups. They learn from each other and build their own support networks, thus minimising dependency on health professionals.

The midwife's role is described by the women in the video as that of a 'facilitator' who makes sure that, each week, a round of introductions starts the group. The midwife running groups such as these develops good listening skills. She needs to know how to ask open-ended questions and how to draw on the expertise of group members. She will make sure that people feel safe to talk or to remain silent and that no one dominates the discussions. She makes sure that newcomers are looked after and that they understand how the group operates. The midwife needs to judge when it is appropriate to interject with information, when to explain things that have arisen and, most importantly, when to keep quiet. Her skill lies in picking up cues from the group's discussion. One woman describes how this process changes the way women learn:

> To have the midwife there to provide some real education as to what it's all about ... bringing in the pelvis and 'baby' [doll] and actually showing how the baby travels down the birth canal ... and that coming up in a sort of organic way as a woman was talking about the birth she'd had last week and how the baby had got stuck somewhere, the midwife showed us. It stayed in my head because it was attached to real people. It wasn't abstract information you were getting. It was associated with women in the group so it got absorbed differently (quotation from video, Leap 1991).

A model of antenatal education and support in which women set the agenda (as opposed to being taught what the midwife has decided they should know about) can have far-reaching consequences for both women and midwives. Such groups are best situated in the community, but have also been run successfully in hospital antenatal clinics as an alternative to classes, and on antenatal and postnatal wards for women who are hospitalised. Anecdotal evidence suggests that antenatal groups offer a powerful tool for exploring the rationale and strategies for keeping birth normal (Reed 2002a,b).

In our reconstructed story, Mary will be able to attend a postnatal group that is run by child health nurses in the same community centre. She will carry on meeting the women she has met in the antenatal group there because she is very motivated to continue these friendships. This will provide a continuity of friendship and support, which the women in the video described as 'a lifeline' in breaking down the isolation of new motherhood.

> Just being able to ring someone up in the middle of the night ... just the fact that you've had a conversation with someone means that you're not there as an island trying to cope on your own.
>
> I think they're probably friends that you'll have for life, even though we're all so different. I would have been very isolated otherwise ... we formed a network of women who met up outside of the group and carried on meeting for years (quotations from video, Leap 1991).

Similar groups to those described in the video have been evaluated in the United States. The 'CenteringPregnancy' program also includes the element of women receiving their antenatal care in groups. This model has been found to be a powerful empowerment tool, especially for young and disadvantaged women (Klima 2003; Schindler Rising 1998). An evaluation of the first pilot program in the United States demonstrated that women enjoyed being with other women in the groups and made plans to continue meeting after their babies were born (Schindler Rising 1998). Another evaluation tested the program in a group of pregnant adolescent women who were identified as being particularly vulnerable. The CenteringPregnancy program was shown to assist these women in terms of empowerment and improved self-esteem (Klima 2003).

Other small studies have also demonstrated positive results in terms of satisfaction and reductions in low birthweight and preterm births (Grady & Bloom 2004). In a matched cohort study of 458 women, most of whom were African-American or Latina, women who received CenteringPregnancy care had larger babies than women having traditional care. This was particularly significant among preterm births: women in the CenteringPregnancy group had babies who were an average 408 grams heavier, and these women expressed higher levels of psychosocial improvements in their lives (Ickovics et al 2003). A similar direction is being noted in a large randomised controlled trial being carried out in the United States at Yale University, funded by the National Institute of Mental Health and nearing completion (Schindler Rising, personal communication 2005).

Building confidence throughout pregnancy

We can return to the reconstruction of Mary and Wayne's story and see how the style of antenatal care they are offered continues to build confidence and social support (see p 287).

Late pregnancy

The 36-week home visit

The 36-week home visit described here was studied by Joy Kemp (2003), who described the initiative as:

> an alternative model of authoritative knowledge, one which acknowledged a role for intervention and technology but placed as central a philosophy of birth as a physiological, transformational and socio-cultural event (Kemp 2003, p 4).

In her research, Joy Kemp (2003) identified a range of productive activities involved in carrying out a 36-week home visit to make plans for labour and the early postnatal period, all of which have implications for promoting physiology:

- involving family members in support in labour and in the early days following birth, with practical suggestions for how this might take place
- discussions about approaches to being with women in pain in labour without rushing to take away pain and to ensure that physiology is promoted
- the use of photographs to encourage discussion about normal birth
- information to reduce premature admission to hospital and choice about place of birth in labour.

Kemp's (2003) study portrayed the 36-week birth talk as an integral part of the ongoing dialogue and relationship of

Scenario

Building confidence and support

Mary has established a group of friends through attending the antenatal groups. She has heard many stories of women's births and looks forward to the day when it will be her turn to come to the group and tell her story. Wayne has met some new fathers too and heard some of their experiences of being at labour, so he is feeling less anxious.

Mary and Wayne have been introduced to all the midwives in the group practice when they went to the community centre for their antenatal care. Sarah has been assigned to them as their second midwife and they have met her at the practice for alternate antenatal check-ups. As Fiona is their primary midwife, she is most likely to be there when their baby is born, but if she is having days off when Mary goes into labour, Mary and Wayne will be very happy to have Sarah be with them as they have come to know her too. Fiona has taken responsibility for keeping the overview of their pregnancy; she made sure that all Mary's tests were completed and explained the results to her.

At 36 weeks, Fiona and Sarah go to Mary and Wayne's home to talk about support in labour and in the early days following birth. At Fiona's instigation, all the relatives and friends who will be supporting Mary come to that meeting. Fiona and Sarah talk about practical support in the first weeks following birth. They suggest rosters for bringing in food, taking away washing, shopping and walking the dog.

Fiona and Sarah also talk to the gathered people about how best to support Mary in labour. They show photos of births and talk about pain. They explain that the midwives will not be rushing to try and take away Mary's pain, that pain is purposeful, and that it would not be helpful to keep asking her if she wants something to take away the pain. They give Mary's supporters ideas about how they can minimise disturbance to help Mary withdraw into her body so that her own opiates can come into play. They talk about noise, moving around, transition and early breastfeeding—in effect, they explain why it is important to promote physiology and give plenty of suggestions about how best to facilitate this. Fiona and Sarah know that if they do not engage in these discussions, Mary's labour supporters are likely to expect them to offer pain relief during Mary's labour, in their distress pestering the midwives to 'do something' about the pain.

Fiona and Sarah also explain about 'pre-labour' or early labour and the importance of not going into hospital too soon. They talk through what to do if the baby comes in a hurry before the midwife arrives, and make sure they know where this is written in Mary's notes.

Fiona and Sarah tell the support people that if Mary's labour is going well, the midwives will offer her the opportunity to stay at home to have her baby, as they always carry all the equipment with them needed for a safe birth. They explain that if Mary needs 'help' they can go to hospital, but otherwise the best place to enable physiology to flourish is in a woman's own home.

The midwives also explain that the majority of white women having first babies do not go into labour until they are at least a week to 10 days after the 'due date'. They talk about the possibility of 'pre-labour' contractions and the importance of Mary eating, drinking and getting lots of sleep while labour gets established. This advice includes when to call the midwives, with clear messages to avoid the hours between midnight and 7 am unless they are worried or the contractions are coming every two to three minutes, lasting about a minute and Mary can't talk through them.

Mary is keen to use water in labour. She has heard stories in the group of how helpful women have found being in a deep tub. Fiona explains to everyone that if Mary's labour is progressing well and she wants to stay in the tub to give birth, this is a safe option.

By the end of this visit, everyone is clear about their possible roles in supporting Mary. The photographs of a labour sequence have helped to promote discussion about the sorts of things to expect, and everyone is excited about approaching labour with an open mind. The midwives have imparted an important message that they trust in Mary's ability to give birth to her baby and to cope well with whatever events unfold.

mutual trust that occurs between a woman and her midwife throughout pregnancy, where the same midwife or midwives are going to be with the woman during labour. The concept is thus directly related to continuity of care that includes an intrapartum component. It is also one element of a midwifery model that aims to focus on birth as a social, rather than a technocratic, event (Kitzinger 2000).

Evidence about strategies during pregnancy

Evidence relating to strategies that keep birth normal in late pregnancy is limited. However, the following principles have been suggested as important (Enkin et al 2000):

- midwifery care for women who do not have serious risk factors
- effective interdisciplinary collaboration
- giving women as much information as they want

- respecting women's choice of birthplace
- encouraging women to organise for companions to support them during labour
- not offering induction of labour until after 41 weeks of pregnancy
- external cephalic version at term for women whose babies are breech.

We return to Mary's story when she is 41 weeks pregnant. For the sake of argument, we will assume that where Mary and Wayne live, home birth is not yet a publicly funded option, nor is there a birth centre nearby.

Promoting physiology during labour

Throughout this reconstruction of the birth of Jason Smith, the midwives have adopted an evidence-based approach to supporting Mary in making decisions that promote physiological birth. They have also made a conscious effort

Scenario

Jason's birth

On a Sunday evening, a week past her due date, Mary starts having some low, period-type pains. She thinks her waters may have broken. She phones Fiona and describes what has happened and tells her that the baby is wriggling around as usual. Fiona is very excited for Mary and Wayne, and offers to call in and see them. She visits, carries out a reassuring check and confirms that Mary is draining clear liquor. Fiona explains the evidence from studies comparing a waiting approach with accelerating labour and together they make a plan to wait and see how events unfold. Mary will keep in touch by telephone if she has any concerns, if her temperature rises or if labour gets under way. Otherwise Fiona will visit again the next day.

Mary manages to get some sleep overnight, although by 6.30 in the morning the contractions are beginning to get stronger and closer together. She lets Wayne sleep, makes herself some breakfast and potters around the house. By the time Fiona visits again at midday, Mary's contractions are coming every three minutes and are lasting about a minute. Mary's Mum Jenny is helping Wayne to rub Mary's back during contractions and is making sure that she is sipping plenty of water. Mary's friend Linda, who has had two babies and was also present at the 36-week home visit, is making sure that everyone has enough to eat and drink. After performing some routine checks to ensure that Mary and her baby are responding well to labour, Fiona watches quietly; she can tell that Mary is in strong labour. She tells Mary this and suggests that this would be a good time to think about going into hospital if this is still what she wants to do. Mary is clear that she does want to have the baby in hospital, so they make plans for the journey.

Fiona goes ahead to the hospital and arranges to meet Mary, Wayne, Jenny and Linda there in the next hour or so. She prepares a room in the birthing suite to make it as cosy as possible, takes the mattresses off the bed and places them in the corner, making a little nest of cushions and bean bags. She pushes the bed up against the wall; it is no longer the centre of

attention in the room. The lights are dimmed, there is possibly some ambient music playing very softly and the room smells good. Fiona is wearing her own clothes—some loose track pants and a T-shirt.

Soon after Mary arrives at St Average, her labour progresses well and she roams around the room, gets in and out of the deep bath and makes loud moaning noises. Fiona keeps a watchful eye, using an unobtrusive Doppler to monitor the baby's heartbeat. She offers Mary a birthing ball, and heated wheat packs for comfort. As Mary's contractions get stronger and closer, she becomes withdrawn. Fiona quietly reassures her that she's doing well after each contraction and when Mary pleads that she 'can't do it', Fiona keeps saying that she *can* do it, that this is normal and that she is doing really well.

Mary starts to feel an urge to bear down and soon the baby's head can be seen. Fiona talks Mary through breathing her baby's head out slowly so that she does not tear.

When Mary is giving birth, with her permission, Fiona invites Alexandria, the new resident, into the room to sit in the corner and watch as Mary gives birth to Jason on all fours. Wayne puts his hands next to Fiona's as Jason emerges and helps to pass him through and place him in front of Mary so that she can pick him up and take him to her when she is ready. Mary confirms for everyone that her baby is a boy. She takes him to her and talks to him, exclaiming as she explores his little body, finding family likeness in features—'Look, he's got your ears, Wayne!'. She is amazed at the cord, which is still pulsating.

Fiona gently reminds Mary that soon she will feel a slight fullness in her vagina as the placenta separates. She reassures Mary that pushing out the placenta will be easy, as it is soft, and that as soon as the placenta is out, they will cut the cord. Within a few minutes Mary has delivered her placenta and, with Fiona's help, she cuts the cord herself.

Jason has a first suckle. He is very alert and latches on enthusiastically. Everyone marvels at the placenta and membranes, as Fiona shows them its various wonders. There is much celebration all round.

to address the crucial role that pain plays in keeping birth normal. There is a need to change the culture in institutions around pain in labour through shifting the approach away from one of 'pain relief' to one of 'working with pain in labour' (Leap & Anderson 2004). Women have highlighted the fact that the attitudes of midwives have a profound effect on their experience of giving birth, in particular how they cope with pain in labour (Halldorsdottir & Karlsdottir 1996; Hodnett, 2002; Lundgren & Dahlberg 1998).

Undoubtedly, words of encouragement and reassurance during labour play a vital role in giving women confidence in their ability to cope with pain, and this, in turn, increases women's ability to avoid the side-effects of pharmacological analgesia and their disturbing effect on physiological processes. The role of the midwife in giving quiet encouragement is one of watchfulness and anticipation.

> Our expertise as midwives rests in our ability to watch, to listen and to respond to any given situation with all of our senses. This will include the conscious and subconscious 'knowing' that has been generated from our experience and learning. It also involves a 'cluefullness' as we respond to the overt and covert clues from women and their worlds. The skill lies in knowing when to inform, suggest, act, seek help and, most importantly, when to be still or when to withdraw and remove ourselves (Leap 2000, pp 5–6).

This approach recognises the need for women to have privacy in order to avoid disturbance of the complex neuro-hormonal cascades of labour. Michel Odent (1992) has suggested that it is important to enable women to find a private, quiet, dark, comfortable space in which to labour and give birth. He explains this in terms of promoting prostaglandins, oxytocins and other labour-enhancing hormones that can be inhibited when there is stimulation to the busy thinking part of the brain, the neocortex, or when fear and anxiety lead to excessive catecholamine production. This makes sense to midwives, who often see women 'disappear into their bodies' and enter a state of altered consciousness as labour intensifies.

A wide range of measures that promote physiology during labour are outlined in *The Labor Progress Handbook: Early Interventions to Prevent and Treat Dystocia* (Simkin & Ancheta 2000). Some of these strategies are outlined in Box 17.2.

Building a culture in which physiological birth can flourish

All the strategies to promote physiological birth that have been addressed so far in this chapter will flourish in an environment where there is collegiality and good support for practitioners. In reconstructing the story of the birth of Jason Smith, there is an opportunity to fantasise about an ideal culture that supports practitioners in promoting physiological birth.

Developing a supportive culture in this way is about breaking down hierarchical barriers, enabling safe situations for all practitioners to share their uncertainty as well as their expertise, and recognising different expertise and complementary roles. Such an approach also depends on the most powerful groups—doctors—relinquishing some of their power. Power cannot be given; it can only be taken, and this process involves mutual sensitivity to the dynamics and potential pitfalls surrounding collaboration on the part of both parties.

In units where multidisciplinary efforts are activated to reduce caesarean sections, success may well depend on raising consciousness and awareness of issues and philosophical approaches, plus a concerted effort from all disciplines. It seems that pulling together, a commitment to evidence-based practice, one-to-one support from midwives during labour, managing change and fostering goodwill are important strategies in reducing interference in labour and improving outcomes for women (Ontario Women's Health Council 2002).

BOX 17.2 Promoting physiology in labour

Measures that can promote physiology during labour include:

▷ Encouraging an atmosphere of privacy, calm and safety and the guaranteed presence of the midwife/birth supporters

▷ Offering comfort devices such as heat/ice packs, warm blankets, birth ball, beanbag, bath, shower, tea, music, massage, wiping her face and neck with a cool cloth

▷ Encouraging immersion in water during labour and for birth in a deep tub that allows movement and different positions, including all fours

▷ The continued presence of a female companion, partner or 'doula', who is committed to promoting normal birth

▷ Encouraging the woman to move around, adopt different positions, rest, make noises and eat and drink as she sees fit

▷ Avoiding continuous electronic fetal monitoring (EFM) in uncomplicated labour and using intermittent auscultation instead

▷ Where continuous EFM is necessary, still encouraging different positions, swaying

▷ Staying at home as long as possible when hospital birth is planned

▷ Understanding the anatomy, physiology and psychology of labour, and the techniques that can enhance these.

(based on Simkin & Anchetta 2000)

Conclusion

Changing the wider culture, outside institutions, to one that privileges normal birth is a daunting task in an era when caesarean and epidural rates are rising and these methods of childbirth are increasingly being identified in the media as the obvious choice for women in order for them to make full use of the benefits of modern technology. Promoting

Scenario

An ideal culture . . .

Fiona knows that if she is worried or tired she can ask for help—this may be from another midwife in her practice. It may also be from one of the core midwives who staff the birthing service and support the midwives in the group practices when they bring women to St Average. If Fiona is concerned about Mary's labour she will discuss the situation with one of the doctors, either in person or by phone. Such a supportive culture has been engendered at St Average by a concerted multidisciplinary approach in the last few years. There is also a 'zero-tolerance' approach to dominating behaviour and horizontal violence.

Every day at 2 pm at St Average, there is some form of interdisciplinary get-together or 'in-service' in the meeting room around the corner. This is organised by the Midwifery Consultant, is open to all staff, including midwives in community-based practices, and may be:

▶ a monthly perinatal mortality meeting where midwives as well as doctors present cases for review. This includes reviewing admissions to the Neonatal Unit.

▶ interesting case reviews, led by midwives, doctors or students on a rotational basis

▶ consensus guidelines for practice development— these have replaced protocols. They are evidence-based and incorporate woman-centred approaches to practice.

▶ student project presentations—students are encouraged to present their projects to all staff

▶ topic-based review of putting evidence into practice. These are guided discussion sessions or lively debates. Recent topics include:

- a multidisciplinary approach to reducing the rate of caesarean sections at St Average by encouraging women to entertain VBAC and ECV, selective use of continuous EFM and informing all staff of the evidence about all of these

- changing the culture of 'pain relief' to one of 'being with women in pain in labour'

- regular practice sessions using the mannequins for emergencies—staff are encouraged to attend the ALSO[3] course and continue to practise the 'hands on' simulations and mnemonics.

normal birth in the media is obviously important but a more fundamental approach may be necessary. The promotion of normal birth may have to start in primary schools through visits by pregnant and breastfeeding women and midwives, in order to plant the seeds of thought that will grow into an adult ability to conceptualise birth as a social event with profound meaning for all involved.

This chapter has explored how promoting physiology involves far more than a series of techniques used in labour. It involves the raising of consciousness at every level in our institutions, health services and governments in order to build systems and services that nurture the potential of birth to transform lives and strengthen women, their families and societies.

Review questions

1 In the context of your own practice, how can you enhance a culture that promotes physiological birth?

2 Imagine that you have been asked to visit a primary school to talk about 'having a baby'. What will you say?

3 Using Box 17.2 as a guide, how many of the measures listed there are in place in your place of work? For those that are not in place, how can you introduce them?

4 You have been asked to prepare a 20-minute talk for the multidisciplinary lunchtime meeting. The topic is 'promoting physiological birth'.

How will you defend your argument when the anaesthetists suggest that all women should be offered an epidural during labour?

5 Name some of the underlying power dynamics in your workplace that possibly subvert the efforts of midwives to promote physiological birth.

6 How have the dynamics you described in question 5 evolved over recent centuries? (1000 words)

7 Describe what you understand by the terms 'interventionist' and 'medicalised' in terms of promoting physiological birth.

Review questions—cont'd

8 Internationally, home birth has been shown to be a safe option for a carefully selected group of women. Look up the recommended references on home birth and make a table of the outcomes achieved in three of the studies compared to those achieved in the hospital closest to where you work.

9 You have been asked to prepare a talk on home birth for the local Country Women's Institute. What are the questions you might expect from a group of women who gave birth in the 1960s and 1970s?

10 Describe some of the activities involved in carrying out a 36-week home visit to make plans for labour and the early postnatal period, all of which have implications for promoting physiology.

Online resources

Centering Pregnancy and Parenting Association, Inc., http://www.centeringpregnancy.com

Florence Nightingale School of Nursing and Midwifery, Research Group Project Information, http://www.kcl.ac.uk/teares/nmvc/research/project

Notes

1 Because over 99% of midwives are women, the midwife is referred to as 'she'. The intention is not to exclude men who are midwives.

2 The first publicly funded home birth service in New South Wales was due to commence at the time of writing this textbook (2005).

3 ALSO: Advanced Life Support in Obstetrics

References

Ackermann-Leibrich U, Voegeli T, Gunter-Witt K et al 1996 Home versus hospital deliveries: follow up study of matched pairs for procedures and outcomes. British Medical Journal 313:1313–1318

Anderson R, Murphy P 1995 Outcomes of 11,788 planned homebirths attended by certified nurse–midwives. A retrospective descriptive study. Journal of Nurse-Midwifery 40:483–492

Bastian, H, Keirse, M, Lancaster, P 1998 Perinatal death associated with planned homebirth in Australia: population based study. British Medical Journal 317:384–388

Beech B 1997 Normal birth: does it exist? Association for Improvements in the Maternity Services (AIMS) Journal, 9:4–8

Benjamin Y, Walsh D, Taub N 2001 A comparison of partnership caseload practice with conventional team midwifery care: labour and birth outcomes. Midwifery 17:234–240

Campbell R, Macfarlane A 1994 Where to be born? The debate and the evidence (2nd edn). National Perinatal Epidemiology Unit, Oxford

Chamberlain G, Wraight A, Crowley P 1997 Home births: the report of the 1994 confidential enquiry by the National Birthday Trust Fund. Parthenon, Carnforth

Crotty M, Ramsay A, Smart R et al 1990 Planned homebirths in South Australia 1976–1987. Medical Journal of Australia 153:664–671

Davies J, Hey E, Reid W et al 1996 Prospective regional study of planned home births. Home Birth Study Steering Group. British Medical Journal 313:1302–1306

Davis-Floyd R 2001 The technocratic, humanistic and holistic paradigms of childbirth. International Journal of Gynaecology and Obstetrics 75: S5–S23

Donnison J 1977 Midwives and medical men. Heinemann, London

Downe S, McCormick C, Beech B 2001 Labour interventions associated with normal birth. British Journal of Midwifery 9(10):602–606

Downe S, McCourt C 2004 From being to becoming: reconstructing childbirth knowledges. In: S Downe (Ed) Normal childbirth: evidence and debate. Churchill Livingstone, Edinburgh

Enkin M, Keirse M, Neilson J et al 2000 A guide to effective care in pregnancy and childbirth (3rd edn). Oxford University Press, Oxford

Grady M, Bloom K 2004 Pregnancy outcomes of adolescents enrolled in a CenteringPregnancy program. Journal of Midwifery and Women's Health 49(5):412–420

Green JM, Curtis P, Price H et al 1998 Continuing to care. The organisation of midwifery services in the UK: a structured review of the evidence. Books for Midwives, Hale

Gulbransen G, Hilton J, McKay L 1997 Home birth in New Zealand 1973–1993: incidence and mortality. New Zealand Medical Journal 110:87–89

Halldorsdottir S, Karlsdottir SI 1996 Journeying through labour and delivery: perceptions of women who have given birth. Midwifery 12(2):48–61

Hodnett ED 2002 Pain and women's satisfaction with the experience of childbirth: a systematic review. American Journal of Obstetrics and Gynaecology 186(5): S160–S172

Hodnett ED 2004 Continuity of care givers during pregnancy and childbirth. Cochrane Review, Oxford

House of Commons 2003 House of Commons Select Committee on Maternity Services. HMSO, London

Ickovics JR, Kershaw TS, Westdahl C et al 2003 Group prenatal care and preterm birthweight: results from a two-site matched cohort study. Obstetrics and Gynecology 102:1051–1057

Katz-Rothman B 1996 Women, providers and control. Journal of Obstetrics, Gynaecology and Neonatal Nursing 25(3):253–256

Kemp J 2003 Midwives', women's and their birth partners' experiences of the 36 week birth talk: a qualitative study. Unpublished thesis. Florence Nightingale School of Nursing and Midwifery, Kings College London

Kirkham M 1986 A feminist perspective in midwifery. In: C Webb (Ed) Feminist practice in women's health. John Wiley & Sons, Chichester, pp 35–49

Kitzinger S 2000 Rediscovering birth. Little Brown, Boston

Klima C 2003 CenteringPregnancy: a model for pregnant adolescents. Journal of Midwifery and Women's Health 48(3):220–225

Leap N 1991 Helping you to make your own decisions—antenatal and postnatal groups in Deptford SE London. VHS video. Available from Birth International, www.birthinternational.com.au

Leap N 2000 The less we do, the more we give. In: M Kirkham (Ed) The midwife/mother relationship. Palgrave Macmillan, Hants

Leap N 2002 Identifying the midwifery practice component of Australian midwifery education programs: results of the Australian Midwifery Action Project (AMAP). Australian Journal of Midwifery 15(3):15–23

Leap N 2004 Journey to midwifery through feminism: a personal account. In: M Stewart (Ed) Pregnancy, birth and maternity care: feminist perspectives. Books for Midwives, London, pp 185–200

Leap N, Anderson T 2004 The role of pain and the empowerment of women. In: S Downe (Ed) Normal childbirth: evidence and debate. Churchill Livingstone, Edinburgh

Leap N, Hunter B 1993 The midwife's tale: an oral history from handywoman to professional midwife. Scarlet Press, Gateshead UK

Lee G 1997 The concept of 'continuity'—what does it mean? In: MJ Kirkham, ER Perkins (Eds) Reflections on midwifery. Baillière-Tindall, London, pp 1–25

Lundgren I, Dahlberg K 1998 Women's experience of pain during childbirth. Midwifery 14(2):105–110

Marland H (Ed) 1987 'Mother and child were saved': the memoirs (1693–1740) of the Frisian midwife Catharina Schrader. Rodopi, Amsterdam

Murphy P, Fullerton J 1998 Outcomes of intended home births in nurse–midwifery practice: a prospective descriptive study. Obstetrics and Gynecology 92:461–470

Nixon A, Byrne J, Church A 2003 The Community Midwives Project: an evaluation of the set-up of Northern Women's Community Midwives Project. June 1998–November 2000. Auspiced by Northern Metropolitan Community Health Services, South Australia. Northern Metropolitan Community Health Service, Adelaide, South Australia

Oakley A, Hickey D, Rajan L et al 1996 Social support in pregnancy: does it have long term effects? Journal of Reproductive Health and Infant Psychology 14:7–22

Oakley A, Rajan L, Grant A. 1990 Social support and pregnancy outcome. British Journal of Obstetrics and Gynaecology 97:155–162

Odent M 1992 The Nature of birth and breastfeeding. Bergin & Garvey, Westport CT

Olsen O 1997 Meta-analysis of the safety of homebirth. Birth 24:4–13

Olsen O, Jewell MD 1998 Home birth versus hospital birth. Cochrane Review. Cochrane Library (3). John Wiley & Sons, Chichester

Ontario Women's Health Council 2002 Attaining and maintaining best practices in the use of Caesarean sections. An analysis of four Ontario hospitals. Report of the Caesarean Section Working Group of the Women's Health Council. Online: www.womenshealth–council.com

Page L, Beake S, Vail A et al 2001 Clinical outcomes of one-to-one practice. British Journal of Medicine 9:700–706

Powell Kennedy H 2004 Orchestrating normal: the art and conduct of midwifery practice. Paper presented at the Second International Conference on Normal Labour and Birth, Grange-over-Sands

Reed B 2002a The Albany Midwifery Practice (1). MIDIRS Midwifery Digest 12(1):118–121

Reed B 2002b The Albany Midwifery Practice (2). MIDIRS Midwifery Digest 12(3):261–264

Sandall J 2004 Promoting normal birth: weighing the evidence. In: S Downe (Ed) Normal childbirth: evidence and debate. Churchill Livingstone, Edinburgh

Sandall J, Davies J, Warwick C 2001 Evaluation of the Albany Midwifery Practice: final report. Nightingale School of Midwifery, Kings College London

Schindler Rising S 1998 CenteringPregnancy: an interdisciplinary model of empowerment. Journal of Nurse-Midwifery 43(1):46–54

Simkin P, Ancheta R 2000 The labour progress handbook: early interventions to prevent and treat dystocia. Blackwell Science, Oxford

Thiele B, Thorogood C 1997 Community based midwifery program in Fremantle WA. Centre for Research for Women, Fremantle, WA

Thompson F 2004 Mothers and midwives: the ethical journey. Books for Midwives, Edinburgh

Thorogood C, Thiele B, Hyde K 2002 Second evaluation of the Community Midwifery Program. Centre for Research for Women, Fremantle, WA

Tyson H 1991 Outcomes of 1001 midwife-attended home births in Toronto 1983–1988. Birth 18:14–19

Wiegers T, Keirse M, van der Zee J 1996 Outcome of planned home and hospital births in low risk pregnancies: prospective study in midwifery practice in the Netherlands. British Medical Journal 131: 1309–1313

Wilson A 1995 The making of man—midwifery. Harvard University Press, Cambridge, Mass.

Witz A 1992 Professions and patriarchy. Routledge, London

Woodcock H, Read A, Moore D et al 1990 Planned homebirths in Western Australia 1981–1987: a descriptive study. Medical Journal of Australia 153:672–678

World Health Organization (WHO) 1996 Care in normal birth: a practical guide. Maternal and Newborn Health/Safe Motherhood Unit, Family and Reproductive Health, WHO, Geneva

Zadoroznyj M 2000 Midwife-led maternity services and consumer 'choice' in an Australian metropolitan region. Midwifery 17:177–185

Further reading

Downe S (Ed) 2004 Normal childbirth: evidence and debate. Churchill Livingstone, Edinburgh

Robertson A 2004 The midwife companion: the art of support during birth (2nd edn). Birth International, Sydney

Simkin P, Ancheta R 2000 The labour progress handbook: early interventions to prevent and treat dystocia. Blackwell Science, Oxford

CHAPTER 18

The physiology of conception and pregnancy

Sally Baddock

Key terms

acrosomal reaction, adrenergic, amnion, amniotic fluid, bilaminar disc, blastocyst, blastomere, capacitation, cervical mucus, chorion, chorionic villi, chromosomes, cleavage, conception, corticosteroid, cytotrophoblast, decidua, differentiation, ductus arteriosus, ductus venosus, ectoderm, embryo, embryology, endoderm, endometrium, erythropoiesis, fallopian tube, fertilisation, fetal placental circulation, fetus, foramen ovale, gastrulation, glomerular filtration, gonadotrophins, haemodilution, human chorionic gonadotrophin, human placental lactogen, hypercoagulability, hyperventilation, hypothalamic-pituitary axis, implantation, induction, inner cell mass, intervillous spaces, lung compliance, mesoderm, morula, negative feedback, neural tube, neurulation, notochord, oestrogens, oocyte, oogenesis, organogenesis, ovaries, ovulation, oxygen saturation, placenta, progesterone, renin-angiotensin, semen, signalling proteins, sperm, spermatogenesis, surfactant, synctiotrophoblast, syngamy, teratogen, trilaminar disc, trophoblast, umbilical arteries, umbilical vein, uteroplacental circulation, uterotonic agonists, uterotonic antagonists, uterus, yolk sac, zona pellucida, zygote

Chapter overview

This chapter focuses on the physiological processes associated with conception and pregnancy. This begins with the formation of the gametes in the female and male reproductive systems, and continues with an overview of embryology from fertilisation until birth. It includes the simultaneous development of the placenta to support the embryo, and the changes of pregnancy occurring in the woman. A good understanding of these physiological processes is essential if a midwife is to make informed decisions with regard to monitoring of the woman and fetus and with regard to interpretation of test results. It also enables informed discussion with the woman regarding the changes occurring to her body as the fetus develops, and an understanding of the factors that contribute to a healthy environment for normal embryological and fetal development.

For ease of study, the development of the embryo and placenta, and the changes in the woman through pregnancy, are presented as separate topics, but the processes are interwoven and simultaneous. The scope of this chapter is limited, but further readings are provided at the end of the chapter for a more in-depth exploration of specific topics. Some of the online resources listed provide animations that can help with the understanding of complex anatomical changes.

Learning outcomes

Learning outcomes for this chapter are:

1 To list key events in the continuum of development from gametogenesis to the development of a mature fetus

2 To describe the physiological changes that occur in the reproductive system and other body systems of the woman during pregnancy

3 To discuss the role of hormones in the reproductive process and in the maintenance of pregnancy.

Female and male reproductive systems

The physiological roles of the female and male reproductive systems are to produce and maintain sex cells (gametes), to transport the gametes to the site of fertilisation, and to produce and secrete sex hormones, which control the reproductive process. The female reproductive system has the additional role of supporting the developing fetus. The structures of the female and male reproductive systems underpin these roles.

Anatomy of the female reproductive system

The female reproductive system consists of a pair of female gonads, commonly referred to as the ovaries, as well as a number of accessory ducts, specifically the uterine or fallopian tubes, the uterus and the vagina. The ovaries and the accessory ducts make up the internal female genitalia. The external female genitalia are referred to as the vulva and consist of the mons pubis, labia majora, labia minor, clitoris and vestibule. The mammary glands of the female are also important in the reproductive system following reproduction.

Female internal genitalia

The structures of the female internal genitalia are depicted in Figure 18.1.

The ovaries have two important roles in the reproductive system: to produce female sex cells (oocytes) through the process of oogenesis; and to produce the female sex hormones—the oestrogens (oestradiol, oestrone and oestriol) and progesterone.

The uterine tubes link the ovaries and the uterus, although there is no anatomical connection. The distal ends of the uterine tubes end in fimbriae, which waft the ovulated ovum towards the opening of the tube. Contractions of smooth muscle in the walls of the uterine tubes and the wafting action of cilia lining the walls aid oocyte movement (fertilised or not) to the uterus.

The uterus is a hollow cavity consisting of three regions: the fundus, the body and the cervix. The fundus is the region superior to the uterine tubes. The body is the major portion of the uterus and is the site where implantation occurs. The cervix is the region that connects the uterus with the vagina and consists of the cervical canal, the internal os and external os. The uterus is a thick-walled organ with three layers: the

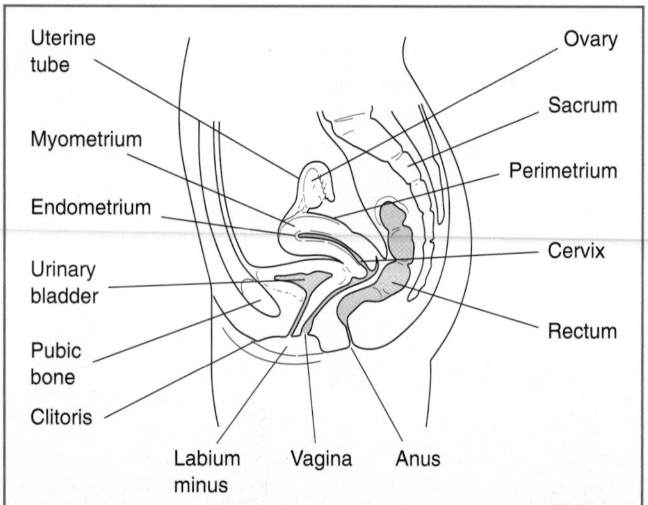

Figure 18.1 Schematic sagittal section of the female pelvic region (based on Moore & Persaud 1998)

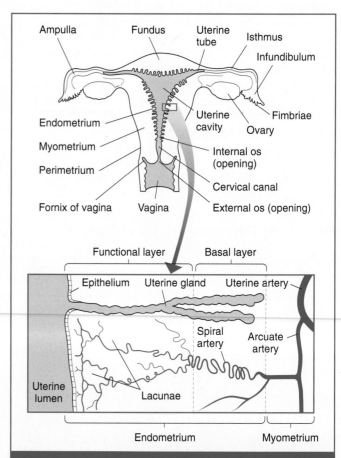

Figure 18.2 Female reproductive organs (based on Moore & Persaud 1998)

perimetrium (outer layer), the myometrium (thick muscle layer) and the endometrium (the inner mucosal lining). The endometrium consists of two layers: the stratum basalis, which lies next to the myometrium, and the stratum functionalis, the outer mucosa that is shed during menstruation (Fig 18.2).

The vagina is often referred to as the 'birth canal' and is the region of the internal female genitalia that connects to the external female genitalia. The vagina is a passage for semen during intercourse and for menstrual blood during menstruation. The epithelial cells that line the vagina produce glycogen, which is metabolised to lactic acid by the vaginal microflora. This results in the vagina having an acidic pH, which protects against foreign microorganisms as well as destroying many sperm cells that enter the vagina.

External female genitalia

The external female genitalia are referred to as the vulva and consist of the mons pubis, labia majora, labia minora, clitoris and vestibule (Fig 18.3).

Mammary glands

The mammary glands or breasts are also present in the male but produce milk only in the female. The breasts are a type of sweat gland (sudiferous gland) positioned over the pectoralis major and serratus anterior muscles and attached by connective tissue. Suspensory ligaments support the breasts and are present between the skin and the deep fascia of the muscle. The areola is the region surrounding the nipple and contains modified sebaceous (oil) glands, which help to keep the tissue supple. Each breast is made up of 15–20 lobes separated by adipose tissue. The amount of adipose tissue determines the size of the breast. The lobes consists of lobules, which are milk-secreting glands commonly referred to as alveoli. The milk is produced in the alveoli and passes into the duct system. Small ducts from each lobule drain into a lactiferous duct that opens onto the nipple surface. The two hormones important in lactation are prolactin and oxytocin. Prolactin is important for milk production and oxytocin is important in the let-down or milk release reflex.

Anatomy of the male reproductive system

The structures of the male reproductive system (Fig 18.4) include the testes, penis, accessory ducts (epididymis, vas deferens (ductus deferens), ejaculatory ducts and urethra) and the accessory glands (prostate, seminal vesicles and bulbourethral glands).

The paired testes each contain coiled seminiferous tubules, which are the site of sperm production. The sperm are moved from the seminiferous tubules to the coils of the epididymis by peristalsis. Secretions from the Sertoli cells, adjacent to the seminiferous tubules, build up pressure and contribute to the movement of sperm (Fig 18.5).

In the epididymis, sperm mature and become motile after approximately 14–21 days. During ejaculation, peristaltic contractions move spermatozoa from the epididymis to the vas deferens, through the ejaculatory duct and into the urethra. The urethra runs from the urinary bladder to the outside of the body, with part of the urethra (spongy urethra) running through the penis. The urethra has the dual role of transporting urine and sperm to exit the body.

During sexual excitement, the three columns of erectile tissue surrounding the urethra become engorged with blood, resulting in erection. This enables the penis to enter the vagina during sexual intercourse. Further stimulation leads to ejaculation of semen (sperm and secretions).

Accessory sex glands and semen

Semen is the alkaline fluid that protects, nourishes and transports sperm during ejaculation. Two to five millitres is ejaculated during orgasm, containing 50–100 million sperm/mL.

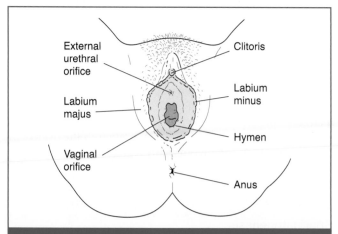

Figure 18.3 External female genitalia. The labia are spread apart to show the external urethral and vaginal orifices (based on Moore & Persaud 1998).

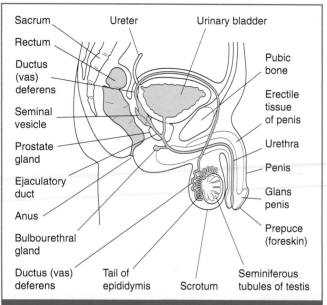

Figure 18.4 Schematic sagittal section of the male pelvic region (based on Moore & Persaud 1998)

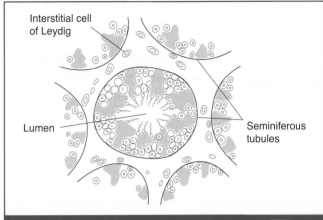

Figure 18.5 The testis in cross-section, illustrating the seminiferous tubules and interstitial cells of Leydig (based on Bray et al 1994)

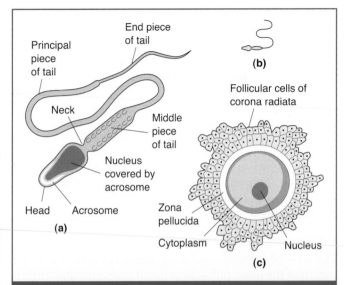

Figure 18.6 Male and female gametes. **(a)** Parts of the human sperm (X 1250). The head, composed mostly of the nucleus, is partly covered by the acrosome, an organelle containing enzymes. The tail consists of three regions: middle piece, principal piece and end piece. **(b)** Sperm drawn to about the same scale as the oocyte. **(c)** Human secondary oocyte or ovum (X 200) surrounded by the zona pellucida and corona radiata (based on Moore & Persaud 1998)

At least 20 million sperm/mL are necessary for fertility. However, 90% of the fluid is made up of secretions from the seminal vesicles, prostate gland and bulbourethral glands.

Seminal vesicles release alkaline secretions into the ejaculatory duct that contain several chemicals, including fibrinogen, fructose and prostaglandins. Fibrinogen helps to coagulate semen just after ejaculation and this contributes to retention of semen in the region of the uterine cervix, until the sperm become motile. Fructose nourishes the sperm, and prostaglandins aid fertilisation by making the cervical mucus more receptive. Prostaglandins also stimulate uterine contractions, which suck semen into the uterus and fallopian tubes, enabling them to reach the ampulla as soon as five minutes after ejaculation, or up to six hours later. These secretions also dilute epididymal inhibitory factor, which is thought to suppress the motility of spermatozoa.

The prostate gland produces an acidic, milky fluid containing citric acid and clotting enzymes that aid coagulation, and this is emptied into the urethra. Bulbourethral (Cowper's) glands produce alkaline fluid that neutralises the acidic urethra along with mucus that lubricates the urethra and protects spermatozoa. Secretions travel through the ducts into the spongy urethra.

Gametogenesis

Fertilisation involves the union of two gametes—an oocyte from the female and a sperm from the male. Gametes are highly specialised sex cells (Fig 18.6). Gametogenesis (formation of the sex cells) necessarily involves halving the number of chromosomes in each cell, by a type of cell division called meiosis, and by altering the shape of the cells. In females this process is termed oogenesis and in males it is spermatogenesis. When the two gametes join at fertilisation, the full number of chromosomes is restored.

Oogenesis

Oogenesis is the process by which mature female sex cells are formed. Much of this process occurs in the fetus prior to birth. Oogonia in the fetus multiply by mitotic division and develop into primary oocytes (containing 46 chromosomes). The first meiotic division also begins before birth, but is arrested until after puberty. Completion of the first meiotic division is linked to the ovarian cycle. Each month, following puberty, several primary oocytes begin to develop but only one matures to complete the first meiotic division 36–48 hours before ovulation (Blackburn 2003). This division results in a large secondary oocyte containing most of the cytoplasm, and a smaller non-functional polar body that soon degenerates. Each has 23 chromosomes (22 autosomes and 1 sex chromosome). At ovulation the secondary oocyte begins the second meiotic division, but the division is only completed if fertilisation occurs. Once again, almost all the cytoplasm goes to one cell, the mature oocyte. The second polar body is non-functional and degenerates. The cellular divisions of oogenesis are outlined in Figure 18.7. The mature oocyte is a large, immotile cell, just visible to the naked eye. Up to two million primary oocytes are usually present in the ovaries of a newborn female infant, but many regress during childhood, leaving about 40,000 at puberty. During the reproductive life of a female, about 400 oocytes mature and are released during ovulation.

Spermatogenesis

Spermatogenesis describes the development of spermatogonia (primitive germ cells) into spermatozoa. This process begins at puberty and continues into old age. At puberty, the

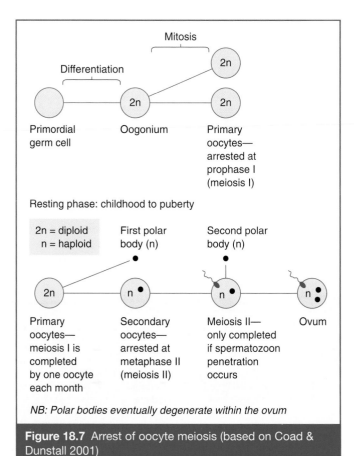

Figure 18.7 Arrest of oocyte meiosis (based on Coad & Dunstall 2001)

spermatogonia increase in number by mitotic division and grow and change to form primary spermatocytes ($2n$ chromosomes). Each primary spermatocyte undergoes the first meiotic division to form two secondary spermatocytes (n chromosomes) and the second meiotic division to result in four spermatids (n chromosomes). Spermatids undergo a considerable change in shape, in a process termed spermiogenesis, to become mature spermatozoa (sperm). The mature sperm has relatively little cytoplasm. It is divided into a head, midpiece and tail, and is motile. The head forms most of the bulk, contains the nucleus with the chromosomes and is covered anteriorly by the acrosome, a structure containing enzymes that facilitate penetration of the ovum at fertilisation. The midpiece is rich in energy-producing mitochondria, which fuel the lashing movements of the tail. Spermatogenesis takes about two months to complete and continues throughout the reproductive life of a male (Moore & Persaud 1998). The sperm move to the epididymis, where they are stored and become functionally mature. A comparison of oogenesis and spermatogenesis is shown in Figure 18.8.

Female reproductive cycles

Females undergo monthly reproductive cycles starting at puberty and continuing through the reproductive years. These cycles are controlled by the hypothalamic-pituitary-ovarian

hormones and result in changes in the ovary that lead to release of one secondary oocyte per month, and changes in the uterus in preparation for implantation of the fertilised ovum. If fertilisation does not occur, the cycle begins again under the influence of the hypothalamic-pituitary hormones. For simplicity, the reproductive cycle is described as an average 28-day cycle. There is considerable individual variation but the cycle length of most women is between 21 and 35 days (Blackburn 2003).

Ovarian cycle

The ovarian cycle (Fig 18.9) includes three phases: the follicular or pre-ovulatory phase, the ovulatory phase or ovulation, and the post-ovulatory or luteal phase.

Follicular phase

In the follicular phase, the ovarian follicles, containing an oocyte, mature. Ovarian follicles are found in the cortex of the ovary and contain a variety of cells, including primary or secondary oocytes, granulosa cells and theca cells. Oocytes are surrounded by a thick membrane, the zona pelucida, and in mature follicles there is a large fluid-filled cavity, the antrum.

Follicles are present in several forms: primordial (the most undeveloped), primary, secondary and Graafian or vesicular follicles (the most mature).

Primordial follicles contain primary oocytes and are the type of follicle present at birth. The first meiotic division has already begun in utero, but the process is arrested partway and does not continue again until puberty, when levels of gonadotrophin-releasing hormone (GnRH), luteinising (LH) and follicle-stimulating hormone (FSH) increase.

The primary follicle is formed in response to the increased level of the hormones mentioned above. The hormones signal the cells surrounding the oocyte to proliferate and form a layer of granulosa cells. These cells allow nutrients and signalling molecules to reach the oocyte.

The secondary follicle is formed when a layer of connective tissue, called the theca folliculi, develops around the follicle and an antrum begins to develop with it. The thecal cells, together with the granulosa cells, produce steroid hormones (mainly oestrogens with small quantities of progesterone). The secondary follicle is also characterised by the zona pellucida, which surrounds the oocyte and is released along with the oocyte at ovulation.

Graafian or vesicular follicles are the final and most mature form of ovarian follicle. This stage of follicular development is characterised by a large antrum and a follicular size of approximately 2.5 cm diameter. Due to its size it bulges from the ovary midway through the ovarian cycle. The completion of meiosis I, in which a secondary oocyte and the first polar body are formed, occurs 36–48 hours before ovulation (Blackburn 2003). Meiosis II continues but is not completed until fertilisation occurs. The process of meiosis results in the total number of genetic material being halved from 46 chromosomes ($2n$) to 23 chromosomes (n).

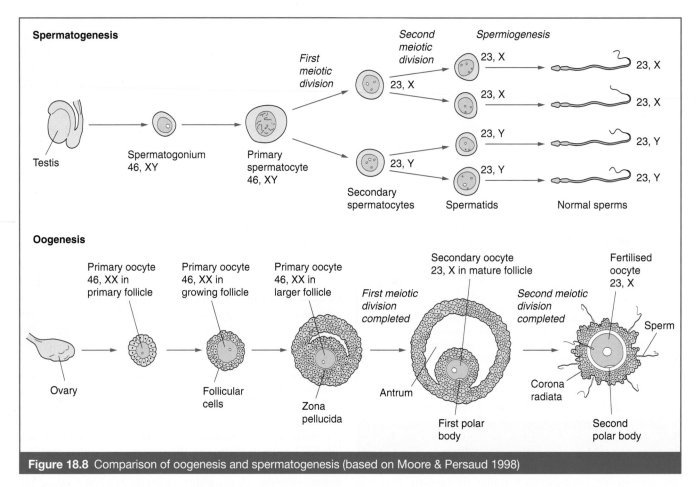

Figure 18.8 Comparison of oogenesis and spermatogenesis (based on Moore & Persaud 1998)

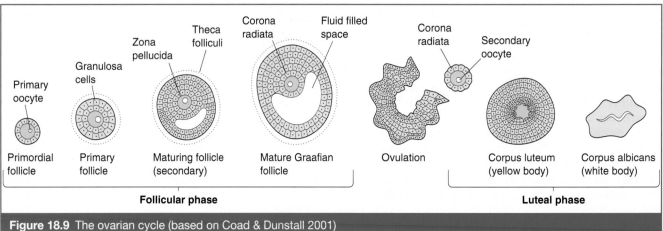

Figure 18.9 The ovarian cycle (based on Coad & Dunstall 2001)

Ovulation

The ovulatory phase begins when oestrogen levels peak and ends when the vesicular follicle ruptures, releasing the secondary oocyte surrounded by the zona pellucida and corona radiata (the crown of granulosa cells around the zona pellucida). Ovulation is under hormonal control, as follows: LH interacts with LH receptors on the granulosa cells, increasing the production of oestrogen by the dominant follicle. The rise in oestrogen levels 12–24 hours before ovulation triggers the LH surge. The high level of LH stimulates production of prostaglandins ($PGF_{2\alpha}$ and PGE_2) and allows the primary oocyte to complete the first meiotic division and become a secondary oocyte. Simultaneously, levels of oestrogen drop and proteolytic enzymes are synthesised, which break down the thecal cells and assist rupture of the vesicular follicle (Blackburn 2003).

Luteal phase

This is the final stage of the ovarian cycle. The ruptured follicle remains in the ovary and the antrum begins to fill with clotted blood. The granulosa and some thecal cells form a structure called the corpus luteum. This is an endocrine structure capable of producing progesterone and smaller amounts of oestrogen. The purpose of the corpus luteum is to provide progesterone until the placenta is adequately formed. If fertilisation does not occur, the corpus luteum degenerates into a corpus albicans and is degraded through lysosomal activity.

Uterine cycle

The uterine cycle occurs in the same timeframe as the ovarian cycle and is similarly controlled by changes to hormonal levels (Fig 18.10). It consists of three stages: the menstrual phase (days 1–5), the proliferative phase (days 6–14) and the secretory phase (days 15–28). The following is a review of each stage.

Menstrual phase

Menstruation is triggered by several factors. The first is the drop in levels of progesterone and oestradiol (one form of oestrogen). The second factor is a change in the ratio of prostaglandins and prostacyclins (hormone-like compounds) that cause vasoconstriction and increased coiling of the spiral arterioles, leading to a decrease in blood flow to the stratum functionalis of the uterus. The cells in the stratum functionalis become ischaemic, necrosed and slough away from the stratum basalis. The straight arterioles dilate, contributing to menstrual flow (Blackburn 2003).

Proliferative phase

In the proliferative phase, the stratum functionalis of the endometrium begins to thicken as endometrial cells proliferate. Arterioles regenerate and endometrial glands develop. These changes occur in response to oestradiol and progesterone. The mucus produced by the cervix also responds to these hormones. The consistency becomes less viscous and less stretchy, showing little or no ferning (spinnbarkeit test), thus becoming more receptive to sperm. Variation in the length of the proliferative phase accounts for most of the variation in uterine cycles (Blackburn 2003).

Secretory phase

The secretory phase occurs following ovulation, when levels of progesterone are high. The influence of progesterone results in further thickening of the stratum functionalis, an increase in the number of blood vessels as well as increased coiling and dilation of blood vessels. Finally, the endometrial glands begin secreting glycogen.

Hypothalamic-pituitary-ovarian (HPO) axis

The female reproductive system is regulated by a variety of hormones produced by the brain (the hypothalamus and the pituitary gland) and the ovaries (Fig 18.11).

Hypothalamus

The hypothalamus produces a peptide hormone called gonadotrophin-releasing hormone (GnRH) within its neurons. This hormone stimulates the release of several hormones from the anterior pituitary gland, specifically FSH and LH.

Pituitary gland

The anterior pituitary gland produces and secretes many hormones, including FSH, LH and prolactin. Luteinising hormone and FSH are glycoproteins that enhance each other's actions (act synergistically) in regulating the ovarian cycle.

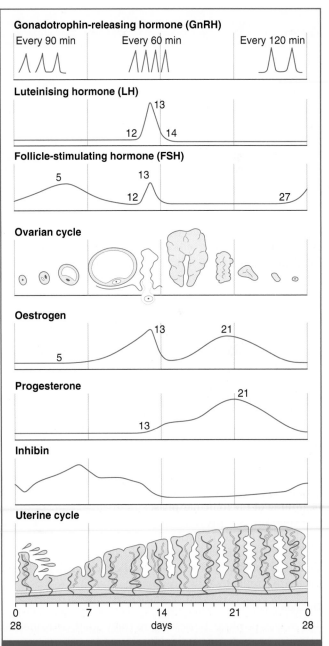

Figure 18.10 Uterine cycle and hormone levels (based on Coad & Dunstall 2001)

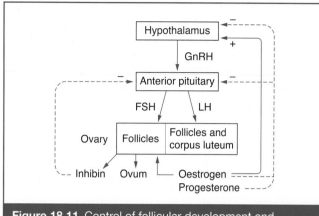

Figure 18.11 Control of follicular development and oestrogen secretion (based on Bray et al 1994)

FSH, along with oestrogen produced by the ovaries, acts on granulosa cells of the follicles to stimulate growth and produce FSH and LH receptors. Luteinising hormone receptors combine with LH during the LH surge to inhibit the growth of granulosa cells and initiate production of progesterone from the follicle. The granulosa cells of a primordial follicle undergo limited growth without FSH. Secretion of FSH peaks mid-cycle at a lower level than the LH surge (Blackburn 2003).

LH acts on thecal cells, instigating the production of androgens that are converted to oestrogens by the granulosa cells. This increases the oestrogen level and inhibits the development of other follicles by inhibiting FSH (negative feedback). At the same time, one follicle becomes dominant and secretes high levels of oestradiol, allowing granulosa cell development in that follicle. As levels of oestradiol increase, the release of GnRH is triggered by positive feedback, allowing increased levels of LH and FSH to complete the maturation of follicles, and an LH surge triggers ovulation within 12–24 hours. Following ovulation, increasing levels of oestrogen and progesterone exert a powerful negative feedback effect, inhibiting the release of GnRH and subsequently LH and FSH. This negative feedback prevents further maturation of follicles—important if the oocyte released at ovulation was successfully fertilised. However, in most cycles, fertilisation does not occur and the corpus luteum degenerates into the corpus albicans, resulting in a decreased level of progesterone. The low progesterone levels cease to inhibit GnRH, which begins to rise, followed by an increase in LH and FSH and the beginning of the follicular phase.

Prolactin is a protein hormone that stimulates milk production. Levels of prolactin rise during pregnancy, but hPL (human placental lactogen) and progesterone prevent the binding of prolactin to receptors in the breast. After delivery, prolactin stimulates milk production.

Ovaries

The ovaries produce the oestrogens (oestradiol, oestrone and oestriol), progesterone and inhibin.

Oestrogens are produced in the ovaries by granulosa cells within the follicles and the corpus luteum. The most abundant oestrogen during a woman's reproductive years is oestradiol, which is responsible for most of the effects of oestrogen in the female reproductive system. However, during pregnancy, oestriol becomes the main oestrogen secreted (Blackburn 2003). The stimulus for oestrogen release is primarily FSH and, to a lesser extent, LH. Oestrogens are responsible for various functions, including:

- development and maintenance of the female reproductive structures such as the endometrial lining of the uterus, and secondary sexual characteristics such as fat content of the breasts, abdomen, mons pubis and hips, voice pitch, broadness of the pelvis, distribution of underarm and pubic hair, and the development of breasts
- fluid and electrolyte balance—by influencing the action of aldosterone, sodium reabsorption in the renal tubules is stimulated and diuresis is reduced
- increasing the rate at which amino acids enter cells, thereby altering protein metabolism, allowing cells to grow and multiply. This action is supported by the influence of growth hormone.
- regulation of oxytocin and adrenergic receptors (Henderson & Macdonald 2004).
- stimulation of uterine tube contractility to assist sperm motility and to retain the ovum (Blackburn 2003).

Progesterone is produced in the ovaries by granulosa cells, primarily of the corpus luteum. Therefore progesterone levels peak in the post-ovulatory phase when the corpus luteum is active, and fall if pregnancy does not occur and the corpus luteum degenerates. LH is the stimulus for progesterone release. Progesterone has various functions, including:

- preparation of the endometrium of the uterus to receive a fertilised ovum
- prevention of sperm entry into the uterus by promoting changes in the cervical mucus
- increasing basal body temperature by influencing the thermostat located in the hypothalamus
- relaxation of the muscle of the uterine tubes during the luteal phase to assist passage of the fertilised ovum to the uterus (Blackburn 2003).

Inhibin is produced in the ovaries by granulosa cells of the follicles and corpus luteum. It exerts negative feedback controls on FSH release during the growth of the dominant follicle and the corpus luteum.

Clinical point

1   Body temperature rises after ovulation, in response to progesterone, and is used in natural family planning to indicate the fertile phases of the reproductive cycle.
2   Hormonal contraceptives contain levels of oestrogen and/or progesterone that cause feedback control on the HPO axis to prevent follicle development and ovulation. Some contraceptives use the cervical mucus-changing properties of progesterone (e.g. the minipill).

Summary: homeostatic control of the reproductive cycle

While the follicular phase of the cycle is characterised by the positive feedback of oestrogen prompting an LH surge, the luteal phase is characterised by negative feedback. GnRH, LH and FSH production is controlled by negative feedback mechanisms linked to the ovarian hormones in the HPO axis (oestrogens, progesterone and inhibin). If the secondary oocyte is not fertilised, the ovum dies in 24 hours and the corpus luteum deteriorates. The levels of oestrogens and progesterone therefore drop, triggering the production of GnRH, LH and FSH, which begins the reproductive cycle (ovarian and uterine cycles) again. If fertilisation and implantation occur (pregnancy), levels of oestrogen and progesterone remain elevated because the blastocyst secretes the hormone human chorionic gonadotrophin (hCG) that maintains the corpus luteum and hormone production. The placenta takes over producing oestradiol and progesterone by 6–10 weeks gestation.

Hypothalamic-pituitary-testicular (HPT) control in the male

Hypothalamic-pituitary-testicular (HPT) control in the male is not cyclical, like the HPO control in the female. The HPT axis regulates physiological changes in the testes from puberty onward. GnRH is secreted by the hypothalamus every 70–90 minutes, which triggers the anterior pituitary to secrete LH and FSH.

LH directly stimulates both the production of testosterone from cholesterol, and the process of spermatogenesis, while FSH primarily facilitates spermatogenesis.

Testosterone is produced by the Leydig (interstitial) cells in the seminiferous tubules (Fig 18.5) and diffuses across the basal membrane to directly influence the spermatogonia and Sertoli cells. Testosterone levels are maintained by negative feedback to the hypothalamus and anterior pituitary, via the HPT axis.

Summary points

- The structures of the female and male reproductive systems are designed to produce and transport gametes: ova and sperm.
- Gametogenesis involves cell divisions that halve the chromosome number: oogenesis produces ova in the ovaries, and spermatogenesis produces sperm in the testes.
- Following puberty, a single oocyte is released from the ovary each month under the control of the hormones of the HPO axis.
- Ovarian hormones stimulate monthly vascular and glandular development of the uterus in preparation for pregnancy.
- Hormones of the HPT axis stimulate sperm production from puberty onwards.
- Sperm are produced in the seminiferous tubules and stored in the epididymis until ejaculation.

- Semen released at ejaculation includes about 200 million sperm and 2–5 mL of secretions from the accessory glands to aid nourishment and support of the sperm.

Embryology

Embryology is described as 'the science concerned with the origin and development of a human being from a zygote to the birth of an infant' (Moore & Persaud 1998, p 2). Moore and Persaud (1998) emphasise that development is a continuum that starts at fertilisation, includes birth—a dramatic event resulting in a change in environment—and continues after birth, with development of teeth, bones, reproductive structures and so on. The process finishes by about the age of 25 years.

This section is limited to antenatal development, which begins with conception. Conception refers to fertilisation that results in pregnancy (Blackburn 2003). The probability of a viable conception has been calculated at only 30% per menstrual cycle (Blackburn 2003), with spontaneous abortions resulting from a range of abnormalities. The processes needed to produce a viable oocyte and a viable sperm have been described earlier in this chapter. This section examines fertilisation and the factors that contribute to successful fertilisation, implantation, development of the embryo and fetus, and development of the placenta.

Fertilisation

Fertilisation normally occurs in the ampulla of the fallopian tube. The beginning of fertilisation occurs when the sperm passes through the zona pellucida and makes contact with the secondary oocyte. This is most likely to occur if sperm enter the vagina just prior to ovulation or when a woman is ovulating, because sperm must undergo capacitation and the acrosomal reaction prior to fertilisation, and these processes require several hours.

Sperm transport

During sexual intercourse, 200–600 million sperm are released into the vagina in about 3 mL of semen. Chemicals present in the semen cause coagulation of the sperm (see accessory ducts above). This may help retain sperm in the vagina and protect against the acidic environment of the vagina. The coagulum is then dissolved in 20–60 minutes by activation of a further enzyme (fibrinolysis) in the semen. The alkaline pH of the semen facilitates sperm motility. Within a minute of sperm deposition, sperm can be detected in the cervix and uterus. However, most sperm are lost through vaginal leakage and never enter the cervix. Those that do survive, may survive in the cervix for hours and be nourished by the cervical mucus. Further progress towards the uterus is dependent on the consistency of the mucus, which is determined by oestrogen and progesterone (see female hormones above). Sperm most likely move both by their own propulsion, and by the action of uterine cilia causing semen to flow through the uterus to the fallopian tubes (Johnson & Everitt 2000).

Capacitation and acrosomal reaction

Capacitation is stimulated by secretions in the oestrogen-dominated uterus and fallopian tubes. As the sperm move through the fallopian tubes, glycoproteins and seminal plasma proteins are removed from the plasma membrane over the acrosome (head of spermatozoa), leading to activation. The capacitated sperm contacts the corona radiata around the secondary oocyte. Enzymes are released from the acrosome (acrosome reaction) and are able to digest a tunnel through the corona radiata and zona pellucida. Tail movements change to wide-amplitude or 'whiplashing' beats that push the sperm forward in vigorous lurches.

Sperm need 4–10 hours in the female reproductive tract before they can fertilise an ovum. Sperm only remain activated for a short time, but a supply of sperm persists for some time as sperm stored in the folds of the mucosa of the cervix trickle gradually through the capacitating uterus to the fallopian tube, where they become activated. This allows a greater time following intercourse in which activated sperm are available to fertilise the ovum (Johnson & Everitt 2000).

The sperm 'bind' with specific receptors (glycoproteins) on the surface of the zona pellucida. Once the spermatozoon penetrates the zona pellucida, it is in the cytoplasm of the ovum. Several hundred sperm can bind on the zona pellucida but only one sperm can penetrate this layer, due to an event called syngamy. This causes changes in the electrical potential and chemical composition of the zona pellucida, which prevents other sperm from penetrating.

The cell membranes of the oocyte and sperm fuse, and the head and tail of the sperm enters the oocyte, leaving the sperm's plasma membrane behind (Fig 18.12). The oocyte completes the second meiotic division, forming a mature oocyte and a second polar body. The nucleus of the mature ovum becomes a female pronucleus and the polar body disintegrates. Within the oocyte, the nucleus of the sperm enlarges to become the male pronucleus and the tail disintegrates. The two pronuclei are morphologically indistinguishable. The membranes of the pronuclei fuse and a zygote is formed. The zygote has 46 chromosomes: 22 autosomes and 1 sex chromosome from each gamete. The zygote is genetically unique, containing a new combination of chromosomes that is different from either of the parents. Fertilisation is completed within 24 hours of ovulation (Moore & Persaud 1998).

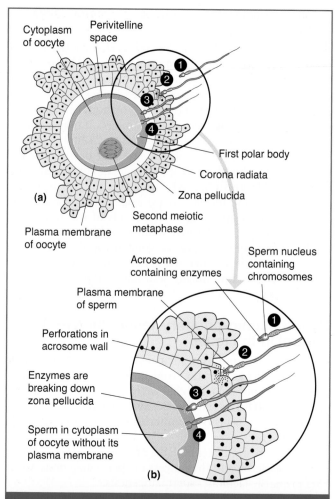

Figure 18.12 Acrosome reaction and sperm penetrating an oocyte. The details of the area outlined in **(a)** are shown in **(b)**. 1 Sperm during capacitation 2 Sperm undergoing the acrosome reaction 3 Sperm digesting a path through the zona pellucida 4 Sperm after entering the cytoplasm of the oocyte (based on Moore & Persaud 1998)

Factors that facilitate fertilisation

The ovum survives for only 12–24 hours after ovulation. Sperm can live up to 72 hours in the female reproductive tract, and require at least 4–6 hours, sometimes 10 hours, in the female reproductive tract to become activated. Sexual intercourse up to 72 hours before and approximately 12 hours after ovulation may result in fertilisation.

Changes in the female reproductive tract mean the female is most receptive to sperm at around the time of ovulation. Increased oestrogen levels at this time have many effects, such as:

- increasing the contractility of the fallopian tube, which assists sperm transport
- decreasing the viscosity of the cervical mucus
- altering the molecular structure of the mucus to form small channels that allow sperm through.

The oocyte secretes a chemical that attracts sperm (Sun et al 2005), and progesterone released after ovulation stimulates the acrosomal reaction (Shah et al 2003). Progesterone also increases the viscosity of the cervical mucus during the luteal phase, preventing further sperm access.

Cleavage and formation of blastomeres

The zygote remains in the ampulla of the fallopian tube for about the first 24 hours and then is swept toward the uterus by ciliary action over the next three to four days (Blackburn 2003). The zygote undergoes repeated mitotic divisions, called cleavage, as it moves towards the uterus. Cleavage increases the number of cells, blastomeres, but not their size, and they are still contained within the zona pellucida. The cytoplasm of the ovum provides the energy and nutrients for the mitotic divisions. The first division into the two-cell stage occurs about 30 hours after fertilisation (Moore & Persaud 1998). Further divisions occur about every 12 to 24 hours. By three days, there are 12 to 15 blastomeres, which now change shape, forming a solid cluster within the zona pellucida, called a morula.

The morula enters the uterine cavity at day 4–5, and as uterine secretions pass through the zona pellucida into the morula, a fluid-filled space, the blastocyst cavity, is formed (Moore & Persaud 1998). As the cavity forms, the surrounding blastomeres separate into two areas:

- the trophoblast—the thin layer of cells around the outside that give rise to the fetal part of the placenta, the chorion
- the inner cell mass—the inner group of blastomeres that give rise to the embryo, yolk sac and amnion.

The conceptus is now called a blastocyst. The blastocyst floats in the uterine cavity for about two days as the zona pellucida disintegrates. This allows more rapid growth of the blastocyst. Uterine secretions containing nutrients, glycogen, mucopolysaccharides and lipids maintain the blastocyst. Approximately six days after fertilisation, the blastocyst attaches to the endometrium and begins to implant (Moore & Persaud 1998). Figure 18.13 summarises the processes of cleavage and implantation during the first week.

Steps of implantation

Implantation of the blastocyst normally occurs in the posterior or anterior wall of the uterine body, with the inner cell mass oriented toward the epithelium of the endometrium. Implantation is essential to maintain nourishment of the blastocyst. The following points detail the steps involved in implantation. This is also illustrated in Figure 18.14.

1　The trophoblast differentiates into two layers: the outer synctiotrophoblast (maternal side of the placenta) and the inner cytotrophoblast (fetal side of the placenta).
2　The cytotrophoblast forms new synctial cells, the chorionic villi and the amnion.
3　The synctiotrophoblast is diffuse tissue with no cell membranes. Projections of the synctiotrophoblast extend

---

BOX 18.1　Assisted reproduction

Examples of assisted reproduction:

▶ *In vitro fertilisation*—ovarian follicles may be stimulated artificially by gonadotrophins. Several secondary oocytes are aspirated from the ovaries prior to ovulation. Sperm and ova are mixed in a laboratory dish, fertilisation and cleavage observed and blastomeres (eight-cell) inserted into the uterus via the cervical canal. Several zygotes may be transferred, to increase the chances of pregnancy.

▶ *In vivo fertilisation*—sperm are deposited in the upper vagina, cervix or uterus by artificial insemination when a woman is ovulating.

---

through the endometrial epithelium and connective tissue (stroma), releasing proteolytic enzymes, which break down the maternal tissues. This allows the blastocyst to burrow into the endometrium. The synctiotrophoblast is not rejected by the mother, possibly because it does not have transplantation antigens (Blackburn 2003). Slight bleeding may occur during this time, and can be mistaken for light menstrual bleeding (Blackburn 2003).

4　The blastocyst is nourished by glycogen and lipids that diffuse from the stromal cells and glands of the eroded tissue.

5　By day 9, degradation by the proteolytic enzymes causes spaces (lacunae) to appear in the synctiotrophoblast. Individual lacunae fuse to form lacunal networks and these fill with fluid from the endometrial glands (Blackburn 2003). Nutrients diffuse from the lacunae to the embryo.

6　Concurrent development of the inner cell mass occurs. At about day 7, a layer of cells, called the hypoblast, forms on the side of the inner cell mass adjacent to the blastocyst cavity (Moore & Persaud 1998). Formation of a bilaminar disc (a two-layered embryo) with a layer of epiblast and hypoblast is complete by day 8. This embryonic disc forms the germ cells that will produce all the tissues and organs of the embryo (described in the next section on embryology).

7　By day 10 the conceptus is completely implanted in the endometrium, covered by a closing plug, and by day 12 the endometrial epithelium has regenerated in the area (Blackburn 2003).

Changes in the endometrium

The uterine endometrium is in the secretory phase during implantation. During this phase there is proliferation of endometrial glands, providing a source of nutrition for the blastocyst. The spiral arterioles form a prolific network of blood vessels supplying the dense capillary bed beneath the epithelial layer of the endometrium.

Following implantation, the endometrium changes in structure and is known as the decidua. Increasing progesterone

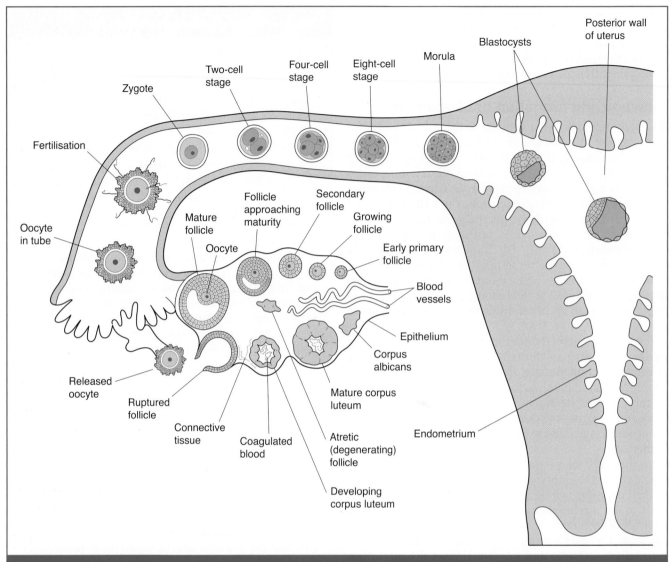

Figure 18.13 Summary of the ovarian cycle, showing cleavage and implantation (based on Moore & Persaud 1998)

facilitates enlargement of the decidual cells and accumulation of glycogen and lipids. These cellular changes, in combination with the vascular changes of the endometrium, are known as the decidual reaction. These structural changes are recognisable during ultrasonography and can be used to diagnose early pregnancy (Moore & Persaud 1998).

Three areas of the decidua are defined by their location relative to the implantation site:

- the *decidua basalis* is the region beneath the site of implantation. This develops into the maternal part of the placenta.
- the *decidua capsularis* is the area covering the implantation site. This disappears as the chorion is formed.
- the *decidua parietalis* (vera) is the remainder of the uterine lining. The chorion and decidua parietalis eventually fuse, obliterating the uterine cavity.

While the posterior wall of the body of the uterus is the most common site for implantation, the blastocyst may implant over the internal os of cervix or cervical canal, resulting in placenta praevia. Extrauterine implantation results in an ectopic pregnancy. The most common site is the ampulla or infundibulum of the fallopian tube.

By the time implantation is complete, at 10–12 days, the inner cell mass has differentiated into a bilaminar disc and the trophoblast has developed into the synctiotrophoblast and the cytotrophoblast. The synctiotrophoblast has formed maternal lacunae and the cytotrophoblast has formed chorionic villi. Further development of the embryo, placenta and fetal membranes occurs simultaneously.

Development of the embryo

The embryonic period refers to the period from the third to the eighth week after fertilisation. During this time the embryo develops from a bilaminar flat disc (Fig 18.14) to an embryo with all the major organ systems and a functioning cardiovascular

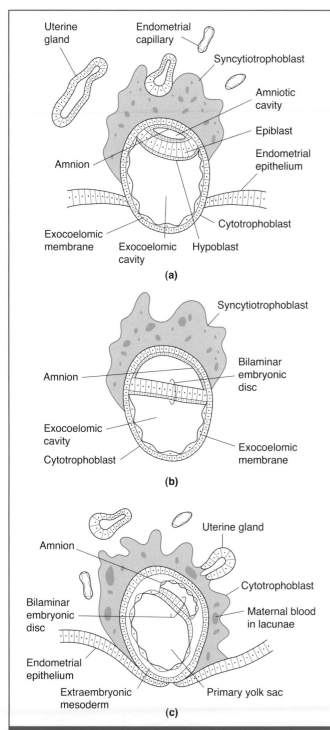

Figure 18.14 Implantation of a blastocyst into the endometrium **(a)** Section through a blastocyst partially implanted in the endometrium **(b)** Slightly older blastocyst after removal from the endometrium **(c)** Section through a blastocyst of about nine days implanted in the endometrium (based on Moore & Persaud 1998)

system. The embryo is vulnerable to developmental disruption from a wide range of teratogens—environmental agents such as infections, hyperthermia, drugs and radiation exposure, nicotine and narcotics exposure, leading to major congenital abnormalities.

It is important to understand embryological development. It explains why a healthy lifestyle prior to conception and during early pregnancy is important in order to provide the best possible environment for normal development of the embryo and why women of reproductive age should avoid potential teratogens at all times. This vulnerable phase of embryological development often occurs before a woman is aware that she is pregnant. Understanding normal embryological development also helps to understand abnormal development (e.g. cleft palate) and has led to the development of processes that can correct some abnormalities.

In considering embryological development, this section reviews changes in the third week and then focuses on the principles that govern development, rather than the detailed development of organ systems, which is beyond the scope of this text. (See the further readings and online resources at the end of this chapter for more detailed accounts.)

The embryo in week 3

Development during the embryonic period is very rapid and this makes it a vulnerable time. Gastrulation is the reorganisation of cells of the bilaminar disc (week 2) to form the trilaminar disc (Moore & Persaud 1998). The notochord and somites also form in week 3, and neurulation begins.

Gastrulation

A line of epiblast cells undergoes very rapid division to form the primitive streak along the midline. Cells from the primitive streak migrate down to form a layer of mesoderm between the epiblast and hypoblast (Fig 18.15), resulting in the trilaminar disc. The primitive streak continues to form mesoderm through the fourth week and then degenerates (Moore & Persaud 1998). All body organs and structures are derived from these three germ layers (ectoderm, mesoderm and endoderm), as shown in Figure 18.16.

Notochord and somite formation

A chord of mesodermal cells migrates to form the notochord, a rigid tube that defines the head–tail axis of the embryo and plays a key role in signalling the development of unspecialised

---

BOX 18.2 Pregnancy test

The developing synctiotrophoblast secretes human chorionic gonadotrophin (hCG) into the maternal circulation to maintain the pregnancy by stimulating the corpus luteum to continue producing oestrogens and progesterone. This hormone is the basis of the pregnancy test. It can be detected by sensitive radioimmunoassays by the end of the second week (four weeks after the beginning of the last menstrual bleeding)—usually well before the woman is aware that she is pregnant.

embryonic cells into specialised adult tissues and organs (Moore & Persaud 1998). The notochord forms the framework for the development of the axial skeleton (bones of head and spinal cord) and the neural plate, which develops into the primitive nervous system. Paired segments of mesoderm also form on either side of the notochord. These are somites, which eventually give rise to the axial skeleton and associated musculature as well as the overlying dermis of the skin. About 38 pairs of somites appear between days 20 and 30, and 42 to 44 pairs are present by the fifth week. They form prominent elevations and can be used to determine an embryo's age at this time.

Neurulation

The notochord induces thickening of the embryonic ectoderm to form the neural plate. A longitudinal groove develops in the plate and neural folds form above this. The folds fuse to form the neural tube—the primordium of the central nervous system (Fig 18.17). Incomplete fusion of the tube results in congenital defects of the central nervous system (e.g. spina bifida).

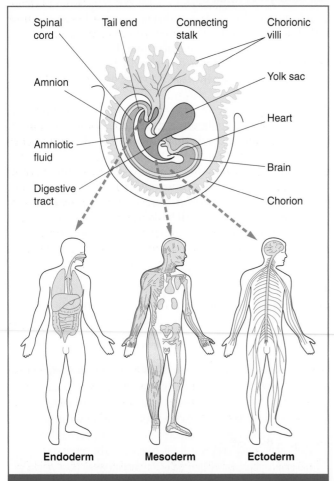

Figure 18.15 Invagination of the cells of the primitive streak to form a trilaminar disc (based on Coad & Dunstall 2001)

Figure 18.16 Organs derived from the ectoderm, mesoderm and endoderm (based on Shier et al 2002)

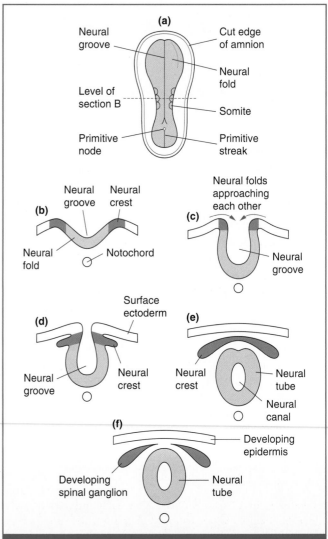

Figure 18.17 Transverse sections through progressively older embryos, showing formation of the neural groove, neural tube and neural crest up to the end of the fourth week (based on Moore & Persaud 1998)

Other changes during the third week include blood vessel formation. By the end of the week, nutrition is delivered by a primitive uteroplacental circulation, the framework for development of the nervous system is present, and the embryo begins organogenesis. A number of fundamental processes guide organogenesis and development of the embryo.

Cellular processes that control embryological development

Embryological development involves growth, differentiation and organisation. Growth involves an increase in cell number and cell size, while differentiation involves the creation of new types of cells and tissues. Organisation describes how the new units become coordinated into functional units (Blackburn 2003). Gene families within the embryo are known to control development. By the 2 to 4 cell stage, activated genes produce intercellular signalling proteins, which regulate cellular activity and development. Environmental factors can interact with groups of genes to turn them on and off at precise intervals.

The mechanisms controlling these processes are complex, but a number of processes have been described that contribute to development. These include: cell differentiation, induction, differential proliferation, programmed cell death, changes in cell size, cell migration, cell recognition and adhesion, folding and differential maturity. The following description of these processes has been adapted from Blackburn (2003).

Cell differentiation

The zygote contains one set of chromosomes, with the blueprint for the development of at least 350 different cell types that make up the body. Initially, cell division produces cells that are identical, but differentiation begins at the end of the first week, when the blastomeres of the morula develop into either cells of the inner cell mass or cells of the trophoblast. Remembering that all cells have the same genetic code, the process of differentiation involves restricting some areas of development while enabling others. This is regulated by gene families, which are switched on to produce specific proteins in a particular order.

Induction

Cells can influence cells in another part of the embryo by induction. Once again this process relies on signalling proteins (from inductors) and the ability of some cells to bind these proteins and respond (inducers). Development of many parts of the embryo is by secondary induction, where one change induces the next and so forth. For example, formation of the structures of the eye involves a series of inductions: the forebrain is induced to form the optic cup, which then induces adjacent tissue to form the lens of the eye, which then induces the surrounding tissue to form the cornea. Interfering with a step in the induction process will prevent the later stages occurring.

Differential cell proliferation

Differential cell proliferation is the process whereby groups of cells grow at different rates. This can give the impression of cells sinking into tissues if adjacent cells proliferate rapidly and build up in one area. This can be seen in the development of the neural groove. Rapid cell proliferation often precedes a period of differentiation. Congenital defects can result if proliferation is inhibited—by teratogenic agents, for example. Proliferation can also be inhibited through lack of space—for example, with a diaphragmatic hernia, the intestinal contents are pushed into the thoracic cavity, where they can inhibit lung growth.

Programmed cell death

Programmed cell death, where cells are destroyed by lysosomal enzymes, is a normal part of embryological development. This is the process whereby hollow tubes are formed (e.g. the trachea and parts of the gut). It also accounts for the disappearance of the webbing between fingers and toes. If the enzyme release is inhibited, congenital malformations such as syndactyly, bowel atresia or imperforate anus may result. Overactive enzymes can produce micromelia (shortened limbs).

Cell size and shape change

Chemical changes in cell microtubules, the skeleton within the cell, are responsible for changing cell shape (e.g. elongation of the cell). The process can be inhibited (e.g. by toxins from microorganisms). Other changes in cell shape (e.g. swelling or shrinking) can be induced by changes in osmotic balance.

Cell migration

Development of structures often involves migration of cells to different areas. This is a controlled process whereby the leading edge of the cell elongates (due to microtubule elongation) and adheres to a new contact point. Contraction of the cell toward the contact point completes the migration. Again, interference with the microtubule enzymes may impede migration—for example, Hirschsprung's disease (a lack of intestinal ganglion cells) results from failure of neural crest cells to migrate. In the central nervous system, at three to six months gestation, there is migration of millions of neurons from their original area in the periventricular area to their eventual location in the cerebrum and cerebellum. Interference with this migration can result in defects in central nervous system function and organisation.

Cell recognition and adhesion

Recognition and adhesion involves interaction of specific substances, such as cell surface enzymes, on one cell with complementary substances or adhesion molecules on another cell. An example of this is when the neural folds meet and fuse to form the neural tube. Adhesion may be prevented if there is interference with cell membrane substrates. This may be the mechanism for cleft palate or neural tube defects.

Folding of the embryo

The embryo starts as a straight line of cells but undergoes folding to adapt to the available space as it grows. Transverse folding results in a cylindrical shape, while longitudinal folding results in the head and tail folds.

Differential maturity

This process refers to the fact that different organ systems mature at different rates; for example, the gut is structurally complete at birth while the alveoli of the lungs and the long bones continue maturation after birth. This explains why different organ systems are vulnerable to damage by toxins at different stages of development.

Any malfunction of these fundamental processes results in impaired development. Understanding the basic principles may help to see why seemingly unconnected pathologies occur as congenital defects. The above processes are responsible for the cascade of changes resulting in organogenesis (development of the organ systems).

Organogenesis: highlights of weeks 4 to 8

All the major organ systems and structures of the body form from the three germ layers of the trilaminar disc. Table 18.1 lists visual highlights of the changes seen in the embryo (adapted from Moore & Persaud 1998). This is a critical period in human development as it is a time of most rapid cell division and the time of greatest vulnerability to teratogens. Different organ systems undergo rapid change at different times and this leads to variable impact of teratogens on different structures. Critical periods for the different organ systems are illustrated in Figure 18.18.

The fetus: from nine weeks to birth

The fetal period is mainly a time of growth and functional maturation. There is rapid body growth, while head growth slows. A fetus is capable of surviving independently at 32–34 weeks gestation, and survival in a neonatal intensive care unit may be possible from 22 to 26 weeks, although survival for babies under 24 weeks gestation is commonly associated with neurological impairment. A survey in Australia of 133 neonatalogists and registered nurses suggested that they would 'almost always' resuscitate an infant of 24 weeks gestation (Oei et al 2000), while health professionals at non-specialist facilities were shown to often underestimate survival of extremely premature infants compared to available Australian data (Gooi et al 2003).

The developmental level at birth may affect adult health. Several studies support a link between low birthweight and increased risk of coronary heart disease, stroke, hypertension and non-insulin-dependent diabetes in adults (Barker 2004; Kajantie et al 2005).

Table 18.2 outlines some visual highlights of fetal development.

The developing embryo and fetus is supported by the development of extraembryonic structures.

Development of the placenta and fetal membranes

The placenta is a feto-maternal organ—that is, it has fetal and maternal regions that develop from the trophoblast region in the blastocyst. Development begins in the second week. The placenta becomes fully established by 8–10 weeks, and full size by the fourth month. The placenta separates the maternal and fetal circulatory systems, yet allows ready exchange of many substances such as respiratory gases and nutrients between the mother and fetus. The placenta is the

TABLE 18.1 Overview of embryonic development from 4 to 8 weeks

Week of gestation	Visual highlight
4	• Embryo straight, C-shape developing • Somites form • Neural tube fusing, but open at rostral and caudal ends • Branchial arches present (develop into primitive face, jaws and neck) • Forebrain prominent • Upper limb buds appear, then lower limb buds • Otic pits present (internal ears) • Tapered tail obvious • Beating heart prominent
5	• Rapid development of brain and head enlargement • Face touches heart prominence • Hand plates develop in upper limbs
6	• Limb buds (especially upper) more differentiated into elbow and wrist • Ridges (digital rays) in hand plates obvious (forerunners of digits) • External ear canal and auricle (pinna) formed • Pigmented eye obvious • Head disproportionately large and bent over • Some straightening of neck and thorax
7	• Umbilical herniation (intestines enter extraembryonic coelom in umbilical cord) • Notches appear between digital rays of hand plates • Liver is prominent
8	• Short, webbed digits of hands gradually lengthen • Notches appear between digital rays of the feet • Stubby tail disappears • Head disproportionately large • Neck apparent • Eyelids more obvious and eyes open • Auricles of external ears are low set • Sexuality of external genitalia not easily determined

(Source: adapted from Moore & Persaud 1998)

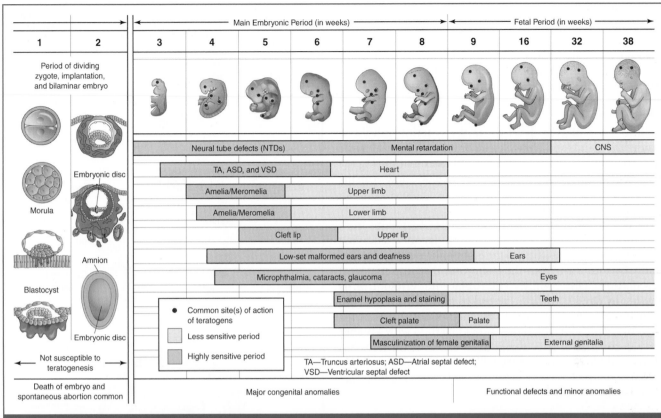

Figure 18.18 Critical periods for the different organ systems (Moore & Persaud 1998)

TABLE 18.2	Overview of fetal development
Week of gestation	**Visual highlight**
9–12	Eyes can close, sex distinguishable externally by 12 weeks, red blood cells produced in liver at first, then mainly in spleen, urine excreted into amniotic fluid
13–16	Head proportionately smaller, ossification of skeleton begins, ovaries differentiated (16 weeks) with primordial follicles containing oogonia, eyes face anteriorly, not laterally now
17–20	Growth slows, lower limbs reach final proportions, quickening felt by mother, brown fat forms (site of heat production), uterus fully formed (18 weeks), vaginal development begun, testes begin descent from posterior abdominal wall (20 weeks)
21–25	Substantial weight gain, body better proportioned, cells in walls of lungs secreting surfactant to keep developing alveoli patent, respiratory system still very immature
26–29	Lungs developed, CNS can direct breathing, bone marrow produces red blood cells by 28 weeks, testes begin descent at 28–32 weeks
30–34	Pupils react to light (31 weeks), white fat 8% body weight
35–38	Firm grasp, circumferences of head and abdomen equal (36 weeks), growth slows, white fat 16% body weight

main site for the production of hormones that maintain the pregnancy, although initially, hormones are supplied from the corpus luteum in the ovary. Secretion of hCG by the trophoblast maintains the corpus luteum until the placenta is able to take over hormone production by 8–10 weeks. The chorioamniotic membrane develops around the fetus and contains the amniotic fluid. It is metabolically active tissue that produces hormones.

Uteroplacental and fetoplacental circulation

Development of the fetal membranes and the placenta, along with development of embryonic blood vessels for transport, enables a more efficient exchange mechanism for the developing embryo than the cell-to-cell diffusion during early development.

Maternal lacunae

Primitive circulation develops as the synctiotrophoblast erodes the glands and blood vessels of the endometrial tissue to form lacunae (spaces). Evidence indicates that during the first trimester, trophoblastic plugs prevent blood flow from the maternal spiral arterioles into the lacunae (Jaffe et al 1997). This means that embryonic development is in a relatively hypoxic environment (Chaddha et al 2004). Secretions from the endometrial glands initially fill the lacunae, allowing nutrients and O_2 to diffuse to the embryonic disc, and wastes and CO_2 to diffuse from the embryonic disc into maternal circulation. This primitive uteroplacental circulation is present by day 13. Towards the end of the first trimester, the lacunar networks develop into the intervillous spaces of the placenta, which fill with blood, providing fluid with a higher oxygen content for fetal exchange. By this time the fetus has developed blood vessels in the villi and mechanisms to cope with the higher levels of oxygen available from the maternal blood (Blackburn 2003).

Chorionic villi

During the second week, the cytotrophoblast invades the areas of synctiotrophoblast between the lacunae and forms finger-like projects called the chorionic villi. Further chorionic villi develop as the synctiotrophoblast continues to invade the decidua. Villus development is stimulated by growth factors and the relatively hypoxic environment (Chaddha et al 2004). Blood vessels develop within the villi by 18–21 days and a primitive fetoplacental circulation operates between embryonic blood in the villi, embryonic vessels and the primitive heart by 20–21 days.

Villi can be two types, anchoring or branch villi, with similar numbers of both. Branch villi facilitate maternal fetal exchange via diffusion, while anchoring villi attach the placenta to the decidua.

Formation of the smooth chorion and amnion

The chorionic villi initially cover the entire surface of the chorionic sac, but during the eighth week they disintegrate in some areas, forming the smooth chorion, and develop in other areas, forming the villous chorion. Degeneration occurs in areas compressed against the decidua capsularis as they lose their blood supply and become the smooth chorion and thus the chorionic membrane. In the area of membrane against the decidua basalis, the villi growing into the endometrium proliferate, and these become the chorionic villi of the fetal placenta (Moore & Persaud 1998).

The amnion is formed from embryonic ectoderm (see embryology section later). Initially the amnion encloses a

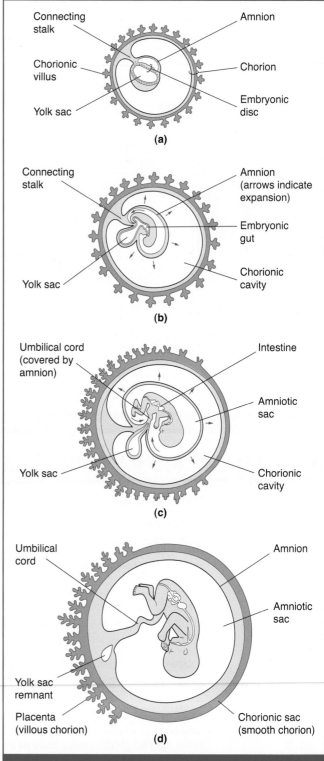

Figure 18.19 Steps showing how the amnion enlarges, fills the chorionic sac and envelops the umbilical cord: **(a)** 3 weeks, **(b)** 4 weeks, **(c)** 10 weeks and **(d)** 20 weeks (based on Moore & Persaud 1998)

small cavity, the amniotic cavity, situated above the embryonic disc, but the membrane and cavity enlarge to surround the embryo (Fig 18.19). The amniotic membrane is pushed against the chorion and they form the chorioamniotic membrane, a double membrane sac surrounding the fetus. The membranes do not fuse, but are separated by 200 mL of amniotic fluid and mucus produced in the amnion. The chorion contains blood vessels that atrophy as pregnancy progresses; the amnion does not have a blood supply, but nutrients pass to it from the chorionic blood vessels. The amnion attachment to the fetus is reduced to the site of the umbilical cord. The membranes continue to grow until the 28th week, after which stretching accommodates the increased fetal size (Blackburn 2003). Connective tissue is heavily interwoven with collagen, allowing stretching and providing strength.

The amnion can rupture independently of the chorion and form amniotic bands of tissue. These bands can constrict and reduce blood supply to fetal parts, sometimes causing amputation (Sentilhes et al 2003).

The fetal membranes have a high metabolic rate, similar to that of the liver. They are active in synthesising many chemicals such as amniotic fluid, nutrients, renin and prostaglandins. The enzyme, phospholipase A2, necessary for prostaglandin synthesis, is found in the membranes and decidua, and the prostaglandin precursor, arachidonic acid, is also found in the membranes. The chorion stores hormones such as progesterone.

Amniotic fluid

Amniotic fluid is contained in the membranes and has several functions. It allows fetal movement and protects the fetus from changes in pressure and temperature. Protection from infection comes from antibacterial factors, such as transferrin (binds iron needed by bacteria), fatty acids (interfere with bacterial membranes), immunoglobulins and lysozymes (destroy bacteria) (Blackburn 2003).

The formation of amniotic fluid relies on diffusion of water and solutes from several sources. Initially there is some secretion by amniotic cells; however, most of the fluid diffuses from the interstitial fluid of the decidua parietalis and from blood in the intervillous spaces of the placenta across the amniochorionic membrane to the amniotic cavity. Exchange also occurs between the fetus and the amniotic cavity. The fetus swallows amniotic fluid and it is excreted by the fetal respiratory tract and fetal renal system (urine present in bladder by 11 weeks). Prior to keratinisation of the skin, which occurs by about 24 weeks, the skin is a major path for exchange of amniotic fluid.

Amniotic fluid is composed of 98–99% water, with the remaining 1–2% comprising electrolytes, creatinine, urea, bile, renin, glucose, hormones, fetal cells, lanugo and vernix. If the volume of amniotic fluid is above or below the expected level for gestational age of the fetus, conditions such as polyhydramnios or oligohydramnios can occur, with both maternal and fetal consequences.

Formation of the yolk sac

As the epiblast migrates to form the amnion, cells from the hypoblast migrate around the blastocyst cavity to form the extracoelomic cavity, which is modified to become the primary yolk sac. The embryonic disc is situated between the amniotic cavity and the yolk sac. The yolk sac is important for nutrient transfer in the second and third weeks. Early blood cell formation occurs in the wall of the yolk sac from the third to sixth week, when the liver takes over this role. During the fourth week, part of it is incorporated into embryo as the primitive gut, and its endoderm develops into the epithelium of the respiratory and digestive tracts. The remainder degenerates by 10 weeks (Fig 18.19).

Placental circulation in the mature placenta

Once embryonic circulation is established, oxygen and nutrients diffuse from the secretions or blood entering the maternal intervillous spaces, through the walls of the branch villi, and then enter the embryonic capillaries in the chorionic villi. Carbon dioxide and waste products are exchanged in the opposite direction. Maternal and fetal blood do not mix unless the placenta tears away from the decidua (Fig 18.20).

The placenta acts as a barrier to very few substances. Some large molecules with a particular shape and charge cannot pass—for example, heparin cannot cross but warfarin can. The placenta becomes thinner as pregnancy advances, and many drugs given to the mother are detected in fetal plasma.

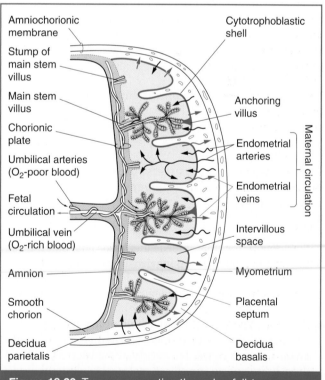

Amniochorionic membrane	Cytotrophoblastic shell
Stump of main stem villus	
Main stem villus	Anchoring villus
Chorionic plate	Endometrial arteries
Umbilical arteries (O₂-poor blood)	Endometrial veins
Fetal circulation	Intervillous space
Umbilical vein (O₂-rich blood)	Myometrium
Amnion	Placental septum
Smooth chorion	Decidua basalis
Decidua parietalis	

Maternal circulation

Figure 18.20 Transverse section through a full-term placenta, showing the relation of the fetal part to the maternal part (based on Moore & Persaud 1998)

Maternal placental circulation

Maternal blood enters the intervillous space from the spiral arteries in the endometrium. Blood spurts towards the roof of the intervillous space and then flows around the villi, allowing exchange of gases and nutrients. Blood then leaves the intervillous spaces via the endometrial veins. Blood flow increases from 50 mL/min at 10 weeks to 600–800 mL/min at term, accounting for 20% of the increased cardiac output (Henderson & Macdonald 2004). The intervillous spaces hold approximately 150 mL of blood, and this is continually replenished. During labour, uterine contractions prevent blood entering the intervillous spaces, but sufficient blood is retained there (150 mL) for fetal exchange of oxygen, nutrients and so on (Fig 18.20).

Fetal placental circulation

The umbilical cord provides circulatory connection between the mother and fetus. Deoxygenated blood leaves the fetus via two umbilical arteries to the placenta and oxygenated blood comes from the placenta via the umbilical vein. Wharton's jelly, consisting of collagen, muscle and mucopolysaccharide, cushions the blood vessels. Fetal blood flow in the placenta is approximately 500 mL/min (Blackburn 2003), and is regulated by several factors, such as fetal heart rate, fetal left-to-right shunts, and systemic and pulmonary vascular resistance (see the section on fetal circulation).

If the blood flow around the villi is compromised (e.g. prolapse of umbilical cord or vasoconstriction of maternal blood vessels due to hypertension), fetal hypoxia occurs. This may be indicated by decelerations in fetal heart rate and can lead to fetal death. A chronic reduction in uteroplacental circulation can result in intrauterine growth restriction due to reduced supply of nutrients and oxygen to fetus.

Placental function

The placenta has four key roles: transport, immunological, endocrine and metabolic. The placenta is also the main route of heat transfer away from the fetus (Blackburn 2003).

Transport role

The embryo, and then fetus, relies exclusively on the placenta for transport of cellular requirements. This includes the transport of:

- respiratory gases, oxygen and carbon dioxide. The rate of delivery is dependent on maternal and fetal blood flow. Any factors that impede uterine or fetal blood flow can lead to fetal hypoxia. Inhaled anaesthetics readily cross the placenta to the fetus, as does carbon monoxide produced from the incomplete combustion of cigarette smoke (Moore & Persaud 1998).
- nutrients. These constitute the bulk of substances transferred. Glucose, water and all vitamins cross rapidly. Small amounts of free fatty acids are transferred, while there is little or no transfer of maternal cholesterol, phospholipids or triglycerides. Transferrin, an iron transport protein, crosses the placenta and delivers iron to the fetus (Moore & Persaud 1998).

- hormones. Steroid hormones cross freely. Protein hormones are generally not transported to the fetus, but small amounts of thyroid hormones cross slowly (Moore & Persaud 1998).
- waste products. Carbon dioxide, urea, uric acid and bilirubin are all transported quickly across the placenta (Moore & Persaud 1998).
- electrolytes, which are freely exchanged. This includes any intravenous fluids given to the mother, which can interfere with fetal fluid balance (Moore & Persaud 1998).

Normal cellular transport mechanisms of simple and facilitated diffusion, active transport and pinocytosis allow movement of these substances between the maternal and fetal circulation. However, many harmful substances can also pass freely by the same mechanisms. These include:

- drugs. Almost all drugs can pass freely and many result in compromise for the fetus; for example, alcohol can cause fetal alcohol syndrome, narcotics may result in heroin addiction in the newborn, sedatives and analgesics such as pethidine used in labour can cause respiratory depression in the newborn. Antibiotics cross the placenta and this may be beneficial.
- infectious agents. Several viruses can cross the placenta and cause fetal infection—for example, rubella, poliomyelitis, measles and HIV. In some cases (e.g. rubella), severe congenital malformations may result (Moore & Persaud 1998).

Figure 18.21 summarises the range of substances that are transported across the placenta.

Increased transport of substances occurs as pregnancy progresses. This is due to a decrease in the distance between maternal and fetal blood as placental development occurs, increased volume of blood transported and greater fetal demands. Many factors can influence placental transport, such as maternal nutritional status or exercise. Disease states that influence maternal nutrient level, such as diabetes mellitus, or influence blood flow, such as hypertension, also affect placental transfer.

Immunological role

The placenta provides an effective barrier against most large bacterial microorganisms; however, most viruses and some smaller bacteria can pass to the fetus. Protection is afforded by maternal antibodies, particularly IgG antibodies, which cross the placenta and provide passive immunity against some diseases, such as measles, diphtheria and smallpox. Maternal antibodies do not protect against chickenpox or pertussis (whooping cough) (Moore & Persaud 1998). Transfer of antibodies can be disadvantageous—an example is transfer of Rh antibodies to a fetus following antibody production by a mother with Rh blood who has been exposed to Rh+ blood. If the fetus is Rh+ this can lead to haemolytic disease of the newborn (erythroblastic fetalis). Despite having a different genetic composition from that of the mother, the trophoblast is protected from generating an immune response in the mother (Gaunt & Ramin 2001; Stables & Rankin 2004).

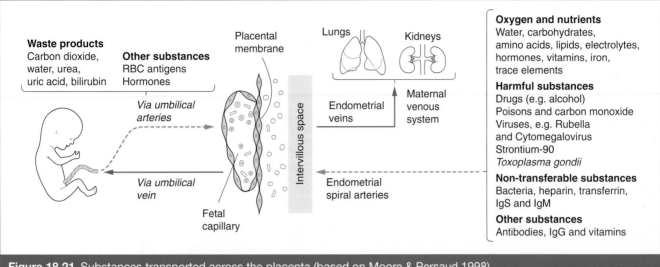

Figure 18.21 Substances transported across the placenta (based on Moore & Persaud 1998)

Endocrine role

Several hormones that maintain pregnancy are synthesised in the placenta: oestrogens, progesterone, hCG and human placental lactogen (hPL). These hormones are discussed later in the section on pregnancy.

Metabolic role

The placenta synthesises glycogen, cholesterol, fatty acids and enzymes, which are used by the embryo/fetus and the placenta. This is particularly important in early pregnancy (Moore & Persaud 1998).

Summary of placental and fetal membrane development

- The placenta begins to form as the synctiotrophoblast invades the endometrium.
- Maternal blood vessels and glands are eroded to form lacunae, and these link over time to form the blood-filled maternal intervillous spaces.
- The cytotrophoblast invades the areas between the lacunae to form the fetal chorionic villi, which are invaded by fetal blood vessels.
- Exchange of nutrients and wastes occurs via cell transport mechanisms such as diffusion and active transport between the blood in the fetal vessels and the secretions or blood in the intervillous spaces. Transport involves crossing the membrane of the chorionic villus and the endothelium of the fetal capillary.
- Maternal blood arrives at the intervillous spaces from the uterine arteries and leaves in the uterine veins. On the fetal side, blood arrives at the placenta from the umbilical arteries and leaves in the single umbilical vein.
- A double membrane develops around the embryo. The outer chorion is formed from the cytotrophoblast, while the inner amnion is formed from migrating ectoderm from the embryonic disc.

- The fetal membranes are metabolically active, producing amniotic fluid and hormones involved in pregnancy.
- The amniotic fluid circulates through the fetus in the digestive, respiratory and renal systems, and is also exchanged across the skin.
- The amniotic fluid protects the fetus from mechanical stress.
- The main functions of the placenta are to provide a transport medium between the fetus and mother, to produce hormones to maintain pregnancy, and to provide some immunological protection to the fetus. It also has a metabolic role.

Fetal circulation

The fetal cardiorespiratory systems have several physiological and structural specialisations that allow survival in a fluid environment. The fetal circulatory system delivers oxygen and nutrients to the fetal tissues and removes metabolic waste products, but the fetus relies on the placenta for oxygenation of the blood, not its own lungs, which remain dormant and fluid-filled until birth. Fetal breathing movements can be detected on ultrasound by week 10 (Blackburn 2003); however, the lungs and associated pulmonary blood vessels do not reach adequate maturity until 28 weeks gestation. Premature delivery with associated immaturity of the lungs and pulmonary vasculature can result in respiratory distress syndrome (RDS).

In the fetus, several structures are present to divert blood from the immature lungs to the placenta for gas exchange: umbilical vein, umbilical arteries, ductus venosus, foramen ovale, and ductus arteriosus. This leads to the mixing of oxygenated and deoxygenated blood in the atria, aorta and vena cava, which lowers levels of oxygen saturation.

Characteristics

Fetal circulation is characterised by fast flow, low vascular resistance (due to the low-resistance umbilical and placental circulations) and high pulmonary vascular resistance. The oxygen content of fetal blood is lower than that of the neonate, but fetal haemoglobin (HbF) has a higher affinity for oxygen, to manage this hypoxic state.

Structures

The fetal structures—umbilical vein, umbilical arteries, ductus venosus, foramen ovale and ductus arteriosus—ensure that the fetal circulation is routed to the placenta for oxygenation and that most of the blood bypasses the lungs, which are non-functional (Fig 18.22). The placenta is a low-resistance pathway, taking 40% of the fetal cardiac output (CO). The umbilical vein carries oxygenated blood from the placenta to the inferior vena cava (IVC), either indirectly via the hepatic portal system, or directly via the ductus venosus. The ductus venosus is a low-resistance pathway that bypasses the liver and takes 40–60% of blood flow, thereby enabling a large amount of the oxygenated blood to reach the heart directly. Deoxygenated blood from the lower part of the fetal body mixes in the IVC with oxygenated blood from the ductus venosus just before the IVC enters the right atrium. The foramen ovale is an opening in the septum between the right and left atria that allows 50–60% of the blood to shunt directly to the left atrium. The rest of the blood flows to the ductus arteriosus via the right ventricle. The ductus arteriosus is situated between the pulmonary trunk and aortic arch, and shunts 60% of the blood away from the pulmonary circulation into the systemic arterial circulation via the aortic arch. The high pulmonary vascular resistance of the deflated lungs allows only 5–15% of the CO from the right ventricle to enter the pulmonary circulation (Blackburn 2003). The umbilical arteries carry deoxygenated blood from the iliac arteries back to the placenta.

Oxygen saturation of fetal blood

The fetus has high oxygen demands for its metabolic needs and this is reflected in the high CO, which is 250 mL/min/kg, compared with the adult value of 85 mL/min/kg. Fetal heart rate is also high at 155 beats/min at 20 weeks and 140 beats/min at 40 weeks (Blackburn 2003).

The highest oxygen saturation occurs in the umbilical vein at 70% (32–35 mmHg), falling to 65% (26–28 mmHg) in the left atrium and ascending aorta. This blood, at 65% saturation, also perfuses the fetal brain and coronary arteries. Blood returning from the lower limbs to the hepatic circulation and from the superior vena cava to the right atrium is very desaturated, at 25% (16–17 mmHg), even less than the 50% (18–19 mmHg) saturated blood returning to the placenta via the umbilical arteries (Fig 18.22).

There is a maternal–fetal oxygen gradient at the placenta (maternal PaO_2 is 33 mmHg, fetal PaO_2 is 28 mmHg), which facilitates oxygen diffusion into the umbilical vein. Fetal blood is uniquely able to maintain oxygen saturation at a

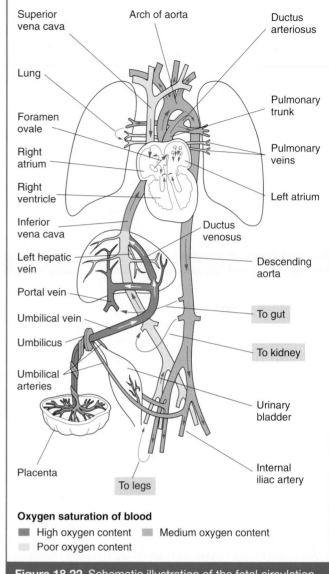

Figure 18.22 Schematic illustration of the fetal circulation (based on Moore & Persaud 1998)

higher level for a given PaO_2 than adult blood. This is due to the increased affinity that fetal haemoglobin (HbF) has for oxygen. This improves saturation and allows more oxygen to reach the tissues.

The fetal oxyhaemoglobin dissociation curve is shifted to the left of the maternal oxyhaemoglobin dissociation curve, and illustrates that HbF binds more oxygen at lower saturations, and equally that very low saturations must be reached before significant oxygen will be released from the HbF (see Fig 18.23).

Development of fetal circulation and lungs

The cardiovascular system is the first embryonic system to start functioning. This facilitates more efficient distribution of oxygen and nutrients around the growing mass of the embryo. An indication of the level of development at various

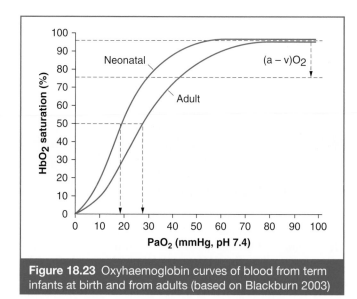

Figure 18.23 Oxyhaemoglobin curves of blood from term infants at birth and from adults (based on Blackburn 2003)

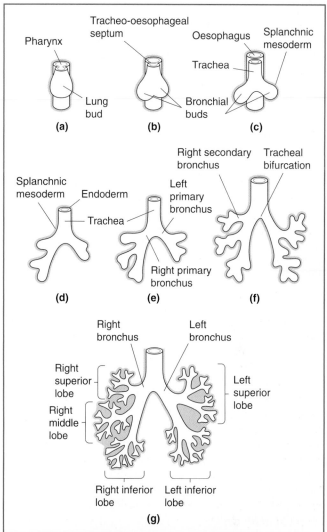

Figure 18.24 Successive stages in the development of the bronchi and lungs: **(a)** to **(c)** 4 weeks, **(d)** to **(e)** 5 weeks, **(f)** 6 weeks, **(g)** 8 weeks (based on Blackburn 2003)

gestational ages follows. (More detail is available from the further readings listed at the end of the chapter.)

By three to four weeks the heart tube, containing one atrium and one ventricle, is beating. Development of the lungs is paralleled by development of the pulmonary circulation, but lungs do not take on a gas exchange function until birth. By three to four weeks a lung bud has appeared at the caudal end of the laryngotracheal tube and blood vessels, which will be the future pulmonary arteries, have formed branches to the lung bud. By eight to ten weeks the heart has four chambers with mitral and tricuspid valves, and bronchi and bronchioles have formed in the lungs (Fig 18.24). Development of pulmonary blood vessels is concurrent with development of the bronchi.

By 20 weeks, pulmonary vascularisation is prominent and development of pulmonary terminal sacs from the respiratory bronchioles is ongoing. Lung fluid secretion begins from the terminal sacs and pulmonary capillaries. Fetal breathing movements are well established. They occur 40–80% of the time, and at a rate of 30–70 breaths/minute (Blackburn 2003).

Fetal breathing movements

Lung fluid is regulated by fetal breathing, and therefore growth of the lungs is affected if breathing is inhibited. For example, maternal alcohol ingestion, hypoglycaemia, accelerated labour and cigarette smoking inhibit fetal breathing movements, the latter for up to an hour. The diaphragm plays an important role in fetal breathing movements, which prepare the lungs for the first breath, and influence differentiation and proliferation of lung tissue (Moore & Persaud 1998).

At 25 weeks, respiration is possible because some primitive alveoli have developed, but severe respiratory insufficiency is likely if the baby is born prematurely. At this time the terminal sacs are sparse, and lined with thick cuboidal epithelial cells; pulmonary capillaries are still developing and there is insufficient surfactant in the alveoli. From 26 to 28 weeks,

terminal air sacs develop and form clusters in conjunction with extensive capillary networks. Terminal sac development continues until birth and beyond, until eight years of age. At 28 weeks, gas exchange during respiration is possible if birth occurs prematurely. This is due to the presence of clusters of thin-walled primitive alveoli (terminal sacs) and pulmonary capillaries. At 32 to 36 weeks, surfactant production by cells within the alveoli, Type II pneumatocytes, begins (Moore & Persaud 1998).

Composition and function of surfactant

Surfactant is a lipoprotein that contains phospholipids. It prevents the formation of an air/water interface, which reduces surface tension in the alveoli. This increases compliance of the lungs, which means they can be inflated for relatively less effort and collapse of the alveoli at the end of expiration is prevented.

The presence of surfactant assists absorption of lung fluid after birth. This amounts to 25 mL/kg body mass that must be absorbed or excreted. If the baby's physiological mechanisms do not change from secretion to absorption of lung fluid, the baby can drown. Labour appears to trigger release of catecholamines (e.g. adrenaline) that enable the switch from secretion to absorption of lung fluid. The sudden change in pulmonary blood flow at birth also helps remove lung fluid in the first few hours.

Glucocorticoid and thyroid hormones enhance surfactant synthesis, the former by increasing glycogen depletion as well as increasing phospholipid synthesis. Glycogen depletion leads to changes in the alveoli, such as thinning and increased size of the alveoli along with increasing the numbers of Type II pneumocytes. If insufficient surfactant is present at birth, ventilation is impaired, resulting in infant respiratory distress syndrome (IRDS). Thyroid hormones increase the rate of phospholipid synthesis (Blackburn 2003).

Clinical applications

Conditions that inhibit glycogen depletion in the lungs, such as insulin-dependent diabetes, may inhibit surfactant synthesis if the condition is not well controlled. Insulin inhibits glycogen breakdown, effectively decreasing the substrate needed for phospholipid synthesis, and the structural changes associated with glycogen depletion are inhibited (Blackburn 2003).

Some conditions accelerate lung maturity by inducing stress in the fetus, therefore increasing secretion of glucocorticoids and catecholamines (e.g. pre-eclampsia, IUGR, premature rupture of the membranes) (Blackburn 2003). Women are often given dexamethasone prior to delivery, which appears to assist surfactant production and prevent RDS. Neonates requiring ventilation may be given surfactant via an endotrachial tube.

Summary of fetal circulation

- Fetal circulation is characterised by fast flow, low vascular resistance, and high pulmonary vascular resistance.
- Fetal structures divert blood from the lungs to the placenta. These are the umbilical vein, umbilical arteries, ductus venosus, foramen ovale and the ductus arteriosus.
- The high oxygen needs of the fetus are met by a high cardiac output. HbF enhances oxygen transfer from maternal blood. This is reflected in a shift to the left of the HbO_2 dissociation curve of the fetus.
- Oxygenated blood from the umbilical vein mixes with deoxygenated blood returning in the vena cava, producing 'mixed blood' with reduced oxygen saturation. This returns to the heart and circulates to the tissues via branches of the aorta. Branches from the internal iliac arteries flow into the umbilical arteries to return to the placenta.
- At 25 weeks gestation, respiration is possible as some primitive alveoli have developed, but the epithelial lining is thick, pulmonary capillaries are sparse and insufficient surfactant is produced.
- At 28 weeks, further development of the terminal air sacs, capillaries and surfactant makes gas exchange possible.
- Fetal breathing movements facilitate development of the lungs.
- Surfactant increases the compliance of the lungs and facilitates fluid reabsorption after birth.

Maternal changes associated with pregnancy

Pregnancy is associated with major physiological changes that enable the woman to support the in utero growth and development of the baby, from the beginnings as a one-celled organism until reaching term as a complex human being. This process takes an average of 266 days (38 weeks) from the time of fertilisation, or 280 days if the time is taken from the first day of the last menstrual bleeding. The maternal physiological changes associated with the growing fetus and with the changes to the maternal body systems are predominantly controlled by hormones, in some instances facilitated by the increase in size of the fetus. The function of these hormones and the subsequent changes to maternal body systems are the focus of this section on pregnancy.

Hormones of pregnancy

There are a vast number of hormones and neurohormones (Reis et al 2001), growth factors and proteins produced by the placenta during pregnancy. The maternal physiological and anatomical changes during pregnancy are largely controlled by the following hormones:
- human chorionic gonadotrophin (hCG)
- human placental lactogen (hPL)
- oestrogens
- progesterone.

Human chorionic gonadotropin

Human chorionic gonadotrophin (hCG) is a glycoprotein, similar in structure to luteinising hormone, secreted by the trophoblast. It can be detected in the blood seven days after fertilisation and in the urine 26 to 28 days after fertilisation (Blackburn 2003). There is a rapid increase in early pregnancy up until nine weeks and then a decrease in levels. hCG forms the basis of the pregnancy test, where hCG antibodies are used to identify the presence of hCG in the woman's urine.

hCG is linked to many maternal changes in the first trimester. Probably most importantly, it prevents the degeneration of the corpus luteum and stimulates it to continue secreting oestrogens and progesterone until the placenta takes over this role. Changes in smell, taste and saliva seem to be correlated with the level of hCG, which has been linked to feelings of nausea in the first trimester. It may also have an immunosuppressant role that reduces maternal rejection of the placenta (Blackburn 2003).

Human placental lactogen

Human placental lactogen (hPL) is a polypeptide, similar to growth hormone, secreted by the synctiotrophoblast. Synthesis begins 5 to 10 days after implantation and levels increase to a peak just before term (Blackburn 2003)—hPL facilitates growth. It changes maternal metabolism to maximise the nutrients available to the fetus in utero. Three key metabolic changes facilitated by hPL are as follows:

- It reduces maternal utilisation of glucose by reducing the response of maternal cells to insulin—it is an insulin antagonist. This raises the maternal blood glucose level and makes more glucose available to the fetus.
- It mobilises maternal lipid stores, releasing fatty acids as the maternal energy source, leaving glucose for fetal uptake.
- It accelerates amino acid transfer to the fetus.

Steroid hormones

The steroid hormones, oestrogen and progesterone, responsible for the maintenance of pregnancy, are initially released from the corpus luteum in the ovaries. The placenta takes over this role at about seven weeks gestation. The synthesis is complex, involving the mother, placenta and fetus, as each lacks the enzymes necessary for independent synthesis. Figure 18.25 illustrates the interconnections in the pathways for synthesis. The common precursor for steroid synthesis is cholesterol. The synthesis of cholesterol is increased in pregnancy to meet the demand for steroid synthesis.

Oestrogens

Three types of oestrogens are synthesised in the ovaries and placenta: oestriol, beta-oestradiol and oestrone. Oestriol, the weaker form, is the most common oestrogen; it increases most significantly during pregnancy. In a non-pregnant woman, oestriol is synthesised from beta-oestradiol and oestrone in the ovaries; however, during pregnancy oestriol synthesis relies on enzymes in the fetal liver and dehydroepiandrosterone sulfate (DHEAS) from the fetal adrenals for synthesis. There is a rapid increase early in pregnancy, which slows between 24 and 32 weeks, and then there is a surge in oestriol at 34–36 weeks. Measurement of oestriol levels were one of the earliest methods of monitoring fetal wellbeing, but this technique is no longer used (Blackburn 2003).

Oestrogens stimulate growth of tissues by increasing protein synthesis. They cause the hyperplasia and hypertrophy of the uterus, the increased vascularisation of the uterus and the development of the mammary ducts and alveolar tissue in the breasts. Oestrogens also cause swelling and softening of connective tissues (e.g. cervix, nipples and ligaments) by increasing the water content in the extracellular matrix and reducing the adhesion of the collagen fibres in connective tissues. Angiotensin and aldosterone levels increase under the influence of oestrogens, leading to fluid retention. Oestrogens increase the sensitivity of the uterus to progesterone and, along with progesterone, they increase the sensitivity of the maternal respiratory centre to carbon dioxide.

These functions of oestrogens contribute to some of the minor discomforts of pregnancy. Water retention mediated by oestrogen can lead to oedema. Pelvic discomfort can result from relaxation of the pelvic ligaments, stretching of the sacro-iliac and sacro-coccygeal joints and the increasing elasticity of the symphysis pubis.

Progesterone

Progesterone is secreted by the corpus luteum initially, and then by the placental synctiotrophoblast. The fetus is not essential for progesterone synthesis, and therefore levels are not indicative of fetal wellbeing. Placental progesterone enters both the maternal and fetal circulations and is broken down and excreted in the urine as pregnanediol.

Progesterone increases the secretory activity of the decidual cells of the uterus, which supply nourishment for the embryo (as discussed in the section on the placenta). Along with other uterotonic inhibitors, progesterone lowers smooth muscle excitability, particularly in the myometrium, to prevent uterine contraction, but also in the ureters, stomach and intestines. It increases the sensitivity of the maternal chemoreceptors to carbon dioxide, thus stimulating ventilation at lower $PaCO_2$

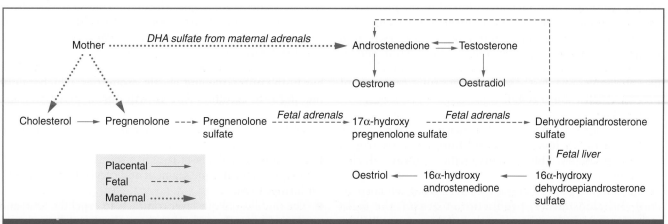

Figure 18.25 Summary of the principal routes by which the human fetoplacental unit synthesises oestrogens (based on Johnson & Everitt 2000)

values than before pregnancy. Progesterone also has a role in implantation, and in helping to suppress the maternal immunological response (Blackburn 2003). Fetal adrenal hormone production relies on progesterone as an essential precursor.

Progesterone-induced relaxation of smooth muscle results in many of the minor discomforts of pregnancy, such as:

- oesophageal reflux (heartburn), due to relaxation of the oesophageal sphincter
- nausea and vomiting, which may be potentiated by reduced peristalsis
- urinary tract infections, which increase in pregnancy due to stasis of urine caused by relaxation of the smooth muscle in the ureters and bladder
- varicose veins and haemorrhoids, due to dilatation of the veins in the legs and rectal region
- postural hypotension, due to venous pooling resulting from reduced peripheral resistance in the blood vessels in the lower limbs.

As well as the smooth muscle relaxation effect, progesterone has a thermogenic effect, increasing body temperature by 0.5°C to 1.0°C, and it stimulates hyperventilation due to the increased sensitivity of chemoreceptors to carbon dioxide.

The level of steroid hormones increases throughout pregnancy, as they mediate maternal changes to facilitate the growth and nourishment of the fetus.

Changes to maternal physiology

Endocrine glands

Pregnancy is associated with an increase in size of the anterior pituitary gland and increases in secretion of adrenocorticotrophic hormone (ACTH). This is likely the result of placental corticotrophic-releasing hormone (CRH) stimulation than hypothalamic CRH stimulation. Placental CRH is present in low levels during pregnancy, but increases twenty-fold at 35 weeks and has a role in the initiation of labour. Increases in prolactin, thyrotropin and melanocyte-stimulating hormone occur and in the third trimester an increase in pituitary beta-endorphin and spinal endorphins is detected. Endorphin increase is linked to the increase in pain threshold in the latter part of pregnancy (Henderson & Macdonald 2004). The posterior pituitary increases secretion of oxytocin but antidiuretic hormone (ADH) levels are similar to non-pregnant levels. However, the osmoreceptors in the hypothalamus are adjusted to the lower osmotic pressure of pregnancy (Blackburn 2003).

Not all hormones are increased. Levels of gonadotrophins (FSH and LH) are depressed via negative feedback due to the increasing levels of steroid hormones (oestrogen and progesterone). This prevents further ovulation during pregnancy.

The adrenal gland increases corticosteroid (glucocorticoid and aldosterone) production. Cortisol, the main glucocorticoid, increases two- to three-fold by term, and the diurnal rhythm of release continues, with higher levels being secreted in the morning than in the evening.

Increases in corticosteroids have been linked to the formation of striae gravidarium or 'stretch marks'. The cause is unclear but may be related to reduced adhesiveness between collagen fibres and decreased collagen synthesis mediated by corticosteroids (Blackburn 2003). Glucocorticoids influence metabolism by stimulating the release of glucose stores into the plasma.

The thyroid gland increases in size in response to low levels of iodine in the blood. During pregnancy, iodine clearance by the kidneys is increased. As iodine is an essential component of the thyroid hormones (thyroxine (T_4) and triiodothyronine (T_3) this stimulates hypertrophy of the thyroid and an associated increase in release of T_3 and T_4. However, there is also increased circulating thyroxine-binding globulin during pregnancy, and therefore there is no actual increase in thyroid hormone activity (Blackburn 2003). In fact, women with preexisting hyperthyroidism may experience some relief of symptoms during pregnancy due to the increased thyroxine-binding globulin (Blackburn 2003). Increased release of parathyroid hormone facilitates increased calcium absorption from the gut and decreased excretion by the kidneys, and therefore increased calcium is available to the fetus.

Changes to the reproductive system

The reproductive system probably undergoes the most obvious changes associated with pregnancy. There is considerable enlargement of the uterus, softening of the cervix, engorgement of the vulva, and growth and development of the breasts. These changes are to accommodate the growing fetus and to prepare for birth and nutrition of the baby.

Uterus

Under the influence of oestrogen, the uterine muscle fibres undergo hypertrophy and hyperplasia, resulting in a spherical, thick-walled (25 mm) uterus by 20 weeks (Blackburn 2003). Following this, the uterus grows by distension as the growing fetus stretches the muscle fibres. During the third trimester, this results in a thinner-walled (5–10 mm) cylindrical-shaped uterus that is easily indented, the fetus is easily palpated and fetal movements are visible. The uterine mass increases from 50 grams pre-conception to approximately 950 grams at term, and the uterine cavity changes from a capacity of 10 mL to 5 L (Blackburn 2003).

The uterine muscle supports and protects the fetus. It has both contractile and elastic properties, which equips the uterus to accommodate growth during pregnancy and to generate tension during labour. The myometrium comprises four layers, which have different roles in preparing for birth:

- The inner, circular layer runs in a spiral around the cornua, lower uterine segment and cervix and stretches during labour.
- The middle, oblique layer contracts to expel the fetus and constrict blood vessels after the placenta is delivered.
- The two outer, longitudinal layers contract and shorten during labour to cause thickening of the upper segment,

which maximises the expulsive force exerted on the baby during labour.

The different layers of muscle have different embryonic origins and may respond differently to uterotonic agonists and antagonists (Blackburn 2003). Uterine muscle is sparsely innervated by adrenergic neurons, which disappear from the myometrium at term.

The lower uterine segment muscles are replaced by connective tissue and this enables stretching in late pregnancy. Uterine blood vessels hypertrophy and become more coiled up until 20 weeks, and then uncoiling occurs as the uterus distends. Stretching of the broad ligament may cause painful sensations during the second and third trimesters. While the myometrium is capable of spontaneous activity, progesterone, relaxin, nitric oxide and prostacyclin exert an inhibitory effect. However, as pregnancy progresses there is an increase in frequency of contractions, about 5% increase per week. Contractions are more common at night and least common in the early afternoon. Contractions in the second trimester are irregular and painless but may become uncomfortable during the third trimester. The changes in character of the contractions are due to structural and functional changes in the myometrium mediated by changing oestrogen and progesterone. Table 18.3 lists some of the key changes that occur as the uterus enlarges.

Cervix

The cervix is primarily composed of connective tissue covered in a thin layer of smooth muscle. Changes occur throughout pregnancy and by the second trimester the cervix becomes swollen as it softens and widens due to the effect of oestradiol, prostaglandins, progesterone, relaxin and nitric oxide on the collagen fibres and water content. These changes culminate in cervical ripening, in preparation for labour. A plug of thick mucus, or operculum, resulting from proliferation of the cervical mucosa and glands, protects the cervix from ascending infection (Coad & Dunstall 2001).

Vagina

Several changes to the vagina occur due to the effects of oestradiol, but primarily there is increased blood flow, leading to venous engorgement. There is marked shedding of superficial mucosal cells, which leads to increased vaginal discharge (leucorrhoea), and normal bacteria of the vagina (bacilli) interact with increased glycogen in the mucosal cells, increasing the acidity of the vagina. This provides protection against some pathogens but encourages *Candida albicans* and *Trichomonas vaginalis* (Stables & Rankin 2004).

Haematological changes

Major alterations to the composition of blood occur during pregnancy. Changes protect against the normal blood loss of around 500 mL that occurs at delivery, maintain cardiac output despite widespread vasodilation, promote rapid haemostasis during placental separation, and increase protection against bacterial infection. These normal changes are reflected in blood screening results.

Haemodilution

Blood volume increases by 30% to 50% (1200 mL to 1500 mL) between about 7 and 34 weeks gestation, but there can be considerable individual variation, as some women have a minimal increase and others up to a two-fold increase (Blackburn 2003). The additional blood volume is accommodated in the uterus, breasts, muscles, kidneys and skin. It is important to note that the plasma increases at a faster rate than the cellular components. This leads to haemodilution, which is reflected in decreased concentration of many elements, such as haemoglobin, immunoglobulins, platelets and plasma proteins.

Plasma volume begins to increase at around seven weeks and increases very rapidly during the second trimester, reaching a 40% to 50% increase by week 28 to 32 (Blackburn 2003). Increasing oxygen demand due to the growing tissues and increased metabolism stimulates erythropoiesis. This

TABLE 18.3	**Stages of uterine development**
Week of gestation	**Characteristic uterine changes**
12	• Uterus rises out of the pelvis in an upright position, often to the right • Cervical isthmus stretches • Fundus can be palpated abdominally above symphysis pubis
20	• Uterus becomes thicker and rounded • Fallopian tubes become more vertically positioned
30	• Lower uterine segment can be identified
36	• Uterus reaches the xiphisternum • Fetus moves down into the lower region of the uterus

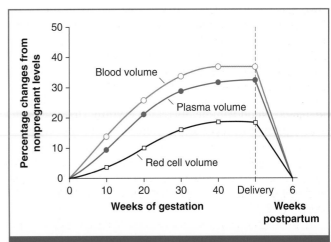

Figure 18.26 Changes in blood volume, plasma volume and red blood cell volume during pregnancy and post partum (based on Blackburn 2003)

increases more slowly and only reaches about a 30% increase in red cell volume (to 1700 mL), thus remaining less than the total plasma increase (Fig 18.26). The resulting haemodilution decreases the blood viscosity by 20%, which has the advantage of decreasing the workload of the heart.

Haemoglobin concentration falls as a result of haemodilution, from a range of 115–160 g/L in a non-pregnant woman to 100–150 g/L in a pregnant woman (Gill et al 2000). Although a decrease in haemoglobin concentration is a normal consequence of haemodilution, there are also increased requirements for iron during pregnancy, to meet the demands of increased erythropoiesis (iron is an essential component of haemoglobin) and the needs of the growing fetus. Plasma iron can be increased by dietary intake, mobilisation of iron stores and increased maternal absorption of iron in the intestines, particularly in the latter stages. This mirrors the increased transfer to the fetus at this time. Serum ferritin levels also fall as stored iron is released from the liver, spleen and bone marrow to boost haemoglobin levels. If a woman's iron stores are not adequate at the start of pregnancy, a deficiency may lead to decreased erythropoiesis, as fetal needs are met at the expense of maternal needs for iron. There is considerable controversy as to whether iron supplements are required to meet the increased demands.

White cell count, particularly the neutrophil count, increases during pregnancy to give more protection against bacterial infections. However, the concentration of immunoglobulins (IgA, IgG, IgM) decreases due to haemodilution and suppression of the immune system.

Plasma proteins also increase but haemodilution lowers the concentration, particularly of albumin, which lowers the osmotic pressure of the plasma. This means there is a greater tendency for fluid movement to the interstitial compartment, and this coupled with the increased water retention mediated by oestrogen leads to an increased possibility of oedema.

Changes to blood coagulability

Clotting factors such as fibrinogen, factors VII, VIII and X increase, and this leads to hypercoagulability of the blood, despite a decrease in platelet count (due to haemodilution). Coagulation times decrease by about 30% near the end of pregnancy (Coad & Dunstall 2001). Coagulation is further enhanced by decreased fibrinolytic activity, which continues until after the birth of the baby.

The haematological changes of pregnancy result in an increased blood volume, increased erythrocytes, leucocytes and coagulation factors, although the greater increase in plasma leads to decreased concentration of many components. Abnormalities in the increases of plasma or cellular constituents may flag underlying pathology; for example, pre-eclampsia is associated with smaller than usual increases in plasma volume (Blackburn 2003).

Cardiovascular system

Plasma volume increases as a result of increased activity of the renin-angiotensin system and of oestrogens, which increase fluid retention by the kidneys. Cardiac output (CO) increases by 30–50% due to this increased blood volume (Blackburn 2003)—an increase from an average of 5 L/min at 10 weeks to approximately 6.5 L/min at 25 weeks. Increased CO is largely determined by increases in stroke volume (30% increase), but the heart rate also increases by 15% (Blackburn 2003). Despite these changes in CO, blood pressure remains the same or drops slightly. This is due to the decrease in total peripheral resistance (TPR) facilitated by the actions of progesterone. Progesterone causes the smooth muscle in the arterial walls to relax, thus enabling vasodilation. Mean arterial pressure is determined by the cardiac output and the total peripheral resistance, and therefore an increase in CO accompanied by a decrease in TPR results in reasonably constant blood pressure. Smooth muscle in the walls of the veins similarly relaxes, increasing the venous capacity by as much as a litre.

Blood flow distribution

As the blood volume increases during pregnancy, it is distributed such that the uterus receives the greatest amount, with an increase from 50 mL/min at 10 weeks to 500 mL/min at term (Blackburn 2003). Eighty per cent of the uterine blood

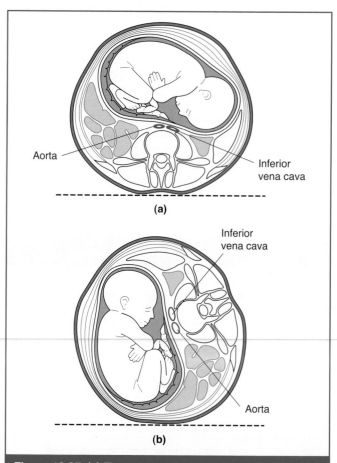

Figure 18.27 (a) The pregnant uterus compressing the aorta and the inferior vena cava. **(b)** Lying on the side changes the position of the uterus and relieves aortocaval compression (based on Blackburn 2003).

supply is directed to the intervillous spaces of the placenta to meet fetal requirements (see section on placental function).

Early in pregnancy there is a significant decrease in the resistance of renal blood vessels, leading to the kidneys accommodating increased CO before the reproductive structures. This decrease in resistance reaches a maximum by eight weeks, and may be under the influence of hCG (Stables & Rankin 2004). Skin and mucous membranes receive up to a 70% increase in blood flow by the 36th week. This can contribute to heat intolerance, sweating and nasal congestion. Nasal congestion and changes in upper airway patency may lead to increased snoring during pregnancy (Izci et al 2005).

The supine position has a marked effect on CO, especially in later pregnancy when the weight of the uterus is greater. By the third trimester, the supine position results in compression of the vena cava by the uterus, leading to decreased venous return and hence CO (Fig 18.27). A change from lying on the side to lying supine can result in a 25–30% decrease in CO (Blackburn 2003).

Respiratory system

Several factors influence ventilation during pregnancy. These include an increase in the basal metabolic rate, leading to increased oxygen consumption (20%) and carbon dioxide production, and increased sensitivity of the chemoreceptors to $PaCO_2$, an effect due to progesterone. The result is an increase in ventilation of 40% from 7 L/min to 10 L/min, contributed mainly by an increase in tidal volume of 25–40%. The increased ventilatory drive from increased chemoreceptor sensitivity leads to hyperventilation—that is, ventilation greater than metabolic need—and this may also account for the sensation of dyspnoea sometimes encountered during pregnancy (Blackburn 2003). Anatomical changes include flaring of the ribs and a raised position of the diaphragm (4 cm) due to uterine enlargement. Functional residual capacity (volume of air left in the lungs at the end of expiration) and residual volume (volume remaining in the lungs at the end of a forced expiration) are both decreased.

During sleep, changes in ventilatory drive and metabolic rate, reduced residual volume and changes in upper airway patency may increase the risk of sleep-disordered breathing. There is currently considerable research interest in Australasia and internationally in a possible link between sleep-disordered breathing, which can be indicated by snoring, and pre-eclampsia (Edwards et al 2002; Guilleminault et al 2000). A greater frequency of snoring has been found among women with pre-eclampsia (controls 32%, pregnant women 55%, women with pre-eclampsia 85%) ($P < 0.001$) (Izci et al 2005).

Renal system

The renal system must handle the increased metabolic wastes of the mother and the wastes from fetal metabolism. Renal function involves the processes of filtration, reabsorption and secretion, all of which are altered to some extent during pregnancy. Glomerular filtration rate (GFR) increases up to 40–50% in the first trimester, and falls significantly in the last three to four weeks (Blackburn 2003). The increase is a result of increased renal blood flow, facilitated by decreased renal vascular resistance. Reabsorption of electrolytes is increased as activity of the renin–angiotensin–aldosterone system increases, due to oestrogen and progesterone stimulation. This prevents excessive loss of sodium and other solutes and may balance the faster excretion rate. Glycosuria is common. Glucose reabsorption depends on a carrier mechanism in the renal tubules. At high glomerular filtration rates this mechanism can become saturated, leaving glucose in the filtrate to be excreted from the body. Proteinuria at levels of 0.3 g/day is also common, probably linked with increased leakiness of the glomerulus. Renal clearance of many substances (e.g. creatinine and iodine) increases, partly due to the increased GFR.

Progesterone is responsible for dilatation and possible kinking of the ureters from 10 weeks. By term the ureters can hold 300 mL of urine. Progesterone also causes dilation of the renal pelvis, with a resultant increased capacity from 12 mL to 75 mL. Relaxation of the smooth muscle in the bladder can lead to urinary stasis and, along with dilatation of the ureters, leads to a greater risk of infection during pregnancy.

Increased frequency of micturition is normal in early pregnancy due to the increased renal plasma flow and increased excretion by the kidneys. It is also normal later in pregnancy due to the pressure of the fetus and uterus on the bladder.

Skeletal system

Progesterone relaxes ligaments and muscles, with maximum effect in the last weeks when the pelvic capacity increases. In particular, the symphysis pubis, sacroiliac and sacrococcygeal joints soften and facilitate widening of the pelvis. The increased mobility of the joints also allows the coccyx to be pushed out of the way during labour.

Integumentary system

Melanocyte-stimulating hormone increases during pregnancy and causes deeper pigmentation of the skin. This can lead to a patchy mask on the face called chloasma, or a pigmented line on the abdomen from the pubis to the umbilicus, called linea nigra. The areola darkens and toughens, as does the perineum, which can also stretch more. In many areas of the body, stretching occurs in the collagen layer of the skin where adipose tissue is most concentrated (e.g. breasts, abdomen and thighs). Stretch marks, striae gravidarium, occur as red stripes and may result from the increased corticosteroids (see earlier section on corticosteroids).

Gastrointestinal system

Pregnancy can result in a number of minor discomforts associated with the digestive system. These are mainly a result of the effect of progesterone.

Gums

Fluid retention in the connective tissue of the gums can lead to a 'spongy' feeling and increased vascularity can result in increased bleeding of the gums during pregnancy.

Effect of progesterone on smooth muscle

Oesophageal sphincter malfunction allows oesophageal reflux of stomach contents, resulting in heartburn. This is exacerbated by higher intra-abdominal pressure in later pregnancy.

Lowered stomach tone and motility (peristalsis) and reduced gastric secretion means food stays in the stomach longer (up to 48 hours during labour). This may be worsened by narcotics. It should be noted that drugs given orally (e.g anticonvulsants) may not be absorbed adequately.

Nausea and vomiting may result from a combination of effects, such as decreased peristalsis and increased intra-abdominal pressure. High levels of hCG and sex steroids may also play a role by stimulating the vomiting centre receptors in the medulla.

A lower rate of peristalsis in the intestines facilitates increased absorption of nutrients, but the increased transit time and subsequent increased water reabsorption in the large intestine may lead to constipation. Compression and displacement of the bowel by the enlarging uterus may aggravate the situation.

Summary of maternal changes in pregnancy

- Maternal changes associated with pregnancy are largely mediated by the steroid hormones, initially from the corpus luteum maintained by hCG, and later from the placenta.
- Other hormones such as hPL, cortisol and aldosterone, mediate many changes.
- Under the influence of oestrogen and progesterone the uterus increases in size, with increased glandular secretions and increased vascularisation. Spontaneous myometrial contractions are largely suppressed by progesterone and other uterotonic inhibitors. The cervix softens as adhesion between collagen bundles is reduced and it is infiltrated by water.
- Oestrogen and the renin–angiotensin system increase sodium and water retention throughout pregnancy, increasing the blood volume by 40%. Plasma volume increases more than the red cell volume, resulting in haemodilution.

- Despite increases in haemoglobin, albumin and immunoglobulins etc, there is a decrease in the concentration of these blood components. Decreased albumin concentration results in decreased colloid osmotic pressure and possible oedema. A state of hypercoagulability exists due to increased coagulation factors.
- Progesterone-mediated vasodilation leads to reduced total peripheral resistance and this more than compensates for the effects of increased blood volume. Blood pressure does not normally increase. The increase in cardiac output is due to an increase in both stroke volume and heart rate. A redistribution of blood flow sends approximately 20% of the CO to the uterus, with 80% of this serving the placenta.
- Changes to the ribcage facilitate ventilation. Progesterone and oestrogen increase sensitivity of the respiratory centre to CO_2, resulting in mild hyperventilation. Tidal volume increases to supply increased O_2 to meet increased metabolic needs, and residual volume is reduced.
- Increased GFR leads to increased micturition early in pregnancy. Renin–angiotensin leads to retention of sodium and water. Mild glycosuria, proteinuria and increased clearance of creatinine result from normal changes in renal function. Smooth muscle relaxation, mediated by progesterone, can lead to stasis of urine and increased risk of urinary tract infection.
- Progesterone-mediated smooth muscle relaxation leads to many of the minor discomforts of pregnancy (e.g. oesophageal reflux, constipation, backache). hCG may be linked to feelings of nausea.
- Modifications of the woman's physiology during pregnancy allow her to meet the many needs of the fetus (including cardiorespiratory, nutritional, metabolic and renal) without compromise to her own wellbeing, and to prepare for birth.

Conclusion

Adaptations by the woman's physiology during pregnancy allow her to support the developing fetus to grow into a healthy baby while maintaining her own wellbeing. Near term especially, there are considerable challenges in meeting, in particular, the respiratory, nutritional, metabolic and renal needs of the fetus without compromise to the woman. Pregnancy also prepares the woman and the fetus for birth.

Review questions

Reproductive systems

1 Describe the changes in motility and maturation that occur in spermatozoa, from the time they leave the seminiferous tubules until they are ejaculated.

2 Outline the action of the combined oestrogen/progesterone contraceptive pill with reference to the hypothalamic-pituitary-ovarian (HPO) axis.

3 Outline the steps involved in the change from a primary oocyte to a secondary oocyte.

Conception and implantation

4 List three physiological factors that promote successful fertilisation.

5 Compare a morula with a blastocyst.

6 Compare the synctiotrophoblast with the cytotrophoblast.

Embryology

7 Outline the difference between a blastocyst and an embryo in their susceptibility to teratogenic agents.

8 Describe the process of gastrulation, name the layers of germ cells present in the trilaminar disc and name one function of the notochord.

9 List the key changes in the lungs and pulmonary circulation between 24 and 32 weeks gestation.

Placenta

10 Draw a flow diagram identifying the key steps involved as the trophoblast differentiates into a functioning placenta.

11 Outline the barriers a molecule of O_2 must pass as it diffuses from the maternal lacuna to the fetal chorionic villus.

12 Describe the key anatomical structures that make up the uteroplacental circulation.

Fetal circulation

13 The fetal oxyhaemoglobin curve is shifted to the left of the adult curve. What advantage to the fetus is depicted by this?

14 Describe the factors that enhance fetal oxygen-carrying capacity.

15 Name each of the vessels that transport blood from the fetus to the placental circulation and back, i.e. along the umbilical cord, through the chorionic villi and back to the fetus.

Maternal changes of pregnancy

16 Outline the contribution of the fetus to the synthesis of oestriol.

17 Why is an increased frequency of micturition likely in both the first and third trimesters?

18 Provide a physiological explanation for mild glycosuria and proteinuria that are common in pregnancy.

Synthesis questions

1 Discuss physiological and anatomical aspects of the uterus that make it a suitable organ for supporting and nurturing an embryo/fetus.

2 Explain the advantages to the embryo of developing a circulatory system. How is nutrition provided prior to this?

3 Identify three potential teratogens. Identify the stage of pregnancy at which exposure to the teratogens would be most damaging. Describe the likely congenital abnormalities that would result from this exposure.

4 Draw a labelled diagram illustrating a three-week-old embryo and the associated cavities and membranes.

5 Describe anatomical features specific to the fetal circulation and the contribution they make to effective gas exchange in utero.

6 Summarise the key information that is depicted in an oxyhaemoglobin dissociation curve.

7 Outline the ways in which human placental lactogen (HPL) changes maternal metabolism to facilitate fetal growth.

8 Outline the physiological reasons that women are more at risk of deep vein thrombosis (DVT), a coagulation defect, during pregnancy.

9 Account for the increased blood volume during pregnancy. Outline the effect this has on cardiac function and any other physiological changes that affect blood pressure during pregnancy.

10 Account for the increased glomerular filtration rate that occurs during pregnancy.

Online resources

Arizona Center for Reproductive Endocrinology and Infertility, http://www.infertility-azctr.com/art.html This website offers explanations for common procedures for assisted reproduction.

Bauer B 2002 Hormones of pregnancy, http://www.rnceus.com/course_frame.asp?exam_id=29&directory=hormone This website is a mini-course on hormones and pregnancy. There is a good animation of the female reproductive cycle and another of implantation.

Indiana University, interactive website on fetal and neonatal circulation, http://www.indiana.edu/~anat550/cvanim/fetcirc/fetcirc.html

References

Barker DJ 2004 The developmental origins of chronic adult disease. Acta Paediatrica (Supplement) 93(446):26–33

Blackburn S 2003 Maternal, fetal and neonatal physiology: a clinical perspective (2nd edn). WB Saunders, London

Bray JJ, Cragg PA, Macknight AD et al 1994 Lecture notes on human physiology (3rd edn). Blackwell Scientific, Oxford

Chaddha V, Viero S, Huppertz B et al 2004 Developmental biology of the placenta and the origins of placental insufficiency. Seminars in Fetal and Neonatal Medicine 9(5):357–369

Coad J, Dunstall M 2001 Anatomy and physiology for midwives. Mosby, Edinburgh

Edwards N, Middleton PG, Blyton DM et al 2002 Sleep disordered breathing and pregnancy. Thorax 57(6):555–558

Gaunt G, Ramin K 2001 Immunological tolerance of the human fetus. American Journal of Perinatology 18(6):299–312

Gill M, Ockelford P, Morris A et al 2000 The Interpretation of Laboratory Tests (3rd edn). Diagnostic Laboratory Holdings Ltd, Auckland. Online: http://www.dml.co.nz/hbook/index.htm

Gooi A, Oei J, Lui K 2003 Attitudes of Level II obstetricians towards the care of the extremely premature infant: a national survey. Journal of Paediatric Child Health 39(6):451–455

Guilleminault C, Querra-Salva MSC, Poyares D 2000 Normal pregnancy, daytime sleeping, snoring and blood pressure. Sleep Medicine 1(14):289–297

Henderson C, Macdonald S 2004 Mayes' Midwifery. A textbook for Midwives (13th edn). Baillière Tindall, Edinburgh

Izci B, Martin SE, Dundas KC et al 2005 Sleep complaints: snoring and daytime sleepiness in pregnant and pre-eclamptic women. Sleep Medicine 6(2):163–169

Jaffe R, Jauniaux E, Hustin J 1997 Maternal circulation in the first-trimester human placenta—myth or reality? American Journal of Obstetrics and Gynecology 176(3):695–705

Johnson MH, Everitt BJ 2000 Essential reproduction (5th edn). Blackwell Science, Oxford

Kajantie E, Osmond C, Barker DJ et al 2005 Size at birth as a predictor of mortality in adulthood: a follow-up of 350 000 person-years. International Journal of Epidemiology (in press)

Moore K, Persaud T 1998 Before we are born: essentials of embryology and birth defects (5th edn). WB Saunders, London

Oei J, Askie LM, Tobiansky R et al 2000 Attitudes of neonatal clinicians towards resuscitation of the extremely premature infant: an exploratory survey. Journal of Paediatric and Child Health 36(4):357–362

Reis FM, Florio P, Cobellis L et al 2001 Human placenta as a source of neuroendocrine factors. Biology of the Neonate 79(3/4):150–157

Sadler TW 1990 Longman's medical embryology (6th edn). Williams & Wilkins, Baltimore

Sentilhes L, Verspyck E, Patrier S et al 2003 Amniotic band syndrome: pathogenesis, prenatal diagnosis and neonatal management. Journal of Gynecology, Obstetrics and Biological Reproduction (Paris) 32(8):693–704

Shah C, Modi D, Gadkar S et al C 2003 Progesterone receptors on human spermatozoa. Indian Journal of Experimental Biology 41(7):773–780

Shier D, Butler J, Lewis R 2002 Hole's human anatomy and physiology (9th edn). McGraw Hill, Boston

Stables D, Rankin J 2004 Physiology in childbearing with anatomy and related biosciences (2nd edn). Elsevier, London

Sun F, Bahat A, Gakamsky A et al 2005 Human sperm chemotaxis: both the oocyte and its surrounding cumulus cells secrete sperm chemoattractants. Human Reproduction 20(3):761–767

Further reading

Blackburn S 2003 Maternal, fetal and neonatal physiology: a clinical perspective (2nd edn). WB Saunders, London

Chaddha V, Viero S, Huppertz B et al 2004 Developmental biology of the placenta and the origins of placental insufficiency. Seminars in Fetal and Neonatal Medicine 9(5):357–369

Gaunt G, Ramin K 2001 Immunological tolerance of the human fetus. American Journal of Perinatology 18(6):299–312

Herrler A, von Rango U, Beier HM 2003 Embryo-maternal signaling: how the embryo starts talking to its mother to accomplish implantation. Reproductive Biomedicine Online 6(2):244–256

Moore K, Persaud T 1989 Before we are born: basic embryology and birth defects (3rd edn). WB Saunders, London

Stables D, Rankin J 2004 Physiology in childbearing with anatomy and related biosciences (2nd edn). Elsevier, London

CHAPTER 19

Nutritional foundation for pregnancy, childbirth and lactation

Sandra L Elias

Key terms

body mass index, essential fats, gastro-oesophageal reflux, gestational diabetes mellitus, iron deficiency anaemia, long chain polyunsaturated fatty acids, nausea and vomiting in pregnancy

Chapter overview

This chapter outlines the importance of good nutrition during pregnancy in order to promote the growth and development of the fetus and maternal tissues, and to support the demands of childbirth and lactation. Dietary strategies found to alleviate some of the conditions associated with pregnancy and lactation such as constipation, gastro-oesophageal reflux, nausea, gestational diabetes, food-borne illness and allergy prevention are included. The chapter is intended to provide midwives with an understanding of the role of nutrients in pregnancy, childbirth and lactation, to identify appropriate dietary sources of these nutrients, and to present practical dietary strategies during pregnancy and lactation.

Learning outcomes

Learning outcomes for this chapter are:

1 To recognise the importance of weight gain during pregnancy and the use of body mass index for underweight and overweight women

2 To discuss the role and dietary sources of macronutrients in pregnancy and lactation

3 To discuss the role and dietary sources of key micronutrients essential for pregnancy and lactation

4 To explain how diet can alleviate some of the common conditions experienced in pregnancy, such as anaemia, nausea and vomiting, constipation and gastro-oesophageal reflux

5 To explain the role of nutrition in gestational diabetes mellitus

6 To explain the risk of food-borne illness in pregnancy and to recognise the importance of food safety in pregnancy

7 To recognise the special nutritional needs of pregnant adolescents and multiple pregnancies

8 To emphasise the importance of hydration and nourishment for childbirth and to recognise appropriate foods and drinks to consume in childbirth

9 To discuss the role of energy intake and output and their effects on lactation

10 To explain the role and limitations of allergy prevention during lactation.

Weight gain

A woman's appetite during pregnancy typically governs when she wishes to eat. Although the phrase 'eating for two' is often used as an excuse to eat ad libitum during pregnancy, this may result in unnecessary weight gain leading to maternal complications such as elevated blood pressure and insulin resistance.

Weight gain recommendations for pregnancy are based on women's pre-pregnancy weight. The body mass index (BMI) is typically used as an indicator of body fat and although this measurement is not valid during pregnancy, a woman's pre-pregnancy BMI can be used to recommend total weight gain during pregnancy (Table 19.1).

For women in the healthy BMI range, an average weight gain of 11.5–16 kg is recommended. Women in the healthy BMI range tend to gain an appropriate amount of weight during pregnancy. However, women who are underweight pre-pregnancy have increased rates of pregnancy loss and small for gestational age or low birthweight infants. It has been suggested that these risks are simply due to a lack of maternal energy stores (Rush 2001). Therefore, weight gain for these women tends to be higher than for women with healthy pre-pregnancy BMI (12.5–18 kg). Women who are overweight pre-pregnancy are at increased risk of developing gestational diabetes and hypertensive disorders or undergoing caesarean section, with the accompanying anaesthetic and postoperative risk (Rush 2001). The recommended weight gain for women with a BMI > 25 is less than for women with a healthy pre-pregnancy BMI (7–11.5 kg).

Women who fall below or above the normal BMI range pre-pregnancy should have weight gain monitored to ensure that an appropriate weight gain occurs—one that does not increase maternal or fetal risks.

Macronutrients

Fats

During pregnancy, fat plays an important role not only as an important energy source but also as a contributor of the fat-soluble vitamins (A, D, E and K) and various polyunsaturated fats required for growth and development.

Linoleic acid, an omega-6 fat, and alpha-linolenic acid, an omega-3 fat, are essential fats required for growth and development. These fats cannot be synthesised by the body and therefore must be consumed in our diet from plant foods.

One of the primary functions of these fats is to produce long-chain polyunsaturated fats (LCPs), which are found in particularly high concentrations in the central nervous system and retina. LCPs are also consumed in our diet, particularly in meat, dairy and fatty fish (Table 19.2). Vegetarians who exclude all animal products from their diet must therefore ensure an adequate intake of essential fats in order to produce LCPs.

Each of the essential fats is responsible for producing one or more specific LCPs (Fig 19.1). Two of the LCPs, specifically arachidonic acid (AA) and eicosapentaenoic acid (EPA), are precursors to a group of hormone-like compounds called eicosanoids. Eicosanoids have an important role in maintaining blood pressure and haemostasis, in inflammation and in parturition. The eicosanoids produced from AA promote vasoconstriction, platelet aggregation and inflammation, whereas the eicosanoids produced from EPA promote vasodilation, inhibit platelet aggregation and reduce

TABLE 19.1 Recommended weight gain during pregnancy based on pre-pregnancy BMI

Pre-pregnancy BMI	Recommended weight gain (kg)
Underweight: < 19.8	12.5–18
Healthy: 19.8–26	11.5–16
Overweight: > 26	7.0–11.5

BMI (body mass index) is calculated as weight (kg) / height squared (m^2). (Source: National Research Council 1990)

TABLE 19.2 Dietary sources of essential and long-chain polyunsaturated fats

Fat	Dietary sources
Essential fats	
Linoleic acid (LA)	Seeds and nuts, vegetable oils, soft margarines
Alpha-linolenic acid (LNA)	Canola and flaxseed oil, walnuts, peanuts, pecans
Long-chain polyunsaturated fats	
Arachidonic acid (AA)	Meat, eggs, milk, cheese, yoghurt
Eicosapentaenoic acid (EPA)	Fatty fish (salmon, tuna, mackerel, herring, sardines)
Docosahexaenoic acid (DHA)	Fatty fish (salmon, tuna, mackerel, herring, sardines)

inflammation. During parturition, the eicosanoids produced from AA appear to enhance the breakdown of collagen fibres within the cervix, whereas the eicosanoids produced from EPA tend to inhibit this process (Allen & Harris 2001).

In Northern European countries, where the intake of fatty fish, and therefore EPA, is high, the incidence of preterm birth is low. This has sparked considerable research into the effect of EPA on parturition, specifically in women at risk of preterm labour. The results of these studies suggest that supplementation with EPA or consumption of fish 2–3 times/week may reduce the risk of preterm labour in some groups of women (Olsen et al 2000; Olsen & Secher 2002).

One concern that arises with recommendations to increase fish consumption during pregnancy is the amount of mercury present in some fish species. Larger fish tend to accumulate mercury. Food Standards Australia New Zealand (FSANZ) has specific recommendations regarding fish consumption, mercury levels and pregnancy (Table 19.3) (FSANZ 2004).

Carbohydrates

Carbohydrates are a major energy source during pregnancy and lactation. There are various classes of carbohydrates, including simple sugars and complex carbohydrates. Simple sugars are present in fruit (fructose), milk (lactose), and table sugar (sucrose). Glucose, another simple sugar, is the body's major energy source and the most abundant carbohydrate. Glucose is also the building block for complex carbohydrates or, more specifically, the starches. Starches are a storage form of carbohydrate present in plants such as grains, legumes and root vegetables. In addition to simple and complex carbohydrates, dietary fibre may be considered a type of carbohydrate. Unlike simple sugars and starches, the human body lacks the necessary enzymes required to break down dietary fibre. Dietary fibre can be classified as either soluble or insoluble. Foods rich in soluble fibre include fruits and vegetables, oats, barley and legumes, whereas foods rich in insoluble fibre include wheat, corn, whole grains and most vegetables. The benefits of dietary fibre include increased satiety, regular bowel movements and a reduction in blood cholesterol levels.

Although carbohydrates should account for the majority of energy intake during pregnancy, the type of carbohydrate consumed is also important, to prevent large fluctuations in blood glucose levels. The rate at which dietary carbohydrate, specifically glucose, is absorbed into the bloodstream can be measured and is referred to as the glycaemic index. Some carbohydrates present in food are rapidly digested in the digestive tract, thereby entering circulation quickly. This can result in a large increase in blood glucose followed by a sudden drop in blood glucose. Foods containing these types of carbohydrates are referred to as having a high glycaemic index value. In contrast, some carbohydrates are digested more slowly, allowing for a slow and steady rise in blood glucose that is not followed by a sudden drop in blood glucose levels. Foods containing these types of carbohydrates are referred to as having a low glycaemic index value. For sustained energy, foods with a low glycaemic index value are recommended.

Protein

Protein, like carbohydrate and fat, is a macronutrient and therefore can provide energy. The body, however, spares protein for energy in order to utilise it for its many other roles. These include its role as a structural component of muscle, connective tissue and bone, ensuring fluid balance and blood pressure, enzymatic activity, transporting substances throughout the body, and formation of hormones and antibodies.

During pregnancy the requirement for dietary protein is slightly higher than in pre-pregnancy, to account for the development of maternal and fetal tissues. The protein requirements are based on body weight; for every kilogram of body weight a non-pregnant woman should consume 0.75 g of protein. Pregnant women should include an additional 6 g of protein/day above the recommendation for non-pregnant women (National Health and Medical Research Council (NHMRC) 1992).

TABLE 19.3 Recommendations for fish intake during pregnancy

Country	Recommended intake
Australia[1]	2–3 serves per week of any fish or seafood not listed below (1 serve = 150 g) OR 1 serve per week of orange roughy (deep sea perch) or catfish and no other fish that week OR 1 serve per fortnight of shark (flake) or billfish (swordfish/broadbill and marlin) and no other fish that fortnight
New Zealand[2]	Consume fish but limit intake of the following species to no more than 4 servings per week (1 serve = 150 g): shark (flake), ray, swordfish, southern blue fin tuna, orange roughy, ling, barramundi, gemfish

1. Source: Food Standards Australia and New Zealand 2004.
2. Source: Food Standards Australia and New Zealand 2001.

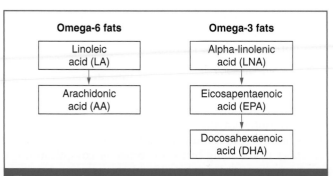

Figure 19.1 Conversion of the essential fats into long-chain polyunsaturated fats (based on Allen & Harris 2001)

Despite limited evidence, high-protein diets have been suggested to help minimise the risk of pre-eclampsia. The World Health Organization does not support these diets and clearly states that in the absence of a protein deficiency, protein supplementation is unlikely to reduce a woman's risk of developing pre-eclampsia (Kramer & Kakuma 2004). Given the high intakes of protein in both Australia and New Zealand, pregnant women are likely to be consuming more than their recommended intake of protein (Australian Bureau of Statistics 1995; Ministry of Health 1999).

Dietary intake of protein is important to ensure that the body has the correct mix of amino acids, the building blocks of protein. There are 20 amino acids, of which nine are considered essential. The body is unable to produce essential amino acids in adequate amounts and therefore they must be obtained from dietary sources. Animal proteins contain all nine essential amino acids, whereas plant proteins are limited in at least one. In the past, vegetarians were encouraged to combine protein sources within a meal to ensure intake of all the essential amino acids. It is now known that the body pools the essential amino acids within a 24-hour period and draws from that pool when needed. Therefore, combining proteins at each meal is not necessary, and by consuming a variety of plant sources such as whole grains, nuts, seeds, legumes and vegetables throughout the day, an adequate intake of essential amino acids should be achieved.

Micronutrients: minerals

There are many minerals that the human body requires to perform a variety of important functions. Only those with a significant role during pregnancy will be highlighted in this chapter.

Iron

Iron is an important mineral present within the haem structure of haemoglobin. In any anabolic condition, such as pregnancy, the increased demands for haemoglobin result in increased demands for iron. During pregnancy, as well as in childhood, intestinal absorption of iron increases to help meet these demands. Despite enhanced absorption during pregnancy, iron deficiency and iron deficiency anaemia still occur in many pregnant women.

Iron is present in food in two forms, haem and non-haem iron. Haem iron is the form present in meat, poultry and fish, as a component of haemoglobin. Non-haem iron is also present in meat, poultry and fish but is the only form found in plant foods, fortified foods and supplements.

Although iron is present in many foods, not all the iron is absorbed and used by the body. Haem iron is more readily absorbed in the intestine than non-haem iron. Up to one-third of haem iron is absorbed, whereas the absorption of non-haem iron can vary from 2% to 20% (Hambraeus 1999). Including foods rich in vitamin C increases the absorption of non-haem iron by keeping iron in a more readily absorbable form, ferrous iron. Consumption of meat, poultry or fish with non-haem iron also enhances iron absorption. In addition to these enhancers or promoters of iron absorption, there are several factors that inhibit iron absorption. Tannins, present in coffee, tea and red wine, have been reported to reduce iron absorption by up to 40%; therefore, it is recommended that these beverages be consumed two to three hours before or after a meal. Another inhibitor of iron absorption are phytates, phosphate-containing molecules present in legumes, nuts and whole grains that bind iron, rendering it unavailable for absorption. Soaking legumes, roasting nuts and fermenting whole grains decreases the phytate content of these foods, thereby decreasing their effect on iron absorption (Hallberg 2002). Finally, high doses of calcium (300 mg) or zinc (15 mg), such as the level present in supplements, consumed with iron-rich foods or iron supplements have been reported to inhibit iron absorption (Sandstrom 2001).

Calcium

Calcium is the most prevalent mineral in our body, with most of it contained within our skeleton. In addition to its structural role, it is involved in neural transmission, haemostasis and muscular contraction. Calcium may also play a role in regulating blood pressure. Several randomised controlled studies have explored the effect of calcium supplementation and incidence of hypertensive disorders in pregnant women. These studies suggest that women with previous pregnancy-induced hypertension or pre-eclampsia, women consuming low intakes of calcium (< 900 mg/day) and adolescents may reduce their risk of pre-eclampsia by 50–65% with daily supplements of 1–2 g of calcium (Atallah et al 2004; Ritchie & King 2000).

Calcium is present in many animal and plant foods (Table 19.4). As with iron, the bioavailability of calcium is much higher in animal foods such as milk, yoghurt and cheese than in plant foods. The calcium present in plant foods may also interact with various inhibitors including phytates, high doses of minerals such as iron, and oxalates. Oxalates are compounds present in foods such as spinach, rhubarb and chocolate. Like phytates, they bind calcium, rendering it unavailable for absorption in the intestinal tract.

Zinc

Zinc is an important component of over 80 enzymes involved in many reactions including cell replication and growth, regulation and expression of genes, optimal immune function and hormone activity. Findings from several observational studies suggest that zinc deficiency during pregnancy increases the incidence of neural tube defects, fetal death and malformations, low birthweight, premature rupture of membranes and increased antenatal and intrapartum complications. Of the 12 randomised controlled trials of zinc supplementation during pregnancy, only six reported an effect in reducing birth outcomes or complications. It has been suggested that zinc supplementation is beneficial in developing countries where zinc deficiency is widespread (King 2000; Shah & Sachhdev 2001).

TABLE 19.4 Dietary sources of iron and calcium		
Mineral	**Animal sources**	**Plant sources**
Iron	• Red meat (beef, venison) • Poultry • Fish and seafood • Eggs	• Legumes (kidney beans, chick peas, lentils, green peas, soy beans) • Tofu and other soy products • Wholegrain or fortified breads and breakfast cereals • Green leafy vegetables (silverbeet, spinach) • Dried fruits • Nuts (cashews, walnuts, peanuts) • Seeds (sunflower and sesame) • Blackstrap molasses • Marmite and Vegemite
Calcium	• Milk • Cheese • Yoghurt • Tinned fish with bones (salmon, sardines)	• Green leafy vegetables (spinach, cabbage, leeks, broccoli) • Peanuts, almonds and sesame seeds • Tofu • Soy milk

Dietary sources of zinc include protein-rich foods such as red meats, seafood, oysters and clams as well as whole grains, legumes, nuts, seeds and wheatgerm. Fruits and vegetables are poor sources of zinc.

Iodine

Iodine is an essential component of triiodothyronine and thyroxine, more commonly known as the thyroid hormones. These hormones regulate body temperature, basal metabolism, reproduction and growth. In pregnancy, iodine deficiency can affect both mother and fetus. Maternal goitre, an enlargement of the thyroid gland, develops when intakes of iodine are habitually low. If iodine deficiency occurs during pregnancy, neonatal cretinism can occur, resulting in stunted growth, mental deficiency, deafness, motor rigidity and possibly hypothyroidism.

Iodine is present in a limited number of foods. Fish, seafood and seaweeds are the richest natural sources of iodine in Australia and New Zealand. In Tasmania and inland regions of New Zealand, the iodine content of soil is very low. Therefore, plants grown in these areas tend to be poor sources of dietary iodine compared to other regions of Australia and New Zealand. In Australia, all table salt is fortified with iodine, whereas in New Zealand fortification of table salt with iodine is not mandatory. All fortified salt is labelled as iodised salt; however, some salts such as rock salt and sea salt do not contain iodine. Most food manufacturers in New Zealand do not use iodised salt and therefore processed foods are an unreliable source of iodine.

Micronutrients: vitamins

Folate

Folate is a generic term used to describe a collection of compounds, of which folic acid is the most stable and absorbable form. Folate is involved in cell replication and division, maturation of erythrocytes and amino acid metabolism. Folic acid also reduces the incidence of neural tube defects when taken prior to and following conception. Folate insufficiency has also been associated with cleft lip, cleft palate, placental abruption, low birthweight, miscarriage and Down syndrome. The recommendations for folate intake in women of childbearing age differ slightly between Australia and New Zealand (Table 19.5).

The term 'folate' is Latin for 'leaf'—one of the major sources of folate is dark, green leafy vegetables such as spinach, silver beet, broccoli and cabbage. Other sources include yeast extracts, whole grains, liver, kidney, asparagus, legumes and wheatgerm. Although folate is found naturally in a variety of foods, only 50–70% is absorbed and used by the body. Folic acid is not found naturally in the food supply but is the form added to breads or cereals as a fortificant and is the form present in supplements. At present, folic acid fortification is

TABLE 19.5 Folate recommendations for Australian and New Zealand women	
Australia	**New Zealand**
All women planning a pregnancy should supplement their diets with 500 µg of folic acid/day beginning one month prior to conception until 12 weeks gestation.	All women planning a pregnancy should supplement their diets with 800 µg of folic acid/day beginning one month prior to conception until 12 weeks gestation.
Women with a previous neural tube defect-affected pregnancy or with close family history of neural tube defect-affected pregnancy should supplement their diet with 5 mg of folic acid/day.	
(Sources: NHMRC 1993; Ministry of Health 1997)	

voluntary in Australia and New Zealand; however, there is a drive towards mandatory fortification as a means of reducing the incidence of neural tube defects.

Vitamin B_{12}

Vitamin B_{12} is involved in folate and fatty acid metabolism, and in the production of myelin. Unlike most water-soluble vitamins, it is stored within the liver for up to five years. A deficiency of vitamin B_{12}, however, can occur with strict vegetarians who eliminate all animal foods from their diet. If untreated, vitamin B_{12} deficiency leads to the degeneration of myelin, resulting in neuropathy and death.

Structures referred to as B_{12} analogues are present in seaweed, spirulina and bacterially fermented soy products such as miso and tempeh. These analogues have a similar structure to vitamin B_{12} but do not have the same metabolic function and therefore are not reliable dietary sources of vitamin B_{12}. Reliable dietary sources of vitamin B_{12} include meats, poultry, fish, seafood, dairy products and eggs. In addition to animal sources, some foods are fortified with vitamin B_{12} including soymilk, yeast extract spreads and nutritional yeasts. Strict vegetarians who consume few vitamin B_{12}-fortified foods should consider B_{12} supplementation.

Vitamin A

Vitamin A is a fat-soluble vitamin essential for vision, cellular differentiation, immune function and bone remodelling. Vitamin A is present in two forms—preformed vitamin A or provitamin A. Preformed vitamin A is present in animal products such as liver, eel, eggs and butter in the form of retinoids, whereas provitamin A, also referred to as carotenoids, is present only in plants. Carotenoids are found in plants of dark green and orange colour, including carrots, apricots, mangoes, pumpkin, silverbeet and spinach.

High intakes of preformed vitamin A from supplements during pregnancy have been associated with birth defects of the cranium, face, heart, kidney, thymus and central nervous system. The liver regulates the conversion of provitamin A into retinol, the body's preferred form of retinoid, based on metabolic need. Therefore, high intakes of provitamin A have not been associated with birth defects (Azais-Braesco & Pascal 2000).

The vitamin A content of most foods is quite low, but liver and liver products have considerably higher levels of this vitamin. Some supplements, such as fish liver oils, may also contain high doses of vitamin A. It is generally recommended that pregnant women avoid liver and liver products, and any supplements that contain more than the recommended nutrient intake of vitamin A, 800 retinol equivalents.

Vitamin D

Vitamin D, another fat-soluble vitamin, is essential for calcium absorption. It is formed in the body when 7-dehydrocholesterol, a steroid present in the skin, is converted to cholecalciferol in the presence of ultraviolet light. Enzymes within the liver and kidney convert cholecalciferol into active vitamin D, commonly referred to as calcitriol.

There are few dietary sources of vitamin D in Australia and New Zealand. Vitamin D is present in small amounts in fatty fish (herring, sardines, tuna and salmon), egg yolks, liver, butter, cheese and milks. It is also added to some full-fat milks and soft margarines. Because vitamin D can be formed by exposure to sunlight, there is no dietary recommendation for dietary vitamin D intake. With high rates of skin cancer, Australians and New Zealanders are encouraged to follow safe sun messages, critical in the prevention of skin cancer. This, however, may also limit production of vitamin D and increase the risk of vitamin D deficiency in some women. Poor vitamin D status has also been reported in dark-skinned and veiled women (Grover & Morley 2001; Nesby-O'Dell et al 2002).

During pregnancy the fetus is dependent on maternal supply for most nutrients, including vitamin D. Because of the role of vitamin D in calcium absorption and therefore skeletal development, it is critical that the mother consumes or produces adequate levels of vitamin D. A Cochrane Review of vitamin D supplementation during pregnancy concluded that there was insufficient evidence to evaluate the requirements and effects of vitamin D supplementation during pregnancy (Mahomed & Gulmezoglu 2004). There is recent concern, however, that the prevalence of vitamin D deficiency is increasing in many countries, including New Zealand. The effect of vitamin D deficiency during pregnancy warrants additional research.

Common conditions of pregnancy

Nausea and vomiting

One of the most common conditions of early pregnancy is nausea with or without vomiting. For most women, nausea and vomiting subsides by 12 weeks gestation; however, some women continue to experience nausea and vomiting throughout pregnancy. Although the aetiology of nausea and vomiting in pregnancy (NVP) is still unknown, there are dietary strategies that may alleviate NVP in some women. Feelings of hunger or dehydration have been associated with nausea and therefore, to prevent this, women are advised to eat small, frequent meals and snacks throughout the day and keep hydrated. A deficiency in vitamin B_6 and zinc has also been suggested to enhance NVP, although there is limited evidence to suggest that supplementation with these nutrients alleviates NVP. Consuming a variety of protein-rich foods will ensure adequate intakes of vitamin B_6 and zinc. The use of ginger, in powdered or syrup form, has been promoted as a safe and effective way to alleviate NVP (Fischer-Rasmussen 1991; Keating & Chez 2002).

Constipation

One of the consequences of elevated progesterone levels during pregnancy is enhanced smooth muscle relaxation. This occurs throughout the digestive system, reducing peristalsis and therefore intestinal motility. The prolonged transit time results in an increase in both electrolyte and water absorption, thereby reducing faecal water content and producing compact stools. In addition, the large intestine is compressed due to the growing uterus, which may contribute to increased pressure and strain during defecation. Dietary strategies to alleviate constipation include increased dietary fibre intake from wholegrain cereals and breads, dried fruits, fruit and vegetables with skin, brown rice and pasta, and legumes. Increasing dietary fibre without adequate fluid intake, however, can enhance the effects of constipation. Therefore, it is important to consume approximately two litres of fluid daily to promote regularity. In addition to diet, physical activity such as walking, housework, gardening and swimming may stimulate peristalsis, thereby alleviating constipation.

Gastro-oesophageal reflux

Gastro-oesophageal reflux (GOR), also referred to as heartburn, is a common condition in pregnancy. Due to elevated progesterone levels, the smooth muscle of the lower oesophageal sphincter is more relaxed than in non-pregnant women. This, along with increased intra-gastric pressure from the growing uterus, may result in the reflux of stomach contents into the oesophagus. Dietary strategies to alleviate GOR focus on reducing stomach volume and further relaxation of the lower oesophageal sphincter and increasing gastric motility. To reduce stomach volume, avoid eating and drinking at the same time, and consume small, frequent meals and snacks throughout the day. Some foods have been associated with GOR by decreasing gastric motility, thereby enhancing intra-gastric pressure, or enhancing relaxation of the lower oesophageal sphincter. These include fatty foods, milk, chocolate, spearmint, peppermint, caffeine, citrus fruits and juices, tomato products, pepper seasoning and alcohol.

Anaemia

As highlighted earlier, iron is an essential mineral required in the formation of haem. With increased tissue growth, the requirement for haemoglobin and therefore iron also increases. Despite an increased production of haemoglobin, the effects of haemodilution—an increase in plasma volume—results in lowered haemoglobin values. This is referred to as physiological anaemia and is normal in pregnancy. Further reductions in haemoglobin, however, may continue, indicative of poor iron intake and may lead to iron deficiency and iron deficiency anaemia (IDA).

Iron deficiency is characterised by the presence of low iron (ferritin) stores, and if untreated can lead to IDA. Iron deficiency anaemia, a reduction in circulating iron, is the most common form of anaemia worldwide. It is referred to as microcytic, hypochromic anaemia because of the presence of small, pale erythrocytes. Although there is evidence to suggest that IDA leads to poor birth outcome, such as low birthweight and increased infant mortality, not all trials have reported similar results.

Assessing iron status in pregnancy is important in order to prevent IDA. A drop in ferritin represents a fall in iron stores and is the first step towards IDA. Once ferritin levels fall, transport iron begins to drop, indicating a reduction in erythropoiesis. Finally, circulating haemoglobin falls, indicating IDA.

In some countries, such as the United States, routine iron supplementation is recommended during pregnancy. However, in Australia and New Zealand, iron supplementation in pregnancy is based on a woman's iron status. Good dietary advice should always be encouraged during pregnancy to promote good iron status (refer to Iron section); however, even with intense individual counselling, women with iron deficiency may experience difficulties in increasing iron status through diet alone (Heath et al 2001; Patterson et al 2001). Therefore, supplementation along with dietary advice may be necessary for some women. The Australian Iron Advisory Panel has developed general guidelines for assessing iron status in pregnancy (Table 19.6). These guidelines include the use of biochemical parameters (ferritin and haemoglobin) and various risk factors to assess a woman's risk for IDA in pregnancy. Suggestions regarding dietary advice and iron supplementation are provided based on a woman's risk factors.

Although IDA is the most common form of anaemia, another type of anaemia can develop in response to folate and/or vitamin B_{12} deficiency. This type of anaemia is characterised by large, pale erythryocytes and is referred to as megaloblastic anaemia. Folate deficiency is unlikely to occur in individuals who consume a varied diet, whereas a B_{12} deficiency may develop in individuals who follow strict vegetarian diets devoid of all animal products. A diet rich in dark green, leafy vegetables, whole grains and animal products should provide adequate intakes of these vitamins.

Cravings

Some women report dietary cravings during pregnancy that disappear following birth. For the most part, these cravings do not have a great impact on nutrient intake. In some cultures, however, the consumption of non-food items such as dirt, clay or ice is common in pregnancy. This practice is referred to as pica. Some have theorised that pica is the consequence of nutrient deficiencies; for example, women with iron-deficiency anaemia consume clay or dirt, a source of iron, to correct their nutrient deficiency. Others speculate that the iron deficiency anaemia is a consequence of pica rather than the cause (Horner et al 1991).

Pica has been associated with lead poisoning (Klitzman et al 2002), hypokalaemia (Ukaonu et al 2003) and lower maternal haemoglobin levels at birth (Rainville 1998). Although the true prevalence of pica in pregnancy is unknown and may be difficult to ascertain, it is important to be aware of the potential consequences of pica as it relates to pregnancy.

TABLE 19.6 **Recommendations for iron supplementation during pregnancy**

Stage of pregnancy	Biochemical parameter	Adequate level	At increased risk
Early pregnancy	Haemoglobin	> 115 g/L	105–115 g/L[1] 105–115 g/L and one major risk factor, or ≥ two other risk factors[2]
28 weeks	Haemoglobin Ferritin	> 105 g/L > 16 µg/L	< 105 g/L < 16 µg/L[3]

Risk factors

Major:
- Previous iron deficiency
- Current or recent history of blood donation

Other:
- Poor socio-economic status
- Previous post-partum haemorrhage
- Short gap between pregnancies
- Heavy periods

(Source: adapted from Australian Iron Status Advisory Panel 2004)
1. Dietary advice to increase iron status and reassess at 28 weeks.
2. Supplement with 30 mg/day of elemental iron, provide dietary advice to increase iron status and reassess at 28 weeks.
3. Supplement with 100 mg/day of elemental iron and provide dietary advice to increase iron status.

Gestational diabetes mellitus

In response to elevated progesterone, pregnancy-related lactogen and oestrogen, some degree of insulin resistance during pregnancy is normal. In women, particularly those who are overweight, the pancreas is unable to produce adequate insulin levels to counteract this resistance. Elevated blood glucose levels in pregnancy may result in the development of *gestational diabetes mellitus* (GDM).

Although there is no specific diet for women with GDM, good nutrition can improve blood glucose control. Eating small meals and snacks often, consuming low-fat rather than high-fat foods, and incorporating plenty of foods rich in dietary fibre to promote enhanced satiety, can help regulate blood glucose levels. In addition to these nutrition guidelines, consuming at least one low-glycaemic index food at each meal or snack can also be useful in regulating blood glucose levels (Clapp 2002; Dornhorst & Frost 2002). Similar to the American Diabetes Association guidelines (2001), Diabetes Australia and Diabetes New Zealand discourage large intakes of artificial sweeteners, although moderate amounts may be consumed during pregnancy. Stevia, a herbal sugar replacement, is promoted in health food stores as a safe alternative to artificial sweeteners. Food Standards Australia New Zealand has not approved its use in foods, and due to insufficient research on its toxicological effects it is not recommended by diabetes organisations worldwide.

Food safety and pregnancy

Food safety is an important issue that is often overlooked in pregnancy. Some microorganisms responsible for food-borne illness can cross the placenta, resulting in serious consequences including fetal death.

Listeria

Listeria monocytogenes is a gram-positive bacterium found naturally in soil and vegetation. In healthy, non-pregnant women, an infection with *L. monocytogenes* results in non-specific symptoms similar to a mild flu (fever, diarrhoea and sore throat). In pregnant women, however, *Listeria* can be passed to the fetus through the maternal–fetal circulation or through the vagina during birth. The effects of listeriosis on the fetus include spontaneous abortion in early pregnancy, stillbirth or premature birth in late pregnancy, or damage to the brain and meninges.

The incidence of listeriosis in Australia and New Zealand is relatively low. In Australia in 2002, 62 cases of listeriosis were reported, of which two were in pregnant women. This represented a rate of 0.8 cases/100,000 live births (OzFoodNet Working Group 2002). The incidence of listeriosis in New Zealand is reported to be approximately 15 cases/year (Bremer et al 2003).

Despite the low incidence of listeriosis, general food safety principles should be promoted particularly during pregnancy, to further reduce a woman's risk. Both raw and processed foods are a potential source of *Listeria*. Foods that have been cooked and then chilled are ideal breeding grounds for this bacteria; therefore, foods stored in the refrigerator longer than 12 hours may contain *Listeria*. Fortunately, high heat destroys this pathogen; therefore, reheating foods can significantly reduce one's risk of contracting listeriosis. Publications by the New Zealand Food Safety Authority titled *Food Safety in Pregnancy*, and by FSANZ, titled *Listeria and Pregnancy*, have further information related to reducing one's risk of listeriosis.

Pregnant adolescents

Adolescence is a stage in life characterised by rapid growth and development. Therefore pregnant adolescents are at increased risk of nutritional inadequacies due to the additional nutritional requirements of pregnancy. Adequate weight gain is important for pregnant adolescents, to ensure not only the growth of the fetus but also that of the adolescent. The recommendations for weight gain in pregnant adolescents are based on pre-pregnancy BMI, aiming for gains at the higher end of the recommendations (National Research Council 1990).

In addition to the energy demands of adolescent pregnancy, requirements for iron and calcium are also increased. During adolescence, total blood volume increases, and therefore adolescents who become pregnant have a substantial increase in blood volume, more so than in adult women (Beard 2000). An adequate intake of iron is critical to prevent iron deficiency and iron deficiency anaemia. Depending on their dietary intake and iron status, adolescents may benefit from iron supplementation early in the pregnancy. The adolescent skeleton is growing rapidly, and therefore sufficient calcium is necessary to promote peak bone mineral density of the adolescent while ensuring skeletal growth of the fetus (National Research Council 1997).

Furthermore, adolescence is a time of exploration and independence. Issues such as body image may result in dietary restriction or altered eating patterns that may have a negative effect on dietary intakes. It is critical to emphasise the importance of good nutrition to pregnant adolescents for their health and that of their unborn child.

Multiple pregnancies

Although the need for additional energy and nutrients in multiple pregnancies would seem obvious, there has been limited research in this area. Recommendations for weight gain in multiple pregnancies aim to optimise pregnancy outcomes, primarily birthweight. The weight gain recommendation for twin pregnancies, 16–20.5 kg, is higher than for singleton pregnancies (National Research Council 1990). A weight gain of 2–3 kg in the first trimester may be beneficial in multiple pregnancies to promote intrauterine growth. This is important, considering the high risk of preterm delivery in multiple pregnancies (Brown & Carlson 2000).

As with pregnant adolescents, multiple pregnancies also require additional iron and calcium to accommodate an increased blood volume and to support the growth and development of the fetal skeleton (Okah et al 1996; Worthington-Roberts 1998). An increase in essential fats has been suggested, based on lower levels of plasma essential fats reported in women with multiple pregnancies (Zeijdner et al 1997).

Summary: pregnancy

Nutrition plays an important role in pregnancy. Plenty of energy from carbohydrate, fats and protein is required to facilitate the growth and development of maternal and fetal tissues. An adequate intake of iron, calcium, zinc, iodine, vitamin B_{12} and folate is particularly important in pregnancy, whereas excess intake of some nutrients such as vitamin A may be detrimental to the fetus. Dietary advice can also help to alleviate common conditions in pregnancy, including constipation, heartburn and nausea, and may be useful in managing gestational diabetes mellitus and avoiding food-borne illness such as listeriosis. Pregnant adolescents and multiple pregnancies are considered high-risk with respect to nutrition, due to increased nutrient and energy demands.

Nutritional foundation for childbirth

Childbirth is an energy-demanding process that requires adequate energy and hydration. The actual energy demands for labour have been estimated to be between 2.9 and 4.2 MJ per hour. However, some researchers disagree with these figures, stating that smooth muscle requires significantly less energy than skeletal muscle, on which the original estimates were based (Champion 2002). Without adequate energy intake, body stores of glycogen and adipose tissue will be used to sustain energy requirements. As the period of fasting increases, ketones begin to appear in the blood. It is largely accepted that some amount of ketosis during childbirth is

Critical thinking exercise

A 22-year-old woman (para 1, gravida 0) has indicated to you that she is vegetarian. She consumes dairy products but no other animal foods. She has followed this diet for six years and is keen to continue the diet during pregnancy.
1 What other questions about her diet might you ask her and why?
2 What nutrients might you be concerned about with her diet and why?
3 How would you follow up with this client to ensure that her diet meets the energy and nutrient requirements of pregnancy?

normal. However, as ketones begin to spill into the urine, the body becomes depleted of sodium and potassium, resulting in dehydration, which may lead to maternal or fetal acidosis. It is important, therefore, to ensure adequate nutrition and hydration to prevent such large aberrations in acid/base balance.

Since the mid-1900s, many hospitals worldwide have implemented policies on restricting oral intake during childbirth. The primary rationale for this restriction was to lower the risk of pulmonary aspiration in women who required anaesthetic during labour. Some countries, including the United Kingdom, do not restrict oral intake in early labour and have very few cases of pulmonary aspiration. Of nine million births in the United Kingdom in the past 12 years, only four maternal deaths occurred due to maternal pulmonary aspiration (Cooper et al 2002).

It is well documented that eating in labour increases gastric volume, thereby increasing the risk of pulmonary aspiration; however, fasting in labour does not always guarantee decreased gastric contents (Scrutton et al 1999). Various factors tend to inhibit gastric emptying, particularly narcotic analgesia. Other factors such as the osmolarity and macronutrient composition of oral intake also affect gastric emptying. Isotonic drinks appear to reduce maternal ketosis (Kubli et al 2002) without increasing gastric volume, whereas fatty foods, and foods containing dietary fibre, tend to slow down gastric emptying, thereby increasing gastric volume. Similarly, liquids are emptied more rapidly than solids from the stomach and are therefore preferable in reducing gastric volume (Table 19.7) (Champion 2002).

Summary: childbirth

Nutrition and hydration are important during childbirth to ensure an adequate energy intake and to maintain normal fluid and electrolyte balance of mother and child. Although large gastric volumes increase the risk of pulmonary aspiration, restricting oral intake during labour does not necessarily result in reduced risk of aspiration. Isotonic fluids and

TABLE 19.7 Appropriate foods and drinks for women in labour	
Foods	**Fluids**
White bread or toast (low-fibre) with low-fat spreads, jam or honey	Low-fat yoghurt drinks
	Ice blocks
	Fruit juices
Low-fibre breakfast cereal with low-fat milk	Clear broths
	Diluted squash drinks
Creamed rice	Water
Plain biscuits	Sports drinks (Lucozade, Gatorade, Powerade)
Low-fat yoghurt	
Fruit (tinned or fresh)	
(Source: adapted from Champion 2002)	

Critical thinking exercise

A 36-year old woman (para 3, gravida 2) currently 37 weeks gestation has asked you whether it is important to eat and drink throughout the entire labour.

Outline the pros and cons of eating and drinking in labour, and the rationale for each.

foods that enhance gastric emptying are best suited for early labour.

Nutritional foundation for lactation

The nutritional needs of a woman change after pregnancy. These needs are based on the nutritional needs of lactation, which in fact exceed those of pregnancy. Lactation, like pregnancy, is an anabolic state and therefore requires adequate energy to support milk production.

The energy costs for lactation have been estimated as additional 650 kilocalories (2720 kilojoules) per day. Taking into consideration the additional energy stores formed during pregnancy, the recommended energy intake is estimated at 500 kilocalories (2100 kilojoules) per day (Picciano 2003).

Because of the energy demands associated with breastfeeding, weight loss is often reported to occur with breastfeeding. Further weight loss often results when breastfeeding mothers restrict caloric intake and/or begin physical activity. Although dieting while breastfeeding is not generally recommended, dieting with or without aerobic exercise does not appear to affect either the quality or quantity of breast milk (Lovelady et al 2000; McCrory 2001; McCrory et al 1999).

The nutritional quality of breast milk is fairly constant regardless of maternal diet. The micronutrient content of breast milk, specifically the minerals calcium, iron and zinc, is tightly regulated (Lonnerdal 2000). Several nutrients present within breast milk, however, can be altered by maternal diet. These include vitamins B_6, B_{12}, A and D, and fatty acid content.

The amount of vitamin B_6 transferred from maternal blood into breast milk is minimal, and therefore recommended intakes are slightly higher than for non-lactating women. The levels of vitamin B_{12}, vitamin A and long-chain polyunsaturated fats in breast milk reflect maternal intake. It is critical, therefore, that vegan breastfeeding mothers ensure an adequate intake of B_{12} and essential fats (Makrides & Gibson 2000; Picciano 2001; Sanders 1999). One nutrient found in low levels in breast milk is vitamin D. Vitamin D levels in breast milk have been reported to fluctuate depending on maternal sun exposure, with higher levels in summer than in winter (Hollis & Wagner 2004).

A non-nutritional advantage to breastfeeding is the immunological protection it affords the infant, which reduces risk of allergy development. Although the true prevalence of food allergy in children is unknown, it has been estimated to be as high as 4–6% in some countries (Zeiger 2003). Some infants, however, are more susceptible to allergies, particularly those born to parents with allergies or whose siblings have an existing allergy.

Despite the immunological benefits of breast milk, sensitisation, an initial exposure to an allergen, can occur during lactation. A subsequent exposure to the same allergen will then result in an allergic reaction. For infants with a parent or sibling who have a confirmed food allergy, it may be advisable for breastfeeding mothers to avoid the major food allergens (nuts, fish and shellfish), to reduce the chance of sensitising the infant. It has been suggested that sensitisation occurs in utero; however, the American Academy

of Pediatrics (AAP) and the European Society for Pediatric Gastroenterology, Hepatology and Nutrition (ESPGHAN) do not recommend maternal allergen avoidance during pregnancy, due to a lack of supporting evidence to suggest otherwise (Zeiger 2003). Women with infants who have a confirmed food allergy should be encouraged to breastfeed; however, elimination of the infant's food allergy in their diet is advised. To ensure that the allergic infant and mother receive adequate nutrition, they should be seen by a dietitian who specialises in food allergies.

Conclusion

Pregnancy, childbirth and lactation are all energy- and nutrient-demanding events. For optimal maternal and fetal health, adequate intakes of nutrients are required, including iron, calcium, zinc, iodine, vitamin B_{12} and folate. Of particular consideration are individuals with higher nutrient demands, such as pregnant adolescents and women with multiple pregnancies. Nutrition plays an important role in alleviating some common conditions associated with pregnancy, including constipation, heartburn and nausea. Similarly, dietary strategies can assist in managing gestational diabetes mellitus, in preventing food-borne illnesses, in maintaining adequate fluid and electrolyte levels during childbirth, and in reducing the development of food allergies in the breastfed infant.

Critical thinking exercise

A 29-year old woman (para 2, gravida 1) is at 34 weeks gestation and is very concerned about her newborn developing food allergies. Her first child has been diagnosed with cow's milk allergy. She has been avoiding all dairy products throughout her pregnancy in an attempt to prevent sensitising her unborn child.

1 What are some potential strategies you might discuss with her for reducing the risk of allergy development in her second child?

2 What advice would you provide her with if she becomes pregnant again?

Review questions

Pregnancy

1 How can body mass index be used as a tool for midwives?

2 What is the importance of each macronutrient in pregnancy?

3 What impact do specific vitamin and mineral deficiencies or excesses have in pregnancy?

4 What preventive dietary strategies would you recommend for the effects you listed in question 3?

5 What dietary strategies would you suggest to a pregnant adolescent or to a woman expecting twins?

6 Why is food safety important during pregnancy?

Childbirth

7 Why are energy intake and hydration important during labour?

8 What types of foods are suitable to consume during labour?

Lactation

9 What nutrients in breast milk reflect maternal diet or lifestyle, and why?

10 What advice would you give to a breastfeeding woman who is concerned that her infant may develop a food allergy?

Online resources

Australasian Diabetes in Pregnancy Society, http://www.adips.org/

Australia New Zealand Food Authority, http://www.foodstandards.gov.au and http://www.foodstandards.govt.nz

Australian Government Department of Health and Ageing, http://www.health.gov.au/

Australian Iron Status Advisory Panel, http://www.ironpanel.org.au/AIS/AISdocs/index.html

Glycaemic Index Symbol Program, http://www.gisymbol.com.au/pages/index.asp

New Zealand Food Safety Authority, http://www.nzfsa.govt.nz/

New Zealand Ministry of Health, http://www.moh.govt.nz

References

Allen KG, Harris MA 2001 The role of n-3 fatty acids in gestation and parturition. Experimental Biology and Medicine 226(6):498–506

American Diabetes Association 2001 American Diabetes Association Clinical Practice Recommendations 2001: gestational diabetes mellitus. Diabetes Care 24(S1):S77–S79

Atallah AN, Hofmeyr GJ, Duley L 2004 Calcium supplementation during pregnancy for preventing hypertensive disorders and related problems (Cochrane Review). Cochrane Library (3). John Wiley & Sons, Chichester

Australian Bureau of Statistics 1995 National Nutrition Survey, nutrient intakes and physical measurements, Australia. ABS, Canberra

Australian Iron Status Advisory Panel 2004 Iron and pregnancy recommended guidelines. Online: http://www.ironpanel.org.au/AIS/AISdocs/pregdocs/pregtitle.html, accessed 1 May 2004

Azais-Braesco V, Pascal G 2000 Vitamin A in pregnancy: requirements and safety limits. American Journal of Clinical Nutrition 71(suppl 5):S1325–S1333

Beard JL 2000 Iron requirements in adolescent females. Journal of Nutrition 130(suppl 2):S440–S442

Bremer PJ, Fletcher GC, Osborne C 2003, *Listeria monocytogenes* in seafood. New Zealand Institute for Crop and Food Research, Christchurch

Brown JE, Carlson M 2000 Nutrition and multifetal pregnancy. Journal of the American Dietetic Association 100(3):343–348

Champion P 2002 Labouring over food: the dietician's view. In: P Champion, C McCormick (Eds) Eating and drinking in labour. Butterworth-Heinemann, Oxford

Clapp JF 2002 Maternal carbohydrate intake and pregnancy outcome. Proceedings of the Nutrition Society 61(1):45–50

Cooper GM, Lewis G, Neilson J 2002 Confidential enquiries into maternal deaths. British Journal of Anaesthesia 89(3):369–372

Dornhorst A, Frost G 2002 The principles of dietary management of gestational diabetes: reflection on current evidence. Journal of Human Nutrition and Dietetics 15(2):145–156

Fischer-Rasmussen W, Kjaer SK, Dahl C et al 1991 Ginger treatment of hyperemesis gravidarum. European Journal of Obstetrics, Gynecology and Reproductive Biology 42(2):163–164

Food Standards Australia and New Zealand (FSANZ) 2004 Mercury in fish. Online: http://www.foodstandards.gov.au/mediareleasespublications/factsheets/factsheets2004/mercuryinfishfurther2394.cfm, accessed 10 May 2004

Food Standards Australia and New Zealand (FSANZ) 2001 Mercury in fish advisory statement for pregnant women. Online: http://www.foodstandards.gov.au/mediareleasespublications/factsheets/factsheets2001/mercuryinfishadvisor1415.cfm, accessed 10 May 2004

Grover S, Morley R 2001 Vitamin D deficiency in veiled or dark-skinned pregnant women. Medical Journal of Australia 175(5):251–252

Hallberg L 2002 Advantages and disadvantages of an iron-rich diet. European Journal of Clinical Nutrition 56(suppl 1):S12–S18

Hambraeus L 1999 Animal- and plant-food-based diets and iron status: benefits and costs. Proceedings of the Nutrition Society 58(2):235–242

Heath AL, Skeaff CM, O'Brien SM et al 2001 Can dietary treatment of non-anemic iron deficiency improve iron status? Journal of the American College of Nutrition 20(5):477–484

Hollis BW, Wagner CL 2004 Assessment of dietary vitamin D requirements during pregnancy and lactation. American Journal of Clinical Nutrition 79(5):717–726

Horner R, Lackey CJ, Kolasa K et al 1991 Pica practises of pregnant women. Journal of the American Dietetic Association 91(1):34–38

Keating A, Chez RA 2002 Ginger syrup as an antiemetic in early pregnancy. Alternative Therapies in Health and Medicine 8(5):89–91

King, JC 2000 Determinants of maternal zinc status during pregnancy. American Journal of Clinical Nutrition 71(suppl 5):S1334–S1343

Klitzman S, Sharma A, Nicaj L et al 2002 Lead poisoning among pregnant women in New York City: risk factors and screening practises. Journal of Urban Health 79(2):225–237

Kramer MS, Kakuma R 2004 Energy and protein intake in pregnancy (Cochrane Review). Cochrane Library (3). John Wiley & Sons, Chichester

Kubli M, Scrutton MJ, Seed PT et al 2002 An evaluation of isotonic 'sports drinks' during labour. Anesthesia and Analgesia 94(2):404–408

Lonnerdal B 2000 Regulation of mineral and trace elements in human milk: exogenous and endogenous factors. Nutrition Reviews 58(8):223–229

Lovelady CA, Garner KE, Morono KL et al 2000 The effect of weight loss in overweight, lactating women on the growth of their infants. New England Journal of Medicine 342(7):449–453

Mahomed K, Gulmezoglu AM 2004 Vitamin D supplementation in pregnancy (Cochrane Review). Cochrane Library (3). John Wiley & Sons, Chichester

Makrides R, Gibson RA 2000 Long chain polyunsaturated fatty acid (LCPUFA) requirements during pregnancy and lactation. American Journal of Clinical Nutrition 71(suppl 1):S307–S311

McCrory MA 2001 Does dieting during lactation put infant growth at risk? Nutrition Reviews 59(1):18–21

McCrory MA, Nommsen-Rivers LA, Mole PA et al 1999 Randomized trial of the short-term effects of dieting compared with dieting plus aerobic exercise on lactation performance. American Journal of Clinical Nutrition 69(5):959–967

Ministry of Health 1999 New Zealand food: New Zealand people. Key results of the 1997 National Nutrition Survey. Ministry of Health, Wellington

Ministry of Health 1997 Code 4147 Planning for pregnancy. Folic acid and spina bifida. Ministry of Health, Wellington

National Health and Medical Research Council 1992 Recommended dietary intakes for use in Australia. AGPS, Canberra

National Health and Medical Research Council (NHMRC) 1993 Revised statement on the relationship between dietary folic acid and neural tube defects such as spina bifida. NHMRC, Canberra

National Research Council 1990 Food and Nutrition Board, Committee on Nutrition Status During Pregnancy and Lactation, National Academy of Sciences. Nutrition during pregnancy. Institute of Medicine, Washington DC

National Research Council 1997 Food and Nutrition Board, Standing Committee on the Scientific Evaluation of Dietary Reference Intakes. Dietary reference intakes for calcium, phosphorus, magnesium, vitamin D, and fluoride. National Academy Press, Washington DC

Nesby-O'Dell SS, Scanlon K, Cogswell M et al 2002 Hypovitaminosis D prevalence and determinants among African American and white women of reproductive age: Third National Health and Nutrition Examination Survey, 1988–1994. American Journal of Clinical Nutrition 76(1):187–192

Okah FA, Tsang RC, Sierra R et al 1996 Bone turnover and mineral metabolism in the last trimester of pregnancy: effect of multiple gestation. Obstetrics and Gynecology 88(2):168–173

Olsen SF, Secher NJ, Talbor A et al 2000 Randomised clinical trials of fish oil supplementation in high risk pregnancies. British Journal of Obstetrics and Gynaecology 107(3):382–395

Olsen SF, Secher NJ 2002 Low consumption of seafood in early pregnancy as a risk factor for preterm delivery: prospective cohort study. British Medical Journal 324(7335):1–5

OzFoodNet Working Group 2002, Foodborne disease in Australia: incidence, notifications and outbreaks. Annual report of the OzFoodNet network, 2002. Communicable Diseases Intelligence 27(2)

Patterson AJ, Brown WJ, Roberts DCK et al 2001 Dietary treatment of iron deficiency in women of childbearing age. American Journal of Clinical Nutrition 74(5):650–656

Picciano MF 2001 Nutrient composition of milk. Pediatric Clinics of North America 48(1):53–67

Picciano MF 2003 Pregnancy and lactation: physiological adjustments, nutritional requirements and the role of dietary supplements. Journal of Nutrition 133(6):S1997–S2002

Rainville AJ 1998 Pica practices of pregnant women are associated with lower maternal haemoglobin level at delivery. Journal of the American Dietetic Association 98(3):293–296

Ritchie LD, King JC 2000 Dietary calcium and pregnancy-induced hypertension: is there a relation? American Journal of Clinical Nutrition 71(suppl 5):S1371–S1374

Rush D 2001 Maternal nutrition and perinatal survival. Nutrition Reviews 59(10):315–326

Sanders TA 1999 Essential fatty acid requirements of vegetarians in pregnancy, lactation and infancy. American Journal of Clinical Nutrition 70(suppl 3):S555–S559

Sandstrom B 2001 Micronutrient interactions: effects on absorption and bioavailability. British Journal of Nutrition 82(suppl 2): S181–S185

Scrutton MJ, Metcalfe GA, Lowy C et al 1999 Eating in labour. A randomised controlled trial assessing the risks and benefits. Anaesthesia 54(4):329–334

Shah D, Sachdev HPS 2001 Effect of gestational zinc deficiency on pregnancy outcomes: summary of observation studies and zinc supplementation trials. British Journal of Nutrition 85(suppl 2): S101–S108

Ukaonu C, Hill DA, Christensen F 2003 Hypokalemic myopathy in pregnancy caused by clay ingestion. Obstetrics and Gynecology 102(5):1169–1171

Worthington-Roberts B 1998 Weight gain patterns in twin pregnancies with desirable outcomes. Clinical Nutrition 7(5):191–196

Zeiger RS 2003 Food allergen avoidance in the prevention of food allergy in infants and children. Pediatrics 111(6):1662–1671

Zeijdner EE, van Houwelingen AC, Kester AD, Hornstra G 1997 Essential fatty acid status: plasma phospholipids of mother and neonate after multiple pregnancy. Prostaglandins, Leukotrienes and Essential Fatty Acids 56(5):395–401

Further reading

Morgan JB, Dickerson JWT (Eds) 2003 Nutrition in early life. Wiley, Guildford, UK

Worthington-Roberts BS, Williams SR (Eds) 1997 Nutrition in pregnancy and lactation. McGraw-Hill, Boston

APPENDIX: Daily recommended nutrient intakes for pregnancy and lactation

Nutrient	RDI Australia[1,2,3]		RDI United States / Canada[4]	
	Pregnancy	Lactation	Pregnancy	Lactation
Vitamin A (mg RE)	750	1200	770	1300
Vitamin C (mg)	60	75	85	120
Vitamin D (IU)	No dietary recommendation		200	200
Vitamin E (mg)	7.0	9.5	15	19
Vitamin K (μg)	No dietary recommendation		90	90
Thiamin (mg)	1.0	1.2	1.4	1.4
Riboflavin (mg)	1.5	1.7	1.4	1.6
Niacin (mg)	15	18	18	17
Vitamin B_6 (mg)	1.0–1.5	1.6–2.2	1.9	2.0
Folate (μg)	400	350	600	500
Vitamin B_{12} (μg)	3.0	2.5	2.6	2.8
Calcium (mg)	1100	1200	1000	1000
Iodine (μg)	150	170	220	290
Iron (mg)	22–36	12–16	27	9
Magnesium (mg)	300	340	350–360	310–320
Phosphorus (mg)	1200	1200	700	700
Potassium (mg)	1950–5460	1950–5460	4700	5100
Selenium (μg)	80	85	60	70
Sodium (mg)	920–2300	920–2300	1500	1500
Zinc (mg)	16	18	11	12

RDI: Recommended Dietary Intake
1. Source: National Health and Medical Research Council 1992 Recommended Dietary Intakes for use in Australia. AGPS, Canberra.
2. New Zealand uses the Australian RDIs.
3. At the time of publication, Australia and New Zealand were considering the adoption of the Dietary Reference Intakes used by the United States and Canada
4. Dietary Reference Intakes based on 19–50 years of age (Food and Nutrition Information Center. Online: http://www.nal.usda.gov/fnic/etext/000105.html)

CHAPTER 20

Working with women in pregnancy

Celia Grigg

Key terms

active decision-making, antenatal education, antenatal visits, assess baby's wellbeing, assess women's wellbeing, assessment and screening, blood pressure (BP) measurement and monitoring, blood screening, booking visit, care plan, constipation, current health review, 'decision point' framework, estimated due date (EDD), evidence-informed midwifery practice, exercise in pregnancy, fetal movement (FM), health promotion and education, heartburn, historical health review, holistic midwifery, information sharing, initial contact, last menstrual period (LMP), nausea and vomiting, palpation, physiological changes, risk markers, urine screening

Chapter overview

This chapter discusses antenatal care within the context of the midwifery model. It provides a broad overview of the issues of antenatal care, and considers some of the core technical components of clinical practice. Where possible, this discussion is based on reviewed research, in order to promote evidence-informed midwifery practice. The dearth of published research that meaningfully addresses midwifery questions is an ongoing problem in this regard. The chapter establishes a framework for understanding the *way* of doing things, as much as it provides instruction on *what* to do. As such, it seeks to interpret routine care with reference to the following set of guiding principles, which are fundamental for midwives working within the midwifery model:

- partnerships with women—women-centred, negotiated relationships

- continuity of care in the holistic process of pregnancy, birth and early parenting

- support and empowerment of childbearing women

- promotion of holistic wellness

- assessment and screening, which includes risk identification, knowledge/understanding and choices

- information sharing as a two-way process

- promotion of active, informed decision-making by women

- health promotion and education within an appropriate 'adult learning' approach.

In this chapter, antenatal care is discussed within a broad practice model of midwife-led continuity of care. While this model characterises New Zealand's maternity services, it is also becoming increasingly available in Australia and is the model to which Australian midwifery aspires. The key components of routine antenatal care are identified using the New Zealand College of Midwives (NZCOM) 'decision points' as a framework (NZCOM 2005). Some of these components are further developed in the explanatory sections that follow. The decision points refer to relevant issues raised in other chapters of this book, and readers are also referred to other reading and research activity where appropriate. Notwithstanding the model of care in which a midwife may practise, the aspects of antenatal care described in his chapter are applicable to any setting.

Of necessity, this chapter discusses antenatal care as a discrete entity, and it may be tempting to consider it as such. However, antenatal care is but a small part of a woman's experience of the broader process of pregnancy, and cannot be separated from childbearing as a holistic process, which includes pregnancy, birth and the postnatal period. Further, the meaning and effect of antenatal care is totally dependent on the individual woman and her personal context.

Learning outcomes

Learning outcomes for this chapter are:

1   To discuss the organisation and form of antenatal care within the context of the midwifery model

2   To illustrate a way in which evidence may be used to inform midwifery practice

3   To describe the essential components of antenatal care

4   To explain the purpose and process of the initial contact and booking visits

5   To describe and explain the concept of 'decision points' as a framework for organising care

6   To discuss the history and processes of establishing the estimated date of delivery

7   To list and describe routine antenatal blood screening, blood pressure and urine screening tests

8   To explain the purpose and process of abdominal palpation of pregnant women

9   To describe the assessment and significance of fetal movements

10   To explain the nature and provision of antenatal education and exercise programs in pregnancy

11   To discuss some of the physiological changes of pregnancy, with specific reference to nausea and vomiting, constipation and heartburn.

Antenatal care: what is it?

Defining antenatal care as a conceptual entity, or even in terms of a list of discrete clinical components, is difficult. Definitions of antenatal care can vary markedly, depending on one's beliefs or understanding of the childbearing process, be it from a midwifery or medical perspective. The underpinning assumptions of these perspectives have been discussed elsewhere in this book, but it is important to recognise how the midwife's perspective will influence the aims, scope and content of the antenatal care she provides, and the way in which she provides this care.

From a midwifery perspective, antenatal care is not an independent entity. It is an integral part of the whole childbearing experience. It usually represents the beginning of the journey that midwives and women will make together, which includes the time before, during and after the birth of the baby. For midwives working from a midwifery model, it is a time of forming and building a relationship with each woman and those who are important to her. It is a time when a partnership is negotiated, roles and responsibilities are identified, information is shared, options are discussed, and choices are made and supported. It is also a time when notions of wellness and normality within the context of pregnancy are supported and promoted.

Each woman and each midwife bring their respective knowledge and expertise together in this new relationship. A woman brings her knowledge of her past and present physical wellness (and that of her family), her personal, social, emotional and cultural realities, her experiences of pregnancy (present and sometimes previous), and her plans for her birth and mothering. A midwife brings her knowledge

of the childbearing process, supports its normality, identifies risks, and shares information that enables the woman to make informed decisions throughout.

However, much of what constitutes contemporary antenatal care throughout the world remains strongly rooted in the 'medical' model within which it developed. Widespread, institutionalised, routine antenatal care began less than eighty years ago, as a mass screening program, with the aim of reducing maternal and perinatal mortality, and brought 'pregnancy' under medical supervision and control for the first time in human history (Wagner 1994). The history and politics of antenatal care will not be discussed here. It is well articulated by many authors, such as Oakley (1984), Strong (2000), Katz Rothman (1989), Donnison (1988) and, in New Zealand, Donley (1998). What is of significance in this context are the beliefs and assumptions that continue to underpin the structure and content of various aspects of antenatal care. Traditionally, and in many contemporary contexts, antenatal care consists of a prescribed set of acts based around the clinical monitoring and screening of all pregnant women, regardless of their health or risk status. This establishment of routine antenatal care was based on the notion that pregnancy is a state of pathology, rather than of normal physiology. Oakley (1984) argues that 'the most characteristic aspect of modern antenatal care is the clinical insistence on the probability of pathology in all childbearing' (p 2). Over the past eighty years, technological advances have brought an ever-increasing array of screening tests and treatments, 'most often . . . without proper scientific evaluation and concrete evidence of benefit' (Villar et al 2004, p 2), although 'few of the procedures commonly undertaken have a major impact on morbidity or mortality, and some may have no effect' (Villar et al 2004, p 2). Further, some have been found to cause physical, emotional or social harm (Wagner 1994). Hall (2001) contends that there are 'remarkably few antenatal measures [which] are known to be effective: these are screening for and prevention of [some] infections; prevention, detection and treatment of anaemia; detection of malpresentations so that external cephalic version can be offered; and detection, investigation, and treatment of pregnancy hypertension' (p 1546). These measures clearly illustrate the scope of antenatal care from a medical perspective, and the outcomes of value that are expected from it.

Some might argue that routine antenatal care fails to meet reasonable expectations of its relevance and effectiveness. If this is indeed the case, then it may be possible to mount a case to abandon it. However, such a proposition would be inappropriate from a midwifery point of view. Maternal and perinatal morbidity and mortality are not the only outcome measures of value. There is substantial evidence that midwifery-provided continuity of care has beneficial effects on other outcome measures, such as reduced anxiety, a greater sense of control (Oakley 1992), reduced use of drugs for pain relief in labour, reduced likelihood of the need for newborn resuscitation, and greater satisfaction with antenatal, intrapartal and postnatal care (Hodnett 2004; McCourt & Page 1996; Page et al 1999). It is extremely important that all those who provide care clearly articulate the scope and limitations of the screening and diagnostic tests used in antenatal care.

The key point here is that antenatal care is a process that consists of more than just a series of medical tests and monitoring procedures. While some of these tests may form part of the process, in the midwifery context they are not of themselves the essence of antenatal care—that is, they do not *define* it. Midwives need to claim and promote the potential of holistic midwifery care, and put this potential into practice in their work. For midwives, antenatal care is fundamentally about a relationship between two actively participating individuals (and the woman's support people), who bring their respective expertise together and work to maximise the health and wellbeing of the woman and her unborn child, and to prepare for labour, birth and parenting. From the midwifery perspective, the term 'routine antenatal care' is perhaps a misnomer, as there is no such thing as a 'routine' woman. Every woman is different, and each of her pregnancy experiences is unique.

Organisation of care

The provision of antenatal care in Australia and New Zealand has traditionally been based on a medically defined, controlled and provided system of assessment, screening and monitoring of pregnant women, which was initiated in Britain and established in the 1920s (Hall 2001). In Australia this remains largely unchanged, although there are increasing examples of alternative models (Reiger 2001; Tracy 2005). In New Zealand, an alternative organisation of care was introduced in 1990, which enabled women to choose, and midwives to provide, full and complete maternity care for well women without referral

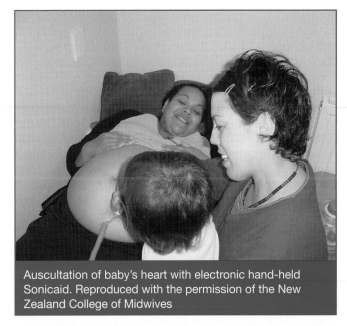

Auscultation of baby's heart with electronic hand-held Sonicaid. Reproduced with the permission of the New Zealand College of Midwives

or deferral to doctors. Today, antenatal care in New Zealand is founded on the concept of a primary caregiver, known as a lead maternity carer (LMC), providing the majority of care and organising referral when care is outside the scope of practice of the LMC.

The antenatal visit

Antenatal visits are the main mechanism for the provision of antenatal care. They are negotiated and agreed upon between the woman and the midwife, and occur at prearranged times and locations, and at regular intervals throughout the woman's pregnancy. They are multidimensional and include several components, such as information sharing, assessment and screening, active decision-making, and health promotion and education. Aspects of these dimensions will be illustrated and discussed throughout this chapter.

The number and timing of visits follow a pattern, which was established when the concept of antenatal care was introduced in the 1920s (Candy et al 2003). This traditional pattern of antenatal visits—four-weekly from booking until 28 weeks, fortnightly until 36 weeks and weekly until birth—remains the standard of antenatal care today in Australia and New Zealand. This format has no particular scientific, medical, social or midwifery foundation, and has recently been the subject of debate and challenge. This challenge arose from the concept of 'evidence-based practice' and has led to the evaluation of this aspect of antenatal care (Enkin et al 2000).

Determining the 'optimal' number of visits in routine antenatal care is extremely difficult. This is due to the complexity of the process of pregnancy itself, the diversity of childbearing women, and the context-bound, multidimensional nature of antenatal care in general (Strong 2000). Attempts to specify a particular number of visits have been based on research which measures only biomedical outcomes, such as incidence rates of pre-eclampsia, low birth weight, urinary tract infections, postpartum anaemia and perinatal mortality, although some studies have surveyed maternal satisfaction (Candy et al 2003; Carroli et al 2001; Petrou et al 2003; Villar et al 2004). Current recommendations, based on these studies and other similar research, are for a schedule with a reduced number of antenatal visits. The British National Institute of Clinical Excellence (NICE) guidelines (2003) and the Australian Three Centres Consensus Guidelines on Antenatal Care Project (ATCCGACP)(2001) both opt for a routine, for well women, of ten visits for women having their first baby (primiparas) and seven for those having their second or subsequent baby (multiparas). It is notable, however, that a reduction in women's satisfaction with fewer visits, as reported in research that studied this issue, has been minimised and largely ignored in these guidelines. Arguably, this illustrates the continuing dominance of the medical model as the foundation of contemporary antenatal care.

In New Zealand, there appears to have been some change in the number of antenatal visits from the traditional pattern, but no research has been published which identifies whether this is woman- or caregiver-led. According to a recent nationwide survey completed by 2909 women, 93% of women had had more than five antenatal consultations and 65% had had more than ten, with 91% agreeing or strongly agreeing that they had had the right number of visits with their lead maternity carer (Ministry of Health 2003).

Issues concerning the length and location of antenatal visits are context-bound in the same way as those associated with the number of visits, and the alternative options offered are equally constrained within socio-political limits. In the New Zealand model, the woman and midwife negotiate the length and location of visits, with each party making her respective personal and practice choices clear prior to any agreement to work together. Although there is no set optimal length for visits, enough time needs to be set aside to include discussion, assessment, decision-making and documentation of the issues, such as those included in the 'decision point' framework set out in this chapter. The time taken for visits will vary according to the practice styles of individual midwives, differences in the needs and personalities of women, the stage of the woman's pregnancy and her health status.

It is also important that the location of visits be one in which both the woman and the midwife feel relaxed and comfortable, and be available at the time most convenient to them. It needs to be safe, both personally and culturally, and afford appropriate privacy. The ideal location will be accessible and have appropriate facilities. If possible, it is valuable for the midwife to provide some of the antenatal care in the woman's home. This may help to restore the traditional power balance between care provider and receiver, and also provides valuable insight for the midwife into the woman's personal and social context.

Initial contact

Initial contact between a pregnant woman and a midwife is generally by phone. This call may simply be little more than an inquiry about the availability of the midwife. It may, however, evolve into a process of establishing more substantial contact between the two, either as a continuation of the phone call, or at a face-to-face meeting. This will represent the first meaningful exchange between the midwife and the pregnant woman. It is an opportunity for the woman to gain a first impression of the midwife—what she sounds like, her ways of practice and her availability. For the midwife, it is an opportunity to help the woman clarify what she is seeking, to share information about how she practises, and to talk about the choices that are open to the woman.

There is no common understanding about the nature of this contact, in terms of what it involves, or what its outcomes are expected to be. Women perceive its purpose in different ways. Some women are better informed about the process of arranging their care than others, and are very clear about what they want. Others have no clear understanding about the process or what will come out of it. It is the midwife's obligation to assist the woman through this initial contact by providing a framework for understanding the exchange, and a pathway through it.

There is no standard terminology for or description of this initial contact. It may be referred to as the 'options' or 'check-out' visit or contact (to 'check out' meaning to gain a first impression or initial understanding of a person or a situation), and many midwives will have their own term for it. It is not the same thing as a 'booking' visit. The key feature differentiating this contact from a booking is that during the initial contact process, the woman and midwife share information that will enable a decision to be made about whether they will work together. The booking visit, by contrast, occurs as a result of that decision having been made.

There is also no standard format for the process itself. While individual midwives will perceive and prioritise its various stages and content differently, it needs to include certain elements in order to be meaningful to childbearing women. For women having their first baby, the system and process are new and unknown. They will often require specific information from the midwife, and will frequently

MIDWIFE'S STORY

When I arrived at the woman's home, I was surprised to find an ashtray in every room—including the toilet! She had told me previously that no one who lived in the house smoked. She hadn't mentioned that her grandmother, who lived close by, spent most of her time at her house, and smoked heavily. It was a delicate situation, with family relationships at stake, and required the full duration of the pregnancy to support the woman in negotiating smoke-free spaces in her own home. Visiting her at home and meeting her family gave me valuable insight into how to support the woman in making changes which would have a positive impact on her own health and that of her baby, without fracturing family relationships.

be dependent upon guidance from her. They often don't know what they need to know, in order to make an informed decision. It is the midwife's role to facilitate informed decision-making by women, which includes the choices they make regarding their caregiver. For a list of questions that women should have answered by a prospective caregiver, see Box 20.1 or go to the New Zealand College of Midwives (NZCOM) website (www.midwife.org.nz).

The overall intention of this process is to identify the level of compatibility between the woman and her potential midwife, in order to determine whether they can establish a constructive working relationship. Without this, effective communication can be difficult, which can lead to a breakdown in the relationship between them, and in turn create the potential for a negative impact on social or clinical outcomes. Compatibility needs to occur at three levels—the interpersonal, the professional and the practical.

The interpersonal level

Each woman and midwife pair needs to feel that there is a comfortable personal connection between them. This is first and foremost a professional relationship, and not one based on shared personal experiences or a common background. The interpersonal dynamic is about a sense of relaxation and trust, and the ability to speak a social 'language' that the other feels comfortable with and understands. Different midwives will suit different women, and sometimes this initial discussion

will result in a decision not to work together. This may be due to character and personality variables, about which we should not be surprised. This process is about establishing an effective human relationship (even if it is professional in nature) and so it should not be regarded as a sign of failure that a woman chooses not to work with a particular midwife.

Cultural factors are also key aspects of compatibility. It is important for women to have the opportunity to evaluate the cultural awareness and sensitivity of a midwife, and be confident that the midwife will be able to advocate for her culture-specific needs or desires.

The professional level

There is variation in the context and scope of practice among midwives. This variation is due in part to differences in belief and understanding of the nature of pregnancy, birth and parenting, and reflects the midwifery philosophy that underpins their practice. Midwives may also feel more or less comfortable in a range of settings. Some work comfortably with women in an obstetric setting, while others are most comfortable in the primary, community or home birth context. The way in which midwives practise professionally will vary according to these beliefs as well as their levels of experience, personal confidence and comfort zones, and their skills or knowledge base.

There is also variation among women in their views, beliefs and understandings of the nature of pregnancy, birth and

---

BOX 20.1   Questions to ask a midwife

Pregnancy

- Are you a member of the Australian/New Zealand College of Midwives?
- Is your practice reviewed annually, through the College Standards Review process? (New Zealand)
- How many women do you 'book' each month?
- Who is your back-up midwife? How do you work together?
- When will I meet her? Will I have the opportunity to get to know her?
- If I require consultation with an obstetrician or other specialist, what are my options?
- Under what circumstances would my care be transferred to hospital staff?
- Where do you provide antenatal visits?
- Between visits, are you available for me to phone you for advice?
- Do you work with or refer to other health professionals or support groups?
- What are your beliefs about pregnancy and birth?

Labour and birth

- Do you offer home birth? Do you have access to small birthing centres in the area?
- What hospitals do you have access to?

- What birthing options do you offer (e.g. water birth)?
- Do you come to my home when I am in labour?
- In labour, if I need care from an obstetrician, how will it be arranged?
- If this happens, what role will you play in my care?
- Under what circumstances would my care be transferred to hospital staff?
- If my labour is long, who will relieve you and provide my care?

After the birth

- How often do you visit after the birth?
- If I need or choose to be in hospital after the birth, will you visit me there?
- What will your role be and what care will you provide, in that situation?
- For how many weeks do you provide care?
- Between visits, are you available for me to phone you for advice?
- Do you work with or refer to other health professionals or support groups?
- What are your beliefs about breastfeeding?

(Source: Adapted from the New Zealand College of Midwives pamphlet, 'Questions to ask when you choose a midwife' (undated publication))

MIDWIFE'S STORY

When Ana and I first met, she was eight weeks pregnant with her first child. She told me of her plan to have an elective caesarean section. She came from a country that offered this option to all women. When asked why she feared vaginal birth so much, she recounted stories of traumatic vaginal births of women she knew. None of these were normal births. I informed her that one of my professional boundaries was to decline to work with women planning a caesarean section with no clinical indication. We talked through my reasoning. Our initial visit ended with the option of us working together on the basis of planning a normal birth, or her choosing to work with someone else. The following week she attended her pre-arranged appointment with an obstetrician and, after considering her options, called me to ask me to provide her maternity care. We began a journey together which eventually included a normal birth.

parenting. This will influence the expectations they have and the priorities they set for the type of care their midwife will provide. For example, before choosing a caregiver, a woman planning a home birth will want to know whether her choice will fit within the scope of practice of, and be genuinely supported by, a midwife.

The practical level

There are a number of practical details of care that will need to be discussed. The first of these is the availability of the midwife to provide care for the woman's pregnancy, birth and postnatal period. This is focused on the estimated due date (EDD).

It is appropriate for midwives to inform women about arrangements for back-up when they are unavailable to provide care, such as during regular time off or illness, or when they are with another woman. In some practices, midwives work together in loose 'partnerships' and arrangements may or may not be made for women to meet their back-up midwives; in others, visits with the back-up midwife are an integral part of the care. There is also a moral obligation on midwives to inform women about their plans for holidays during the period of care.

A second major issue is the time and place of antenatal care. Women and midwives need to identify whether they can organise antenatal visits at a time and place that suits. This is affected by the context in which care is provided, and by the personal choices made by individual midwives. Some midwives provide clinic-based antenatal care on set days of the week. Others may negotiate with women to visit them in their home for some or all of the antenatal care.

Summary

The main purpose of the initial contact is to establish a two-way partnership between the woman and the midwife.

Both are active decision-makers in this process, and negotiate their respective roles and responsibilities. Both need to have the opportunity to make choices about whether or not they will work together.

During the initial contact, the midwife learns about the plans, beliefs and concerns the woman has about her pregnancy, childbirth and postnatal care. She also learns a little about her social, cultural and physical history and context. The midwife identifies issues that may make it inappropriate for her to provide care, such as when a woman has specific social or cultural needs, or an underlying medical condition that requires care and knowledge that is beyond the midwife's personal scope of practice.

The woman learns about the midwife's personal beliefs and scope of practice, her professional boundaries, and the practical arrangements that may affect the woman's choice of caregiver. She develops a sense of the midwife's personality and practice, and decides whether she can trust the midwife to provide the kind of care that she wants.

This process should function as a positive screening process for both the woman and the midwife. Each has the right to *choose* to work with the other, as it is important that this relationship begins as it is to go on—with both woman and midwife sharing information, and actively participating and making decisions in a negotiated partnership.

The booking visit

The booking visit is essentially the beginning of the care relationship between the midwife and the woman and her family. It is an important part of the whole context of midwifery care, and of the antenatal care component in particular. It occurs early in the pregnancy and at the woman's home where possible, and includes the midwife, the woman, and whomever else she chooses to have with her—partner, mother, sister or friend. The purpose of this visit is to formalise the arrangements for care, and to establish a foundation for the partnership. In other words, it is about defining the nature of the relationship between the woman and the midwife, and the context and meaning of antenatal care for both of them. It will:

- have a holistic focus
- be a two-way process of information sharing and decision-making
- review the past, identify the present, and plan the future
- include the identification of health, known ill-health, and risk markers for potential ill-health, for the woman or her baby
- include practical arrangements of care, in terms of frequency, time and place.

The booking visit happens as a result of a decision being made by the woman and midwife to work together. At this point, they will have already spoken by phone, and may have met, and will know a little about each other. If the initial contact or 'check-out' visit was not done face to face, it is preferable that the booking visit be held off until they have

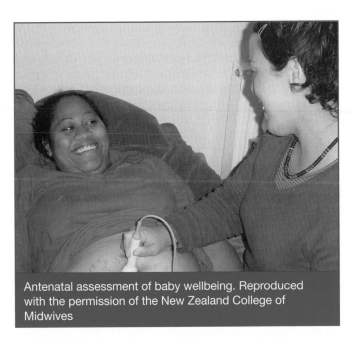

Antenatal assessment of baby wellbeing. Reproduced with the permission of the New Zealand College of Midwives

had an opportunity to meet. Alternatively, the visit could begin as a check-out opportunity for both, with a clearly identified end point for the meeting, in order to give some time and space for the woman to consider whether or not she would like to work with that midwife. If both are comfortable with each other, they may decide to formally begin the relationship at that point.

The booking visit represents the beginning of a shared journey. It is the beginning of a relationship that will last for about ten months (in the first instance), and encompass a special, powerful and life-changing period for the woman and her family. It is a time when many personal and private aspects of a woman's life will become shared with the midwife. As such, the booking is a great opportunity for the midwife to *get to know* the woman she will be working with. The woman's home is the ideal venue for this visit, as it is in her place and space, which can help to moderate the traditional hierarchical power dynamic between 'health professional' and 'patient', to that of a more equitable partnership between midwife and woman.

Having the booking visit at the woman's home can also give the midwife important information about the woman's personal and social context. The midwife will be able to gain valuable insight into the woman's personality and outlook, her understanding of pregnancy and childbirth, and her life situation and lifestyle choices, when discussing her history and her present and future plans. There is as much to be learned from the *way* in which the woman talks about these things and the way she responds to new information or options, as from *what* she says. During the discussion, the midwife can develop a sense of how the woman perceives her own role in the birth process—as an active 'doer', or a passive 'receiver' of care—as well as her understanding of health issues and the concept of risk in pregnancy.

Learning about *who* a woman is, in a holistic sense, is a central and integral component of the midwifery model. It is not an optional extra to the 'real' physical or clinical aspects, but an imperative for midwifery care, if an effective working relationship is to develop. Having this understanding helps the midwife to tailor the way she shares information with the woman, so that it may be meaningful for her. Midwives cannot identify what is appropriate for women if they know nothing of their personal, social or cultural 'self'. Sharing information or making recommendations that are irrelevant or inappropriate to their personal, social or cultural circumstances will be ineffectual, can be offensive, and may have a negative impact on the woman and the outcomes.

The booking visit and the process of establishing a partnership is not about 'becoming friends' or 'being nice'. It is about developing an effective working relationship at a professional level, between human beings.

Reviewing the past

The quality and quantity of information shared during the booking visit depends on a number of factors. The specific questions asked by the midwife, the way in which they are asked, and the timing of them (in terms of when in the booking process they are asked), may influence a woman's responses, particularly when they relate to sensitive information such as that regarding sexually transmitted infections, abortions or abuse.

It is also important to recognise that a woman's knowledge of her family's health history and that of her own childhood illnesses or operations may be limited, perhaps due to poor access to those details, possibly as a result of family separation or dislocation or such like. Some women may also have limited understanding of the details of treatments or the nature of medical procedures they have undergone. For example, the detail, meaning or significance of differing cervical treatments (such as loop surgery, cone biopsy, laser treatment, and the associated terminology such as 'CIN I, II or III') are sometimes not known or understood by women. This means that women, understandably, are sometimes unable to provide the level of detail sought by midwives.

The midwife identifies risk markers from the woman's history, and discusses them with her. This discussion may include options for testing, screening, treatment, self-care, referral for consultation with situation-appropriate specialists, support and further information gathering. (See Ch 32 for discussion on screening, assessment and consultation options, and Ch 33 for discussion on risk markers and potential complications in pregnancy.)

Research findings suggest that midwives who use a 'structured paper history' incorporating a cue sheet (see Appendix A) are likely to get 'more and better information' than those using an unstructured format (cited in NICE 2003). Documentation of shared information is very important for both the woman and the midwife. During the care, it is appropriate for the woman to carry her own maternity notes (see NICE 2003). Upon completion of care, the midwife also needs to keep a copy of these documents, in order to meet her respective professional and legal requirements.

Identifying the present

As part of the booking visit, the midwife also undertakes a 'current health review' (see Appendix B) and an initial examination, in order to establish baseline information and facilitate the process of planning the care. All the issues identified in the 'current health review', and those raised in the aforementioned historical health review, have the potential to influence the process or outcome of pregnancy, although some are more significant than others. They should provide the midwife with cues as to the nature and detail of any physical examination that may be required.

Currently, there is no consensus as to the detail, make-up and content of a 'routine' initial physical examination of a well pregnant woman. Chan and Kean (2004) state that 'there is very little to be gained from a full formal physical examination' (p 80). They suggest that 'routine auscultation for maternal heart sounds in asymptomatic women with no cardiac history is unnecessary', and that neither formal breast examination nor routine pelvic examination is appropriate (p 80). The NICE (2003) guidelines do not address the issue of cardiac examination, but support the recommendation against routine breast and pelvic assessments. In contrast, Frye (1998) recommends a full medical examination including the above checks and details such as assessment of lymph nodes, reflexes, mouth, eyes and lungs, in addition to the 'vital signs'. It is debatable whether such an examination is indicated, or within the scope of midwifery practice. Certainly, midwives generally work with well women, and should have sound knowledge of normal anatomy and physiology, and organ and hormone function, as well as signs of dysfunction, but a *routine* full examination may be both inappropriate and outside the midwifery scope of practice. To date, there is limited evidence available which addresses this issue to any significant degree.

It is important to distinguish between something that is offered routinely, and that which is offered in response to risk markers. For example, offering vaginal swabs as a screening test routinely is not currently recommended, but for a woman with a history of chlamydia and ongoing unsafe sex practice, screening may well be indicated. In such cases it is appropriate to discuss the option of carrying out a diagnostic test to identify whether there is a current infection, along with issues of self-care, and the potential risks from such an infection to the woman's health and wellbeing and that of her baby.

Planning the future

Working through the relevant aspects of the woman's past and present health status enables a foundation to be established which facilitates effective planning for the future care of the woman. The midwife and the woman are now in a position to make decisions about the relevance or appropriateness of particular screening or diagnostic tests, and to determine whether there is a need for referral for specialist consultation. This may be to any one or a number of specialists, such as an obstetrician, dietician, physiotherapist, psychiatrist, sexual health specialist or geneticist. They are also in a position to make decisions about those other matters that are outlined in Decision point 1 (see page opposite).

Decision points

Decision points are a significant new initiative in the organisation of antenatal care. They provide a systematic framework for organising care, and are articulated in their primary form in the New Zealand College of Midwives *Midwives' Handbook for Practice* (2005). A modified and expanded version of these decision points was developed for this chapter, a key theme of which is a holistic midwifery approach to antenatal care.

The decision points are based on eight time frames, which are loosely tied to gestation periods through the course of pregnancy. They consist of four categories of cues that provide a guiding form and structure for care. These cues alert the midwife to the components of what is currently considered appropriate and necessary in the provision of comprehensive antenatal care. The four categories include cues about information sharing, assessment and screening, active decision-making and health promotion and education. These categories are intended to assist the midwife to consider the various dimensions of care, beyond the purely clinical aspects of it, and reflect a holistic understanding of the care process, without being overly prescriptive. It is important that the midwife actively considers each aspect of care raised in the decision point framework with reference to the social, emotional, physical and cultural realities of each woman.

Each decision point contains references to other chapters in this book, and to following explanatory sections (called 'explanations' in the decision point boxes) where a range of components of routine antenatal care are described and discussed in further detail. These explanatory sections cover:

- estimated due date (EDD)
- routine antenatal blood screening
- routine blood pressure screening
- routine urine screening
- palpation—hands-on learning, identification and assessment
- fetal movement (FM)
- antenatal education
- exercise in pregnancy
- physiological changes of pregnancy.

DECISION POINT 1: the booking visit (before 12 weeks)

1 Information sharing

Choices for maternity care

Inhformation on community groups and agencies

Woman's:

▶ plans regarding pregnancy, birth and early parenting (care plan)

▶ experience of pregnancy

▶ physiological changes (see Explanations)

▶ social, emotional, medical, physical, cultural situation

Midwife's practice—support, time-off, how to contact, confidentiality

Folic acid supplementation

Options for:

▶ antenatal education (see Explanations)

▶ place for birth

▶ midwifery student involvement, if relevant

2 Assessment and screening

Review history (see Appendix A):

▶ maternity, medical, social, physical, psychological

▶ identify and discuss alerting factors or risk markers

Review current health status (see Appendix B):

▶ physical, social, emotional and cultural

▶ identify and discuss alerting factors or risk marker

▶ establish EDD (see Explanations)

Initial antenatal screening—routine (with informed consent)

▶ Blood
   — routine (see Explanations)
   — options from risk markers—STIs, TB, HIV, Hep C

▶ Urine—MSU and dipstick urinalysis and/or microscopy and culture (see Explanations)

Screening options if risk markers from history or current health review

▶ blood tests, scan (nuchal translucency), CVS or amniocentesis

3 Active decision-making

LMC—decided prior to 'booking' process

Screening options—routine and options due to 'risk markers'

Referral—if indicated and wanted—for 'specialist' input (e.g. obstetrician, dietician, physiotherapist)

Meeting/involvement of midwifery student

Time, place, frequency of antenatal care

4 Health promotion and education

Lifestyle affirmation, or review 'readiness' for change

Diet, exercise, self-care, employment

Safety—physical, emotional, cultural

Avoiding infections—listeria, toxoplasmosis, STIs, etc

DECISION POINT 2: 16 to 20 weeks

1 Information sharing

Decisions made since last visit—re screening, care plan, lifestyle changes

Results from screening or diagnostic tests, and implications discussed

Normal physiological changes (see Explanations)

Expectations re first fetal movements—timing range, initial irregularity

Options re employment and parental leave

2 Assessment and screening

Assess woman's wellbeing—discuss options re physiological changes

Screen:

▶ Urinalysis (glucose and protein), blood pressure

▶ Discuss option of fetal anomaly scan (18–20 weeks) timing, expectations, limitations, information, diagnostic and decision options

▶ Family violence (routine)

Assess baby's wellbeing

▶ size (fundal height—see Explanations)

▶ growth, movements, heart rate (Doppler)

3 Active decision-making

Scan (decision may be made after visit, form given if requested, self-booked)

Antenatal education decision made—classes booked if desired

Plans re infant feeding

4 Health promotion and education

Breastfeeding promoted—information, resources and support options

Self-care and lifestyle—diet, exercise, support re healthy changes, employment issues

Pelvic floor exercises

DECISION POINT 3:   20 to 24 weeks

1 Information sharing

Normal physiological changes (see Explanations)

Relationship issues—changes, support, involvement of partner/ friends

Results from and experience of anomaly scan (if done)

2 Assessment and screening

Assess woman's wellbeing—discuss options re physiological changes

Screen—urinalysis (glucose and protein), blood pressure

Assess baby's wellbeing—size (fundal height), growth, movements, heart rate (Doppler)

3 Active decision-making

Place for the birth (if decided)—if hospital: booking forms and arrange visit

Any follow-up from anomaly scan indicated

4 Health promotion and education

Discussion re woman's own wellbeing and preparation for parenthood

Diet, exercise, support, stress minimisation, employment—as relevant/appropriate

DECISION POINT 4:   24 to 28 weeks

1 Information sharing

Signs of premature labour and when to call midwife

Signs of baby's wellbeing—expectations re movements (see Explanations)

Normal physiological changes (see Explanations)

Discuss emotional and social situation—feelings re pregnancy, financial changes, career/employment implications and plans (timing of work reduction/finishing)

2 Assessment and screening

Assess woman's wellbeing—discuss options re physiological changes

Screen:

▶ Urinalysis (glucose and protein), blood pressure

▶ Routine blood screen (option discussed)—CBC, blood group antibodies

▶ Review risk markers for gestational diabetes—discuss option of screening, information, limitations, expectations, diagnostic and decision options

▶ Family violence (routine)

Assess baby's wellbeing—size (fundal height), growth, movements, heart rate (Pinard/Doppler)

3 Active decision-making

Continue developing care plan—antenatal education start date, if appropriate, or alternative arrangements (books/videos, resources, support)

Preparations for change of life with new baby:

▶ emotional, social, practical

▶ car seat (bought or booked for hire), clothing and bedding

4 Health promotion and education

Postnatal sleeping arrangements—appropriate bed sharing, and risk markers re SIDS

Self-care and support networks (check knowledge re community groups and agencies)

DECISION POINT 5:   30 to 32 weeks

1 Information sharing

Check that the woman, and her family, is comfortable with planned place for birth and birth plan discussed, including expectations of midwifery care

Discuss options for working with pain in labour (see Chs 22 and 23)

Discuss signs of pre-eclampsia, and when to contact midwife

Discuss family's expectations and preparations for life with a new baby

Discuss postnatal care plan—re vitamin K and newborn metabolic screen test

2 Assessment and screening

Assess woman's wellbeing—discuss options re physiological changes (see Explanations)

Screen—urinalysis (glucose and protein), blood pressure

Assess baby's wellbeing—size (fundal height), growth, movements, heart rate

3 Active decision-making

Postnatal care and support—community groups and agencies (Well Child services)

Plans for placenta

Plans for working with pain in labour

Plans for feeding baby—check knowledge, resources, support

4 Health promotion and education

Childcare arrangements (if applicable) for end of pregnancy, labour, early postnatal days

Support and resources for postnatal days

Self-care:

▶ review employment arrangements, emotional and social situation

▶ review woman's feelings about birth and parenting—support options

DECISION POINT 6: 34 to 36 weeks

1 Information sharing

Discuss signs of labour, expectations, support, beliefs and feelings about labour

If hospital birth planned:

▶ check that all know where it is, check cultural needs

▶ discuss policies which may affect the woman's choices

If home birth planned—discuss appropriate environment and gear needed

Physiological changes and expectations (see Explanations)

2 Assessment and screening

Assess woman's wellbeing—discuss options re physiological changes

Screen:

▶ urinalysis (glucose and protein), blood pressure

▶ consider blood screen of Hb (if woman taking iron or symptomatic) and Rh antibody screen (if woman Rh negative)

Assess baby's wellbeing:

▶ size (fundal height), growth, movements, heart rate

▶ presentation—if not cephalic, discuss referral options (36 weeks)

3 Active decision-making

Birth plans identified

Preparation of other child(ren) for changes with new baby

Practical arrangements made for early postnatal days—meals in freezer or support as appropriate

Plans made for labour:

▶ support people, child care, resources (food, comfort measures)

▶ home birth gear together, or bag packed for hospital

4 Health promotion and education

Self-care—diet, exercise and lifestyle changes for this stage of pregnancy

Review emotional and social situation, review employment plans

DECISION POINT 7: 38 to 40 weeks

1 Information sharing

Review signs of labour, expectations, support, beliefs and feelings about labour

Recognising labour, and when and how to contact midwife

Review woman's knowledge of risk markers:

▶ fresh vaginal blood loss

▶ reduced fetal movements

▶ signs of pre-eclampsia

▶ ruptured membranes (without contractions, meconium stained liquor)

Physiological changes and expectations of timing of labour (discuss normal range)

Review blood results (if appropriate)

2 Assessment and screening

Assess woman's wellbeing—discuss options re physiological changes (see Explanations)

Screen:

▶ urinalysis (glucose and protein), blood pressure

▶ family violence, antenatal depression

Assess baby's wellbeing:

▶ size (fundal height), growth, movements, heart rate

▶ presentation, descent in the woman's pelvis, liquor volume

Review EDD—check and confirm expected dates

3 Active decision-making

Support networks arranged for labour, birth and postnatal

Confirm postnatal care plan re:

▶ vitamin K

▶ newborn metabolic screening test

4 Health promotion and education

Review self-care:

▶ adjustments to life without paid work (if relevant)

▶ support, opportunities

▶ diet, exercise, sleep, emotions, self-esteem

Review partner and/or family readiness, support, resources, arrangements for time off work

Discuss first breastfeed and importance of skin-to-skin contact for some women

---

DECISION POINT 8: 41 to 42 weeks

1 Information sharing

Discuss wellbeing of woman and baby, family support

Discuss issues and options re 'post dates' (see Ch 33)

Discuss option of vaginal exam and membrane sweep/cervical massage

Discuss option of obstetric referral and timing and process of induction of labour

2 Assessment and screening

Assess woman's wellbeing:

▶ discuss options re physiological changes (see Explanations)

▶ screen—urinalysis (glucose and protein), blood pressure

Assess baby's wellbeing:

▶ size (fundal height), growth, movements, heart rate

▶ presentation, descent in the woman's pelvis, liquor volume

▶ screen—discuss option of CTG or scan, to assess baby's wellbeing if indicated

▶ discuss risk markers—reduced fetal movements, low liquor volume

3 Active decision-making

Set plan re assessment of baby and woman's wellbeing—referral for consultation

4 Health promotion and education

Additional care and support options

Check support networks and resources

Explanatory sections

Estimated due date

Dating in history and Naegele's rule

Women have been calculating their menstrual cycles and pregnancies using lunar months for 'tens of thousands of years' (Frye 1998). However, the method based on a set number of days following the last menstrual period (LMP) was proposed by Professor Boerhaave in 1709 and popularised by, and subsequently attributed to, Dr Naegele (Baskett & Naegele 2000). Boerhaave proposed that gestation be calculated 'by counting one week after the last period and by reckoning the nine months of gestation from that time' (cited in Baskett & Naegele 2000, p 1433). Neither man specified whether it is the first or last day of the LMP that is the start point.

The first day of LMP is currently taken as the starting point, to which nine months and seven days are added. The inherent variability in the length of different months has been negated with the conversion of the formula into pregnancy calculators as LMP plus 280 days. This rule has *all* women ovulating at the same time within a cycle, having a cycle of the same length (which is set at 28 days), and taking the same length of time to gestate. Some individual variation is allowed for in this formula by altering the estimated due date (EDD) by the regular cycle length. This is recommended by the British Confidential Enquiry into Stillbirths and Death in Infancy (CESDI), with 'EDD = LMP + 280 days + length of cycle − 28 days' (cited in Stenhouse et al 2003). This formula is in contrast to dating by ultrasound scanning, which uses universally standardised measurements for dating. Contradicting such a notion, midwives' knowledge and common sense support inherent differences in human size and gestation. Research has also variously identified maternal height, ethnicity, parity and age as potentially influential in the length of gestation, although not with predictive reliability (Rosser 2000).

While it is estimated that only five per cent of women give birth on their EDD (Frye 1998), the date has taken on new significance in the contemporary context, with decisions regarding medical screening and interventions demanding 'exact' or standardised dating. Several authors have argued that ultrasound dating is more 'accurate' and that calculating EDD from women's LMP should be abandoned (e.g. Tunon et al 1996).

Standardisation with medicalisation

In reviewing the literature on the topic, Olsen and Clausen (1997) found the 280-day 'rule' to be consistently three days too short—that is, the most common gestation length is 283 days. They also report ultrasound dating to be consistently two days too long. They challenged the accuracy of both the Cochrane Review and the MIDIRS (Midwives Information and Resource Service) 'informed choice' leaflet, which both accept the contention that ultrasound scans provide a more accurate EDD than the use of a calendar and LMP (Olsen & Clausen 1997). The 'improved' accuracy relates primarily to the reduced 'post-dates' induction of labour rates when scan dating is used. Menticoglou and Hall (2002) have convincingly challenged the evidence used for the guideline on routine post-dates induction of labour (IOL) at 41 weeks. Altering Naegele's rule to 283 days, rather than discarding it, will achieve the same outcome, and is supported by others (Nguyen et al 1999; Savitz et al 2002; Smith 2001; Yang et al 2002).

Scan dating and research

Recently, evidence has been published which exposes systematic errors in scan dating that have the potential to lead to compromised care and outcomes (Källén 2004; Nakling & Backe 2002; Nguyen et al 2000). Källén (2002) reviewed 571,617 women's records at the Swedish Medical Birth Registry and found male babies to be judged on average to be 1.5 days 'older' than females at 16–18 weeks, on the basis of their slightly bigger comparative size. She reports that 'similarly, the fetuses of young women, multiparous women, smokers and women with low educational level were at increased risk of being smaller than expected at ultrasound examination in early pregnancy' (Källén 2002, p 558). Källén (2004) (reviewing over 700,000 Swedish women) and Nguyen et al (2000) (reviewing 16,469 Danish women) found increased adverse outcomes when scan dating re-dates women's pregnancies by more than seven days, with significantly more stillbirths, pre-term and intrauterine growth retarded (IUGR) babies and perinatal deaths. This contradicts earlier reports by others who suggest that there are no adverse effects of scan dating (Tunon et al 1999). Rather than being more 'accurate', it is possible that 'the erroneous adjusted dates may be due to incorrect measurements or systematic bias (e.g. gender), but they are also likely to reflect early growth restriction' (Källén 2002, p 558). Although first trimester scan dating may be less affected by such differences, variability still occurs, and evidence regarding its 'accuracy' and the impact on clinical outcomes is lacking to date.

Pregnancy calculators

Pregnancy calculators are the most common tool for midwives identifying women's EDD. They are subject to both intra- and inter-calculator variability (Ross 2003), and so should be checked against each other and the most reliable chosen. New computer software is available free from the Gestation Network website (www.gestation.net/main.htm), although it does not allow for variance in cycle length, and works on the 280-day rule.

Midwifery practice

When working with women to identify their EDD, midwives should:
- identify the first day of LMP, if known
- ask if it was a normal period in timing, length and volume
- ask about the normal cycle—length and regularity
- ask about contraceptive use prior to conception
- use Naegele's rule or the pregnancy calculator to get an EDD (consider using 283 days)
- discuss variability and expectations regarding the actual timing of the birth
- review the signs, symptoms and experiences and compare with expected dating
- ask if they can palpate the woman's abdomen to compare uterine size with dates
- consider the option of a scan if the woman has no idea of LMP or timing of conception, and date-specific screening is to be undertaken; or if her uterine size is significantly mismatched with estimated EDD on palpation.

Routine antenatal blood screening

The use of blood tests as a screening tool is routine in antenatal care, although there is variation in the tests included or offered between states and countries (Hunt & Lumley 2002; Three Centres Consensus Guidelines on Antenatal Care Project 2001; Ministry of Health 2002). Currently, both Australia and New Zealand include the following tests as routine:
- blood group and rhesus factor
- rhesus antibodies

> ### Critical thinking exercise
>
> Jenny is pregnant. She is not sure when her baby is due. The first day of her LMP was 15 February 2005. She has a regular cycle, which lasts five days, every 30 days.
> 1 Calculate the EDD using three different pregnancy calculators.
> 2 Calculate the EDD manually using Naegele's rule.
> 3 Calculate the EDD using the computer software mentioned above.
> 4 Compare the EDDs from each method, and consider the implications of any potential variation.
> 5 What information would you share with Jenny regarding her EDD?

- full blood count
- syphilis
- hepatitis B
- rubella antibodies.

For detailed discussion on the conditions being screened for, see Boyle (1995) and Frye (1998). The issues of the nature of screening itself, informed choice and the politics regarding antenatal screening are addressed in Ch 32 of this book; and elsewhere, for example, Broclain et al (2003), Grimes & Schulz (2002), National Health Committee (2003), Oats (2000), Searle (1997) and Strong (2000).

Debate continues over the appropriateness of universal versus risk-based, and opt-in versus opt-out, screening for the following conditions:
- human immunodeficiency virus (HIV)
- hepatitis C (HCV)
- fetal aneuploidy (focused on neural tube defects and Down syndrome)
- gestational diabetes
- haemoglobinopathies (e.g. sickle cell and thalassaemia)
- tuberculosis (TB).

See Chapter 32 for discussion on these conditions and contemporary screening options offered. Gates (2004) addresses some of the political issues involved, as do Parker et al (2002) and Santalahti et al (1998).

Iron levels, measures and supplementation

In the context of routine antenatal care, the midwife uses the results from the complete blood count as part of the process of screening for iron deficiency anaemia. Anaemia is potentially a significant threat to the health and wellbeing of women and their babies. Physiological changes induced by pregnancy may expose underlying anaemia, or it may develop during pregnancy (Coggins 2001). Haemoglobin levels are used as a primary measure of anaemia, as 'about 70% of iron in the body is in haemoglobin' (Jordan 2002, p 268). Serum ferritin levels have been used as markers of anaemia as an adjunct to haemoglobin in recent times, although currently there are no reference ranges available that are specific to

---

Critical thinking exercise

Mai is 14 weeks pregnant with her first child when she first seeks maternity care. She is 24 years old, and a recent immigrant of West African ethnic origin. She and her partner Ahut are well educated and have good English-language skills.

1   What tests would be carried out if you ordered 'routine' initial blood screening for Mai?

2   Describe what is being tested, and its potential significance.

3   What additional blood screening tests might you consider discussing with Mai and Ahut, and what information would inform this discussion?

4   What written information is available for them in your region, on either 'routine' or 'additional' blood tests?

---

pregnancy. Parameters for normal physiological changes in serum ferritin and their clinical significance are yet to be established (Chandler 2000). There is also ongoing debate over the appropriate reference ranges for haemoglobin during pregnancy; and the boundaries between physiological changes and pathological changes requiring intervention in the form of supplementation are not well defined or understood (Baston 2002; Bluck et al 1990; Coggins 2001; Mohamed 2004). No single measure should be taken in isolation, or without reference to the past and present context of the individual woman.

Potential signs and symptoms of anaemia include tiredness, dizziness, tinnitus, feeling cold, dry or itchy skin, infections, palpitations or breathlessness, tachycardia, headaches, pallor, glossitis and koilonychias (Coggins 2001; Jordan 2002). It is important to note that many of these signs and symptoms could also be those of other conditions, so a definitive diagnosis of anaemia by means of further blood tests is required.

For further discussion on anaemia and related issues, see Chapter 32 for screening and guidelines, Chapter 33 for risk factors and effects for women and their babies, Chapter 19 for details of dietary options and Chapter 29 for pharmacological options.

Routine blood pressure screening

Blood pressure measurement and monitoring is a core feature of routine antenatal care. Blood pressure (BP) may be defined as 'the force exerted against the arterial walls when the heart pumps', and 'the blood pressure reading is a reflection of how hard the heart must work to adequately circulate the blood' (Frye 1998, p 420). Taking blood pressure is essentially a screening test for hypertension, and careful measurement is important as the technique used can significantly affect the accuracy of the reading. Blood pressure should be taken using a regularly calibrated sphygmomanometer and an appropriate-sized cuff, and the woman should be seated and rested, with her elbow at heart level and her arm straight.

The cuff should be inflated to 20 mmHg above the systolic BP palpated at the brachial artery, and deflated slowly (about 2 mmHg/second). Both the systolic (Korotkoff I) and diastolic (Korotkoff V) pressures should be recorded. See the guidelines in the Australasian Society for the Study of Hypertension in Pregnancy (ASSHP) Consensus Statement (Brown et al 2000) or Taylor (2004) for detailed instructions. The ASSHP (Brown et al 2000) recommend that BP be taken on both arms at the first assessment, with significant difference in readings being an indication for specialist consultation.

Sustained elevated blood pressure beyond normal values is referred to as hypertension, which presents some risk to the wellbeing of women and their babies. The ASSHP (Brown et al 2000) defines hypertension in pregnancy as a systolic BP of ≥ 140 mmHg and/or a diastolic BP (KV) of ≥ 90 mmHg (p 2). The group identifies four classifications of hypertension, namely gestational hypertension (GH), pre-eclampsia (pre-eclampsia), chronic hypertension (CH) and pre-eclampsia superimposed on CH (Brown et al 2000). Pre-eclampsia, if unrecognised, may develop into eclampsia, which is a major cause of maternal and perinatal morbidity and mortality (NICE 2003). Pre-eclampsia is a multi-system disorder which is unique to pregnancy, and remains a condition that is difficult to predict, prevent or treat (see discussion in Ch 33). It affects between two and ten per cent of childbearing women, with the incidence varying with 'the population studied and the criteria used to diagnose the disorder' (NICE 2003, p 99). The diagnostic criteria for P-E have changed in recent years, with the inclusion of a urine protein/creatinine ratio and the exclusion of oedema. The ASSHP criteria are as follows:

Hypertension arising after 20 weeks gestation and the new onset after 20 weeks gestation of one or more of:
- Proteinuria— ≥ 300 mg/24h or spot urine protein/creatinine ratio ≥ 30 mg/mmol
- Renal insufficiency—serum/plasma creatinine ≥ 0.09 mmol/L or oligouria
- Liver disease—raised serum transaminases and/or severe epigastric/right upper quadrant pain
- Neurological problems—convulsions (eclampsia); hyperreflexia with clonus; severe headaches with hyperreflexia; persistent visual disturbances (scotomata)
- Haematological disturbances—thrombocytopenia; disseminated intravascular coagulation; haemolysis
- Fetal growth restriction (ASSHP 2000, p 4).

Numerous risk markers have been identified over the years, although none reliably predict who will develop pre-eclampsia, or when or how unwell they will become. The risk markers currently associated with pre-eclampsia include women who are having their first baby (or first baby with a different partner), are over forty years old, have a family history of pre-eclampsia, have a personal history of pre-eclampsia, have a body mass index (BMI) at or above 35, have a multiple pregnancy or have pre-existing vascular disease (e.g. hypertension or diabetes) (Brown et al 2000; NICE 2003). In the contemporary Australasian context, this group of women may well represent the majority of the total childbearing population, yet only a fraction of the actual total will develop pre-eclampsia, and the majority of women in every one of the above groups will remain well and go on to give birth to a healthy baby.

While we cannot predict or prevent the development of pre-eclampsia, current routine antenatal BP screening does help identify some women who may be showing signs or experiencing symptoms that signal the need for closer monitoring or diagnostic testing, which may facilitate detection of pre-eclampsia prior to it causing morbidity or mortality (Enkin et al 2000). The distinction between isolated hypertension (be it chronic or gestational) and pre-eclampsia is an important one, with many more women having hypertension than those who go on to develop pre-eclampsia. 'Chronic hypertension and mild or moderate pregnancy-induced hypertension carry little risk to the mother or the fetus, unless severe hypertension, pre-eclampsia, or eclampsia ensue' (Enkin et al 2000, p 123).

Midwives have an important role in sharing information with women about the symptoms of pre-eclampsia, such as severe headaches, visual disturbances (not caused by postural hypotension), epigastric pain (not heartburn), or sudden marked swelling of the face, hands and feet. This information needs to be presented in a way that enables women to recognise and respond to symptoms appropriately, rather than frightening them into a hypersensitive state of anxiety. It is important that midwives and women maintain a sense of perspective regarding the actual incidence of this condition, as it is rare, affecting less than 5% of the childbearing population.

Routine urine screening

Urine screening is offered routinely throughout pregnancy, although there is variation in both the method and markers used, and no consensus about what constitutes best practice. The aim of urine screening is the detection of proteinuria (as a marker for pre-eclampsia and urinary tract infection) and glycosuria (as a marker for gestational diabetes). Some practitioners also screen for asymptomatic bacteriuria early in pregnancy, using a microscopy and culture test. The dipstick urinalysis used routinely at every antenatal visit is easy to use, gives immediate results that are assessed by the midwife, and is markedly cheaper than laboratory microscopy and culture. Unfortunately, it has consistently been found to have poor

sensitivity and predictive value for all of the variables it is used to test (see reviews by TCCGACP 2001, NICE 2003, Smaill 2004 and Waugh et al 2004).

Screening for proteinuria as a marker for pre-eclampsia

It is routine practice for midwives to ask women to pass urine at every antenatal visit, and to use a dipstick to assess the level of protein present, as part of the diagnosis of pre-eclampsia. There is mounting evidence, however, that calls into question the accuracy of this test. A recent review of dipstick detection of proteinuria by Waugh et al. (2004) concluded that 'significant proteinuria, with point-of-care urine dipstick analysis, cannot be accurately detected or excluded at the 1+ threshold and is not recommended for diagnosing pre-eclampsia. Further research is necessary to determine the prediction of proteinuria using higher dipstick thresholds' (p 776). It is currently recommended that a dipstick measure of proteinuria be requested from women with hypertension. The ASSHP states that 'dipstick testing for proteinuria is a screening test only, with very high false positive rates' (Brown et al 2000, p 4). They recommend that 'all hypertensive pregnant women with any level of positive dipstick proteinuria should be . . . confirmed with either: a 24-hour urine collection ≥ 300 mg/day [an abnormal level] or a spot urine protein/creatinine ratio ≥ 30 mg protein/mmol creatinine [an abnormal level]. Urinary tract infection should also be excluded'. Clearly, a single mid-stream urine (MSU) sample for the protein/creatinine ratio and culture is likely to be chosen by women, over the 24-hour urine collection option. A protein/creatinine dipstick measure is currently being developed, although assessing its sensitivity and predictive accuracy is expected to take some time (Waugh et al 2004).

Screening for asymptomatic bacteriuria

Proteinuria on dipstick is also used to screen for asymptomatic bacteriuria in routine antenatal care, although some practitioners use dipsticks with additional measures for blood, leucocytes and nitrites for this purpose. The aim of screening is to identify those with asymptomatic bacteriuria and to offer (prophylactic) antibiotic treatment to reduce the incidence of pyelonephritis. Asymptomatic bacteriuria is defined as 'the persistent bacterial colonisation of the urinary tract in the absence of specific symptoms and is usually diagnosed as > 100,000 bacteria/mL on a single voided midstream urine' (TCCGACP 2001, p 24). Asymptomatic bacteriuria is reported to occur in between two and ten per cent of women, with significant variation between countries and communities, and greater incidence in women of low socio-economic status (SES) (NICE 2003). It is 'generally benign' for those who are otherwise well and not pregnant (Smaill 2004). It is the risk of these women developing pyelonephritis, and its association with preterm labour, that makes it of interest during pregnancy. The physiological changes in the urinary tract during pregnancy make acute pyelonephritis much more likely. In the Cochrane Review, Smaill (2004) states, in the background section of the report, that '20–30% of pregnant women will develop pyelonephritis', but the evidence reviewed identified an 'overall incidence of pyelonephritis in the untreated group [of] 19%, but [this] ranged from 0% to 29%' (p 4).

Asymptomatic bacteriuria is also associated with a two-fold increase in preterm labour, although a causal link is yet to be proved, as confounding factors such low SES potentially influence outcomes (Ovalle & Levancini 2001). Smaill (2004) identifies the 'number needed to treat' (NNT) ratio as 7:1, resulting in an approximately '75% reduction in the incidence of pyelonephritis' (p 4). To date, none of the studies identified in any of the reviews cited above have addressed the issues relating to antibiotics themselves, such as 'allergic reactions, yeast infections, gastrointestinal side-effects and the development of bacterial resistance' (Smaill 2004). Smaill (2004) considers it 'unlikely that the expected side effects from a short course of antibiotics would be of sufficient significance to warrant reconsideration of the recommendation to routinely treat asymptomatic bacteriuria' (p 4). Nor have the issues of the information and options given to, and choices made by, women been addressed in the research available on the topic.

Contemporary medical literature recommends routine screening in early pregnancy (NICE Guidelines 2003; Smaill 2004; TCCGACP 2001). The Australian guideline (Three Centres Consensus Guidelines on Antenatal Care Project 2001) suggests two options for screening women for asymptomatic bacteriuria:

- MSU and laboratory microscopy and culture
- MSU and dipstick test for blood, protein, nitrites and leucocytes, which is sent to the laboratory if there is a positive result in any of the four categories.

The British guidelines (NICE 2003) recommend that routine MSU culture be offered to all pregnant women. They suggest that the four-category dipstick option 'will detect 50% of women with asymptomatic bacteriuria', and consider that inadequate (p 80). Midwives need to provide information regarding the screening and treatment options available, including potential antibiotic risks and efficacy rates, in the context of the risks of women developing pyelonephritis, to facilitate active and informed decision-making by women.

Screening for glycosuria as a marker for gestational diabetes mellitus

Although glycosuria is screened for routinely at every antenatal visit currently, it is not considered to be the primary screening test for gestational diabetes mellitus (GDM). Its presence is interpreted as a potential sign of GDM. Blood glucose screening tests are offered for women with risk markers or symptoms of GDM (see Ch 32). Glycosuria is not an independent or reliable marker of GDM. Glycosuria can reflect a lowered renal threshold, which is a normal physiological change of pregnancy (Watson 1990). The only recent review published states that 'urine testing has low sensitivity and is a poor screening test for GDM' (NICE 2003, p 97).

There is much ongoing debate regarding routine antenatal screening for GDM. The New Zealand College of Midwives Consensus Statement (2003), the British NICE guidelines (2003) and Enkin et al (2000) all recommend against *routine* screening for GDM. These recommendations are generally referring to blood glucose screening tests. However, urine screening, in the form of dipstick glycosuria, is a poorer screening test than blood glucose and its usefulness in routine antenatal care is debatable.

Summary

The practice of routine screening (i.e. for *all* pregnant women) of urine for protein and glucose may be reviewed in the light of an increasing body of evidence which has found both screening tests to have poor sensitivity and predictive values (see references cited above). Currently, the Australian Three Centres Consensus Guidelines on Antenatal Care Project (2001) state that the 'use of dipstick measurement for routine screening of proteinuria in low risk pregnant women is not recommended' (p 49). The New Zealand College of Midwives (2003), the NICE guidelines (2003) and Enkin et al. (2000) recommend against routine urine testing as a screening test for gestational diabetes.

These tests may be maintained for women with risk markers or signs or symptoms of pre-eclampsia or diabetes, as an adjunct to other assessments, screening and diagnostic tests. It is important for midwives to be aware of the limitations of these tests, and understand that they cannot be relied upon in themselves. The whole clinical and personal context of each woman needs to be considered when screening options are discussed and care choices are made. See Chapters 32 and 33 for fuller discussion on risk markers, screening and response to pre-eclampsia and gestational diabetes. See Chapters 32 and 33 for details of the signs, symptoms and treatment options for urinary tract infection or pyelonephritis.

Palpation: hands-on learning, identification and assessment

Palpation, or examination by touch, is a process of the 'hands-on' identification and assessment of the position, growth and

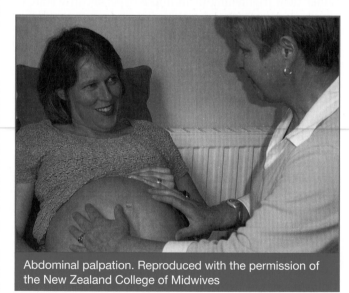

Abdominal palpation. Reproduced with the permission of the New Zealand College of Midwives

wellbeing of the baby. It is an integral part of every antenatal visit, and is an acquired and highly valued midwifery skill. Each midwife has her own style, with the whole process being more than the sum of the parts described here. The process involves the gathering of small pieces of information, using the senses of hearing, seeing and touching, to put together an invisible four-dimensional 'puzzle'. It is also a significant time for two-way sharing of information. It is important for the midwife to discuss her plans with the woman, to explain the reasons for doing the examination, and to acknowledge the limitations of palpation (see Enkin et al 2000). She must seek the woman's consent, leaving open the option for her to decline, and check out any personal and cultural safety issues surrounding this intimate and exposing experience. The midwife asks about and listens to the woman's experience of her baby's growth and the nature and pattern of movements, and listens to the baby's heartbeat. She looks at the size and shape of the woman's abdomen, and notes her responses to palpation and to the baby's movements. The midwife uses touch to estimate the size and position of the baby, and its response to contact and voice. She also assesses the fluid volume and may identify other unexpected findings such as uterine fibroids. Observation and 'hands-on' practice are the best way to learn the art and skill of effective palpation.

Context and preparation

The context within which the palpation occurs is a significant feature of the process. The comfort, privacy and safety of the physical environment are as important as meaningful communication between the midwife and the woman. The midwife should strive to ensure that the environment is appropriate, which will include a comfortable place on which the woman can lie down. This may be the floor (if in the woman's home), or a bed or sofa (couch), which is firm, wide and low enough to be used with comfort.

Equipment

The midwife should ensure that she has the necessary equipment for the palpation. This includes:

- Pinard stethoscope and (possibly) Doppler ultrasound, conductive gel, tissues

- watch with a second hand
- privacy/modesty sheet
- tape measure (if used).

Preparation

Prior to the palpation, the midwife should:

- have clean, warm hands (and short fingernails)
- affirm the woman's active role in the process
- caution her, if the palpation is occurring in later stages of pregnancy, about the possibility of hypotension while lying on her back
- ensure that the woman's privacy and modesty are protected and respected.

In preparation for the palpation, the woman should:

- be encouraged to empty her bladder
- lie down on her back, with her abdomen exposed or accessible for palpation
- be comfortable, with her head supported and perhaps her knees bent, with or without support under them.

During the palpation, the midwife should:

- take care not to focus exclusively on the woman's abdomen—maintain frequent verbal and eye contact
- tell the woman (and those with her) what she is doing/feeling for/finding
- encourage the woman to tell of any discomfort caused by palpating
- not palpate when the uterus is contracting—wait until it is relaxed
- guide the woman (include her partner, if she wishes) in palpating herself.

Techniques and methods

Palpation may be divided into five stages.

1 Initial visual assessment

Purpose: The purpose of this relatively brief stage in the process is to form an initial impression of the progress of the growing baby. It also provides an opportunity for discussion of the visible physiological changes; for example, she may have a linea nigra, increased hair growth or stretch marks.

Technique: Begin by establishing eye contact, once the woman is lying down. Ask her about her experiences of the baby's growth, movements and position as you look at her abdomen and begin the palpation. Check the size, shape and contours of the uterus, and consider these in relation to gestation, presentation and position. Match visible scars with your knowledge of her history. Note bruising or other signs of physical violence and, once she is upright again and if she is alone, ask about her experience and safety. Alternatively, follow up at another time, as appropriate.

2 Fundal assessment

Purpose: Fundal assessment identifies the uppermost part of the uterus and baby, from which the size and 'lie' of the baby are first distinguished, and initial information as to the 'presentation' is gained. The 'lie' of the baby is the position of the baby's spine relative to the woman's spine, and is described

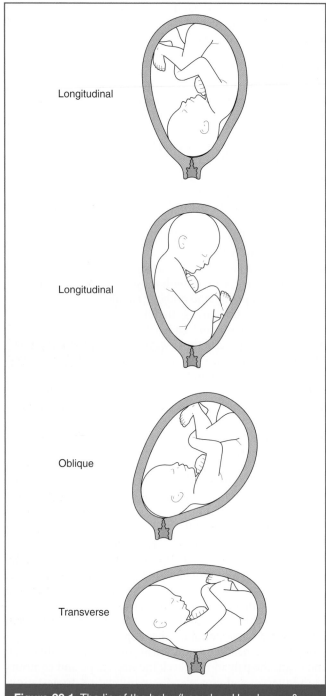

Figure 20.1 The lie of the baby (based on Henderson & Macdonald 2004)

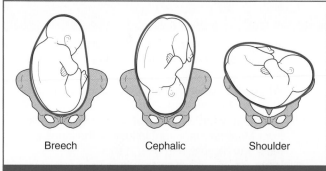

Figure 20.2 The presentation of the baby (based on Henderson & Macdonald 2004)

difficult to palpate, and its mobility makes identification of the lie or presentation irrelevant.

The second aspect of fundal assessment is the estimation of the size of the baby, which is compared with the expected size for the gestation. There are two methods used for comparing fundal height with gestation. Both have limitations, as fundal height varies with the position of the baby, the volume of liquor, and the size and shape of the woman. Assessing growth using fundal height, by landmark or measurement, is vulnerable to subjectivity and variability in technique between assessments and assessors. To date, neither method has been shown to be more effective than the other at detecting growth abnormalities at a level that improves outcomes (NICE 2003). Certainly there is a poor record of detecting IUGR babies with current traditional Western routine antenatal care (McGeown 2001). Babies that are small for gestational age (SGA) or IUGR are known to have high rates of morbidity and mortality (Enkin et al 2000), which presents an ongoing challenge for midwives. These two methods are described and discussed below.

● *'Landmark' guided fundal height assessment* is well-established practice, and is included in possibly every midwifery text. The 'landmarks' used are the symphysis pubis, umbilicus and xiphisternum (see Fig 20.3). The growth of the fundus is expected to approximate this pattern, although there is variability between women and babies, as described above. McGeown (2001) notes that 'there is no scientific foundation for the use of the umbilicus as a landmark to indicate a specific gestational age, i.e. umbilicus = 22/24/26 weeks gestation, dependent on which text one reads' (p 191). This does not mean that it is not a useful guide. It may be just that it has not been subject to scientific evaluation.

● *Measurement of the fundal height* is also common practice. Fundal height measurement is taken using the uppermost part of the baby as the starting point. A tape measure is held on the fundus, with the centimetre markers on the underside (to reduce bias), and laid on the skin along the longitudinal axis of the baby, to the symphysis pubis (Perinatal Institute 2004). The traditional 'standardised' guide is said to be for the fundal height measurement in centimetres (cm) to

as longitudinal, oblique or transverse (see Fig 20.1). The term 'presentation' distinguishes the part of the baby that is lying lowest in the uterus, with cephalic, breech or shoulder the most common (see Fig 20.2). Cephalic presentations can be divided into vertex, brow or face; and breech presentations divide into frank, complete, footling or incomplete. In the first two trimesters, the fundal height is the primary palpation measure used to assess fetal growth, as the baby's small size makes it

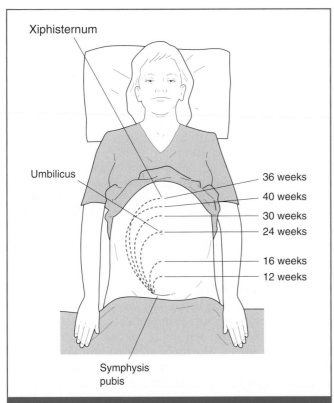

Figure 20.3 Landmarks of fundal height

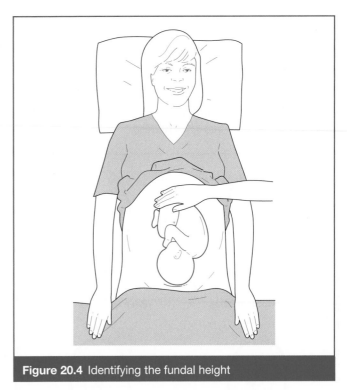

Figure 20.4 Identifying the fundal height

approximately equal the weeks of gestation, after 24 weeks. For example, a woman who is 34 weeks would be expected to have a fundal height measurement of approximately 34 cm. The 'customised growth charts' recently developed in England by the West Midlands Perinatal Institute (Gardosi et al 2000) calculate an optimal birth weight range adjusted for 'the physiological variables of maternal height, weight in early pregnancy, parity, ethnic group and by excluding known pathological variables such as smoking' (McGeown 2001). The software is available free from the Perinatal Institute website (www.wmpi.net), and includes a New Zealand version. At the time of writing, there is no Australian version. The charts may facilitate better detection of SGA/IUGR babies. With limited data to date, improved outcomes have not yet been demonstrated. The charts may, alternatively, further medicalise antenatal care without improving outcomes. They are 'customised' to include four potentially influential factors, but cannot be 'individualised' to include many other potential influences. Conscientious midwifery care provided within the midwifery model and context of continuity, arguably has the potential to improve outcomes, but it also lacks current data.

Technique: First, find the fundus by working from the woman's chest towards her pelvis, using your finger pads (not tips) pressing firmly enough to feel the increased resistance of the uterus relative to the other abdominal organs. The pressure required varies between women, with those having tight abdominal muscles or significant fat needing firmer pressure, but not so much as to cause pain (see Fig 20.4).

Once the fundus is found, cup your hand around it to define the shape and overall size of the uterus and the baby. The shape and height of the uterus help with identification of the lie of the baby. From approximately 28 weeks gestation, it is usually possible to identify the presentation of the baby by using the fingers, palm and heel of your cupped hand, or fingers and thumb extended, to identify which part of the baby is in the upper part of the uterus. You may use both hands, with one on either side of the part of the baby's body, to help with identification. The head feels hard and round, and is ballottable. The buttock may be firm in earlier gestations, but is never ballottable, as it is the extension of the torso/back.

Possible causes of discrepancies between the expected fundal height and gestation include:
- large or small baby
- multiple pregnancy
- molar pregnancy
- poly/oligohydramnios
- errors in gestational age estimation
- oblique or transverse lie.

3 Lateral assessment

Purpose: Lateral assessment involves palpation of the central part of the uterus. In the third trimester, it facilitates confirmation of the lie and presentation, and identifies the 'position' of the baby. The 'position' refers to the combination of the lie and presentation with the orientation of the baby—be it anterior, lateral or posterior. While the terminology used to define the baby's 'position' describes the position of the lowest part of the baby (the denominator) in relation to points on the woman's pelvis, it is primarily assessed by the location of the baby's back on palpation. Although there are more than 36 possible positions (see Frye 1998), in practice only the positions relating to the most common cephalic and breech presentations are used in the context of antenatal palpation (see Fig 20.5). Other more unusual positions are generally described only by lie and presentation.

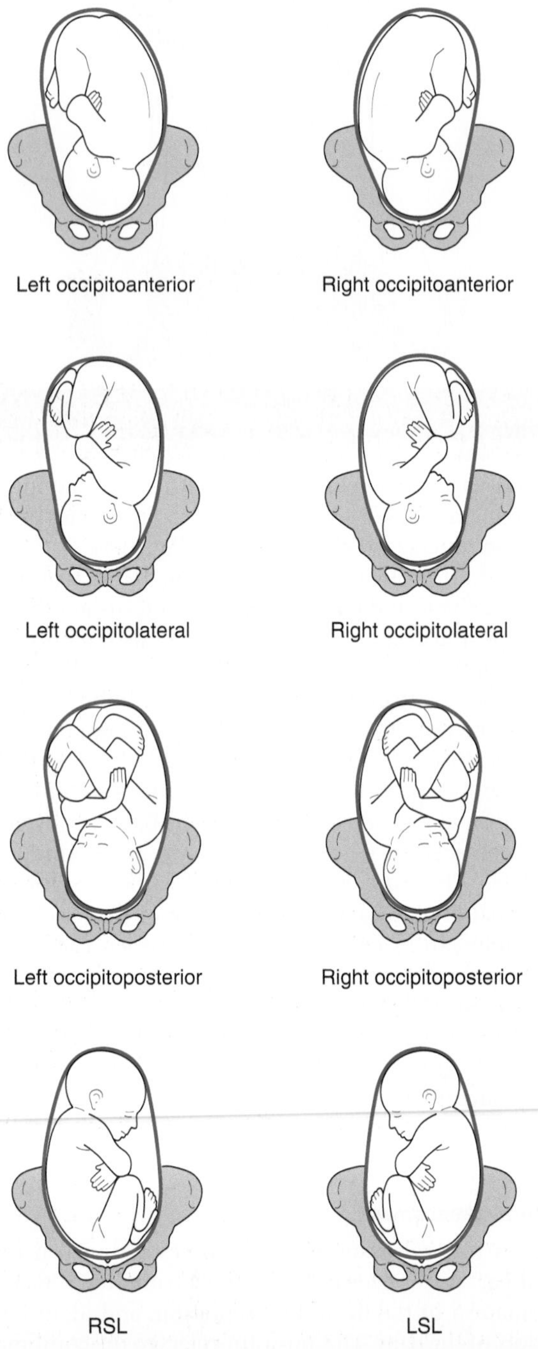

Technique: There are two main techniques used for lateral palpation. The first involves 'walking' both hands across the woman's uterus and back again, using the pads of your fingers and keeping both hands close together, taking small 'steps' (see Fig 20.6). The second involves the use of one hand as an 'anchor' lying along the length of one side of the woman's uterus, while the other hand is used to examine the other side; then changing to use the other hand as 'anchor' (see Fig 20.7). Apply as much pressure as is needed to feel the baby, without causing discomfort to the woman—be aware of the possibility of causing discomfort and responsive to any signs of this. Effective communication will help both the woman and the midwife. Some women develop a sensitive spot, or experience generalised tenderness. It is worthwhile considering how important it is to gather detailed information at any one antenatal visit. For example, at 32 weeks it is not important to identify more detail than the presentation and which side the back is on. If the baby wakes and moves prior to your finding the presentation or position, it can be helpful to spread both of your hands over the woman's uterus and feel the site and nature of the movements.

The back feels firm and can be 'tracked' for most of the length of the uterus. The limbs are small and knobbly and more likely to move during the palpation. If the baby is lying longitudinally and you cannot feel the back initially, broaden your search, by bringing your hands to the woman's side closer to her back, as the baby's back may be tucked in closer to the woman's back, in a posterior position. If only the baby's limbs are palpable, the back will be in the opposite quadrant. For example, if limbs are felt in the right anterior area, the back

Left occipitoanterior

Right occipitoanterior

Left occipitolateral

Right occipitolateral

Left occipitoposterior

Right occipitoposterior

RSL

LSL

Figure 20.5 The most common positions of the baby (based on Fraser & Cooper 2003)

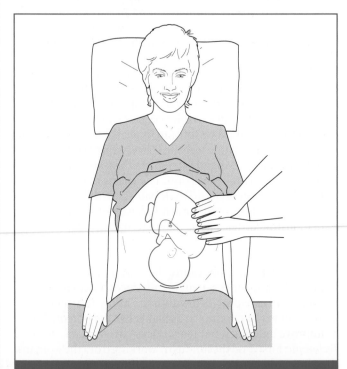

Figure 20.6 Lateral palpation: finding the back—'hand walking'

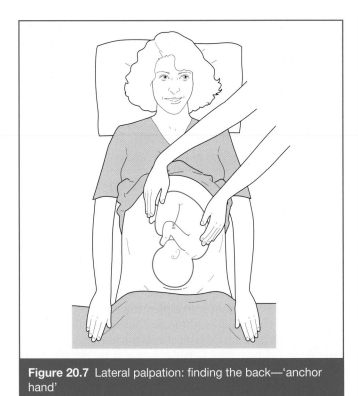

Figure 20.7 Lateral palpation: finding the back—'anchor hand'

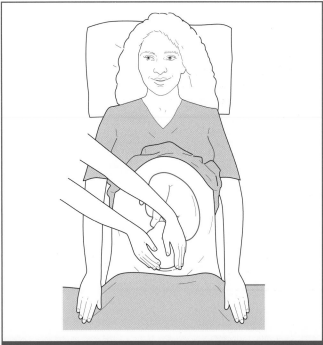

Figure 20.8 Pelvic palpation—feeling for the head using two hands

will be in the left posterior position—check that area again to confirm this.

Once the position of the back is identified, cup the fundus once more, to confirm the presentation by assessing the relationship between the top fetal pole (mostly the buttock) and the back. Consider whether the top part moves when the back is pressed. It will move if it is the buttocks.

The amount of amniotic fluid or liquor can also be estimated during this part of the process. When palpating for the back, take note of how freely the baby is 'floating' in the uterine space. If there is reduced liquor (oligohydramnios), there will be minimal cushioning between the baby and the walls of the uterus. If there is excess liquor (polyhydramnios), the baby can be difficult to palpate, as it floats about (see Ch 33 for discussion on the detail and significance of these conditions).

4 Pelvic palpation

Purpose: Palpating the lower part of the woman's uterus, just above the pelvic bones, is the final stage of the process. It serves to identify the part of the baby lying lowest (the 'presenting part'), and should confirm your impressions from the fundal and lateral stages. It also enables the midwife to assess the descent of the presenting part into the pelvis. This may be more uncomfortable for the woman than the rest of the palpation, so use communication and sensitivity to manage this. If you work together, so that you press in with her out breath, it may be less uncomfortable for her.

Technique: There are two techniques used for pelvic palpation. The first involves using both hands, initially placed midway between the woman's side and centre line, with fingertips

touching the pubic bone (see Fig 20.8). Let the woman know when you are about to begin, then move the tips of your fingers towards the woman's back just above the pubic bone, feeling for the outer boundaries of the presenting part. The second technique (known as Pawlik's manoeuvre) uses one hand, with the heel of your hand beginning resting on the pubic bone and the thumb and fingers extended to reach either side of the presenting part (see Fig 20.9). The head feels hard on both sides, while the buttock is irregular and soft on one or both sides. If the head is very well down in the pelvis, it may not be palpable, and the shoulder can feel like the buttocks, so it is worth re-checking the upper fetal pole.

Once the presenting part is identified, the next step is to assess its descent into the woman's pelvis. When palpating, you need also to assess the mobility of the presenting part (usually the head). If it is immobile, you need to assess the shape of the part that you can feel, considering whether it is broadening or narrowing from the top of the pubic bone. You are judging how much of the head has gone in, by how much of it is left above the pubic bone, and expressing it in fifths (see Fig 20.10). For example, if the head is immobile but broadening as you track its shape towards the torso, it may be one-fifth or two-fifths into the pelvis. It is defined as 'engaged' once the broadest part (the bi-parietal diameter) has descended below the pelvic rim. When documenting the descent, clearly note whether you are recording that which is palpable, or that which has descended (i.e. '2/5ths up/↑' or '3/5ths down/↓').

There are other measures of the baby's position, which note the angle, 'flexion' or 'attitude' of the head, but they are not usually significant in the context of antenatal care (see Frye 1998). Of potential significance for a primiparous woman is

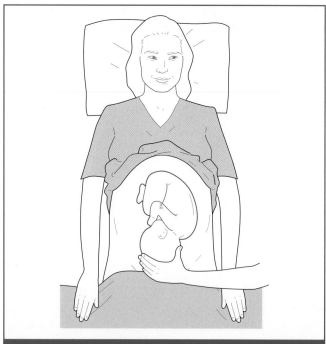

Figure 20.9 Pelvic palpation—ballotting the head with one hand

whether the baby's head is engaged by 40 weeks. If it is not, the possibility of cephalo-pelvic disproportion (CPD) should be considered and discussed with the woman. Non-engagement for a primiparous is not definitive of CPD and evidence to date shows that pelvic assessment or changed management, such as early induction of labour, does not improve outcomes (Enkin et al 2000).

5 Listening or auscultation

Purpose: Listening to the baby's heart rate (HR) serves to identify whether the baby is alive. The NICE guidelines (2003) suggest that it has 'no other clinical or predictive value' (p 107). This does not mean that it may not have personal or social value for pregnant women and their families, particularly those who have miscarried previously.

It appears that the option to use technology, in the form of portable Doppler ultrasound, has been taken up by the

vast majority of pregnant women and midwives where it is available. Its ability to give instantaneous audible access to the baby's heartbeat from approximately 12 weeks gestation facilitates assessment of the wellbeing of babies, before their movements can be felt, and before the HR can be heard via a Pinard stethoscope (24–28 weeks).

Technique: Whether listening to the baby's heartbeat using a Pinard stethoscope or a Doppler, the basic technique is similar. Once the fundal height and/or position of the baby are identified, the instrument is placed on the woman's abdomen external to the baby's back. For example, if the baby is lying in a left occipitoanterior (LOA) position (see Fig 20.5), the Pinard or Doppler should be placed in the lower left quadrant of the woman's abdomen. It is an acquired skill to hear the baby's heartbeat with a Pinard, as the experience is closer to feeling vibrations than hearing sound, and quite different from the sound that the Doppler produces. See Cronk (2002) or Wickham (2002) for more detailed instructions on the use of the Pinard.

Fetal movement

Women who are having their first baby may feel its first movements from around 18 weeks gestation, although some may not feel them until as late as 21 weeks. Women having their second or subsequent baby may feel movements as early as 15 or 16 weeks. These movements are often referred to as 'flutters' or 'quickening', and are variously described as feeling like butterflies or bubbles. They are initially felt fleetingly, intermittently and irregularly. By 22 to 24 weeks, most women will be feeling many movements per day, and these will reflect a fairly regular sleep–wake pattern.

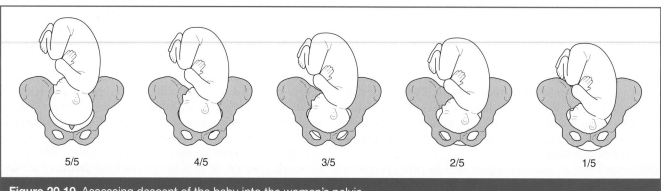

5/5   4/5   3/5   2/5   1/5

Figure 20.10 Assessing descent of the baby into the woman's pelvis

From about 28 weeks, fetal movements (FMs) may be regarded as a fairly significant and reliable marker of a baby's wellbeing. It is in fact 'the oldest technique for assessing fetal wellbeing' (Christensen et al. 2003, p.118). Since the 1970s, when routine formalised charting of FMs was advocated, it has been the subject of contradictory research and much debate (see comprehensive literature reviews in Frøen 2004, and Fisher 1999). The focus has been on the efficacy of the routine counting and charting of FMs as a predictor of fetal compromise, in time to prevent a stillbirth. There is a key difference between requesting that all pregnant women complete FM charts all the time, and informing women of signs of compromise and recommending selective use of charts when they are concerned. Frøen (2004) identified 24 studies addressing the issue, all of which 'suggest that the increased vigilance to maternal perception of FMs caused by performing a study significantly reduced stillbirth rates' (p 23), in contrast to one randomised controlled trial (Grant et al. 1989, cited in Frøen 2004).

Frøen (2004) identified several key points from the research:
- Reduced FMs are predictive of perinatal mortality in women with high- or low-risk pregnancies.
- The use of FM charts was more effective than 'spontaneous' reporting.
- The format of the chart does not matter, as they are 'only tools for information'.
- Although the lower limits of 'normal' FMs have not been identified, if a woman experiences her baby moving ten times over a twelve-hour period, it is unlikely to be at risk (excluding other causes of intrauterine death (IUD) such as cord accidents).
- Women need to be given information regarding expectations of FMs and what to do if these are not met.
- Health professionals need to respond to women's concerns and provide appropriate assessment and follow-up.

Fisher's (1999) review of the literature notes that 'it is well documented that maternal perception of fetal activity varies greatly' (p 706). She identified issues of pattern and perception that may influence women's experience of FM, and reports research to date:
- More FM is experienced when a woman is 'recumbent'.
- There are conflicting reports regarding the influence of increased maternal weight, parity, anterior placental position, and anxiety or psychological issues.
- Women experience different types of movements variably, with greater perception when 'more than one fetal part was involved'.
- There is 'individuality in patterns of fetal activity/sleep'.
- The nature and pattern of movements change as pregnancy progresses.
- Caffeine increases activity.
- Cigarette smoking, sedatives, narcotics, methadone and alcohol suppress FM.
- 'Gross' FM are not affected by maternal exercise.
- Women eating meals does not affect FM, although 'glucose levels do ... increase fetal breathing'.

> ## Critical thinking exercise
>
> Belinda is having her third baby and is 16 weeks pregnant.
> Liz is 26 weeks into her first pregnancy.
> Ella is 37 weeks pregnant with her first baby.
> 1   What would you ask each of these women about their babies' movements?
> 2   What differences would you expect in the frequency, pattern and nature of their babies' movements?
> 3   What factors might influence the women's understandings, expectations and experiences of the movements of their babies?

Clearly, the role of midwives as 'individualised information sharers' and listeners is critical in this context. Individualised care, planning and response are required, with each woman's personal and clinical situation and past experience being important issues for inclusion. If women have good knowledge of appropriate expectations of FM, and they 'tune in' to their baby's movement pattern and routine, they are likely to be better able to identify and communicate marked changes in FM that may be significant to their baby's wellbeing. Fetal movement counting is arguably not a screening 'test', but one tool in shared awareness, knowledge and understanding. Midwives are able to affirm women's experience and knowledge of their baby's wellbeing, most of the time.

Antenatal education

Antenatal education is an integral part of the formal process of antenatal care in New Zealand, Australia and the rest of the Western world. Defining its aims, scope, role and efficacy, however, is not straightforward, as programs vary with the beliefs, expectations and frameworks of those who provide it (Health Department Victoria 1990; Nolan & Hicks 1997). For a discussion of the history and politics of antenatal education see Oakley (1984), Nolan (1999, 2000) or Robertson (2001, 2004).

What is antenatal education?

The term 'antenatal education', when used generically, refers to information sharing between childbearing women (and their partners or friends) and caregivers, which is intended to facilitate informed choices and decision-making by the women about their pregnancy, childbirth and early postnatal period. It encompasses health promotion and preparation for childbirth and early parenting. As such, it is integral to midwifery-provided antenatal care. It is not usually used to describe the active or passive learning that comes from books, the Internet or other media, or which occurs between women and their friends or family.

During the past fifty years, however, 'antenatal education' has become the term used more specifically to describe group sessions run by various providers, which are additional to and separate from antenatal care per se. These courses are typically run for women in their third trimester, on the basis of weekly classes for approximately two hours, often over five to eight weeks. Topics covered also vary considerably, but are likely to include at least some of the following aspects (Cole, undated personal correspondence; Ministry of Health 2002):

● *health promotion*—nutrition, exercise, relaxation and stress reduction; minimisation of alcohol, smoking and other 'hazardous substances'; 'pelvic awareness' and self-help for physiological changes of pregnancy
● *childbirth preparation*—signs and process of normal labour (expectations and coping skills); choices for labour and birth, such as place and pain management; unexpected outcomes, interventions (risks and appropriate use); role of support people and self-help strategies
● *parenting preparation*—establishing breastfeeding, care and safety of the newborn, appropriate clothing and equipment for babies, family and personal adjustments, support, expectations and coping strategies.

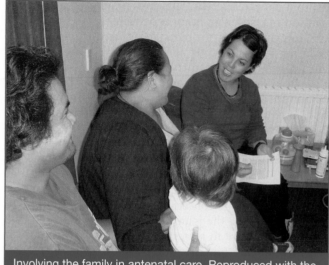

Involving the family in antenatal care. Reproduced with the permission of the New Zealand College of Midwives

Who provides antenatal education and who are its consumers?

At an organisational level, providers of antenatal education can be divided into three broad groups:

● those associated with care provision, such as those run by hospitals or home birth groups
● those run by community groups, such as Parents Centre or Marae based courses (New Zealand), or the Childbirth Education Association (Australia)
● those working as autonomous individuals offering private classes.

At the classroom level, the providers of antenatal education vary greatly, with trained childbirth educators, health workers and midwives being the main leaders or facilitators. There is also considerable variation in the level and nature of training within and between these groups. Many classes have additional input from other health professionals or special-interest consumer groups, such as physiotherapists, lactation consultants or La Leche League leaders, doctors, psychologists, or consumers who have recently given birth. Traditionally, these classes have been used by white, middle- and upper-SES heterosexual couples having their first child, and not by indigenous peoples, teenagers, low-SES or gay couples, single women or those from ethnic minorities or other socially marginalised groups (Health Department Victoria 1990; Lumley 1993).

What are the objectives of antenatal education, and how is it evaluated?

There is ongoing debate regarding the objectives, role, scope and potential impact of antenatal education. A commonly expressed aim is to build women's confidence in their ability to give birth and care for their babies (Nolan 1999). It may also serve to build personal and social relationships, and develop shared experiences. These aims are not always realised, however, and research has identified numerous discrepancies

between theory and practice in antenatal education. These include differences between the experiences and perceptions of women and those of providers, in terms of needs, desired outcomes, and the role and efficacy of antenatal education overall (Health Department Victoria 1990; Lumley 1993; Nolan 1999; Weiner 2002).

Evaluation of antenatal education beyond internal 'satisfaction' surveys or informal feedback is rare and potentially difficult. 'Because of their complex, often disparate goals and ideologies, one cannot make general statements about the effects of antenatal classes as if they were a single entity' (Enkin et al 2000, p 24).

What is the role of the LMC midwife in antenatal education?

At the generic level, antenatal education is a core midwifery role. Throughout the antenatal period the midwife gets to know the woman and her supporters, and learns about her knowledge base and the beliefs, fears, plans and dreams she

---

Critical thinking exercise

Peter and Sue are in their mid-thirties, Summer is 18 years old, and Aaliya and Hamsa are Somali refugees with fairly good English-language skills. All are having their first babies.

1 What antenatal education options are available in your region for these families?
2 What is the format, content and aim of the classes which are offered?
3 Who runs them, at both organisational and classroom levels?
4 How might you work with these families in order to see if any of the classes available might meet their needs?

has about childbirth and caring for a baby. It is the midwife's role to share her belief in the woman's ability and in the process of childbirth. It is also her role to participate in health promotion and the preparation of the woman for birth and early parenting.

In relation to antenatal education classes, it is the midwife's role to inform women of the options available to them, and to discuss the various formats, content and underpinning philosophies of these. In order to do this, midwives should familiarise themselves with the local programs on offer. Midwives need to work with women for whom existing programs are inappropriate, to facilitate them accessing information and support which is more suited to their needs.

Exercise in pregnancy

Exercise in pregnancy has different meanings for different people. For some, it means gentle stretching exercises done as preparation for labour and birth, and is sometimes incorporated into group antenatal education (Brayshaw 2003). For others, it means recreational sport or general physical fitness, in the form of aerobic exercise such as swimming, cycling, walking or team sports (Howells 2002; Kramer 2004).

There is ongoing debate about exercise in pregnancy. See Brayshaw (2003), Howells (2002) and Goodwin et al. (2000) as examples—they address issues including:

- the role of exercise in improving or maintaining the health of women and their babies
- its benefits (physical, psychological, social and clinical)
- appropriate 'safety' boundaries (the type, frequency and intensity of exercise)
- the contraindications for exercise in pregnancy (underlying medical conditions).

Historically, beliefs about exercise in pregnancy have varied with the social, cultural and political context of the time, with 'advice for physical activity reflect[ing] activities and behaviour deemed to be socially acceptable' (Rankin et al 2000, p 764). Arguably, this continues today. Although caregivers have been advising women about appropriate exercise in pregnancy for centuries (Ranking et al 2000), our knowledge about its psychological and physiological effects is still limited (Kramer 2004).

Medical literature has focused on the physiological aspects of exercise (see recent reviews: Jones 2000; Kramer 2004; Wolfe & Weissgerber 2003). The Cochrane Review concludes that 'regular aerobic exercise during pregnancy appears to improve (or maintain) physical fitness and body image. Available data are insufficient to infer important risks or benefits for the mother or infant' (Kramer 2004, p 1). 'Regular aerobic exercise' is defined by Kramer (2004) as 'vigorous exercise that results in a rise in oxygen consumption (to 50 to 85% of maximum) and heart rate (to 60 to 90% of maximum) and maintains that level for at least 15 to 20 minutes...at least two to three times per week' (pp 1–2). Evidence with regard to the effect of frequent (≥ 5 times/week) and vigorous exercise is contradictory, with some research finding an association with low birth weight and shorter gestations, and others finding no significant

Reflective exercise

1   What are your personal beliefs about physical exercise?
2   How might these influence the way in which you discuss the place of exercise during pregnancy with pregnant women?
3   Spend some time talking with pregnant women and practising midwives about their beliefs and behaviours with regard to the place of exercise during pregnancy.

differences in outcomes measured between groups of women who exercise in this way, and those who exercise moderately (Wolfe & Weissgerber 2003). Carrying out research on this issue is difficult, given the many confounding variables involved, which include underlying wellness and fitness levels, physiological and psychological changes induced by pregnancy, and the potential bias within any group of women who agree to participate in research on exercise.

Midwifery literature has explored some of the psychological and social aspects of exercise. For example, Clarke & Gross (2004) and Symons Downs & Hausenblas (2004) found that:

- many women discontinue regular pre-pregnancy exercise during pregnancy
- many women perceive that rest and relaxation are more important than exercise
- magazines and books were important sources of information initially
- friends and family strongly influence exercising behaviour
- the most common exercise beliefs were that exercise improves mood
- physical limitations (e.g. nausea) obstructed participation in exercise.

The attitudes, beliefs and behaviours women have about exercise are rooted within their personal, social and cultural context, and cannot be addressed in isolation. As with any other issue of health promotion, a complex process is involved, and requires midwives to work in partnership with women, and use effective communication, support and affirmation skills (Crafter 1997).

Physiological changes of pregnancy

Pregnancy brings about many changes within a woman's body. Almost all of these physiological changes are experienced as unwelcome and unpleasant, and some are very distressing and debilitating (see Box 20.2). They are commonly referred to as 'minor' discomforts or disturbances, which does not reflect the impact that some of these conditions have on many women and their families. The fact that they are common, natural and not 'pathological', and generally resolve as spontaneously as they arise, appears to contribute to the dismissal or minimisation of them by many caregivers.

There are marked differences in the incidence and severity of these changes, both between different women, and for the same woman during different pregnancies. There are also significant variations in the experiences, perceptions and responses of women to the changes caused by pregnancy. The socio-cultural context within which women (and midwives) live also influences the way in which they respond. Arguably, in contemporary Western society, there is a lower tolerance for discomfort or pain among many, and an increased expectation that the negative aspects of physiological changes can be alleviated (without risk to the health of woman or baby), whether by the use of 'medicated' pharmacological remedies or by 'alternative' remedies. Further, contemporary lifestyles including diet, exercise and work patterns (paid and unpaid) may exacerbate these changes, and changing these factors can be difficult during pregnancy. Unfortunately, the very nature of physiological changes, as expressions of the normal physiology of pregnancy, makes them difficult to resolve with 'treatment' of any type. The focus is therefore on understanding the physiology and minimising the discomfort of these changes.

Responses to physiological changes vary widely, and a vast array of 'therapies' are used by women today. They include herbal medicine, homeopathy, acupuncture/acupressure, osteopathy, aromatherapy, reflexology, massage, reiki, hypnotherapy, bach flower remedies, shiatsu and 'conventional' Western medicine. Additionally, there are numerous dietary and exercise approaches advocated by various health professionals and lay people. Among them are those who advocate strongly for their particular therapies (both conventional and alternative), but evidence to date is very limited as to the efficacy and safety of many interventions for the alleviation of pain or discomfort caused by these changes. It is beyond the scope of this chapter to include a description or an evaluation of the range of therapeutic options for the physiological changes to be discussed, beyond the brief exemplar given on nausea and vomiting. See Balaskas (1998), Jamil & Evennett (2000) and Tiran (2001) for further reading.

All interventions, including 'conventional' and 'alternative' medicines or remedies, should be treated with due respect and caution when being considered as treatments for physiological changes. (See the case relating to nausea and vomiting, below.) It should not be assumed that because something is 'natural' or 'alternative' that it is therefore any safer, lower risk or more effective than 'conventional' options. It is appropriate for midwives to carefully review the available evidence regarding the safety and efficacy of any intervention option they offer women. Midwives should recognise the limits of their knowledge and training, and when discussing options and alternatives, be able to refer on to those who are trained, accredited and accountable within their own profession, when these therapies are outside their scope of practice.

When women describe discomfort or pain they are experiencing, midwives must take care to differentiate between physiological and pathological symptoms. For example:

BOX 20.2 Physiological changes of pregnancy

Circulatory—related to changes in blood vessels or lymph system
▸ oedema
▸ carpal tunnel
▸ fainting and dizziness
▸ palpitations
▸ varicose veins—leg, vulval or anal (haemorrhoids)
▸ bleeding gums or nose

Muscle and ligament
▸ leg cramps
▸ 'ligament' pain (abdominal)
▸ back pain
▸ sciatica
▸ symphysis pubis dysfunction
▸ incontinence
▸ uterine cramps—'irritable' uterus, Braxton Hicks contractions

Digestive
▸ nausea and vomiting
▸ constipation
▸ heartburn and indigestion
▸ ptyalism
▸ bloating and excessive 'wind'
▸ diarrhoea

Breast —tenderness, growth, colour and size of areola, 'leaking'
Vagina—increased discharge, pH (thrush susceptibility)
Urinary—frequency, UT dilation, shortening (UTI susceptibility)
Sleep—pattern, nature, insomnia, dreams
Nose—congestion, bleeds, hay fever
Hair—growth on skin (abdomen, face), loss from head
Skin—itching, pregnancy rash (PUPP), acne, chloasma, linea nigra, stretch marks
Dietary—hypersensitivity to taste and/or smell, pica, appetite and metabolism changes
Sexuality—libido changes
Emotional—volatility and mood swings
Headaches and/or migraines
Tiredness/fatigue increased (1st and 3rd trimesters)

● vomiting may be physiological or pathological, and caused either by bacterial or viral infection, or by hyperemesis
● indigestion needs to be distinguished from epigastric or chest (cardiac) pains
● normal physiological increase in vaginal discharge needs to be differentiated from infections, such as chlamydia or thrush.

The physiological changes listed in Box 20.2 are the most common, and three of these will be discussed briefly here, as limited space does not permit a discussion of each and every one.

Nausea and vomiting (morning sickness)

Nausea and vomiting is a common, very unpleasant, yet not well understood condition of pregnancy. 'Nausea is the conscious recognition of subconscious excitation of the vomiting centre or an area close to it in the medulla. Vomiting is a complex series of movements which rids the gut of its contents when any part of it is irritated or distended' (Jordan 2002, p 121). While it is associated with raised levels of human chorionic gonadotropin (hCG) hormone and changes in blood sugar levels, variability in incidence, severity and response to treatments are indicative of a multifactorial state. Box 20.3 is a summary of a range of statistics on the occurrence and severity of nausea and vomiting. These statistics have been sourced from Chandra et al (2003), Frye (1998), Jewell & Young (2004), and NICE (2003).

Nausea and vomiting occurs predominantly in the first trimester. It is notoriously difficult to treat, in part because of the potentially greater harm that treatment poses to the baby during this critical developmental time, compared with other periods of pregnancy. Many treatments have been tried: Jewell and Young (2004) cite a 1968 report that identified thirty treatments 'in addition to the traditional dietary interventions' (p 2). Conventional medications in use currently include antihistamines, antipsychotics, gastro kinetics and vitamin supplements (Jordan 2002). (See also Ch 29 for prescription options.) The history of conventional pharmaceutical medications for nausea and vomiting is notably marked by the tragic consequences of the use of the drug thalidomide, which caused severe limb defects in babies (Frye 1998). This situation illustrates the point that the widespread use of medications should not be interpreted as proof of sound evidence of safety or efficacy. For example, the NICE guidelines (2003) state that the commonly prescribed drug metoclopramide 'has insufficient data on safety to be recommended as a first-line agent' (p 54). Vitamin B6 (pyridoxine) has also recently been introduced as a treatment for nausea and vomiting, and once again, evidence of its safety or efficacy is limited and not robust (NICE 2003). Questions regarding safety levels and potential toxicity at high doses are unresolved, with 10 mg/day set as the safe upper limit by the Committee on Toxicity of Foods in the United Kingdom, and doses of '25–75 mg up to three times daily' used in the research trials (NICE 2003).

It is also appropriate to be cautious about the use of alternative herbal medications. An example of these is powdered ginger in capsules, which is currently popular, but also poorly evaluated (Wilkinson 2000). Wilkinson's (2000) literature review found a dearth of evidence and contradictory advice regarding the use of ginger for nausea and vomiting, with 16 per cent of sources citing it as 'unsafe for use in pregnancy' (p 226). The NICE guidelines (2003) also cite very weak evidence in support of their recommendation for the use of ginger as an appropriate 'non-pharmacological' intervention. In common with many conventional medications, its mechanism of action in the relief of this condition is not understood— 'one proposed mechanism is inhibition of thromboxane synthetase, described in rat models, which has the potential to affect . . . differentiation of the fetal brain' (Barclay & Lie 2004, p 2). Its use as a medication in capsule form may cause unforeseen problems due to the increased dosage

> **BOX 20.3 Incidence and severity of nausea and vomiting**
>
> **Incidence**
> ▶ 80–85% of pregnant women experience it; 52% of these vomit
>
> **Severity**
> ▶ varies greatly—most women have symptoms by eight weeks (94%)
> ▶ one-third have symptoms by 4 weeks gestation
> ▶ resolved by 12–14 weeks for the majority of women
> ▶ resolved by 16–20 weeks for most (90%)
> ▶ not confined to the morning for most (80–90%)
> ▶ causes lost work time (at least 25% in paid and unpaid work time)
> ▶ causes increased weight gain for some (frequent snacking to feel better) and weight loss for others (decreased appetite with moderate vomiting)
> ▶ emotional, social and psychological impact can be marked
> ▶ 1% of women with nausea and vomiting will develop the pathological condition of hyperemesis gravidarum

that capsules facilitate, above that which might have been ingested traditionally in its natural state as fresh root ginger, eaten or taken in a tea. Further research is required on both conventional and herbal treatments for nausea and vomiting (Enkin et al 2000).

Alternative intervention for the treatment of nausea and vomiting, in the form of acupressure is showing promising results in most trials (Enkin et al 2000; NICE 2003), and its 'chemical-free' nature arguably makes it a lower-risk option. Each of the alternative forms of therapy mentioned in the introduction earlier offer therapeutic options for nausea and vomiting which women may wish to consider, and midwives need to be able make referrals as appropriate for the woman concerned.

Self-help responses to nausea and vomiting include lifestyle and dietary changes, which may provide some relief from this sometimes debilitating condition, which is recognised as having 'a profound impact on women's general sense of wellbeing and day-to-day life activities' (Smith et al 2000). They include the following sourced from the Auckland Home Birth Association (1993), Balaskas (1998), Chandra et al (2003), Frye (1998) and Jamil & Evennett (2000):

● Increase rest periods.
● Minimise work and home stressors.
● Eat carbohydrate (and wait 20 minutes) before getting out of bed in the morning.
● Eat protein before going to bed, or if up during the night.
● Do low energy/impact exercise, such as walking or yoga, after eating.
● Have regular small snacks of high protein and unprocessed carbohydrate (2–3 hourly).
● Avoid refined, fried and spicy foods.
● Eat foods rich in B group vitamins.
● Eat five to six small 'meals' a day, rather than three large ones.

- Increase fluid (water, milk or juice) intake.
- Reduce coffee and tea intake if > 3 per day.

Constipation

'Constipation may be defined as a delay in the passage of food residue, due to the accumulation of hard, dry stool, associated with painful defaecation, abdominal distension and a palpable mass' (Jordan 2002, p 290). Normal patterns for bowel movements vary significantly between women, and have been defined as anything from three per day to one every three days (Jordan 2002). It is therefore not the frequency of bowel motion per se, but the discomfort and difficulty in passing one that is more significant in defining constipation.

Constipation is caused by hormonal changes (which result in slowed bowel motility and changes in absorption patterns), changes in food and fluid intake (volumes, times and types), and for some, by reduced rates of exercise (Frye 1998; Walsh 2001). Constipation is common during pregnancy, possibly occurring in forty per cent of women (NICE 2003). It is difficult to establish incidence rates, due to disclosure issues for women, and to other confounding variables, such as the effects of routine iron supplementation at the time the abovementioned research was carried out.

Dietary and lifestyle changes are the primary response to constipation during pregnancy. Both herbal and pharmaceutical laxatives should only be used as a short-term (one to two weeks) last resort while dietary changes are made, as they can cause flora, fluid and electrolyte imbalances in the bowel and reduced gut motility and absorption of nutrients (Jordan 2002).

Dietary changes include increased fibre intake, such as grains (whole or bran form), beans and lentils, brown rice, nuts and seeds and dried fruits. Fresh fruit and vegetables are an excellent source of fibre and have the advantage of providing both fibre and fluid together, as well as valuable nutrients. As most fibre absorbs fluid during digestion, it is important that women increase both fibre and fluid intake, or the increased intake of some types of fibre can aggravate rather than resolve constipation. Fluid intake is very important. There is no 'right' number of cups of fluid to have each day, but if a woman is constipated she is unlikely to be having enough fluid, either in foods or in liquid form. It is important that women drink plenty of fluid daily and not just when constipated. Prunes and kiwifruit, as fruit or juice, are excellent, but many women do not like or have access to them. Tea and coffee worsen constipation by acting as diuretics, so fluid is passed out as urine, not leaving enough in the intestine to keep the stool soft. The midwife should work individually with women, acknowledging their personal, social and cultural context, to find high-fibre foods and appropriate fluids that they might include in their diet. Regular consumption of these foods and fluids is important, rather than in response to constipation, as the bowel works best in a regular pattern or routine.

It is also worthwhile discussing issues of bowel motion pattern and technique with women. During pregnancy it may take longer to pass a motion, due to slowed peristaltic action. It is important for a woman to take note of her body's natural urge to go to the toilet when it occurs and not put it off or hold on, as it may be some hours or the next day before another urge occurs, and by then more fluid has been absorbed from the faecal mass and greater compaction has occurred. If a woman has lost the natural regular urge to pass a bowel motion, she should be encouraged to make a regular time each day for trying, after meals being the best time, given the natural peristalsis that occurs with the intake of food. Positioning on the toilet and pushing technique can also affect ease or speed of passing a motion. Women should:

- sit on the toilet with knees higher than their hips (a foot stool helps)
- have their legs hip-width apart
- lean forward with forearms resting on their knees (leaning back to push presses the stool against the posterior vaginal wall/pelvic floor and tenses the pelvic floor, when relaxation is needed)
- keep their back fairly straight, not rolled over
- let their tummy drop forward
- with the first push (using diaphragm), lift their heels and feel widening of the waist
- breathe out and push/grunt, relax, breathe deeply and try again
- try not to strain with prolonged pushes
- allow time for the peristaltic action, if it does not come
- try massaging their abdomen in a clockwise direction, starting at the right hip (possible until about 20 weeks gestation).

Heartburn

Heartburn (or gastro-oesophageal reflux) is a common experience for pregnant women, with different research citing incidence rates of between 72 and 85 per cent (NICE 2003). It is a very unpleasant condition in which stomach acid enters the lower oesophagus causing a 'burning sensation' in the chest or back of the throat (Frye 1998). It is caused by hormonal changes, which slow gastric motility and promote sphincter relaxation, and physical pressure from the growing uterus (Jordan 2002). It tends to worsen as pregnancy progresses (Jewell & Young 2004), and can cause major physical discomfort for women. It can interfere with content and pattern of eating, interrupt physical activity and sleeping, and result in considerable emotional and psychological distress for some women.

Numerous self-help measures for the relief of heartburn are listed below. Some will appeal to or work for one woman but not another, and some women find that something that helps initially may become ineffective as pregnancy progresses. Self-help measures for heartburn include the following:

- identifying foods which cause heartburn and avoiding them
- avoiding fried, fatty or spiced foods (for some women, bread causes heartburn)
- avoiding coffee, tea, alcohol and cigarettes, all of which worsen heartburn
- chewing food thoroughly and eating slowly

- eating apple, pineapple, papaya or kiwifruit with meals, as they have digestive enzymes which speed the breaking down and digestion of food
- eating four to six small meals a day, rather than three large ones (dividing the main meal onto two small plates and eating the second portion the next day reduces 'snack food' intake)
- eating the last meal of the day at least two hours before bedtime
- drinking plenty of fluid, but *not* with meals (they dilute digestive juices; wait thirty minutes)
- drinking milk or eating yoghurt (alkaline)
- drinking orange juice (acidic)
- chewing raw almonds or cashew nuts.
  Other non-food-related strategies may include:
- checking posture, especially while sitting—slouching will worsen heartburn
- trying exercises that stretch the upper torso while sitting or standing (not lying)
- staying upright for two hours after eating—walking may help
- sleeping with upper body elevated, with bricks under the bed legs, or several pillows (Balaskas 1998; Frye 1998; Jamil & Evennett 2000).

There are numerous herbal remedies available, in addition to the options from all the other therapies described earlier. There are also a number of medicated pharmaceutical options, which have varying levels of efficacy, and are variably supported by evidence (see Jordan 2002).

Conclusion

This chapter has sought to provide an introduction to the care of pregnant women. It has presented an overview of the purpose and provision of antenatal care within the context of the midwifery model. A primary aim of the chapter has been to outline the key components of antenatal care, and describe a framework for organising these components in a relatively systematic and coherent way. These components include:

- the nature and process of establishing a relationship with a pregnant woman and her support people
- the principles involved in and assisting or supporting a woman to make appropriate decisions regarding her pregnancy, and developing an individualised and effective care plan
- the assessment and monitoring of the health and wellbeing of a pregnant woman and her baby.

A framework of eight decision points has been presented, which comprise a set of four categories of cues, including

Reflective exercise

1 Consider the potential impact of physiological changes on the physical, psychological and social lives of pregnant women.
2 Identify your own scope of practice regarding interventions for treating or managing the physiological changes associated with pregnancy.
3 Identify referral options for 'out-of-scope' treatments.

information sharing, screening and assessment, decision-making, and health promotion and information. They are intended to prompt the midwife to consider the holistic nature of antenatal care. While this framework strives to provide a clear structure to antenatal care, it is intended to act primarily as a set of cues for the midwife rather than a strict prescription. The partnership between a pregnant woman and her midwife is a unique one, and it is incumbent on the midwife to facilitate an effective process that meets the woman's individual needs and reflects her personal reality.

The chapter has also discussed some of the knowledge and skills a midwife might apply in the provision of antenatal care. These include:

- establishing an estimated due date
- abdominal palpation
- blood pressure measurement
- routine blood and urine screening options
- describing the nature and significance of fetal movements
- antenatal education and exercise during pregnancy
- the concept of physiological changes associated with pregnancy, and issues related to the management of them.

A second objective of the chapter has been to argue for, and model the use of reviewed research to promote, evidence-informed midwifery in the provision of antenatal care. Much of what has traditionally been included in routine antenatal care has been based on anecdote and happenstance, rather than clear evidence that supports or refutes these practices. A good deal of the research reviewed to date either does not address issues of concern to midwives and childbearing women, or is weak, or is primarily applicable to the type of antenatal care which is provided within the medical model. This has limited the extent to which the concept of evidence-based practice has been applied within this chapter. It is to be hoped that in the future, midwives will be able to use evidence to inform their practice within the context of the midwifery model of care.

Review questions

1 What methods for establishing EDD are used in your region?

2 What antenatal blood tests are considered to be 'routine' in your region, and what are the 'normal' reference ranges for them?

3 Describe the physical, personal, social and emotional implications of positive blood screening tests for pregnant women and their families.

4 What are the contemporary diagnostic criteria for pre-eclampsia?

5 What are the essential components of measuring blood pressure?

6 What are the aims of routine antenatal urine screening, and what evidence is there for the accuracy and efficacy of contemporary urine screening tests?

7 What are the basic palpation techniques, and what information can be gained from abdominal palpation in antenatal care?

8 How might midwives help women to experience palpation positively?

9 What is the significance of fetal movements over the course of a woman's pregnancy, and how might a woman and her midwife monitor these?

10 What antenatal education and/or exercise classes are available in your region?

11 What place does exercise have in influencing the emotional and physical wellbeing of pregnant women, and what impact might social, personal or cultural factors have on exercise patterns?

12 List ten physiological changes associated with pregnancy, and identify the following:
   - the nature of the condition
   - the cause (if known)
   - its incidence (frequency and timing during pregnancy)
   - its natural course and resolution
   - the potential for pathology
   - relevant self-help measures.

Online resources

Australian College of Midwives, http://www.acmi.org.au

Australasian Society for the Study of Hypertension in Pregnancy 2000 Consensus Statement: The detection, investigation and management of hypertension in pregnancy, http://www.racp.edu.au/asshp/asshp.pdf

Perinatal Institute (UK), http://www.perinatal.nhs.uk

Medical Journal of Australia, http://www.mja.com.au

MIDIRS (Midwives Information and Resource Service), http://www.midirs.org

National Institute for Clinical Excellence (NICE) 2003 Antenatal care: routine care for the healthy pregnant woman. Royal College of Obstetricians and Gynaecologists, http://www.rcog.org.uk

New Zealand College of Midwives, http://www.midwife.org.nz

Radical Midwives Website, http://www.radmid.demon.co.uk

Robertson A 2004 A new approach to prenatal education. Birth International, http://www.acegraphics.com.au/articles/andrea04.html

Three Centres Consensus Guidelines on Antenatal Care Project 2001 Mercy Hospital for Women, Southern Health and Women's & Children's Health, Melbourne, http://www.dhs.vic.gov.au/maternity/anteguide.pdf

West Midlands Perinatal Institute, http:// www.wmpi.net and http://www.gestation.net

References

Auckland Home Birth Association 1993 A Guide to healthy pregnancy and childbirth. Auckland Home Birth Association, Auckland

Australasian Society for the Study of Hypertension in Pregnancy 2000 Consensus Statement: The detection, investigation and management of hypertension in pregnancy, http://www.racp.edu.au/asshp/asshp.pdf

Balaskas J 1998 New natural pregnancy (2nd edn). Sandstone, Leichhardt

Barclay L, Jones L 1996 Midwifery: trends and practice in Australia. Churchill Livingstone, Melbourne

Barclay L, Lie D 2004 Ginger helpful for nausea and vomiting of pregnancy. Online:http://www.medscape.com/viewarticle/466746_print, accessed 24 June 2004

Baskett T, Naegele F 2000 Naegele's rule: a reappraisal. British Journal of Obstetrics and Gynaecology 107:1433–1435

Baston H 2002 Antenatal care—blood tests in pregnancy. The Practising Midwife 5(11):28–32

Bluck R, Dixon M, Ramage C et al 1990 A reference range for the haematological changes of pregnancy. New Zealand Journal of Medical Laboratory Technology 44(4):103–106

Boyle M 1995 Antenatal investigations. Books for Midwives, Cheshire

Brayshaw E 2003 Exercises in pregnancy and childbirth:a practical guide for educators. Books for Midwives, London

Broclain D, Jepson R, Moumjid Ferdjaoui N 2003 Influence of comprehensive versus partial information on consumers' screening choice. (Protocol for a Cochrane Review) In: The Cochrane Library, Issue 4, John Wiley, Chichester

Brown M, Hague W, Higgins J et al 2000 Australasian Society for the Study of Hypertension in Pregnancy Consensus Statement: The detection, investigation and management of hypertension in pregnancy. Online:www.racp.edu.au/asshp/asshp.pdf, accessed 14 June 2004

Candy B, Clement S, Sikorski J et al 2003 Antenatal visits. In S Wickham (Ed) Midwifery Best Practice. Books for Midwives, London, pp 34–37

Carroli G, Villar J, Piaggio G et al 2001 WHO systematic review of randomised controlled trials of routine antenatal care. The Lancet 357:1565–1570

Chan K, Kean L 2004 Routine antenatal management at the booking clinic. Current Obstetrics and Gynaecology (14):79–85

Chandler D 2000 The relationship between iron levels during pregnancy and birthweight. Thesis submitted for Master of Health Sciences, University of Otago, Dunedin

Chandra K, Magee L, Einarson A et al 2003 Nausea and vomiting in pregnancy: results of a survey that identified interventions used by women to alleviate their symptoms. Journal of Psychosomatic Obstetrics and Gynecology 24(2):71–75

Christensen F, Olsen K, Rayburn W 2003 Cross-over trial comparing maternal acceptance of two fetal movements charts. Journal of Maternal–Fetal and Neonatal Medicine 14(2):118–122

Clarke P, Gross H 2004 Women's behaviour, beliefs and information sources about physical exercise in pregnancy. Midwifery 20:133–141

Coggins J 2001 Iron deficiency anaemia: a complication of pregnancy or a foregone conclusion? A midwife's view. MIDIRS Midwifery Digest 11(4):469–474

Crafter H 1997 Health promotion in midwifery: principles and practice. Arnold, London

Cronk M 2002 Me and my Pinard's. Midwifery Matters (94). Online: www.radmid.demon.co.uk/pinard.htm, accessed 28 June 2004

Donley J 1998 Birthrites: natural versus unnatural childbirth in New Zealand. The Full Court Press, Auckland

Donnison J 1988 Midwives and medical men: a history of the struggle for the control of childbirth. Historical Publications, London

Enkin M, Keirse M, Neilson, J et al 2000 A guide to effective care in pregnancy and childbirth (3rd edn). Oxford University Press, Oxford

Fisher M 1999 Fetal activity and maternal monitoring methods. British Journal of Midwifery 7(11):705–709

Fraser D, Cooper M 2003 Myles textbook for midwives (14th edn). Churchill Livingstone, Edinburgh

Frøen J 2004 A kick from within—fetal movement counting and the cancelled progress of antenatal care. Journal of Perinatal Medicine 32:13–24

Frye A 1998 Holistic midwifery, Vol. I: Care during pregnancy. Labrys Press, Portland

Gardosi J, Mongelli M, Wilcox M et al 2000 Gestation related optimal weight (GROW) program. Software version 3. West Midlands Perinatal Institute, Birmingham, www.gestation.net

Gardosi J, Vanner T, Francis A 1997 Gestational age and induction of labour for prolonged pregnancy. British Journal of Obstetrics and Gynaecology 104(7):792–797

Gates E 2004 Communicating risk in prenatal genetic testing. Journal of Midwifery and Women's Health 49(3):220–226

Goodwin A, Astbury J, McMeeken J 2000 Body image and psychological well-being in pregnancy: a comparison of exercisers and non-exercisers. Australian and New Zealand Journal of Obstetrics and Gynaecology 40(4):442–447

Grant A, Elbourne D, Valentin L et al 1989 Routine formal fetal movement counting and risk of antepartum late death in normally formed singletons. Lancet 2:345–349

Grimes D, Schulz K 2002 Uses and abuses of screening tests. Lancet 359:881–884

Hall M 2001 Rationalisation of antenatal care. The Lancet 357:1546

Health Department Victoria 1990 Having a baby in Victoria: final report of the Ministerial Review of Birthing Services in Victoria. Health Department Victoria, Melbourne

Henderson C, Macdonald S 2004 Mayes' midwifery (13th edn). Baillière Tindall, Edinburgh

Hodnett E 2004 Continuity of caregivers for care during pregnancy and childbirth (Cochrane Review). In: The Cochrane Library, Issue 2. John Wiley, Chichester

Howells D 2002 Exercise in pregnancy. The Practising Midwife 5(4):12–13

Hunt J, Lumley J 2002 Are recommendations about routine antenatal care in Australia consistent and evidence-based? Medical Journal of Australia 176:255–259

Jamil T, Evennett K 2000 The alternative pregnancy handbook. Judy Piathus, London

Jewell D, Young G 2004 Interventions for nausea and vomiting in early pregnancy (Cochrane Review). In: The Cochrane Library, Issue 2, John Wiley, Chichester

Jordan S 2002 Pharmacology for midwives. Palgrave, Basingstoke

Källén K 2002 Mid-trimester ultrasound prediction of gestational age: advantages and systematic errors. Ultrasound in Obstetrics and Gynecology 20:558–563

Källén K 2004 Increased risk of perinatal/neonatal death in infants who were smaller than expected at ultrasound fetometry in early pregnancy. Ultrasound in Obstetrics and Gynecology 24(1):30–34

Katz Rothman B 1989 Recreating motherhood: ideology and technology in a patriarchal society. Norton, New York

Kramer M 2004 Aerobic exercise for women during pregnancy (Cochrane Review). In: The Cochrane Library, Issue 2, John Wiley, Chichester

Lumley J 1993 Attenders and nonattenders at childbirth education classes in Australia: how do they and their births differ? Birth 20(3):123–130

McCourt C, Page L 1996 Report on the evaluation of one-to-one midwifery practice. Wolfson School of Health Sciences. Thames Valley University

McGeown P 2001 Detecting fetal growth abnormalities. MIDIRS Midwifery Digest 11(2):09–193

Menticoglou S, Hall P 2002 Routine induction of labour at 41 weeks gestation: nonsensus consensus. British Journal of Obstetrics and Gynaecology 109:485–491

Midwifery News 2003 (28):5 **(to come)**

Ministry of Health 2002 Maternity services: Notice pursuant to Section 88 of the New Zealand Public Health and Disability Act 2000. Ministry of Health, Wellington

Ministry of Health 2003 Maternity services consumer satisfaction survey: 2002 Ministry of Health, Wellington

Mohamed K 2004 Iron supplementation in pregnancy (Cochrane Review). In: The Cochrane Library, Issue 3. John Wiley, Chichester

Nakling J, Backe B 2002 Adverse obstetric outcome in fetuses that are smaller than expected at second trimester routine ultrasound examination. Acta Obstetrics and Gynecology Scandinavia 81(9):846–851

National Health Committee 2003 Screening to improve health in New Zealand. Ministry of Health, Wellington

National Institute for Clinical Excellence (NICE) 2003 Antenatal care: routine care for the healthy pregnant woman. Royal College of Obstetricians and Gynaecologists, London, www.rcog.org.uk

New Zealand College of Midwives 2003 Consensus statement on gestational diabetes (1996). New Zealand College of Midwives, Christchurch

New Zealand College of Midwives 2005 Midwives handbook for practice (3rd edn). The New Zealand College of Midwives, Christchurch

Nguyen T, Larsen T, Engholm G et al 2000 A discrepancy between gestational age by last menstrual period and by parietal diameter may indicate an increased risk of fetal death and adverse pregnancy outcome. British Journal of Obstetrics and Gynaecology 107(9):1122–1129

Nguyen T, Larsen T, Engholm G et al 1999 Evaluation of ultrasound-estimated date of delivery in 17,450 spontaneous singleton births: do we need to modify Naegele's rule? Ultrasound Obstetrics and Gynecology 14(1):23–28

Nolan M 1999 Antenatal education: past and future agendas. The Practicing Midwife 2(3):24–27

Nolan M 2000 The influence of antenatal classes on pain relief in labour. The Practicing Midwife 3(5):23–26

Nolan M, Hicks C 1997 Aims, processes and problems of antenatal education as identified by three groups of childbirth teachers. Midwifery 13:179–188

Oakley A 1984 The captured womb. Blackwell, Oxford

Oakley A 1992 Social support and motherhood: the natural history of a research project. Blackwell, Oxford

Oats J 2000 Routine antenatal screening: a need to evaluate Australian practice. Medical Journal of Australia. Online:http://www.mja.com.au/public/issues/172_07_030400/oats/oats.html

Olsen O, Clausen J 1997 Routine ultrasound dating has not been shown to be more accurate than the calendar method. British Journal of Obstetrics and Gynaecology 104:1221–1222

Ovalle A, Levancini M 2001 Urinary tract infections in pregnancy. Current Opinion in Urology 11(1):55–59

Page L, McCourt C, Beake S et al 1999 Clinical interventions and outcomes of 'one-to-one' midwifery practice. Journal of Public Health Medicine 21(3):243–248

Palasathiran P, Starr M, Jones C 2002 Management of perinatal infections. Australasian Society for Infectious Diseases, Sydney

Parker M, Forbes K, Findlay I 2002 Eugenics or empowered choice? Community issues arising from prenatal testing. Australia and New Zealand Journal of Obstetrics and Gynaecology 42(1):10–14

Perinatal Institute 2004 Customised growth charts. Online: http://www.perinate.org/growth/fhm.htm, accessed 10 May 2004

Petrou S, Kupek E, Vause S et al 2003 Antenatal visits and adverse perinatal outcomes: results from a British population-based study. European Journal of Obstetrics, Gynecology and Reproductive Biology 106(1):40–49

Rankin J, Hillan E, Mutrie N 2000 An historical overview of physical activity and childbirth. British Journal of Midwifery 8(12): 761–764

Reiger K 2001 Our bodies, our babies: the forgotten women's movement. Melbourne University Press, Melbourne

Robertson A 2001 Prenatal education:time to lift our game. The Practicing Midwife 4(1):38–39

Robertson A 2004 A new approach to prenatal education. Birth International. Online: http://www.acegraphics.com.au/articles/andrea04.html, accessed 14 Aug 2004

Ross M 2003 Circle of time: errors in the use of the pregnancy wheel. The Journal of Maternal–Fetal and Neonatal Medicine 14(6): 370–372

Rosser J 2000 Calculating the EDD: which is more accurate, scan or LMP? The Practising Midwife 3(3):28–29

Santalahti P, Aro A, Hemminki E et al 1998 On what grounds do women participate in prenatal screening? Prenatal Diagnosis 18:153–165

Savitz D, Terry J, Dole N et al 2002 Comparison of pregnancy dating by last menstrual period, ultrasound scanning, and their combination. American Journal of Obstetrics and Gynecology 187(6):1660–1666

Searle J 1997 Routine antenatal screening: not a case of informed choice. Australian and New Zealand Journal of Public Health 21(3):268–274

Smaill F 2004 Antibiotics for asymptomatic bacteriuria in pregnancy (Cochrane Review). In: The Cochrane Library, Issue 3, John Wiley, Chichester

Smith G 2001 Use of time to event analysis to estimate the normal duration of human pregnancy. Human Reproduction 16(7): 1497–1500

Smith C, Crowther C, Beilby et al 2000 The impact of nausea and vomiting on women: a burden of early pregnancy. Australia and New Zealand Journal of Obstetrics and Gynaecology 40(4):397–401

Stenhouse E, Wright D, Hattersley A et al 2003 How well do midwives estimate the date of delivery? Midwifery 19:125–131

Strong T 2000 Expecting trouble: what expectant parents should know about prenatal care in America. New York University Press, New York

Symons Downs D, Hausenblas H 2004 Women's exercise beliefs and behaviors during their pregnancy and postpartum. Journal of Midwifery and Women's Health 49(2):138–144

Taylor R 2004 Correct technique for blood pressure measurement—why bother? Midwifery News 32:23

Three Centres Consensus Guidelines on Antenatal Care Project 2001 Mercy Hospital for Women, Southern Health and Women's & Children's Health, Melbourne. Online: www.dhs.vic.gov.au/maternity/anteguide.pdf, accessed 15 May 2004

Tiran D 2001 Natural remedies for morning sickness and other pregnancy problems. Quadrille Publishing, London

Tracy S 2005 The quality review of Ryde Midwifery Group Practice. Final report. Northern Sydney and Central Coast Health, NSW

Tunon K, Eik-Nes S, Grottum P 1996 A comparison between ultrasound and a reliable last menstrual period as predictors of the day of delivery in 15,000 examinations. Ultrasound in Obstetrics and Gynecology 8(3):178–185

Tunon K, Eik-Nes S, Grottum P 1999 Fetal outcome when the ultrasound estimate of the day of delivery is more than 14 days later than the last menstrual period estimate. Ultrasound in Obstetrics and Gynecology 14(1):17–22

Villar J, Carroli G, Khan-Neelofur D et al 2004 Patterns of routine antenatal care for low-risk pregnancy (Cochrane Review). In: The Cochrane Library, Issue 2, John Wiley, Chichester

Wagner M 1994 Pursuing the birth machine: the search for appropriate birth technology. Ace Graphics, Sydney

Walsh L 2001 Midwifery: Community-based care during the childbearing year. WB Saunders, Philadelphia

Watson W 1990 Screening for glycosuria during pregnancy. Southern Medical Journal 83(2):156–158

Waugh J, Clark T, Divakaran T et al 2004 Accuracy of urinalysis dipstick techniques in predicting significant proteinuria in pregnancy. Obstetrics and Gynecology 103(4):769–777

Wickham S 2002 Pinard wisdom: tips and tricks from midwives (Part 1). The Practising Midwife 5(9):21

Wiener A 2002 The brick wall of labour. The Practicing Midwife 5(2):38–39

Wilkinson J 2000 What do we know about herbal morning sickness treatments? A literature survey. Midwifery 16:224–228

Wolfe L, Weissgerber T 2003 Clinical physiology of exercise in pregnancy: a literature review. Journal of Obstetrics and Gynaecology Canada 25(6):473–483

Yang H, Kramer M, Platt R et al 2002 How does early ultrasound scan estimation of age lead to higher rates of preterm birth? American Journal of Obstetrics and Gynecology 186(3):433–437

Further reading

Balaskas J 1998 New natural pregnancy (2nd edn). Sandstone, Leichhardt

Boyle M 1995 Antenatal investigations. Books for Midwives, Cheshire

Brayshaw E 2003 Exercises in pregnancy and childbirth: a practical guide for educators. Books for Midwives, London

Donley J 1998 Birthrites: natural vs unnatural childbirth in New Zealand. The Full Court Press, Auckland

Enkin M, Keirse M, Neilson, J et al 2000 A guide to effective care in pregnancy and childbirth (3rd edn). Oxford University Press, Oxford

Frye A 1998 Holistic midwifery, Vol. I: Care during pregnancy. Labrys Press, Portland

Hunt J, Lumley J 2002 Are recommendations about routine antenatal care in Australia consistent and evidence-based? Medical Journal of Australia 176:255–259

Jamil T, Evennett K 2000 The alternative pregnancy handbook. Judy Piathus, London

Jordan S 2002 Pharmacology for midwives. Palgrave, Basingstoke

Katz Rothman B 1989 Recreating motherhood: ideology and technology in a patriarchal society. Norton, New York

Ministry of Health 2002 Maternity services: Notice pursuant to Section 88 of the New Zealand Public Health and Disability Act 2000. Ministry of Health, Wellington

New Zealand College of Midwives 2005 Midwives handbook for practice (3rd edn). The New Zealand College of Midwives, Christchurch

Nolan M 1999 Antenatal education: past and future agendas. The Practicing Midwife 2(3):24–27

Oakley A 1984 The captured womb. Blackwell, Oxford

Reiger K 2001 Our bodies, our babies: the forgotten women's movement. Melbourne University Press, Melbourne

Strong T (2000) Expecting trouble: what expectant parents should know about prenatal care in America. New York University Press, New York

Tiran D 2001 Natural remedies for morning sickness and other pregnancy problems. Quadrille Publishing, London

Wagner M 1994 Pursuing the birth machine: the search for appropriate birth technology. Ace Graphics, Sydney

APPENDIX A: Historical health review

Maternity: midwifery and obstetric

Gravida—number of pregnancies (includes living children, miscarriage, termination of pregnancy, ectopic pregnancy, stillbirth, neonatal death)

Parity—number of babies born at or beyond 20 weeks, preterm (< 37 weeks), post term (> 42 weeks)

Contraceptive history

Past pregnancy(ies)—date, place, pregnancy complications, labour spontaneous/induced, gestation, duration of complications, outcome, name, sex, weight, breast/artificial feeding, postnatal complications, S/E/C issues

Risk markers

Chronic hypertension—genetic hypertension or pre-eclampsia (degree), gestational diabetes

Multiple pregnancy—congenital abnormalities, antenatal anaemia (Hb < 90)

Preterm birth (< 37 weeks)—small baby (IUGR/SGA), APH

Post term birth (> 42 weeks)—large baby (> 4500 g), shoulder dystocia

Assisted birth (forceps/vent.)—lower-segment caesarean section, vaginal birth after caesarean section, postpartum haemorrhage (>1000 or treated)

Rh sensitisation/ABO incompatibility—perinatal infection

Antenatal or perinatal depression/psychosis

Other

Medical

Essential hypertension, diabetes, heart disease

Asthma, TB/pulmonary disease, thyroid disease

Neurological disorder (epilepsy), musculoskeletal disease

Renal/urinary tract disorder

Haematology disorder, liver disease, digestive disorder

STI, infertility, cervical abnormality/treatment

Polycystic ovaries, fibroids, endometriosis

Allergies, infections, vaginal/urinary tract abnormality/treatment

HIV status risk (high/low)

MRSA risk (high/low)

TB risk (high/low)

Medical examination

Surgery (what, when, complications)

Blood transfusion

Physical, sexual, psychological abuse

Other

Mental health

Depression, eating disorder, other

Family health

Maternal—diabetes, hypertension/pre-eclampsia, multiple pregnancy, asthma, intellectual disability, haemoglobinopathy, allergies, other

Congenital abnormalities (maternal and/or paternal)—chromosomal, limb deformity, metabolic, neural tube defect, cardiac defect, cleft palate, dislocated hip(s), severe infant morbidity, SIDS, other

APPENDIX B: Current health review

Physical

General health

Any underlying/ongoing health concerns

Medical examination (as appropriate)

Cervical smear screen—when

Any sign of current infection (review risk re STI)

BP, pulse, MSU

Height (cm), weight (kg), BMI

Diet (details), exercise (details)

Smoking (what, how much, readiness to reduce/stop)

Alcohol, drugs (what, how much, readiness to reduce/stop)

Safety from violence (if woman alone or maybe wait until visit with woman alone)

Medications and supplements (details), folic acid

Emotional

General health

Feelings about pregnancy and having a baby

Planned/unplanned and welcome/unwelcome pregnancy

Social

Autonomy, support, resources, employment, community 'belonging' or isolated

Is there a current relationship—partner, husband? Is it stable and supportive?

Cultural

Identity, integration/isolation, support, resources, needs

Safety issues

Spiritual

Any religious beliefs that may influence needs/choices/care options

Current pregnancy: establish EDD

LMP (sure/unsure), known conception date

EDD (consider 283-day option)

Positive pregnancy test

Menstrual cycle—regular/irregular/frequency, contraception, last cycle and menstruation normal (Y/N (details))

CHAPTER 21

Physiological changes during labour and the postnatal period

Sally Baddock and Lesley Dixon

Key terms

acid–base balance, breathing patterns, cellular barrier, cervical ripening, dilatation, diuresis, effacement, energy needs, fetal responses, fetal wellbeing, hormones, hypercoagulable state, involution, lochia, mechanism of labour, myometrial activation, onset of labour, placental separation, regeneration, smooth muscle tone, uterine contractions, uterotonins, water and electrolyte balance

Chapter overview

This chapter focuses on the physiological processes associated with birth and the postnatal period. This begins in the final weeks of pregnancy as changes occur to the uterus and cervix in preparation for birth, and continues through the processes associated with the birth of the baby. It concludes by examining the changes during the six to eight weeks following birth, when the reproductive organs return to a non-pregnant state, and lactation is started. Understanding the underlying physiology is essential if a midwife is to make informed decisions about the progress of labour and adequately assess the wellbeing of the woman and baby throughout labour and the postnatal period. It also enables informed discussion with the woman throughout these times of significant physiological change.

The chapter is divided into two major sections—the physiology of labour and the physiology of the postnatal period—although physiologically the division is not so clear, as one process leads into the next.

The physiology underlying labour and the changes of the postnatal period include many physical and chemical processes controlled by hormones. Before labour begins, hormones mediate the preparatory changes that occur in the uterus and cervix. The actual mechanisms that initiate labour are not clear, but they are associated with fetal, placental and maternal hormones. Progress in labour is largely mediated by hormones that govern uterine contractions. Effective contractions first lead to dilatation of the cervix and then generate the pressure to birth the baby. The mechanism of labour describes the manipulations the baby must make to negotiate the narrow pelvis and birth canal. Following the birth of the baby, the placenta separates from the uterus and may be delivered without intervention, while continuing uterine contractions minimise blood loss from the placental site. Labour is a physically demanding time that is supported by changes to metabolism and probably changes to all body systems to maximise the efforts of the woman. During labour the fetus is normally exposed to considerable stress.

The postnatal period is defined as the period up until six to eight weeks after birth, when the genital organs return to a non-pregnant state, and lactation is started. Many of the physiological, anatomical and endocrine changes in this period occur in the first 10 to 14 days; for example, some hormone levels drop significantly, whereas others involved in lactation rise. Involution is the process that reduces the size of the uterus, cervix and vagina. In non-lactating women this includes reduction in the size of the breasts.

These processes are the focus of this chapter. Further readings are provided at the end of the chapter for a more in-depth exploration of specific topics.

Learning outcomes

Learning outcomes for this chapter are:

1 To outline the changes involved in myometrial activation and cervical ripening

2 To discuss the physiological factors that may be responsible for initiating labour

3 To outline the role of hormones in the maintenance of labour

4 To describe the physiology underlying the three stages of labour, including the physiology of effective uterine contractions, the mechanism of second stage and the steps involved in placental separation in third stage

5 To discuss physiological changes that occur to other systems to support labour

6 To describe fetal responses and measures of fetal wellbeing during labour

7 To describe the change in maternal hormone levels following the birth of the baby

8 To describe the processes of involution and of healing at the placental site

9 To provide a physiological rationale for blood and fluid loss during the puerperium

10 To describe the changes that occur in the cervix, vagina and vulva in the puerperium

11 To compare oxygen consumption during labour and the puerperium

12 To compare physiological changes in the maternal body systems during pregnancy and during the postnatal period, particularly the renal, haematological and cardiovascular changes

13 To identify physiological vulnerability during the puerperium

14 To outline the hormonal control of lactation during pregnancy and the pueperium.

Physiology of labour

Labour is a process in which regular and coordinated muscular contractions of the uterus lead to gradual effacement and dilatation of the cervix, followed by expulsive contractions that result in the birth of the baby and placenta. For simplicity, the physiological changes that occur during this process can be divided into three stages. Stage one describes the time when uterine contractions are of sufficient frequency, intensity and duration to cause effacement and dilatation of the cervix. Stage two begins with the complete dilatation of the cervix and ends with the birth of the baby, and stage three involves the delivery of the placenta. Physiologically there is no abrupt transition between the stages of labour or between the end of pregnancy and the onset of labour. The events leading to the onset of labour build gradually during the last weeks of the pregnancy, and there is overlap of physiological changes between the stages of labour.

The exact mechanisms that initiate and control labour are still not well understood. It is an extremely complex physiological process involving positive feedback and negative feedback loops and interconnections between maternal and fetal processes. Before exploring the physiology of labour it is important to review the changes that occur in the uterus and cervix prior to active labour.

Uterine changes in preparation for labour

The myometrium consists of bundles of non-striated muscle fibres, intermixed with connective tissue, blood and lymph vessels and nerves. Throughout pregnancy the uterus is preparing for labour and there is an enormous increase in the bulk of the myometrium due to hypertrophy and hyperplasia of the cells. Myometrial cells are smooth muscle cells and therefore are capable of spontaneous activity independent of external stimuli. Low-amplitude activity occurs even in a non-pregnant uterus (Challis 2001). During pregnancy, however, contractions are largely prevented by uterotonic inhibitors, such as progesterone, nitric oxide and prostacyclin, and those that do occur tend to be mild, irregular and non-synchronised. Women are generally not aware of these contractions. As pregnancy progresses, contractions gradually increase in intensity and frequency, until in labour, strong, synchronous, effective contractions occur.

Changes in the structure of myometrial cells enable them to contract more strongly and to maintain this through labour. The initial changes are termed 'activation'. Four main events occur during activation: the ratio of hormones changes, electrical activity increases, myometrial cells become more responsive and there is an increase in ion channels. This occurs in the last few weeks of pregnancy as uterotonic inhibitors decrease and oestrogen and contraction-associated proteins

(CAPs) increase. Contraction-associated proteins include gap junction proteins, myometrial oxytocin receptors and prostaglandin receptors, and calcium and sodium channels (Blackburn 2003). Increased gap junction formation facilitates the spread of electrical activity over the myometrium, and increased prostaglandin and oxytocin receptors enhance the responsiveness of target tissues to these uterotonins. Increased sodium ion channels facilitate sodium movement into the cells. This is required for electrical excitation. Increased calcium ion channels enable increased calcium movement into the cells. Calcium is required for binding of myosin to actin during contraction.

Cervical changes in preparation for labour

Another region of the uterus that undergoes changes is the cervix. During pregnancy, the cervix is important in retaining the fetus in the uterus. Stretching of the cervix is resisted due to its high connective tissue content, which is made up of collagen-fibre bundles embedded in a proteoglycan matrix. Before effacement and dilatation can occur, the cervix must change structure and soften or 'ripen' and this occurs towards the end of pregnancy (Winkler et al 1999). The softening process is characterised by an infiltration of leucocytes, an increase in water and a decrease in collagen content of the cervix. Infiltration of the cervix by leucocytes and macrophages leads to the release of proteolytic enzymes that cause collagen degradation. Increases in hyaluronic acid and changes in blood vessel permeability increase the water content of the cervix. Increases in glycoaminoglycans reduce the ability of collagen fibres to bind together (Johnson & Everitt 2000; Winkler et al 1999). The changes associated with cervical ripening are independent of myometrial contractions (Blackburn 2003).

The process of cervical ripening is complex and depends on the hormones present at the end of pregnancy. Increases in the oestrogen-to-progesterone ratio and increases in relaxin promote collagen degradation. Nitric oxide in the cervix increases near term and may act with prostaglandin E_2 to induce vasodilation and facilitate neutrophil infiltration (Ledingham et al 2000). Stretching of the cervix results in the local release of prostaglandin $F_{2\alpha}$ ($PGF_{2\alpha}$) and the release of oxytocin from the posterior pituitary (the Ferguson reflex), which in turn increase uterine activity (Blackburn 2003). It is worth noting that, clinically, prostaglandin E_2 and $PGF_{2\alpha}$ are used for softening of the cervix prior to induction of labour because of their localised effect on cervical softening (Johnson & Everitt 2000; Tenore 2003). Once the cervix is prepared physiologically and structurally, labour can begin.

What initiates labour?

In a number of mammalian species the onset of labour is timed primarily by the fetus via secretions of the adrenal cortex that increase oestrogen levels and subsequently $PGF_{2\alpha}$ in the uterus. Prostaglandin $F_{2\alpha}$ activates myometrial contractions and cervical ripening (Johnson & Everitt 2000). In humans, it is likely that maternal as well as fetal mechanisms are involved,

although the final pathway appears to involve activation of the fetal hypothalamic-pituitary-adrenal axis (Norwitz et al 1999).

Mechanisms leading to labour are mediated by changes in hormone levels. It is important to realise that hormone effectiveness is changed not only through increased synthesis and release of hormones, but also by reduction in the concentration of hormone-binding proteins or, alternatively, by an increase in numbers of receptors on target tissues. Therefore the plasma concentration of a hormone may not reflect the degree of hormone binding at the local site.

It is known that increases in placental uterotonic hormones are linked to maturation of the fetal adrenal glands and the mechanical stretching of the uterus due to the growing fetus. Maternal adrenal glands and other endocrine or neural mechanisms may also play a role (Johnson & Everitt 2000).

A growing number of placental hormones have been identified, although their exact function in labour is not yet clear (Reis et al 2001). The roles of some of the key hormones and chemical mediators that contribute to labour, such as corticotrophin-releasing hormone, prostaglandins, oxytocin, oestrogen, progesterone, relaxin and nitric oxide are outlined below.

Corticotrophin-releasing hormone

It is suggested that placental corticotrophin-releasing hormone (CRH) plays an important role in the onset of labour (Challis 2001; Grammatopoulos & Hillhouse 1999), along with maturation of the fetal hypothalamic-pituitary-adrenal system. CRH is a neuropeptide produced by the hypothalamus, placenta, decidua, chorion and amnion. CRH receptors are found in the decidua and fetal membranes and in the myometrium. The complexity of control is highlighted by the fact that CRH appears to have a dual role: during pregnancy it promotes uterine quiescence; during labour, under the influence of oxytocin, it binds to different receptor types and promotes uterine contraction (Grammatopoulos & Hillhouse 1999).

There is strong evidence for the role of CRH in the initiation of labour. For example, placental CRH levels increase markedly after 35 weeks gestation, partly due to a 60% decrease in protein binding of the hormone, and then CRH levels decrease by 50% within 20 to 30 minutes of birth. Longer duration of labour has been associated with lower levels of CRH (Chrousos, cited in Blackburn 2003). Additionally, CRH levels are increased in pregnancies complicated by pregnancy-induced hypertension and intrauterine growth restriction (Petraglia, cited in Grammatopoulos & Hillhouse 1999), which may lead to preterm labour.

Grammatopoulos and Hillhouse (1999) proposed that placental CRH initiates labour via mechanisms that increase placental oestriol (active form of oestrogen) production and fetal cortisol production. The pathways for this are shown in Figure 21.1. Corticotrophin-releasing hormone stimulates the fetal adrenal gland to produce cortisol and the oestrogen precursor, dehydroepiandrosterone sulfate (DHEAS). Fetal cortisol exerts positive feedback to increase placental CRH

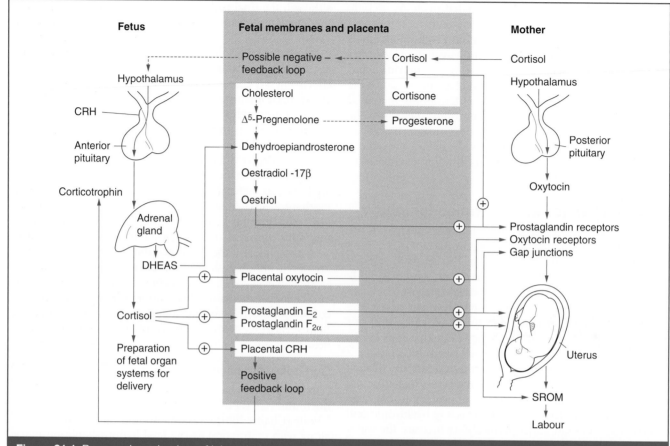

Figure 21.1 Proposed mechanism of labour induction at term (based on Blackburn 2003)

and increases prostaglandin and oxytocin synthesis. DHEAS is an essential precursor to placental oestrogen synthesis, particularly oestriol, which drives other mechanisms associated with the initiation of labour. The specialised fetal adrenal cells responsible for DHEAS production atrophy after birth.

Although cortisol appears to have a role in the initiation of labour, some evidence suggests labour may still progress when levels of fetal cortisol are low. For example, neither fetal anencephaly, where there is an absence of adrenocorticotrophic hormone (ACTH), nor adrenal hypoplasia, where cortisol production is reduced, necessarily result in prolonged labour (Johnson & Everitt 2000). Other clinical evidence indicates that although maternal corticosteroid administration results in a decrease of fetoplacental oestrogen production, it does not delay the onset of labour (Johnson & Everitt 2000) as would be expected.

In summary, placental CRH behaves differently to hypothalamic CRH. Placental CRH may promote uterine quiescence during pregnancy and then enhance contractility during labour. It is suggested that, via the production of fetal cortisol and DHEAS, CRH leads to increased oestrogen production in the placenta, which drives the other mechanisms of labour such as an increase in oxytocin receptors, gap junctions and prostaglandins.

Prostaglandins

Prostaglandins are lipids that are synthesised in tissues throughout the body. They are local hormones (paracrine hormones), which act at or near the place where they are synthesised. Prostaglandins are uterotonins directly responsible for uterine contraction. Two prostaglandins are particularly important in labour: PGE_2 and $PGF_{2\alpha}$. These prostaglandins stimulate smooth muscle fibres to contract, stimulate the formation of gap junctions in myometrial tissue and increase calcium levels in myometrial cells. As mentioned previously, prostaglandins also have a role in softening the cervix, enabling effacement and dilatation (Johnson & Everitt 2000).

Levels of PGE_2 and $PGF_{2\alpha}$ in the amniotic fluid are known to increase before and during labour; however, evidence for an increase of these hormones in maternal plasma before labour begins, is not conclusive (Johnson & Everitt 2000).

Prostaglandin synthesis has a complex pathway. During labour, prostaglandins are synthesised by the decidua, cervix, placenta and fetal membranes. The pathway for synthesis of prostaglandins is outlined in Figure 21.2. Arachidonic acid is the common precursor of both PGE_2 and $PGF_{2\alpha}$. Arachidonic acid is produced by the action of phospholipase A2 on phospholipids in the fetal membranes and the decidua. Phospholipase A2 is stored within lysosomes, which release the enzyme in the presence of oestrogen, and retain the

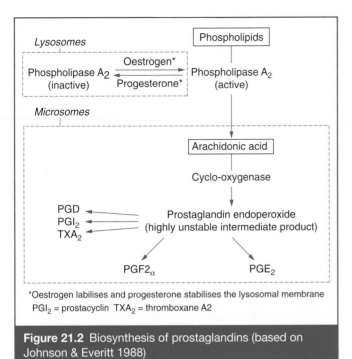

Figure 21.2 Biosynthesis of prostaglandins (based on Johnson & Everitt 1988)

enzyme in the presence of progesterone. Consequently, a rise in the oestrogen-to-progesterone ratio results in increased phospholipase A2, leading to increased production of arachidonic acid and prostaglandin synthesis. Oxytocin also promotes prostaglandin release.

Other evidence that prostaglandins contribute to the initiation of labour comes from the finding that inhibitors of prostaglandin synthesis, such as the anti-inflammatory drug indomethacin, are effective at reducing preterm labour (Enkin et al 2000).

Oxytocin

Another hormone essential for labour is oxytocin. Oxytocin is released into the sytemic circulation from the posterior pituitary in response to tactile stimulation of the reproductive tract, particularly the cervix. This is known as the Ferguson reflex and is outlined in Figure 21.3. There is also a local (paracrine) release of oxytocin from the fetal membranes, decidua and placenta (Reis et al 2001). There is little evidence that oxytocin initiates or is the primary uterotonin of labour, and it can only be used clinically to induce labour if the cervix is ripe (Tenore 2003). Plasma oxytocin levels do not increase physiologically until the second stage of labour, although

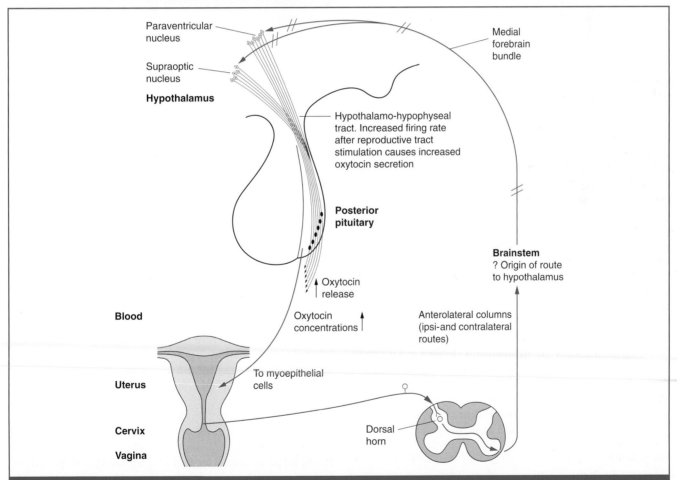

Figure 21.3 The neuroendocrine reflex (Ferguson reflex), underlying oxytocin synthesis and secretion (based on Johnson & Everitt 1988)

local concentrations may increase before this. The importance of oxytocin for labour is demonstrated by the increase of oxytocin receptors in the decidua during pregnancy, reaching a 300-fold increase by term (Zeeman, cited in Blackburn 2003; Takemura, cited in Reis et al 2001). Oxytocin binds to these decidual receptors, stimulates the release of prostaglandins from the decidua and stimulates uterine pacemakers.

Oestrogen

Oestrogen has a primary role in initiating many changes that are essential for labour, and levels begin to rise at about 34 weeks gestation. Oestrogen increases the sensitivity of the myometrial oxytocin receptors during pregnancy (Blackburn 2003) and thus facilitates myometrial contractility. Oestrogen promotes the formation of CAPs and prostaglandin synthesis via increases in phospholipase A2 release from lysosomes (Johnson & Everitt 2000). The synthesis of oestriol (the active oestrogen in pregnancy) relies on the fetal adrenal precursor DHEAS as outlined earlier (see Fig 21.1). Therefore maternal serum oestriol levels are an indicator of fetal hypothalamic-pituitary-adrenal maturity and elevated levels of oestriol levels are associated with the onset of labour (Norwitz et al 1999).

Progesterone

Progesterone is also a pregnancy hormone and, like oestrogen, it is produced in the placenta. However, in contrast to oestrogen, it is not reliant on fetal precursors for synthesis and its role is in suppressing uterine excitement. Progesterone does this by promoting the uptake of intracellular calcium into the sarcoplasmic reticulum of the myometrium, and works with nitric oxide to inhibit the production of CAPs (Challis 2001). Progesterone also has a role in decreasing oxytocin binding during pregnancy, and it is understood that removal of this effect at the onset of labour could facilitate myometrial contractions (Thornton et al 1999). Maternal plasma progesterone does not decrease at parturition, as it does in some animals (Norwitz et al 1999), but there may be local decreases in progesterone activity through increased progesterone-binding protein. The decreased availability of progesterone and increased synthesis of oestrogen produce an increased oestrogen-to-progesterone ratio, allowing the uterotonic effects of oestrogen to dominate, enabling contraction of uterine muscle.

Relaxin

Relaxin, like progesterone, supports quiescence of the uterus. Relaxin is produced by the myometrium, decidua and placenta. Its levels are highest in the first trimester, but are measurable throughout pregnancy. Relaxin has a role in enhancing cervical ripening; although exogenous application of relaxin promotes cervical ripening, the implications of clinical use of the hormone are not clear (Kelly et al 2001).

Nitric oxide

Nitric oxide (NO) is important in maintaining myometrial quiescence (Longo et al 2003). It is produced by the decidua, fetal membranes, and fetal and placental vascular epithelium.

Nitric oxide is believed to interact with progesterone to inhibit the production of CAPs (Challis 2001). Levels of NO in the myometrium decrease near term but increase in the cervix. Nitric oxide production is dependent on the enzyme nitric oxide synthetase (NOS), which has three forms. There is an increase in the expression of one form, iNOS, in the cervix prior to the onset of labour, suggesting that nitric oxide contributes to cervical ripening (Ledingham et al 2000).

Summary of hormonal contribution to labour

- Plasma levels of hormones are not representative of local changes that may initiate and maintain labour.
- During pregnancy, hormones such as progesterone, relaxin and nitric oxide maintain the uterus in a quiescent state.
- Prior to labour, changes in the oestrogen-to-progesterone ratio facilitate activation of the uterine muscle, and ripening of the cervix occurs under the influence of prostaglandins, relaxin and nitric oxide.
- Following activation of myometrial cells and cervical ripening in the uterus, the myometrium responds to the uterotonins, oxytocin and prostaglandins.
- Initiation of labour probably involves fetal and maternal influences.

First stage of labour

During the first stage of labour, myometrial contractions lead to effacement and dilatation of the cervix. The first stage is often divided into two phases, latent and active.

In the latent phase, uterine contractions occur but cervical dilatation is slow. The timeframe for this phase varies considerably (Enkin et al 2000). In the active phase, strong, effective contractions lead to cervical dilatation. Cervical dilation of 3 cm is sometimes regarded as an indicator of active labour (Johnson & Everitt 2000).

Uterine contractions during first stage

For contractions to be effective and result in effacement and dilatation of the cervix, several processes must occur. The cervix must be softened, as described earlier; contractions must be coordinated so that all regions of the myometrium contract in unison under the influence of pacemaker cells, and there must be a descending gradient of uterine activity such that contractions are stronger at the uterine fundus and lessen towards the lower uterine segment. This gradient of activity allows retraction of the upper uterine segment to mediate the processes of effacement and dilatation. Control of myometrial contractions is via the changing concentrations of placental hormones (prostaglandins, oxytocin, oestrogens, progesterone and relaxin) as described earlier.

Uterine muscle cells undergo some unique changes. For example, pacemakers, located in each cornua of the uterus, initiate contractions under the influence of local hormones. Gap junctions between the myometrial cells facilitate the rapid spread of electrical activity downward over the muscle cells, facilitating almost synchronous contraction of the myometrium so that maximum tension is generated in all myometrial cells at the same time. However, as expected, the strength of contraction is greater in the fundus and less in the lower uterine segment, due to the relatively low muscle and high connective tissue content in the lower region of the uterus. Along with synchronous contraction, smooth muscle can also maintain tone between contractions, a characteristic called retraction. Due to retraction, the smooth muscle

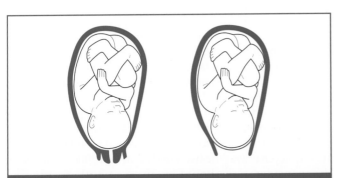

Figure 21.4 The uterus, showing dilatation of the cervix and the formation of the lower uterine segment (based on Henderson & Macdonald 2004)

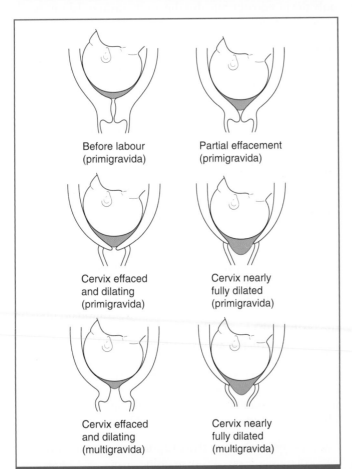

Before labour (primigravida)

Partial effacement (primigravida)

Cervix effaced and dilating (primigravida)

Cervix nearly fully dilated (primigravida)

Cervix effaced and dilating (multigravida)

Cervix nearly fully dilated (multigravida)

Figure 21.5 Effacement and dilatation of the cervix (based on Henderson & Macdonald 2004)

cells of the upper segment never fully relax and thus each contraction causes the muscle cells to become progressively shorter and fatter. Retraction of the upper segment enables shortening of the lower uterine segment so that the cervix becomes continuous with the lower uterine segment— that is, effacement. The process is illustrated in Figures 21.4 and 21.5.

As contractions of the upper uterine segment of the uterus continue to pull on the lower segment, dilatation of the external os is achieved. Full dilation of the cervix is measured at 10 cm. In the multigravida woman, effacement and dilatation tend to occur as a single process. During the early stages of dilatation, the operculum or mucous plug that was formed during pregnancy, under the influence of progesterone, is lost. This may appear as a bloodstained mucoid 'show'. The blood is due to the detachment of the chorion from the dilating cervix.

There is a relationship between the pressure generated in the uterus during labour and the level of pain encountered at each phase. Generally, the uterus has a resting tone of approximately 10 mmHg between contractions, and intrauterine pressure rises to 30–50 mmHg during contractions, but it may reach 100 mmHg in second stage during a Valsalva manoeuvre. Abdominal palpation can detect contractions generating pressure greater than 10–20 mmHg and a woman can perceive contractions around 15–20 mmHg. Pain is usually felt when contractions generate pressures more than 25 mmHg, but there is considerable variation among women (Blackburn 2003). These intrauterine pressures are shown in Figure 21.6. The pain may be due to ischaemia that occurs in muscle fibres during active contraction (visceral pain), and due to stretching of the vaginal, perineal and pelvic tissues caused by the pressure of the presenting part (somatic pain) during second stage.

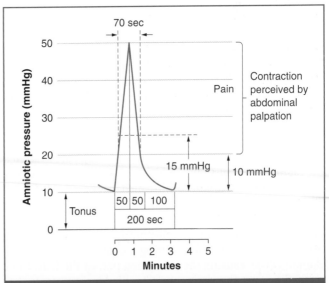

Figure 21.6 Correlation between abdominal palpitation and intrauterine pressure tracing (based on Blackburn 2003)

Uterine contractions and the fetus

Effective myometrial contractions are needed to push the fetus downward towards the vagina. This process induces a positive feedback mechanism because as the upper uterine segment shortens and thickens, and the fetus is pushed downward, the pressure on the cervix initiates the reflex release of oxytocin (Ferguson reflex). The more pressure, the greater the release of oxytocin, which further facilitates uterine contractions.

There are other effects involving the fetus. For example, during contractions the force is transmitted to the upper pole of the fetus, down the long axis of the spine, causing increased flexion of the head and ensuring that the smallest circumference of the head is presented to the cervical os.

Also, as the fetal head is forced against the cervix, a small amount of amniotic fluid (the forewaters) is trapped in front of the head, separated from the remainder of the amniotic fluid (the hindwaters). This separation protects against ascending infection as long as the membranes are intact. There is another advantage to the fetus of intact membranes—the pressure of contractions is spread over the amniotic fluid, rather than being applied directly to the fetus, and thus facilitates fetal oxygen delivery during contractions (Stables & Rankin 2004). Eventually, spontaneous rupture of the membranes occurs under the force of the uterine contractions. Artificial rupture of the membranes is sometimes performed to increase the progress of labour; however, this exposes the fetus to increased risk of infection and greater direct pressures during uterine contraction. Evidence suggests that routine amniotomy in the first stage of labour is not justified (Bricker & Luckas 2002; Enkin et al 2000).

The first stage of labour ends with full dilatation of the cervix, then there is a transition phase before the second stage commences. This phase is associated with very intense feelings, perhaps irritability and panic for the woman. There is no clear timeframe for transition and intervention is not necessary in a normal pregnancy.

Second stage of labour

The second stage of labour results in the birth of the baby. During the second stage of labour, uterine contractions are assisted by abdominal muscles and result in expulsive forces that move the baby through the pelvis and birth canal. There is a variable time until the presenting part of the fetus is visible (crowned) at the vulva. Crowning occurs once contractions force the fetus down and cause the presenting part to stretch the vagina and tissues of the pelvic floor. Crowning is generally associated with the urge to 'push', which may be overwhelming. The 'pushing urge' recruits the voluntary skeletal muscles of the abdominal wall and diaphragm. During this time, several changes result. Spontaneous pushing usually occurs for about 5–6 seconds, several times during a contraction (Stables & Rankin 2004), causing the presenting part of the fetus to be pushed against the perineum. The bladder is protected as it is pushed up into the abdominal cavity, and the rectum is flattened against the sacral curve, causing defecation of any contents. The effort of the second stage of labour causes sweating due to increased heat generated by muscle activity, and a rise in pulse rate in the woman. There are also pressure sensations on the rectum, and/or radiating pain in the thighs, due to pressure on the sacral plexus and the obturator nerve (Stables & Rankin 2004).

As well as the spontaneous desire to push that occurs during the second stage of labour, women are sometimes directed to push. There are reasons to question this practice. Evidence suggests that directed pushing may compromise fetal wellbeing by causing abnormalities in fetal heart rate (above 160 or below 110 bpm) and reduced Apgar scores (Enkin et al 2000; Roberts 2002). Also, mean umbilical arterial pH has been shown to be lower where women are subjected to sustained pushing (Enkin et al 2000). The reduction in pH may indicate fetal acidaemia caused by reduced blood flow to the placenta. (The physiology underlying fetal acidosis is described later, in the section on fetal responses during labour.) Similar results are obtained when women labour in the supine position, as this can also restrict placental blood flow due to maternal vena cava constriction (Enkin et al 2000). Therefore, due consideration should be given to both positioning and abstaining from directed pushing when supporting a labouring woman.

If the second stage of labour is to be fully understood, not only the physiology but also the mechanism of labour needs to be explained.

Mechanism of labour

Two issues complicate the birth of a human fetus: the curvature of the spine—a consequence of human upright posture—and the large size of the fetal head. In a normal birth, the head presents downward. As the fetus descends through the pelvis, it changes position so that the fetal head can be accommodated by the widest diameter of the woman's pelvis—the transverse diameter of the pelvic inlet, and the anteroposterior diameter of the pelvic outlet. During descent, the fetal head flexes to allow it passage through the pelvic inlet, with subsequent engagement in the pelvic cavity. The stages in the mechanism of labour are illustrated in Figure 21.7. Following engagement, internal rotation of the fetal head aligns it with the anteroposterior diameter of the pelvic outlet. This occurs due to several influences: pressure exerted on the fetus by the uterine contractions, the shape of the pelvic floor and the presence of the ischial spines. The head is born by extension (it is pushed upwards) and by flexion. Restitution occurs after the birth of the head, when the head returns to its original position. External rotation occurs when the shoulders turn to fit the widest diameter of the pelvis (anteroposterior), causing the head to rotate. Then the anterior and posterior shoulders are born (Stables & Rankin 2004). After the birth of the baby there may be some blood loss due to the contraction of muscle fibres, which retracts the uterus to a 20-week size.

Factors that influence the progress of second stage

Several factors influence the length of the second stage of labour: the bony pelvis, the fetal lie and presentation, and the pelvic floor muscles.

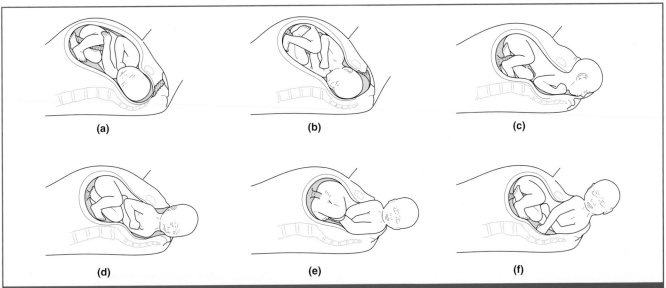

Figure 21.7 Normal labour, showing **(a)** engagement and flexion of the head, **(b)** internal rotation, **(c)** delivery by extension of the head after dilation of the cervix, and **(d–f)** sequential delivery of the shoulders (based on Johnson & Everitt 1988)

- Bony pelvis—the relationship of the woman's bony pelvis to the size and lie of the fetus may affect progress. Very rarely, cephalopelvic disproportion may impede the progress of labour. The diameters of the pelvic brim and outlet can be measured by pelvimetry but this does not accurately predict labour outcome (Enkin et al 2000). Various other unusual bony structures may slow the progress of labour (e.g. protruding sacral promontary, enlarged ischial spines).
- Fetus—the lie and presentation of the fetus influence progress. A longitudinal lie with head presentation is most common, then longitudinal lie with breech. A transverse lie with shoulder presentation, however, could not result in a vaginal birth. Passage through the vagina is facilitated by moulding of the fetal skull, which is made possible by the fontanelles and the unfused sutures of the fetal skull.
- Pelvic floor muscles—the vagina passes through the muscles of the pelvic floor. As the fetus descends through the vagina, the levator ani muscles are pushed downward and thin out, and the perineal body is stretched. In nulliparous women these muscles are being stretched for the first time, and this can lead to spasms and resistance against the descending fetus. Hence nulliparous women may have a longer second stage than multiparous women.

Midwives should be aware that the duration of second stage should be related to the progress of the labour and the satisfactory condition of woman and fetus, not an arbitrary timeframe (Enkin et al 2000). Once the baby is delivered, second stage is complete.

Third stage of labour

This is the stage when separation and delivery of the placenta and membranes occurs, and mechanisms are initiated that minimise bleeding from the placental site. Separation usually begins with the contraction that delivers the baby (Stables & Rankin 2004). This stage may be managed passively (physiologically) or actively (with intervention). Passive management is a 'hands off' approach, where the infant is encouraged to suckle to induce uterine contraction (Tenore 2003), and the woman maintains an upright position to use the effect of gravity to deliver the placenta. The cord is not clamped in physiological management. Active management involves the administration of oxytocics, cord clamping and controlled cord traction. Oxytocics (e.g. Syntocinon) induce uterine contraction. Randomised case control studies in the hospital setting have shown that active management is associated with decreased maternal blood loss, decreased incidence of postpartum haemorrhage and decreased duration of third stage. It is also associated with increased maternal side-effects of nausea and vomiting (Prendiville et al 2000). Once active management has begun, cord clamping and controlled cord traction are necessary (see below).

Normally, the process of placental separation follows a particular pattern of events.

Mechanism of separation of the placenta

The placenta separates from the decidua basalis as a result of uterine contractions that cause retraction of the uterus, and a 75% reduction in the area of the placental site. Blood in the intervillous spaces is forced back into the decidua basalis, causing congestion. Some of the blood trapped in the uterine muscles is pumped back into the baby via the pulsating cord. The placenta buckles and the arteries and veins of the intervillous spaces tear, leading to retroplacental haemorrhage, with the formation of a retroplacental clot and further placental separation. The weight of the placenta strips the membranes off the uterine wall and the placenta and membranes descend into the vagina and out of the body (Fig 21.8) (Coad & Dunstall 2001). It is normal to lose blood vaginally during the third stage due to retroplacental haemorrhage and separation of the placenta, but a loss greater than 500 mL is regarded as a postpartum haemorrhage (Stables & Rankin 2004). The uterus retracts further and the criss-cross arrangement of muscle fibres (termed 'living ligatures') strangle the blood vessels, including the spiral arterioles supplying the placental site. This prevents further blood loss, as shown in Figure 21.9. Fibrin plugs deposited in the torn ends of blood vessels further reduce blood loss.

Cord clamping

Interventions such as cord clamping can interrupt the normal mechanism of third stage and if oxytocics are not administered, cord clamping should not be necessary. If the mother suckles her baby, a reflex release of oxytocin occurs that stimulates

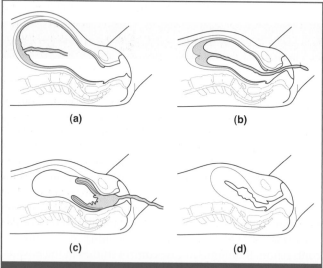

Figure 21.8 The mechanism of placental separation (based on Henderson & Macdonald 2004)

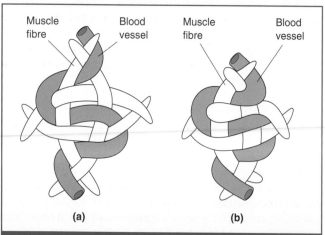

Figure 21.9 How the blood vessels run between the interlacing fibres of the uterus **(a)** Muscle fibres relaxed **(b)** Muscle fibres contracted (based on Henderson & Macdonald 2004)

uterine contractions (Tenore 2003). In the umbilical cord, vasoconstriction of the umbilical arteries occurs at birth in response to increasing partial pressure of oxygen (PaO_2). This prevents blood flow from the baby to the placenta, but blood flow can occur from the placenta to the baby via the umbilical vein, which does not constrict. This occurs to a greater extent if the baby is held below the level of the placenta. A placental transfusion of 80 mL can occur—a significant increase to the baby's total blood volume of 70–80 mL/kg body weight. On the other hand, if the cord is clamped early, this extra blood can be trapped in the uterine muscles and prevented from reaching the baby. However, by three days of age the difference in blood volume between infants with late or early clamping of the cord has disappeared (Blackburn 2003).

If an oxytocic is given, the uterine muscles contract more vigorously than normal and cord clamping prevents over-infusion of the baby with the extra blood and reduces the likelihood of transient polycythaemia.

Other maternal body systems during labour

Along with significant physiological changes that occur in the woman's reproductive system during labour, there are also changes to other body systems and processes. Metabolism alters to meet the increased energy demands of labour, along with changes to the respiratory and cardiovascular systems. Haematological changes maximise blood-clotting mechanisms and reduce the chances of haemorrhage. Water and electrolyte balance may be more difficult to maintain during labour.

Metabolism

Energy needs increase during labour, mainly due to the demands of both uterine and cardiac activity. Glucose is the prime energy source but if the woman's intake is insufficient, then oxidation of body fat (triglycerides) occurs to provide energy. Ketone bodies are produced through beta-oxidation of fats, and if excessive this can cause ketoacidosis, which may interfere with myometrial action (Liu, cited in Stables & Rankin 2004). Ketones can cross the placenta to the fetus and, because of their acidic nature, may depress fetal pH (Foulkes & Dumoulin, cited in Coad & Dunstall 2001). It is normal for maternal blood pH to fall 0.05 units but it usually remains within the range 7.3–7.4.

Respiratory system

Normal breathing patterns are overridden by events in labour that prompt hyperventilation or hypoventilation, leading to changes in acid–base balance. This is at a time when increased oxygen is required to support strenuous myometrial contractions.

Mild respiratory alkalosis occurs as a result of hyperventilation during late first stage of labour. Hyperventilation tends to increase if the woman is in pain or anxious. Excessive hyperventilation leading to a decreased $PaCO_2$ and alkalosis can be potentially hazardous to both the mother and the fetus. Extremely low $PaCO_2$ levels result in cerebral vasoconstriction and may reduce intervillous perfusion and blood flow (Blackburn 2003). The resulting alkalosis shifts the oxygen–haemoglobin curve to the left and impairs the release of oxygen from the maternal blood to the fetus. This is during a time when oxygenation of the fetus may already be impaired during uterine contractions. Hyperventilation may also lead to dizziness and tingling in the mother due to the low $PaCO_2$ levels. Encouraging the woman to slow her respiration rate and promoting deep breathing between contractions can help reduce alkalosis (Blackburn 2003).

Another factor to be aware of with respect to respiration during labour is the level of oxygen consumption, which increases with contractions. If there is insufficient time between contractions for replenishment of the blood supply, myometrial hypoxia may occur, with associated increases in pain. With insufficient oxygen available, anaerobic metabolism is stimulated and may lead to metabolic acidosis, most likely near the end of first stage labour. Respiratory alkalosis, which normally occurs during labour, can compensate to some extent for mild metabolic acidosis. During second stage labour, breath-holding during pushing results in respiratory acidosis and increased $PaCO_2$. This may reduce the uptake of CO_2 from the fetal circulation and result in fetal respiratory acidosis.

Cardiovascular system

Several changes occur in the cardiovascular system due to the increased blood volume that is returned to the systemic circulation from the uterus with each contraction (300–500 mL). This increases cardiac output by about 30% during contractions. Systolic blood pressure may rise about 35 mmHg during contractions in first stage and even more in second stage (Blackburn 2003). As there is little change in total peripheral resistance, the increase in blood pressure must be largely due to the increase in cardiac output. An increase in heart rate is usual but a heart rate greater than 100 beats/min may indicate ketoacidosis. Cardiopulmonary blood volume also increases but this increased load is not normally a problem unless a woman has cardiac complications.

Haematological changes

Birth of the baby is associated with blood loss (approximately 500 mL with a vaginal delivery) and rapid coagulation to compensate. The hypercoagulable state of pregnancy is increased in labour and this facilitates clot formation at the placenta. The release of thromboplastin during placental separation activates the extrinsic coagulation pathway. Immediately after delivery there is an increased risk of coagulation disorders due to the hypercoagulable state. Other changes include an increase in haemoglobin concentration due in part to increases in erythropoiesis, but also due to haemoconcentration associated with dehydration. There is an increase in leucocytes, particularly neutrophils, possibly due to stress (Blackburn 2003).

Renal function

Maintaining water and electrolyte balance during labour is influenced by increased aldosterone secretion, which stimulates sodium retention, and by loss of water through sweating and increased respiration. A labouring woman can quickly become dehydrated, particularly if there is excessive blood loss. Fluid intake must be maintained to prevent dehydration. If administration of intravenous fluids is necessary, they must be monitored to avoid water intoxication. Oxytocin has an antidiuretic action and if added to the IV fluid it can increase the possibility of water intoxication. Careful monitoring is required.

Fetal responses during labour

While the woman is undergoing major changes associated with labour, the fetus is also experiencing major changes. The fetus is exposed to considerable stress during labour. Although this is necessary to provoke respiration and other processes, monitoring of fetal wellbeing is essential. Fetal heart rate monitoring provides a measure of fetal wellbeing during labour although interpretation remains an inexact science. Monitoring can be via intermittent auscultation or continuous electronic monitoring, but the evidence is strongly against routine use of continuous monitoring in a normal labour (Thacker & Stroup 2003). Neonatal outcomes such as metabolic acidosis, low Apgar scores and admission to neonatal units are not improved with continuous electronic monitoring and continuous monitoring is associated with increased obstetric interventions (Goddard 2001). Fetal heart rate is normally in the range of 110 to 160 beats per minute (bpm), with an average baseline of 140 bpm (King & Parer 2000). Factors that reduce oxygen delivery to the fetus, such as hyperactivity of the uterus, Valsalva pushes during second stage, and maternal supine position, may lead to fetal hypoxia and a drop in fetal heart rate.

Control of the fetal heart rate

An understanding of the control of fetal heart rate is important in interpreting fetal heart rate changes in labour. Fetal heart rate is controlled by the autonomic nervous system, and the cardiovascular centre in the medulla oblongata of the brain. The medulla receives feedback from baroreceptors, chemoreceptors and inputs from higher cerebral centres. Efferent output to the heart is via the sympathetic and parasympathetic nerves. Heart rate variability, changes in timing from beat to beat, is the result of the multiple inputs and is an indicator of fetal wellbeing (King & Parer 2000). Fetal heart rate patterns and baseline readings are influenced by factors such as fetal blood supply and oxygen and carbon dioxide content of the blood, and therefore can also be used to indicate fetal wellbeing.

Baroreceptors in the aortic arch and the carotid arteries detect blood pressure. An increase in blood pressure will cause a rapid reflex drop in heart rate (mediated by parasympathetic nerves). This could occur during umbilical cord compression, because as flow within the umbilical vein is slowed, pressure in the fetal arterial circulation increases (King & Parer 2000).

Chemoreceptors detect oxygen and carbon dioxide levels in the blood. Receptors are located in the aortic arch and central nervous system. Increases in carbon dioxide and decreases in oxygen in the fetus are mainly detected by the central receptors and cause a reflex decrease in heart rate, mediated by parasympathetic nerves. Decreased placental perfusion during uterine contractions may impair fetoplacental gas exchange and result in a gradual drop in arterial oxygen. Detection by the chemoreceptors results in a more gradual decrease in fetal heart rate—a late deceleration. In a well-oxygenated fetus, heart rate variability is maintained during the contraction, and after the contraction, normal metabolism resumes and the bradycardia resolves (King & Parer 2000).

Non-asphyxial events can also influence heart rate variability and baseline levels (e.g. central nervous system depressants, beta sympathomimetics, congenital neurological abnormalities, defective cardiac conduction).

Finally, it is important to note that bradycardiac events in the fetus may cause hypoxia or be the result of hypoxia. Bradycardic events in second stage occur secondary to fetal head compression and vagal (parasympathetic nerve) stimulation. The fetus can tolerate these bradycardic events as long as the heart rate remains above 80 bpm and variability is maintained. If severe or prolonged, bradycardias resulting from impaired placental blood flow are likely to lead to fetal acidosis.

Fetal responses to hypoxia

During times of decreased placental blood flow, the fetus has mechanisms to maintain normal aerobic metabolism. Blood flow can be redistributed to supply the vital organs (heart, brain and adrenals) at the expense of flow to the gut, kidneys and limbs; and secondly, myocardial oxygen consumption can be reduced by reducing the heart rate (King & Parer 2000). If these mechanisms are not sufficient to meet metabolic needs, the fetus may change to anaerobic metabolism. Anaerobic metabolism produces energy, in the form of adenosine triphosphate (ATP), less efficiently than aerobic metabolism, and results in lactic acid production. Lactic acid is slow to cross the placenta, and may accumulate to cause metabolic acidosis in the fetus. Fetal heart rate is a useful monitor of fetal acid–base status (King & Parer 2000).

Summary

- Before labour begins, myometrial activation occurs. This involves structural and chemical changes to the smooth muscle cells of the myometrium to enhance electrical transmission and contractility of the uterus. The process is controlled by hormones, particularly oestrogen.
- Cervical ripening must also occur before labour will proceed. This involves an inflammatory-like response that results in loss of collagen, increase in water content of the cervix and loss of collagen binding. This is mediated by oestrogen, relaxin, nitric oxide and prostaglandins. Stretching of the cervix leads to release of prostaglandins.
- The physiological factors that may be responsible for initiating labour include an increase in placental corticotrophic-releasing hormone, maturation of the fetal hypothalamic-pituitary-adrenal axis, an increase in placental oestriol, synthesised from fetal precursors, an increase in prostaglandins and a decrease in the effectiveness of the anti-uterotonics, progesterone, relaxin and nitric oxide. Pressure from the fetus against the uterus and cervix stimulates release of prostaglandins and oxytocin.
- Maintenance of labour depends on the presence of the uterotonic hormones, in part stimulated by the Ferguson reflex.
- The first stage of labour involves effacement and dilatation of the cervix. This only occurs if myometrial contractions are effective. Contractions must be coordinated and show a decreasing gradient of activity with fundal dominance. They must generate sufficient pressure, last for sufficient time and be frequent enough to bring about progressive dilatation of the cervix until it is fully dilated at 10 cm.
- Second stage of labour begins at full dilatation of the cervix and ends with the birth of the baby. The woman feels the urge to push, leading to contractions of the abdominal muscles for 5–6 seconds several times during each very strong, expulsive contraction of the uterus.
- The mechanism of labour describes the manipulations the baby must make to negotiate the narrow pelvis and birth canal. Progress during the second stage depends on effective expulsive contractions and is influenced by the shape of the bony pelvis, the lie and orientation of the fetus and the resistance of the pelvic floor.
- Following the birth of the baby, uterine contractions separate the placenta from the uterus. The placenta may be delivered without intervention or by active management, involving administration of an oxytocic drug, cord traction and clamping of the cord. Continuing uterine contractions minimise blood loss from the placental site and are facilitated by reflex oxytocin release due to suckling of the baby.
- Labour is a physically demanding time that is supported by metabolic changes. If glucose intake is insufficient, fatty acid oxidation provides energy. If excessive, this can result in ketone formation and ketoacidosis.
- Hyperventilation or hypoventilation during labour can lead to changes in acid–base balance. Hyperventilation with the resulting respiratory alkalosis can impair oxygen release from the maternal blood to the fetus. Maternal respiratory acidosis can reduce fetal transfer of CO_2 to the maternal circulation and lead to fetal respiratory acidosis.
- Maternal cardiac output increases with contractions as blood in uterine vessels is squeezed into the systemic circulation, and therefore during contractions blood flow to the placenta is reduced.
- Haematological changes facilitate blood coagulation, but also increase the risk of coagulation disorders immediately after birth. Changes to aldosterone levels and increased water loss due to sweating may interfere with water and electrolyte balance during labour.

- During labour the fetus is normally exposed to stress. Heart rate is controlled by baroreceptor and chemoreceptor input and input from higher centres to the medulla oblongata. Asphyxial and non-asphyxial events can influence fetal heart rate and fetal heart rate variability.
- Monitoring fetal heart rate and fetal heart rate variability provides indicators of fetal wellbeing. During times of decreased blood supply, the fetus can maintain energy requirements by redistribution of blood flow to vital areas, reduction of heart rate and oxygen needs, and if necessary switch to anaerobic metabolism, although this is less efficient and leads to lactic acid production.

Physiological changes in the postnatal period

The postnatal period is also known as the puerperium. This is the time following the birth, when the woman's body adapts to a non-pregnant state. This involves recovery from the physical effects of pregnancy, labour and birth and a longer-term physiological adjustment as the changes that maintained and supported pregnancy and labour are no longer required. This is also the phase when infant-feeding practices and mother–child relationships are established. The physiology underpinning these changes is presented in this section. Body systems are described separately, but it should be remembered that systems do not work in isolation but are integrated in a complex manner.

Hormonal changes

The placental hormones human placental lactogen (hPL), human chorionic gonadotrophin (hCG), the oestrogens and progesterone, control maternal physiology in pregnancy to provide an optimal environment for fetal development. The return of the body systems to a non-pregnant state is largely governed by the removal of the placental hormones. Following expulsion of the placenta, metabolism of circulating hormones and hormone stores results in a rapid drop in placental hormone levels. These changes are illustrated in Figure 21.10. Human placental lactogen is absent from the plasma within two days, HCG is not detected in the urine by seven to ten days and oestrogens and progesterone reach basal levels by seven days (Blackburn 2003). After birth, prolactin levels also drop significantly but are maintained above normal for three to four weeks even in non-breastfeeding women (Johnson & Everitt 2000).

Involution of the uterus

The uterus reduces in size immediately following birth, due to myometrial contractions, and then continues to reduce in size over the next few days and weeks, until it returns to being a pelvic organ. This process is termed involution. During this time the height of the fundus usually decreases by about 1 cm/day, and by 10 days the fundus cannot be

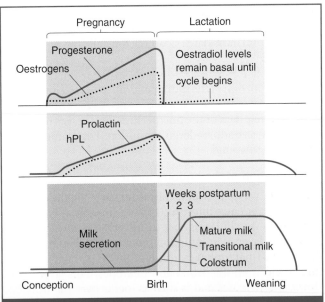

Figure 21.10 Sequence of hormone changes in the maternal circulation that underlie the onset of lactation in women (adapted from Johnson & Everitt 2000)

palpated abdominally as the uterus has descended into the pelvis (Blackburn 2003).

Oxytocin continues to be released from the posterior pituitary after the delivery of the placenta and membranes. It stimulates strong intermittent contractions of the uterus, which lead to collapse of the uterine cavity, which no longer contains the fetus, and realignment of the uterine walls in apposition to each other (Coad & Dunstall 2001). This aids the process of haemostasis and also reduces the size of the uterus immediately following birth.

The uterus decreases from 1 kg to about 350 g in the first two weeks and then decreases more slowly over the next six weeks to approximately 60 g (Blackburn 2003). This process involves a reduction in the thickness of the myometrium, a shedding of the decidua and regeneration of the endometrium. Although the exact mechanisms involved are unclear, the rapid withdrawal of the placental hormones appears to facilitate the changes (Stables & Rankin 2004).

Changes to the myometrium

Changes in the collagen and elastin content of the cells, along with water and protein loss, aid the process of involution (Coad & Dunstall 2001; Stables & Rankin 2004). Withdrawal of oestrogen reduces protein synthesis in the muscle fibres. Blood flow is reduced to the myometrium as the uterus contracts and compresses the uterine blood vessels. The resulting ischaemia aids in destruction of myometrial cells. Proteolytic enzymes digest superfluous actin and myosin protein in the muscle cells by a process termed autolysis. The size of the muscle cells is reduced, rather than the number of cells (Blackburn 2003). The products of autolysis as well as excess fibrous and elastic tissue are engulfed by macrophages—a process called phagocytosis. A proportion of fibrous and elastic tissue remains within the uterus and increasing amounts may remain following further pregnancies; thus the uterus never returns to the pre-pregnant state (Coad & Dunstall 2001).

Shedding of the decidua

The upper portion of the spongy endometrium is sloughed off with delivery of the placenta and is shed as part of the lochia in the first few days of the puerperium. This assists the uterus to reduce in size and undergo involution. The placental site is left as a large wound.

Regeneration of the endometrium

In the first two to three days following the birth, the epithelial lining differentiates into two layers: a superficial layer and a basal layer. A cellular barrier to infection is formed by the superficial layer of granulation tissue and by the invasion of leucocytes (macrophages and lymphocytes) that enter the area to clean up the debris and microbes. This layer breaks down and necroses and is shed as lochia over the next four to six weeks. Regeneration of the decidual layer surrounding the placental site takes two to three weeks, and by 16 days this layer is similar to the non-pregnant endometrium in the proliferative phase of the menstrual cycle (Blackburn 2003). The placental site involutes very rapidly over 24 hours and then less rapidly over the next six to seven weeks (Coad & Dunstall 2001; Stables & Rankin 2004). Large blood vessels that supplied the intervillous spaces are blocked by invading fibroblasts. Healing occurs by exfoliation without the formation of scar tissue. Endometrial tissue heals inwards from the edges of the placental site and upwards from the endometrial glands.

Afterpains

Contraction of the uterine muscles is felt as 'afterpains' for four to seven days and is strongest 12–24 hours post partum, especially in multiparous women. Suckling stimulates the release of oxytocin and aids uterine contractions and involution.

Lochia

Lochia refers to the discharge from the vagina that continues over the three to six weeks following birth. Lochia changes in appearance over time, and between 150 mL and 400 mL of lochia can be lost in total (Blackburn 2003).

Red lochia (lochia rubra) is described as red or dark brown with a fleshy smell and is discharged for the first one to three days on average. This lochia contains mainly blood and pieces of chorionic villi from the placental site, shreds of amnion and chorion, leucocytes, epithelial cells, vernix, lanugo and meconium. Pink lochia (lochia serosa) is the pinkish-brown discharge from day 4 to day 10, and this contains blood, mucous, erythrocytes, leucocytes, microorganisms and superficial decidual cells. Following this, white lochia (lochia alba), a whitish-yellow discharge, continues until three to six weeks post partum. It is similar in composition to pink lochia but does not contain erythrocytes (Blackburn 2003).

Lochia is sterile until it reaches the vagina. However, it is an excellent medium for the growth of bacteria. Puerperial infection may result from the invasion of endogenous organisms, those that are normally present in the woman's body, or from exogenous organisms, introduced to the woman's body from elsewhere (e.g. from another person). The woman is particularly vulnerable to infections during the puerperium due to the open wound at the placental site, the tissue trauma associated with labour and the excellent culture medium provided by the decidua and lochia (Stables & Rankin 2004).

Soft tissue damage and healing

Soft tissue damage occurs to the genital tract with the birth of a baby, and healing takes place in the days and weeks following the birth. This involves an immediate inflammatory response, which acts to isolate the damaged tissues and reduce the spread of any infection. Vasodilation occurs in the surrounding blood vessels, facilitating the transport of white blood cells such as neutrophils and monocytes to the area. These blood cells invade the damaged tissue and engulf bacteria and necrotic tissue by the process of phagocytosis. Following this inflammatory response, mesenchymal cells migrate to the area, form fibroblasts, and form a scab over the open wound site. Blood vessels grow into the area and granulation tissue grows from the base of the wound up. Following this is a phase of proliferation where the epithelial cells grow rapidly under the scab. Finally, as the new cells become mature, the scab is shed from the wound (Coad & Dunstall 2001).

The soft tissues of the cervix and vagina undergo healing during the puerperium.

Cervix

Immediately after vaginal delivery, the cervix appears stretched, swollen and bruised, with several lacerations. The cervix loses its bruised, swollen appearance within 48 hours and the cervical os, while constricted, is still partially dilated 3–4 cm (two fingers). This reduces to approximately 1 cm (one finger) dilatation by 10–12 days and the external os is a small slit by four weeks. Normal consistency returns within the first three to four days (Blackburn 2003).

Vagina and vulva

The elevated progesterone level during pregnancy causes increased vascularity of the vagina and vulva. These structures and the perineum are susceptible to bruising and oedema during labour. Immediately post partum, the vaginal wall is stretched, bluish and swollen but regains tonicity rapidly. Rugae reappear by three to four weeks. The vaginal mucosa is fragile for the first few weeks, but generally heals by six to ten weeks (Blackburn 2003). Submucosal venous congestion can take the entire puerperium to clear up. Small lacerations heal quickly but larger ones may need sutures to prevent haemorrhage and to aid healing. The perineal tissues will be stretched and may have lacerations. If the perineum is torn or cut (episiotomy), sutures may be inserted. Unsutured lacerations can make micturition extremely uncomfortable for 24–48 hours. During the first week, marked healing usually occurs in the perineal area (Stables & Rankin 2004). Sexual intercourse can be very uncomfortable in the first weeks due to perineal trauma and reduced lubrication of the vagina (Blackburn 2003).

While involution of the uterus, regeneration of the endometrium and healing of the cervix and vagina take place in the puerperium, major changes also occur to non-reproductive structures and body systems. Key changes to the renal, cardiovascular, respiratory and gastrointestinal systems are described in the next section. Readers are referred to the list of further readings for more in-depth explanations.

Renal system

Following the birth and with the loss of progesterone, the renal system is able to revert to non-pregnant anatomy and physiology. The dilatation of the renal tract is resolved and peristaltic action returns to normal. The bladder returns to its non-pregnant position—although there can be a loss of tone due to the displacement and stretching during labour (Stables & Rankin 2004).

With the removal of oestrogen from the system there is an increase in diuresis of circulating fluid. This usually occurs between two and five days after birth (Coad & Dunstall 2001). There is some evidence that it is more likely to occur sooner after birth in women who have obvious oedema in late pregnancy (Howie 2001). The other parameters of the renal system, such as the renal plasma flow, glomerular filtration rate and plasma creatinine, return to pre-pregnant levels by approximately six weeks post partum (Coad & Dunstall 2001).

Urinary tract

In the first few hours after delivery, micturition may be difficult due to several factors. Reflex suppression of detrusor muscle activity—that is, loss of muscle tone in the bladder—can reduce bladder emptying. Urethral sphincter spasm due to traumatised levator ani muscles and oedema caused by bruising of the bladder base and urethra during labour can interfere with normal micturition.

Dilatation of the urinary tract clears within six weeks in most women, though some may take 12 weeks. Urinary tract infection is more likely in the latter group (Blackburn 2003). Over-stretching of the pelvic floor muscles during birth can lead to damage to nerves and ligaments, which can lead to prolapse or urinary or faecal incontinence. Pelvic floor exercises post partum assist in re-toning muscles and may reduce incontinence problems (Salvesen & Morkved 2004).

Cardiovascular and respiratory systems

Cardiac output increases significantly immediately after delivery, as blood is returned to the systemic circulation from the uterus as it contracts, and the placenta as it buckles. Venous return to the maternal heart also improves after birth with

the relief of inferior vena cava compression. This results in autoinfusion into the systemic circulation. Immediately after birth there is an increase in cardiac output to approximately 60–80% of pre-labour levels but then a sharp decline within 10 minutes, to levels that are maintained over the next days and weeks. The cardiac output returns to non-pregnant levels between two and four weeks post partum (Blackburn 2003). This remains elevated for longer if the woman is breastfeeding. However, if there is a greater blood loss than normal (e.g. postpartum haemorrhage or caesarean) or if dehydration is present, then the cardiac output may not increase.

The extra blood volume acquired during pregnancy compensates for blood loss at the birth and it is estimated that women can lose up to one litre before haemoglobin concentration is affected (Letsky, cited in Coad & Dunstall 2001). There is a transient increase in haemodilution of both haemoglobin and plasma proteins. Haemoglobin levels return to pre-pregnant levels at about four to six weeks following the birth (Coad & Dunstall 2001). The number of platelets increases in the first few days, then gradually falls to non-pregnant levels.

In the last four weeks of pregnancy, the levels of fibrinogen, plasminogen and coagulation factors II, VII, VIII and X rise significantly, resulting in a state of hypercoagulability. This facilitates rapid blood clotting at delivery and reduces the risk of haemorrhage. With the delivery of the placenta, fibrinolytic inhibitors are removed, and after one to three hours fibrinolytic activity (breakdown of blood clots) increases to normal (Blackburn 2003). Lysis of fibrin deposited in the placental bed leads to a rise in fibrin degradation products (FDPs). As FDPs interfere with the formation of stable blood clots, there is an increased risk of coagulation disorders immediately after birth. There is also a secondary increase in various clotting factors (fibrinogen, factor V and factor VIII) during the first week, which enhances coagulability. All clotting factors gradually return to pre-pregnant levels over the first two weeks, but changes to flow velocity and diameter of the deep veins may take up to six weeks to return to pre-pregnant levels. Overall there continues to be an increased risk of thromboembolism through the puerperium.

Oxygen consumption increased 15–25% during pregnancy to meet fetal and placental needs and the demand from increased maternal tissues, and then increased by 300% during each contraction during labour. Oxygen consumption drops back to normal levels once the fetus and placenta are delivered and more gradually as maternal tissues return to normal. During pregnancy, progesterone increased the sensitivity of chemoreceptors to carbon dioxide and thus stimulated some degree of hyperventilation. Dyspnoea and hyperventilation disappear in the puerperium as progesterone levels drop.

Gastrointestinal system

Following the birth and with the drop in circulating progesterone, the smooth muscle tone throughout the body returns, the woman's appetite is increased and gastric tone and motility return (Stables & Rankin 2004). Heartburn and constipation resolve, although in the first few days there can be an increase in gas distension due to the reduced gastrointestinal muscle tone and motility (Stables & Rankin 2004). Often prior to labour or during the birth, the rectum has been evacuated and the first bowel movement can take two to three days to occur following the birth, as the effects of the progesterone diminish (Coad & Dunstall 2001). Haemorrhoids will take some time to disperse and can become more oedematous immediately in the first few days, due to pressure on the rectum and anus during the birth (Coad & Dunstall 2001).

Lactogenesis

The puerperium also sees the initiation of lactation. A brief account of the underlying hormonal changes is presented here.

In breastfeeding women, nipple stimulation during suckling initiates the neuroendocrine reflex, which stimulates the secretion and release of prolactin from the anterior pituitary gland and oxytocin release from the posterior pituitary gland. Although prolactin levels increase throughout pregnancy, lactogenesis is prevented by the presence of oestrogens and progesterone. With the drop in level of these hormones following placental expulsion, prolactin is effective at stimulating milk synthesis (Johnson & Everitt 2000). Oxytocin stimulates myometrial contraction and ejection of milk during lactation. Within one minute of breast stimulation there is a rise in the blood levels of oxytocin, which remain elevated throughout the stimulation and then fall to normal levels about six minutes after stimulation ceases. This rise and fall in oxytocin continues throughout a feed and throughout the course of lactation (Riordan 2005).

Suckling the infant immediately following birth may facilitate involution of the uterus (Blackburn 2003).

Return of menstruation and ovulation

There is considerable variation among women as to when menstruation and ovulation return, but it is generally found that breastfeeding delays the resumption of the reproductive cycle (Campbell & Gray 1993). Ovulation seldom occurs prior to 10 weeks, but may occur as early as 35 days—even in lactating women (Blackburn 2003). Prolactin reduces the effectiveness of GnRH released from the hypothalamus, which in turn decreases the release of FSH and LH from the anterior pituitary. Prolactin also reduces the sensitivity of ovarian follicles to FSH and LH. Although lactation is associated with decreased fertility, it may not be a reliable method of contraception (Blackburn 2003). Several studies suggest that menses returns to most non-lactating women between seven and nine weeks after birth (Blackburn 2003). Menses is not a reliable indicator of ovulation. Some women ovulate prior to the resumption of menses, while others experience anovulatory menstrual cycles (Blackburn 2003).

Thus by six to eight weeks, involution of the uterus and associated structures of the reproductive system has occurred and maternal physiology has largely changed to a non-pregnant state. Physiological and anatomical adjustments continue to support lactation.

Summary of key learning points

- The postnatal period (puerperium) is the six to eight weeks following the birth when the woman's body adapts to a non-pregnant state.
- Anatomical and physiological changes of the puerperium are largely governed by the removal of the placental hormones hCG, hPL, oestrogens and progesterone.
- The process by which the uterus reduces in size to being a pelvic organ is called involution. This involves a reduction in protein synthesis due to the removal of oestrogen, destruction of actin and myosin fibres by autolysis and removal of the products of autolysis by phagocytosis.
- A cellular barrier to infection is formed at the placental site by a superficial layer of granulation tissue. Regeneration of the decidual layer surrounding the placental site takes two to three weeks and at the placental site takes six to seven weeks.
- Lochia is the 150–400 mL discharge from the vagina that continues over the three to six weeks following birth. Over time it changes in composition and appearance.
- Healing of soft tissue damage to the cervix, vulva and vagina also occurs during this time.
- Body systems other than the reproductive system also undergo changes during the puerperium.
- Dilatation of the renal tract and peristaltic action return toward normal as progesterone levels decrease, but micturition may continue to be difficult in the hours following the birth. Removal of oestrogen leads to diuresis.
- Blood loss of 500–1000 mL may occur at birth. Autoinfusion into the systemic circulation occurs with contraction of the uterus and relief of vena cava compression. A state of hypercoagulability continues during the first two weeks as the levels of coagulation factors remains high. High levels of FDPs increase the risk of coagulation disorders.
- Oxygen consumption returns to normal as demands reduce and as progesterone levels decrease.
- Functioning of the gastrointestinal system returns to a non-pregnant state as progesterone levels drop.
- Prolactin levels increase throughout pregnancy; however, lactogenesis is prevented by oestrogens and progesterone. With the drop in level of these hormones following placental expulsion, prolactin is effective at stimulating milk synthesis. Nipple stimulation results in release of prolactin and oxytocin. Oxytocin stimulates the milk let-down reflex.
- Breastfeeding, although not a reliable method of contraception, is associated with decreased fertility. Prolactin reduces the effectiveness of GnRH released from the hypothalamus which in turn decreases the release of FSH and LH from the anterior pituitary.

Review questions

1   Differentiate between the hormones that promote uterine quiescence and those that promote contractions.

2   Outline the changes in myometrial structure that occur during activation to facilitate the forceful contractions of labour.

3   Describe the hormonal control of cervical ripening.

4   Describe one probable fetal and one probable maternal contribution to the onset of labour.

5   Present reasons why it may or may not be appropriate to extrapolate findings from animal research about the initiation of labour to explain the process in humans.

6   Identify two examples of abnormal fetal or maternal hormone function that have added to knowledge about possible mechanisms that contribute to the initiation of labour.

7   Identify two different stimuli that initiate the release of oxytocin from the posterior pituitary gland.

8   List three physiological features that contribute to effective uterine contractions.

9   Briefly define or describe each of the following, and identify at what stage of labour each would occur: effacement, retraction, the urge to push, crowning, contraction of voluntary muscles, state of hypercoagulability.

10   Place the following terms in the correct order to describe the movements of the baby in the second stage of labour: engagement, flexion, descent.

11   Outline the physiological effects of inadequate water and nutrient intake during labour.

12   Explain why oxytocin administered during second stage of labour can affect water and electrolyte balance.

13   Explain in physiological terms why hyperventilation can lead to respiratory alkalosis.

14   Explain the link between anaerobic metabolism and metabolic acidosis.

15   Outline physiological implications for the fetus if the mother lies in a supine position during labour.

16   Describe the normal physiological mechanisms that protect a woman from postpartum haemorrhage following the separation of the placenta from the uterine lining. What implications, if any, do these physiological mechanisms have for the woman in the immediate postpartum period?

17   Explain the physiology underlying separation of the placenta in a normal birth.

18   Outline the reflex responses of the fetus to a decrease in PaO_2.

19   Suggest some situations that may result in a decrease in fetal PaO_2.

20   Suggest some physiological advantages and disadvantages of anaerobic metabolism compared to aerobic metabolism in the fetus.

21   Draw a timeline to illustrate the changes in the level of hormones once the placenta is delivered and provide a brief explanation of why the changes in the levels of hormones occur.

22   In regard to healing at the site of placental separation, explain what is meant by the term 'cellular barrier'. Outline a consequence if the barrier was to fail.

23   Outline the process of healing at the placental site.

24   Describe how you would explain to a woman why micturition may be difficult following birth.

25   Provide a physiological explanation for the increased risk of thrombosis during the first two weeks of the puerperium.

26   Following delivery, the oxygen needs of the woman decrease, yet cardiac output increases. Account for the increase in cardiac output and outline the mechanism that returns cardiac output to non-pregnant levels.

27   Explain why 'thirst' and 'constipation' are associated with the early puerperium.

28   The withdrawal of which hormone allows skeletal and smooth muscle fibres of the pelvic floor, perineum, vagina, and urinary tract to return to normal tone?

29   Choose three systems and compare the physiological changes that occur in pregnancy with those that occur during the puerperium.

30   Name the hormone that is responsible for milk production. Explain why milk production does not occur during pregnancy.

Online resources

Power M, Schulkin J (Eds) 2005 Birth, distress and disease: placental-brain interactions (excerpt), Cambridge University Press, http://assets.cambridge.org/052183/1482/excerpt/0521831482_excerpt.pdf

Rai J, Schreiber J 2005 Cervical ripening, emedicine, http://www.emedicine.com/med/topic3282.htm

Steer P, Flint C 1999, ABC of labour care physiology and management of normal labour. British Medical Journal 318(7186):793–796, http://www.pubmedcentral.nih.gov/articlerender.fcgi?artid=1115220

References

Blackburn S 2003 Maternal fetal and neonatal physiology: a clinical perspective (2nd edn). WB Saunders, London

Bricker L, Luckas M 2002 Amniotomy alone for induction of labour. Cochrane Database of Systematic Reviews (2), CD002862

Campbell OM, Gray RH 1993 Characteristics and determinants of postpartum ovarian function in women in the United States. American Journal of Obstetrics and Gynecology 169(1):55–60

Challis JRG 2001 Understanding pre-term birth. Clinical and Investigative Medicine 24(1):60

Coad J, Dunstall M 2001 Anatomy and physiology for midwives. Mosby, Edinburgh

Enkin M, Keirse M, Neilson J et al 2000 A guide to effective care in pregnancy and childbirth (3rd edn). OUP, Oxford

Goddard R 2001 Electronic fetal monitoring. British Medical Journal 322(7300):1436

Grammatopoulos DK, Hillhouse EW 1999 Role of corticotropin-releasing hormone in onset of labour. Lancet 354(9189):1546

Henderson C, Macdonald S 2004 Mayes' midwifery. A textbook for midwives (13th edn). Baillière Tindall, Edinburgh

Howie P 2001 The physiology of the puerperium and lactation. In: G Chamberlain, S Steer (Eds) Turnbull's obstetrics (3rd edn). Churchill Livingstone, London

Johnson MH, Everitt BJ 1988 Essential reproduction (3rd edn). Blackwell Scientific, Oxford

Johnson MH, Everitt BJ 2000 Essential reproduction (5th edn). Blackwell Scientific, Oxford

Kelly AJ, Kavanagh J, Thomas J 2001 Relaxin for cervical ripening and induction of labour. Cochrane Database of Systematic Reviews (2), CD003103. DOI: 003110.001002/14651858.CD14003103

King T, Parer J 2000 The physiology of fetal heart rate patterns and perinatal asphyxia. Journal of Perinatal and Neonatal Nursing 14(3):19

Ledingham M, Thomson A, Young A et al 2000 Changes in the expression of nitric oxide synthase in the human uterine cervix during pregnancy and parturition. Molecular Human Reproduction 6(11):1041

Longo M, Jain V, Vedernikov Y et al 2003 Effects of L-type Ca2+-channel blockade K+ATP-channel opening and nitric oxide on human uterine contractility in relation to gestational age and labour. Molecular Human Reproduction 9(3):159–164

Norwitz E, Robinson J, Challis J 1999 The control of labor. New England Journal of Medicine 341(9):660

Prendiville WJ, Elbourne D, McDonald S 2000 Active versus expectant management in the third stage of labour. Cochrane Database of Systematic Reviews (3), CD000007

Reis FM, Florio P, Cobellis L et al 2001 Human placenta as a source of neuroendocrine factors. Biology of the Neonate 79(3/4):150–157

Riordan J 2005 Breastfeeding and human lactation (3rd edn). Jones and Bartlett, Boston

Roberts JE 2002 The 'push' for evidence: management of the second stage. Journal of Midwifery and Women's Health 47(1):2–15

Salvesen KA, Morkved S 2004 Randomised controlled trial of pelvic floor muscle training during pregnancy. British Medical Journal 329(7462):378

Stables D, Rankin J 2004 Physiology in childbearing with anatomy and related biosciences (2nd edn). Elsevier, London

Tenore JL 2003 Methods for cervical ripening and induction of labor. American Family Physician 67(10):2123–2128

Thacker SB, Stroup DF 2003 Revisiting the use of the electronic fetal monitor. Lancet 361(9356):445–446

Thornton S, Terzidou V, Clark A et al 1999 Progesterone metabolite and spontaneous myometrial contractions in vitro. The Lancet 353(9161):1327–1329

Winkler M, Fischer DC, Ruck P et al 1999 Parturition at term: parallel increases in interleukin-8 and proteinase concentrations and neutrophil count in the lower uterine segment. Human Reproduction 14(4):1096

Further reading

Bemal AL 2001 Timing of parturition. Lancet 358:S51

Blackburn S 2003 Parturition and uterine physiology. Ch 4. In: Maternal fetal and neonatal physiology: a clinical perspective (2nd edn). London: WB Saunders Co

Campbell OM, Gray RH 1993 Characteristics and determinants of postpartum ovarian function in women in the United States. American Journal of Obstetrics and Gynecology 169(1):55–60

Coad J, Dunstall M 2001 Physiology of parturition. Ch 13. In: Anatomy and physiology for midwives. Mosby, Edinburgh

Coad J, Dunstall M 2001 The puerperium. Ch 14. In: Anatomy and physiology for midwives. Mosby, Edinburgh

Johnson MH, Everitt BJ 2000 Parturition. Ch 12. In: Essential reproduction (5th edn). Blackwell Scientific, Oxford

King T, Parer J 2000 The physiology of fetal heart rate patterns and perinatal asphyxia. Journal of Perinatal & Neonatal Nursing 14(3):19

Norwitz E, Robinson J, Challis J 1999 The control of labor. New England Journal of Medicine 341(9):660

Stables D, Rankin J 2004 The onset of labour. Ch 36. In: Physiology in childbearing with anatomy and related biosciences (2nd edn). Elsevier, London

Stables D, Rankin J 2004 The first stage of labour. Ch 37. In: Physiology in childbearing with anatomy and related biosciences (2nd edn). Elsevier, London

Stables D, Rankin J 2004 The second stage of labour. Ch 39. In: Physiology in childbearing with anatomy and related biosciences (2nd edn). Elsevier, London

Stables D, Rankin J 2004 The third stage of labour. Ch 40. In: Physiology in childbearing with anatomy and related biosciences (2nd edn). Elsevier, London

Stables D, Rankin J 2004 The puerperium. Ch 56. In: Physiology in childbearing with anatomy and related biosciences (2nd edn). Elsevier, London

CHAPTER 22

Supporting women in labour and birth

Juliet Thorpe and Jacqui Anderson

Key terms

afterpains, artificial rupture of membranes, continuity of carer, controlled cord traction, partnership, postpartum haemorrhage, normal physiological birth, vaginal examinations, women-centred care

Chapter overview

This chapter takes a women-centred approach to the midwifery care of women in physiological labour at term. Labour and birth are considered a single continuous process, from the beginning of labour until two hours following the birth, although the traditional divisions into stages of labour are discussed. Using the New Zealand College of Midwives 'Decision Points for Midwifery Care' as a framework, a midwife's work, 'with women', through labour and birth is examined (NZCOM 2005). Underpinning this work is the midwife–woman relationship, assessment skills, decision-making and the provision of supportive care that facilitates and enhances the normal physiological process of labour and birth. Key midwifery principles of partnership, continuity of caregiver and the promotion of physiological birth also underpin this chapter.

Learning outcomes

Learning outcomes for this chapter are:

1 To explain labour and birth as a continuum that integrates physical, psychological, emotional, social and spiritual processes

2 To demonstrate awareness of the impact of the labour and birthing environment and relationship with carers, on each woman's experience

3 To explain the importance of women-centred care based on the midwifery principles of partnership, continuity of carer and holism

4 To identify evidence-informed care appropriate to the individual needs of each woman and her baby.

Developing the woman–midwife relationship

A midwife's role in supporting women in labour begins in the antenatal period with the establishment of the relationship between each midwife and each woman (Guilliland & Pairman 1995). For a midwife to be able to provide effective and individualised care, she must spend time with each woman, getting to know her and her desires and dreams for the birth of this baby. Spending time getting to know each other also enables trust to develop, and anxieties, fears and misconceptions to be acknowledged before labour starts. Unexplored fears and issues can exacerbate the challenges that occur in labour, and without this understanding a midwife will find it more difficult to provide women-centered care.

The midwifery definition of labour relies on each woman's perceptions and will always be unique to the individual woman and therefore difficult to define in an exact way. Within the midwifery model of care, the woman is the focus and therefore her perceptions are the governing factors when providing care in labour (Gould 2000).

The knowledge that a midwife gains through the partnership relationship established with each woman guides her ability to support the woman to use her own strength to labour and birth her baby. As the woman moves through the various stages of her labour, the midwife's role in facilitating and promoting normal physiological labour and birth relies on her ability to be 'with the woman' (Daellenbach 1999; Pairman 1998). The ability to provide supportive midwifery care in labour is a multifaceted skill. The parameters of normal labour and birth are individual to each woman. To be able to recognise what is 'normal' for each woman, a midwife needs to be available to her and alert to the ebbs and flows of that woman's experience. By truly being 'with' the woman, the midwife is able to recognise and acknowledge the complexity of a process that is at once emotional, spiritual and physical (Chapman 2003). With this acknowledgement comes understanding of the factors that may affect labour and birth both positively and negatively. The combination of the birth environment, relationships with partners and carers, the physiological processes of labour and birth, and psychological influences, can have a profound effect on the progress of a woman's labour (Walsh 2001).

Decision points for midwifery care in labour and birth

Throughout this chapter, decision points are identified to provide a framework for provision of midwifery care. Developed by the New Zealand College of Midwives (NZCOM) in 1993 and revised in 2005, the decision points identify those times when a midwife ought to make a midwifery assessment, although it is recognised that assessments are based on individual need (NZCOM 2005). The decision points outline what information needs to be shared between each woman and midwife at each assessment point as well as the health information and midwifery care that should be provided.

The continuum of labour and birth

Labour has traditionally been separated and compartmentalised into arbitrary stages, unimaginatively labelled first, second, third and, more recently, fourth stages. For midwives and women the reality is that labour and birth are a continuous process (McCormick 2003; Wickham 2003). Even so, as a woman moves into and through her labour process, there are recognisable emotional and physical changes. As a part of midwifery assessment it is important to understand and recognise these changes, to identify normal progress. Reorienting thinking about labour to acknowledge the physiological process as experienced by women has led some researchers to define labour as consisting of:

- latent phase to the onset of active phase
- active phase to onset of transition
- transition to birth
- birth to skin-to-skin (Downe 2000).

This chapter reflects this understanding of labour and birth as a continuum, and discusses midwifery care from the perspective of a midwife providing continuity of care.

Recognising labour

Normal labour occurs between 37 and 42 weeks gestation (McCormick 2003). As a woman approaches the end of the pregnancy she will often experience an increase in intensity of Braxton Hicks contractions and commonly an increase in vaginal discharge/mucus. Other signals indicating that labour may be imminent include further descent of the baby into the pelvis and bouts of strengthening uterine activity. The advent of approaching labour can elicit intense emotional responses in some women, ranging from acute apprehension to excited anticipation. Midwives must be sensitive to these feelings and changes, and be able to reinforce the normality of these responses.

During the antenatal period, a midwife will have discussed with the woman the signs and symptoms to aid recognition of the beginnings of labour (see Clinical point). She will identify

---

Clinical point

Signs of labour

- Increasingly intense contractions that become painful
- Increasingly regular and more frequent contractions
- Vaginal discharge of bloodstained mucus (called a 'show'); may occur before contractions commence
- Vaginal discharge of clear fluid if membranes rupture spontaneously; can occur before contractions and is considered a sign of labour if accompanied by contractions and cervical dilatation

with the woman when to make contact and what information will be sought at this initial contact. It is helpful to summarise this discussion in the woman's notes so that she can remind herself of these points later and as reassurance for her and her family.

Labour: latent phase to onset of active phase

The latent phase is recognised as a valid phase of labour but is difficult to define and poorly understood (Enkin et al 2000; Walmsley 2003). It has been described as the start of uterine contractions until progressive dilatation of the cervix commences (Enkin et al 2000). Confusing the latent phase with a poorly progressing active phase can lead to inappropriate and unnecessary interventions that may affect the outcomes for mother and baby. This can occur because duration of the latent phase varies from woman to woman. There is no consensus in the literature on what constitutes the length of a normal latent phase. Definitions vary from 6–8 hours up to 24–36 hours (Enkin et al 2000; Stables 1999; Walmsley 2003).

Some women may not experience the latent phase of labour, but for those who do, it can be a confusing time. It is common for women to need time, support and reassurance for labour to establish and become progressive. Viewing labour and birth as a normal process enables a woman to find her own way through her own unique experience. Encouraging her to listen and trust her body, and to rest and fuel her body, enables the process of birth to happen at its own pace. Rest, food and fluids, supportive, professional midwifery care, and the avoidance of unnecessary interventions will assist most women through this time (Simkin & Ancheta 2000). It is important to remember that slow progress in the first stage of labour does not necessarily mean the presence of a problem or abnormality (Enkin et al 2000; Simkin & Ancheta 2000).

> # First decision point in labour:
> ## when the woman or her support person first informs the midwife that she is in labour

At this stage a woman begins to notice signs that she may be in labour, and makes contact with her midwife to inform her that she may be in labour. A midwife will need to ask questions in order to assess whether the woman is in labour and whether she needs a physical assessment and attendance by the midwife. A midwife will need to gather information about the woman's general state and how she is coping, and review the woman's history to this stage. The following questions should be asked of the woman:

- Is she having discomfort/pain? When did this start? The midwife needs to ascertain whether the pain is caused by uterine activity/contractions.

> ## Clinical point
>
> ### Characteristics of the latent phase
> ▶ The contractions are short, irregularly spaced and easily interrupted by inactivity and distractions (e.g. the woman's other children, unexpected visitors, loud noises, taking a bath).
> ▶ The woman may be able to sleep for short periods.
> ▶ The woman will often still feel hungry.
> ▶ The woman will still be connected to what is going on around her (e.g. she will join in on conversations and may be able to talk during a contraction).

- What are her contractions like? Where does she feel them? How often do they come? How long do they last?
- Can she talk through them? Does resting or being active change their pattern?
- How is she feeling? Who is there to support her?
- Has she had any vaginal discharge? If so, what does it look like (e.g. bloodstained mucus or watery discharge)?
- Does she think her membranes have ruptured? If so, what colour is the liquor (clear, pink, green or brown/black)?
- Has her baby been moving in the last few hours?
- Does she want the midwife to attend?

On the basis of this assessment, a midwife will decide whether to visit the woman at home. Sometimes a woman can be reassured by phone that she is in the latent phase of labour and asked to contact the midwife again when the contractions become more regular, frequent and painful, or if there are any other signs that labour is progressing. If a midwife is not certain of the progress of labour, then a home visit should be made before a woman is advised to come into the maternity unit. Research shows that women who are reviewed in early labour have shorter labours, fewer epidurals, less syntocinon augmentation and more positive birthing experiences (Walsh

> ## Critical thinking exercise
>
> Michelle is expecting her third baby. She is not planning to have any more babies after this one and has really enjoyed being pregnant. Michelle is at 41 weeks and five days gestation and has had a full night of irregular painful contractions. Although she has not slept, Michelle is not in established labour. Her two children, aged two years and five years, are due to wake soon, and her mother, sister and best friend have arrived to be with her in the expectation that she will have her baby today. Michelle's two previous children were born in hospital and she is planning to have this baby at home. Her mother thinks she should be in hospital with a doctor.
> 1   What issues may influence what happens next?
> 2   What is the midwife's role in facilitating a supportive environment for Michelle?

TABLE 22.1 Factors that can affect the progress of labour	
Supportive influences	**Unsupportive influences**
• Trust in the woman's body and the birthing process • Sensitive, nurturing, appropriate supporters • Comfortable environment—a feeling of safety, privacy, familiarity • Knowing that other children are well cared for • A known, trusted midwife who supports the birth plan • Opportunities for rest periods, able to eat and drink as she desires	• Unexplored fears and distrust of labour and birth • Inappropriate, insensitive supporters • Environment uncomfortable, noisy, distracting, lack of space and privacy • Woman's concern about her children or other family members • A midwife who is unfamiliar with and/or unsupportive of the birth plan • Tiredness and hunger

2000a). The key assessment is whether the woman is in latent or active labour; if she is in latent labour she should be encouraged to stay at home.

If a visit is made, the midwife should make a full assessment of the woman and her baby and document this (see details of assessment later in the chapter). An abdominal examination to define the position of the baby and listen to the baby's heart rate gives the midwife and the woman information to reassure and guide further advice. If the baby isn't in an optimal position, recommendations can be made regarding strategies for the woman to work with (Sutton 2003). Vaginal examinations, while not generally warranted at this stage, may assist in the diagnosis of the latent phase, as minimal dilatation will have occurred (Chapman 2003). Observing the woman's behaviour will help the midwife differentiate between latent and active labour.

If the woman is in latent labour and is well supported at home by friends and family, it may then be appropriate to leave her and return when she requires additional midwifery support and/or labour becomes active. The woman needs to know that the latent phase is normal and may be lengthy, and that it is not the time for clock watching (Baston 2004). The woman should continue with her usual activities but ensure that she continues to eat, rest and sleep so that she can find the focus and energy required when labour does establish.

At home, women can work with the latent phase by being able to rest in their own bed, walk in their garden, lean against their kitchen bench, kneel into a bean bag or take a warm bath. Women planning to birth in hospital should try to use all the resources available to them at home before going into the hospital environment, which does not favour the latent phase (Walsh 2000a). Being confined to one room and exposed to the sounds of other women in active labour does nothing to

support the woman or give her confidence when she still has many hours of labour ahead of her.

Before leaving, the midwife needs to ensure that the woman knows how and when to make contact with her.

Second decision point in labour:
when the woman wants intermittent support from the midwife

At this stage a woman contacts her midwife because she feels labour is progressing or changing and she wants more support, or the midwife may have contacted the woman to ask about how she is feeling and how labour is progressing. As with the first decision point, a key assessment is to ascertain whether the woman is still in latent labour or if she is in established labour, and if so, what progress she is making. The woman should be visited at home and the following assessments and discussions should be considered:

- Assess the woman's wellbeing, including her emotional and behavioural responses.
- Assess the adequacy of her food and fluid intake, and her ability to rest.
- Consider physical assessments including abdominal palpation, strength, length and frequency of contractions, blood pressure, and the baby's wellbeing, including heart rate.
- If her membranes have ruptured, assess the liquor.
- Discuss the relevance of a vaginal examination at this point.

If the woman is still in the latent phase, then midwifery care and advice will continue as before. If the woman has progressed into early labour, she may feel the need for intermittent support from the midwife. If the woman is well supported at home by friends and family, then the midwife may be able to leave for periods of time, always ensuring that she can be contacted if required and clearly stating when she will return for a further assessment. The woman is advised to eat and drink and move about as she wishes. Once labour establishes, the woman is likely to want continuous support from her midwife.

Clinical point

When doing home visits to women in labour, bring a full birth kit in case of unexpected or unplanned homebirth—see Table 22.2.

Note that it is sensible to keep a birth kit in your car when visiting women at home at any time, so that you are prepared for unexpected situations.

Labour: active phase to onset of transition

Active labour is characterised by contractions that increase in intensity, length and frequency. The pattern of contractions tends to be more regular and is less affected by external influences than those that characterise the latent phase. The active pattern of contractions causes effacement and dilatation of the cervix and promotes the descent and rotation of the baby through the pelvis. The individuality of each woman's experience means that the frequency of contractions in active labour may vary, for example, from every three minutes for some women, to every 10 minutes for others.

Traditionally, normal progress has been identified by a cervical dilatation rate of 1 cm/hour in active labour. This definition was based on the work of Friedman in the 1950s and has been universally adopted to assess the parameters of 'normal' progress (Friedman 1954). (For more detailed information on this aspect of labour progress, see Ch 34.) However, in reality, many midwives and women know that what is slow progress for one woman may be acceptable for another. There is continued debate about what actually constitutes a normal cervical dilatation rate. Much of the research undertaken to identify 'normal' progress in labour

---

TABLE 22.2 What to bring to a home birth

| Preparation for home birth | Equipment for assessment and care of the woman and her baby | |
	Woman	Baby
• A strong and well-founded belief in birth as a normal physiological process • An in-depth understanding of the physiology of normal birth • A continuous and unobtrusive presence that is eternally vigilant • A means of monitoring the wellbeing of the woman and her baby during labour, birth and the post-birth period • A copy of the woman's birth plan • A set of well-developed midwifery skills, including emergency skills • A list of telephone numbers for emergency assistance • A second midwife (present during late second stage and birth) • A set of clearly identified notes in which to record the details of events as they unfold • Birth notification documents • Prescription pad, referral pad	• Watch with a second hand • Stethoscope and sphygmomanometer • Thermometer, bath thermometer • Vaginal assessment swabs and solution (used if membranes have ruptured) • Sterile gloves for vaginal assessment/s and conduct of birth • Amnihook • Birth pack, large plastic sheet/ incontinence sheets • Woman's own container for placenta or plastic bag • Container bags for soiled equipment/swabs • Torch with adequate light for suturing (a headlamp works well) • Suturing material: 20 cc syringe, 22–gauge needle, 1% plain lignocaine (20 mL ampoule) • Sterile vaginal swabs • Drugs: syntocinon 5 and 10 unit ampoules (keep refrigerated and use a cold storage container for transport) and syntometrine 1 mL syringes and needles • Oxygen available with Hudson mask • Cannulation equipment (16- and 14-gauge cannulae) and tourniquet • Normal saline and/or Ringers Lactate/ Hartmans and IV giving set • Sharps disposal unit	• Pinard stethoscope and/or Doppler sonicaid (one that is safe to use in water) • Suction equipment for the baby • Cord clamp (or traditional cord ties according to cultural practice) • Infant Laerdahl bag and mask, and infant airways • Oxygen cylinder and gauge, tubing • Baby scales (weight conversion chart) • Tape measure • Vitamin K

For further information contact:
- Homebirth Aotearoa (NZ); New Zealand College of Midwives (www.midwife.org.nz)
- Australian College of Midwives Inc for a copy of the Application for Accreditation as an Independently Practising Midwife. This contains prompts for the midwife to consider skills in perineal repair, neonatal resuscitation, maternal resuscitation. In addition this asks the midwife to determine what she or he has available in terms of equipment for fetal monitoring and resuscitation, maternal assessment and care including resuscitation, drugs and communication equipment.

(Source: This table was prepared by Maralyn Foureur 2005.)

has been undertaken in medicalised settings and has focused mainly on the rate of cervical dilatation while ignoring other physiological changes and influences (Philpott & Castle 1972; Seitchik 1987; Studd 1973). More recent work challenges these findings and encompasses a holistic approach to labour assessment that centres on the woman and baby's wellbeing rather than the length of labour (Albers 1999; Crowther 2000). Albers (1999), in her study of the duration of labour in low-risk women, found that normal labour for these women lasted longer than many clinicians expect. This research suggests that a cervical dilatation rate of 0.3–0.5 cm/hr may be more appropriate and recommends the revision of criteria determining normal labour progress.

Clinical point

Characteristics of the active phase

▷ Contractions are of increasing regularity, strength, length and frequency.

▷ The woman needs to move about and cannot rest in one position for long.

▷ The woman will be less connected to what is going on around her and increasingly will not be able to talk through contractions; increasingly she will go 'into herself' as the labour 'takes her over'.

▷ The woman may not feel like eating.

▷ On abdominal palpation, the baby is felt to have moved down further into the pelvis.

▷ On vaginal assessment of the cervix, increasing effacement, softening and dilatation is felt, and the baby's head descends lower into the pelvis.

Third decision point in labour:
when the woman wants continuous support from a midwife

As a woman becomes established in labour she will usually want continuous support from her midwife. The active phase of labour demands complex midwifery care as the midwife works in partnership with the woman. The midwife's role is to help the woman and her family and supporters to follow their birth plan while at the same time making regular assessments of progress and determinations as to whether the progress is 'normal' for this woman and her baby. As labour advances, the woman will often require more support and encouragement to help her work through the challenges ahead.

Clinical research

Women's recognition of the spontaneous onset of labour

Reported signs & symptoms	No. (%)	
	Nulliparae	Multiparae
Recurrent pain	62 (32.8)	80 (44.4)
Non-recurrent pain	51 (27.0)	41 (22.8)
Watery loss	30 (15.9)	17 (9.4)
Bloodstained loss	17 (9.0)	16 (8.9)
Gastrointestinal symptoms	8 (4.2)	2 (1.1)
Emotional upheaval	8 (4.2)	14 (7.8)
Sleep disturbance	6 (3.2)	5 (2.8)
Other	7 (3.7)	5 (2.8)
Total	189 (100)	180 (100)

A study was undertaken to assess how women experience spontaneous onset of labour at term. The authors found that:

No single test, clinical or otherwise, can determine the onset of labor, both objectively and with a reasonable degree of precision. Caregivers should listen to women and listen carefully instead of applying arbitrary measures as to how and when labor started ... The right questions, as indicated by our data, are not 'When did the contractions start?' or 'When did contractions become regular?' but 'When did your labor start?' and 'How did you know?' ... This is especially important, since spontaneous onset of labor rarely occurs in controlled environments, such as maternity units, hospitals, or research settings (p 270).

(Source: Mechthild et al 2003)

Staying with the woman is an essential midwifery role. Being 'with the woman' requires not only the physical presence of the midwife but also her focus and attention. Women identify that the quality of the 'presence' of the midwife is directly related to the midwife's energy and commitment to her (Baston 2004). The midwife can also encourage the woman's support people to be as involved as the woman needs. The midwife needs to recognise that support people may have their own anxieties during the labour, which may impinge on their ability to support the woman. The midwife can guide support people to participate in nurturing the woman to maintain a positive environment.

If the woman is planning to have her baby in a maternity facility, she will need to be transferred to the facility once she is in the active phase of labour. The midwife needs to be alert to the possible impact of this new environment on the woman and her support people (Cluett 2000) (see the Clinical point below).

Facilitating a supportive labour environment

Wherever a woman is birthing, it is important to assess the labouring and birthing environment to take into account the wishes of the woman and the factors that will enhance and support her normal physiological labour. These include ensuring adequate open spaces to move around, a nearby toilet, comfortable furniture, low or adjustable lighting, support people, and, for many women, privacy and quiet (Newburn 2003). Assisting the woman to make use of these 'tools' will help her to use her intuition and instinct to find the right place and positions for effective, active labour.

The birth space needs to feel safe for that woman. This concept of a 'safe place' incorporates both physical and psychosocial/spiritual safety that cannot be imposed on the woman (Parratt & Fahy 2004). Most women appear to labour most effectively when there is an atmosphere of calm and the focus is on her and her experience. Some women, however, feel self-conscious and prefer to be left alone or to have the distraction of her supporters' conversations, the television, her favourite music or even her children being busy around her. It is therefore important to talk to the woman to find out what she wants. Taking into account cultural preferences is also imperative in facilitating an appropriate environment for effective labour. For example, it may be inappropriate for there to be men (including the father of the baby) present or it may be that the woman's entire family, including aunts, uncles and grandparents, are to be actively involved.

Most women who begin their labour spontaneously will do so at home. It is well documented that women should be encouraged to stay at home when in early labour, and that women are more relaxed and have more options in their own environments (Baston 2004). For those women who choose not to birth at home, the timing for transfer to hospital is crucial. If too soon it may disrupt the flow of labour and slow progress, thus risking unnecessary intervention. If too late there is the risk of birthing somewhere unplanned, such as at home or, worse, in a car, where the environment may carry risks for the mother or baby.

Once the woman is in hospital, creating a calm, positive, welcoming atmosphere will assist in reducing tension and anxiety (Page 2000). This can be a challenge when confined to one room. If the midwife arrives at the hospital before the woman, she should ensure that there is something available for the woman to drink, the lighting is dimmed and the room is warm. To make adequate space for the woman to be active in labour, consider placing the bed against the wall (or removing it from the room) and using beanbags, pillows and soft mats if available. This will signal to the woman when she arrives that there is not an expectation that she lie on the bed.

Research has shown that lying supine is not only uncomfortable for women but also does not aid the descent and rotation of the baby through the pelvis, and can contribute to fetal distress. Supine positions can compromise the uterine blood flow during labour and have been shown to decrease the intensity and frequency of contractions (Enkin et al 2000). The physical layout of the labour environment will have a significant influence on what positions a labouring woman adopts, and if a woman is given many options this will have a positive impact on the birth outcome (Hodnett 2003). The culture of the birthing facility will influence a woman's behaviour in labour, and if there is an expectation that the bed is to be used then she may feel pressured to do so.

Women who labour at home are rarely at a loss as to where to go or what to do next. Given the freedom of their own space, most women will adopt a variety of positions and use a number of rooms throughout their labour. If a woman is able to move freely at will and rest when her body tires, she will find the right places to labour in. The midwifery role is to be willing to support her wherever it is that she chooses to be, and to offer advice and suggestions when required.

Clinical point

What to consider when moving from home to hospital

▶ Visit at home to assess progress and discuss transfer to hospital with woman.

▶ Check the birth plan. Did the woman think she would feel more comfortable transferring in early or more established labour? How does she feel now?

▶ If unable to assess progress from observations and discussions with the woman, consider vaginal examination.

▶ Distance from the woman's home to the hospital— i.e. consider transfer time.

▶ Mode and availability of transport, comfort during transfer.

▶ Collect 'tools' to take into hospital—e.g. supporters, own pillow, wheat bag, food, drink, music, massage oils, car seat and clothes for baby, fresh clothes for the woman.

▶ Ensure equipment is available in case of unexpected, unplanned home birth.

Very few women at home will lie on their bed except when trying to rest or sleep, so when women move to the hospital environment from home the midwife needs to positively encourage and support women to continue moving freely and adopt different positions. By trying to make the labour room more home-like, midwives will assist in minimising disturbance to the flow of a woman's labour and this will be of significant benefit to a woman and her baby (Hodnett 2003). This requires skill, effort and thought. As a woman's contractions increase in strength and intensity, the midwife needs to be constantly thinking ahead about what position changes, ideas and strategies she may need to suggest, to support and encourage the woman through the challenges ahead.

Eating and drinking in labour

Women experiencing normal labour should be free to eat and drink as their body demands. Labour is a physically challenging process and requires as much fuel as any other strenuous activity. Most women will still feel able to snack on light foods in early labour, but as the contractions intensify may feel less inclined to eat (Enkin et al 2000). It is useful to talk with the woman and her supporters prior to labour about what she thinks she may like to eat, and ensure that those foods are available to her. Most hospitals do not provide a particularly wide range of food, so if the woman is planning to birth in hospital she may need to bring her own food with her. Some institutions have protocols that require labouring women to fast. For many women this may not present a problem, as they are already unwilling to eat when in active labour. But for others, enforced hunger becomes an extremely unpleasant experience. It may also lead to ketosis and poor progress in labour (Micklewright & Champion 2002). Having the freedom to eat whenever and whatever she chooses allows a woman to be in control, and reinforces the concept that labouring women know what their bodies need (Pengelley 2002).

Women should be encouraged to drink according to their thirst but may sometimes need prompting to drink when the labour becomes all-consuming. If a woman's fluid intake is inadequate or she is experiencing episodes of vomiting, she will soon become dehydrated, especially if the physical demands of her labour cause her to sweat excessively (Micklewright & Champion 2002). This is particularly the case if the woman is labouring in a bath or birthing pool. One of the first symptoms of dehydration is fatigue and this can disrupt the progress of labour and make it difficult for the woman to feel motivated and active. Decreased urine output may also be an indication for the need to increase fluid intake. If women are enabled to follow their inclinations about drinking, they are unlikely to become dehydrated (McCormick 2003).

Working with contractions

When each woman experiences contractions, a midwife needs to observe their length, strength and frequency, the body language of the woman and the impact on the contractions of the positions she adopts. Many women who experience lower back and sacral pain will adopt a leaning forward position or be on their hands and knees. Squatting or soaking in a warm bath may help those with intense supra pubic pain. Sitting on the toilet is an ideal place to be when the contractions' intensity builds, and this position also assists in widening the pelvic outlet. A woman's instinct is to find a position that assists her in dealing with the contraction, and often this action also allows the baby to rotate into a more favourable position (Sutton 2003).

Much has been written about the 'labour dance' (Kitzinger 1997; Vincent 2002). As a midwife it is a privilege to watch a woman unrestricted by technology, rules and expectations of others, listening and responding as her body tells her. The dance may be evident by rhythmic rocking, hip circling and adjustments of position as the contractions exert their energy and power. As the labour moves forward, each woman's dance will adapt to the physiological changes that are occurring in her body. For example, a woman who has previously been pacing and swaying with contractions may suddenly need to be rocking backwards and forwards on her hands and knees. For others who have found the birthing pool or bath soothing, it may now be more comfortable to be leaning against a wall with pressure applied to the sacrum. The use of moist heat can be particularly effective. This can be provided by soaking hand towels in very hot water, then wringing them out and applying them at the start of a contraction. Where they are placed depends on where the woman is feeling her contractions most. An attentive support team will soon recognise the signs that a contraction may be beginning, and have the heat available before the contraction has reached its full intensity. The use of heat provides comfort and a positive sensation, which may assist a woman as she works with her contractions.

Midwifery support in labour is about reading the cues and suggesting positions and actions that will assist the constant shifts in each woman's experience. This may require the active involvement of supporters and the midwife by the provision of touch, massage, acupressure and physical support. It is also about trusting that the woman will find her own way and supporting, with patience, the time that the woman needs to do this.

Physical assessment in active phase of labour

Throughout labour, midwifery assessment relies on integration of the following aspects:

- observing the woman—her demeanour, length and frequency of contractions, how she responds to them and the positions she adopts, interactions with support people
- listening to the woman—how she relates her labour story so far, fears or concerns, vocal/breathing responses during contractions
- assessing the environment—the effect of those present, lighting, temperature, general atmosphere
- physical assessment—baseline parameters of uterine

activity (length, strength and frequency of contractions, cervical dilatation and descent of the baby), baby's reaction to labour (heart rate, reactivity, variability), vaginal loss, maternal responses to labour (pulse, temperature, blood pressure, level of hydration, level of pain, urinalysis).

In all labours, a midwife carries out continuous assessment of each woman she works with. Assessment and familiarity with the physiological signs that labour is progressing enables a midwife to determine that labour is progressing normally or to identify signs that complications may be developing and that other interventions must occur. There are several specific physical assessments that will be made by midwives with varying regularity throughout labour. These are measurement of contractions, assessment of vaginal loss, abdominal palpations, vaginal examinations, auscultation of baby's heart rate and assessment of maternal urine, temperature, pulse and blood pressure and fluid balance. From time to time midwives may use interventions such as artificial rupture of membranes but these should be viewed with caution.

Contractions

Each woman will exhibit her individual pattern of contractions through her labour. However, in active labour that is progressing, contractions will increase in strength and intensity and in length and frequency. A midwife can assess tone, length and frequency of contractions by placing her hand on the woman's fundus and holding it there through several cycles of contraction and relaxation. The contraction can be timed from its beginning to end, and the length and frequency in each 10-minute period determined. It is useful for a student midwife to place her hand on a woman's fundus for 10-minute periods in order to become familiar with assessing contractions. The student will be able to feel the contraction beginning, often before the woman feels it as pain. In this way, student midwives will become familiar with the range of contractions felt and observed for different women.

When the pattern of contractions changes, this may be a sign that labour is slowing because of a problem such as maternal exhaustion or poor positioning of the baby, or it may be that the woman has reached a plateau in labour that is normal for her and her labour will recommence in time. Where there is a change from an expected pattern, a midwife needs to make further assessments to determine the cause and possible midwifery actions. Usually such a diagnosis can only be made through the integration of several assessments of wellbeing of mother and baby and the progress of labour.

Vaginal loss

Vaginal loss can provide signs of labour progressing, although the amount and type of loss will vary between women. A small amount of bloodstained mucus can indicate detachment of the membranes as the cervix dilates. Midwives must record when membranes rupture and check the liquor for colour, amount and odour. Clear liquor is normal, while a greenish tinge indicates meconium staining and may be associated with fetal distress. Often the membranes will rupture as the cervix nears full dilatation, but this can occur earlier. A heavy, bloodstained mucus loss may also indicate full dilatation of the cervix. However, frank bleeding is always abnormal and must be further assessed and managed appropriately.

Abdominal palpation

Alongside the assessment of uterine activity, an abdominal palpation is very important (Stuart 2000). Palpation of the baby's position, presentation and descent into the pelvis early in the labour provides a baseline for ongoing assessment of the progress of the labour and auscultation of the baby's heart rate. Asking a woman about her impressions of her baby's position and movements during labour will assist the midwife

> ### Clinical point
>
> **Revision of palpation**
> Review Chapter 20, Working with women in pregnancy.
> ▶ Consider:
>   — consent from woman
>   — maintaining privacy and dignity for the woman
>   — religious and cultural considerations
>   — hand washing
>   — comfort measures:
>   — encourage her to empty her bladder prior to examination
>   — assist her to get into a comfortable position
>   — wait for time between contractions to palpate
>   — gentle touch.
> ▶ Abdominal palpation involves:
>   — visual assessment
>   — fundal assessment
>   — lateral assessment
>   — pelvic palpation
>   — auscultation.
> ▶ Identify:
>   — lie
>   — presentation
>   — position
>   — engagement
>   — descent
>   — optimum position to hear and count baby's heart rate.
> ▶ Does the baby feel to be appropriate size for its gestation? Is the baby presenting head first? Is the head flexed? What position is the baby? Is descent appropriate for stage of labour and position of baby? Is the fetal heart rate within normal range?
> ▶ Compare descent of presenting part on abdominal palpation with descent of presenting part as assessed by vaginal examination.
> ▶ Assess tone, length and frequency of contractions.
> ▶ Share findings with woman and document fully in notes.

Clinical point

Reasons to consider performing a vaginal examination in normal labour

▶ Woman's request
▶ Assessment of cervical effacement and dilatation
▶ Confirmation of presentation, position and descent of the baby through the pelvis

Clinical point

Reasons to consider avoiding a vaginal examination in normal labour

▶ Woman's consent declined
▶ History of sexual abuse
▶ Potential for introduction of infection
▶ Disruption to woman's focus and confidence

(Sources: Chapman 2003; Enkin et al 2000; McCormick 2003; Walsh 2004)

Clinical point

Definitions

▶ *Effacement*: shortening and thinning of the cervical canal as the internal os dilates and forms part of the lower uterine segment (see Fig 22.1).
▶ *Dilatation*: the external os (os uteri) increasingly dilates as a result of the contraction and retraction of the uterine muscles. In primigravidae, effacement of the cervix usually precedes dilatation but in multigravidae effacement and dilatation normally occur simultaneously. Full dilatation has been achieved when the os uteri has dilated sufficiently to allow the baby's head to pass through.
▶ *Position*: comparison of the position of the fontanelles and sutures of the baby's head in relation to the woman's pelvis. In occipito-anterior positions, the posterior fontanelle is felt towards the anterior part of the pelvis. In occipito-posterior positions, the anterior fontanelle will be felt anteriorly. The position of the sagittal suture in relation to the oblique diameters of the woman's pelvis further clarifies the position. For example, when the sagittal suture lies in the left oblique diameter of the pelvis (from the left posterior quadrant to the right anterior quadrant) and the posterior fontanelle anteriorly to the right, the position is the right occipito-anterior (see Fig 22.2)
▶ *Station*: the relationship of the presenting part to the ischial spines of the maternal pelvis (see Fig 22.3).

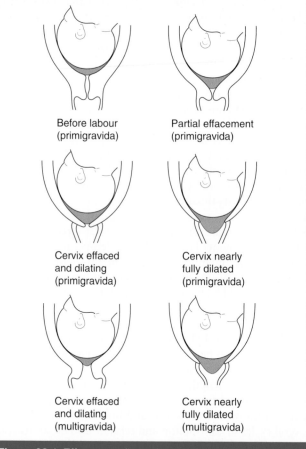

Before labour (primigravida)

Partial effacement (primigravida)

Cervix effaced and dilating (primigravida)

Cervix nearly fully dilated (primigravida)

Cervix effaced and dilating (multigravida)

Cervix nearly fully dilated (multigravida)

Figure 22.1 Effacement (based on Henderson & Macdonald 2004)

in gaining valuable information prior to abdominal palpation (Banks 2003). When undertaking an abdominal palpation, a number of factors need to be considered and assessed (see the Clinical point). Abdominal palpation is a useful tool for assessing the progress of labour by defining descent and flexion of the presenting part and thereby avoiding unnecessary vaginal examinations.

Vaginal examinations

Routine vaginal examinations (VE) are a common intervention in labour (Crowther 2000; Walsh 2000a). They have become accepted as the definitive gauge of progress in labour, but the literature indicates that they are subjective and invasive, and that their benefit in normal labour is unproven (Crowther 2000). Even so, they are an important skill that midwives need to use judiciously. As part of a woman's individualised care, a vaginal examination may be appropriate. It is important for a midwife to have a sound rationale for why she would perform a vaginal examination and what information she hopes to obtain. While some women find vaginal examinations unnecessarily intrusive, others may find the information gained valuable and be happy to have a vaginal examination performed if it is carried out sensitively. Developing the skills required for vaginal examination is an important part of being

Clinical point

Performing a vaginal examination

Preparation:

▶ Explain to the woman the rationale for VE, what is involved, what she can expect to feel and how long it may take; gain consent.

▶ Reassure the woman that the midwife will immediately discontinue the examination at the woman's request.

▶ Maintain privacy and dignity for the woman.

▶ Recognise and discuss religious and cultural considerations with the woman.

▶ Comfort measures:
  – encourage her to empty her bladder prior to examination
  – comfortable position
  – wait for time between contractions to examine
  – sensitive touch.

▶ Perform an abdominal palpation first to obtain comparative information, particularly in relation to descent of the baby

▶ Position woman in semi-reclining position with knees raised and abducted (can also be performed with woman lying on her side or on hands and knees, but student should gain experience with semi-recumbent position first).

▶ Explain all actions throughout the procedure.

▶ Wash hands and wear gloves; maintain sterile field and aseptic technique if the woman's membranes have ruptured.

▶ Observe vulva for any unusual features or any discharge, e.g. vulval varicosities, previous scarring, lesions (warts).

▶ Apply lubricant to forefinger and middle finger and gently insert into vagina.

▶ Note tone of vaginal muscles and pelvic floor, moisture (dryness may indicate pyrexia).

▶ Identify cervix and note consistency, effacement, position and dilatation.

▶ Identify presenting part, feel for sutures and fontanelles to determine position of head in relation to pelvis, feel for moulding or caput succedaneum.

▶ Feel for spines and assess station of presenting part in relation to spines; feel for membranes—intact? Bulging forewaters or smooth?; note application of cervix to presenting part; note any unusual or abnormal features such as umbilical cord pulsation or vessels in the membranes.

▶ After VE listen to the baby's heart and count the rate.

Information gained:

▶ Assessment of vulva and vagina, identifying any abnormalities of tissues or discharge.

▶ Cervix—position (anterior, central, posterior, lateral)
  – consistency (soft, thick, firm, thin, stretchy)
  – effacement (non-effaced, partial or fully effaced)
  – dilatation (os closed, 1–9 cm dilated, or fully dilated)
  – application of the cervix to the baby's head (loosely, moderately or well applied).

▶ Presenting part—cephalic:
  – position (anterior, lateral, posterior)
  – station in relation to ischial spines
  – presence/degree of caput/moulding

▶ Membranes—intact or ruptured, bulging
  – presence of liquor, colour, amount.

Findings from vaginal examination that, in conjunction with other midwifery assessments, indicate that labour is progressing normally:

▶ increasing descent, flexion and rotation anteriorly of baby's head in relation to the pelvis

▶ continued softening, effacement and dilatation of the cervix

▶ increasing application of the cervix to the presenting part.

Following the examination, the findings should be discussed with the woman and the fetal heart rate assessed. Documentation would include all information gained from the procedure.

---

able to provide appropriate and effective midwifery care. The decision to perform a vaginal examination must be made in discussion with the woman and her consent documented along with the rationale for the examination.

Artificial rupture of the membranes (amniotomy)

Sometimes artificial rupture of the membranes (ARM) is recommended in an attempt to accelerate labour (Fraser et al 2004). The supposition is that, with the membranes ruptured, the baby's head descends onto the cervix, causing more frequent and stronger contractions. Artificial rupture of the membranes also enables visualisation of the colour of the liquor (Baston 2004). However, what commonly occurs is that the baby's head moves down and loses the manoeuvrability

Critical thinking exercise

Consider how you will share information with a labouring woman prior to possible amniotomy.

▶ What is the rationale used for amniotomy in normal labour?

▶ What is the evidence for and against this practice?

---

it once had with the support of the liquor-filled membranes. If the baby isn't in an optimal position, amniotomy may exacerbate this. It may also cause an increase in the intensity of the contractions, making them more difficult to cope with

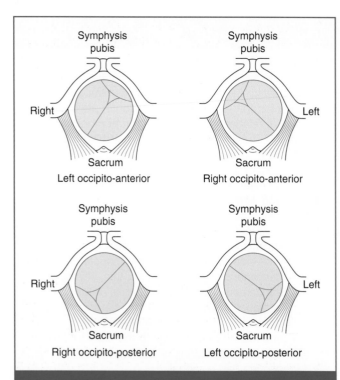

Figure 22.2 Position of the fontanelles and sutures of the baby's head in relation to the woman's pelvis (based on Henderson & Macdonald 1988)

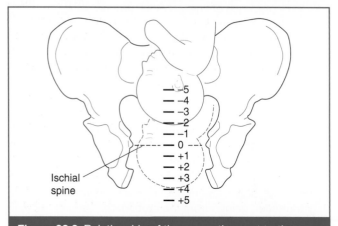

Figure 22.3 Relationship of the presenting part to the ischial spines of the maternal pelvis (based on Henderson & Macdonald 2004)

(Enkin et al 2000). Research shows that there is an increase in fetal distress and caesarean section following amniotomy in early labours, and one systematic review concluded that amniotomy should be reserved for labours that are not progressing normally (Enkin et al 2000; Fraser et al 2004; Goffinet et al 1997).

Listening to the baby's heart rate

The baby's heart rate is listened to during labour to confirm its presence, rate and how it responds to the labour process. It is important to identify any indicators of hypoxia in the baby. In normal labour, the appropriate method for listening to the baby's heart rate is intermittent auscultation (NICE 2001). Intermittent auscultation is achieved by listening at intervals using a monaural stethoscope (Pinard) or a hand-held Doppler device (Sonicaid). This is most effective with the constant presence of an attentive midwife who is able to assimilate information regarding the woman and her baby's wellbeing through a combination of assessments. Using a Pinard stethoscope, the heart rate can be heard as a contraction is finishing. This will confirm the rate and detect any slow recovery back to the baseline. For some women, using a Pinard to listen throughout a contraction may be uncomfortable, and the heart sounds may not be audible. A Doppler device can be used during a contraction and the heart rate can be heard without requiring the woman to adjust her position. A Doppler can also be used for women labouring in water (if the transducer is water-resistant). Intermittent auscultation enables regular, direct contact between the midwife and the woman. It provides an opportunity for the midwife to reassure the woman and her supporters, and provides encouragement (Page 2000).

The baby's heart rate should be counted over a minute, to ascertain beat-to-beat variability. Variability of more than five beats per minute (bpm) is normal throughout labour. The baseline heart rate refers to the heart rate present between periods of acceleration or deceleration and is considered normal between 110 and 160 bpm. The heart rate will usually remain steady or accelerate during contractions. Decelerations of the heart rate during contractions may be associated with

> ## Clinical point
>
> ### Recommended monitoring in an uncomplicated pregnancy
> For a woman who is healthy and has had an otherwise uncomplicated pregnancy, intermittent auscultation should be offered and recommended in labour to monitor fetal wellbeing.
>
> In the active stages of labour, intermittent auscultation should occur (with the woman's permission) after a contraction, for a minimum of 60 seconds, and at least:
> - every 15 minutes in the first stage
> - every 5 minutes in the second stage.
>
> Continuous EFM should be offered and recommended in pregnancies previously monitored with intermittent auscultation:
> - if there is evidence on auscultation of a baseline less than 110 bpm or greater than 160 bpm.
> - if there is evidence on auscultation of any decelerations
> - if any intrapartum risk factors develop.
>
> Current evidence does not support the use of admission cardiotocography (CTG) in low-risk pregnancy and it is therefore not recommended. (Source: NICE 2001)

umbilical cord compression or compression of the baby's head as it descends through the pelvis. McCormick (2003) suggests that this may be more likely when the membranes are not intact. Decelerations where the heart rate returns to the baseline immediately the contraction ceases are not generally associated with hypoxia (Enkin et al 2000; Page 2000). Counting the heart rate during and immediately following a contraction provides the midwife with a clear indication of the baby's response to the labour (see Clinical point).

There are no studies that confirm the frequency of auscultation necessary to maintain safety. The National Institute for Clinical Excellence recommends 15-minute intervals during active labour (NICE 2001). It also suggests listening after every contraction and pushing effort once the cervix is fully dilated. Many midwives consider that 15 to 30 minute intervals during labour are more realistic, especially when they are providing continuous care in active labour and making comprehensive assessments. Increased monitoring is recognised as being appropriate from the transition phase until the birth of the baby. The midwife will document her assessment of the baby's wellbeing, including the heart rate, each time she listens. The frequency of monitoring the baby's

heart rate throughout the labour in relation to outcome is not widely researched and there is a need for further studies in this area. The NICE Guidelines (2001) appear to have been accepted as a baseline but they stress that consideration should be given to maternal preference and priorities.

There are often variations in a baby's heart rate during the different phases of labour. These may be due to, for example, maternal position, dehydration, overheating, and baby's head compression during transition and the pushing stage. The midwife needs to take these into consideration and, if possible, institute changes and re-check the heart rate response. Any persistent abnormal recordings are an indication for more frequent observations, which may include continuous electronic monitoring and consultation with another midwife or an obstetric specialist. (For more detail about electronic fetal monitoring see Ch 35.)

Maternal responses to physiological changes of labour

Assessment in active labour includes baseline urinalysis, blood pressure, temperature and pulse recordings and fluid balance. While research indicates that there is little value in routinely monitoring these recordings in a normal labour, having baseline information is useful for ongoing comparison, particularly if the labour develops complications (Enkin et al 2000). For example, ketones in urine and increasing pulse and temperature may indicate that the woman is becoming dehydrated; if not addressed, dehydration can lead to alterations in contractions and a slowing of labour. Fluid balance does not need to be formally recorded but the midwife needs to be alert to keeping the woman hydrated through labour and preventing dehydration. Where a woman is not passing urine frequently, the midwife should consider whether the woman has been drinking sufficiently.

Despite the lack of evidence about frequency of these assessments, most midwifery texts recommend regular observations at a variety of intervals and more frequently if problems present (McCormick 2003; Sinclair 2004). This may be due to the fact that, in most countries, midwifery care is fragmented and the midwife and woman are unlikely to have already established a relationship in pregnancy. Continuity of carer allows a more individualised approach to physical assessment and recordings.

Nevertheless, there are some situations in normal labour that may warrant more frequent monitoring. These include:
- pre-labour rupture of membranes
- recent history of vaginal infections
- invasive procedures, including vaginal examinations, bladder catheterisations
- irregularity of fetal heart rate (Enkin et al 2000; NICE 2001; Walsh 2004).

Ongoing assessment of progress in labour

Having facilitated a supportive environment, taking into account the wishes of the labouring woman and the physical

---

Clinical point

Listening to the fetal heart rate (FHR): what to listen for

The use of intermittent auscultation minimises the risk for iatrogenic interventions associated with continuous electronic fetal monitoring (EFM).

Listen immediately after a contraction for 60 seconds to ascertain the absence of the following markers of possible hypoxia or acidaemia in the fetus:

▶ recurrent decelerations of any type defined as decelerations occurring > 50% of the time or with 50% of the contractions in two consecutive 10-minute windows
▶ prolonged decelerations
▶ sustained fetal bradycardia (60 bpm or less)
▶ persistent fetal tachycardia greater than 180 bpm
▶ an audibly unchanging/fixed baseline FHR.

A non-reassuring fetal heart rate occurs when the lower level is equal to or below 110 beats per minute and above or equal to 160 beats per minute (Okosun 2005).

When these patterns are identified by auscultation, studies suggest that the use of EFM can help in evaluating the accompanying baseline FHR variability. Note:

▶ Continuous EFM should be reserved for the mother and/or fetus at risk.
▶ A sustained bradycardia may indicate a prolapsed cord or complete placental abruption. When the FHR is reduced to 60 bpm or less, a significant fetal acidosis can develop quickly.

(Sources: Fox et al 2000; Okosun & Arulkumaran 2005)

context of where she will birth, assessment of her progress in labour will require the midwife to be present and 'with' the woman. We have already discussed the importance of viewing each woman's labour as particular to her, rather than trying to 'fit' her labour into a standardised format. The holistic nature of midwifery care means constantly assessing the environment for its impact, as well as watching, talking with and listening to the woman. As labour advances, her contractions will change. From being able to talk through some contractions and having a connection with what is going on around her, a woman in a progressing labour will begin to concentrate with each deeper sensation and may require support to work through each contraction. If her movements are unrestricted she should be encouraged to adopt positions in which she feels most comfortable. Encouraging her to empty her bladder regularly will aid her comfort as well as providing an opportunity for finding alternative positions. Women who have the choice to be upright will have greater contraction intensity and efficiency and are less likely to require pharmacological pain relief (Enkin et al 2000). However, it is important to keep a balance between rest and activity. Some women will need periods of inactivity

during the not-uncommon plateaus of labour to recharge and refocus their energy levels (Page 2000).

Documentation

It is important that the midwife collates and documents comprehensive assessments of the woman and baby's health and wellbeing (NZCOM 2005). This serves three main purposes:

● to be able to review and assess the progress of labour
● to provide an accurate diary of events for the woman to read, refer to and keep
● to provide a legal document that illustrates the information and care given, and the subsequent events and outcomes.

For the midwifery notes to assist in assessment of progress they should be a time-based diary of events permitting a detailed documentation of all assessments of the woman and her baby. Documentation provides evidence of midwifery decision-making and as such they should contain as much information as possible. In contexts where partograms are used routinely (Australia), additional information must be recorded, as the partogram does not provide enough on its own.

Partograms

Partograms have been shown to be an efficient means of exchanging information about labour progress between teams of caregivers. However, in a continuity of carer setting, the partogram has little value. Partograms provide a visual display of only part of the woman's progress in labour and they assume that there will be vaginal examinations and charting of cervical dilatation (Chapman 2003). They are a structured graphical representation (with alert and action lines) and may rely too much on a strict protocol of action. Partograms can be an agent for regimenting labour rather than supporting the woman's individual process (Chapman 2003; Enkin et al 2000). Observational studies have shown improved outcomes with the use of partograms when the labour is not progressing normally (Enkin et al 2000; Lavender et al 1998). However, there is a need for research into the efficacy of the use of partograms in physiologically normal labour. Albers (1999) suggests that the parameters of normal labour need to be researched and redefined to increase midwifery knowledge by more accurately reflecting women's actual experiences.

Woman-centred midwifery notes

The comprehensive nature of the labour notes means that they need to clearly document and describe midwifery care, advice and consultations. They should be written in a narrative style that is woman-centred and provides the story of events as they unfold. The notes will outline information discussed with the woman and the rationale for the decisions made. The story of the labour and birth is an invaluable aid for later reflection on the birth with the woman. Professional midwifery care requires reflection on practice, and comprehensive notes

---

Clinical point

Facilitating a woman's ongoing labour

▶ Check how the woman is feeling about the labour and what form of support she wants from you.
▶ Avoid arbitrary time limits.
▶ Follow the birth plan in consultation with the woman as appropriate.
▶ Assess her wellbeing, including her emotional and behavioural responses.
▶ Check blood pressure, temperature, pulse and urinalysis—look for signs of dehydration and take appropriate action.
▶ Discuss the need, or not, for a vaginal examination. If VE is done, look for increasing dilatation, anterior position of baby, continual descent and rotation through pelvis.
▶ Assess contractions, lie, presentation and descent of the baby—look for signs of continual progress and follow up any indication of delay such as lack of descent of baby, slowing of contractions.
▶ Assess baby's wellbeing, including heart rate— look for continual reassuring signs and follow up any non-reassuring patterns such as decelerations, tachycardia or bradycardia.
▶ If membranes have ruptured, check colour of liquor—follow up any non-reassuring signs such as meconium.
▶ Facilitate partner/supporter's involvement as per care plan.
▶ Encourage the woman to move into whatever positions she feels comfortable in.
▶ Encourage the woman to drink regularly and to eat if she wishes.

support this process. Although some may view constant and concurrent documentation as time consuming and tedious, it need not be.

Tips for documentation

- Involve the supporters in the woman's care to free you for short periods to document events.
- Write something every 15 minutes—e.g. how the woman is feeling, the positions she is using, frequency/strength/length of contractions, vaginal discharge, input from supporters, baby's heart rate.
- If you use abbreviations, explain their meaning when first used and keep the notes in a form that can be understood by the woman and her family.
- If at times you are unable to write full notes, jot down brief reminders and times of significant events—e.g. rupture of membranes, vaginal examinations, fetal heart rate recordings—and update more comprehensively as soon as possible.
- Clearly note references to the woman's care plan and whether there are any changes to this plan. Document details of the discussion with the woman, and the rationale and consent for any decisions or birth plan changes.

Labour: transition phase to birth

Most labouring women and midwives are aware of a transitional period between the first stage of labour and the time when active maternal pushing efforts begin (Downe 2003). Changes in the woman's behaviour, body language and vocal responses towards the end of the active phase of labour may indicate this transition stage. This often tumultuous period can challenge the woman and her supporters, and the midwife needs to guide and support them through the intensity of this time.

A woman's responses to this change in her labour may include increasing restlessness, breathing rhythm changes, shaking, vomiting, a feeling of panic and of being engulfed by the process. The contractions relentlessly roll from one into the next, giving the woman no time to focus as she had earlier. Often at this time, women will vocalise that they 'can't do this any more' and plead to the midwife and supporters to 'help me'. Supportive midwifery care can help the woman by continually reassuring her that she is safe and that these feelings are normal and a sign of labour progress. The midwife's confidence and belief in the woman's ability helps to strengthen the woman and her supporters to meet the challenges of this part of normal labour. She will need to use all of her strength and experience to provide support and encouragement. The midwife needs to acknowledge that this process is taking the woman to the edge of her ability to cope. The constant presence and reassurance of the midwife will reduce the chance of resorting to the use of pharmacological interventions at a time when the woman is at her most vulnerable.

Clinical point

Characteristics of transition to full dilatation of the cervix
- The woman may feel she has lost control and have feelings of panic.
- She may say she cannot carry on, and ask for help.
- She may ask for pain relief.
- She may vomit or feel nauseous and be shaking.
- There may be a heavy 'show' of bloodstained mucus.
- She may have beginning sensations of pressure in her bottom or the urge to push—can be variable.
- For some women, labour slows down and she can rest or may even sleep.

There is no clear timeframe for the transition period. For some women it can be a few hours and for others a matter of just a few contractions. Occasionally women find that the contractions begin to ease off and will benefit from this sudden calm in their labour and may even sleep. It is once again important to reassure the woman that this lull in her labour is very normal and that it is her mind and body preparing her for the next stage and the birth of her baby. If this happens it is often a good time for the supporters to get a break, get some fresh air, go to the toilet, eat and drink before they are needed again. Midwives may often feel a need to 'do something' when the labour slows after a torrent of strong contractions and, as is also the case in misunderstood latent phase, it can be a time when unwarranted interventions are introduced, such as ARM and VE. Patience and trust are the hallmarks of an effective midwife and as long as mother and baby are both well they should not be interfered with. As the woman's cervix becomes fully dilated and the baby descends further, the woman's contractions and her responses give cues to the midwife that the woman is moving closer to the birth of her baby (Walsh 2000b).

Fourth decision point in labour: second stage or birth to skin-to-skin

At this stage there will be a number of signs that the woman is ready to birth her baby. These cues may include the following:
- a pushing urge at the peak of a contraction
- the urge to push accompanied by deep, throaty sounds
- the woman tells you that she is feeling pressure or wants 'to push'
- bloodstained vaginal mucous discharge
- anal dilation
- possible spontaneous rupture of membranes

● perineal distension caused by pressure from the presenting part and/or intact membranes.

If a woman is experiencing urges to push and the other cues do not become apparent, it would be appropriate to consider a vaginal examination to confirm descent and position of the presenting part and dilatation of the cervix.

These sensations are often very intense and can be challenging for the woman. This is a time for the midwife to reassure the woman and explain what is happening for her and her baby. It is important for the midwife to communicate calmly and clearly with the woman. Helping the woman to focus on and trust what her body is telling her enables the woman to work with these powerful sensations and find the positions that help her most effectively.

As the contractions become increasingly expulsive, most women will experience stronger urges to push. Urges to push may vary in frequency and intensity. Supporting spontaneous, involuntary pushing means that the woman pushes only when the contraction has built up and she is unable to resist the pushing urge. Spontaneous pushing is characterised

---

Clinical point

Advantages of being upright for birth

▶ Reduced risk of aorta-caval compression, which means maximising oxygen availability for the woman and baby.

▶ Gravity assists the baby into the optimal position and aids descent through the pelvis.

▶ Stimulates stronger and more efficient uterine contractions.

▶ Increases the diameter of the pelvic outlet.

(Source: Albers et al 1997; Gould 2000; MacLennan et al 1994).

Clinical point

Effective positions/places for pushing

▶ Squatting—using support people and/or furniture

▶ Kneeling—using cushions, mats, beanbags

▶ Sitting on the toilet or birthing stool

▶ Standing—leaning against furniture, wall, people, tree

▶ Use of pool or bath—buoyancy of water supports upright positions

---

Critical thinking exercise

Consider the labour environments in which you are with women.

1   What can you do to facilitate upright positions for women in labour?

2   What equipment is available to you and how could you adapt it to support the woman to be upright?

---

by short periods of breath holding (for no more than six seconds) followed by expiratory grunts (Sleep et al 2000). This is often referred to as non-directed pushing, and has been found to result in shorter second stages, a reduction in maternal fatigue and fetal distress, and less intervention (Walsh 2000b).

Upright positions for pushing are most effective in assisting women to birth their babies. Using upright positions enables women to remain mobile and they often prefer them (Gupta & Hofmeyr 2004). There are a number of physiological advantages in being upright (Rosser 2003).

This part of labour has traditionally been compartmentalised and subjected to strict timeframes in the mistaken belief that this will benefit the mother and baby. Focus on the purely physical aspects of birthing denies recognition of the complexities involved. This has led to a variety of interventions in response to the urgency that has developed around the birthing process. These interventions include directed or coached pushing, vaginal examinations, ARM, episiotomy and assisted or operative delivery. Arbitrary timeframes have not been found to improve outcomes and have subjected women and their babies to procedures that may have been unnecessary and at times caused harm (Walsh 2000b). Previous studies have investigated the outcomes for well women and their babies where the pushing stage has exceeded the traditional timeframes. These traditional limits have restricted primiparous women to two hours and multiparous women to one hour to birth their babies. Research shows that women and babies come to no harm where pushing efforts have exceeded these time limits (O'Connell et al 2003; Sleep et al 2000).

Facilitating a supportive birthing environment

The midwife has an important role in facilitating the birth of the baby by ensuring that the environment is appropriate and supportive of this physiological process. It is necessary to consider the following:

● the woman's plan, desires and dreams for the birth of her baby

● privacy—phone off the hook, doors closed, curtains pulled, note on the door saying 'not to be disturbed'

● warmth—room temperature, warm towels for the baby, pool temperature at 37°C

● comfort—positional techniques, hot towels, warm compresses, encouraging words

● a space in which to use a variety of positions and props (e.g. pool, bath, mats, pillows, beanbags, birth stools, mirror)

● involvement of partner and supporters—supplying drinks to the woman, cool cloth for her face, massage or acupressure, applying hot towels, physical support for the woman, encouraging words

● unobtrusive presence of a second midwife who is known to the woman, is supportive of her birth plan and familiar with the safety equipment

- preparation of birthing and safety equipment—oxygen, suction, infant Ambubag, oxytocics, cord ties/clamps, scissors, availability of intravenous cannulation equipment and fluids.

Facilitating effective pushing efforts means that the midwife recognises when it is appropriate to make suggestions for the woman to try a variety of positions. This may be in response to recognition that efforts so far have resulted in little change in the descent of the presenting part of the baby. Identifying a lack of progress usually results from a combination of assessments. These may include:

- the woman stating that 'Nothing has changed'
- no obvious anal dilatation or perineal distension, and no presenting part visible
- abdominal palpation to identify the degree of descent of the presenting part in relation to the pelvic brim
- VE to confirm presentation, assess cervical dilatation, define position, assess station and the development of caput and moulding.

If lack of progress has been identified, sometimes simple changes to the woman's position may be all that is required to enable the labour to advance. The midwife can then guide the woman into more upright, open positions to enhance rotation and descent of the baby. This can be achieved, for example, by the use of supported squatting, sitting on the toilet or birth stool, or standing. Enabling the woman to see the effect of her pushes using a mirror can be very encouraging and energising as the presenting part becomes visible.

As the presenting part descends with contractions, it advances with the assistance of expulsive pushing efforts. It will initially advance, then recede between contractions. This process is necessary to enable the woman's tissues to accommodate the presenting part and also support gentle moulding of the baby's head. The use of hot compresses on the perineum and vulva can provide some soothing comfort at this time and is associated with lower rates of perineal trauma (Jackson 2000). As the presenting part distends the vulva and perineum and then doesn't recede, the woman may experience intense burning and stretching. Hot compresses may provide some relief, and the midwife's calm, clear reassurance will be helpful. At this time the woman and her supporters will benefit from a relaxed, calm and unhurried atmosphere as the birth becomes imminent.

The midwife can encourage the gradual birth of the baby's head by suggesting that the woman breathes gently, pants or gives gentle, small pushes (Chapman 2003). With the intention of reducing perineal trauma, the midwife may have her 'hands on' or 'hands poised' to prevent rapid extension of the baby's head (McCandlish et al 1998). Traditionally, midwives have been taught to apply digital pressure to the occiput to maintain flexion and reduce tissue damage. There is no evidence to support this practice at every birth; however, a midwife must be poised to support the baby's head if it appears to be advancing rapidly or if there is an indication of possible perineal trauma.

Once the baby's head is born there can be a resting period before the next contraction. Midwives have routinely used

---

Clinical point

When is the optimal time to clamp the cord?

The optimal time for clamping the umbilical cord at birth is unclear. Delaying clamping may facilitate transfusion of blood between the placenta and the baby (Rabe et al 2004). In a review of the literature, more than 500 term infants enrolled in randomised controlled trials and controlled trials (Mercer 2001) whose cords were clamped between 3 and 10 minutes or when pulsations ceased, showed no adverse outcome. Benefits are clearly documented for preterm infants (Rabe et al 2004) and suggested for term infants. There is no evidence that early cord clamping is better, and evidence is lacking regarding long-term harm from immediate or delayed cord clamping. Until we have sufficient appropriate evidence showing otherwise, it is better to mimic nature than to interfere with the intricate, complex, and only partially understood design of the physiological neonatal transition.

Level at which the infant is held

Delaying cord clamping and keeping the infant at the level of the introitus for 45 seconds results in an 11% increase in blood volume, but a 24% increase in oxygen-carrying red blood cells (Yao & Lind 1969). Raising the infant significantly (30–60 cm) delays placental transfusion, and lowering the infant 30–60 cm speeds the transfusion of blood from the placenta from 3 minutes to 1 minute (Yao et al 1969).

(Sources: Mercer 2001; Rabe et al 2004; Yao & Lind 1969; Yao et al 1969)

---

this time to check whether there is a nuchal cord. There is ongoing debate regarding the usefulness of this procedure and women can find it extremely painful (Wickham 2003). If the cord is present it can be looped over the baby's head or rolled down over the baby's shoulders as the baby is born (Downe 2003). If the cord is wound tightly around the neck it has been common practice to clamp and cut the cord to release it. As this severs the baby's oxygen supply this practice is being increasingly questioned and should be used with caution. Tight nuchal cords have been associated with shoulder dystocia, and depriving the baby of its vital oxygen supply will only aggravate an already serious situation (Iffy et al 2001). Clamping and cutting the cord before the baby is born also alters the physiology of placental separation and commits the woman to active management procedures.

With the next contraction, the baby's shoulders rotate into the anterior/posterior diameter of the outlet of the pelvis and the baby's head will turn to be in alignment with the body (restitution). As the woman pushes, the shoulders are birthed and the rest of the body follows. The degree of hands-on support and guidance the midwife needs to provide will depend on the woman's wishes, her birth plan and the

TABLE 22.3 The Apgar score

	0	1	2
Heart rate	Absent	Slow (< 100)	Fast (> 100)
Respiratory effort	Absent	Slow and irregular	Good and crying
Muscle tone	Limp	Some flexion of extremities	Active
Reflex irritability	No response	Grimace	Cry/cough
Colour	Pale	Body pink, extremities blue	Pink

(Source: Levene & Tudehope 1993)

position she is in. The woman may wish to reach for her baby and lift it to her or have the baby placed gently against her warm skin. It is not unusual for some women to need time before they touch and hold their baby. It is important that the baby is kept warm by skin-to-skin contact and gentle drying with warm towels, to maintain the baby's temperature and stimulate respirations. The towels should be replaced as soon as they are damp. These first few minutes of relief, exhilaration and delight are precious. The midwife, however, needs to be alert to the wellbeing of the mother and baby. An effective, skilful midwife is able to make careful assessments without interfering in these moments.

Assessments should include:

- baby's colour, heart rate, initiation of respiration, muscle tone, reflex irritability (Apgar score at 1, 5 and 10 minutes) (see Table 22.3)
- observing the woman's response to her baby
- observing the woman's general wellbeing and ensuring her comfort
- maintaining observations of blood loss and signs of separation of the placenta.

The Apgar score was devised by Virginia Apgar in 1953 and has since become the most commonly used quantitative measuring tool for assessing the wellbeing of the newborn baby (Levene & Tudehope 1993).

Enabling the new family to savour the moments after the birth involves supporting the woman and her family to take the time they need as they greet their new baby. This time also allows the woman's physiological responses to continue unimpeded. The woman holding her baby close encourages the release of oxytocin to facilitate the separation of the placenta and membranes. As the baby adjusts to the new environment, she or he may begin to look around, nuzzle the breast and display signs of being interested in suckling. It is important not to force this process but to observe for these cues. The baby may bring her hands to her mouth and start mouthing or rooting for the breast. There is no specific timeframe for this to occur but it is important that when the baby is ready, she has the opportunity to latch to the breast. An unhurried, non-interfering approach best achieves this.

Fifth decision point in labour: the third stage

A supportive, warm environment, low lighting, attention to the woman's comfort, and having the baby close to or feeding at the breast have all been found to encourage the spontaneous birth of the placenta (Odent 1999). The birth plan developed by the woman and her midwife will have identified preferences for the birth of the placenta and membranes. Where the labour and birth have proceeded normally with no intervention, it is reasonable to expect that the birth of the placenta and membranes will follow the physiological process uninterrupted. This is referred to variously as expectant, physiological or natural care (Long 2003). It is important for the midwife to be alert to the amount of vaginal blood loss and its effects on the wellbeing of the woman. Usually there is very little blood loss until the placenta begins to separate from the wall of the uterus.

Physiological management of third stage

This process facilitates the birth of the placenta physiologically and without interference. The midwife waits for the following signs of separation:

- uterine contractions
- slowing and cessation of umbilical cord pulsations
- lengthening of the umbilical cord
- gush of fresh blood or clots per vaginam
- placenta visible at the introitus of the vagina.

With the separation of the placenta, the woman will commonly experience low pelvic pain and heaviness as the placenta descends into the lower segment of the uterus. With contractions the woman may feel a pushing urge. She may find it helpful to be in an upright position to assist her to birth the placenta. The use of gravity and pelvic opening positions can facilitate this. It may be helpful to reassure the woman that the sensations when birthing the placenta won't be as intense as birthing the baby. Palpation of the uterus and/or application of traction to the umbilical cord are contraindicated during this process, as they are implicated in the potential for increased bleeding and retention of the placenta (Sinclair 2004). As the placenta descends into the vagina, the midwife can assist the woman to birth her placenta gently so that trailing membranes can be eased out and not trapped or torn. As part of the midwifery assessment of the woman's wellbeing it is important to monitor vaginal bleeding and uterine contractility immediately after the placenta's birth. Women at this time will often experience a great sense of relief and comfort. When physiological management has been chosen, the therapeutic use of uterotonic drugs, oxytocin and/or ergometrine are only indicated where there is increased or unexpected blood loss before or after the birth of the placenta or where the uterus is atonic.

BOX 22.1 Lotus birth

Some families choose to leave the placenta attached to the baby until the cord separates. This is known as a lotus birth. The cord is not cut, and once the placenta is born it is dried, salted and wrapped in pre-prepared leak-proof material. The wrapping is changed as needed and some also choose to place fresh rosemary or lavender next to the placenta. The cord dries within 24 hours and separates (with the placenta) from the baby within two to five days. Reasons for choosing a lotus birth include the following:

▸ The family must carry both the baby and the placenta, and so will tend to stay at home and rest.

▸ The cord falls off in a shorter time than when cut and requires no extra care.

▸ Some claim the baby is calmer and more in tune with her or his surroundings.

▸ It is thought to provide the baby with a natural, gentle transition to extra-uterine life from being connected to the mother.

(Source: Rachana 2000)

The timing of cutting the umbilical cord after pulsation ceases can be influenced by:

● the birth plan
● a short cord interfering with the woman's ability to hold the baby close to the breast
● waiting until the placenta is born
● plans for a lotus birth (see Box 22.1)
● the woman's request to change position in order to birth the placenta.

Active management of third stage

Early cord clamping, the administration of uterotonic drugs and the application of controlled cord traction (CCT) are used to shorten the time between the birth of the baby and the birth of the placenta and membranes. This is referred to as active management and the impetus for this is the prevention of postpartum haemorrhage (PPH) (Prenderville & Elbourne 2000).

If uterotonic drugs are used during labour, it is important to continue with the active management procedures of cord clamping and CCT, as the physiological process has been interfered with. Mixing active and physiological care has been associated with adverse effects for the woman and her baby (Rogers et al 1998).

The research concerning management of the birth of the placenta and membranes has been conducted in obstetric settings where physiological management is not necessarily understood. There is a need for studies to be undertaken in a variety of birth settings that investigate third stage practices and outcomes where practitioners are more familiar with physiological management.

Midwives should be aware that blood loss is often minimal in active management. However, it is often the case that when the woman gets up for a shower after the birth, she passes a large clot, and may feel faint and exhibit signs of blood loss. Often this hidden blood loss is not

---

TABLE 22.4 Management of third stage

Physiological management	Active management
1 Observe for signs of separation.	1 Administer oxytocic after birth of anterior shoulder or after birth of the baby (if midwife is alone).
2 Continuously observe blood loss.	
3 Assist the woman into a comfortable and upright position for birthing placenta.	2 Clamp and cut the cord.
	3 Feel for uterine contraction.
4 Encourage the woman to push the placenta out.	4 Apply controlled cord traction by winding fingers around cord and applying sustained downward traction; when the placenta is visible, apply upward traction to follow the curve of the birth canal.
5 Ease the placenta and membranes out.	
6 Note the time.	
7 Clamp and cut the cord after it has stopped pulsating.	5 While traction is applied, counterpressure can be provided with the other hand placed above the symphysis pubis.
8 Palpate the uterus to ensure it is contracted.	6 Note the time of delivery of the placenta.
9 Estimate the blood loss.	7 Palpate the uterus to ensure it is contracted.
10 Complete the documentation.	8 Estimate the blood loss.
	9 Complete the documentation.

Note: Do not mix methods; do not stimulate the uterus by 'fundal fiddling' as this may lead to partial separation of the placenta and blood loss.

recorded and is not recognised in the literature about active management.

Examination of the placenta and membranes

Careful and thorough inspection of the placenta and membranes will need to be undertaken soon after the birth. If there is evidence of retained products, it is important to be aware of this as it may predispose the woman to bleeding or infection. During the examination of the placenta it is ideal to include the woman and her family in this fascinating exploration and to explain your findings with them. The aim is to identify the following:

- condition of the placenta and membranes
- number of vessels in the cord, insertion site and presence of knots
- signs of absence of cotyledons, including vessels through the membranes
- completeness of the membranes.

Assessing injury to the woman's labial, vaginal and perineal area

Episiotomy should be avoided during a normal birth and every effort should be made to minimise perineal injury and discomfort (Karacam & Eroglu 2003). Sometimes, however, a tear to the woman's perineum, vagina or labial area is unavoidable and it is the midwife's role to make a careful assessment of the degree of trauma to this area. The assessment does not need to be done immediately, as every effort should be made to establish bonding between the woman and her baby and to give them time to explore each other and initiate breastfeeding. (Ch 25 provides information about assessment of perineal trauma and repair.)

Ongoing assessment

Following the birth of the placenta and the perineal assessment and repair, the midwife needs to estimate the blood loss sustained and its effect on the woman. This is calculated by measuring actual blood loss and making a visual assessment of bloodstained linen, combined with assessment of the woman's wellbeing, including measurements of pulse and blood pressure. The actual amount of blood loss estimated is subjective. Each woman's individual response will need to be carefully assessed by the midwife. Palpation of the uterus and assessment of the fundal height to confirm that it is contracted and central assures the midwife that the woman's body is responding appropriately. Encouraging the woman to palpate her own uterus and recognise when it is well contracted or otherwise enables her to take responsibility for her wellbeing and know when to ask for assistance.

Examination of the baby

Assessment of the baby occurs from the moment she or he is born. Observing the baby in her mother's arms, her body movements, colour and alertness, allows the midwife to ensure that the baby has made an effective transition from unborn to newborn. The first hour or so of the baby's life will be spent in skin-to-skin contact with her mother and feeding at the breast. At some stage following this it is appropriate for the midwife to examine the baby and to discuss her findings with the parents. It is important that the room is warm and that the baby does not become cold during this assessment. Wrapping the baby in soft warm towels and exposing only the part of the baby you are examining not only keeps the baby warm but also helps to keep the baby calm. It is important to remember that she has just come from the warm, confined space of her mother's uterus. Babies will often cry if unwrapped and left naked, and this can be distressing for the baby and the parents. (Information about full examination of the newborn baby can be found in Ch 27.)

Ongoing care in the first few hours

The woman has expended an enormous amount of effort and will need to eat and drink to help restore her energy. Some families may have a special meal ready to celebrate the birth, others may have cultural preferences about the type of food first consumed after the birth of a baby and yet others know they are hungry but can't think what they would like to eat. Offering light food and fluids is helpful, and organising this can enable the midwife to give the new family some time to themselves.

When the woman is ready, she may like to have a shower or bath. It is important to assist the woman and ensure that she is feeling able to manage; she should not be left alone but given the privacy that she requires. A wash in bed may be more helpful for a woman who is tired and lacking energy. A seat in the shower can provide support if the woman is feeling weak and tired. This is also a useful time for the woman to try to empty her bladder. Encouraging the woman to empty her bladder within an hour or two of the birth is important for a number of reasons:

- It confirms that the woman can empty her bladder and that there are no issues of retention of urine possibly caused by trauma and/or oedema.
- A full bladder can impede effective uterine contractions and therefore increase the potential for bleeding.
- It reduces discomfort.
- Being upright can assist the expulsion of any clots that may have collected in the vagina/cervix.

As the birth process can sometimes result in a loss of bladder sensation initially, encouraging the woman to empty her bladder regularly, every two to three hours, in the first 12 hours or so after the birth, assists the uterus to remain contracted. It also enables the woman to recognise that her bladder is filling. Emptying her bladder regularly, especially just prior to breastfeeding, can help reduce the severity of the 'afterpains' that many women experience in the early postpartum period.

Afterpains (postnatal uterine contractions) are more commonly associated with multiparous women and with breastfeeding, but women can experience afterpains whether or not they have had a baby before and regardless of how they are feeding their baby. There has been a tendency to dismiss these as a mild inconvenience. However, there is a wide variation in women's experiences of afterpains. Some women feel the afterpains to be mildly uncomfortable and others describe them as excruciating or not dissimilar to labour pains. As the uterus contracts there is also usually a concurrent increase in bleeding and this may include some clots. The oxytocin release resulting from breastfeeding can strengthen afterpains and cause women to be fearful when latching their baby. It is helpful to explain to women what the afterpains are and what they achieve. For many women, afterpains settle after a few days but they can last up to a week or so for others. In the initial period after the birth, applying heat to the lower abdomen can be comforting. Ensuring the bladder is empty and not creating pressure on the uterus will also help. Acknowledging that afterpains can be distressing is important for women who may be worried that something is wrong.

Documentation

Documentation of the labour and birth process and the ongoing care provided is intended to give a comprehensive and accurate account of the woman and her baby's experience and wellbeing. Any plans, decision points and actions taken, as well as their outcome, should be recorded. The aim when documenting is to provide a contemporaneously written record of events as they occur. As mentioned previously, this may not be possible at all times but relevant times and events should be noted for further elucidation later. All documentation written retrospectively should be acknowledged as such. In the first few hours after the birth there is often opportunity for the midwife to complete the appropriate documentation. This will include:

- an accurate description of the labour and birth events, actions taken and outcome
- the woman's and baby's responses to the birth and each other
- description of the birth of the placenta and membranes, the examination and any findings—either normal or abnormal, blood samples taken and estimation of the woman's blood loss
- description of the assessment of perineal and vaginal trauma, and the process of any repair undertaken, including suture material and technique used
- assessment of the woman's and baby's wellbeing, including the results of any examinations undertaken, with attention drawn to any concerns and the midwife's actions in response to this
- timing of any drugs given, reason for administration and response

- completing any requirements for notification of birth, newborn records, maternity facility documentation
- midwife's assessment of the woman's and baby's wellbeing prior to the midwife leaving the woman's home, handing care to postnatal ward staff or the woman going home
- any specific plans for the next 12 hours or so regarding rest, breastfeeding, self-care and contacting/accessing caregivers.

Conclusion

The essence of being able to provide midwifery support for women in physiological labour involves a number of beliefs, attitudes and practices. The importance of the midwife–woman relationship and its development over time cannot be overestimated. This relationship enables the woman and the midwife to learn to understand one another, and the midwife to come to know what and who are important for this particular woman. This 'knowing' can enable the midwife to be 'with woman' in the full sense of the term.

Understanding the physiological process of labour and birth enables the midwife to recognise that each woman will respond in her own way. This encompasses the physical, psychological, emotional and spiritual dimensions. What is normal for one woman may be abnormal for another. Being present, and the quality of that presence, enables the midwife to support the woman in the way that is most appropriate for that situation. Not all women wish for a constant presence but when they want the midwife they want her to be 'there'. Being in the room is not enough: it is important to listen and attend to the woman and her supporters. This is most easily achieved through continuity of care provided by a known carer. Words of praise, comfort, encouragement and reassurance are all valuable tools of the midwife who actually means them (Page 2000).

Midwives can support women through labour and its ebbs and flows, by being available to the woman, encouraging and comforting her and helping her support people to do the same. Labour and birth are challenging for most women and they require understanding and belief to work through the challenge. Labours can be affected by a multitude of issues, and the midwife who recognises the potential impact of these issues will be in a position to assist the woman.

There are a variety of assessment tools that midwives can use to identify that labour is progressing. The skilful midwife will use these tools in combination with her observations and knowing of the woman. Understanding the effect of mobility, positions, gravity and environment can enable the midwife to assist the woman through her labour, especially when it is hard work. Knowledge of what supports and what may adversely affect the physiological process are key skills for a midwife.

Review questions

1 What elements is it important to include in a birth plan to enable the midwife to provide effective support during labour?

2 What impact might the birthing environment have on a woman's ability to labour and birth normally?

3 How would a midwife distinguish between latent and active labour?

4 What support does a midwife require to be able to provide a continuous, attentive presence during a woman's childbirth experience?

5 What are the signs that a woman in labour is dehydrated?

6 What key information is gained from a vaginal examination?

7 Describe how to monitor the fetal heart effectively in a normal labour.

8 List the signs of a non-reassuring fetal heart rate.

9 What are the signs of lack of progress in labour?

10 What are the differences between physiological management and active management of the third stage of labour?

Online resources

Active Birth Centre, http://www.activebirthcentre.com/pb/index.shtml
Homebirth Aotearoa, http://www.homebirth.org.nz
La Leche League, NZ, http://www.lalecheleague.org/LLLNZ/
MIDIRS website, http://www.midirs.org/
Midwifery Today, http://www.midwiferytoday.com/
National Institute for Health and Clinical Excellence, http://www.nice.org.uk
New Zealand College of Midwives, http://www.midwife.org.nz/
World Health Organization, Care in normal birth, http://www.reproductive-health/publications

References

Albers L 1999 The duration of labour in healthy women. Journal of Perinatology 19(2):114–119

Albers L, Anderson D, Cragin L 1997 The relationship of ambulation in labour to operative delivery. Journal of Nurse-Midwifery 42(1):4–8

Banks M 2003 Utilizing the unborn baby's in-labour movements. New Zealand College of Midwives Journal 29:6

Baston H 2004 Midwifery basics: care during labour. The first stage of labour. The Practising Midwife 7(1):32–36

Chapman V 2003 The midwife's labour and birth handbook. Blackwell Science, Oxford

Cluett E 2000 The onset of labour. 2: Implications for practice. The Practising Midwife 3(7):16–19

Crowther C 2000 Monitoring progress in labour. In: M Enkin, M Keirse, J Neilson et al (Eds) A guide to effective care in pregnancy and birth. Oxford University Press, Oxford

Daellenbach R 1999 Midwifery partnerships: a consumer's perspective. New Zealand College of Midwives Journal 21:22–23

Downe S 2000 A proposal for a new research and practice agenda for birth. MIDIRS Midwifery Digest 10(3):337–341

Downe S 2003 Transition and the second stage of labour. In: D Fraser, M Cooper (Eds) Myles textbook for midwives. Churchill Livingstone, London, pp 487–506

Enkin M, Keirse M, Neilson J et al 2000 A guide to effective care in pregnancy and birth. Oxford University Press, Oxford

Fox M, Kilpatrick S, King T et al 2000 Fetal heart rate monitoring: interpretation and collaborative management. Journal of Midwifery and Women's Health 45(6):495–507

Fraser W, Turcot L, Krauss I et al 2004 Amniotomy for shortening spontaneous labour. The Cochrane Library (2), Oxford

Friedman E 1954 The graphic analysis of labour. American Journal of Obstetrics and Gynaecology 68:1568–1575

Goffinet F, Fraser W, Marcoux S et al 1997 Early amniotomy increases the frequency of fetal heart abnormalities. British Journal of Obstetrics and Gynaecology 104(5):548–553

Gould D 2000 Normal labour: a concept analysis. Journal of Advanced Nursing 31:418–427

Guilliland K, Pairman S 1995. The midwifery partnership (monograph series: 95/1). Victoria University, Wellington

Gupta JK, Hofmeyr G 2004 Positions for women during second stage of labour. Cochrane Database of Systematic Reviews (2): CD002006

Henderson C, Macdonald S (Eds) 1988 Mayes midwifery. A textbook for midwives (11th edn). Ballière Tindall, Edinburgh

Henderson C, Macdonald S (Eds) 2004 Mayes midwifery. A textbook for midwives (13th edn). Ballière Tindall, Edinburgh

Hodnett E 2003 Home-like versus conventional institutional settings for birth (Cochrane Review). Cochrane Library (4). John Wiley & Sons, Chichester

Iffy L, Vavadi V, Papp E 2001 Untoward neonatal sequelae deriving from cutting of the umbilical cord before delivery. Medical Law 20(4):627–634

Jackson K 2000 The bottom line: care of the perineum must be improved. British Journal of Midwifery 8(10):609–614

Karacam Z, Eroglu K 2003 Effects of episiotomy on bonding and mother's health. Journal of Advanced Nursing 43(4):3843–3894

Kitzinger S 1997 Authoritative touch in childbirth. In: RE Davis-Floyd, CF Sargent (Eds) Childbirth and authoritative knowledge: cross cultural perspectives. University of California Press

Lavender T, Alfirevic Z, Walkinshaw S 1998 Partogram action line study: a randomised trial. British Journal of Obstetrics and Gynaecology 105(19):976–980

Levene M, Tudehope D 1993 Essentials of neonatal medicine. Blackwell Science, Oxford

Long L 2003 Defining third stage of labour care and discussing optimal practice. MIDIRS Midwifery Digest 13(3):366–370

McCandlish R, Bower U, van Asten H et al 1998 A randomised controlled trial of care of the perineum during the second stage of normal labour (HOOP Trial). British Journal of Obstetrics and Gynaecology 105:1262–1272

McCormick C 2003 The first stage of labour. In: D Frazer, M Cooper (Eds) Myles textbook for midwives (14th edn). Churchill Livingstone, London, pp 445–469

MacLennan A, Crowther C, Derham R 1994 Does the option to ambulate during spontaneous labour confer any advantage or disadvantage? Journal of Maternal and Fetal Medicine 3(1):43–48

Mechthild M, Gross T, Haunschild T et al 2003 Women's recognition of the spontaneous onset of labor. Birth 30(4):267–271

Mercer JS 2001 Current best evidence: a review of the literature on umbilical cord clamping. Journal of Midwifery and Women's Health 46(6):402–414

Micklewright A, Champion P 2002 Labouring over food: the dietician's view. In: P Champion, C McCormick (Eds) Eating and drinking in labour. Reed, London, pp 29–45

National Institute for Clinical Excellence (NICE) 2001 Guideline C. The use of electronic fetal monitoring: the use and interpretation of cardiotocography in intrapartum fetal surveillance. NICE, London

New Zealand College of Midwives (NZCOM) 2005 Handbook for practice. NZCOM, Christchurch, NZ

Newburn M 2003 Culture, control and the birth environment. The Practising Midwife 6(8):20–25

O'Connell MP, Mussain J, Maclennan FA et al 2003 Factors associated with a prolonged second stage of labour: a case-controlled study of 364 nulliparous labours. Journal of Obstetric Gynaecology 22(3):253–257

Odent M 1999 The scientification of love. Free Association Books, London

Okosun H, Arulkumaran S 2005 Intrapartum fetal surveillance. Current Obstetrics and Gynaecology 15(1):18–24

Page L 2000 Keeping birth normal. In: L Page, P Percival (Eds) The new midwifery. Science and sensitivity in practice. Churchill Livingstone, London, pp 105–121

Pairman S 1998 Women-centred midwifery: partnerships or professional friendships? New Zealand College of Midwives Journal 19:5–10

Parratt J, Fahy K 2004 Creating a 'safe' place for birth: an empirically grounded theory. New Zealand College of Midwives Journal 30:11–14

Pengelley P 2002 Eating and drinking in labour: the consumer's view. In: P Champion, C McCormick (Eds) Eating and drinking in labour. Reed, Oxford, pp 111–123

Philpott R, Castle W 1972 Cervicographs in the management of labour on primigravidae 1. The alert line for detecting normal labour. Journal of Obstetrics and Gynaecology of the British Commonwealth 79:592–598

Prendiville W, Elbourne D 2000 The third stage of labour. Ch 33. In: M Enkin, M Kierse, J Neilson et al (Eds) A guide to effective care in pregnancy and childbirth (3rd edn). Oxford University Press, Oxford

Rabe H, Reynolds G, Diaz-Rossello J 2004 Early versus delayed umbilical cord clamping in preterm infants. Cochrane Database of Systematic Reviews (3)

Rachana S 2000 Lotus birth. Greenwood Press, Victoria

Rogers J, Wood J, McCandlish R et al 1998 Active versus expectant management of the third stage of labour: the Hitchingbrook randomised controlled trial. Lancet 351:693–699

Rosser J 2003 Women's position in second stage: a Cochrane database review. In: S Wickham (Ed) Midwifery: best practice. Books for Midwives. Elsevier, Edinburgh

Seitchik J 1987 The management of functional dystocia in the first stage of labour. Clinical Obstetrics and Gynaecology 30(1):42–49

Simpkin P, Ancheta R 2000 The labour progress handbook. Blackwell Science, Oxford

Sinclair C 2004 A midwife's handbook. Saunders, Missouri

Sleep J, Roberts J, Chalmers I 2000 Second stage of labour. In: M Enkin, M Keirse, J Neilson et al (Eds) A guide to effective care in pregnancy and birth. Oxford University Press, Oxford

Stables D 1999 Physiology in childbearing with anatomy and related biosciences. Baillière Tindall, London

Stuart C 2000 Invasive actions in labour. Where have all the 'old tricks' gone? The Practising Midwife 3(8):30–33

Studd J 1973 Partograms and nomograms of cervical dilatation in management of primigravid labour. British Medical Journal 4: 411–455

Sutton J 2003 Occipito-posterior positioning and some ideas about how to change it. In: S Wickham (Ed) Midwifery best practice. Books for midwives. Elsevier Science, London

Vincent P 2002 Babycatcher—chronicles of a modern midwife. Scribner, New York

Walmsley K 2003 Caring for women during the latent phase of labour. In: S Wickham (Ed.) Midwifery: best practice. Books for midwives, Elsevier Science, London

Walsh D 2000a Part three: assessing women's progress in labour. British Journal of Midwifery 8(7):449–455

Walsh D 2000b Part six: limits on pushing and time in the second stage. British Journal of Midwifery 8(10):604–608

Walsh D 2001 Are midwives losing the art of keeping birth normal? British Journal of Midwifery 9(3):146

Walsh D 2004 Care in the first stage of labour. In: C Henderson, S Macdonald (Eds) Mayes midwifery. A textbook for midwives (13th edn). Ballière Tindall, Edinburgh

Wickham S 2003 To feel or not to feel? Checking the nuchal cord. The Practising Midwife 6(2):27

Yao AC, Lind J 1969 Effect of gravity on placental transfusion. Lancet 2(7619):505–508

Yao AC, Moinan M, Lind J 1969 Distribution of blood between infant and placenta after birth. Lancet 2(7626):871–873

Further reading

Davis E, Harrison L, Arms S 1997 Heart and hands: a midwifes' guide to pregnancy and birth (3rd edn). Celestial Arts, Berkeley, California

Downe S (Ed) 2004 Normal childbirth: evidence and debate. Churchill Livingstone, London

Frye A 2004 Holistic midwifery. Vol II. A comprehensive textbook for midwives in homebirth practice; care of the mother and baby from the onset of labour through the hours after birth. Labrys Press, Oregon

Gaskin I 2003 Ina May's guide to childbirth. Random House, NY

Halldordottir S, Karlsdottir S 1996 Empowerment or discouragement: women's experience of caring and uncaring encounters in childbirth. Healthcare for Women International 17(4):361–379

Hodnett E 2001 Caregiver support for women during childbirth. Cochrane Library (4). Update Software, Oxford

Robertson A 1997 The midwife companion. ACE Graphics, Sydney

Thompson F 2004 Mothers and midwives. The ethical journey. Books for midwives. Elsevier Science, London

CHAPTER 23

Working with pain in labour

Nicky Leap and Stephanie Vague

Key terms

'being with' women, control, empowerment, labour pain, midwife–woman relationship, non-pharmacological pain relief

Chapter overview

This chapter explores the midwifery art of being with women in pain with labour. The advantages of promoting women's confidence in their ability to cope with pain are discussed in relation to evidence that supports this approach. Historical, psychosocial, cultural and feminist perspectives on pain in labour are presented in order to inform and highlight exemplary midwifery practice.

Learning outcome

The learning outcome for this chapter is to encourage midwives to consider how they engage with women around in labour in order to promote women's sense of confidence, ability and self-esteem

Introduction

This chapter is concerned with the midwifery art of being with women in pain in labour. As such, it explores the rationale for engaging with women and their families[1] around the role of pain in normal birth. While acknowledging that midwives must be prepared to support all women in labour, including those who choose to use pain medication (van Hoover 2000), it is not the intent of this chapter to give midwives information about specific methods of 'pain relief' and their administration; there are comprehensive textbooks about pain in childbirth that cover this more fully than is possible here.[2]

There are also handbooks that explore the practicalities of supporting labouring women using 'active birth' techniques (Robertson 1994; Simkin & Anchetta 2000). The authors of this chapter are assuming that midwives will be aware of the benefits of providing supportive strategies such as encouraging women to move around, find positions that feel right and make noise if they wish. It is essential that midwives have these skills if they are to work with women in pain and encourage normal birth. In a culture where epidural anaesthesia is increasingly being promoted, it is also important that midwives are able to articulate why there is value in working with pain in labour, as opposed to taking away pain (Leap & Anderson 2004). This is especially important because, although there has been an increase in numbers of women wanting to use epidurals, there has also been an increase in those wanting to avoid all kinds of analgesia (Henry & Nand 2004; Horrowitz et al 2004).

It has been suggested that anticipation of labour pain causes intense anxiety for many women (Coombes & Schonveld 1992; Lowe 1989; Shearer 1995) and that this can have a negative effect on their experience of birth (Green et al 1988). This chapter offers an overview of the evidence that midwives can draw on in order to engage with women around pain in labour, with a view to addressing these anxieties and enabling situations in which women can feel more powerful and confident as a result of their experiences of pregnancy and birth. In order to achieve this, it is imperative that midwives explore and appreciate the various meanings that may be associated with labour pain for individual women and their families (Mander 2000). An understanding of how perspectives on the physiology of pain and the culture of 'pain relief in labour' have evolved over the past century in industrialised countries will provide a starting point.

Historical perspectives on pain in labour

A comprehensive history of the development of pain theories can be found in Melzack and Wall's *The Challenge of Pain* (1988). The traditional theory of pain is known as 'specificity theory'. Pain is seen as no more than a particularly complex signal, broadcast over nerves leading from the site of injury to the brain, as first suggested by Descartes in 1664 and modified by Muller in 1842 and von Frey in 1894. Various theories on pain were developed in the first half of the twentieth century but a major breakthrough occurred in 1965 when Melzack and Wall proposed the 'gate control theory of pain'; this provided a conceptual framework for understanding how pain messages are filtered and facilitated or inhibited through a 'gate' in the spinal cord that modulates reception and responses (Melzack & Wall 1965). In recent years, Melzack (1999) has proposed the 'neuromatrix' theory of pain, which retains key elements of the 'gate theory', but includes additional inputs from the brain. Memory, emotion, cultural factors, stress regulation, immune systems and past experiences play a role in how the brain processes and synthesises genetic and sensory nerve impulses. The neuromatrix theory of pain can be used to enable understandings about the complexity of responses to pain and may also provide a framework for exploring the beneficial effects of non-pharmacological methods of pain relief in labour (Trout 2004).

The notion of a systematic approach to 'pain control' in labour begins in Edinburgh with the experimental work of James Young Simpson in the 1840s (Caton 1999). Simpson's introduction of inhalation anaesthesia in childbirth spawned a series of campaigns led by middle-class women demanding access to this resource. Such demands played a significant role in the move from home to hospital birth in the twentieth century. Debates and concerns about the advisability of analgesia and anaesthesia in terms of safety and possible physical and psychological consequences have changed little since Simpson's day. The potential harmful side-effects of drugs and the social value of pain versus the preservation of meaning in childbirth when pain is removed continue to be hotly debated issues (Caton 1999) that affect how women approach labour pain.

In the early 1930s, Grantly Dick-Read published *Childbirth without fear: the principles and practice of natural childbirth* (Dick-Read 1933). This book launched the concept of eliminating the cycle of 'fear, tension and pain' through counteractive education and training. Gentle, coached breathing and relaxation, with the emphasis on collaboration with a coach, were to play a vital role in keeping the woman on course in the teachings of the natural childbirth movement and later the 'psychoprophylaxis' movement in Europe and North America. In the latter decades of the twentieth century, the mechanistic focus of psychoprophylaxis increasingly gave way to the psychosexual approach, a model that sees acceptance of labour as purposeful within the highly charged, significant act of giving birth, with its far-reaching sequel for women's lives (Kitzinger 1962, 1987). This approach became incorporated into that of the active birth movement (Balaskas 1983), which drew on activities and philosophies associated with the yoga tradition in teaching women to develop 'all of their bodily resources for giving birth, to follow their own instincts and to take full control of the childbirth experience' (Balaskas 1992, back cover).

In the 1980s, a new dimension to understanding pain in labour, incorporating neuro-hormonal physiology, was provided by Michel Odent (1984), who proposed that intrinsic opiates, such as the endorphins released by marathon runners, enable labouring women to enter a state of consciousness that enhances the progress of labour as well as providing a way of coping with pain. Odent drew on the work of Newton and colleagues (Newton et al 1966, 1968) in suggesting that privacy, intimacy and non-disturbance are required to enable the delicate balance of hormonal cascades to interact and promote effective physiological processes. Odent (1984, p 14) described the 'virtually ecstatic state' induced by endogenous opiates where women labour undisturbed as something that has always been sensed. This 'sense' of women having some 'inbuilt' coping mechanism has probably always been familiar to midwives in the absence of any physiological explanations, as described here by a retired midwife who practised in the 1930s in Britain:

> I think myself that the system has a certain amount of sedative in itself that it releases at a time like that. I'm sure it has, because I've seen people that looked as if they were half sozzled—and they didn't have anything! Just looked like somebody 'gone'—and they hadn't had any dope (Leap & Hunter 1993, pp 168–9).

The familiarity of women disappearing into their own world in strong labour meant that midwives and childbirth educators embraced the theory of the body's own pain-modifying substances as 'Nature's reward' (Ginesi 1996, p 9). A full scientific description of the role of endogenous opioids in spontaneous labour is needed if 'endorphin' theory is to be given widespread credence. However, it is thought that incoming impulses of pain stimulate the release of encephalins, dynorphins and endorphins in the dorsal horn of the spinal cord and that these opioid-peptides have the ability to inhibit the sensations of pain carried by neurons to the brain.

Overall, in the past few decades, challenges to the concept of managing labour pain with anaesthesia and analgesia in industrialised societies have tended to concentrate on 'non-pharmacological methods of pain relief' (Simkin 1989) and have therefore often upheld the basic concept of controlling and minimising pain. Midwives who have written about the role of the midwife in relation to pain in labour have continued this trend by focusing on the skills needed to facilitate 'pain relief' (Moore 1994). With the development of antenatal education came a belief that midwives should be preparing women for labour by giving them 'informed choice' about all the 'methods of pain relief', the benefits and disadvantages of each.

In recent years, the offering of what Leap (2000b) has referred to as the 'menu' of various methods of 'pain relief' has been associated with the notion of a woman's right to make 'informed choices' about all aspects of her care (Department of Health 1993; NHMRC 1996). This approach requires practitioners to adopt a systematic approach to explaining the advantages and disadvantages of each method 'on the menu' so that the woman may make appropriate choices, usually in advance of labour. Many practitioners and women therefore assume that some form of pain relief in labour is necessary. This assumption also underpins most research in

the area. In contrast, midwives are increasingly articulating an approach that contributes to positive birthing experiences through building women's confidence in their ability to find ways to deal with labour pain through drawing on their own resources (McCrea et al 2000). The rationale for this 'working with pain' approach rests in a belief that pain is purposeful in promoting normal birth and that the 'triumph' women experience after a drug-free labour can have far-reaching consequences for how they feel about their capabilities as women and as mothers (Anderson 2000; Leap 2000b; Leap & Anderson 2004). Listening to women's ideas and experiences concerning pain in labour reinforces this theory.

Women's perspectives on pain in labour

Labour pain is complex and it is thought that the experience of pain itself may be mediated by physical, psychological, spiritual and cultural factors such as tradition, anxiety, emotional associations, the position of the baby in utero, and levels of preparation and support (Mander 1998). Importantly, effective forms of pain relief are not necessarily associated with greater satisfaction when women evaluate their experience of birth (Heinz & Sleigh 2003; Hodnett 2002; Morgan et al 1982; Ross 1998). Studies have repeatedly shown that the quality of support and the caregiver relationship are so important to women that they override the influences of age, socioeconomic status, ethnicity, childbirth preparation and the physical birth environment; the influence of pain, pain relief and intrapartum medical interventions on subsequent satisfaction are not as obvious, direct or powerful as the influence of the attitudes of the caregivers (Hodnett 2002).

Women have identified that support for coping with labour pain and access to different ways of reducing or relieving pain is important to them (Chamberlain et al 1993; Lundgren & Dahlberg 1998, 2002). The quality of these supportive interactions is more important to women than the level of pain per se (Callister et al 2003) and the attitudes of midwives have a profound impact on how women feel about their labours (Kitzinger 2000). It has been suggested that a form of reconstruction occurs after birth, when memories of labour pain are based on recall of the remembered emotional and behavioural consequences of the pain (Terry & Gijsberg 2000) and the meanings ascribed to the pain (Mander 2000).

In a number of studies, women have expressed satisfaction with the midwifery care they received when the midwife was 'present' in offering support and information (Hodnett 2002). They also valued feeling respected, and commented on the sense of trust that evolved, even when they had often not met the midwives prior to labour (Berg et al 1996). Culturally diverse groups of women have described childbirth as a difficult but empowering experience leading to a sense of achievement and a feeling of pride in their ability to cope with intense pain (Callister et al 2003; Dickenson et al 2003; Halldorsdottir & Karlsdottir 1996; Lundgren & Dahlberg

1998; Niven & Murphy-Black 2000). In contrast, women who have had obstetric intervention, particularly those who had unknown attendants, describe increased anxiety and pain, and place less emphasis on their active participation in birth (Callister et al 2003).

The rise in epidural and elective caesarean section rates has been apportioned to women making choices that help them deal with uncertainty and the fear of pain in labour (Silverton 2001). However, practice regarding epidurals, narcotics and elective caesarean section varies greatly regionally, between different maternity units and according to practitioner employment status, with particularly high rates in the private obstetrics sector (Roberts et al 2000). Variations appear often to be related to institutional or professional opinion factors rather than population factors or individual women's choices (Hodnett 2002).

Women who express a desire to have a normal birth often cite concerns about the side-effects associated with the use of narcotics and epidurals in labour as a major source of motivation (Henry & Nand 2004; Souter 2004). Such concerns sit within wider debates about the potential public and psychological health impact of rates of intervention that are above those indicated by current evidence (Johanson et al 2002).

Although epidural analgesia is very effective in reducing pain, it is associated with increased risks of prolonged labour, fetal malposition, augmentation and instrumental vaginal birth (Anim-Somuah et al 2005; Howell 2002; Howell et al 2001; Mayberry et al 2002). Controlled observational studies also indicate a possible association with higher caesarean section rates, and although these findings must be viewed with caution due to methodological challenges, there is sufficient evidence to warrant concern. There has also been a suggestion that the rate of crossover in trials is masking the relationship between epidurals and caesarean section (Lieberman 2004). The only uncontaminated randomised controlled trial to demonstrate an association between epidural and caesarean section was published over 12 years ago (Thorpe et al 1993). This small trial showed that women having first babies who were randomised to have an epidural were 11.4 times more likely to have a caesarean due to dystocia than women who were randomised to have narcotic analgesia. The trial was discontinued on the grounds that it was unethical to continue to randomise women to have an epidural. Concerns have been raised that supportive midwifery care may be jeopardised by the monitoring activities associated with epidural analgesia in hospitals where there are high epidural rates; these concerns are particularly acute in terms of women's ability to care for women who choose non-pharmacological pain relief (Mayberry et al 2002).

The use of narcotics, such as pethidine, in labour is associated with harmful effects on the mother's birth experience, longer labours, compromise of the baby and difficulties initiating breastfeeding (Heelbeck 1999; Hunt 2002). Furthermore, while such drugs induce sedation and may therefore give caregivers the impression of having relieved pain, women overwhelmingly report on how ineffective narcotics are in

providing pain relief (Bricker & Lavender 2002; Olofsson et al 1996).

Studies comparing different types of pain have identified the severity of labour pain for the majority of women (Melzack & Wall 1965). However, the National Birthday Trust Fund Pain Relief in Labour Study (Chamberlain et al 1993) found major differences between the perceptions of over 1000 women and those of their birth attendants with regards to the experience of pain and the effectiveness of pain relief methods. Professionals' concepts of pain relief tended to be restricted to pharmacological methods—less so with midwives than with doctors—and they were more likely to agree with each other about the efficacy of different methods than with the women. This difference is understandable if one considers that, although today, books for women about childbirth tend to be illustrated throughout with personalised accounts of births, this is not generally the case with textbooks for professionals. Arney and Neill (1982) have suggested that professionals need to listen to the subjectivity of individual women's experience in order to move away from the one-dimensional approach based on anatomy and physiology. Like Bendelow and Williams (1995) and Martin (1987), they stress the importance of learning from narratives in order to make more appropriate responses to those in pain.

The particular quality of labour pain

The Association of Radical Midwives has always paid tribute to the value of learning from women's accounts of their births and, since its inception in 1978, its newsletter has consistently published birth stories written by women. An example is the moving account by Agnes Kotreba (1994), who gave birth after a fast labour, before the midwives arrived. Her account acknowledges aspects of loneliness, potential death, images of water, and the physical and mental challenges of pain that are common themes elsewhere.

> Dear God, how many more hours? I especially don't let myself panic or drown in this tidal wave which breaks my entrails and comes from a distance like the sound of a plane, intensifying until it gets intolerable, and then nothing—nothing, no pain whatsoever. I'm like cleansed, surprised, pulverized—Will I have the strength to endure the next attack? . . . I twist myself in pain . . . I think I emit a sound . . . so far I am unable to show my suffering, it's my business, my biggest intimacy, my most complete and total nudity (Kotreba 1994, pp 16–17).

When listening to such accounts, Kelpin (1992) suggests that it is not useful to compare labour pain to any other pain. She also questions the validity of fragmenting our understanding by analysing the pain of labour within different theories such as physical, psychological, sociological and cultural perspectives. She suggests that such approaches militate against the understanding of the nature of 'painfulness' as lived by women and mothers and that the inwardness of the birth experience is an opportunity to be attentive to:

> the deep significance of the momentous quality of the pain . . . As we are surrounded by the deep sense of inwardness, we are forced to recognize our independence, our loneliness, our selfhood. To

be conscious of our own existence. This actual self-consciousness exposes to us our wholeness, our strengths and our endurance (Kelpin 1992, p 101).

The pain of labour is constructed by Kelpin as an expression of 'the narrow gateway leading to release in the expanse of life' (p 101). The release she describes with the birth of the baby is given the significance of change from 'self-as-world' to 'baby-as-world' where a new pain comes with the awe of focusing on a new being. She quotes Phyllis Chesler (1979, p 281): 'Being born with motherhood is the sharpest pain I've known' and uses words like 'relief', 'disbelief', 'joy' and exhilaration to describe the excitement and poignancy of the new baby's presence (p 102). This exhilaration usually masks the ability to recall the exact nature of pain.

> But who can remember the pain [of childbirth], once it's over? All that remains of it is a shadow, not in the mind even, in the flesh. Pain marks you but too deep to see. Out of sight, out of mind (Atwood 1987, p 135).

Attempts to describe pain reinforce the elusive nature of pain but also the crossing of borders between the emotional and physical way it is experienced. Pain has a common language, as this passage illustrates:

> Pain … is stark and unyielding to decoration, pain fills the world to the hilt, bursting its edges in an unseemly way; pain doesn't admit anything else—it usurps all the space available (Kassabova 1999, p 52).

The pain described above is the pain expressed by a young woman who has had to leave her homeland and flee far across the world to a place of safety. Such is the universal nature of pain that it could equally well be describing the pain of a heart attack or the pain of labour. However, it should be noted that many women say that labour pain is quite different from any pain that is associated with injury or trauma but that this is hard to explain in concrete terms.

In her important study of pain, Elaine Scarry (1985) states that the person in pain may experience pain as 'the most vibrant example of what it is to have certainty': pain is 'effortlessly grasped', while for the onlooker, the other person's pain is so elusive that it could be seen as 'the primary model of what it is to have doubt'; here 'what is effortless is not grasping it' (Scarry 1985, p 4).

> Pain can be seen as capable of bringing about an absolute split between one's own sense of reality and that of another person, even when in close proximity [as during labour] (Scarry 1985, p 4).

This concept is significant for midwives who sit alongside women in pain; they can respond to cues given by the woman in order to offer support and suggestions but primarily the midwife's role is to help the woman identify her own spontaneous coping strategies (Escott et al 2004) and to be alert to aspects of care and the environment that disrupt these (Spiby et al 2004).

Studies have suggested that midwives consistently underestimate the intensity of pain experienced by women in labour (Chamberlain et al 1993; Niven 1994). This may be a coping mechanism on the part of midwives as the onlookers of pain. Scarry's reading of the role of the physician in hearing the fragmentary language of pain, 'coaxing it into clarity' in order to interpret it, could be applied to the role of the midwife, who equally needs not to bypass the person in pain as an 'unreliable narrator' since doubting people in pain amplifies their suffering (Scarry 1985, pp 6–7). However, recognising the severity of pain that a woman is suffering during labour does not necessarily equate to the need to offer pain relief. In fact, women identify that when they are in pain, any offer of pain relief is irresistible and undermines their confidence in their ability to cope without using pharmacological pain relief:

> I didn't really want an epidural. That wasn't what I was saying. What I wanted was something magic that no one's ever thought of before, that you were going to quickly invent right then to make it all better. But I really didn't want an epidural. It was an expression of my pain (Leap 1997, p 49).

Midwives have talked about the significance of the particular nature of pain in labour: its rhythms, the fact that it has a positive, finite goal and that it stops as soon as the baby is born and then cannot be recalled.

> Afterwards, I'm still emotionally and physically wrecked and they've moved on completely. It's like, through a fog they can remember the time they were pleading for an epidural but they've moved on. So that's been significant for me just in terms of women's ability to recover or move on or have a different agenda in a very short space of time. And that's given me enormous confidence to … just be there … and not see pain as long-term damage (Leap 1997, p 48).

Cultural perspectives on pain in labour

> Pain is never the sole creation of our anatomy and physiology; it emerges only at the intersection of bodies, minds and cultures. (Morris 1991, p 1)

New Zealand and Australia are multicultural societies and, as such, the midwife is likely to be involved in the care of women from a range of backgrounds, including Maori, Polynesian, Asian, Middle Eastern, African and European descent. She needs to be mindful that different cultural practices may be employed to help women cope with pain during labour. For some women, prayers may be read by family members or songs sung to provide support and to welcome a new member of the family. For some Maori women, these would be in the form of *karakia* or *waiata*.

Cultural perceptions and expressions of pain vary widely. Women from some European cultures, such as Greece and Italy, for example, tend to vocalise pain in an uninhibited fashion, while those from other cultures, such as Polynesian women, often appear to value stoicism. Samoan and Tongan women, therefore, may appear very calm during labour, with little outward show of their pain.

Midwives must be aware, however, of the potential pitfalls associated with ethnic stereotyping, and it is important never to assume that a woman will respond to labour pain in a culturally determined way. A book describing Maori women's experiences of pregnancy and birth, *Ukaipo* (Rimene et al 1998) highlighted communication as an area where possible misunderstandings could arise. One woman pointed to the fact that nodding the head after receiving information from a midwife does not necessarily indicate understanding. Sometimes it is merely an effort to try to please or just to acknowledge that the information has been heard.

Holroyd and colleagues' (1997) study of Hong Kong Chinese women's perception of support during labour from midwives describes how the cultural reluctance of women to express emotions meant that the midwives found it very difficult to interpret non-verbal expressions of pain, even though they were from the same ethnic background. Sometimes clues about the pain women are experiencing and the progress they are making can be as subtle as beads of perspiration on the upper lip, or a slight frown.

Bowler (1993) showed how midwives are in danger of stereotyping women according to their cultural background. In her study, she demonstrated how midwives dismissed Asian women in pain as 'making a fuss about nothing' because they were perceived to have a low pain threshold. This assumption led to women having pain relief withheld and receiving different treatment from that received by other women. The racist notion that all women who share a particular culture are the same can mask the needs of individual women and lead to poorer service provision.

While the pain of other peoples' bodies may be unknowable and indescribable, again, it is through listening to women that professionals may develop an understanding of the complex meanings that women attribute to pain. This may be significant in how midwives engage with women, and facilitate the way they approach pain in labour and how they reflect on it afterwards (Mander 2000). In particular, there is the potential to address issues related to power and control for individual women.

Enabling a sense of control

Enabling women to feel in control during labour is important if they are to feel confident and satisfied with the childbirth experience (Lavender et al 1999; McCrea et al 2000). A sense of control is of great significance to labouring women, although their definition of personal control is complex. For some women, control is associated with feeling in control of their emotions and behaviour in labour (Green et al 1998; Niven 1994). For others, control involves some participation in the decisions that are made about the management of their labour and birth (Berg et al 1996; Bluff & Holloway 1994; Green et al 1988; Halldorsdottir & Karlsdottir 1996; Hundley et al 2001; Niven 1994). However, as Green and colleagues (1988) found, choice can prove threatening for a woman because she is asked to assume responsibility for decisions or because she is overwhelmed by a plethora of options. Bluff and Holloway's important study (1994) coined the phrase 'They know best' where women and their partners believed that the midwife

knew what care was best, even when their own specific wishes were disregarded. This study clearly demonstrates a need for midwives to acknowledge the inequality and power dynamics within the relationship. The midwife is seen to hold much 'expert' knowledge and the potential exists for her to abuse the trust placed in her professional judgement. Conversely, the midwife can use the authoritative trust that is placed in her knowledge and experience to encourage women to believe that they can cope with pain in labour, even when the woman has lost confidence in her ability to do so. This often requires courage on the part of both. Resisting women's pleading for pain relief and insistence that they 'can't do it anymore' requires the midwife to be very clear that this is normal labour pain and that as soon as it stops, the woman is going to be very pleased that she 'did it all herself'.

The psychosocial dynamics of pain in labour

> To separate sense from emotion, body from mind is hardly useful when we are trying to understand the whole of female experience, and in particular a function—childbirth—so charged with unconscious and subjective power, and so dramatic in its sensations (Rich 1977, p 157).

Raphael-Leff (1986) has drawn on psychotherapeutic practice in suggesting that conscious and unconscious attitudes or 'orientations' to pregnancy, labour and motherhood will affect whether women see labour as a 'natural event' or a 'depleting, medical event' and that this in turn will affect their experience of labour pain. She encourages midwives to identify the psychological factors that may assist them in recognising and acknowledging individual women's needs in labour. However, it has been shown that stereotyping can occur when midwives attempt to apply an understanding of the psychological factors that may influence an individual's experience of pain in labour (Bowler 1993; Green et al 1990; Niven 1994). Experienced midwives are aware of the pitfalls in deciding who will or will not cope with the pain of normal labour.

> Women constantly shock me and I think I've learnt from those women. You could sit there and think, 'She's a hopeless case, she said her pain threshold's really low'—and all you've got to do is tell her she's doing well, that it's normal and allow her to get on with it in her own way, and I think she will (Leap 1997, p 44).

There has been a questioning of the tendency for midwives to feel that they should work out the deep psychological processes affecting the women they care for and that they should identify and help women get rid of the 'baggage' that might impede the process of childbirth (Leap 2000a; Oakley 1980). Concerns have been expressed about the disempowering effect that such approaches can have on women where there is a shift in the midwife's role from empathetic listener to a more interventionist psychological role (Gosden 1996; Gosden & Saul 1999). Midwives have described the fallacy of predicting how women might cope with pain in labour within a culture where such predictions are a regular feature of informal discussions dominated by 'psychological' value judgements (Leap 2000a).

Feminist perspectives on pain in labour

Adrienne Rich (1976) points out that metaphors of pain in childbirth can be related to wider feminist issues.

> The pains of labour have a peculiar centrality for women and for women's relationship—both as mothers and simply as female beings—to other kinds of painful experience (Rich 1976, p 158).

Rich describes uterine contractions in terms of 'pressing the self out of us' (p 158). She questions whether physical pain can be distinguished from alienation and fear, and poses the notion of 'creative' versus 'destructive' pain. She draws on the work of Simone Weil (1951) in highlighting the difference between the destructive affliction of powerlessness, which can be avoided, and the potentially creative power of pain that can lead to growth and enlightenment:

> where it is unavoidable, pain can be transformed into something usable, something which takes us beyond the limits of the experience itself into a further grasp of the essentials of life and the possibilities within us ... this insight illuminates much of the female condition, but in particular the experience of giving birth (Rich 1976, p 158)

Rich warns against labelling as 'pain' the complexity of each individual woman's physical experience of labour. Such reductionism can lead to the avoidance of pain through analgesia and anaesthesia, a process that Rich describes as:

> a new kind of prison for women—the prison of unconsciousness, of numbed sensations, of amnesia, and complete passivity ... a dangerous mechanism which can cause us to lose touch not just with our painful sensations but with ourselves. (Rich 1976, pp 158–9).

However, Rich advises caution when it comes to the metaphor of 'I am a woman giving birth to myself'. For most women there has always been a distinct lack of choice and very little consciousness around childbirth, let alone personal growth. Historically, women have always been told how they should feel about labour pain from the classic victimisation of 'Eve's curse' to the 'ecstatic fulfillment' of the natural birth movement (p 156). Rich makes a plea for us to view childbirth as a challenge rather than pain, 'as one way of knowing and coming to terms with our bodies, of discovering our physical and psychic resources' (p 157) as 'one experience of liberating ourselves from fear, passivity and alienation from our bodies' (p 184). She suggests that there are far-reaching implications in highlighting the need for women to be attended by midwives who respond to a woman's distressing labour as a cry for active care and support, not as a demand to have pain taken away or numbed.

> As long as birth—metaphorically or literally—remains an experience of passively handing over our bodies to male authority and technology, other kinds of social change can only minimally change our relationship to ourselves, to power, and to the world outside our bodies (Rich 1976, p 185).

Pain in labour and the notion of empowerment

> To have experienced birthing pain offers the possibilities of self knowledge, knowledge of our limitations and capabilities, knowledge of new life, as mother and of our place in the mysterious cycle of human life: birth, death and rebirth. As we birth our children, we, in a sense, birth ourselves. We are mothers, like our mothers, and our daughters after us (Kelpin 1992, p 103).

The notion of women 'being born' with their babies is described by one respondent in a study of single women who developed strategies in order to have children. In spite of an extremely traumatic labour and birth, she reported:

> It was about the best thing I ever experienced. I was totally amazed. The labour was like I had died ... I had just died. The minute she came out, I was born again. It was like we'd just been born together (Lewin 1985, p 135).

This young woman described how the birth led her to make significant changes in her life, in particular in relation to her own parents.

Robertson (1996, p 19) sees the universality of pain in labour as a bond between women, 'a fundamental truth that confirms our special biological role and affirms the importance of our contribution to society'. Feminists may have difficulty with Robertson's biological reductionism, especially when she refers to women's bodies as 'designed to be as efficient as possible' and describes 'the very few failures ... necessary to ensure reproductive success amongst strong breeding stock' (Robertson 1996, p 19). Robertson makes an impassioned plea for reclaiming pain in labour. She sees its role as vital in stimulating hormonal responses that allow a biological function to take place with optimum efficiency while at the same time promoting the 'innate sexuality' of the experience of labour. The body's 'natural painkillers' can be released and a positive emotional climate is ensured for the meeting of mother and child (Robertson 1996, p 19). Robertson (1994) describes 'transition' (the name given to the end of the first stage of labour, when women are generally expressing most difficulty with pain) as 'the moment of truth' and suggests that 'it may be very important to allow women to have the experience of conquering an overwhelming personal crisis, to promote confidence and self-esteem in the new mother' (Robertson 1994, p 92).

> Submission to the all-consuming and overwhelming nature of birth and the weathering of the inherent pain of labour is an empowering process for a woman, and one that should not be denied unless critical for her own well-being or that of her baby (Robertson 1994, p 88).

Martin (1987, p 202) suggests that the potential joy expressed by one respondent—'the joy will take away from the pain and I'm willing to face the pain'—stood as a lone image among others where women are passively being 'done to', where the concept of the 'involuntary uterine contractions' referred to in childbirth texts and classes creates a culture where women end up feeling a sense of alienation from their bodies:

> We are still a long way from seeing quintessentially female

functions as acts women do with body, mind and emotional states working together or at least affecting one another (Martin 1987, p 204)

Kathryn Allen Rabuzzi (1994) was originally inspired to write about the potential 'ecstasy' of birth after an unanticipated 'natural' birth in the late 1950s which left her with a quest to find out more about the extraordinary and unanticipated feelings of 'dying, being born, and giving birth' and the accompanying sensations of 'outward and inward expansion' (Rabuzzi 1994, p vii). She claims that in order for women to reframe the deeply acculturated belief that childbirth is painful and dangerous, they need to see pain as something to conquer, rather than something posing a threat to conquer us. This way, she suggests, its meaning, though not its intensity, may change, although she recognises that there is a potential problem with reconceptualising around 'control' when many midwives propose a 'letting go' approach to labour (Rabuzzi 1994, pp 98–105).

Pain in labour and the midwife–woman relationship

There is strong evidence that continuity of caregiver through-out pregnancy, labour and birth reduces the amount of pain relief women have during labour, and increases their satisfaction with their maternity care, particularly where women give birth at home (Hodnett 2003). This may be due to the relationship of trust that develops and the ability of midwives to enable situations where both women and midwives feel confident and positive when approaching birth (Reed 2002a,b; Walsh & Newburn 2002). In situations where there is not necessarily a midwifery relationship that has developed through pregnancy, women who have continuous support from a female caregiver who is not a professional during labour are less likely to use pharmacological pain relief and are more likely to have a spontaneous vaginal birth (Hodnett 2003). It may be that midwives who work in situations involving fragmented care are more likely to have to deal with the demands of the institution; they are less likely to be able to concentrate on intensive support of the woman than a lay person, such as a 'doula', who knows the woman and is focused on helping her to find her inner resources in coping with pain without resorting to pharmacological pain relief (Hodnett 2003).

Midwives enjoy a special position where they work with women throughout pregnancy, labour and the postnatal period. They begin to work with pain in labour during the antenatal period during discussions with a woman about the potential challenges of that pain. The midwife's interpretation of pain is a key factor in working with a woman before labour. She strives to convey the message that the pain of labour is a safe and purposeful pain that heralds the birth of the baby.

Midwives have the opportunity to help a woman prepare for her pain by exploring the particular nature of labour pain. It can be argued that this is different from other types of pain because it is of a positive nature. The pain is bringing a baby; it therefore has a different meaning for women (Soutter 2004). In industrialised societies, pain generally has negative connotations—it represents trauma, disease or stress, something fearful, to be avoided or alleviated—and it is therefore a challenge for midwives to help women (re)frame their understanding of pain. Given the high rates of epidural anaesthesia in Australia and New Zealand, the task of enabling situations where women embrace the pain of labour as part of a normal, physiological event is particularly challenging (Fenwick et al 2005).

Where a midwife is able to provide continuity of care through pregnancy, she also has the opportunity to engage with the people the woman has chosen to support her during labour, and explain to them the rationale for not automatically trying to take away pain in labour. This is particularly effective where midwives are able to visit the woman's home towards the end of pregnancy and make plans for the labour and birth, possibly sharing photographs of women in labour (Kemp 2003). This visit to the woman's home provides an ideal opportunity to talk about how being alongside the woman in pain might affect her supporters. The concept of decision-making about the place of birth during labour can be explored, with a clear message that it is safe to stay at home when labour is progressing well and where the midwife is well supported to provide this service by staff in a referral hospital.

Pain and the place of birth

Kitzinger (1991) has argued that the environment and relationships of those present at birth have a profound effect on the way a woman perceives and interprets pain. In a content analysis of letters describing 40 births at home and 40 births in hospital, she concluded that women giving birth at home feel more in control of the process and report less pain. This is in keeping with other studies that have concluded that women perceive home birth as less painful than hospital birth (Chamberlain et al 1997; Chamberlain et al 1993; Morse & Park 1988; Sandall et al 2001).

In making her decision about where to give birth, a woman often confronts her own beliefs and attitudes about the pain of labour. For some women, a hospital will be chosen because she expects that she will need pharmacological pain relief. This perception may reflect the attitudes and experiences of her family and friends who have also given birth in a hospital. Her choice may also be made because she is unaware of any alternatives to hospital birth.

Andrea Robertson (1996, p 20) sees pain as a biological tool to inform women when they are going into labour so that they can 'retire to a safe place while the process unfolds'. She decries the fact that 'of all the animal species on earth, human beings are the only ones who make their nests in one place, then trek elsewhere to give birth' (p 20) and suggests that this disruption may explain the difficulties experienced during birth by Western women. Helman (1990, p 203) suggests that the rituals associated with hospitalisation cause the patient to enter 'a state of limbo characterized by a sense of vulnerability and danger'. Shizuko and colleagues (1977, p 8) see this state as induced by entering 'a highly politicized area . . . the home terrain of the staff . . . who make and enforce the basic rules which prevail'.

During the antenatal period, decisions about where to give birth allow for discussions about managing pain and the implications of a woman's choice. This midwife describes the importance of thinking ahead about the place of birth in this context:

> If they're opting to have their babies at home . . . they have made it very clear what their perception of managing pain is and that's enormously helpful. They have made a statement about where they're coming from and also indicated that they are resourceful and prepared to rise to the challenge in a way that often women who choose to have their babies in hospital don't (Vague 2003, p 61).

Midwives know that women who choose to birth at home have consciously addressed the issue of how they will manage the pain of labour. They have faith in the ability of their body to birth the baby and trust in their own inner strength to allow this to happen. Where a woman chooses to give birth at a birthing centre or in hospital, she can be encouraged to anticipate spending a significant part of her labour at home. In this familiar environment she is likely to be more relaxed and therefore more able to cope with pain.

The culture of hospital settings creates expectations that women should be offered what Leap (2000b) describes as 'the menu' of pain-relief options. This is particularly acute where women are making noise. There is an unspoken pressure on the midwife sometimes to suggest pain relief to a labouring woman in order to quieten her rather than because she is actually requesting it, as this midwife describes:

> If you're looking after a client in hospital, there's the expectation that you're a good midwife if you keep her quiet and have control. If a woman is making a lot of noise there's a perception that you're not being a good midwife if you are not taking that pain away and helping her to be nice and quiet and appearing to be managing the labour (Vague 2003, p 73).

Labour and birth support

Women have identified that the midwife plays a crucial role in supporting them during labour and birth (Lundgren & Dahlberg 1998). Halldorsdottir and Karlsdottir (1996) studied labour using the metaphor of a journey. Midwives were categorised by women as either 'an indispensable companion' or an 'unfortunate hindrance'. There appeared to be no middle ground in their eyes. Of particular importance was the midwife's ability to make herself emotionally available to address fear and anxiety. This involved being fully 'present' to the woman.

As identified earlier, continuous one-to-one support during labour by midwives and women supporters has been found to reduce the likelihood of analgesia and operative birth and to increase women's satisfaction with their childbirth experience (Hodnett 2003). Common elements of this care include emotional support, information about labour progress and advice regarding coping techniques, and comfort measures. In fact, continuous support has been viewed in itself as a form of pain relief, specifically as an alternative to epidural anaesthesia (Dickenson et al 2003) because of concerns about the deleterious effects of epidural anaesthesia on labour progress.

Support for labour and birth also comes from another important source—the woman's chosen support people. Often a woman's partner will be a vital source of comfort and encouragement and can augment the midwife's supportive role. Increasingly, women are inviting additional family members or friends to provide support at this time too. They can be very helpful, not only to the woman but also in supporting her partner. This midwife sounds a note of caution about expectations that men will always be capable of supporting a woman without back-up:

> Sometimes I think men have their needs and they override what their role is in terms of being there for that woman. Sometimes you are giving the epidural for the partner who's really unhappy and uncomfortable and feels very anxious about their loved one. I'm not talking about all men . . . some are just absolutely fantastic at being brilliant support and as effective as a strong form of pain relief. But I think men often do need to have support and that helps them put things in perspective a bit because the responsibility is not 100% theirs. I think that's where they crumble often and they see what women are doing in labour as a reflection on them as opposed to it just being a normal process (Vague 2004, p 23).

Whoever the woman chooses to be present to support her, she needs to feel comfortable and safe with them. They need to have had their roles clearly explained by the woman. Principally, their job is to focus on the woman and her needs, either physical or emotional. They need to take their cues from her behaviour. Sometimes they will need to just sit quietly because the woman has turned inward on her labour and needs no overt support. Their presence is sufficient, with their unspoken yet unwavering commitment to her and belief in her ability to cope with labour. At other times, they may need to be much more actively involved, with encouraging words, massage, soothing cold flannels for flushed face, cold drinks, assistance in changing position. This is not the time for them to relive their birth experience or to discuss the latest sports results, unless the woman seeks that form of distraction.

Other useful tasks that support people can perform include running baths and making cups of tea or getting light snacks for others, including the midwife. They can keep other family members and friends informed of progress and help care for a woman's other children if necessary.

Working with pain in labour

For any woman, the onset of labour can be a time of conflicting emotions. There is usually excitement that labour is here and that soon she will meet her baby, tinged with apprehension about what it will be like, how long it will last and whether she will be able to cope. Early elation can begin to fade as contractions become increasingly frequent and more demanding. Doubts can begin to crowd in. She may be tired after a lost night's sleep and a little frightened of this force that has taken over her body and gives no indication of stopping for an unknowable period stretching ahead of her.

The midwife can help by reminding her of the physiology of labour's first stage and reinforcing the notion that everything she is feeling is entirely normal and appropriate. Many women benefit from praise and the expression of quiet confidence that all is well. This 'midwifery muttering' (Leap & Anderson 2004) can have a steadying effect on women, particularly when they are doubting their ability to cope. Women can be encouraged to 'tune out' and concentrate on meeting each contraction and then seeing it off rather than interacting too much with their surroundings.

The way in which this midwife sees labour and birth in the context of a normal life event is evident in her words:

> I think [the first part of the labour] is often the most difficult part because they're very intellectually 'there'. They are having to mastermind and intellectualise the process and cope with it on that level. Once they get further up the track in their labour, then they go into 'dozy land' when the endorphins are released and I think it's an easier phase. They capitulate to the process, whereas at the beginning they are often intellectually trying to mastermind it. Once they capitulate and allow the process to go, then I think they usually deal with it a lot better. I often say 'You are not alone. There will be hundreds of women out in the world doing exactly what you are doing right now. This is a really big journey in your life but it is a journey women have made since time began' (Vague 2003, p 74).

A woman who has previously had a straightforward labour is usually more confident because she has an idea of what lies ahead and believes in her body's ability to birth. Generally, successive labours are shorter than the first and that fact, combined with the knowledge that she has already negotiated a birth, adds to a woman's resolve when her next labour starts.

If the previous labour and birth were not a good experience, however, the woman may be harbouring many fears and traumatic memories. These feelings may not have been addressed prior to labour and may cause a woman's perception of pain to be considerably heightened. Clearly this presents a challenge to a midwife. In an ideal situation, the midwife would have already met the woman antenatally and have had a chance to build a relationship of trust. There would have been

Reflective exercise

Consider the following questions in relation to your own practice.

1. How do I discuss labour pain with pregnant women and their families?
2. What messages might I be giving about the advantages of coping with pain in labour and their ability to cope?
3. Am I clear about the evidence regarding the potential unwanted side-effects of pharmacological pain relief?
4. How do I respond when women in complicated labour plead for an epidural?
5. How do I explore women's experiences of pain in labour in order to inform my practice?

an opportunity to review her previous labour and possibly obtain her maternity records in order to gain a clear picture of what happened, in order to construct a birth plan that reflected the woman's wishes for a safer and more satisfying outcome in this labour.

The midwife in this story describes such an occasion:

> I had a lady who'd had a very bad experience with her first birth—very, very frightened. I spent a lot of time with her antenatally talking through [her labour experience] . . . When she arrived in labour this time . . . she was still frightened. She started to say that she needed an epidural. I said 'No, you're just saying that because that's where you were last time when you had the epidural. You don't need one. Just trust me. You're fine. Your body is doing it, you're just great. Don't fret, just relax'. And about an hour later, she delivered. She was totally rapt. It's so exciting to see women do that (Vague 2003, p 96).

The force of this midwife's belief that everything was progressing well and that the woman could do it resonates through this story. These feelings were just as strongly felt by the woman because, despite her fears, she was able to place her trust in the midwife and her skilled support.

Conclusion

Midwives have an important role to play in fostering women's belief that they will be able to cope with the pain of normal labour, and this has important consequences for women in terms of empowerment. Where women choose pharmacological pain relief, or if an epidural is necessary due to complications, the way in which the midwife engages with the woman around her experience of labour is equally important. It seems that the experience of being in pain in labour—particularly the kind and unkind things that people say—is never forgotten (Leap & Hunter 1993; Simkin 1999).

Review questions

1 Describe in your own words what you understand as the 'components of labour pain'.

2 Describe ten ways in which you would assist a woman to 'cope' with labour pain.

3 Much has been written about pain in labour. Can you describe some of the different accounts of labour pain?

4 How would you explain the concept that 'pain in labour keeps you safe'?

5 How would you explain the way you observe pain in labour in order to help you understand the progress a woman is making?

6 What are endorphins?

7 What research is there on the effect of the place of birth on pain in labour?

8 Give five examples of the way in which pain in labour has been interpreted historically.

9 Can you describe a way of perceiving pain in labour that is based on a different cultural expectation of pain in labour?

10 What physiological pathways are implicated in pain in labour? How do these differ from those involved in post-surgical pain?

Notes

1 'Families' is used in this chapter in a similar way to the New Zealand concept of 'whanau' to mean the network of significant people to whom the woman turns for support during her experience of pregnancy, birth and new motherhood.

2 See, for example, Mander (1998), Moore (1997) and Yerby (2000).

Online resources

MIDIRS online service provides a series of standard and advanced searches on topics related to pain and pain relief in labour, www.midirs.org

References

Anderson T 2000 Feeling safe enough to let go: the relationship between a woman and her midwife during the second stage of labour. In: M Kirkham (Ed) The midwife–mother relationship. Macmillan, London, pp 92–119

Arney W, Neill J 1982 The location of pain in natural childbirth: natural childbirth and the transformation of obstetrics. Sociology of Health and Illness 7:375–400

Atwood M 1987 The handmaid's tale. Virago, London

Balaskas J 1983 Active birth. Unwin Paperbacks, London

Balaskas J 1992 Active birth: the new approach to giving birth naturally. Harvard Common Press, Harvard

Bendelow GA, Williams SJ 1995 Transcending the dualisms: towards a sociology of pain. Sociology of Health and Illness 17(2):139–165

Berg M, Lundgren I, Hermansson E et al 1996 Women's experience of the encounter with the midwife during childbirth. Midwifery 12:11–15

Bluff R, Holloway I 1994 'They know best': women's perceptions of midwifery care during labour and childbirth. Midwifery 10:157–164

Bowler I 1993 Stereotypes of women of Asian descent in midwifery: some evidence. Midwifery 9:7–16

Bricker L, Lavender T 2002 Parenteral opioids for labour pain relief: a systematic review. American Journal of Obstetrics and Gynecology 186(5):94–109

Callister LC, Khalaf I, Semenic S et al 2003 The pain of childbirth: perceptions of culturally diverse women. Pain Management in Nursing 4(4):145–154

Caton D 1999 What a blessing she had chloroform: the medical and social response to the pain of childbirth from 1800 to the present. Yale University Press, New Haven

Chamberlain G, Wraight A, Steer P (Eds) 1993 Pain and its relief in childbirth: the results of a national survey conducted by the National Birthday Trust. Churchill Livingstone, Edinburgh

Chamberlain G, Wraight A, Crowley P 1997 Home births: the report of the 1994 confidential enquiry by the National Birthday Trust Fund. Parthenon, Carnforth

Chesler P 1979 With child: a diary of motherhood. Thomas Y Crowell, New York

Coombes G, Schonveld T 1992 Life will never be the same again— learning to be a first–time parent: a review of antenatal and postnatal education. Health Education Authority, London

Department of Health 1993 Changing childbirth (Cumberledge Report). Department of Health, HMSO, London

Dickenson J, Paech M, McDonald S et al 2003 Maternal satisfaction with childbirth and intrapartum analgesia in nulliparous labour. Australian and New Zealand Journal of Obstetrics and Gynaecology 43(6):463–469

Dick-Read G 1933 Childbirth without fear: the principles and practice of natural childbirth. Heineman, London

Escott D, Spiby H, Slade P et al 2004 The range of coping strategies women use to manage pain and anxiety prior to and during first experience of labour. Midwifery 20(2):144–156

Fenwick J, Hauck Y, Downie J et al 2005 The childbirth expectations of a self-selected cohort of Western Australian women. Midwifery 21:23–35

Ginesi L 1996 Physiology and birth—a personal view. Midwifery Matters: Journal of the Association of Radical Midwives (68): 8–11

Gosden D 1996 Dissenting voices: conflict and complexity in the home birth movement in Australia. MA Honours Thesis. Anthropology Department, Macquarie University, Sydney

Gosden D, Saul A 1999 Reflections on the use of psychotherapy in midwifery. British Journal of Midwifery 7(9):543–546

Green JM, Coupland VA, Kitzinger JV 1988 Great expectations: a prospective study of women's expectations and experiences. Child Care and Development Group, University of Cambridge, Cambridge

Green JM, Kitzinger J, Coupland V 1990 Stereotypes of childbearing women—a look at some of the evidence. Midwifery 6:125–132

Green JM, Curtis P, Price H et al 1998 Continuing to care. The organisation of midwifery services in the UK: a structured review of the evidence. Books for Midwives, Hale

Halldorsdottir S, Karlsdottir SI 1996 Journeying through labour and delivery: perceptions of women who have given birth. Midwifery 12(2):48–61

Heelbeck L 1999 Administration of pethidine in labour. British Journal of Midwifery 7:372–377

Heinz SD, Sleigh MJ 2003 Epidural or no epidural anaesthesia: relationships between beliefs about childbirth and pain control choices. Journal of Reproductive Health and Infant Psychology 21(4):323–333

Helman CG 1990 Culture health and illness (2nd edn). Butterworth-Heinemann, Oxford

Henry A, Nand S 2004 Women's antenatal knowledge and plans regarding intrapartum pain management at the Royal Hospital for Women. Australian and New Zealand Journal of Obstetrics and Gynaecology 44(4):314–317

Hodnett ED 2002 Pain and women's satisfaction with the experience of childbirth: a systematic review. American Journal of Obstetrics and Gynaecology 186(5):S160–S172

Hodnett ED, Gates S, Hofmeyr GJ et al 2003 Continuous support for women during childbirth. Cochrane Library (3). Update Software, Oxford

Holroyd E, Yin-King L, Pui-yuk LW et al 1997 Hong Kong Chinese women's perception of support from midwives during labour. Midwifery 13:66–72

Horrowitz E, Yogev Y, Ben-Haroush A et al 2004 Women's attitudes toward analgesia during labour—a comparison between 1995 and 2001. European Journal of Obstetrics and Gynecology and Reproductive Biology 117(1):30–32

Howell CJ 2002 Epidural versus non-epidural analgesia for pain relief in labour. Cochrane Library (2). Update Software, Oxford

Howell CJ, Kidd C, Roberts W et al 2001 A randomised controlled trial of epidural compared with non-epidural analgesia in labour. BJOG: An International Journal of Obstetrics and Gynaecology 108(1):17–33

Hundley V, Ryan M, Graham W 2001 Assessing women's preferences for intrapartum care. Birth 28(4):254–263

Hunt S 2002 Pethidine: love it or hate it? MIDIRS Midwifery Digest 12(3):363–365

Johanson R, Newburn M, Macfarlane A 2002 Has the medicalisation of childbirth gone too far? British Medical Journal 324:892–895

Kassabova K 1999 Renaissance. Penguin, Auckland

Kelpin V 1992 Birthing pain. In: J Morse (Ed) Qualitative health research. Sage, London, pp 93–103

Kemp J 2003 Midwives', women's and their birth partners' experiences of the 36 week birth talk: a qualitative study. Unpublished thesis. Florence Nightingale School of Nursing and Midwifery, Kings College, London

Kitzinger S 1962 The experience of childbirth. Victor Gollancz, London

Kitzinger S (Ed) 1987 Giving birth: how it really feels. Victor Gollancz, London

Kitzinger S 1991 Childbirth and society. In: I Chalmers, M Enkin, M

Keirse (Eds) Effective care in pregnancy and childbirth. Oxford University Press, Oxford, pp 99–109

Kitzinger S 2000 Rediscovering birth. Little Brown, Boston

Kotreba A 1994 The birth of my child: Monday 9th November 1992 at home. Midwifery Matters: Journal of the Association of Radical Midwives (60):16–17

Lavender T, Walkinshaw SA, Walton I 1999 Psychosocial factors influencing personal control in pain relief. International Journal of Nursing Studies 37: 493–503

Leap N 1997 A midwifery perspective on pain in labour. Unpublished MSc Dissertation. South Bank University, London

Leap N 2000a The less we do the more we give. In: M Kirkham (Ed) The midwife/mother relationship. Palgrave Macmillan, Hants

Leap N 2000b Pain in labour: towards a midwifery perspective. MIDIRS Midwifery Digest 10(1):49–53

Leap N, Anderson T 2004 The role of pain and the empowerment of women. In: S Downe (Ed) Normal childbirth: evidence and debate. Churchill Livingstone, Edinburgh

Leap N, Hunter B 1993 The midwife's tale: an oral history from handywoman to professional midwife. Scarlet Press, Gateshead UK

Lewin E 1985 By design: reproductive strategies and the meaning of motherhood. In: H Homans (Ed) The sexual politics of reproduction. Gower, London

Lieberman E 2004 Epidemiology of epidural analgesia and caesarean delivery. Clinical Obstetrics and Gynecology 47(2):317–331

Lieberman E, O'Donaghue C 2002 Unintended effects of epidural analgesia during labour: a systematic review. American Journal of Obstetrics and Gynecology 186(5):S31–S68

Lowe B 1989 Vaginal breech delivery: inaccurate reporting. New Zealand Medical Journal 102(866):202–208

Lundgren I, Dahlberg K 1998 Women's experience of pain during childbirth. Midwifery 14(2):105–110

Lundgren I, Dahlberg K 2002 Midwives' experience of the encounter with women and their pain during childbirth. Midwifery 18:155–164

McCrea H, Wright M, Stringer M 2000 Psychosocial factors influencing personal control in pain relief. International Journal of Nursing Studies (37):493–503

Mander R 1998 Pain in childbearing and its control. Blackwell Science, Oxford

Mander R 2000 The meanings of labour pain or the layers of an onion? A women-orientated view. Journal of Reproductive Health and Infant Psychology 18(2):133–141

Martin E 1987 The woman in the body: a cultural analysis of reproduction. Open University Press, Milton Keynes

Mayberry LJ, Clemmens D, De A 2002 Epidural analgesia side effects, co-interventions, and care of women during childbirth: a systematic review. American Journal of Obstetrics and Gynecology 186(5):S81–S93

Melzack R 1999 From the gate to the neuromatrix. Pain (82):S121–S126

Melzack R, Wall P 1965 Pain mechanisms: a new theory. Science 150:971–979

Melzack R, Wall P 1988 The challenge of pain. Penguin, London

Moore S 1994 Pain relief in labour: an overview. British Journal of Midwifery 2(10):483–486

Moore S (Ed) 1997 Understanding pain and its relief in labour. Churchill Livingstone, Edinburgh

Morgan BM, Bulpitt CJ, Clifton P et al 1982 Analgesia and satisfaction in childbirth. Lancet ii:808–810

Morris D 1991 The culture of pain. University of California Press, Berkeley

Morse JM, Park C 1988 Home birth and hospital deliveries: a comparison of perceived painfulness of parturition. Research in Nursing and Health 11:175–181

Newton N, Foshee D, Newton M 1966 Experimental inhibition of labour through environmental disturbance. Obstetrics and Gynaecology 27(3):371–377

Newton N, Peeler D 1968 Effect of disturbance on labour. An experiment with 100 mice. American Journal of Obstetrics and Gynaecology 101(8):1096–1102

NHMRC 1996 Options for effective care in childbirth. AGPS, Canberra

Niven C 1994 Coping with labour pain: the midwife's role. In: S Robinson, A Thompson (Eds) Research and Childbirth. Chapman & Hall, London

Niven C, Murphy-Black T 2000 Memory for labor pain: a review of the literature. Birth 27(4):244–253

Oakley A 1980 Women confined: towards a sociology of childbirth. Martin Robertson, Oxford

Odent M 1984 Birth re-born: what birth can and should be. Souvenir Press, London

Olofsson C, Ekblom A, Ekman-Ordeberg G 1996 Lack of analgesic effect of systematically administered morphine or pethidine on labour pain. British Journal of Obstetrics and Gynaecology 103: 968–972

Rabuzzi KA 1994 Mother with child: transformations through childbirth. Indiana University Press, Bloomington

Raphael-Leff J 1986 Facilitators and regulators: conscious and unconscious processes in pregnancy and motherhood. British Journal of Medical Psychology 59:43–55

Reed B 2002a The Albany Midwifery Practice (1). MIDIRS Midwifery Digest 12(1):118–121

Reed B 2002b The Albany Midwifery Practice (2). MIDIRS Midwifery Digest 12(3):261–264

Rich A 1976 Of woman born: motherhood as experience and institution. Virago, London

Rimene C, Hassan C, Broughton J 1998 Ukaipo: The place of nurturing Maori women and childbirth. University of Otago, Dunedin

Roberts C, Tracy S, Peat B 2000 Rates for obstetric intervention among private and public patients in Australia: population based descriptive study. British Medical Journal 321:137–141

Robertson A 1994 Empowering women: teaching active birth in the 90's. ACE Graphics, Sydney

Robertson A 1996 The pain of labour. Midwifery Today 37:19–42

Ross A 1998 Maternal satisfaction with labour analgesia. Baillière's Clinical Obstetrics and Gynaecology 12(3):499–512

Sandall J, Davies J, Warwick C 2001 Evaluation of the Albany Midwifery Practice: final report. Nightingale School of Midwifery, Kings College, London

Scarry E 1985 The body in pain: the making and unmaking of the world. Oxford University Press, Oxford

Shearer EL 1993 Caesarean section: medical benefits and costs. Social Science and Medicine 37(10):1223–1231

Shizuko Y, Fagerhaugh S, Strauss A 1977 Politics of pain management: staff-patient. Addison-Wesley, San Francisco

Silverton L 2001 Why women choose caesarean section. RCM Midwives Journal 4(10)

Simkin P 1989 Non-pharmacological methods of pain relief during labour. In: I Chalmers, M Enkin, M Keirse (Eds) Effective care in pregnancy and childbirth. Oxford University Press, Oxford

Simkin P 1999 Just another day in a woman's life? Women's long term perceptions of their first birth experience. Part 1. Birth 18:203–210

Simkin P, Ancheta R 2000 Labor progress handbook: early interventions to prevent and treat dystocia. Blackwell Science, Oxford

Soutter C (writer) 2004 Labour pain. VHS video. New Zealand. Online: www.birthinternational.com.

Spiby H, Slade P, Escott D et al 2004 Selected coping strategies in labour: an investigation of women's experiences. Birth 30(3): 189–194

Terry R, Gijsberg K 2000 Memory for the quantitative and qualitative aspects of labour pain: a preliminary study. Journal of Reproductive Health and Infant Psychology 18(2):143–152

Thorpe JA, Hu DH, Albin RM et al 1993 The effect of intrapartum epidural analgesia on nulliparous labour: a randomized, controlled, prospective trial. American Journal of Obstetrics and Gynecology 169(4):851–858

Trout KK 2004 The neuromatrix theory of pain: implications for selected nonpharmacologic methods of pain relief for labor. Journal of Midwifery and Women's Health 49(6):482–488

Vague S 2003 Midwives' experiences of working with women in labour: interpreting the meaning of pain. Unpublished Masters thesis. Auckland University of Technology, Auckland

Vague S 2004 Midwives' experiences of working with women in labour: interpreting the meaning of pain. New Zealand College of Midwives Journal (31):22–26

van Hoover C 2000 Pain and suffering in childbirth: a look at attitudes research and history. Midwifery Today (55):39–42, 69

Walsh D, Newburn M 2002 Towards a social model of childbirth. Parts 1 & 2. British Journal of Midwifery 10(8):476–481

Yerby M (Ed) 2000 Pain in childbearing: key issues in management. Baillière Tindall, Edinburgh

CHAPTER 24

Using water for labour and birth

Robyn Maude and Shea Caplice

Key terms

anxiety, continuity of caregiver, pain perception, partnership, physiological birth, relaxing effect, water immersion

Chapter overview

This chapter provides an overview of the use of water immersion for labour and birth. It tracks the history and development of the use of water immersion for labour and birth over the past two decades, reviews some of the most recent literature that informs practice, and explores the physiology, potential problems and issues related to practice. We have included women's perspectives on their experiences of using water for labour and birth, and provided recommendations for the safe use of water immersion in labour and water birth.

The key principles of a midwifery model of care that underpin this chapter are that:

- pregnancy and childbirth is a normal life event for most women

- midwifery care is woman-centred

- continuity of care should be provided throughout the entire childbearing experience

- the woman–midwife relationship is a partnership based on:
    - trust, reciprocity and respect for the expertise of both the woman and the midwife
    - the woman's personal knowledge of her health history being considered as important as that of the midwife's
    - both partners having equal status and shared meaning through mutual understanding
    - the sharing of knowledge and power between the partners.

Learning outcomes

Learning outcomes for this chapter are:

1   To describe some of the history of using water for labour and birth

2   To integrate the literature that informs safe evidence-based care for women using water for labour and birth

3   To describe the principles and guidelines for using water for labour and birth

4   To support the use of water for labour and birth as a means of enabling midwives to be 'with women' and supporting physiological birth.

Introduction

Since the early 1980s, when water immersion during labour and birth was used predominantly by women birthing at home, many questions have been asked about efficacy and safety for both the woman and the baby. Globally, women, midwives, doctors and researchers have attempted to answer these questions, and the inquiry continues. The use of water immersion in labour and the phenomenon of water birthing are closely associated with the act of physiological birth, which is widely supported by women and midwives in many countries. However, controversy between professionals has surrounded its use, with much debate over the perceived benefits and potential risks.

The role of water birth in supporting physiological birth

As midwives, we are increasingly searching for the best available evidence to challenge and change many of the practices in obstetrics that are 'routine' and/or based on the risk management processes of institutions and some maternity care providers. Midwives recognise that practice wisdom comes from many sources and use evidence from scientific inquiry and the shared stories that have informed our practice over time. We need to validate the advice we give to women by exploring and sharing the research findings and practice wisdom in order to facilitate the woman and her family making informed decisions about their care, based on this information. Women are entitled to receive thorough,

Clinical point

Avoiding pharmacological pain relief
Increasingly, women want to find ways to manage the pain of labour naturally, thereby reducing the likelihood of requiring pharmacological pain relief, but are unsure about their ability to go through a labour without some help, especially women having their first baby. 'I didn't want to use drugs if I could help it but then I'm such a "wuss" when it comes to pain' (Linda, in Maude 2003).

Women and midwives have come to see water immersion as a means of achieving this. These women are encouraged to use other methods to promote comfort and support until labour is established and they are able to get into the pool. Being with the woman, supporting and encouraging her through the sometimes difficult transition phase and honouring her choices has meant that many nulliparous women are able to birth in the pool without interventions.

unbiased information about choices for care, place of birth and caregiver, so that they can make informed decisions about their care.

Women know that they should avoid drugs and harmful substances during their pregnancies, yet the protocols for active management of labour subject them to a range of drugs and practices that often start a cascade of intervention, resulting in operative delivery. Wagner (cited in Hall & Holloway 1998, p 31) suggests that 'Many midwives and the women in their care are becoming advocates of more natural forms of childbirth and demand care that is sensitive to the psychological needs of the individual and her family'.

The option to use water is one way of supporting women in labour without drugs, along with continuity of caregiver and the availability of private and peaceful surroundings in which to labour and birth. The demand for water immersion in labour and water birth has grown rapidly throughout the world over the past two and a half decades. Hall and Holloway (1998) suggest that this may be one reaction against medical control of childbirth. This is supported by Kitzinger (1996), who says that the use of warm water also seeks to change the dynamics of the care of labouring and birthing women, to give control back to them. She says warm water immersion and water birth are not just another 'trendy' technique but rather an approach to childbirth that enables the birthing woman to have autonomy, by changing the environment and the quality of interactions between all those involved in the care.

The history of water birth

The first documented birth in water was reported in a French medical journal in 1805, when a woman, exhausted after a 48-hour labour, climbed into a warm bath to relax, giving birth to her child into the water shortly afterwards (Church 1989, cited in Richmond 2003a). In the following 150 years, the subject of water birth was rarely broached in the medical literature. Igor Tjarkovsky, the Russian water birth enthusiast, generated much interest in this method of birth in the 1960s, both within his own country and around the world, through claims that birth in water improved the psychic abilities of the baby (Zimmerman 1993, cited in Richmond 2003a). There are no data, however, to support this theory.

In 1975, Leboyer's book, *Birth Without Violence*, described the use of water as a healing therapy for babies. His work was based on the idea that birth has a profound effect on the future development of the baby, and stressed the need for peace, quiet and gentleness at the time of birth. Leboyer proposed the use of water immediately after birth as a gentle introduction for the baby, minimising harsh stimuli such as light and sound.

In France in the 1970s, Dr Michel Odent observed that women were attracted to the use of the shower or bath when in labour. As with most practitioners new to water birth, Odent's initial experience was with a woman so completely relaxed in the bath that the baby was born before she was able to get out (Lichy & Herzberg 1993). After that first experience

Odent began to offer water birth to all women who had long labours. In 1983, Odent published in *The Lancet* the summary of the outcomes of 100 water births at his alternative-birthing unit in Pithiviers, France. Odent's article was one of the first major medical publications dealing with birth in water. While Tjarkovsky was concerned with the baby and its development, Dr Odent was more concerned with the labouring woman.

Following on from the work of Tjarkovsky, Leboyer and Odent, the practice of labouring and birthing in water gathered momentum in the 1980s within the home birth community and the practice of domiciliary midwives. With the emergence of a spiritual movement that supported the notion of the dolphin and human connection and rebirthing, there was an increased demand for 'water babies' (Sidenbladh 1983). Inspired by enthusiastic women and midwives, labouring and birthing in water spread into birth centres and hospital maternity units in the 1990s. Its growing popularity is largely attributable to the women and families who have experienced the benefits of birthing this way.

The first water births in New Zealand and Australia

The first of the modern water births in New Zealand, believed to be the first in the southern hemisphere, occurred at Estelle

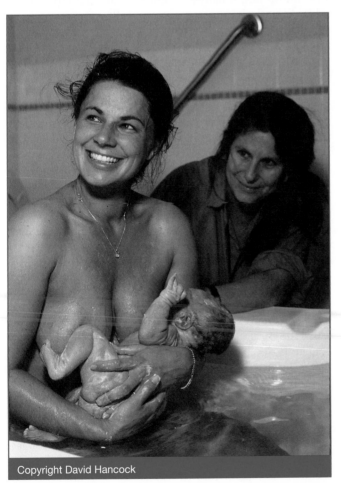

Copyright David Hancock

> ### Clinical point
>
> **The first water births in Indigenous Australia and New Zealand**
> There is little early documented evidence of the practice of water birthing among the Indigenous women of Australia, although Odent (1990) says that some Aboriginal women on the western coast of Australia first paddled in the sea, then gave birth on the beach. There are stories of traditional birthing practices among the Maori of New Zealand where water was used. It was common for babies to be born on beaches in the Te Kaha area (Binney & Chapman 1986; Irwin & Ramsden 1995) and Makereti records the use of water to facilitate birth of the whenua (placenta) when it was delayed (Makereti 1986).

Myer's Rainbow Dolphin Centre in Tutukaka in the north of the North Island on 17 March 1982. The baby's mother had read an article on water birth and the underwater birth experiments of Igor Tjarkovsky. She drove her house bus and three children to Tutukaka, intent on birthing in water. Estelle, friends, a midwife and a nurse attended the woman during her birth. The baby, weighing 3.6 kg, was born in the bath, in a posterior position (her second persistently posterior baby) after two and a half hours of labour. Similarly, a few years later in 1985, Estelle supported a Russian woman who birthed her son into water in Sydney. There were six midwives present to observe this new practice, and hence the water birth movement in Australia was born.

In New Zealand, to date there are no national data available as to water birth rates and how women use pools and baths during labour and birth. Individual practice or facility audits report a 65–75% rate of pool use in labour (Banks 1998; Cassie 2002) and a 25–38% water birth rate (Banks 1998; Fenton 2004). In New Zealand, Wanganui Hospital's maternity unit led the country by openly using water immersion for birth. The first documented water birth at Wanganui occurred in November 1989. Between July 1991 and December 2000 there were 916 water births in the maternity unit (Young 2001).

Similarly, there is generally a lack of published data in Australia regarding the use of water for labour and birth, which is not indicative of its widespread usage. Labouring in water and births in water have been occurring at planned home births attended by home birth midwives since the early 1980s (Lecky-Thompson 1989) and within hospital-based birth centres in Sydney and Melbourne since the early 1990s (Caplice 1999; Page 1994). Currently the hospital facility audits report a water birth rate of 35–44% of total births at the Royal Hospital for Women in Sydney, which represents a steady increase since the inception of the practice in 1992. In addition, Australian independent midwives report a water birth rate of around 60–80% of total births (Caplice 2004).

Using water for labour and birth: the evidence

A review of the literature reveals research documenting the history and development of the use of water for labour and birth, and also a progression of thinking and sophistication, based on the outcomes of the research. When looking at the research into the use of water for labour and birth, it is important to understand the methodology and methods used in the research. This is because research is weighted according to the traditional hierarchy of evidence. The hierarchy of evidence is a standard notation for the relative weight carried by different types of study when decisions are made about the effectiveness of clinical interventions. The randomised controlled trial (RCT) is considered the 'gold standard' and represents the only true means of evaluating the effectiveness of an intervention (in this case, water immersion) in improving outcomes such as operative delivery or exogenous pain relief.

Qualitative studies using techniques such as a grounded theory approach, phenomenology or narrative inquiry are not placed high in the traditional hierarchy of evidence. There are important and valid studies of the use of water for labour and birth that use qualitative methodologies that should be considered alongside the studies employing quantitative methodologies. It should be understood that quantitative designs attempt to answer questions as to 'what works', which is a result that can be measured. Qualitative designs ask 'What is going on?', 'How does it work?', 'How can we understand the factors that affect people?' and 'How do individuals feel and behave the way they do?'.

The Cochrane Database of Systematic Reviews (February 2004) updated reports on eight trials (2939 women) examining the effects of water immersion during labour. The only trial that researched birth in water was too small to determine outcomes for women and babies, and so was not included. Nor were any studies of the third stage of labour in water. The reviewers concluded that there was a statistically significant reduction in women's pain perception, and that the rate of epidural analgesia is reduced, which suggests that water immersion during the first stage of labour is beneficial to some women (Cluett et al 2004a).

There was no evidence that the benefits were associated with adverse outcomes for babies or longer labours. To date there is insufficient evidence about the use of water immersion during second stage to enable the formation of firm conclusions about the safety and effectiveness of giving birth in water. Water immersion during the first stage of labour can be supported for low-risk women (Cluett et al 2004a).

To date there are no significant or multicentred RCTs comparing birth in water with land birth, even though numerous authors have called for such rigorous testing. A commonly held belief has been that the ethical considerations of an RCT for water birth make the prospect of such a study unlikely (Woodward & Kelly 2004). However, a recent pilot study conducted by Woodward and Kelly (2004) to assess the feasibility of an RCT and the willingness of women to participate in such a trial has produced some positive results. The study proves that women are willing to enrol in an RCT comparing water birth with land birth and that randomisation does not necessarily affect women's satisfaction with their birth experience. This research paves the way for the organisation of a multicentred RCT to evaluate the differences between land and water births with large enough numbers to produce statistical significance.

In the meantime, however, there is some good-quality descriptive research that gives us information to consider. This review will attempt to provide an overview of the current debates about birthing in water. Most of the studies reviewed refer to the use of water immersion in labour rather than water immersion during birth, unless otherwise specified.

Physiological effects

The calming and relaxing effect that water immersion has during labour and birth is well recognised. How this helps women to birth without exogenous pain relief and other forms of interventions was first described by Odent (1983). Church (1989) also proposed that water immersion decreases anxiety in the woman and that this works to reduce adrenaline levels, thereby encouraging the uninhibited flow of natural oxytocins and endorphins. A natural balance of pain and relaxation is achieved, and labour progresses normally.

Much of the research to date has attempted to quantify the absolute effect of pain relief afforded to the woman by water immersion during labour and birth. Women in trials have been asked to rank their level of pain using a visual analogue scale. The prospective RCT by Cammu and colleagues (1994) found no statistical difference between the absolute values of labour pain between the two groups of women in their trial. They reported that bathing provided no objective pain relief, but did have a temporal pain stabilising effect, possibly mediated through the improved ability to relax in between contractions. This was supported in the historical cohort study by Aird and colleagues (1997), who found that labouring in water allowed greater relaxation of the mother during the first stage of labour, thereby allowing her to reach the second stage better prepared to give birth without assistance. The pain relief effect of warm water immersion is probably associated with a reduced level of endorphins and catecholamines, as 'there is a tendency to fall asleep in a comfortable tub' (Odent 1997, p 415). The explanation for this effect is related to the 'soothing warmth', 'support of the body' and 'pleasurable sensation' of water, the effect of which stimulates the closing of the gate for pain at the level of the dorsal horn, and supports the notion that water provides women with a temporal stabilising effect (Cammu et al 1994).

The hydrothermic effect relates to the conduction of heat from the warm water through the skin, leading to peripheral vasodilation. The resultant release of muscle spasm contributes to the reduction in pain (Brown, cited in Richmond 2003a). The hydrokinetic effect refers to the feeling of weightlessness often described by women (Deschennes 1990). The combined effect of warmth and weightlessness contributes to women feeling more relaxed and less anxious (Ginesi & Neiscierowicz 1998). The vasodilation of the peripheral blood vessels and the redistribution of blood flow when women are immersed in warm water during labour have been observed to contribute to a reduction in blood pressure (Church 1989; Nightingale 1994). A common concern has been that vasodilation and relaxation of uterine muscles might lead to an increased possibility of postpartum haemorrhage. However, numerous audits in units that use immersion in water for labour and birth do not support this (Caplice 2004; Garland 1994; Rosenthal 1991). It would seem that the natural processes already in place in the body are sufficient to counteract this theoretical problem (Richmond 2003a).

What women say about water immersion

Reviewing the qualitative research on birthing in water revealed strong themes, including the following:
- Women feel more in control. Water reduces their anxiety about pain and about the process of childbirth itself.
- Women use water to cope with pain, not necessarily to remove or diminish it.
- Women feel more relaxed and the water promotes their comfort.
- Women feel sheltered and protected in the water, which promotes privacy.
- Women are able to move around more easily and feel supported by the water (Hall & Holloway 1998; Maude 2003; Richmond 2003b).

Stories of women's experiences of using water for labour and birth have broadened our understanding of the meaning they make of the experience, and have demonstrated that the efficacy of water immersion goes beyond measurable outcomes. Being in water during labour and birth is not the end product; it is not the water itself that makes a difference. It is a shared philosophy and a shared belief in birth as a normal life event that supports women to use water. It is also the planning, preparation, education and anticipation of using water for labour and birth, supported by safe and judicious

use, that creates an environment that promotes relaxation, privacy and a release that enables and empowers women to maintain control. It appears that it is not necessary for women to actually give birth in the water to achieve these benefits (Maude 2003).

Safety and efficacy of using water

Water immersion during labour and water birth is widely practised globally by practitioners who employ a holistic approach to birth and support women to birth physiologically. While most health professionals involved in the care of women during pregnancy and birth now agree that there is adequate evidence to support labouring in water, there continues to be tension between health professionals concerning its safety, particularly birth under water. This section examines the literature relating to some of these issues.

Water temperature

The temperature of water used in labour and for birth has caused concern in relation to fetal outcomes. In the late 1980s, this concern focused on the potential dangers of temperatures below 37°C, with a suggestion that low temperatures may stimulate the baby to breathe (Gradert et al 1987; Lecky-Thompson 1989; Lenstrup et al 1987). Subsequently, attendants erred on the side of caution, maintaining pool temperatures at levels around 37–38°C. However, in 1994, maternal hyperthermia became an issue when two babies were born with perinatal asphyxia after the mothers were immersed in water for some hours during labour, as it was thought that the temperature of the water had been a contributing factor (Rosser 1994). This assumption was never proved.

Johnson (1996) explains that, as the baseline fetal temperature is normally 0.5–1°C above maternal temperature, the fetus is placed at risk when the mother experiences hyperthermia. The fetal oxygen demands increase, making the baby susceptible to fetal distress. In response to this information, guidelines have been set to reduce the risk of birth asphyxia in water: the recommended temperature of the water is no higher than 37.5°C, which is normal body temperature (Deans & Steer 1995; Duley 2001; Richmond 2003a). In contrast, in a paper on fetal hyperthermia, Charles (1998) explains that a maternal temperature rise of up to 1°C may be beneficial to the baby as there is an increase in oxygen transfer across the placenta; however, this research does not define temperature thresholds that might be considered too hot.

Geissbuehler and colleagues (2002) measured maternal and neonatal temperatures of women who birthed in water and compared them with those of women and babies who birthed on land. The authors concluded that birth in water did not pose a thermal risk to either mother or baby. Furthermore, they assumed that women self-regulate their body temperature according to changes in the water temperature and that this mechanism of self-regulation of core body temperature would be far superior to any water temperature guideline. There is no reason for practitioners to adhere to protocols that recommend keeping the water at a set temperature, other than the mother's physical comfort. More recently, in support of Geissbuehler's proposition, Tricia Anderson (2004) suggests that practitioners give up their obsession with the temperature of the water and instead focus on ensuring that the woman has control over her environment and on facilitating her comfort. It would seem therefore more appropriate to check the woman's temperature before she enters the pool and during the time that she is in the pool, while regularly checking with her about the temperature of the water. It is useful to also have supplies of cool water or ice chips and access to a fan.

Immersion and duration of labour

Studies investigating a reduction in the duration of labour in relation to water immersion have been inconclusive. In 1994, Garland and Jones analysed data from 209 primiparous women and 220 multiparous women and demonstrated a median and mean reduction in labour length, but since then other studies have been unable to replicate these findings. Schorn and colleagues' (1993) prospective RCT of the use of warm water immersion by 93 women could not demonstrate a shortening of labour; however, the immersion was only for an average of 30–45 minutes. Other retrospective comparative studies show small decreases in length of labour. More recently, Cluett and colleagues (2004b), in their RCT comparing water immersion with standard management for labour dystocia, reported water immersion as being of benefit, but the mean duration of labour was similar in both groups.

Use of analgesia in labour

Being immersed in water does not necessarily take the pain away. What it does appear to do, and this is supported in the literature, is provide a release from the pain in the form of warming, soothing, comforting and relaxing. For women who want to avoid pharmacological pain relief and for midwives who support these women, judicious use of water immersion may offer the means to achieve this. One historical cohort study of the effects of immersion in warm water during labour found that the requirement for both pethidine and epidural analgesia was significantly reduced among women having their first baby (Aird et al 1997). The Cochrane Review (Cluett et al 2004a) reports that there is evidence that water immersion during the first stage of labour reduces the use of analgesia and reported maternal pain, without adverse outcomes on labour duration, operative delivery or neonatal outcomes.

Most maternity care providers and facilities accept that the use of water immersion during labour significantly reduces pain. However, recent research suggests that the role of the birthing pool may be even more important than care providers realise. Cluett and colleagues (2004b), from Southampton Hospital in England, have discovered that women with labour dystocia who use water immersion during the first stage of labour are less likely to need analgesia or an operative delivery. The research compared women who used water immersion during labour with those who had standard augmentation for dystocia and demonstrated that the women who used the birthing pool had significantly fewer epidurals, needed less assistance with giving birth and had fewer obstetric interventions.

The women in a study by Taha (2000) also reported less pain when using water immersion in labour. Two qualitative

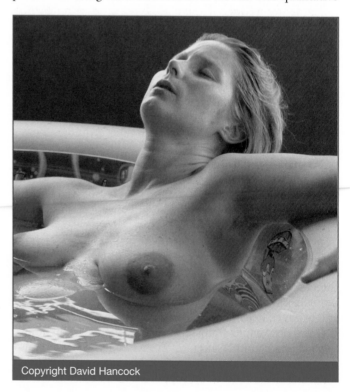

Copyright David Hancock

studies on women's experiences of water immersion report that in addition to the pain-relieving effects of water, the therapeutic qualities of water helped the women to cope better with the pain of labour and birth (Maude 2003; Richmond 2003b).

Perineal trauma

The findings regarding perineal trauma associated with birth in water consistently show a higher intact rate in the water birth group and a higher rate of sustained perineal trauma in the land birth group (Aird 1997; Burke & Kilfoyle 1995; Geissbuehler & Eberhard 2000). The most startling evidence is the reduction in episiotomy rates, demonstrating the protective aspect of water birth against intervention. In Geissbuehler and Eberhard's (2000) study, the episiotomy rate in the water birth group was 12.8% compared with 35.4% in the land birth group. One could argue, however, that there is no place for episiotomy in the practice of water birth, because if you are performing an episiotomy out of concern for the condition of the baby then you should not be continuing with a birth in water!

Risk of infection

The theoretical risk of infection to either the woman or her baby has often been put forward as an argument against the use of water for labour and birth, particularly for women with ruptured membranes. Waldenstrom and Nilsson (1992) conducted a non-randomised controlled study at the Stockholm Birth Centre comparing women who used the bath after ruptured membranes with women who had ruptured membranes but did not use the bath. The authors concluded there was no statistically significant difference between the groups with regard to infection, infant respiratory problems or symptoms of amnionitis in the mother. More recently, Robertson and colleagues (1998) conducted a medical review that examined the association between the use of water immersion in labour and the development of chorioamnionitis and endometritis, and found no significant association. Similarly, Geissbuhler and Eberhard (2000) analysed 7508 births and reported no statistically significant difference in infection rates between infants born in water and those born on land.

Michel Odent (2001) discussed bacteriological colonisation of babies at birth. He explained the concept of the 'race to the surface' used by bacteriologists, meaning that the first bacteria to reach a bacteria-free surface will be the likely rulers of the territory. Babies are born sharing the immunoglobulin G (IgG) antibodies of their mothers and therefore it is beneficial for a baby to be colonised by the mother's bacteria. From a microbiological perspective, it would seem that birth in water is a positive action, in line with skin-to-skin contact. It is when babies come in contact with unfamiliar bacteria from caregivers and hospitals that the bacteria they are colonised by become potentially dangerous. This theory supports the idea that caregivers should stay out of the water unless absolutely necessary, but partners and siblings should not be discouraged,

as they are likely to have similar bacterial colonisations to those of the mother.

The literature indicates that if pools/baths are adequately cleaned, there is no increase in neonatal or maternal infection (Global Maternal/Child Health 2000, cited in Harper 2000). Infection risks to babies appear to be caused primarily by gram-negative organisms that colonise pump systems of spa baths and filling and draining hoses, and by inadequate bath-cleaning procedures (Vochem et al 2001).

The issue of blood-borne viruses such as HIV and hepatitis B and C was discussed at the First International Waterbirth Conference in London in 1995. It was concluded that the water diluted such viruses to the point where they became impotent and posed much less of a threat than the blood splashes that may occur in a land birth (Beech 1996). In researching the risk of work-related HIV exposure or infection to midwives attending water births, Colombo and colleagues (2000) took pool water samples from 14 different water births and measured the haemoglobin content to estimate the viral load the liquid would be carrying. The authors concluded that because of the diluting effect of the water, the potential risk for HIV-exposure to intact skin was minimal and unlikely to have consequences. However, in their opinion, the risk of nosocomial hepatitis B infection is significantly higher, and they recommend wearing gauntlet gloves and ensuring that all healthcare workers are vaccinated.

Third stage and blood loss

There have been no documented cases of complications in relation to the third stage being conducted in the bath. In 1983, Odent proposed a theory that water embolism could be a risk factor. This has now been largely dismissed, and Odent himself has withdrawn the hypothesis, admitting that it was unfounded and a mythical concept.

Richmond (2003a) hypothesises that there is an increased potential for postpartum haemorrhage associated with water birth. Her rationale for this is based on the hyperaemia induced by warm water and the relaxing effect it has on uterine muscles. However, in the many audits in units practising water birth this has not proved to be a problem (Caplice 2004; Garland 2002; Garland & Jones 1997).

Effects on the baby

Johnson (1996) describes in depth the physiology of fetal breathing in utero and the main factors that inhibit breathing in the newborn until she or he is lifted into air. Fetal breaths in utero are intermittent isometric movements with very little inspiration of amniotic fluid. Approximately 24–48 hours prior to birth, in response to the increase in prostaglandin E_2 levels from the placenta, the fetal breathing movements slow down or cease. This decrease in fetal breathing movements allows more blood flow to the vital organs, including the brain. At birth, when the prostaglandin level is still high, the baby's breathing response is still slow—this is the first inhibitory response.

A second inhibitory response is related to acute hypoxia in the newborn. Babies are born experiencing a lack of oxygen in response to the birth process. This normal inhibition of breathing may be overridden if the baby becomes compromised in utero. Acute hypoxia causes apnoea and swallowing, but if severe and prolonged, it will cause breathing and gasping (Fewell & Johnson 1983).

Another important inhibitory component is the 'dive reflex'. Central to the physiology of the dive reflex is the larynx, which is covered with chemoreceptors (like taste buds). With application of foreign stimuli such as water to the larynx, these chemoreceptors initiate the closure of the glottis so that the water is swallowed and not inhaled (Harding et al 1978). Johnson (1996) reports that while substances such as water, non-species milks, isotonic alkalis and ammonia initiate the full diving response, physiological saline, amniotic fluid, lung and gastric fluids, urine, blood, meconium and milk from the same species at body temperature illicit little response when instilled to the larynx.

The last main factor thought to inhibit the newborn from initiating a breathing response while in water is environmental temperature. Johnson (1996) reports that the fetus is co-dependent on maternal temperature control and with the fetal core temperature 0.5–1°C above the mother's, there are important implications for practice. Maternal hyperthermia and the resultant hyperthermia in the fetus may override the inhibition to breathe. Therefore it is advisable that strategies be put in place to avoid maternal hyperthermia or overheating. However, the issue of keeping the water at maternal body temperature and no less in order to maintain the inhibitory effect needs to be reconsidered in light of births taking place in oceans, where the babies are reported to be born with no adverse effects (Harper 2002).

Perinatal mortality and morbidity/adverse outcomes

In England and Wales, an extensive survey was conducted of the extent to which women were labouring or giving birth in water. In addition, the survey assessed the problems reported following births in water (Alderdice et al 1995). Of the 4834 births in water from 1992 to 1993 it was reported that there were six stillbirths/neonatal deaths, none of which could be attributed to the use of water. The estimated mortality rate was 1.24 per 1000 live births. Women giving birth in water are generally perceived as low risk, and therefore this figure needs to be viewed accordingly.

In 1999, Gilbert and Tookey compared the perinatal morbidity and mortality rates for babies born in water with those for babies born on land in the British Isles, England and Wales. The key message from this study was that perinatal mortality and risk of admission to special-care baby units is similar for babies delivered in water and for low-risk deliveries that do not take place in water (Gilbert & Tookey 1999).

Polycythaemia

In 1997, an isolated case of neonatal polycythaemia following a birth in water was reported in *The Lancet*. The labour and birth were uneventful and the mother remained in the water for 30 minutes following the birth. There was a delay in clamping and cutting of the cord for a further 10 minutes. At two days of age, the baby was diagnosed as severely polycythaemic and an exchange transfusion was performed. The baby developed normally and the interpretation was that the warm water prevented the normal vasoconstriction of the cord when exposed to air (Austin et al 1997). As an isolated case, the implications for practice are minimal.

Cord snapping

Gilbert and Tookey's (1999) surveillance study and postal survey of perinatal mortality and morbidity among babies born in water identified that delivery in water may have contributed to snapped umbilical cords in five babies (out of a total of 4032 births in water). One of the five babies required a blood transfusion. The snapped cords were probably the result of cord traction when bringing the baby to the surface rapidly.

Cro and Preston (2002) report on an audit conducted following an instance of cord snapping at a water birth. They identified four cases of snapped umbilical cord out of 100 water births between September 1996 and March 2001. In three instances the cord was noted to have snapped while bringing the baby to the surface, and the ends were immediately clamped with no adverse effects for the babies. In the fourth case, the snapped cord was discovered when it was noted that the baby was becoming paler and making reduced respiratory effort. A lot of blood was noted in the water. The baby required a blood transfusion and was discharged from hospital after three days. Follow-up at eight weeks found the baby to be developing normally.

There is no way of knowing how many umbilical cords snap during birth under water, nor indeed is there any research on cord snapping during birth in air. Some authors have suggested lowering the level of the water just prior to second stage; however, this is not thought to be wise as it decreases the advantages of water immersion (comfort, buoyancy, hydrostatic pressure and freedom of movement). The baby's being born completely under water can only be assured when the water is high enough to ensure the woman's comfort (at the level of the breasts while sitting). Midwives supporting women who birth in water should be aware of and prepared for this rare event. It is recommended that the baby be brought to the surface slowly, to avoid undue traction on the cord. The midwife is advised to check the cord as soon as possible after birth.

Neonatal resuscitation

An RCT in Australia comparing outcomes of women who used water immersion during the first stage with those who did not concluded primarily that there was no reduction in the use of pharmacological pain relief for the water immersion group. The secondary finding was that the babies in the water immersion group required more resuscitation than those in the control group, which is an unexpected finding, particularly when the trial did not include any actual births in water

(Eckert et al 2001). This publication caused some clinicians and services to rethink the practice of water immersion in labour. The flaws in the research, however, limit its reliability and clinical applicability. The short time that some women spent in the bath (times varied from 5 to 360 minutes) causes the reader to question the commitment of the midwives to the practice of immersion in water. It is unrealistic to believe that five minutes in the bath would have any analgesic effect or significant effects on the baby.

The large number of women who 'crossed over' from their allocated group is a concern. This high crossover level may have directed the groups to have similar outcomes because the intervention essentially became the same. Furthermore, it is difficult to see how some of the outcomes could be convincingly linked to the intervention—being allocated to a room with a bath.

Another concern with this study identified by Homer (2004) is the choice of analysis and the conclusions reported. In spite of stating at the outset that the neonatal outcomes studied would be clinical and laboratory signs of infection, antibiotic use, and nursery care, the authors use resuscitation at birth as a significant outcome. Resuscitation at birth is considered a 'soft' outcome that is directly related to the experience of the attending clinicians and their individual assessment of the baby's condition. In addition, the type of resuscitation used in the study was described as waving oxygen around the baby's face, a practice that one could argue might be directly related to practitioner anxiety with regard to the use of water immersion.

Potential near-drowning

More recently, Nguyen and colleagues (2002) reported, in *Pediatrics*, four cases of babies admitted to the neonatal unit following birth in water at other hospitals and at home. These babies presented to hospital with moderate to severe respiratory distress and were reported to have water aspiration and subsequent pulmonary oedema. With clinical support, all the babies improved over a 24-hour period. This article highlights a concern about potential near-drowning associated with birth in water, and the authors call for all water births to be prospectively audited.

Similarly, Bowden and colleagues (2002) report, in *Pediatrics*, on four admissions to a neonatal intensive care unit after birth in water. The first case was suspected to have water inhalation; however, his discharge diagnosis was respiratory distress syndrome. The second baby developed seizures at eight hours of age and his discharge diagnosis was probable water intoxication after birth in water. The third baby had a congenital abnormality diagnosed on day two. The fourth baby was admitted at four days of age with Group B streptococcal meningitis not directly attributable to birth in water.

In response to the concerns raised by their paediatric colleagues regarding the effects of birth in water on the neonate, Pinette and colleagues (2004) conducted a retrospective review of the literature regarding possible complications associated with birth in water. They identified 16 citations that reported

> ### Clinical point
>
> **Key messages from research**
> - Women are highly satisfied with using water for labour and birth.
> - Women feel more in control of the process of birth, which ultimately leads to a more positive experience.
> - Outcomes and risks are similar for low-risk women who labour and birth in water, and those who labour and birth in air.
> - There is a need to continue to audit the practice in combination with comments on experiences from women and midwives. Research into the effects on the baby of birth underwater is recommended.
> - Research evidence should continue to inform practice.

on complications with neonates that could be attributed to birth in water. The possible complications included freshwater drowning, neonatal hyponatraemia, hypoxic ischaemic encephalopathy, and death. The authors, however, state that the rates of these complications are likely to be low.

Conclusions about adverse outcomes need to be considered in relation to the small sample sizes of all the trials reviewed. Women contemplating birth in water need to know the possibility of adverse effects on the baby, in order to make an informed decision. However, because of insufficient data, the evidence for attributable risk associated with water birth is unclear. The literature informs us that there are occasional poor outcomes that may be associated with birth in water.

There is a continuing call to research birth in water and to monitor the outcomes for both mother and baby. All maternity facilities, birthing units and independent practitioners offering water immersion and birth should be collecting prospective outcome data. In light of Woodward and Kelly's (2004) pilot study, it seems that a multi-centred RCT comparing birth in water with birth on land is now more feasible.

Using water for labour and birth: the practice

Women and midwives have used water for labour and birth, at home births, for decades. At home, women use their domestic bath, portable birth pools and sometimes inflatable paddling pools bought especially for the purpose. Women birthing at home actively seek to avoid any intervention into their birth process and are largely very well informed and knowledgeable about the benefits of using water for labour and birth. Home birth midwives have explored, with women, the means of birthing physiologically. The use of water is one method used to achieve this. To this end, home birth midwives generally have become knowledgeable and experienced in water immersion and water birth.

Globally, and not just at home births, there has been an increase in the number of women seeking to use water for labour and birth. In response to the increasing demand from women and midwives it has become more common to find water-immersion facilities in maternity units at all levels. This is an attempt by institutions to provide a home-like environment that supports a more holistic approach to birth. Hodnett 2000 has found that women who were allocated to care in home-like settings were less likely to use pharmacological pain relief measures during labour, less likely to have labour augmented with oxytocin, less likely to be immobile during labour, less likely to have fetal heart abnormalities, and were happier with their care, than women who received standard care. Hospitals and birth units have spa baths/birth pools that vary widely in size, shape, depth, place and position in the birth room.

Ideally, women will have antenatal preparation and education regarding, amongst other things, the use of water for labour and birth. This education is best provided by the midwife who provides care throughout pregnancy, labour and birth and postnatally. Continuity of caregiver supports informed decision-making. However, not all midwives are able to practise as the lead maternity carer, enabling continuity of care and the formulation of a midwifery partnership. This places greater challenges on the midwife, especially in the maternity facility where the midwife may not have met the woman until she is in labour, to ensure that the women she recommends water to are fully informed of all the possibilities.

In the studies reviewed, women had made an informed decision to use water immersion for labour and birth. They were therefore strongly motivated to labour without pain relief and medical intervention. Furthermore, the presence of a midwife throughout the labour and birth potentially affects the research, given that constant support of a female companion has been shown by a large number of studies to decrease both the length of labour and the need for pain relief (Hodnett 1999).

Subsequently, one needs to ask whether the women in the studies had such straightforward labours because of

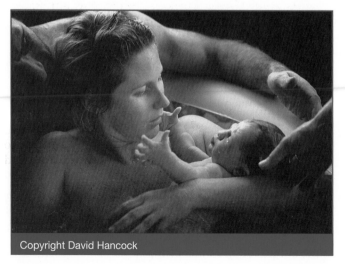

Copyright David Hancock

> ### Clinical point
>
> **Continuous support in labour**
> Research supports the need for a continuous supportive presence with women during labour. This by itself has been shown to reduce the likelihood of medication for pain relief, a caesarean section or a forceps delivery. For the women in this study, to be able to labour and birth in water meant that they were required to form a relationship with a midwife who was philosophically in tune with them and would support their choices. There is a need for partnership and teamwork between women and midwives.

this constant companionship and the environment, rather than any benefits associated with water, or whether it was a combination of all these components. In addition, most of the studies do not give any clear indication of the attitudes of the midwifery staff towards the use of water immersion during labour and birth. This will surely affect the outcome for women. Midwives who are unfamiliar or opposed to water immersion for labour and birth may become more sensitive about potential problems and are therefore more likely to use resuscitation and initiate unnecessary interventions such as directing the woman to leave the water. Midwives need to be educated in how to support women during labour and birth in water, as well as having the opportunity to witness water labour and birth before they attend one, and to have ongoing professional development.

Guidelines and principles for the use of water for labour and birth

The principles that underpin midwifery practice are the belief that pregnancy and childbirth are normal life events for most women, that midwifery care is woman-centred and continuity of care is desirable throughout the entire childbearing experience. These philosophies provide midwives with the opportunity to support physiological birth. One of the strategies used by midwives in support of physiological birth is the use of water during labour and birth. Midwives recognise that warm water immersion changes the dynamics of labour and birth and empowers women, in most instances, to birth without intervention.

While guidelines will vary in each location, there are general principles that can be drawn from the literature regarding the benefits and considerations of using water for labour and birth.

Benefits of labour and birth in water

For the woman:
- Warm water cradles, supports, relaxes, comforts and soothes, thereby reducing anxiety.
- It enables instinctive behaviour and increases the feeling of being in control, which in turn leads to a high degree of postnatal wellbeing.

- There is less operative delivery and perineal trauma.
- It provides buoyancy and increased mobility, reduces pressure on muscles and vena cava (reduces BP).
- It reduces the need for pharmacological pain relief.
- It provides a protected, secure birthing space.

For the baby:
- The reduced maternal need for pharmacological pain relief reduces the side-effects on the baby.
- Theoretically, the baby's first breath is gentle, as the air above the water is warm and humidified.
- Theoretically, it provides a smooth, trauma-free transitory passage for the baby.

For the midwife:
- It provides the increasingly rare opportunity to witness and facilitate physiological birth.
- It develops and enhances the fundamental skill of working in partnership with women.
- It enables her to extend her knowledge base and participate in research into the use of water for labour and birth.

Important considerations for attending labour and birth in water

Two important considerations are:
- the birthing family's attitude and expectations. Education regarding the use of water for labour and birth is important antenatally to prepare women and their families. A woman's fear/anxiety about birthing in water is a contraindication.
- the midwife's attitude, experience and confidence in supporting women to use water for labour and birth. Women who labour and birth in water should expect practitioners who have appropriate skills.

Who can use water for labour and birth?

Because each woman is an individual and her pregnancy unique, her care should be individually negotiated by a known midwife. The midwife uses her clinical judgement as to the suitability of using water for each woman. Many maternity facilities have developed water immersion and water birth criteria that are too prescriptive, inhibit autonomous midwifery practice and are more to do with facility risk management than what women want.

Criteria:
- low-risk pregnancy > 36 weeks (no adverse factors noted in maternal or fetal wellbeing during pregnancy or labour)
- the woman's choice to use water for labour and birth
- established labour
- no specific requirement for continuous fetal heart rate monitoring.

Some reasons why it may *not* be advisable for a woman to use the birth pool include the following:
- maternal temperature > 37.5°C
- thick meconium staining of liquor
- recent use of a systemic opioid for analgesia.

Most practitioners consider breech presentations and multiple pregnancies unsuitable for underwater birth; however, there is anecdotal evidence that these do occasionally occur both in hospitals and at home.

Equipment

- purpose-built birthing pool, portable birth pool, spa bath or inflatable paddling pool with firm sides
- a continuous supply of hot and cold water (temperature can be maintained by immersion heater or continuous supply of temperature-regulated water)
- adequate supply of dry linen, especially towels
- sieve—for keeping water as free of faecal contamination as possible
- light source (e.g. waterproof torch or headlamp)
- mirror
- protective clothing (personal choice or according to hospital guidelines)
- plastic waterproof support pillow or a rolled-up towel for head or arm support
- portable delivery pack, oxygen and suction, oxytocics
- waterproof Doppler and a Pinnard
- portable nitrous oxide/entonox as appropriate, though generally not at a home birth
- foot stool
- fan
- bed or mattress nearby.

Occupational health and safety considerations

- back care—midwife awareness
- protective clothing:
  - long latex gauntlet gloves
  - knee pads or low stool
  - plastic aprons
- infection control:
  - Hoses and jets in the pool are not recommended. However, when hoses are required for filling pools, especially at home births, two different-coloured hoses, one for filling and one for emptying pools must be used.
  - an agreed policy for cleaning the birth pool (and hoses)—chlorine agents are most effective against HIV, hepatitis B and C
- non-slip flooring/mats in pool
- electrical equipment kept away from 'wet' areas
- adequate room ventilation
- promotion of the safety and wellbeing of all, particularly children.

Care of woman and baby

During labour:
- Advise and assist the woman to wait until she is in active labour before entering the pool.
- The water in the pool should be filled to the level of the woman's chest while she is sitting in the pool.
- Maintain the water temperature according to the woman's comfort.
- Do routine labour observations and FHR recording.

- Encourage the woman to drink as desired while in the water.
- As much as possible keep faecal contamination of the water to a minimum.
- Encourage the woman to explore different positions in the pool.

During a birth in water:

- The woman should not be left alone when in water, and during the second stage the midwife should remain in the room.
- Attend to routine second-stage observations.
- Encourage physiological pushing. Physiological or non-directed pushing is less likely to tire the woman and her baby (Paine & Tinker 1992).
- A 'hands-off' technique by the midwife is advised when appropriate, supported by verbal guidance.
- A hands-off technique keeps tactile stimulation to a minimum (Johnson 1996).
- The practice of checking for nuchal cord is to be avoided.
- In most cases the nuchal cord can be loosened and disentangled as the baby is born (Burns & Kitzinger 2000).
- The baby should be born completely under the water and brought gently to the surface, being careful to minimise unnecessary cord traction. In the surveillance study reported by Gilbert and Tookey (1999), the incidence of five snapped cords highlights the importance of minimising traction on the cord during birth. If the cord is short, then the woman is instructed and assisted to stand out of or above the water to receive her baby.
- Following the birth, do *not* allow the baby's head to re-submerge. It is important to communicate to the woman the need for the baby's head to remain above the water once born, and for the midwife to ensure that while in the woman's arms the baby does not inadvertently slip back into the water.
- Carry out routine observations and Apgar score on baby. Experienced water birth practitioners observe that babies born in water appear more relaxed and quiet at birth, which may affect the one-minute Apgar score.
- Maintain the baby's temperature by using a woollen bonnet and keeping the baby's body under the warm water. There is a need to maintain a neutral thermal zone for the baby and minimise oxygen consumption by reducing heat loss. Babies lose a lot of heat from their heads. Replace wet blankets with warm, dry ones as needed.
- Conduct a physiological third stage, where the cord is left unclamped until the placenta and membranes are born. This is encouraged wherever possible. Active management may be used if indicated. When a midwife is judicious in conducting a physiological third stage, there is no increase in postpartum haemorrhage. There is no evidence to suggest that third stage must be conducted out of the water (Burns & Kitzinger 2000; Levy 1990).
- The woman is assisted from the pool to a nearby couch or bed, as required, when she is ready.
- Ensure the baby's warmth by drying thoroughly and maintaining skin-to-skin contact with the woman, as appropriate.

Complications

The midwife's use of wise clinical judgement is of paramount importance.

As with all aspects of care during pregnancy, labour and birth, there is an expectation that the midwife will have discussed the full range of possibilities and actions with the woman in her care. A woman who is fully informed will trust the midwife's judgement and immediately heed her advice to leave the water if there are any concerns for her safety or that of the baby. It is important for midwives to acknowledge that 'uneasy' feeling they may have even though it may not appear clinically justified. Experienced midwives often describe acting on intuition that, on reflection, was very predictive of outcome. Be honest with the woman regarding your feelings—she may be feeling the same!

- *fetal distress—FHR irregularity/abnormality*. Where there is any non-reassuring fetal heart rate, the midwife should advise the woman to birth out of the water (Johnson 1996).
- *grade II meconium staining*. Grade I meconium is considered normal. The woman is requested to leave the water if time permits and she is able when > Grade I meconium is present. If she is unable to exit the water in time, continue with the birth and suction the baby's airways when the baby's head is above the water. Thick meconium is the most ominous sign and requires the woman to exit the water immediately (Enkin et al 2000).
- *slow progress in labour (any stage)*. Sometimes the water slows the labour down. Often simply assisting the woman from the water will remedy this situation (Eriksson et al 1997). Ask the woman to have some time out of the water (advising her to go to the toilet to pass urine is useful), thereby allowing gravity to help contractions to re-establish. Going back into the water is still an option.
- *use of narcotic analgesia*. Women who have used a systemic opioid for pain relief in labour need to be carefully assessed due to the sedating effect of the medication on her and her baby.
- *tight nuchal cord*. In the rare event that the cord needs to be cut, the mother is asked to stand out of the water. The cord must not be cut and clamped under water (Burns & Kitzinger 2000).
- *maternal hyperthermia*. This may lead to the overriding of the baby's normal inhibition to breathe (Johnson 1996).
- *episiotomy*. The most common indication for episiotomy is fetal distress, and therefore one could argue that there is no place for it in the practice of water birth because if the midwife is worried about the wellbeing of the baby, the mother should be assisted out of the water to birth on land (Cluett et al 2004a).
- *shoulder dystocia*. This is considered an obstetric or

midwifery emergency. When shoulder dystocia is diagnosed, the woman is assisted to stand up and place her leg on the side of the pool (this encourages hyperflexion of the leg, as in the McRoberts manoeuvre). The over-stimulation from the manipulation of the baby may initiate respirations or fetal distress in the baby and subsequent gasping under water. Often the act of changing position alone dislodges the shoulders.

- *postpartum haemorrhage*. Blood loss is assessed as > 500 mL or < 500 mL due to the difficulty of accurate estimates in water. A useful guide is how dark the water is getting and whether you can still assess the skin colour of the woman's thighs. It is wise to assist the woman out of the water sooner rather than later, when her condition may be compromised (Harper 2000).

Conclusion

History and over two decades of research and literature have informed midwives' practice around the use of water for labour and birth. From the most recent Cochrane Database Systematic Review of immersion in water in pregnancy, labour and birth, the reviewers have concluded that there is evidence that water immersion during the first stage of labour reduces the use of analgesia and reported maternal pain, without adverse outcomes on labour duration, operative delivery or neonatal outcomes. Water immersion during the first stage of labour can be supported for low-risk women (Cluett et al 2004a).

Generally, there is a lack of published data in Australia and New Zealand on the use of water for labour and birth, and this is not indicative of its widespread usage. To date there is insufficient evidence regarding the use of water immersion during second stage to enable firm conclusions to be drawn about the safety and effectiveness of giving birth in water, and researchers and practitioners have called for further research and prospective auditing.

In response to the increasing demand from women and midwives, it has become more common to find water-immersion facilities in maternity units. This is an attempt by institutions to provide a home-like environment that supports a more holistic approach to birth.

Women report that the use of warm water changes the dynamics of labouring and birthing and gives control back to them. Women also report that being immersed in water does not necessarily take the pain away. What it does appear to do, and this is supported in the literature, is to provide a release from the pain in the form of warming, soothing, comforting and relaxing. For women who want to avoid pharmacological pain relief and for midwives who support these women, judicious use of water immersion may offer the means to achieve this.

For midwives, the option to use water is one way of supporting women to birth physiologically and to experience the skill of being 'with woman'.

Review questions

1   What are the key principles of a midwifery model of care that supports women in using water for labour and birth?

2   What do women like about using water for labour and birth?

3   The Cochrane Database of Systematic Reviews, updated February 2004, reports on eight trials (2939 women) examining the effects of water immersion during labour. What conclusions did the reviewers reach?

4   What are the main mechanisms that inhibit breathing in utero to prevent the inhalation of water during a water birth?

5   What is the current thinking on the recommended temperature of the water during labour and birth?

6   Who can use water for labour and birth? When is it *not* advisable?

7   Discuss the research evidence associated with perineal trauma and the use of water immersion for labour and birth.

Review questions—cont'd

8   Describe the occupational health and safety considerations for the woman and the baby during a water birth.

9   Discuss a midwife's care of a woman and a baby during a water birth.

10   Describe how a midwife would assess a woman's blood loss during a water birth.

Online resources

Gentlebirth, http://www.gentlebirth.org/archives/watrbrth.html

MIDIRS leaflets for professionals and women, http://www.infochoice.org

Sheila Kitzinger website, http://www.sheilakitzinger.com/WaterBirth.htm

Waterbirth International, http://www.waterbirth.org

References

Aird IA, Luckas MJM, Buckett WM et al 1997 Effects of intrapartum hydrotherapy on labour related parameters. Australian and New Zealand Journal of Obstetrics and Gynaecology 37(2): 137–142

Alderdice F, Renfrew M, Marchant S et al 1995 Labour and birth in water in England and Wales: a survey report. British Journal of Midwifery 3(7):375–382

Anderson T 2004 Time to throw the water birth thermometer away? MIDIRS Midwifery Digest 14:3

Austin T, Bridges N, Markiewicz M et al 1997 Severe neonatal polycythaemia after third stage of labour underwater. Lancet 350(9089):1445

Banks M 1998 Water birth pools—the essential labour aid! In: Water birth: debunking the myths. Seminar Booklet, Hamilton, NZ

Beake S 1999 Water birth: a literature review. MIDIRS Midwifery Digest 9(4):473–477

Beech BL 1996 Water birth unplugged. Proceedings of the First International Water birth Conference. Books for Midwives, Cheshire

Binney J, Chapman G 1986 Nga Morehu—the survivors. Oxford University Press, Auckland

Bowden K, Kessler D, Pinette M et al 2002 Underwater birth: missing the evidence or missing the point? Pediatrics 112(4):472–473

Burke E, Kilfoyle A 1995 A comparative study: water birth and bedbirth. Midwives January:3–7

Burns E, Kitzinger S 2000 Midwifery guidelines for use of water in labour. OCHRAD, Oxford Brookes University

Cammu H, Clasen K, van Wettere L et al 1994 'To bathe or not to bathe' during the first stage of labor. Acta Obstetricia et Gynecologica Scandinavica 73:468–472

Caplice 2004 Birth and water. Presented at Birthing Normally Conference, Royal Hospital for Women, Sydney, August 2004

Caplice S 1999 Birth in water: waving not drowning. NSW Midwives Association Annual Conference. NSW Midwives Association Inc., Sydney

Cassie F 2002 Water birth—a midwife's viewpoint. New Zealand Midwifery News 25:4–6

Charles C 1998 Fetal hyperthermia risk from warm water immersion. British Journal of Midwifery 6(3):152–156

Church L 1989 Water birth: one birthing centre's observations. Journal of Nurse–Midwifery 34(4):165–170

Cluett ER, Nikodem VC, McCandlish RE et al 2004a Immersion in water in pregnancy, labour and birth. Cochrane Library (2). The Cochrane Collaboration

Cluett ER, Pickering RM, Getliffe K et al 2004b Randomised controlled trial of labouring in water compared with standard augmentation for management of dystocia in first stage labour. British Medical Journal 328(7435):314–317

Colombo C, Pei P, Jost J 2000 Water births and the exposure to HIV. Pflege Germany 13(3):152–159

Cro S, Preston J 2002. Cord snapping at waterbirth delivery. British Journal of Midwifery 10(8):494–497

Deans AC, Steer PS 1995 Temperature of pool is important. British Medical Journal 311:390–391

Deschenes L 1990 Hydrotherapy in midwifery. Nursing Quebec 10(3):49–53

Duly LMM 2001 Birth in water. Royal College of Obstetricians and Gynaecologists. Statement on behalf of the Guidelines and Audit Committee of the RCOG. Oxford

Eckert K, Turnball D, MacLennan A 2001 Immersion in water in the first stage of labor: a randomised controlled trial. Birth 28:84–93

Enkin M, Keirse M, Neilson J et al 2000 A guide to effective care in pregnancy and childbirth. Oxford University Press, Oxford

Eriksson M, Mattsson LA, Ladfors L 1997 Early or late bath during the first stage of labour. Randomised study of 20 women. Midwifery 13:146–148

Fenton 2004 Pukekohe Maternity Unit waterbirth audit 2002. Midwifery News 32:24–25

Fewell JE, Johnson P 1983 Upper airway dynamics during breathing and during apnoea in fetal lambs. Journal of Physiology 339:495–504

Garland D 2002 Collaborative waterbirth audit: supporting practice with audit. MIDIRS Midwifery Digest 12(4):508–511

Garland D, Jones K 1994 Waterbirth: first stage immersion or non-immersion? British Journal of Midwifery 2(3):113–120

Garland D, Jones K 1997 Water birth: Updating the evidence. British Journal of Midwifery 5(6):368–372

Geissbuehler V, Eberhard J, Lebrecht A 2002 Water birth: water temperature and bathing time—mother knows best! Journal of Perinatal Medicine 30:371–378

Geissbuehler V, Eberhard J 2000 Water birth: a comparative study. A prospective study on more than 2000 water births. Fetal Diagnosis and Therapy 15:291–300

Gilbert R, Tookey 1999 Perinatal mortality and morbidity among babies delivered in water: surveillance study and postal survey. British Medical Journal 319:483–487

Ginesi L, Niescierowicz R 1998 Neuroendocrinology and birth 1: stress. British Journal of Midwifery 6(10):659–663

Gradert Y, Hertel J, Lenstrup C et al 1987 Warm tub bath during labour. Acta Obstetrica et Gynaecologica Scandinavica 66:681–683

Hall SM, Holloway IM 1998 Staying in control: women's experiences of labour in water. Midwifery 14:30–36

Harding R, Johnson P, McClelland M 1978 Liquid sensitive laryngeal receptors in the developing sheep, cat and monkey. Journal of Physiology 277:409–422

Harper B 2000 Water birth basics: from newborn breathing to hospital protocols. Midwifery Today 54:20–28

Harper B 2002 Taking the plunge: re-evaluating water birth temperature guidelines. MDIRS Midwifery Digest 12(4):506–507

Hodnett E 1999 Caregiver support for women during childbirth (Cochrane Review). Cochrane Library (4). Update Software, Oxford

Hodnett E 2000 Caregiver support for women during childbirth (Cochrane Review). Cochrane Library (4). Update Software, Oxford

Hodnett E 2001 Continuity of caregivers for care during pregnancy and childbirth (Cochrane Review). Cochrane Library (3). Update Software, Oxford

Homer C 2004 Immersion in water during first stage of labour (letter to the editor). Birth 29(1):76–77

Irwin K, Ramsden I (Eds) 1995 Toi wahine. The worlds of Maori women. Penguin, Auckland

Johnson 1996 Birth under water—to breathe or not to breathe. In: BA Beech (Ed) Water birth unplugged. Proceedings of the First Water Birth Conference. Books for Midwives, Cheshire

Kitzinger S 1996 In: BA Beech (Ed) Water birth unplugged. Proceeding of the First International Water Birth Conference. Books for Midwives, Cheshire

Leboyer F 1975 Birth without violence. Mandarin, London

Lecky-Thompson M 1989 Water birthing. Celebrating a revolution in birth. Proceedings of the Tenth National Homebirth Conference. Homebirth Access, Sydney, pp 115–122

Lenstrup C, Schantz A, Berget A et al 1987 Warm tub during delivery. Acta Obstetrica et Gynecologica Scandinavica 66: 709–712

Lepori B 1994 Freedom of movement in birth places. Children's Environments 11(2):81–87

Levy V 1990 The midwife's management of the third stage of labour. In: J Alexander, V Levy, S Roch (Eds) Midwifery practice: intrapartum care. A research-based approach. Macmillan, Basingstoke

Lichy R, Herzberg E 1993 The water birth handbook. Gateway Books, Bath

Makereti 1986 The old-time Maori. New Women's Press, Auckland

Maude R 2003 It's beyond water: stories of women's experience of using water for labour and birth. Unpublished masters thesis. Victoria University

Ngugen S, Kuschel C, Teele R et al 2002 Water birth—a near drowning experience, Pediatrics 110(2):411–413

Nightingale C 1994 Water birth in practice. Modern Midwife 4(1): 15–19

Odent M 1983 Birth under water. Lancet 24(31):1476–1477

Odent M 1990 Water and sexuality. Penguin, London

Odent M 1997 Can water immersion stop labour? Journal of Nurse-Midwifery 42(5):414–416

Odent M 2001 The scientification of love. Free Association Books, London

Page A 1994 A midwives' perspective of water birth. Unpublished study, Melbourne

Paine LL, Tinker DD 1992 The effects of maternal bearing down efforts on arterial umbilical cord pH and length of the second stage of labour. Journal of Nurse Midwifery 37(1):61–63

Pinette M, Wax J, Wilson E 2004 The risks of underwater birth. American Journal of Obstetrics and Gynaecology 190:1211–1215

Richmond H 2003a Theories surrounding water birth. The Practising Midwife 6(2):10–13

Richmond H 2003b Women's experience of water birth. The Practising Midwife 6(3):26–31

Robertson Huang LJ, Croughan-Minihane MS, Kilpatrick SJ 1998 Is there an association between water baths during labor and the development of chorioamnionitis or endometritis? American Journal of Obstetrics and Gynaecology 178(6):1215–1221

Rosenthal MJ 1991 Warm water immersions in labour and birth. The Female Patient 16:35–44

Rosevear SK, Fox R, Marlow N et al 1993 Birthing pools and the fetus. Lancet 342: 1048–1049

Rosser J 1994 Is water birth safe? The facts behind the controversy. MIDIRS Midwifery Digest 4(1):4–6

Schorn M, McAllister JL, Blanco JD 1993 Water immersion and the effect on labor. Journal of Nurse-Midwifery 38(6):336–342

Sidenbladh E 1983 Waterbabies. Adam and Charles Black, London

Taha M 2000 The effects of water on labour: a randomised controlled trial. Unpublished thesis. Rand Afrikaans University, South Africa

Vochem M, Vogt M, Doring G 2001 Sepsis in a newborn due to pseudomonas aeruginosa from a contaminated tub bath. New England Journal of Medicine 345:378–379

Waldenstrom U, Nilsson CA 1992 Warm tub bath after spontaneous rupture of the membranes. Birth 19(2):57–63

Woodward J, Kelly SM 2004 A pilot study for a randomised controlled trial of water birth versus landbirth. British Journal of Obstetrics and Gynaecology 111:537–545

Young L 2001 The Wanganui experience of waterbirth from July 1991 to December 2000 (unpublished clinical audit)

Further reading

Balaskas J 2004 The water birth book. Unwin Hyman, London

Garland D 2000 Waterbirth. An attitude to care. Books for Midwives, London

Harper B 1995 Gentle birth choices. Healing Arts Press, Rochester, Vermont

Lichy R, Herzberg E 1997 The waterbirth handbook. A guide to the gentle art of water birthing. Gateway Books, Bath

Napierala S 1994 Water birth—a midwives' perspective. Bergin and Garvey, Westport, Connecticut

Video

The art of birth 2002 The story of four gentle births in water. Producers S Caplice, T Dusseldorp. Australia

CHAPTER 25

Maintaining the integrity of the pelvic floor

Sue Hendy

Key terms

episiotomy (midline, mediolateral), first-degree tear, fourth-degree tear, pelvic floor exercises, perineal suturing, perineal trauma, postnatal pain, second-degree tear, third-degree tear, urinary incontinence

Chapter overview

The *pelvic floor* is the term given to the structures that fill the outlet of the bony pelvis. These muscles have extensive functions, and disruption to their integrity can have serious consequences for a woman's physical, social and sexual health. Their main function is to support the internal pelvic and abdominal organs and maintain the integrity of bladder, uterus, vaginal and rectal function. They are also important for sexual function. During pregnancy and birth, the structure of these muscles is altered, and it is crucial for the midwife to have an understanding of the anatomy of the pelvic floor in order to minimise trauma

and prevent long-term morbidity. The midwife's role in the education of women in the antenatal and postnatal periods can ensure that they avoid long-term incontinence and sexual dysfunction. This chapter outlines the anatomy and physiology of the pelvic floor, methods for prevention of damage based on the latest evidence, surgical repair, and care and advice.

Learning outcomes

Learning outcomes for this chapter are:

1 To identify the structures of the pelvic floor and its importance in midwifery practice

2 To discuss best available evidence in the prevention of damage to and repair of the pelvic floor

3 To discuss health promotion advice that can be given to women in the antenatal and postnatal periods that will reduce damage and provide optimal health outcomes for women post birth.

Anatomy and physiology of the pelvic floor

This section describes the main structures of the pelvic floor, and its functions.

Structures of the pelvic floor

Pelvic peritoneum

The pelvic peritoneum lies over the uterus and ovaries. The front aspect forms the uterovesical pouch and this covers the upper surface of the bladder. At the back, it dips behind the posterior vaginal fornix and forms the Pouch of Douglas prior to passing over the rectum.

Pelvic fascia

The pelvic fascia consists of connective tissue that fills the spaces between the pelvic organs and forms strong ligaments to support the uterus (see Fig 25.1).

Broad ligaments

The peritoneal covering of the uterine tubes are called the broad ligaments but they do not have a supportive function.

- Transverse cervical ligaments (Cardinal or Mackenrodt's ligaments) (2) are attached to the sides of the cervix and extend laterally in a fan-like structure and adhere to the walls of the pelvis.
- Uterosacral ligaments are attached to the upper portion of the posterior wall of the cervix and extend upwards and back, encircling the rectum before attaching to the anterior part of the sacrum.
- Pubocervical ligaments (3) originate in the cervix, pass under the bladder and attach to the pubic bone. They suspend the uterus at the level of the supra-vaginal cervix. Their function is to aid mobility of the uterus but they also act as a hammock to assist in the prevention of prolapse.
- Round ligaments are two bands of fibrous tissue enclosed in the peritoneum that originate near the fundus of the uterus. They pass between the folds of the broad ligament to the sides of the pelvis, through the inguinal canal and fuse with the labia majora. Their function is to maintain the uterus in the anteflexed (bent on itself) and anteverted (tilted forward) position.

Deep muscle layer

The deep muscle layer is composed of two levator ani muscles. These originate from the back of the pubic bone, follow the obturator fascia and the ischial spine. They pass backwards and downwards to meet in the perineum around the anal canal. They insert into the coccyx and lower sacrum. This anatomical structure provides the hammock of strong muscle that supports the vaginal walls and uterus. The levator ani muscles also provide some support to the bladder and anal canal, and are critical to maintenance of the integrity and

strength of the pelvic floor. They are divided into three muscles (see Fig 25.2):

- The pubococcygeus muscles form the anterior section of the levator ani. Originating from the posterior aspect of the pubic bone, they pass backwards on either side of the urethra and the lowest part of the vagina and anal canal, terminating into the coccyx and anococcygeal body.
- The iliococcygeus muscles arise from the white line of pelvic fascia, pass downwards and inwards to the coccyx and anococcygeal body. This is the broader muscle section of the levator ani.
- The ischiococcygeus muscles originate at the ischial spines and pass downwards and inwards to be inserted into the coccyx and lower sacrum.

Superficial muscle layer

Although these muscles are small and contained in the superficial layer of the pelvic floor, they are critical to the

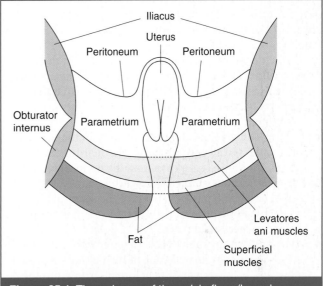

Figure 25.1 Tissue layers of the pelvic floor (based on Davis and Geck)

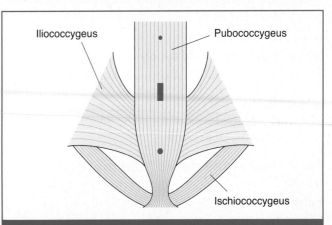

Figure 25.2 Deep muscles of the pelvic floor (levator ani muscles) (based on Davis and Geck)

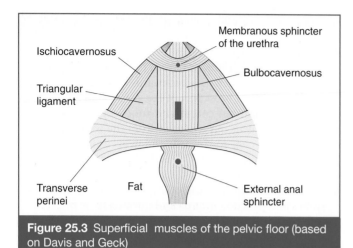

Figure 25.3 Superficial muscles of the pelvic floor (based on Davis and Geck)

overall function and strength of the pelvic floor. These muscles extend from the perineal body around the vagina to the clitoris (see Fig 25.3). They strengthen the sphincter action of the vagina and urethra, and play a part in sexual function.

- The ischiocavernosus muscles (2) originate in the ischial tuberosities and terminate in the clitoris. They are part of the triangular ligament across the pubic arch that supports the neck of the bladder and prevents urinary incontinence.
- The transverse perineal muscles pass from the ischial tuberosities to the perineal body and their function is to provide additional support across the perineal region.
- The external anal sphincter muscle encompasses the anal opening and passes in front of the perineal body before attaching posteriorly to the coccyx. It controls the passage of faeces and flatus.
- The membranous sphincter of the urethra are two bands of muscle that originate at one of the pubic bones, pass above and below the urethra before inserting into the other pubic bone.
- The bulbocavernosus muscles (2) arise in the centre of the perineum and pass on either side of the urethra and vagina, encircling the orifices before inserting into the pubic bones.

Nerve, lymph and blood supply

The third and fourth sacral nerves and the pudendal nerve supply the pelvic floor. Lymph drainage is via the internal iliac glands, and the blood supply is from the internal iliac arteries and veins. The final layer of the pelvic floor is composed of superficial fascia, fat and skin.

Functions of the pelvic floor and perineal body

Pelvic floor

As noted earlier, pelvic floor is the term given to the structures that fill the outlet of the bony pelvis. Their main function is to provide support for the internal pelvic and abdominal organs, which include the bladder, uterus, vagina and rectum. When intra-abdominal pressure is increased (during sneezing, coughing etc), the pelvic floor works to balance the pressure. These muscles have extensive functions, and disruption to their integrity can have serious consequences for a woman's physical, social and sexual health. Pregnancy and birth pose an enormous challenge to these structures, weakening them and causing stress incontinence (involuntary leakage of urine). This is a common complication of childbirth—some studies cite 20% of women experiencing stress incontinence many months after birth and one in four adult women being affected (Herbert 1998).

Under the influence of pregnancy-initiated hormones, the pelvic floor relaxes during pregnancy. This is to enable the structures to expand considerably during birth to allow passage of the fetus through the birth canal. Paradoxically, this process also assists practitioners in performing vaginal examinations, as the musculature is less rigid and the woman less uncomfortable. Due to the elasticity and complex structure of the pelvic floor, it is possible for a woman to gain full control and function of her muscles within a short time after the birth. The midwife has a crucial health promotion role here. During the late antenatal period, women should be advised not to undertake any high impact exercises, as these increase stress on the pelvic musculature, which has already been adversely affected by pregnancy hormones and the gravid uterus (Dunkley 2000). However, the midwife should include education for women about pelvic floor strengthening to prevent urinary incontinence.

Perineal body

The perineal body is a triangular structure located between the lowest part of the vaginal introitus and the anal canal (see Fig 25.4). This is the point at which the levator ani muscles and superficial muscles unite and is the structure that stretches to a large extent during crowning of the baby's head. The core strength of the pelvic floor is contained within this structure. It is made up of skin, and the superficial and deep muscles of the pelvic floor:
- bulbocavernosus
- transverse perinei
- pubococcygeus.

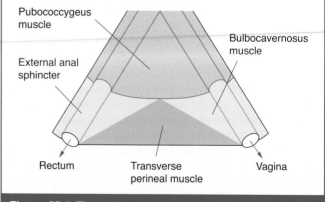

Figure 25.4 The perineal body (based on Davis and Geck)

The nerve supply is from the perineal branch of the pudendal nerve, lymphatic drainage is via the inguinal and external iliac glands, and blood supply is from the pudendal arteries and veins. Its chief function is control of defecation and childbirth. The perineal body varies in size and can be absent in some women. There is an association between a small perineal body and severe perineal trauma.

It is important for the midwife to understand the underlying anatomy and physiology of the pelvic floor, to assist in maintaining its integrity during childbirth. A clear anatomical understanding is vital for repair of the pelvic floor, to achieve optimal outcomes for women. The following sections outline the types of perineal trauma, and management during and after birth.

Perineal trauma

Perineal trauma can be caused by perineal laceration or episiotomy. Cervical lacerations can cause significant brisk bleeding after birth and these are also briefly discussed.

Perineal trauma can be classified as first-, second-, third- or fourth-degree (see Table 25.1).

Further definition of third- and fourth-degree tears are provided by a recent clinical guideline:
● Third: injury to perineum involving the anal sphincter complex:
  ● 3a less than 50% of external anal sphincter (EAS) thickness torn
  ● 3b more than 50% of EAS thickness torn
  ● 3c internal anal sphincter (IAS) torn.
● Fourth: injury to perineum involving the EAS and IAS and anal epithelium (RCOG 2004).

Labial lacerations

Labial lacerations are very superficial tears that generally do not require sutures unless haemostasis cannot be achieved. Like skin grazes they can be very painful in the first few days after birth, particularly on micturition (passing urine). Women should be advised to keep the area clean and dry, and to use a douche when urinating. Analgesia can be given and if pain persists, the midwife must exclude infection and deeper trauma. The use of an alkaliniser such as Ural® for the first couple of days can make the urine sting less when urinating.

Vaginal and cervical lacerations

Vaginal and cervical lacerations can cause serious postpartum haemorrhage. Both structures are very vascular and careful inspection should be carried out after birth to exclude trauma, which can precipitate excessive blood loss. Once detected, suturing should occur without delay. Caution is required, and the midwife may need to seek advice to avoid the formation of a vaginal haematoma. An experienced obstetrician should carry out cervical suturing to avoid excessive bleeding and cervical complications in subsequent pregnancies.

TABLE 25.1	Classification of perineal trauma
First degree	Involves only skin of the fourchette and/or vaginal mucosa
Second degree (episiotomy)	As above, with involvement of skin of perineal body and muscles: • superficial—bulbocavernosus, transverse perinei • deep—pubococcygeus. The rectal mucosa is not involved.
Third degree	As for second degree, with involvement of the anal sphincter
Fourth degree	Third-degree tear that extends into the rectal mucosa

Prolapse

When the perineal muscles are overdistended, the musculature is unable to provide appropriate support for the organs, resulting in a prolapse of the pelvic organs. Those most at risk are grand multiparous women or women who have had a long, difficult labour with vaginal birth of a large baby. Types of prolapse are:
● uterovaginal prolapse—the vaginal wall is weak and the uterus protrudes down into the vagina
● cystocele—the bladder bulges into the vagina due to a weakened upper anterior vaginal wall
● rectocele—the rectum bulges into the vagina due to a weakened posterior vaginal wall
● cervical prolapse—the cervix protrudes into the lower half of the vagina.

Depending on the severity, most prolapses require surgical intervention. The mode of delivery for subsequent pregnancies would need to be carefully considered, to prevent further damage.

Episiotomy

An episiotomy is an incision through the perineum and perineal body that is performed immediately prior to birth. It enlarges the vaginal outlet to expedite the birth of the baby. The presenting part should be distending the perineum and analgesia should be given. This is usually in the form of local anaesthetic (see below). A midwife is trained to infiltrate the perineum and perform an episiotomy. The use of episiotomy is restricted to the following indication:
● to expedite birth when the presenting part is distending the perineum and there is evidence of non-reassuring fetal heart rate pattern.

Further consideration can be given to the following situations:
● maternal exhaustion
● to reduce maternal effort if cardiac disease, epilepsy or hypertension is present
● rigid perineum—in some cases, increased rigidity of the

perineal musculature causes a prolonged delay in the second stage.
● 'button holing' of the perineum.
● to prevent perineal trauma associated with a history of surgical repair of the pelvic floor, bladder repair or fistula.

Women should be fully informed about the need for an episiotomy and give consent to the procedure. This issue should be discussed in the antenatal period so that women can understand the criteria that would require a midwife to seek permission to perform an episiotomy. This is then noted on the birth plan. Unexpected changes to a woman's birth plan in labour need to be fully discussed so that the woman understands the need to perform an episiotomy and can fully consent. This is then documented in the notes.

Performing an episiotomy

There are two types of episiotomy (see Fig 25.5):
● Mediolateral—the incision starts in the midline of the fourchette and runs backwards to a point between the ischial tuberosity and the anus. This type of incision appears to be less likely to extend to involve the anal region and helps prevent damage to the Bartholin's gland.
● Midline—the incision is from the fourchette directly down towards the anus. It is easier to repair and has been associated with less pain and bleeding, although there is an increased risk that it will extend to a third- or fourth-degree tear.

The structures involved when performing an episiotomy include the skin of the fourchette, posterior vaginal wall and perineal muscles (superficial and deep).

Infiltration of the perineum

Prior to performing an episiotomy, analgesia should be considered. This is usually achieved by infiltration of the area with local anaesthetic such as lignocaine 0.5% or 1% (10 mL). The baby's head should be distending the perineum so that the muscles are thinning. The area should be cleaned with an antiseptic solution. The midwife inserts two gloved fingers into the vagina to protect the baby's head. The needle is inserted into the muscle layer in the area of the incision. The plunger of the syringe is withdrawn to ensure that the needle is not in a blood vessel. If blood is seen in the syringe then the needle should be withdrawn slightly and another area tested. The anaesthetic should never be put into a blood vessel. Once clear of blood vessels, the anaesthetic is inserted into the muscle as the needle is withdrawn from the tissue (approximately 3–4 mL). Just prior to the needle being completely withdrawn, the needle is reinserted to the side of the incision site, where 2–3 mL of local anaesthetic is discharged and this is repeated on the other side. Each time, the midwife must check to avoid blood vessels. This provides a fan-like cover of the area. The infiltration should be performed three to five minutes prior to the incision, to ensure adequate analgesia. However, lignocaine transfer to the fetus is quite rapid and so caution should be exercised with local anaesthetic (ALSO 2000).

Women with epidurals need to be assessed carefully, especially if the anaesthetic effect has worn off and may require extra cover with infiltration. An obstetrician sometimes performs a pudendal block for episiotomy prior to instrumental birth. Very little research has been carried out in the area of pain experienced by women undergoing episiotomy, but many women are not given adequate analgesia for this procedure, some being offered nothing or the use of nitrous oxide (Maunders 1998).

Once anaesthesia is achieved, the midwife inserts the same two fingers into the vagina to protect the baby's head. An episiotomy is performed using blunt-ended Mayo scissors. These are now opened and one blade is placed between the fingers and the other blade along the area where the lignocaine was introduced. A single, confident cut, approximately 4 cm long, is made, preferably during a contraction, to minimise pain. A thin, well-stretched perineum is also less likely to bleed. Remove the scissors quickly and prepare for the imminent birth of the baby's head. It is critical to control the birth of the

---

BOX 25.1 Episiotomy

History and clinical practice
Perineal lacerations have been documented throughout history, with reference to them even in ancient times. It is estimated that, even with a restricted episiotomy policy, approximately 51–77% of women sustain sufficient trauma to the perineum during birth to require suturing (Beckmann & Garratt 2005). During the early part of the twentieth century, a new surgical procedure was introduced, called *episiotomy* (cutting of the perineum to enlarge the vaginal opening). This procedure, which was used to speed up birth of the baby, quickly gained popularity, particularly during the medicalisation of childbirth in the 1950s and 1960s. Midwives and doctors readily accepted the procedure as good practice, without any scientific evaluation, until it became the most commonly used surgical procedure after cutting of the umbilical cord.

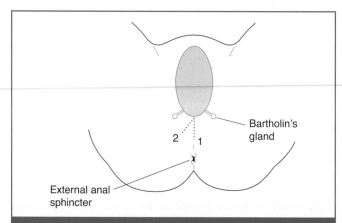

Figure 25.5 Types of episiotomy: 1 midline, 2 mediolateral (based on Davis and Geck)

head, as rapid expulsion could extend the episiotomy. If the baby is not born, the midwife will need to apply pressure to any bleeding points in the incision to minimise blood loss.

Episiotomy for vaginal birth

The claimed benefits of universal use of episiotomy were that it prevented severe tearing of the perineum, aided suturing by avoiding ragged edges, prevented long-term damage and protected the baby by expediting birth. In the early 1980s, midwifery students were taught at least nine indications, which included abnormal presentation, preterm birth, instrumental delivery, rigid perineum and fetal and maternal distress. The lack of research to evaluate the policy continued until Sleep's seminal work (1984), which revolutionised practice in the United Kingdom. Previously, the only controversy was concerning the type of incision rather than the benefits. In a review of all available trials, Sleep concluded that:

> Liberal use of episiotomy is associated with higher overall rates of perineal trauma. There is no evidence that this policy [liberal use of episiotomy] reduces the risk of serious perineal or vaginal trauma (Sleep et al 1987).

After publication of this research, a restrictive use of episiotomy was advocated. This meant that only fetal or maternal distress were used as indications for episiotomy. More recently, a Cochrane Review has supported this practice while noting an increased risk of anterior perineal trauma (Carroli & Belizan 2005). However, as the presence of an anterior tear did not significantly contribute to overall suturing, there are suggestions that anterior tears are less severe than posterior tears (Hartmann et al 2005). This review also states that women who have had an episiotomy have reduced pelvic floor muscle strength at three months post partum compared to women with tears. Certain risk factors have been identified, with rates particularly high in nulliparous women (see below). Episiotomy is known to be the greatest risk factor for a third- or fourth-degree tear (ALSO 2000). These tears require suturing in theatre under general anaesthetic by an experienced obstetrician. The stress of undergoing this procedure, as well as pain and fear, can prevent women enjoying the birth of their baby. Previous experience of severe perineal trauma and long-term morbidity can create enormous anxiety in a woman embarking on a subsequent birth. The woman should be offered counselling prior to or during pregnancy and supported to make an informed choice about mode of birth and the likelihood of recurring damage. Caesarean section may be an option for some of these women.

Even with a restrictive policy, rates of perineal trauma requiring suturing remain high at 51–77% (Kettle & Johanson 1998). Wide variations in practice exist between midwives and obstetricians, with place of birth, training and public or private status affecting episiotomy rates. These persistent wide variations in clinical practice suggest that episiotomy use is 'heavily driven by local professional norms, experiences in training and individual practitioner's preference rather than variations in the needs of individual women at the time of vaginal birth' (Hartmann et al 2005). This systematic review

identified 26 articles outlining the best available evidence in relation to the use of restrictive versus routine use of episiotomy. Synthesis of these studies reported more pain and delayed healing, increased rates of third- and fourth-degree tears, no difference in rates and duration of urinary incontinence, and an increase in dyspareunia (painful sexual intercourse) at three months post partum with the use of routine episiotomy. There was also no reported benefit in respect of preserving pelvic floor integrity and decreasing the incidence of stress incontinence when using episiotomy. It is suggested that an episiotomy rate of 15% or less with spontaneous births is achievable and should be implemented immediately, and that this would clear the way for study of other techniques aimed at decreasing perineal trauma. The authors conclude that:

> Our systematic review finds no benefit from episiotomy . . . Indeed, routine use is harmful to the degree that some proportion of women who would have had a lesser injury instead had a surgical incision . . . In the absence of benefits and with a potential for harm, a procedure should be abandoned . . . The time has come to take on the professional responsibility of setting and achieving goals for reducing episiotomy use (Hartmann et al 1995).

In the current era of midwifery, many students do not get the opportunity to perform an episiotomy. It is important that students and midwives do acquire and maintain this skill, as judicious use of episiotomy is still an important aspect of contemporary midwifery care.

Risk factors for severe perineal trauma

- routine episiotomy (midline more likely than mediolateral)
- birth in lithotomy position
- operative birth, particularly forceps delivery
- experience of accoucheur
- prolonged second stage and use of oxytocin
- nulliparous women
- malposition (e.g. occipito transverse or posterior position)
- anaesthesia (local and epidural)
- increasing fetal head circumference and weight > 4 kg
- ethnicity (some ethnic groups are at higher risk).

Prevention of damage

There is a potential for perineal trauma with significant morbidity after vaginal birth, and some of these women may seek a caesarean section in subsequent pregnancies to alleviate their anxiety and pain. This is of concern in an era of increasing operative delivery rates. What role can the midwife play in reversing this trend, and what advice can be given to women to decrease their likelihood of sustaining significant perineal trauma? Perineal massage has been shown to increase the likelihood of an intact perineum when commenced at 34 weeks in nulliparous women but has no effect in subsequent pregnancies (Labrecque et al 1999). As nulliparous women are at an increased risk of severe perineal trauma, this may be an effective intervention to promote during antenatal care. Further reviews of evidence are currently under way (Beckmann & Garratt 2005). Perineal massage can be carried out during pregnancy using a pure vegetable oil such as almond. The woman or her partner should insert a thumb into the lower vagina and massage the skin gently externally to improve elasticity.

It has been suggested that ethnicity, age tissue type and nutritional state in pre-pregnancy years influence extent of trauma to the perineum (Renfrew et al 1998). Nutritional advice, including prevention of anaemia, will aid healing of any trauma in the postnatal period.

A meta-analysis of randomised controlled trials showed evidence that spontaneous vaginal birth or vacuum extraction reduced the incidence of perineal trauma (Eason et al 2000). There is no clear evidence or consensus about guarding the perineum in the second stage of labour, maternal position in labour (apart from the avoidance of lithotomy) or perineal massage in the second stage of labour (Beckmann & Garratt 2005; Enkin & Keirse 1999; Stamp et al 2001). It has been suggested that adopting a squatting position during labour evenly distributes vaginal and perineal pressure, maximising perineal stretching (McKay 1984). Use of a birthing chair has been associated with increased rates of postpartum haemorrhage, although this may be due to improved accuracy of estimation of blood loss. However, it has been suggested that use of the birth chair may increase blood loss from perineal trauma due to obstructed venous return as a result of pressure on the buttocks and perineum. Excessive perineal oedema and haemorrhoids have been reported in women who are upright in birth for long periods. Hands and knees or all-fours position is associated with less perineal trauma, although it may increase the risk of anterior tears and vulval trauma (Enkin & Keirse 1999). Warm pads applied during the second stage have also been used, but to date this technique has not been fully evaluated. The warm pack trial is now complete and awaiting publication (Stamp et al 2001)

It is important for the midwife to allow time for perineal thinning during crowning of the head and to seek assistance from the woman at this time to facilitate a slow, controlled birth of the head. An uncontrolled expulsion of the baby's head will not only risk perineal trauma but can also cause trauma to the baby's brain.

Birth can be an overwhelming and frightening experience for women, particularly during the second stage. A midwife's role is to support the woman and provide her with information to assist in ensuring that the birth has the best possible outcome. Working with women in this way can greatly assist in reducing perineal trauma and subsequent postnatal pain for the mother.

Perineal suturing technique and materials

Continuity of care includes completion of the birth process by suturing the perineum if required. This may also mean that the suturing is attended to promptly rather than having to wait for a medical colleague. Immediately after birth, the sensation in the perineal area is often diminished and so it is preferable to complete any suturing then. A midwife who has undergone training and is competent to do so may suture perineal trauma. However, a midwife must always be aware of her own level of expertise and seek advice and medical support as required. In Australia each health service will have a policy concerning authority to suture perineal trauma. Severe perineal trauma, excessive bleeding or problems with haematoma formation should always be referred to a senior medical colleague. Verbal consent should be sought from the woman, with a full explanation of what the procedure entails.

Controversy exists over non-suturing of perineal lacerations in terms of pain, infection rates and healing (Maunders 1998). Minor lacerations and labial tears are often a matter of personal choice for the woman. Trauma that involves more than superficial perineal muscles requires suturing. The practice of leaving first- and second-degree tears unsutured is associated with poorer wound healing but no significant difference in short-term pain outcomes (RCOG 2004). A woman's health status, hygiene and understanding may necessitate suturing of minor tears as well. The type of suture material, technique of repair and skill of the operator are the main three factors that influence perineal repair outcome (RCOG 2004).

The use of absorbable synthetic sutures such as polyglycolic acid and polyglactin 910 (Dexon or Vicryl) is associated with less perineal pain, analgesia use, dehiscence and resuturing, but increased suture removal, compared with catgut (ALSO 2000; RCOG 2004). Polyglactin 910 is associated with a significant decrease in pain and suture removal and is rapidly absorbed. It is the most appropriate material for perineal repair at present (RCOG 2004). Subcuticular sutures also disperse oedema through the whole stitch rather than being concentrated at each suture site.

Perineal repair

After delivery of the placenta, the midwife must make a through inspection of the vagina and perineum to ascertain the extent of the trauma. If an episiotomy has been performed, it is essential to identify the apex of the incision on the post vaginal wall. Failure to do so can result in haematoma formation and postpartum haemorrhage. Similarly, bleeding points should be identified and haemostasis achieved. Placing a pack or pad in the vaginal vault and leaving for a while can sometimes resolve superficial bleeding. It is essential that this be removed prior to transfer to postnatal. This procedure must be documented, including removal of the pack. If control of haemorrhage is not generally achieved within half an hour, suturing will be required.

Once a thorough inspection is complete and the midwife is satisfied that the suturing is within her capabilities, the repair is carried out under aseptic conditions. A good light is essential and the woman should be positioned appropriately to maximise the visual field. A lithotomy position is not generally required for suturing as long as inspection is easily managed and the woman is comfortable. The area is swabbed with an antiseptic solution or warm water. Sterile drapes are used as required before insertion of a local anaesthetic such as lignocaine (0.5–1%, 10–30 mL) or bupivicaine 0.25% with adrenaline 1:400,000. This is injected under the skin into the perineal muscles in a similar fashion to that used before an episiotomy. It is very important to wait for this to work, which normally take four to five minutes. Women should be advised that inserting the local can sometimes be uncomfortable. The addition of sodium bicarbonate to anaesthetic will reduce pain on infiltration (1:20 solution, e.g. 1 mL sodium bicarbonate to 20 mL lignocaine). Also, local anaesthetic with adrenaline added will help with vasoconstriction of a bleeding wound. It also prolongs the action of the anaesthetic. If the woman has an epidural it should be topped up prior to suturing, otherwise local anaesthetic is required. A woman who is pain-free will be able to relax, which makes suturing much easier. Prior to commencing, test with a needle to ensure the local is effective.

A taped tampon is sometimes inserted into the vagina to prevent vaginal loss obscuring the wound. Bleeding points are identified and sutured to prevent haematoma formation. It is important to repair the muscle layer competently, to prevent dead spaces that can also fill with blood. The repair is planned, and at each stage progress is evaluated by ensuring that edges are coming together and that the finished product realigns the anatomical structures. Perineal trauma is traditionally repaired in three layers:

1 The suture at the apex of the wound is very important, as it provides the anchor for the procedure. The vaginal epithelium is closed with a continuous running suture, which starts at the apex of the wound and finishes at the fourchette, which is then taken through into the deeper muscle layer.

2 The deep and superficial muscle layers are closed with three or four interrupted sutures aimed at approximating the muscles—continuous running sutures may also be used. Care is taken not to bite too deep into the muscle, as this may cause the rectal mucosa to be involved.

3 Finally, the skin is closed with interrupted or continuous subcuticular sutures. The continuous subcuticular technique of perineal repair has been associated with less perineal pain in the immediate postpartum period than interrupted sutures (RCOG 2004). The sutures are placed in the subcutaneous tissue instead of in the nerve-rich superficial skin.

It is important to ensure that the tension of the sutures is just right. Too tight will cause unnecessary pain and too loose will not align the structures appropriately, impairing healing and decreasing integrity of the pelvic floor. An overly tightened introitus may lead to dyspareunia.

On completion of the suturing, the vaginal tampon is removed and the vaginal vault inspected. A finger is then inserted into the rectum to ensure that no sutures have been placed in this area. This can be uncomfortable, so an explanation should be given.

Accurate documentation of the procedure should be completed, including anaesthetic used, insertion and removal of the vaginal tampon, extent of the wound and layers repaired, suture material used and advice given to the woman. All sponges and needles *must* be counted before the procedure and after the procedure before leaving the room.

Severe perineal trauma

An experienced obstetrician should suture third- and fourth-degree tears under general anaesthetic or epidural. Faecal incontinence and vesicovaginal fistula formation (where a hole is present between the bladder or urethra and vagina) are serious complications of severe perineal trauma and can have long-term physical and psychological effects. A full explanation is given and a broad-spectrum antibiotic prescribed to reduce the incidence of infection. Continuous drainage of the bladder is necessary for two to three weeks to enable the fistula to close spontaneously. If this does not happen, operative closure will be required. Hydration, diet and aperients are used to prevent constipation. Postnatal follow-up with a medical practitioner is important to detect and prevent long-term sequelae. Assessment of urinary and anal integrity via ultrasound and urodynamic tests should be performed. Counselling should be provided prior to another pregnancy.

Pelvic floor exercises

Urinary incontinence and childbirth are inextricably linked, and antenatal, postnatal and lifelong pelvic floor exercises have been shown to have a protective effect (Dunkley 2000). Midwives have an important role in providing education and advice for women in this area. Kegel (1948) was the first to advocate the promotion of pelvic floor exercises after birth to prevent stress incontinence (the involuntary loss of urine on sneezing, coughing etc). It is estimated that as many as one in four women suffer from incontinence after birth, and many women think this is a normal consequence of pregnancy and vaginal birth. Caesarean section has been shown to reduce the incidence of incontinence. However, coupled with the risks of

Scenario

Massive PPH from perineal trauma
A primigravida had given birth after a prolonged labour due to a persistent occipitoposterior position (POP). The midwife performed an episiotomy due to a non-reassuring fetal heart rate pattern and maternal distress. After the birth the woman had a 2500 mL PPH despite appropriate management, which included prompt suturing of the episiotomy. She was taken to theatre for an examination under anaesthetic (EUA), where it was discovered that the apex of the episiotomy had been missed during repair. The woman required blood replacement and intensive care as a result.

How would you document this and what information would you give to the woman about the outcome?

injury to the bladder during surgery and the other significant morbidity associated with operative birth, caesarean section is a radical step when pelvic floor exercise can cure incontinence (NICE 2004). Recent studies have continued to find significant benefits to women who are taught pelvic floor exercises, particularly in the antenatal period. Midwives should use the antenatal period to educate women about urinary and faecal incontinence and to raise awareness of this previously taboo subject (Dunkley 2000). It is important that women do not see incontinence as a normal event after pregnancy, regardless of their culture or societal background. The midwife will need to direct questions that enable women to be frank and open about any problems. Asking women if their bladder and bowel functions are 'normal' or 'okay' is ineffective communication (Scowen 1996).

Perineal trauma (prolonged second-stage, third-degree and episiotomy) and parity greater than four have been linked with the problem of stress incontinence, although women with an intact perineum and post caesarean section can also have stress incontinence. Therefore the mechanism is not fully understood, but it is believed that overstretching of the pelvic floor muscles and damage to the pudendal nerve may be risk factors. Another study compared caesarean section, parity and obesity and urinary incontinence at three months post birth. Operative birth was excluded, but parity and obesity were significant risk factors (Wilson et al 1996).

Teaching pelvic floor exercises

It is important for the midwife to explain to women the anatomy and physiology of the pelvic floor, as many women do not understand the location and structures of this important area of their body. The use of diagrams is advisable. Their use during childbirth should be outlined, as well as their long-term function.

Two types of muscles control continence: slow-twitch and fast-twitch. Both sets must be exercised to ensure effective control. Slow-twitch muscles make up 70% of the pelvic floor and are designed to be more durable in strength as their main function is to support the pelvic organs. The levator ani muscles are fast-twitch, as they react quickly to acute changes in intra-abdominal pressure such as during coughing or sneezing. This muscle group fatigues quickly. For total control, both sets of muscles must be exercised. Despite education, some women may still not contract the correct muscles. There are two ways to ensure that the right method is employed. A woman can place two fingers into the lower vagina, and should feel the muscles pull away from her fingers as she contracts the muscles.

Alternatively, she can stop and start the flow of urine mid-stream. This method enables a woman to locate the pelvic floor but must *not* be used to exercise the muscles, as it can lead to damage of the sensitive nerve fibres in the bladder. Once a woman understands the location and feel of the muscles, the midwife can teach effective exercises (see Box 25.2).

This ensures that both sets of muscles are exercised. Ideally this should be done five times a day and increased as strength is gained. Women often get discouraged from continuing

---

BOX 25.2   Pelvic floor exercises

1 Squeeze your back passage (anus) together as if you are stopping yourself from passing wind.
2 Squeeze your front passage (urethra) together as if you need to stop the flow of urine.
3 Lift both together and count to 10.
4 Repeat 10 times.
5 Repeat 1 and 2 and release quickly, 10 times.

---

these exercises after birth because they may not be able to hold on and the muscles release involuntarily. There *will* be progress and this can be demonstrated by recording the length of discernible contraction and time until fatigue sets in. All women should be taught these exercises and encouraged to do them regardless of mode of birth.

Care of the perineum and postnatal pain

A major issue for many women in the postnatal period is vulval and perineal pain, particularly after suturing. Perineal pain can cause considerable distress for women and can dominate the postnatal period. It can negatively affect breastfeeding, and cause maternal exhaustion and depression. This pain is often underestimated, and women may suffer in silence. As mentioned earlier, since Sleep's Berkshire Trial in 1984, there has been very little comprehensive research to guide practice. Sleep's comprehensive study found that 20% of women still had perineal pain at 10 days and that 7.5% of women still had problems at three months post birth.

It is important to educate the woman about the extent of the perineal trauma. Even with an intact perineum, labial lacerations can be very uncomfortable, particularly when passing urine in the first few days. Women can be advised to douche the area with warm water the first couple of times they pass urine, and then pat dry. This can prevent stinging. Care should be taken to ensure that dysuria is caused by lacerations rather than a urine infection. General care consists of mild analgesia (e.g. paracetamol), bathing and inspection of the perineal area to exclude infection, haematoma and so on (WHO 1998). Hygiene is very important during the healing period. Although the Berkshire trial found no benefit from adding salt or antiseptics to baths in relation to improved healing or effective pain relief, 93% of women still felt that bathing reduced perineal pain. Women often worry about

---

BOX 25.3   HIPS

A midwife's guide to perineal care and repair
Hygiene—keep clean and dry
Ice—first 48–72 hours
Pelvice floor exercises—after first 48 hours
Support—all the time
(source: Dahlen 2001)

opening their bowels after birth, and sensation and control are often altered. Constipation should be avoided. Women should be advised that absorbable suture material might break off during the healing process, which can take several weeks to complete.

Other methods of pain relief include the use of an ice pack enclosed in a soft cloth (to prevent ice burns), which has been commonly used. There has been some concern in the literature that ice packs can delay healing (Grundy 1997). However, Low and Reed (2000) have identified that initial vasoconstriction followed by vasodilatation will increase vascularity and promote healing. Application of witchhazel to the perineum to promote healing, and the use of homoeopathic drugs such as arnica to reduce bruising, have not been fully evaluated.

Ultrasound and pulsed electromagnetic energy have also been used but again are unproven. Application of lignocaine gel or aqueous 5% lignocaine spray are recommended in the literature, as long as they do not contain steroids, which can cause wound breakdown (Grant & Sleep 1989). Intense pelvic floor exercise has also been associated with a decrease in perineal pain (Henderson & McDonald 1998, p 481).

Conclusion

Childbirth and perineal trauma are linked, and the midwife has an important role in providing advice and education to women in the antenatal, intrapartum and postnatal periods to decrease trauma and prevent long-term morbidity. Midwives who are skilled in perineal repair can provide holistic care to women. It is important for midwives to understand the anatomy of the pelvic floor and its role in childbirth. Although the use of episiotomy is restricted, midwives should be proficient in performing an episiotomy when required. Urinary incontinence must not be viewed as a consequence of childbirth, and the midwife must be proactive in educating women about pelvic floor exercises and prevention of long-term morbidity.

Review questions

1 Succinctly describe the structure of the pelvic floor.

2 List the structures of the pelvic floor.

3 Describe the function of the pelvic floor.

4 Explain the importance of the perineal body and its relationship to the pelvic floor.

5 Explain the effects of perineal trauma caused by perineal laceration or episiotomy.

6 Provide a definition for each of the following: first-, second-, third- and fourth-degree perineal trauma.

7 List the main types of prolapse of pelvic organs.

8 Illustrate the different types of episiotomy.

9 Describe the role of the midwife in teaching women pelvic floor exercises after the birth of their baby.

10 Discuss methods of pain relief that midwives can provide for women who experience perineal pain after their baby is birthed.

Online resources

American Academy of Family Physicians: perineal repair guide: http://www.aafp.org/afp/20031015/1585.html
Royal College of Obstetricians and Gynaecologists: methods and materials used in perineal repair: http://www.rcog.org.uk/resources/Public/pdf/perineal_repair.pdf

References

ALSO (American Academy of Family Physicians) 2000 Advanced life support in obstetrics course syllabus (4th edn). American Academy of Family Physician, Kansas
Beckmann MM, Garratt AJ 2005 Antenatal perineal massage for reducing perineal trauma (protocol). Cochrane Database of Systematic Reviews (1). Update Software, Oxford
Carroli G, Belizan J 2005 Episiotomy for vaginal birth. Cochrane Database of Systematic Reviews (3). Update Software, Oxford
Dahlen H 2001 A midwife's guide to perineal care and repair, part two. Midwifery Matters December

Davis and Geck Education Centre, 88 Christie St, St Leonards, NSW 2065
Dunkley J 2000 Health promotion in midwifery practice: a resource for health professionals. Baillière Tindall, London
Eason E, Labrecque M, Wells G et al 2000 Preventing perineal trauma during childbirth: a systematic review. Obstetrics and Gynecology 95(3):464–471
Enkin M, Keirse MJ (Eds) 1999 Effective care in pregnancy and childbirth, Vol 2. Oxford University Press, Oxford
Grant A, Sleep J 1989 Relief of perineal pain and discomfort after childbirth. In: L Chalmers, M Enkin, M Keirse (Eds) Effective care in pregnancy and childbirth, Vol 2. Oxford University Press, Oxford, p 1351
Grundy L 1997 The role of the midwife in perineal wound care following childbirth. British Journal of Nursing 6(10): 584–588
Hartmann K, Viswanathan M, Palmieri R et al 2005 Outcomes of routine episiotomy: a systematic review. Journal of the American Medical Association 293(17):2141–2148

Henderson C, McDonald S (Eds) 1998 Mayes midwifery: a textbook for midwives (12th edn). Baillière Tindall, London

Herbert J 1998 Overcoming the pelvic flaw: exercise for continence. In: J Dunkley (Ed) 2000 Health promotion in midwifery practice: a resource for health professionals. Baillière Tindall, London

Kegel A 1948 Progressive resistance exercise in the functional restoration of the perineal muscles. In: J Dunkley (Ed) 2000 Health promotion in midwifery practice: a resource for health professionals. Baillière Tindall, London

Kettle C, Johanson RB 1998 Continuous versus interrupted sutures for perineal repair. Cochrane Database of Systematic Reviews (1). Update Software, Oxford

Labrecque M, Eason E, Marcoux S et al 1999 Randomised controlled trial of prevention of perineal trauma by perineal massage during pregnancy. American Journal of Obstetrics and Gynecology 180(3):593–600

Low J, Reed A 2000 Electrotherapy explained. Principles and practice (3rd edn). Butterworth-Heinemann, Oxford

Maunders R 1998 Pain in childbearing and its control. Blackwell Science, Oxford

McKay S 1984 Squatting: an alternative position for the second stage of labour. American Journal of Maternal-Child Health Nursing 9:181–183

National Institute of Clinical Evidence (NICE) 2004 Caesarean section: clinical guideline. National Institute of Clinical Excellence. RCOG Press, London

Renfrew MJ, Hannah W, Albers L et al 1998 Practices that minimise trauma to the genital tract in childbirth: a systematic review of the literature. Birth 25:143–160

Royal College of Obstetricians and Gynaecologists (RCOG) 2004 Methods and materials used in perineal repair. Royal College of Obstetricians and Gynaecologists Guideline 23: Revised. June 2004. RCOG, London

Scowen P 1996 Childbirth and continence. In: J Dunkley (Ed) 2000 Health promotion in midwifery practice: a resource for health professionals. Baillière Tindall, London

Sleep J 1987 West Berkshire perineal management trial: a three-year follow up. British Medical Journal 295(6601):749–751

Sleep J, Grant A, Garcia J et al 1984 West Berkshire perineal management trial. British Medical Journal 289(6445):587–590

Stamp G, Kruzins G, Crowther C 2001 Perineal massage in labour and prevention of perineal trauma: randomised controlled trial. British Medical Journal (clinical research edition) 322(7297):1277–1280

World Health Organization (WHO) 1998 Postpartum care of the mother and newborn: a practical guide. Maternal and Newborn Health/Safe Motherhood Unit. WHO, Geneva

Wilson P, Herbison R, Herbison GP 1996 Obstetric practice and the prevalence of urinary incontinence three months after delivery. In: J Dunkley (Ed) 2000 Health promotion in midwifery practice: a resource for health professionals. Baillière Tindall, London

CHAPTER 26

Supporting women becoming mothers

Lesley Dixon

Key terms

afterpains, anti-D gammaglobulin, baby blues, backache, constipation, debriefing, deep vein thrombosis, direct Coombs', dyspareunia, endometritis, episiotomy, fatigue, fourth trimester, haemorrhoids, headaches, involution, Kleihauer test, lochia alba, lochia rubra, lochia serosa, lochia, micturition, perineum, postnatal period, puerperium, pulmonary embolism, pyrexia, secondary postpartum haemorrhage, tachycardia, thromboembolism, tiredness

Chapter overview

This chapter discusses the midwife's role in assessing maternal health and wellbeing in the postnatal period. In a partnership model of midwifery care there will be continuity of care and a holistic approach to assessing a woman's health, with equal emphasis on the physical, emotional and social aspects of a woman's wellbeing. Midwifery support and care that recognises a woman's cultural heritage, existing knowledge, practices and values will enable the woman to have a positive experience in becoming a mother.

Learning outcomes

Learning outcomes for this chapter are:

1 To identify normal responses to changes in the postnatal period, and assess maternal wellbeing

2 To recognise the integration of physical, emotional and social aspects as women adapt to motherhood

3 To discuss the importance of support for each woman in the postnatal period

4 To explore the role of the midwife during the postnatal period.

Introduction

The glow of having our baby remained with me during those first few days when I rested on the couch. My husband did everything for us and the baby lay snuggled with me. We didn't have to drive anywhere and didn't have to report to anyone. Everything in my home was there for me, the food I liked, the view out my window to the mountains as I dozed on the couch in front of the fire, a short walk in the garden when I was strong enough, a shower and to sleep in my own bed. That first morning after our baby was born, I woke early with excitement and leant over just to see him, to be near him ... I feel like it carries forward so far, the feelings about the birth and even now I go back through it in my mind when I look at my little baby and it gives me a glowing feeling. I recall the rushes of love, the reverence of the moment there in front of the fire. I didn't expect to find the confidence in myself and my own body that I now know. Perhaps in my heart and my body, I always knew how to have a baby, I just didn't know I knew. So our midwife didn't direct me how, she just showed me that I knew how. What a wonderful, inspiring gift. I am grateful. And confident.

(Extract from *Bea's Story*, In *Having a Great Birth in Australia*, Vernon 2005, p 63)

Giving birth is a major life change for each woman, affecting her personal identity and social role, and there is need for emotional, physical and social support during this time (Percival & McCourt 2000). Support can make a difference to the emotional wellbeing and coping ability of each individual, and family, friends, professional helpers and social institutions can all provide it in various ways (Ball 1994). In most societies throughout the world, women have traditionally helped each other by providing care and support following a birth. This help could be with domestic chores, care of existing children, or personal care (Goldsmith 1990; Marchant 2004; Podkolinski 1998).

Following the birth of a baby there is a period of adjustment and recovery for the mother from both the pregnancy and the birth. This adjustment period involves physical, emotional and social changes, and may take weeks or months. The six-week period following the birth has been referred to as the puerperium or the postnatal period. However, Coad and Dunstall (2001) suggest that the puerperium should be seen as a transitional phase, which begins at the birth of a child and ends with a return to fertility, although a woman does not return to the same physiological and anatomical state as before pregnancy. Davis (1997) discusses the postnatal period as the fourth trimester, suggesting that the first three months following birth are transformative and culminate in the reintegration of women as mothers into society.

The parenting role requires adjustments to behaviour, lifestyle and relationships in the weeks and months following the birth (Percival & McCourt 2000). How women will react to motherhood does not become apparent until after the birth, so the continuity and support of the midwife in the first few weeks can have a significant contribution and influence on a woman's coping process (Ball 1994).

The midwife and postnatal care

In the nineteenth century, because of high levels of maternal mortality due to postpartum infection, formalised postnatal care was instituted in order to identify poor health and pathological conditions in women (Donnison 1988; Marchant 2004). In the United Kingdom, legislation (in 1902) set 10 days as the time for 'lying in' after a birth when the woman was expected to rest, and a midwife would visit daily to ensure her physical recovery (Ball 1994, p 15). The midwife was expected to perform a complete examination of the woman's physical health during the postnatal visit (Sweet 1989).

Since the nineteenth century, maternal mortality has dropped significantly, due to the development of antibiotics and other new treatments for pathological conditions; however, there continue to be significant physical and psychological health problems following birth, many of which are not reported or identified (Brown & Lumley 1998; Glazener et al 1995).

Women's health following childbirth has not been a focus of research until recently. This may be a reflection of the low status attributed to postpartum care by both society and health professionals (Wray 2003). Many obstetric and midwifery textbooks emphasise only physical aspects of postnatal care, particularly abnormal or ill health, and ignore the emotional and psychological aspects of the transition to motherhood (Beischer & Mackay 1991; Bennett & Brown 1999; Sweet 1989). Ball (1994) suggests that the aim of maternity care should be to help women become successful mothers, and that to achieve this there needs to be as much emphasis placed on the psychological and emotional processes as on the physiological processes. Ball (1994, p 117) has defined three objectives of postnatal care:

- to promote the physical recovery from the effects of pregnancy, labour and birth
- to establish good infant-feeding practices and foster good maternal–child relationships
- to strengthen the mother's confidence in herself and her ability to care for her baby in her own social, cultural and family situation.

In New Zealand, a consensus workshop on postnatal care in 1993 suggested that the following were desired outcomes of care:

- The mother is comfortable, free of pain and physiologically stable, in an environment that provides safety, rest and nourishment.
- The mother feels in control of the pace and framework of events.
- The mother is given information specific to her culture and knows when and how to get help for herself or her baby.
- Information is shared between the mother, family and care providers.
- The transition to motherhood is individual but each mother goes through naturally occurring phases at her own pace. Good-quality care recognises this and

provides guidance and intervention as appropriate (National Advisory Committee on Core Health and Disability Support Services (NACCHDS) 1993).

Infant feeding and transition to parenthood are discussed in Chapters 9 and 28, so this chapter focuses on supporting women during the postnatal period. It includes discussion of a woman's response to the physiological changes of the postnatal period, and practical aspects of assessment and support. Caring for women during the postnatal period involves being aware of the physical, emotional and social adaptations that women make and how these are interrelated. The postnatal period can be seen as the time of maximum change and growth for women and families as they complete the transition to parenthood.

Assessment of women's health

The midwifery partnership model, which encompasses continuity of care, enables the building of a supportive relationship between a midwife and a woman and her family throughout pregnancy and childbirth (Guilliland & Pairman 1995). This relationship continues to be important during the postnatal period, when there is a time of physical recovery and emotional adaptation to parenthood. Assessment of a woman's health includes assessment not only of her physical recovery but also of her emotional responses to the demands of parenthood and the social supports that she has to help with these changes. Ussher (2004) argues that depression following childbirth is an understandable response to the difficulties of motherhood. She suggests that having good social support, realistic expectations of the difficulties of the mothering role, and practical help with child care can reduce the likelihood of becoming depressed following birth (Ussher 2004).

A midwife is able to assess a woman's health holistically, sharing her own knowledge and experience and encouraging the woman to monitor her own health. The impact of the woman's culture, beliefs, values and previous experiences with parenting must be recognised and respected.

In New Zealand, the minimum specifications for postnatal care have been defined (Box 26.1) and each woman is entitled to at least this level of care (Ministry of Health 2002a). There are no similar specifications for minimum levels of care in Australia; care varies across all states and territories depending on the models of maternity and midwifery care available to women.

Phases of the postnatal period

Regional workshops were held throughout New Zealand in 1993 to achieve consensus agreement on the level of care of a

---

BOX 26.1 Postnatal care in New Zealand

As described in Chapter 1, all pregnant women within New Zealand are expected to choose a practitioner as their lead maternity carer (LMC). The LMC is responsible for ensuring the following services after the birth:

▶ Visits to assess and care for the mother and baby in a maternity facility and at home until four to six weeks after the birth. These visits include the following:
  — a detailed clinical examination of the baby within the first 24 hours of birth
  — a daily visit while the woman is receiving inpatient postnatal care, unless agreed otherwise with the woman and the maternity facility
  — a total of five to ten home visits by a midwife (and more if clinically needed)
  — a minimum of seven postnatal visits as an aggregate of home and postnatal facility visits
  — one home visit within 24 hours of discharge
  — a detailed clinical examination of the baby within seven days of birth
  — a detailed clinical examination of the baby prior to transfer to the well child provider
  — a postnatal examination of the mother at a clinically appropriate time and prior to discharge from LMC services.
▶ Assistance with and advice about breastfeeding and the nutritional needs of the woman and baby

▶ Assessment for risk of postnatal depression and/or family violence, with appropriate advice and referral
▶ Provision of Ministry of Health information on immunisation
▶ Provision of or access to services, as outlined in the Well Child Tamariki Ora National Schedule
▶ Advice regarding contraception
▶ Parenting advice and education.
  A plan of care should be documented, reviewed and updated with progress, care given and outcomes in the maternal notes. If the woman is receiving inpatient postnatal care, then the maternity facility should have a copy of this care plan.

The Maternity Facility Service Specifications are the national documents that describe the services that maternity facilities are required to provide to women and their families (NZCOM 2004). There is an expectation that women will be ready to go home within 48 hours of the birth. The LMC, in discussion with the woman and the facility, may identify clinical reasons for a longer length of stay. The reasons may include:
▶ breastfeeding problems
▶ postoperative recovery
▶ ongoing medical problems
▶ psychological problems
▶ babies with special needs
▶ geographical isolation.

mother and baby following a normal birth. These workshops included lay experts as well as health professionals and identified the following phases of the postnatal period:

- phase 1—the first few hours
- phase 2—the early days
- phase 3—the early weeks
- phase 4—completing the transition to parenthood (NACCHDS 1993).

Each phase has different characteristics and each woman will go through these phases at her own pace (NACCHDS 1993).

In phases 1 and 2, physical recovery is a main focus of concern for most women, along with caring for and being able to breastfeed the baby. Women need to be reassured regarding their physiological wellbeing, supported in a comfortable environment, and be pain-free. High levels of physical discomfort can cause emotional distress and lessen the ability to cope with the physical and emotional changes. At this time the midwife needs to be aware of normal physiology and be able to give practical help and advice.

Women should be encouraged to spend time holding, touching and breastfeeding the baby, as this will increase levels of oxytocin and prolactin. Oxytocin acts to keep the mother relaxed and calm, and there are indications that it is involved in tolerance and adaptation, and feminine responses such as 'tending' and 'befriending' (Buckley 2004, p 205). Prolactin is produced during lactation and stimulates breast milk production (Riordan & Auerbach 1993). Buckley (2004) suggests that it also reduces the stress response, alters sleep patterns and stimulates natural hormonal analgesia.

During phase 3, as a woman's physical recovery and breastfeeding abilities progress, she will gain confidence in her ability to care for herself and her baby. At some point the emotional aspects of the changes to her social world will start to have an impact. A woman will begin to realise and understand the significant changes that have occurred to the family dynamics, since becoming a mother. Being able to talk about how she feels is an important part of the coping process; listening, understanding and reassuring may be of more value to the woman than physical assessment. A supportive partner, family and friends can make a lot of difference to how a woman feels about herself and her baby. A midwife will need to discuss support and, if necessary, help the woman to identify where support can be obtained, perhaps from groups that are culturally appropriate. Each interaction that a midwife has with a woman and her family should be seen as an opportunity to enhance the woman's self-knowledge and learning, as well as promoting health, confidence and independence.

Phase 4, the completion of the transition to parenthood, involves a woman and her family accepting the change in family dynamics and shared responsibility for the baby. In most cases this will occur during the six-week postnatal period and signals a time when a midwife is no longer needed because the woman and her family are independent. Completing the midwifery relationship is discussed fully in Chapter 30 and will not be discussed here.

Frequency of midwifery visits

In New Zealand the minimum number of visits that a midwife should make for postnatal care is specified (see Box 26.1), but this is not the case in Australia, where opportunities for postnatal visiting in the woman's home after discharge from hospital are limited according to models of care and funding. Ideally a midwife would decide, on an individual basis with each woman, the frequency and length of visits that are required and when these visits should cease (Ministry of Health 2002a). There are many aspects of a mother's or baby's health that may indicate the need for more frequent visits.

The New Zealand College of Midwives *Midwives Handbook for Practice* (2005) outlines decision points that can be used to help identify times when there should be full midwifery assessments during the postnatal period. Each decision point summarises the assessments that should be made, investigations that should be performed, possible treatments, legal requirements and health information and education that should be shared. The timing of decision points should be based on individual need but the first decision point should occur within the first 24 hours of the birth (NZCOM 2005). Subsequent decision points should be every 24–48 hours until the woman is confident in her home environment (NZCOM 2005) (see Box 26.2).

Munday (2003) suggests that postnatal care should include time for physical assessment as well as a discussion of the socio-emotional issues important to women. She contends that midwives should facilitate continued contact with the woman for as long as the woman feels that the contact is of benefit (Munday 2003). Different countries have individual legislation and expectations regarding the timeframe for formal postnatal care, as well as differences in frequency of home visits, so it is difficult to make comparisons about what constitutes the correct amount of postnatal care. However, it seems unlikely that a woman would complain about too many visits, and much more likely for concerns to be raised about insufficient visits. A survey of 2909 women who gave birth in New Zealand during February and March 2002 found that women were generally positive and satisfied with their postnatal care, although some 23% received conflicting breastfeeding advice while in hospital and 36% stated that they received fewer than the required minimum of five postnatal home visits (Ministry of Health 2002b).

Emotional responses to change

The transition from pregnancy through the birth to becoming parents is a challenging time for a mother and the wider family (Percival & McCourt 2000). A range of emotions are felt in the postpartum period, and many women describe relief, euphoria, joy, pleasure, and also despair, fear and concern. These emotions will vary depending on the woman, the

---

BOX 26.2 Decision point

Decision point up to and including the first 24 hours post partum

Reflect on the birth experience with the woman and assess the health and wellbeing of the woman and her newborn baby.

Information shared:

- identify and discuss ongoing support
- discuss general wellbeing
- identify assistance required with breastfeeding.

Examination

Full physical assessment of woman, including:

- involution of the uterus and blood loss
- perineum
- breasts.

Full physical assessment of baby, including:

- heart sounds
- hip check
- weight and measurements when appropriate.

Possible tests:

- blood group for Rh factor and direct Coombs'/Kleihauer

Possible treatment

Respect the birth plan, developed antenatally with the woman, in relation to:

- vitamin K for baby
- anti-D gammaglobulin
- hepatitis B vaccine and gammaglobulin for baby
- facilitate BCG vaccination for baby.

Health information and education:

- Facilitate mother–baby relationship. Give opportunity for peace, quiet and breastfeeding if that is the woman's choice.
- Facilitate rest and ongoing support if at home.
- Education for self-care related to:
  — uterus
  — blood loss
  — perineum
  — breasts
  — bladder
  — bowels
  — emotional wellbeing
  — social support.
- Identify when and how to call for assistance.

- Guide and assist with breastfeeding as required.
- Information given for baby care related to:
  — feeding
  — breathing
  — passing urine and meconium
  — umbilical cord
  — crying, warmth
  — safety.
- National Immunisation Register
- Information concerning development of parenting skills, including feeding.

Legal requirements

- birth notification—BDM 9

Subsequent decision points in postnatal period every 24–48 hours until woman feels confident in her home environment

The timing provides the opportunity to promote the woman's independence while ensuring the wellbeing of the woman and baby.

Information shared:

- Discuss woman's health status, both physical and psychological.
- Discuss lactation and ongoing feeding.
- Discuss parental and baby's wellbeing.

Examination:

- full physical assessment to ascertain recovery from birth process, including breast examination and perineal examination if required
- full physical assessment of baby

Tests:

- Guthrie test
- consider SBR

Possible treatment:

- rubella vaccination
- red eye reflex

Health information and education:

- opportunity for rest and ongoing support
- parenting including feeding
- self-care for self and family
- other support agencies.

(Source: NZCOM 2005)

---

birth, her own life experiences, family roles and history, all of which will influence her adjustment to the new or expanded responsibilities of becoming a mother. In the first days and weeks following the birth there are disruptions to previous routines as the needs of the baby become dominant. Disrupted sleep, lack of freedom, lack of social life, and changes to relationships with partners and other family members add to the emotional rollercoaster of the first few weeks and months following the birth of a baby (Ussher 2004). Ussher (2004) discusses the paradox of motherhood: the need to be with your child but also the wish to have time alone; the wish to be selfish and independent but also to enjoy the needs and dependency of the baby. She discusses the overwhelming love between mother and child but also the exhaustion, frustration and relentless hard work, and says, 'It involves endless sacrifice, patience and self-control and when that is impossible (for no one can be patient and calm at all times), the ability to forgive oneself, for not being perfect' (Ussher 2004, p 107).

Birth stories

In the first few days following birth, most women will tell their family and visitors about their labour and birth. Often

Reflective exercise

1 Think about a time in your life where there were major changes. How did you feel? What helped you to cope? Who provided the most support?

2 Think about women you have worked with during the postnatal period. What range of emotions did you observe? What coping mechanisms did these women use?

the story is told repetitively and with incredible detail as the woman sorts out what happened and when. These birth stories are retained for many years and will be told at different times around pregnancy and births of friends and relatives. It is important that a midwife is aware of women's need to assimilate the events of their births and takes time to discuss with each woman her perceptions of the birth, what was said and done, who was present, and the order of events by which each woman builds a picture of her birth. Ideally the midwife

who attended the birth will talk through the birth with the woman, but if this is not possible, another midwife can assist a woman with this by reference to notes and giving the woman time to talk. In building her picture of the birth, a woman draws on her own experiences, comments and discussions with the people who were present during her labour and birth, and the documentation and timelines provided for her by her midwife through the midwifery notes. Lyons (1998) suggests that in writing notes and in talking through birth stories, a midwife should focus on the positive qualities shown by the mother, especially in situations where the mother may have a sense of failure or disappointment. Lyons (1998) takes talking through birth stories one step further, to a more formal process of debriefing, and suggests that the primary aim of psychological debriefing is to 'provide the person with as much information as possible to enable the person to assimilate and emotionally adjust' (Lyons 1998, p 137). She contends that in the postnatal context it provides a mother with the opportunity to tell her own story and access information about the birth from health professionals, as well as allowing mental processing, in which the mother sorts out the sequences of the events (Lyons 1998). Debriefing may be used as a screening process when there are

MIDWIFE'S STORY

The importance of talk

Cindy was a late referral for booking, and when I went to see her she was bubbling with happiness. She was 35 years old and had been married for many years but had remained childless. Following investigations for infertility, which found no cause for her inability to conceive, she had given up hope of having a family (her husband was not keen on adopting) and had planned to change her career by going back to college. She went to see her GP to discuss her issues about weight gain, digestive and bowel problems, which were thought to be due to irritable bowel syndrome. The doctor palpated her abdomen and said, 'I think you're about six months pregnant'. He organised a scan, which found that she was 28–30 weeks pregnant *with twins*! Cindy and her partner were astounded but very pleased and started to re-plan their lives. During what would have been early pregnancy, Cindy had had a laparoscopy and had also been taking various medications. She was now concerned about harmful effects on the pregnancy. A detailed scan reassured her that both babies appeared well and normal.

About two months later (38 weeks), Cindy went into labour and had an emergency caesarean section. She gave birth to two lovely little girls, who were both well. At the time, as a community midwife, I didn't visit women at the hospital, only when they were discharged home. Two days after Cindy's birth I received a phone call from the ward staff, who were concerned about Cindy's behaviour, which was unusual, in that she couldn't seem to stop talking. She seemed unhappy, and would talk non-stop when a midwife or anybody entered the room. They asked if I would visit

her to see if this would help. This was an unusual request from the hospital midwives. When I went to see Cindy she was very happy to see me and explained that nobody really understood how difficult it was for her. Three months ago she had had no expectation of having a family and now here she was having just given birth to twins. She said other women had nine months to get used to becoming a mother, whereas she had had two months! She needed to tell everybody about this so that they would understand why she wasn't able to look after her babies like other mums were able to. That first visit I was there for two hours as she talked and talked. I went every day until she was discharged home and we just talked. I helped her with breastfeeding her twins if needed but my main task was just to be there for her to talk to and support her in this environment, so that she was able to come to terms with becoming a mother. When Cindy went home I continued to visit her at home, but by this time my visits were a lot shorter and she was coping really well and had good support from her partner and family.

On reflection I realised that Cindy had needed to talk in order to be able to come to terms with the enormous life change that she was going through. Talking to anybody and everybody about it was her way of vocalising her need to have others understand this as well as helping her to organise her thoughts and feelings about becoming a mother.

I saw Cindy when the twins were 18 months old, and she was the happy, bubbly person that I'd first met. She told me proudly that things were going well and that she was still breastfeeding her twin girls.

concerns for post-traumatic stress disorder. (This is discussed more fully in Ch 37.)

Hormonal influences or 'baby blues'

Following the birth, many women feel high or elated; often they get very little sleep and are very happy to socialise with their visitors, friends and relatives. This high mood often turns to a low mood on about the third to fifth day post partum, and the characteristic tearfulness, anxiety and irritability are often called the 'baby blues'. Despite a great deal of research, the cause is still unknown, although one theory is that it occurs because of the decrease in oestrogen and progesterone, and changes in the blood electrolyte balance and in the balance of serotonin and dopamine (neurotransmitters) (Stables 2000). It is estimated that 50–80% of women experience this mood swing, which is generally transient and lasts only a few days (Dennis & Kavanagh 2004). Paradice (2002) cites studies in which there were similar mood changes in groups of men and women following surgery, and argues that the blues could be a normal response to a stressful event rather than a response that is unique to postpartum women. Postoperatively it occurs immediately after surgery and is recognised as an understandable response to stress and part of normal recovery (Paradice 2002).

For women who do experience the blues there is a tendency to cry for no reason, feel overwhelmed, tired, and for everything to ache or feel sore. It often coincides with the onset of full lactation and unsettled behaviour in the baby. Women need help to achieve physical comfort as well as emotional support and reassurance at this time (Sweet 1999).

Physical assessment of maternal health

In the early postpartum period, a midwife needs to ask specific questions related to physical recovery, in order to establish whether there are any problems or concerns that may otherwise not be voiced. Following the birth, the baby is often the focus of attention and a woman's health can become secondary. Childbirth is a time when intimate areas of a woman's body become a focus of attention and some women may feel uncomfortable with this and reluctant to volunteer information about their private body functions. Taking time to talk about a woman's health and feelings is an important way of reinforcing the need for the woman to look after herself and of the normality of the physiological changes she is experiencing. While there is little evidence to support the routine taking of temperature, pulse and blood pressure on a daily basis, there should always be individual decision-making regarding the necessity of these physical observations. Women who have previously had raised blood pressure in pregnancy should have regular postpartum assessment of blood pressure. Temperature and pulse should be taken if there are concerns regarding postpartum infection.

Breasts and feeding

As part of the postnatal assessment there should be a discussion about the breasts, breastfeeding and any breast discomfort. (For more information see Ch 28.)

Involution of the uterus

A midwife will normally palpate the uterus shortly after the expulsion of the placenta, to ensure that there is a reduction in size of the uterus and an overall contraction of the uterus. The uterus can be felt as a hard round or ovoid structure at about the level of the woman's umbilicus or sometimes just below. The fundus of the uterus should be central and feel firm to the touch.

It is common practice for the midwife to palpate a woman's uterus to check for involution on a regular basis after birth and until the fundus is no longer palpable outside the pelvis. A tender uterus can be a sign of infection or retained products of conception, as can slow involution, which is known as subinvolution (Coad & Dunstall 2001). The uterus can also be tender to the touch and slower to involute following a caesarean section (Coad & Dunstall 2001).

Previously, midwifery textbooks have discussed the rate of involution and suggested that the height of the uterus should decrease at a rate of 1 cm a day with an expectation that the uterus will be within the pelvis and no longer palpable at 10 days post partum (Coad & Dunstall 2001; Howie 1995; Stables 2000). However, Cluett and colleagues (1997), in a small study of 28 women, found considerable variability in the pattern of involution within the normal puerperium. Measurements of the height of the fundus of the uterus were undertaken daily and showed that most women had an episode of slow decline (less than 1 cm over three or more days) and that for most women the uterus ceased to be palpable between 11 and 16 days, while a small group (three women) took 19 days. All the women had normal postnatal recovery. As this research was undertaken in the United Kingdom, there were several midwives providing postnatal care. Having a midwife who knows the woman and is able to discuss the woman's understanding and perceptions of her health would probably give more insight into problems than physical observations alone (Cluett et al 1997).

Marchant and colleagues (2003) looked at midwives' records in the United Kingdom to determine how involution was described and recorded within the midwifery notes. They found marked differences in how midwives in two different health districts recorded the involution of the uterus. These records varied from measurements, with or without a description, to some form of abbreviation or symbols used. The researchers identified the need for improved and consistent record keeping, arguing that there is little point 'in undertaking and recording an observation if the record cannot be unambiguously understood by others and used to construct an accurate chronological picture of events' (Marchant et al 2003, p 139).

Marchant and colleagues (2003) suggest that women could self-assess the condition and involution of their uteri in the postpartum period. They argue that women often touch their enlarging abdomen during pregnancy, but after the birth there appears to be little interest in the reducing uterus. They asked women as part of the larger Blood Loss in the Post Partum (BliPP) study (1999) whether they had felt for their own uterus since the birth of the baby. The majority of women had not done so (67%) but 31% had tried to feel their own uterus; some had been unable to find the uterus (15%), whereas others had tried but were unsure what they were feeling (49%) and 36% were able to describe the position, size and texture.

A continuity-of-care model ensures that in most circumstances one midwife will provide care within the postpartum period, thus increasing consistency of physical assessments and the identification of potential morbidity. Palpation of a woman's uterus provides an opportunity to show her what is being done and discuss the signs that involution is normal. Advising women on how to palpate their own uterus early in the postpartum period promotes an understanding by women of their own bodies and returns the ability to monitor their own health to each woman. The midwife will need to judge on an individual basis whether assessing her own uterine involution is a viable option for each woman. Descriptions or measurements, when done, need to be consistently and accurately recorded, whether recorded by the midwife or the woman during the postpartum period.

Vaginal blood loss

Many textbooks refer to the blood loss following birth as the 'lochia' and suggest that there are three types of lochia (Howie 1995; Stables 2000; Sweet 1999). These are known as lochia rubra, lochia serosa and lochia alba. However, research by Marchant et al (1999) found that these colour changes were not supported by the majority of women's experiences and that women reported vaginal loss to be more predominantly red/brown in colour. Marchant (2003) argues for the term 'lochia' to be abandoned and replaced with 'postpartum vaginal blood or fluid loss' as this is language that is familiar to women and therefore of more value to both the woman and the midwife. She contends that as women are used to blood loss during menstruation, they are able to identify the colour and consistency of vaginal loss quite clearly after the birth (Marchant 2003).

It is important for a midwife to discuss with the woman the blood loss following birth. Excessive bleeding or infection (endometritis) is detrimental to maternal health but precise definitions and the incidence of either problem are not consistent (Bick et al 2002). Excessive bleeding is regarded as a secondary postpartum haemorrhage if it occurs after 24 hours and before six weeks post partum (Bick et al 2002). If there were concerns regarding excessive blood loss at any time, the midwife should check the blood pressure and pulse; a rapid pulse and low blood pressure would confirm that the blood loss is affecting the maternal physiology.

Assessing normal vaginal blood loss is subjective and the volume of blood loss is difficult to measure when it occurs over

several days and weeks. Immediately after the birth, women should expect the vaginal blood loss to be heavy and this may continue for the first few days (Bick et al 2002). It is also normal for blood loss to be heavier following breastfeeding. The amount of blood loss should start to diminish over the first few days but the duration of blood loss is variable (Bick et al 2002). It is not unusual for women to pass blood clots as part of vaginal fluid loss; the size and frequency of these clots need to be described as these may be related to excessive or prolonged bleeding. Marchant (2003) suggests that using familiar items to identify and record the size of clots can be a useful guide in assessing the extent and size of blood clots and the extent of postpartum bleeding. Another method of determining the extent of postpartum blood loss is by how frequently a woman changes her sanitary pad, although this has to be interpreted with some caution, as some pads are more absorbent than others and some women will change pads more frequently depending on their hygiene requirements. Changing sanitary pads frequently due to full pads (several times in an hour) would be an indication of heavy, possibly excessive, vaginal bleeding.

As each woman is individual and will have different expectations of vaginal blood loss following the birth, the midwife needs to use and integrate all these methods to obtain an overall picture of the woman's blood loss and to assess whether it is a problem for that woman.

The BliPP study undertaken by Marchant and colleagues (1999) was a prospective survey of women's experiences and the duration, amount and colour of vaginal loss after childbirth. The objective of the research was to describe the range of normal vaginal loss as reported by women from 24 hours after birth until three months post partum. There were 524 women recruited to the survey, and these were asked to keep a record of the amount and colour of their vaginal loss daily until the tenth postnatal day, and then at 14, 21 and 28 days post natal. Findings showed that women report a more varied duration, type and quantity of vaginal loss than has been described in textbooks, although the overall trend was for the amount of vaginal loss to decrease from the time of birth. Two women reported no loss after two days and a few had no loss after one week, but for the rest there was considerable variation in patterns over the first month. Of these, 17% recorded no loss or a small loss on day five but subsequently experienced moderate or heavy loss again. By the 28th day postpartum, 48% of the sample reported no loss, 47% reported a small or variable loss and 5% reported a moderate or heavy loss. Women were also asked to record the frequency and size of blood clots, and again there was wide variation reported, although the presence of blood clots rarely led to any further problems (Marchant et al 1999). In this study 2% (7) of the women were unaware that there would be a blood loss following the birth.

As many women may be reluctant to discuss vaginal loss it is important for midwives to discuss the subject during postnatal visits and to reassure women if they are concerned about the amount or continuation of blood loss. Asking women to describe their vaginal loss and listening to concerns related to the amount of blood loss is useful in determining whether the amount of vaginal blood loss is extensive and life-threatening or within normal expectations. Documentation of the nature of the blood loss needs to be reflective of the woman's words and experiences. Recording the blood loss in the woman's words will also increase the participation of the woman in monitoring her health, as well as aiding in the detection of ill health (Marchant 2003).

An increase in blood loss along with uterine tenderness and/or raised temperature could indicate endometritis or retained products of conception, and would require referral to a medical practitioner. If a woman is feeling unwell and an infection is suspected, the midwife should always remember to take the temperature and pulse to check for pyrexia and tachycardia.

Afterpains

Many women have afterpains following birth; these are common in multiparous women but can also be experienced by primiparous women. Afterpains are contractions, of varying intensity, of the uterine myometrium following birth. Theories on the cause are that the pain is due to the ischaemia of the uterus following the birth (Sine & Cameron 1968), or that because the tone of the uterine muscle becomes more relaxed and for longer with each pregnancy, more forceful contractions are required to keep the uterus contracted (Waite 2002). Afterpains can cause a significant level of pain that can be debilitating and distressing for many women (Phipps 2003). Descriptions range from 'like going into labour all over again' to 'like a dull backache that starts in my hips and around my back, then becomes like a strong period pain' (Phipps 2003, p 121). Uterine pain is normally more intense in the first 12 hours but will often continue for two to three days following the birth. Acknowledging this pain and discussing ways of alleviating the pain is an important aspect of providing care and support.

The relief of afterpains has not been a focus of recent research. Sine and Cameron (1968) suggested practical methods of easing afterpains that arose from observation and experience. These included keeping the bladder empty, massaging the uterus to aid expression of clots and applying pressure to the abdomen (Sine & Cameron 1968).

Critical thinking exercise

The information provided in the list above (at top right) has been accumulated through practice experience and has not been evaluated. Midwives and women have found these measures helpful as a means of alleviating afterpains. Further research is required to ascertain the most effective methods of alleviating afterpains. How would you undertake research to investigate this area further? What research designs could be used?

An audit undertaken at Rangiora Hospital (New Zealand) highlighted midwives' concerns about how to provide adequate practical help and pain relief for women experiencing afterpains. A pamphlet was developed which advises the following (Waite 2002):

- frequent emptying of the bladder
- regular oral analgesia
- gentle massage of the fundus by the mother
- a heat pack applied to the abdomen
- applying pressure to the abdomen by the mother lying on her stomach with a pillow against the lower abdomen
- homeopathic remedies such as arnica—following discussion with a suitably qualified practitioner.

Perineal healing

Following birth, many women will experience some pain, swelling or tenderness in the perineum. The intensity of the pain will be subjective but women who have had some degree of perineal trauma such as a tear or episiotomy are more likely to have higher levels of pain in the perineum (Bick et al 2002). A painful perineum can have a negative impact on a woman, as she is unable to move freely, sitting can be uncomfortable and caring for her baby becomes more difficult, marring her enjoyment of the early motherhood experience. Longer-term problems may arise when sexual intercourse is resumed, as dyspareunia (pain or discomfort during sexual intercourse) can also occur. Avoiding damage to the perineum and appropriate repair is the best way of avoiding and alleviating high levels of pain (Hedayati et al 2004).

When there has been trauma, perineal pain is generally more severe in the first few days but discomfort can continue for up to two weeks for some women and for up to three months for a small number (Hedayati et al 2004). Recognition and acknowledgement that perineal pain is distressing is important, along with discussion about different methods of alleviating the pain and support of the choice that is culturally valid for the woman. Many women who have had perineal trauma are concerned about urinary, bowel or future sexual function; discussion and reassurance will help to relieve these concerns (Marchant 2003). Most perineal trauma will heal within seven to ten days of birth (Marchant 2003). (For a fuller discussion of perineal pain and healing see Ch 25.)

Where trauma has occurred, midwives should check the perineum and assess the healing regularly until they are sure that full healing has occurred. Marchant (2003) suggests that the level of perineal discomfort experienced or degree of anxiety exhibited by women may mirror the progress of healing. If perineal pain is unchanged or diminishing, there is unlikely to be infection or haematoma development (Marchant 2003). Increased pain may indicate the development of inflammation or infection. In a continuity-of-care model the midwife will know the woman and the type of birth, which will assist in assessing the need for and frequency of perineal examination. A physical assessment of healing and exclusion of haematoma should always be considered, if perineal pain is increasing or the woman is anxious.

Bladder function

Immediately following the birth, a full bladder will prevent the uterus from fully contracting and can cause heavier vaginal blood loss and increase severity of afterpains. Women should be encouraged to pass urine as soon as possible after the birth and to micturate every two to three hours in the first day or two. There may be stinging during micturition due to grazes around the vulval area or perineal damage. There may also be some oedema around the urethra, giving the woman less control when passing urine or making it difficult to pass urine. Asking women about frequency and control will identify urinary problems and will often lead to discussion of pelvic floor exercises, perineal healing and adequate fluid intake.

Gastrointestinal system

Food is often associated with caring and nurturing as well as social occasions. Women need to be well nourished following the birth, so regular meals and fluids will help to promote health and a feeling of wellbeing. Most women will resume eating their normal diet and should eat when hungry. Breastfeeding requires an increase in calories, so women will often have an increased appetite during lactation. Bowel movement can occur within 24 hours of the birth but can also be delayed for up to three days following the birth. This is due to the pregnancy hormones aiding bowel evacuation prior to labour. Constipation can continue to be a problem for some women, but increased dietary fibre is recommended, with laxatives prescribed only when fibre and dietary interventions have failed (Bick et al 2002).

Haemorrhoids are the result of swollen veins around the anus becoming prolapsed and causing pain (Bick et al 2002). Following birth, haemorrhoids can become worse due to pressure and can take some time to resolve. There is an increased incidence of haemorrhoids following a forceps birth, a longer second stage and vaginal births of heavier babies (Bick et al 2002). Hartley (2003) suggests that pain caused by haemorrhoids in the postnatal period is drastically underestimated and that midwives rarely ask about haemorrhoids, assuming that pain in that area is due to perineal trauma and healing. There are a variety of treatments ranging from topical applications to homeopathy, herbal remedies, hot or cold compresses, and acupuncture (Hartley 2003). There are no trials to show which of these treatments are most effective. Avoidance of constipation is important as it can make haemorrhoids more extensive and painful. Some midwives advise women to gently push the haemorrhoids back into place while having a warm bath or by using a lubricant such as KY Jelly or olive oil (Hartley 2003). As the effects of progesterone decrease, haemorrhoids should improve, but for a small number of women haemorrhoids can continue for up to a year after the birth and will often recur and be worse with subsequent pregnancies (Bick et al 2002).

Cardiovascular system

The cardiovascular system returns to a near pre-pregnant state rapidly following the birth. If there has been excessive bleeding at any time, an assessment of haemoglobin level would be useful in determining whether iron therapy is required. Women who are rhesus-negative, and their babies, should be assessed for anti-D gamma globulin through the direct Coombs' test (level of maternal antibodies in cord blood) and the Kleihauer test (number of fetal cells in maternal blood). If indicated, anti-D should be administered to the mother within 72 hours of the birth. It can also be administered antenatally to women who are Rhesus-negative and the National Institute for Clinical Excellence (NICE) supports its routine administration prophylactically for these women (NICE 2002).

Pregnancy and birth can predispose to venous thrombo-embolism because of the increased coagulability of the platelets. Early ambulation helps to reduce the risk of deep vein thrombosis or pulmonary embolism. The midwife needs to be aware of the signs and symptoms of both these complications and refer to a medical practitioner if she has any concerns. It is usual to check for pain, redness or swelling in the legs on a regular basis to rule out deep vein thrombosis and thrombophlebitis. This assessment will often lead to discussions regarding ankle oedema and promotion of health through exercise and reduced levels of smoking for those women who smoke.

Assessment of general health and common discomforts

Fatigue

Many women will express concern about being tired in the postpartum period and this often lasts for many months after the birth. Tiredness and fatigue are thought to be part of a continuum and are difficult to define (McQueen & Mander 2003). Tiredness can be defined as a temporary state that can be helped by resting or sleep, while fatigue is an unrelenting overall condition that interferes with the ability to function normally (McQueen & Mander 2003).

Fatigue is felt following prolonged activity and is a protective mechanism where the body slows down or stops, so that overuse is prevented and regeneration of the body can happen (Bick et al 2002). It is individual and is affected by psychological and environmental factors, although it is expected following physical exertion or long periods without sleep (Bick et al 2002). Most women are aware that high levels of tiredness can be expected following the birth because of the physical activity of giving birth followed by interrupted sleep patterns due to the needs of the baby. When tiredness becomes overwhelming, to the point of exhaustion, there can also be a strong association with anxiety and depression (Bick et al 2002). Extreme tiredness can affect how women care for their babies, and how they relate to their partners and other children (McQueen & Mander 2003).

Tiredness and fatigue can be caused by physical factors such as anaemia (which can be remedied with iron therapy once diagnosed) or infection, thyroid disorder or depression

(Bick et al 2002). Discussing the woman's feelings about her fatigue and what she thinks may be the cause can be helpful in identifying ways to reduce it. In their review of tiredness and fatigue, McQueen and Mander (2003) suggest that postnatal adjustment could be enhanced if childbirth education focused more on realistic expectations of motherhood. They suggest that women should seek help from support people for routine household tasks and activities in the postpartum period (McQueen & Mander 2003).

Backache

Backache is a common disorder among the general population and it can be a common complaint during pregnancy that often continues into the postpartum period. It is difficult to assess whether there is an increase in complaints about backache following childbirth (Bick et al 2002). An acute onset of backache should be referred to an appropriate practitioner for investigation immediately. For ongoing postpartum backache, women can be advised to remain active and try localised applications of heat and mild oral analgesia (Bick et al 2002). If the backache does not improve or continues for up to six weeks, referral to an appropriate practitioner such as a GP, physiotherapist, osteopath or chiropractor is advised (Bick et al 2002).

Headaches

Observational studies have found that headaches are relatively common after childbirth, although headaches are also common among the general population (Bick et al 2002). No comparative studies have yet been undertaken to determine whether headaches are more common in the postpartum period (Bick et al 2002). Headaches may be due to tension, lack of sleep and increased stress; or women who previously suffered from migraine headaches may find these recurring in the postnatal period (Bick et al 2002). Methods of alleviating tension and ensuring sufficient sleep need to be explored if headaches become more frequent, and analgesia such as paracetamol may be helpful.

The importance of support after the birth

Podkolinski (1998) researched women's experiences of postnatal support from a feminist perspective and using questionnaires, interviews and diaries from 10 women. She asked the women to comment on who had supported them during the postnatal period, how they had been supported, what they felt about the support they had received, whether they had felt special because of it and whether there was anything they would have liked that they did not receive. In this study, which was set in the United Kingdom, the majority of women received a daily visit from a midwife until 10 days post partum. Podkolinski (1998) found that the women's main source of support was a combination of their partner and their mother, although all women identified the midwife

Critical thinking exercise

You are visiting Kelly, who is three days post partum following a normal birth at the local birthing unit. She was discharged home this morning and appeared to be recovering well until today. During your visit she is tearful and upset. She says she feels tired and aches 'everywhere'. The baby is feeding frequently and isn't settling between feeds. Kelly's partner has gone out to get some food and do some other errands.

1. What are the issues causing Kelly to be upset?
2. What is the midwife's role in this situation?
3. When will you plan to visit again?

BOX 26.3 Helping women in a maternity facility

Practical ways of helping women within a maternity facility environment:

- Promote a restful and caring atmosphere from all staff.
- Ensure regular meals and drinks are provided; have snacks readily available.
- Promote maternal and family contact with the baby.
- Control noise so that women can sleep/rest at appropriate times (Ockenden 2003).
- Provide consistent help and advice regarding baby care; use positive feedback.
- Provide consistent help and advice regarding breastfeeding (Ockenden 2003).
- Discuss pain and provide appropriate help with pain whether it be pharmacological or non-pharmacological management (Ockenden 2003).
- Give frequent praise and reassurance.
- Promote a family-friendly facility, and encourage family and friends to visit and provide extra support.
- Many women when stressed, tired or in pain find a warm bath relaxing and refreshing. Lavender oil in the bathwater appears to aid this relaxation and may be helpful as a way of reducing stress, helping to alleviate muscle fatigue and promoting the feeling of being cared for. Research suggests that having a bath can relieve perineal discomfort and other aches and pains, but that it does not reduce high levels of pain or improve healing of the perineum (Bick et al 2002). Adding salt or a disinfectant to the bath has not been proved to have any more benefits than bathing in water alone (Bick et al 2002).

as an important source of support both in the hospital and at home. The type of support the women received from midwives included information and practical advice on baby care, advice on how to cope with a crying baby, encouragement and advice on breastfeeding, and advice about pain relief and self-care. Midwives also gave praise and reassurance, which helped to increase the women's confidence. This aspect of support

---

BOX 26.4 Helping women at home

Practical ways of helping women at home:

▶ Ask friends, partners and family to help with household tasks; foster the idea that this should be normal within our society (Bick et al 2002; McQueen & Mander 2003).

▶ Be flexible about visits but ensure they are regular, giving a date and time for next visit.

▶ Have sufficient time set aside to listen, understand, reassure and give positive feedback.

▶ Discuss types of social support—how much does she have, is it enough and if not, how can she recruit more.

▶ Encourage the woman to accept a lower standard of tidiness and cleanliness within the house.

▶ Discuss the benefits of exercise, which can improve mood level and reduce tension and anxiety. A short walk every day or several times a week can be helpful (Bick et al 2002).

▶ Encourage women to have frequent short rests during the day (Bick et al 2002).

▶ Encourage healthy eating and ensure that dietary needs are being met (Bick et al 2002).

▶ Encourage discussion of problems or other concerns, such as finances, family relationships, lack of personal time. These may affect how a woman feels and copes (Symon et al 2003).

▶ Explain that 'perfect mothers' are a myth and that she only needs to be 'good enough'.

---

was highly valued by the women. When discussing what makes support good or bad, the women stated that it was the way in which support was offered and given. Perceptions of support were individual but support was felt to be intrusive and inappropriate when assumptions were made or when women did not feel listened to or treated as an individual. Podkolinski (1998) found that women sought emotional support from other women, whether friends, relatives or health professionals. It was the sense of a shared experience and reassurance that gave the women support and made them feel that they were not alone or different. It was these supportive relationships that women valued highly (Podkolinski 1998).

McCourt and colleagues (2000) suggest that one of the concepts of care and support is feeling that you are the centre of care and that people are interested and concerned with you and your welfare. They suggest that women expect good care, support, practical help and good communication from midwives (McCourt et al 2000).

Podkolinski (1998) identified that while all the women in her study needed support, the length of time and type of support needed by each woman varied. She suggests that midwives should help women establish their own support networks as well as trying to make women feel special, nurtured and cared

for. Ockenden (2003) agrees and suggests that midwives can support women by trying to make motherhood a special time in which a new mother feels valued and cared for, by providing care based on individual need with a balance between support and physical monitoring.

Munday (2003) undertook a phenomenological study of women's experiences of the postnatal period following a home birth. The women participants commented on the positive effect the home birth had had on their partners and family, but were concerned by the lack of practical assistance in the home and with looking after other children. Because a home birth was seen as 'normal', the woman and family were not seen as needing any practical help.

Conclusion

The postnatal period is the final transition, a time of major life change and of potential stress as a woman becomes a mother and a couple become a family. Support from family, friends and health professionals is important and can affect the emotional wellbeing and coping ability of each individual. How a woman adjusts to her new role will depend on her previous experiences, her family and social roles as well as the birth itself. Postnatal care should help women achieve a smooth transition into motherhood with as much attention given to women's psychological and emotional adaptations as to their physical recovery.

Assessment of maternal wellbeing is based on knowledge of the physiological, psychological and social changes in the postnatal period and how these may affect the woman's recovery. Sharing knowledge and experience with women enables and supports them to monitor their own health. There is need for flexibility, sensitivity and understanding from midwives when providing postnatal care.

Women have traditionally helped each other following childbirth by helping with domestic chores or caring for other children. There should be a focus on encouraging women to seek practical help and support at home from family, friends and community support groups, so that women are not expected to manage alone. As women go through each phase of the postnatal period in their own time, the focus of the midwives' visits will change. Providing support to women is about giving practical help, advice, positive feedback and praise. It needs to be done in a sensitive and caring way, which is individual to each woman and her family. Women value the support of a midwife whom they know and who has established their confidence and trust.

Becoming a mother is challenging, exciting and difficult; it involves physical, social and emotional changes that women can manage successfully when provided with good care and support.

Review questions

1 Identify and describe the physiological changes that occur during the postpartum period.

2 What are the aims of postnatal care?

3 How can a midwife promote these aims?

4 How often should a midwife visit during the postnatal period?

5 Identify and describe the four phases of the postpartum period.

6 Discuss the physical assessment that a midwife should undertake during a postnatal visit.

7 Describe the range of emotions that could be felt by a woman in the postpartum period.

8 Identify the emotional and social adaptations that a woman and her partner make in the first few weeks after the birth of a baby.

9 What is support?

10 How can midwives support women during the postnatal period?

Online resources

NICE, postnatal care, http://nice.org.uk/page.aspx?o=63357

Parents Centres New Zealand Inc, http://www.parentscentre.org.nz/parenting

WHO, publications on maternal and newborn health, http://www.who.int/reproductive-health/publications/maternal_newborn.en.html

References

Ball J 1994 Reactions to motherhood. The role of postnatal care (2nd edn). Books for Midwives, Cheshire

Beischer N, Mackay E 1991 Obstetrics and the newborn. An illustrated textbook (2nd edn). Saunders, Sydney

Bennett V, Brown L 1999 Myles textbook for midwives (13th edn). Churchill Livingstone, London

Bick D, MacArthur C, Knowles H et al 2002 Postnatal care: evidence and guidelines for management. Churchill Livingstone, Edinburgh

Brown S, Lumley J 1998 Maternal health after childbirth: results of an Australian population based survey. British Journal of Obstetrics and Gynaecology 105:156–161

Buckley S 2004 Undisturbed birth—nature's hormonal blueprint for safety, ease and ecstasy. MIDIRS Midwifery Digest 14(2):203–208

Cluett E, Alexander J, Pickering R 1997 What is the normal pattern of uterine involution? An investigation of postpartum uterine involution measured by the distance between the symphysis pubis and the uterine fundus using a paper tape measure. Midwifery 13:9–16

Coad J, Dunstall M 2001 Anatomy and physiology for midwives. Mosby, London

Davis E 1997 Heart and hands. A midwife's guide to pregnancy and birth. Celestial Arts, Canada

Dennis C, Kavanagh J 2004 Psychosocial interventions for preventing postpartum depression. Cochrane Library (2). John Wiley & Sons, Chichester

Donnison J 1988 Midwives and medical men: a history of the struggle for the control of childbirth. Historical Publications, London

Glazener C, Abdalla M, Stroud P et al 1995 Postnatal maternal morbidity: extent, causes, prevention and treatment. British Journal of Obstetrics and Gynaecology 102:282–287

Goldsmith J 1990 Childbirth: wisdom from the world's oldest societies. East West Health Books, New York

Guilliland K, Pairman S 1995 The midwifery partnership. A model for practice. Monograph Series: 95/1. Victoria University, Wellington

Hartley J 2003 Piles: ideas on how to reduce the pain from haemorrhoids. In: S Wickham (Ed) Midwifery best practice. Elsevier Science, London

Hedayati H, Parsons J, Crowther C 2004 Topically applied anaesthetics for treatment of perineal pain after childbirth. Cochrane Library (2). John Wiley & Sons, Chichester

Howie P 1995 The physiology of the puerperium and lactation. In: G Chamberlain (Ed) Turnbull's obstetrics (2nd edn). Churchill Livingstone, Edinburgh

Lyons S 1998 Post-traumatic stress disorder following childbirth: causes prevention and treatment. In: S Clement (Ed) Psychological perspective on pregnancy and childbirth. Churchill Livingstone, Edinburgh

McCourt C, Hirst J, Page L 2000 Dimensions and attributes of caring: women's perceptions. In: L Page (Ed) The new midwifery: science and sensitivity in practice. Churchill Livingstone, London

McQueen A, Mander R 2003 Tiredness and fatigue in the postnatal period. Journal of Advanced Nursing 42(5):463–469

Marchant S 2003 The puerperium. In: D Fraser, M Cooper (Eds) Myles textbook for midwives. Elsevier Science, London

Marchant S 2004 Transition to motherhood: from the woman's perspective: In M Stewart (Ed) Pregnancy, birth and maternity care; feminist perspectives. Books for Midwives, London

Marchant S, Alexander J, Garcia J et al 1999 A survey of women's experiences of vaginal loss from 24 hours to three months after childbirth (the BliPP study). Midwifery 15:72–81

Marchant S, Alexander J, Garcia J 2003 How does it feel to you? Uterine palpation and lochia loss as guides to postnatal recovery. In: S Wickham (Ed) Midwifery best practice. Churchill Livingstone, London

Ministry of Health 2002a Maternity Services Notice pursuant to Section 88 of the New Zealand Public Health and Disability Act 2000, Issued by the Crown

Ministry of Health 2002b Maternity services consumer satisfaction survey. MOH, Wellington

Ministry of Health 2003 Report on maternity 2000 and 2001. MOH, Wellington

Munday R 2003 A phenomenological study of women's experiences of the postnatal period following planned homebirth. MIDIRS Midwifery Digest 13(4):519–523

National Advisory Committee on Core Health and Disability Support Services (NACCHDSS) 1993 Care of mother and baby after normal delivery. NACCHDSS, Wellington

National Institute for Clinical Excellence (NICE) 2002 Technology appraisal guidance no. 41: guidance on the use of routine antenatal anti-D prophylaxis for rhesus negative women. NICE, London

New Zealand College of Midwives (NZCOM) 2004 What should your local maternity facility be offering? Midwifery News 33:25–28

New Zealand College of Midwives (NZCOM) 2005 Midwives handbook for practice (2nd edn). NZCOM, Christchurch

Ockenden J 2003 After the birth is over … rest and support for the new mothers. In: S Wickham (Ed) Midwifery best practice. Elsevier Science, London

Paradice R 2002 Psychology for midwives. Mark Allen, Wiltshire, UK

Percival P, McCourt C 2000 Becoming a parent. In: L Page (Ed) The new midwifery. Science and sensitivity in practice. Churchill Livingstone, London

Phipps F 2003 Pain in the early puerperium. Women's experiences following normal vaginal delivery. In: S Wickham (Ed) Midwifery best practice. Elsevier Science, London

Podkolinski J 1998 Women's experience of postnatal support. In: S Clement (Ed) Psychological perspectives on pregnancy and childbirth. Churchill Livingstone, Edinburgh

Riordan J, Auerbach K 1993 Breastfeeding and human lactation. Jones and Bartlett, Boston

Sine I, Cameron J 1968 Relief of afterpains. A deliberative nursing approach. Nursing Clinics of North America 3(2):327–335

Stables D 2000 Physiology in childbearing with anatomy and related biosciences. Baillière Tindall, London

Sweet B 1989 Mayes' midwifery. A textbook for midwives (11th edn). Baillière Tindall, London

Sweet B 1999 Mayes' midwifery. A textbook for midwives (13th edn). Baillière Tindall, London

Symon A, Glazener CM, MacDonald A et al 2003 Pilot study: quality of life assessment of postnatal fatigue and other physical morbidity. Journal of Psychosomatic Obstetrics and Gynaecology 24:215–219

Ussher J 2004 Depression in the postnatal period: a normal response to motherhood. In: M Stewart (Ed) Pregnancy, birth and maternity care: feminist perspectives. Books for Midwives, London

Vernon D (Ed) 2005 Bea's story: having a great birth in Australia. Australian College of Midwives, Canberra, Australia

Waite J 2002 Report on Rangiora Hospital after pains audit; feedback on a midwifery-led initiative. New Zealand College of Midwives Midwifery News 24:28

Wray J 2003 Postnatal care: is it an afterthought? The Practising Midwife 6(4):4–5

Further reading

Coad J, Dunstall M (Eds) 2001 Anatomy and physiology for midwives. Mosby, London

Kirkham M (Ed) 2000 The midwife–mother relationship. Macmillan, London

Page L (Ed) 2000 The new midwifery science and sensitivity. Churchill Livingstone, London

Stables D 2000 Physiology in childbearing with anatomy and related biosciences. Baillière Tindall, London

Stewart M (Ed) 2004 Pregnancy, birth and maternity care. Feminist perspectives. Books for Midwives, London

Wickham S (Ed) Midwifery best practice. Elsevier Science, London

Acknowledgement

I would like to thank midwives Coral Moir and Cathy Whyte for their help and support during the writing of this chapter.

CHAPTER 27

Supporting the newborn infant

Jackie Gunn

Key terms

Barlow's test, birthmarks, brown adipose tissue, centile charts, core temperature, developmental dysplasia of the hips, ductus arteriosus, fetal breathing movements, fetal haemoglobin, foramen ovale, grasp reflexes, hyperthermia, hypogastric arteries, hypoglycaemia, hypothermia, hypoxia, immunisation, jaundice, lung fluid, meconium, neonatal examination, neurological examination, non-shivering thermogenesis, Ortolani's test, plagiocephaly, skin variations, sleep–wake state, thermogenesis, thermoregulation, vitamin K deficiency bleeding

Chapter overview

This chapter provides an overview of neonatal physiology and the transition to extrauterine life. It explains the knowledge and skills that midwives need for assessing neonatal wellbeing, including puerperal assessment. It concludes with an overview of the most common minor complications that affect the neonate's health.

Learning outcomes

Learning outcomes for this chapter are:

1 To promote understanding of neonatal physiology and the transition to extrauterine life

2 To promote understanding and assessment of physiological and social development of babies in the first weeks after birth

3 To develop assessment skills to monitor infant health, wellbeing and responses to physiological changes (including neonatal screening tests)

4 To enable midwifery practice that informs, educates and supports the baby's mother related to normal baby behaviour patterns, daily care and the minor complexities of the neonatal period

5 To promote understanding of evidence for midwifery care that supports the newborn infant

6 To describe how to undertake a comprehensive physical assessment of the newborn infant

7 To explain specific examination techniques

8 To outline the normal ranges for growth and development of newborns

9 To discuss the assessment of infant wellbeing and how to recognise a sick baby

10 To explain the minor complexities of the neonatal period

11 To discuss how to assist mothers to identify and manage baby emergencies.

Introduction

The neonatal (or newborn) period lasts from birth until 28 days of age (London et al 2003). Midwives care for women and their new babies for up to six weeks post partum. In Australia the period of postnatal midwifery care varies between states and between urban and remote settings. In New Zealand, women and babies are generally discharged from midwifery care at four weeks post partum, although visits may continue up to six weeks if there is a clinical requirement. Initial and ongoing monitoring of the health and wellbeing of the newborn infant is one of the primary purposes of ongoing midwifery care.

While much midwifery care for newborn infants involves information sharing, maternal support and day-to-day observations of normal growth and development, there are times when individual babies show behaviours or signs that are not quite as expected. At these times, midwives must use professional knowledge and judgement to assess the baby and to implement care that may include continued observation, midwifery intervention and/or referral to a medical practitioner. Women and their families expect that the midwife's practice and the information they receive is current and supported by available evidence.

Midwives are part of families' lives for a very short period. One of their major roles is to support and enable women to be confident mothers. Having knowledge of her baby's behaviour and development, understanding how to care for her baby, and reinforcement that she is a capable mother, all help to engender the mother's confidence.

Caring for newborn babies is not always part of young women's experiences before they have their own children, and therefore midwives are often in the position of supporting and guiding women as they learn to care for their new infant. In these circumstances, it is tempting for professionals to regard the baby as 'theirs' and to give women information in an instructional fashion that relegates the baby's mother to the role of 'outside' caregiver afraid to use her own common sense or to do things for her baby. At all times the midwife's client is the woman. The woman is the baby's mother. She generally knows whether her baby is doing well or not. Midwifery care is provided in partnership with the baby's mother, and therefore all midwifery observation, care, treatment and referral are undertaken only in consultation and agreement with her.[1]

Neonatal physiology and the transition to extrauterine life

This section explores neonatal physiology and the transition to neonatal life, in sections related to body systems.

Respiratory system

While functional at birth, the alveoli continue to mature until about eight years of age (London et al 2003; Michaelides 2004a). A term baby has approximately 8% of the adult numbers of alveoli (Hand et al 1990). Pulmonary, vascular and lymphatic structures differentiate during the first 20 weeks gestation. Alveolar ducts have begun to develop by 24 weeks of pregnancy and primitive alveoli appear by 28 weeks gestation. There are two types of alveolar cells: type I cells necessary for gas exchange, and type II cells for the synthesis and storage of surfactant (London et al 2003).

Surfactant

Surfactant is produced in the lungs in increasing amounts from 32 weeks gestation. It comprises phospholipids and specialised protein molecules that reduce the surface tension of the alveolar fluid at the air/alveolar interface, and contributes to the elasticity of lung tissue (London et al 2003; Varney et al 2004). As gestation increases, the lining of alveoli becomes thinner, increasing the surface area for eventual gas exchange and effectively fusing the capillary endothelium and alveolar basement membranes (Michaelides 2004; Novak 2005a). At term, the alveoli are lined with surfactant. Because surfactant reduces the surface tension in the alveoli, it reduces the tendency of the alveoli to collapse with each breath due to the elastic recoil of the lungs. Surfactant increases lung compliance and thus reduces the pressure required to inflate the lungs for inspiration (Michaelides 2004; Novak 2005; Varney et al 2004). Synthesis of surfactant is thought to be affected by acidosis and/or hypothermia (Michaelides 2004a).

Fetal breathing movements

Breathing after birth can be seen as a continuation of an intrauterine process. From as early as 11 weeks gestation, fetal breathing movements occur in order to develop the chest muscles and diaphragm (London et al 2003). As the fetus grows, the frequency and strength of breathing movements increases, until they reach 30–70 breath movements per minute and are present 40–80% of the time (Davis & Bureau 1987, cited in Michaelides 2004a, p 530).

Lung fluid

Lung fluid is not surfactant. It is a clear fluid that facilitates cell proliferation and differentiation. At birth the lungs' function changes from secretion of fluid to the absorption of gases. It is likely that the catecholamine surge at birth is the final trigger for this change (Milner & Vyas 1982, cited in Michaelides 2004a, pp 529). At birth the remaining fluid is either expelled through the upper airways or absorbed via the pulmonary lymphatic system (Michaelides 2004a). Within two hours of the birth of a healthy term neonate, about 80% of the fluid has been reabsorbed and is completely absorbed from the alveoli within 12–24 hours. The fluid is absorbed from the interstitial tissue into the pulmonary vasculature and lymphatic drainage over the next few days (Novak 2005a).

Clinical point

Monitoring 'wet' lungs

Occasionally audible rales and/or rhonchi may be present at birth. These sounds may be associated with lung fluid that has not yet been reabsorbed. Observation and management:

▶ If:
– the baby is full term, healthy and alert
– respiratory rate is normal
– colour is pink and maintained
– the baby has good muscle tone
– heart rate is within normal range and not increasing,
recheck in 15 minutes.

▶ If the sounds are diminishing in audibility and harshness at this time: continue to check every 15 minutes.

▶ If the baby remains well and the sounds continue to diminish: continue to monitor until they have gone. They should have substantially cleared within an hour of birth.

▶ Refer to a medical practitioner if there are any or all of:
– persistent or fluctuating colour change (dusky, cyanosis)
– tachycardia
– tachypnoea
– reduced muscle tone
– lethargy
– lung sounds getting worse or not clearing.

(Source: London et al 2003)

Note: Transient tachypnoea of the newborn can occur in otherwise healthy babies (see Ch 38).

Clinical research

Oropharyngeal suctioning at birth

Routinely suctioning lung fluid from the baby's nose and oropharynx at birth was abandoned in most places more than a decade ago. However, where meconium is present in the liquor amnii, suctioning is practised, especially before the baby has taken the first breath.

Recent research has shown that even in the presence of meconium, routine suctioning a healthy newborn's oropharynx and nasal passages is contraindicated and may even be harmful (Vain et al 2004) (see Ch 36).

First active breath

Most babies gasp and establish respiration at birth. The lungs are expanded within the first few breaths. Alveolar inflation is complete a few hours after birth, resulting in a fairly consistent

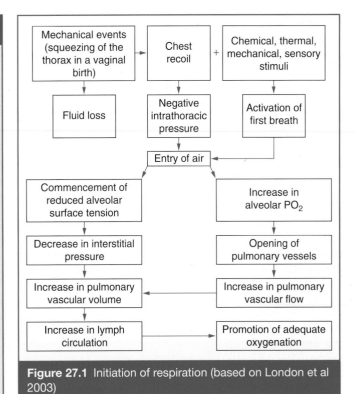

Figure 27.1 Initiation of respiration (based on London et al 2003)

lung volume of 25 mL/kg body weight (Coad & Dunstall 2001; Novak 2005a).

Factors initiating the first breath and lung expansion are:

● *compression of the chest wall during birth and the recoil of the chest wall immediately after birth.* Chest compression and recoil expand intrathoracic capacity, stimulating the baby to take a breath. Lung fluid is displaced through the nose and mouth or across the alveolar walls into the interstitial space, and the mechanism essential for effective respiration and pulmonary gas exchange is triggered (Novak 2005a). Significant negative intrathoracic pressure of up to 9.8 kPa (100 cm of water) is produced as the lung fluid is emptied and the pulmonary tissue and vasculature expand. Much less pressure is needed for subsequent breaths (Farrell & Sittlington 2003a).

● *chemoreceptor stimulation by reduction in oxygen and increase in carbon dioxide in the blood.* Normal labour results in mild hypoxia, hypercapnia and acidosis, which stimulate respiration. Physiological hypoxia and hypercapnia trigger the establishment of the respiratory drive in the respiratory centre in the medulla oblongata (Farrell & Sittlington 2003a; Novak 2005a). The chemoreceptors are less responsive in the first few days after birth (Blackburn 2003), emphasising the major role of chest recoil and absorption of fluid in facilitating the first breaths.

● *other external stimuli* such as cold, light, noise, touch and pain are secondary triggers for the baby to take the first breath.

Neonatal breathing patterns

At birth the respiratory system is immature. Neonates have shallow, irregular breathing and breathe through the nose for the first two to three months. 'Babies are obligatory nose breathers and do not convert automatically to mouth breathing when nasal obstruction occurs' (Farrell & Sittlington 2003a, p 729). On auscultation, breathing may sound noisy and wet during the first one to two hours while any remaining fluid is cleared from the lungs (Varney et al 2004) (see 'wet lungs' Clinical point).

The normal baby has an average respiratory rate of 40 breaths/minute (range is 30–60 breaths/min; see Table 27.1). Breathing is diaphragmatic—the chest and abdomen rise and fall together. Such symmetry confirms that the lungs and diaphragm are functioning correctly. Newborn babies commonly have periods of irregular breathing, particularly during REM sleep. The irregular gaps between breaths are termed apnoea. Apnoea of less than 20 seconds is not usually of clinical concern.

Clinical point

Assessing neonatal respiratory rate
- Record when the baby is quiet or asleep.
- Always count for a full minute.
- Assess the baby's colour
- Observe for any signs of respiratory difficulty (see Table 27.1).

Counting respirations when the baby is clothed can be difficult. The following methods are practical ways to count the rate without disturbing the baby.
- Listen through the diaphragm of a stethoscope held a few centimetres from the baby's nose.
- Feel the rise and fall of the baby's abdomen through a hand placed on the baby's abdomen.

While an elevated respiratory rate is a sign that the baby is unwell, tachypnoea cannot be assessed without taking the baby's other behaviour into account, such as recent crying, feeding or sleeping (Farrell & Sittlington 2003a; Michaelides 2004a). A baby's cry is loud and of medium pitch. Over time, mothers learn to distinguish variations in crying and to attach meaning to them (e.g. hungry, wet, in pain).

Cardiovascular system

Note that respiratory and cardiovascular changes occur simultaneously and are mutually dependent (Farrell & Sittlington 2003a).

Cardiovascular adaptations at birth

Cardiovascular adaptations that occur at birth are outlined in Table 27.2.

Pulmonary oxygenation of blood

In uterine life, 5–10% of cardiac output enters the pulmonary circulation to meet pulmonary cellular growth and nutrition needs. High pulmonary vascular resistance and the patent ductus arteriosus ensure that the remainder of the cardiac output enters the arterial system. At birth, adjustments must be made to the baby's circulation so that deoxygenated blood can go to the lungs for oxygenation. This involves several mechanisms. The expansion of the lungs and lowered pulmonary vascular resistance that occurs with the first breath enables virtually all the cardiac output to enter the pulmonary circulation. The oxygenated blood returning to the heart via the pulmonary veins increases the pressure within the left atrium (Farrell & Sittlington 2003a; Michaelides 2004a).

Closure of foramen ovale

The foramen ovale is an opening in the atrial septum created by a flap of tissue that is kept open in fetal life by the higher pressure of the blood in the right atrium. At birth, the vessels in the umbilical cord constrict, the cord is clamped and the

TABLE 27.1 Neonatal breathing patterns

	Normal variations	Outside normal variations (any or all of these)
Rate	40 breaths/minute average Range 30–60 breaths/min (sleeping or in quiet alert state)	More than 60 breaths/minute (sleeping or in quiet alert state)
Rhythm	Regular and irregular periods Apnoea < 20 seconds	Irregular breathing Apnoea > 20 seconds
Chest/abdominal movement	Synchronised diaphragm and abdominal movement	Subcostal and /or intercostal in-drawing
Nose	Breathes through the nose, no nasal flaring	Flaring of nostrils
Sound	Silent	Expiratory 'grunt'
Colour	Pink	Pale/cyanosis
(See Ch 38 for respiratory distress syndrome.)		

TABLE 27.2	Fetal and neonatal circulation	
System	**Fetal**	**Neonatal**
Pulmonary blood vessels	Constricted, with very little blood flow; lungs not expanded	Vasodilation and increased blood flow; lungs expanded; increased oxygen stimulates vasodilation
Systemic blood vessels	Dilated, with low resistance; blood mostly in placenta	Arterial pressure rises due to loss of placenta; increased systemic blood volume and resistance
Ductus arteriosus	Large, with no tone; blood flow from pulmonary artery to aorta	Reversal of blood flow; now from aorta to pulmonary artery because of increased left atrial pressure. Ductus is sensitive to increased oxygen and body chemicals and begins to constrict.
Foramen ovale	Patent, with increased blood flow from right atrium to left atrium	Increased pressure in left atrium attempts to reverse blood flow and shuts one-way valve.

(Source: London et al 2003)

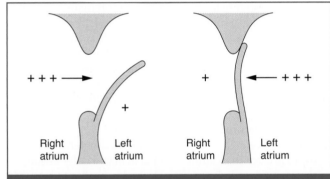

Figure 27.2 Closure of the foramen ovale (based on Coad & Dunstall 2001)

pulmonary vasculature expands. These events result in a fall in right atrial pressure and a rise in left atrial pressure. The pressure alterations, especially the higher left atrial pressure, cause the flap of the foramen ovale to be pressed flat against the septum and therefore to functionally close. Flow murmurs in the first 24–48 hours post partum may be the result of incomplete closure of the foramen ovale and persist until the pressures stabilise and the foramen stays closed. In the first days after birth, closure is reversible; if pulmonary vascular resistance is high—for example, when crying—transient cyanotic episodes may occur as a result of the foramen temporarily reopening. The foramen anatomically closes within the first year of life (Farrell & Sittlington 2003a; London et al 2003).

Closure of the ductus arteriosus

In fetal life, the ductus arteriosus is nearly as wide as the aorta. Blood is shunted directly from the pulmonary artery to the aorta via the ductus arteriosus, thereby avoiding the lungs. At birth, the pulmonary vascular resistance falls and the amount of blood being shunted to the aorta via the ductus arteriosus is substantially decreased. Contraction of the muscular walls of the ductus arteriosus occurs almost immediately after birth. Decreasing levels of maternal prostaglandin

(previously supplied by the placenta) and rising arterial oxygen tension trigger vasoconstriction. The ductus arteriosus is usually functionally closed by 8–10 hours after birth, but not anatomically closed for several months. Before pressures stabilise, a temporary reverse shunt through the ductus arteriosus may persist for a few hours. In some babies the ductus has been shown to be intermittently patent up to three days after birth (Farrell & Sittlington 2003a; Michaelides 2004a; Novak 2005a).

Adaptation of other temporary fetal cardiovascular structures

Clamping the cord causes the foramen ovale and hypogastric arteries to functionally close almost immediately. Anatomical closure occurs within two to three months. The resulting fibrous structures are known as the ligamentum venosum and ligamentum teres. The superior vesical arteries are the vestiges of the hypogastric arteries (Farrell & Sittlington 2003a).

Characteristics of neonatal cardiac function

● Heart rate—in the first week after birth the average heart rate is 110–150 beats per minute in a quiet, healthy, term neonate. However, wide fluctuations occur when the baby is active, feeding or asleep (Farrell & Sittlington 2003a; London et al 2003).

- Peripheral circulation—the healthy term baby's hands and feet are mildly cyanosed (acrocyanosis) for several hours after birth until peripheral perfusion is complete.
- Blood volume and blood pressure—systolic blood pressure varies with gestation, birthweight and neonatal activity such as crying. It is not usually assessed in healthy term infants (London et al 2003). At birth, the total circulating blood volume is 80 mL/kg of body weight (i.e. 280 mL for a 3.5 kg baby) (Blackburn 2003). The relatively low total circulating blood volume means that quite small quantities of blood represent a large blood loss for the neonate (e.g. 10% of adult blood volume is 800 mL; 10% of a 3.5 kg baby's blood volume is 28 mL).

  Attentive concern is required when assessing blood loss from the cord or the amount of blood taken for laboratory analysis.

Heart murmurs

Heart murmurs are sounds that may be heard as blood flow is disturbed as it crosses an abnormal valve, as it flows under pressure through a defect in either the atrial or ventricular septum, or sometimes when there is increased flow as it crosses a normal valve. In neonates, 90% of all murmurs are transient and not associated with anomalies (London et al 2003).

Clinical point

Neonatal heart murmurs
Murmurs are not heard if there is nothing to make the flow turbulent. Many serious cardiac malformations are silent, and therefore midwives need to always be observant for systemic signs of cardiac compromise—colour, respiratory rate, muscle tone, feeding problems and so on (see Ch 38).

Clinical point

Why large cardiac septal defects are usually silent
Flowing fluid does not make a noise if it is not under a lot of pressure. Think of the absence of noise when water flows through a wide-bore hose. When fluid is forced through a small opening, the pressure is raised and the resulting turbulence creates a noise. Think of the way water begins to hiss when pressure is increased by a thumb partially closing the opening of a wide-bore hose. Large defects in the atrial or ventricular septa allow the blood to flow through the defect with little or no change in pressure. Consequently there is no turbulence and no is sound made. Diagnosis of large cardiac anomalies is nearly always made through clinical observation of babies and their behaviour.

Thermoregulation

Newborn babies sustain life within a narrow range of core (internal) body temperature, generally 36.5–37.5°C (Blackburn 2003). The body uses a number of mechanisms to balance heat loss and heat production in order to maintain the core temperature within this range despite a wide range of environmental temperatures. Balancing heat loss and gain is known as thermoregulation. The range of ambient temperature that maintains a baby's core body temperature using minimum oxygen consumption at a minimum metabolic rate is called the thermoneutral range (Blackburn 2003; London et al 2003).

At birth, babies' thermoregulatory mechanisms are not fully developed, although they become progressively more efficient. Limited response to temperature changes in the first 24 hours of life results in babies being particularly susceptible to chilling during this time. By 24–48 hours of age, healthy term neonates are able to increase their heat production up to 2.5 times in response to cold; however, they remain susceptible to environmental temperature changes. Until the mechanisms controlling thermoregulation (and heat loss in particular) stabilise, the thermoneutral range of babies is at a higher environmental temperature than older children and adults. In the first weeks of life, warm rooms, or extra clothing and blankets if outside, are required (Blackburn 2003; Michaelides 2004b; London et al 2003).

Neonatal features contributing to heat loss:
- large surface area to mass ratio (approximately three times greater than adults). In particular, a baby's head, the major heat loss area in a clothed baby, is a larger proportion of the body than is an adult's.
- less subcutaneous fat
- thin epidermis
- blood vessels closer to the skin, so changes in the ambient temperature more readily influence the circulating blood, thereby influencing the temperature-regulating centre in the hypothalamus
- decreased ability to shiver.

Neonatal features contributing to heat production:
- decreased ability to sweat
- flexed posture, which conserves heat by reducing exposed surface area
- non-shivering thermogenesis (Blackburn 2003; London et al 2003; Michaelides 2004b).

Neonatal heat loss

Heat is very easily lost at birth, when autonomic thermo-regulation is at its least efficient and the baby is wet. Hypothermia (a temperature less than 36.5°C) can occur rapidly unless active steps are taken to prevent heat loss.

There are four ways in which babies can lose heat from their body surface:
- Evaporation—heat loss occurs when water evaporates as vapour from the skin. Babies are particularly vulnerable to cooling by evaporation at birth and during bathing if the environmental temperature is too low. A birthing room temperature of at least 25–28° C is needed, to

prevent heat loss at birth. Minimising the time the baby is wet by careful drying also helps to prevent heat loss by evaporation.

- Convection—cooler air passing over a warm baby causes heat loss by convection. Preventive measures include eliminating cool air flows from draughts and air conditioning. Oxygen given by mask or by oxygen catheter can cause heat loss by convection.
- Conduction—coming into direct contact with a colder surface can rapidly cool a baby. Items such as cold hands, clothes and bedding, weighing scale trays and stethoscope diaphragms fall into this category. All such items should be warmed before coming into contact with the baby's skin.
- Radiation—radiant heat loss happens when heat is transferred from the body to cooler objects not in direct contact with the baby; for example, bassinets or cots placed against external room walls or under windows can cause heat loss by radiation (Blackburn 2003; London et al 2003; Michaelides 2004b; Novak 2005b).

Neonatal thermogenesis

Neonates rarely shiver. They generate heat by increasing their metabolic rate using muscular activity such as moving limbs and suckling, and by chemical thermogenesis (heat production), also called non-shivering thermogenesis (Blackburn 2003).

Thermogenesis and brown adipose tissue

Heat production by chemical means involves the metabolism of brown adipose tissue (BAT). Approximately 2–7 % of neonatal body weight is thought to be BAT or brown fat. It begins to be deposited in the fetus from 26 weeks gestation, steadily increasing in amount until two to five weeks after birth. At term, BAT is deposited around the nape of the neck and mid-scapular area, under the clavicles and in the axillae, around the kidneys, adrenal glands and large vessels in the neck and in the mediastinum (London et al 2003; Novak 2005b). Maternal prostaglandins and adenosine prevent non-shivering thermogenesis in utero; BAT is only activated after birth. Brown fat stores are not renewable once they have been used (Michaelides 2004b).

Brown adipose tissue is so-named because of the colour that results from the tissue containing a more extensive blood supply and greater numbers of intracellular organelles such as mitochondria, than white adipose tissue. Neonatal cooling causes noradrenaline, other catecholamines and thyroid hormones to be released so that rapid lipolysis of brown adipose tissue and consequent heat production is induced. Oxygen and glucose are required in the metabolism of brown fat. Brown fat lipolysis uses up to three times as much oxygen as other tissue. Normal oxygen consumption, conservation of brown fat stores and maintenance of core body temperature are promoted by keeping babies in a thermoneutral range. (Blackburn 2003; Farrell & Sittlington 2003a; London et al 2003; Novak 2005b).

Maintaining temperature after birth

At birth, healthy term babies are placed against their mothers' body skin-to-skin, dried and covered with a warm blanket to maintain their temperature. A mother's body conducts direct warmth to the baby, and the blanket traps a layer of warm, insulating air around the baby (Blackburn 2003; Michaelides 2004b). Studies of preterm babies in Colombia and England showed that 'kangaroo care' (skin-to-skin between the mother's breasts) satisfactorily maintains body heat (Sleath 1985; Whitelaw et al 1988).

The following methods are commonly used to conserve heat in newborn infants.

- Place the baby in immediate skin-to-skin contact with the mother.
- Dry the baby immediately.
- Pre-warm any hats, blankets and clothing prior to the birth.
- Pre-warm the resuscitation area.
- Maintain the temperature in the birthing room at > 25°C.
- Replace wet blankets or towels after drying the baby.
- Do not bath the baby until temperature has been stable for two hours.
- Do not place the bassinet against windows, outside walls or doorways.
- In cooler environments, keep the baby's head covered and body well wrapped (McHugh 2004).

Clinical point

Heat loss in preterm and SGA babies
Preterm infants and small for gestational age (SGA) babies have less adipose tissue and a greater surface area to mass ratio than full-term babies. Furthermore, the lower the gestational age, the less brown adipose tissue (BAT) is deposited and the less the body and limbs are flexed. Consequently these babies are extremely vulnerable to hypothermia. They require a higher environmental temperature to maintain a thermoneutral range (London et al 2003).

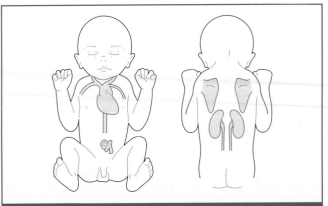

Figure 27.3 Brown adipose tissue (BAT) deposits in the term neonate (based on Stables & Rankin 2005)

Wrapping babies

While warm towels, blankets and clothing are a necessity and many babies appear to prefer being firmly wrapped, overly tight wrapping prevents the movement that generates heat. The baby's clothes should not be too tight. It is better to use several thin layers than one or two thick layers (natural fabrics 'breathe' better than synthetics). Hats, especially for small and preterm infants, have proved effective in reducing heat loss from the head in cool environments or when heat loss is a concern. When transporting small or sick babies, a thermoblanket that retains body heat is used (London et al 2004; Michaelides 2004b).

Hot water bottles and electric blankets

These items are used only for heating fabrics and must never be left in the cot with the baby. This is also true of wheat bags or anything else that retains heat in a similar way, such as gel packs.

Bathing and temperature maintenance

Babies are no longer bathed immediately after birth unless there is a risk of vertical transmission of an infection from the mother, such as hepatitis B or HIV. Bathing soon after birth increases the risk of hypothermia, and therefore it should not be undertaken until the baby's temperature has stabilised (Leveno et al 2003). Breastfeeding is more important, both to initiate feeding and to provide fuel for the baby's metabolic processes, including temperature maintenance. Although babies' thermoregulatory mechanisms become more efficient as the days pass, bathing remains a time when they can be easily chilled. The following precautions should always be taken:

- Bathe the baby in a draught-free room.
- Ensure the ambient temperature is 25–28°C.
- The baby's temperature should be within the normal range.
- Water temperature should be 36.7°C (similar temperature to skin when tested with the inside surface of an adult's wrist).
- Warm the towels and clothing.
- Do not expose the baby unnecessarily (e.g. keep wrapped in a towel while bathing the head).
- Dry the baby promptly and thoroughly, especially the hair and in the folds of the skin (London et al 2003; Michaelides 2004b; Varney et al 2004).

Impaired thermoregulatory control

Neonatal hypothermia

If the neonate's temperature falls below 36.5°C, the baby is at risk of hypothermia. *Prevention is the best treatment.* A mildly hypothermic baby (36–36.5°C) can generally be warmed without difficulty by tucking up skin-to-skin with the mother in a warm (≥ 25°C) room if stable, or by placing in an incubator set at 35–36°C. In the latter situation the baby should be clothed but not under a blanket (Blackburn 2003; London et al 2003; Michaelides 2004; Novak 2005b). Untreated hypothermia can result in generalised vasoconstriction that

---

Clinical point

Neonatal temperature measurement

▶ **Axillary temperature**
This is the preferred site.
Note: In a hypothermic baby, the reading will be higher than the core as the area contains large areas of brown fat (Bliss-Holtz 1991). As this may make recognition of hypothermia more difficult, behavioural and other physiological signs should also be assessed when the temperature is taken.

▶ **Rectal temperature**—It is considered preferable to routinely measure the temperature via the axilla; however, core temperature may be required in individual situations. The rectal temperature *measures the core temperature and is the most accurate.* It is used when the axillary temperature is abnormal; e.g. check rectal temperature if axillary temperature is < 36.5°C.
Measuring a newborn's rectal temperature: The well-lubricated thermometer should be gently inserted no more than 3 cm into the rectum of the term baby and no more than 2 cm in the preterm baby (Blackburn 2003; Fleming et al 1983). The baby's legs need to be held still during this procedure and great care taken to ensure that the rectum is not damaged. For this reason, many institutions prohibit this procedure.

▶ **Tympanic temperature**—As the reading is often affected by environmental temperature, this site is less accurate for newborn babies and *should not normally be used.* Wells et al (1995) showed that readings were 0.5–1.0°C higher than the core temperature when the environmental temperature was > 30°C, and 0.5-1.0°C lower when environmental temperature was < 30°C.

▶ **Skin sites**—For a rapid general assessment of temperature, skin sites can be useful.
  – Feeling the forehead or the back of the neck with the inside of the wrist can provide a quick check, to decide whether the baby needs extra clothing for example.
  – The area between the scapulae, the abdomen and the feet can fulfil the same assessment. However, it needs to be remembered that the feet are cooler than the rest of the body, which makes this assessment less valuable.

▶ **Commercial 'spots' or 'tapes'**—used on the skin these are a non-invasive method for taking the temperature that parents may find useful as the baby grows older.

---

includes the pulmonary vessels. Pulmonary vasoconstriction results in decreased pulmonary perfusion that affects pH, PaO_2 and $PaCO_2$ levels. Increased $PaCO_2$, decreased PaO_2 and pH levels result in respiratory acidosis. Consequently the baby

Clinical point

Relationship between hypothermia, hypoxia and hypoglycaemia in neonates

▶ Healthy neonates have limited stores of glycogen and brown fat and are vulnerable to rapid heat loss.

▶ Preterm infants have less glycogen stores and brown fat and greater vulnerability to heat loss than term babies.

▶ Hypothermia leads to brown fat lipolysis to restore the temperature. The process consumes oxygen and glycogen.

▶ Hypoglycaemia leads to mobilisation of glycogen stores to restore serum glucose levels. The process of converting glycogen to glucose requires oxygen and heat. Glycogen stores are depleted.

▶ Hypoxia leads to anaerobic methods of oxygen production. These inefficient processes require heat and glucose. Glycogen stores are depleted.

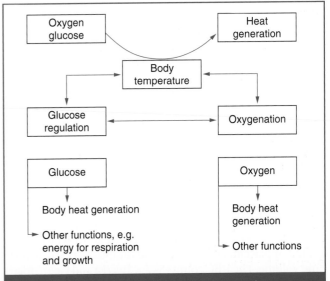

Figure 27.4 Interrelationship between temperature regulation, glucose concentration and respiration (based on Coad & Dunstall 2001)

exhibits signs of respiratory distress (Farrell & Sittlington 2003).

Underscoring the need for active steps to prevent heat loss is the fact that in newborn babies there is an interrelationship between hypothermia, hypoxia and hypoglycaemia, where the development of any one condition puts the baby at risk of the other two conditions.

Neonatal hyperthermia

Hyperthermia is a temperature above 37.5°C and is much less common than neonatal cooling. It can be as harmful as hypothermia if it is ignored. The most common cause of neonatal hyperthermia is under-estimation of the effect of the environmental temperature on the baby (e.g. putting the bassinet next to a heater). Babies can develop hyperthermia in response to an infection, environmental overheating or occasionally an underlying medical condition. Clinically discriminating between environmental factors and an infection can be extremely difficult, as babies with an infection can have a temperature below 37.5°C, while a temperature above 37.5°C can be the result of environmental factors. It is important to assess the whole clinical picture rather than rely solely on temperature as a guide.

Medical consultation is warranted when the temperature is above 37.5°C without an obvious environmental cause, such as direct sunlight in a well-heated room, or when the baby has a lower temperature but is exhibiting other signs of unwellness, such as not feeding. Similar consultation would be made if the temperature has not returned to normal within an hour of correcting an environmental cause (Farrell & Sittlington 2003a; Michaelides 2004b).

In the case of overheating due to an environmental cause, the baby should be slowly cooled by removing bootees and hat, exposing hands to the air and leaving the baby under a

Clinical alert!

Clothed babies who become hypothermic in an appropriately warm environment need *very prompt* medical assessment and investigation, especially for infection. In these circumstances the low temperature is likely to indicate a serious illness (usually an infection) rather than an environmental cause for the hypothermia.

Referral must not be delayed.

A low (or raised) temperature may be the only sign of early onset Group B streptococcal infection. Unexpected hypothermia in an otherwise well baby is *always* abnormal.

single blanket or sheet. Extremes such as removing all covers or cool bathing must be avoided, as rapid cooling can precipitate excessive heat loss and shock (Michaelides 2004b).

Haemopoietic system

Haemoglobin concentration

The fetal circulation enables fetal blood to be oxygenated at the placental site and to be transported to the brain and other vital organs as efficiently as possible. This is assisted by high concentrations of fetal haemoglobin (HbF), a type of haemoglobin that has a higher affinity for oxygen than adult haemoglobin. After birth the neonate is exposed to higher oxygen levels associated with breathing air. As the red cells with fetal haemoglobin are haemolysed, they are replaced by cells containing adult haemoglobin with a lower affinity for oxygen. Neonatal red blood cells have a shorter lifespan than adult cells and as they are destroyed this produces elevated serum bilirubin levels and physiological jaundice in some babies (Johnston et al 2003).

The haemoglobin level is initially high (130–200 g/L), and 50–85% of this is fetal haemoglobin. The levels decrease gradually, with changes apparent in the first week after birth (see Table 27.3), and fall to approximately 120 g/L by three months of age. Conversion from fetal to adult haemoglobin, which is commenced in utero, is completed in the first one to two years of life (Blackburn 2003; Michaelides 2004a).

Red blood cells, haematocrit and leucocytes

After birth the red blood cell (RBC) count gradually decreases as adult-sized red cells replace the larger HbF red cells. Neonatal RBCs have a lifespan of 80–100 days, approximately two-thirds of the lifespan of adult RBCs. In the first days after birth, the haematocrit (PCV) may increase above fetal levels as a result of placental transfusion and diminished extracellular fluid volume. The RBC count ($5–7 \times 10^{12}$/L) and haematocrit levels (55%) decrease gradually during the first two to three months of life. During this time, erythropoiesis is suppressed due to the relatively high hyperoxide environment that the neonate is exposed to after birth. Erythropoietin release is reduced due to lack of hypoxic stimulus (Blackburn 2003; Roberton 1996).

The leucocyte or white blood cell (WBC) count is initially high ($1–25 \times 10^9$/L) but decreases rapidly (Roberton 1996). Immature leucocytes, such as band neutrophils, are present in cord blood but disappear as transitional changes take place.

An elevated level of immature neutrophils is an indicator of infection.

Clotting factors

Colonisation of the intestine by the bacteria that synthesise vitamin K does not occur until milk feeding is established. Therefore, blood clotting is impaired in the first week post partum while levels of vitamin-K-dependent clotting factors II (prothrombin), VII, IX and X are low. Adult levels of platelets are present, but their capacity for adhesion and aggregation is reduced (Blackburn 2003; Michaelides 2004a).

Vitamin K prophylaxis

It is unclear why newborn infants have reduced levels of vitamin K dependent clotting factors; it has been postulated that it may be related to fetal growth regulation (Blackburn 2003). If vitamin K is not administered parenterally, the natural course is for the vitamin K levels to initially decrease as maternally acquired vitamin K is used. Neonatal vitamin K stores then increase gradually over the first month (Blackburn 2003).

Vitamin K deficiency bleeding

In some babies, the decline in vitamin K after birth leads to haemorrhagic disease of the newborn, now called *vitamin K deficiency bleeding* (VKDB). VKDB occurs in an early (< 48 hours), classic (2–7 days) or late (1 week – 6 months) form (Blackburn 2003). The natural prevalence of the classic form is 4–17 per 1000 (Greer 1995; Zipursky 1999).

The risk of late VKDB without and with vitamin K prophylaxis in Europe and Australia is shown in Table 27.4.

Breastfed babies are more at risk of haemorrhagic disease than formula-fed infants because formula contains vitamin K. Unfortunately, it is difficult to predict which babies

---

TABLE 27.3 Normal neonatal blood values*

	Cord blood	Day 1	Day 2	Day 3	Day 4	Day 5–14	Week 2–5
Hb (g/L)	136–196	165–215	165–215	165–215	165–215	150–200	110–185
PCV (haematocrit)	0.46–0.60	0.50–0.70	0.50–0.70	0.50–0.70	0.50–0.70	0.47–0.65	0.31–0.54
MCV	100–120	107–128	107–128	107–128	107–128	93–130	93–130
MCH	33–41	33–41	33–41	33–41	33–41	32–40	31–40
WBC b/L	10–25	10–25	10–25	10–25	10–25	10–25	5–17
Seg. neutrophils (b/L)	2–13	2–13	2–13	2–13	2–13	2–13 (day 5–7) 0.5–0.7 (day 7–14)	0.5–0.7
Band neutrophils	0.06	0.06	0.06	0.06	0.06	0.06	0.06
Lymphocytes	2–85	2–85	2–85	2–85	2–85	2–85 (day 5–7) 2.5–12 (day 7–14)	2.5–12
Platelets	150–500	150–500	150–500	150–500	150–500	150–500	150–500

*All cell counts 10^9/L.
(Source: Diagnostic/Medlab 2000)

TABLE 27.4 Risk of late VKDB		
	Risk (%)	
	Australia	**Europe**
No vitamin K	33.4	–
1 dose oral Konakion®	20	–
2 doses oral Konakion® MM	–	5
2 doses oral Konakion®	4.1	2.6
IM Konakion® at birth	0.2	0
(Source: NZCOM 2001)		

will develop VKDB as babies without specific risk factors can develop classic VKDB (Zipursky 1999). Because of these factors, prophylactic vitamin K at birth is recommended to prevent VKDB (Blackburn 2003; NZCOM 2001).

Routine vitamin K prophylaxis

The need for routine prophylaxis for all babies has been questioned since Golding et al (1990, 1992) published the results of a study that linked administration of intramuscular (IM) vitamin K to increased risk of childhood cancer. Several later reports have not demonstrated the same relationship (McKinney et al 1998; Olsen et al 1994; Passmore et al 1998; Zipursky 1996). While some methodological criticisms have been made of some of these later studies, in places where routine use of IM vitamin K was stopped or replaced by oral doses subsequent to the Golding et al study, the incidence of VKDB increased (Passmore et al 1998; Zipursky 1996). It is probable that vitamin K prophylaxis is not needed at birth by every baby; nevertheless, because it is not possible to identify those who do need vitamin K with any certainty, prophylaxis is policy in most maternity services. The New Zealand College of Midwives Consensus Statement (2001) supports vitamin K prophylaxis. In Australia, most babies are given Konakion®. The NHMRC (2000) recommends that an IMI dose of Konakion® be given to all newborns as prophylaxis against VKDB. A selective policy of vitamin K administration after screening is not appropriate, because a relatively high incidence of late VKDB occurs without prophylaxis. However, there is sufficient evidence to show that oral regimens are effective.

Informed consent

Depending on local policy, IM or oral vitamin K is given at birth. Maternity care providers have a responsibility to provide access to information and discussion. Parents need time to consider the information related to vitamin K prophylaxis. It is preferable that they receive written information and an opportunity to discuss their choices during pregnancy so that their decision can be recorded in their plan of care.

Dosage

After the Golding et al report, several studies were carried out comparing different dosage regimens (Cornelissen et al 1992; Greer et al 1998). The conclusions drawn from these studies are as follows:

- IM or oral vitamin K improves the neonate's coagulation status in the first week (Farrell & Sittlington 2003a).
- A single dose (1 mg) of IM vitamin K at birth effectively prevents classic VKDB.
- The effectiveness of intramuscular vitamin K in the prevention of late VKDB has been established (Loughnan et al 1999, cited in NZCOM 2001).
- The effectiveness of oral vitamin K in the prevention of late VKDB has been not established (Zipursky 1999).
- Local policies relating to the administration of oral vitamin K may differ. The three-dose regimen is common. The doses are usually spread across the first six weeks of life (e.g. at birth, one week and six weeks) (NZMOH 2004).

Immunological adaptations

Functional immaturity of the immune system and lack of exposure to common microorganisms at birth means that babies are very vulnerable to infections, particularly respiratory and gastrointestinal infections. Antibody-mediated and cell-mediated immunity, the inflammatory response and complement factors are different in newborn infants. Neonates cannot localise infections very well, and so an infection is more likely to become systemic. The immaturity of the gut defence mechanism increases the likelihood of both gastrointestinal infection and later development of allergies (Blackburn 2004; Farrell & Sittlington 2003b; Novak 2005b; Varney et al 2004). Both commensal and pathogenic microorganisms begin to colonise the baby during birth. Colonisation occurs first from the maternal genital tract, then from the mother's skin, and finally from other people and the general environment (Novak 2005b).

Specific immune responses

Antibody-mediated immunity

At birth the neonate has 55–80% of the adult total immuno-globulin values (IgG, IgA and IgM) (Blackburn 2003).

- Immunoglobulin G (IgG)—the baby's levels of IgG are equal to or slightly higher than those of the mother as maternal IgG is transferred across the placenta. Transfer increases progressively until term. The maternal IgG gives the baby some degree of passive immunity to the diseases to which the mother has antibodies, for approximately six months. After birth, levels fall gradually as the transferred IgG is used. The baby does not develop significant production of IgG until after six months of age. Adult levels are reached over four to six years (Blackburn 2003; Michaelides 2004a; Novak 2005b).
- Immunoglobulin A (IgA)—newborn levels of IgA and IgM are low, as the molecules are too large to cross the

placenta. IgA is important for localised immunity in the gastrointestinal and respiratory tracts. It is found in saliva, tears, and intestinal mucosa by two to three weeks of age, although adult levels are not reached in the saliva for two months. Maternal secretory IgA is also transferred to the baby in colostrum and breast milk, affording local protection to the gut. IgA levels reach 20% of adult levels by one year (Blackburn 2003; Farrell & Sittlington 2003b; Novak 2005).

- Immunoglobulin M (IgM)—at term the baby's IgM level is 20% of the adult value, which is not reached for two years. In utero, IgM is able to be formed after 19–20 weeks gestation in response to exposure to certain antigens, such as the TORCH organisms. IgM protects against blood-borne infections and is the main immunoglobulin produced in the first four weeks of life. Half the adult value of IgM is reached by six months of age (Blackburn 2003; Farrell & Sittlington 2003b).

Cell-mediated immunity

- Lymphocytes—at birth, T cell numbers are similar to those of adults but their function is decreased for approximately three to six months (Blackburn 2003). 'The thymus gland, where lymphocytes are produced, is relatively large at birth and continues to grow until eight years of age'(Farrell & Sittlington 2003b, p 730).
- Polymorphonuclear neutrophils and complement—immaturity of the polymorphonuclear neutrophils alters the inflammatory response and phagocytosis in neonates. Neonatal polymorphonuclear neutrophils are structurally more rigid, respond more slowly to antigen stimulus, move more slowly to the antigen site and are less efficient at aggregation and phagocytosis. Neutrophil function gradually matures through childhood.

Low levels of complement components contribute to decreased opsonisation capability. Serum complement levels increase to adult values by 6–18 months (Blackburn 2003). Nevertheless, Blackburn (2003) reports that neutrophils act normally in neonates when bacterial numbers are not too large and the baby is not stressed (e.g. by perinatal asphyxia). However, significantly reduced bacteriocidal activity for Gram-positive and Gram-negative organisms has been shown in stressed babies (Blackburn 2003).

Gut defence mechanism

In humans the gastrointestinal (GI) tract is part of the natural immune system. Defences in the GI tract include acidity, digestive enzymes that break down large molecules and secretory IgA that lines the small intestine (Varney et al 2004). At birth, the epithelial lining of the GI tract is immature and relatively permeable. Development of the epithelium and the mucosal surface as an impenetrable barrier against pathogenic microorganisms and other antigens is known as gut closure. Gastric acid, peristalsis and the mechanical barrier properties of the gut mucosal surface are some non-immune factors that contribute to the gut defence mechanism (Blackburn 2003).

Clinical point

Prevention and assessment of neonatal infection

Prevention:

- Practise standard precautions at all times.
- Teach parents to prevent infection through general hygiene measures such as hand washing, keeping equipment used for the baby in closed containers and by encouraging commonsense precautions such as keeping the baby away from people with colds etc.

Assessment:

- Recognise any risk factors for development of infection and monitor for signs of onset.
- Understand the subtle signs of infection in neonates and particularly note that fever is rarely a sign of infection.
- Know and teach parents the signs of illness in their baby.
- Understand normal neonatal laboratory findings and recognise changes that are associated with neonatal infection.

Role of breast milk in gut colonisation

Breastfeeding promotes gut colonisation because it provides a large amount of secretory IgA and stimulates the proliferation of intestinal enzymes. Colostrum and breast milk contribute to the development of protective gut flora by creating an acidic enteral environment, which favours growth of *Lactobacillus* and *Bifidobacterium*, thereby preventing growth of acid-sensitive organisms such as *Bacteroides* and enterobacteria. Breast milk also contains the protein lactoferrin, which binds with unabsorbed iron in the intestine, making it unavailable for bacterial metabolism (Blackburn 2003).

While there are fewer differences in gut colonisation when formula closely resembles breast milk, an alkaline environment is produced when babies are fed formula. In an alkaline environment, enterobacteria outcompete bifidobacteria, resulting in Gram-negative enterococci becoming the dominant organism in the intestine (Blackburn 2003).

Renal system

At birth the kidneys are structurally complete but functionally immature. There are limitations in the glomerular filtration rate capability and the ability to concentrate or dilute urine. Newborn babies have little renal reserve to cope with increased levels of solutes, which may occur in physiologically stressed or ill neonates (Farrell & Sittlington 2003b; Michaelides 2004a; Novak 2005a; Varney et al 2004). The total body water content in newborn babies is a larger proportion of body fluid than in adults. The shift of intracellular fluid into the extracellular compartment after birth results in a diuresis that causes loss of 5–10% of birthweight over the first week (Novak 2005a).

Urine is first passed within 24 hours of birth. Initially the newborn baby excretes only a small quantity of urine; as little as 30–60 mL is passed in the first 48 hours of life. Volume and frequency increases with rising fluid intake. The urine has a low specific gravity, is straw-coloured and odourless. There should be no protein or blood in the urine. Until fluid intake increases, the urine may be cloudy from the presence of mucus or urates. Urates may cause pink or brick-red staining on the nappy. While common in the first few days of life, the presence of urates in the urine of babies more than a few days old may indicate dehydration (Farrell & Sittlington 2003b; Michaelides 2004a; Novak 2005a; Varney et al 2004).

When the bladder becomes full it is palpable abdominally. The kidneys may also be palpable. On micturition the direction and force of the stream of urine should be noted (Farrell & Sittlington 2003; Michaelides 2004; Novak 2005a; Varney et al 2004).

Gastrointestinal system

Mouth

The mucous membrane is pink and moist, and both the hard and soft palate are complete. The teeth are buried in the gums, but occasionally a tooth may be present in the mouth. Small epithelial retention cysts, called Epstein's Pearls, are sometimes found along the midline of the palate and occasionally elsewhere in the mouth. They disappear over time. The sucking pads in the cheeks give a rounded, full appearance to the face (Blackburn 2003; Farrell & Sittlington 2003b; Michaelides 2004a; Varney et al 2004).

Swallowing and sucking

At birth the term baby has mature gag, cough, suck and swallow reflexes. As well as sucking fingers and thumbs, in utero the fetus swallows amniotic fluid from 10–14 weeks gestation to prepare the oesophagus to move food into the stomach by peristalsis. The swallowing reflex is mature at approximately 34 weeks gestation. The mature pattern of coordinated sucking–swallowing–breathing is seen as three to four bursts of sucking–swallowing followed by a pause for breathing. This pattern may not appear fully synchronised for a day or two after birth. The burst–pause pattern of sucking, swallowing and breathing seems to occur earlier in breastfed babies. Neonates cannot draw food from the lips to the pharynx, and therefore the nipple is drawn deeply into the mouth to enable suckling to occur (Blackburn 2003; Farrell & Sittlington 2003b; Michaelides 2004a; Varney et al 2004).

Stomach

At birth the capacity of the stomach is approximately 6 mL/kg of body weight (i.e. 21 mL in a 3.5 kg baby) (Blackburn 2003). However, capacity increases rapidly over the first few weeks. Gastric emptying time averages two to three hours, with breast milk emptying more rapidly than formula. When food enters the stomach, the ileo-caecal valve opens in response to a gastrocolic reflex. The contents of the ileum pass into the large intestine, and rapid peristalsis means that feeding is often accompanied by a bowel motion.

During the first 24–48 hours, gastric emptyin[g] delayed by mucus in the stomach. Older neonate[s] air from the nasal passages when feeding espe[cially by] bottle. The competition for space can cause regurgitation of milk or the appearance of satiety before adequate intake. This can be prevented by release of the air when the baby burps, either spontaneously or as a result of 'winding' by rubbing or patting the back while holding the baby upright. Breastfed babies appear to swallow less air and rarely require winding in the first days of life (Blackburn 2004; Farrell & Sittlington 2003b; Novak 2005b).

At birth the cardiac sphincter and nervous control of the stomach are immature. The cardiac sphincter has transient episodes of relaxation that predispose to possetting (regurgitation). Sphincter muscle tone improves rapidly during the first week, while final maturity may take up to 12 months (Blackburn 2003; Michaelides 2004a). Projectile vomiting, especially appearing from approximately the end of the first week, may indicate congenital pyloric stenosis.

Liver

Physiological immaturity of the liver results in low production of hepatic glucuronyl transferase for the conjugation of bilirubin. This may result in transient physiological jaundice after 48 hours. Glycogen stores are rapidly depleted, and therefore early feeding is needed to maintain normal blood glucose levels and compensate for used glycogen. Liver function and colonisation of the intestine, both of which assist in the formation of vitamin K, are stimulated by feeding (Farrell & Sittlington 2003b).

Digestion

Between 6 and 16 weeks of fetal life, polypeptides that regulate the gastrointestinal tract appear. At term the baby can digest, absorb and metabolise simple carbohydrates, proteins and emulsified fats. After birth, maturation of the gastrointestinal tract is stimulated by specific peptides. Breast milk assists this adaptation as it contains many gastrointestinal trophic factors. Oral feeding stimulates the epithelial cells lining the newborn's small intestine to mature by promoting rapid cell turnover and producing gut enzymes such as amylase, trypsin and pancreatic lipase (Blackburn 2003; Farrell & Sittlington 2003b; Michaelides 2004a). Supporting early feeding aids maturation of intestinal capabilities. Colostrum is non-irritating and enhances the passage of meconium. As well as promoting gut closure, breastfeeding stimulates intestinal enzyme proliferation (Blackburn 2003; Varney et al 2004).

Intestine

Intestinal villi begin developing between 14 and 19 weeks. The gut is sterile at birth but is colonised within hours of birth. Bowel sounds can be heard one hour after birth (Farrell & Sittlington 2003b; Novak 2005). 'Absorption of water by the colon is less efficient than in adults hence the propensity for serious water loss when neonates contract gastrointestinal infections' (Varney et al 2004, pp 68–69).

Alterations to bowel motions

Breastfed babies:

▶ Stool generally has little or no odour.

▶ Day 1 to 2/3: meconium (dark green, sticky and unformed).

▶ Day 2/3 to 3/4: meconium → transitional stool (i.e. copious greenish-brown, loose stool). The baby's mother may need reassurance that this is not diarrhoea.

▶ Day 3/4 to approx 10/12: mustard yellow, very loose, unformed stools, often only yellow fluid containing seed-like solid waste. Passed at almost every feed.

▶ Approx. day 10/12 onward: mustard yellow, soft, loosely formed stools. Solids retain a seed-like appearance.

▶ After the first fortnight, breastfed babies generally pass a bowel motion 2–3 times a day. However, some exclusively breastfeeding babies may only pass a stool once every 3–5 days. As long as the baby is content, gaining weight, feeding well and passing normal amounts of urine, the baby is not constipated. These babies pass a large quantity of soft, non-constipated stool when they do have a bowel motion.

Formula-fed babies:

▶ Stools have a sharp, distinctive odour.

▶ Meconium and transitional stool are passed as for breastfed babies.

▶ From 3–4 days onward, stools are pale yellow, well-formed and solids do not have a seed-like appearance.

▶ Formula-fed babies pass 2–3 stools a day.

▶ They do not exhibit the irregular pattern seen in some breastfed babies. If a formula-fed baby does not pass at least one bowel motion each day, the baby should be assessed for constipation.

Clinical point

Signs of neonatal hypoglycaemia

Signs of neonatal hypoglycaemia are often vague and non-specific. They can include:

▶ jitteriness

▶ cyanosis

▶ apnoea

▶ weak cry

▶ lethargy

▶ lack of muscle tone ('floppiness')

▶ refusal to feed.

(Source: McHugh 2004)

indicates a patent GI tract. Once lactation and breastfeeding are established, soft, yellow stools are passed.

Glucose regulation

During pregnancy the fetus is in an environment in which glucose levels are consistently 60–70% of maternal levels. Glycogen stores are laid down in the third trimester, primarily in the liver. After birth the healthy term baby naturally stabilises glucose levels through feeding and by using glycogen stores. Feeding within an hour of birth conserves glycogen and minimises the risk of hypoglycaemia. While healthy term babies are at low risk of developing hypoglycaemia, any situation before or after birth that has either prevented the accumulation of glycogen stores (e.g. preterm birth or fetal growth restriction), or has caused abnormal consumption of glycogen (e.g. fetal distress or hypothermia), increases the risk of hypoglycaemia. Satisfactory early feeding is particularly important for these babies and blood glucose levels may need to be monitored (see Ch 38).

Neurological system

Nervous system activity develops progressively in fetal life; however, while term babies are able to receive and process stimuli appropriate for neonatal development, the nervous system is still quite anatomically and physiologically immature. The brain is approximately a quarter of adult size and myelination of nerve fibres is incomplete. Such immaturity results in brain stem and spinal reflex activity predominating in the early months. Healthy term babies are capable of social interaction, which continues to develop as the brain continues to grow rapidly (Blackburn 2004; Farrell & Sittlington 2003b; London et al 2003; Michaelides 2004a).

The baby's autonomic nervous system maintains homeostasis; however, temperature instability in the early days and uncoordinated muscle movement reflect the incomplete state of neurological development. The presence of a wide range of reflex activities at varying ages is an indication of the normality and integrity of the neurological and muscular systems (Roberton 1996).

Midwives can gain information about the baby's neurological state from observation and by asking the mother

Bowel motions

Initially all babies pass meconium. Meconium is found in the colon from 16 weeks gestation. It is generally passed within the first 24 hours of life and fully excreted within 48–72 hours. Meconium is an unformed, sticky, greenish-black stool made up of intestinal debris including fatty acids from swallowed amniotic fluid, vernix caseosa, epithelial cells, lanugo, bile and other intestinal secretions. 'Most term infants pass meconium by 12 (69%) to 24 (94%) hours, almost all (99.8%) by 48 hours of age' (Blackburn 2003, p 444). Passing meconium indicates that the baby's lower bowel is patent, although there are exceptions (e.g. an ano-urethral fistula in the presence of an imperforate anus). The bowel motion changes to a greenish-brown colour (transitional stool) as residue from oral food mixes with the meconium. The change to transitional stool

Clinical practice

Collecting a neonatal capillary blood sample

For estimation of blood glucose, serum bilirubin, full blood count, and Guthrie test.

▶ The sample is collected from the heel.

▶ Foot must be lower than body.

▶ Warm the heel by wrapping warmed gauze or muslin cloth around the foot to improve peripheral vascular perfusion and thus prevent falsely low results.

SAFETY ALERT!

▶ *Test* the heat of the gauze/cloth against the inside of the wrist. It should feel a similar temperature to that of the skin.

▶ *Never* put the baby's foot in warm water. It is very easy to seriously scald a neonate's sensitive skin.

Procedure:

1   Clean the heal with an alcohol wipe. Allow to dry. Alcohol-impregnated swabs should never be used prior to collecting a blood sample for a Guthrie test (neonatal screening test) or glucose readings, because the alcohol can affect the accuracy of the results (Johnston & Taylor 2000).

2   Avoid sensitive areas of the heel (see Fig 27.5).

3   Puncture the outer aspect of the heel with a sterile disposable lancet. Automated lancets are preferable to manual ones.

4   Wipe away the first drop of blood with dry sterile gauze.

5   Gently fill the microcapillary collection tube or press collection filter paper against a large drop of blood.

6   Apply gentle pressure with gauze or cotton ball until bleeding stops.

7   Label specimen appropriately and send for analysis.

(Source: Michaelides 2004a)

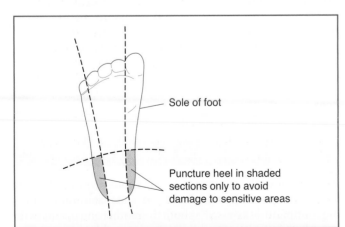

Sole of foot

Puncture heel in shaded sections only to avoid damage to sensitive areas

Figure 27.5 Heel puncture sites for neonatal blood sampling

---

about latching and sucking on the breast, how much the baby cries and sleep–wake patterns (Johnston et al 2003). The term baby lies with the limbs flexed and limb movements are uncoordinated and purposeless. No two newborn babies behave in exactly the same way but there is a broadly predictable pattern of behaviour that is regarded as normal. At first, it is a relatively simple pattern of sleep, wakefulness, semi-purposeful movements and reflex reaction to stimuli such as sucking and swallowing.

Senses and perception

Habituation is the process whereby there is an initial response to a visual or auditory stimulus such as a loud noise, followed by diminishing response with repetition until the response disappears. Being able to ignore a noisy environment is a new-born defence mechanism. Orientation is the neonate's ability to be alert to, follow and fixate on appealing, complex visual stimuli. Self-quieting ability refers to babies' capacity to quiet and comfort themselves (e.g. fist sucking) (London et al 2003).

Vision

Babies are sensitive to bright lights, which make them blink or frown. They focus at a distance of 15–20 cm and show a preference for the shape of the human face and bold black and white patterns. They can briefly track a moving object by the end of the first week and can differentiate their mother's face from a stranger's by two weeks. Over the first two months, interest in colour and variety of patterns develops (Blackburn 2003). Interaction with the mother is developed through eye-to-eye contact.

Hearing

Newborn babies turn towards localised sound. High-pitched sound makes them blink or startle. They are comforted by low-pitched sounds such as the crooning noises mothers make to comfort a crying baby. They prefer the sound of their mother's voice to others' and prefer the human voice over other noise. After a few weeks, neonates mimic the patterns of human speech by moving in response (Blackburn 2003; Farrell & Sittlington 2003b).

Smell, taste and touch

Babies prefer the smell of human milk and can differentiate their mother's milk within a few days. They prefer a sweet taste and turn away from unpleasant smells.

Babies respond to being picked up, stroked and talked to. They can mimic facial expressions and hand movements made by adults by 12 days of age. They enjoy skin-to-skin contact, immersion in warm water, rocking, cuddling and stroking (Blackburn 2003; Farrell & Sittlington 2003b; Michaelides 2004a). 'Pain in babies is expressed by brow bulging, eyelid squeezing, nasolabial furrowing and open lipped crying' (Farrell & Sittlington 2003b, p 732).

Sleep–wake states

From the moment of birth, infants are alert and aware of their surroundings, and able to respond to their carers and the environment. Understanding the baby's sleep–wake state can help both the mother and the midwife to provide care that works with, rather than against, the baby's state of consciousness, thereby conserving energy.

Behavioural observation of sleep–wake states in the newborn:

- Sleep states:
  - deep sleep—eyes closed, no eye movements, respirations regular, hard to wake, occasional jerky movements
  - light sleep—eyes closed, rapid eye movements seen, respirations less regular, may be sucking movements, easier to wake, occasional random movements.
- Awake states
  - drowsy—eyes open or closed, eyelids may flutter, occasional smiling, smoother limb movements but may startle, minimal response to sensory stimulus and minimal motor activity
  - quiet alert—eyes open, alert and focuses on source of stimulus, minimal motor activity, may or may not be fussing
  - active alert—eyes open, alert, generally active and reactive to a variety of stimuli and the surrounding environment, may or may not be fussing
  - crying—actively, may be hard to console, much muscular activity. Difficult to get a response, need to bring baby down to active alert state to feed (Brazelton 1984; Brazelton & Nugent 1995).

Initially the baby is wide-eyed, alert and hungry. Approximately an hour after birth the baby falls asleep for a few minutes or several hours. The importance of initiating breast feeding in the first period of reactivity is evident. Successive sleep–wake patterns are very individual and the baby will take some time to demonstrate a consistent pattern. At first the baby wakes because of hunger, but longer periods of wakefulness unrelated to hunger, that meet the baby's social interaction needs, begin to occur in the succeeding weeks.

At times during the day, the baby will be active and crying, or will lie quietly awake. Newborns sleep for 16–20 hours each day, although the depth and duration of sleep vary considerably from one baby to another. Some wake only to be fed and changed, others are easily disturbed and wakeful even though well fed (London et al 2003; Farrell & Sittlington 2003b; Johnston et al 2003; Michaelides 2004a).

Crying

Term neonates usually cry without tears and generally for reasons of hunger, thirst or discomfort, although sometimes there is no obvious reason. Parents are able to differentiate the cry as they gain experience with their baby. Midwives have a role in supporting parents as they grow to understand the baby's individual pattern of communication and learn to comfort him or her.

Mother–baby relationship

It is important to keep mother and baby together. Emotional care is just as important as physical care for the baby's ongoing health and development. Unless ill and requiring intensive care, the baby should stay with the mother so that she can enjoy and get to know, love and care for her baby (Johnston et al 2003). The mother examines her baby minutely in a predictable pattern at birth. The father is also involved in this early exploration. Apart from their pre-understandings, the parents' response is affected by the baby's appearance and response. Close contact in the first hour after birth fosters the attachment process and promotes later neonatal development. The mother examines the baby first by using her fingertips to explore the baby's head, fingers and toes. She then strokes the baby's body with her hand before cuddling the baby into her arms with the baby facing her. She establishes eye contact and talks to her baby, looking for support from her partner and the midwife. Sometimes the father's overt responses are stronger than his partner's. Some fathers are surprised at the depth of their emotional response to the birth of their baby. They also feel a sense of deep satisfaction and self-esteem, are elated and eager to touch and hold their baby and their partner (Barclay & Lupton 1999; Farrell & Sittlington 2003b).

The baby's responsive behaviours induce further responses from the parents, which calls forth a response from the baby. These interactions develop the bond between parents and child that is essential for the baby's ongoing development (Farrell & Sittlington 2003b).

Fostering the process of attachment

Studies suggest that physical contact between the mother and baby encourages attachment between them, and research evidence shows that the chances of successful breastfeeding are enhanced when the baby is put to the breast immediately after birth (Johnston et al 2003). Midwives can foster the process of parental attachment by keeping the baby with the parents, fostering privacy for the parents to be alone with their baby and to talk with each other, providing information and reassurance about the range of normal baby behaviour, reassuring the parents that attachment to the new baby is not always instant and is commonly a gradual process over the first few months. When the father is encouraged to be involved in discussions and decisions and to share responsibility for baby care, it is thought that the parent's relationship is enhanced. Both parents need opportunities to voice their feelings and reactions about their baby. Sensitive and supportive midwifery care can foster confident parenting for both parents (Farrell & Sittlington 2003b; Johnston et al 2003).

Neonatal assessment

Assessment of the neonate is a continuous process. Many of the assessments undertaken in a formal neonatal examination are continuously assessed by both the mother and the midwife on a daily basis (see Ongoing assessment, this chapter). The general principles that apply to the full neonatal examination also apply to ongoing assessments.

Formal neonatal examination

A full examination of newborn babies is undertaken at birth, at the end of the first week and at discharge from midwifery care. It is generally accepted that it is good practice to undertake a comprehensive physical examination of the baby within 24 hours of birth (Hall 1999). The initial examination allows observation of the baby as a whole, forms the baseline for future checks and provides an alert to areas of concern (Johnston et al 2003). The examination also gives parents an opportunity to ask questions and to express any concerns.

Scope of practice

The formal examination of healthy term neonates is within the midwife's scope of practice. In New Zealand it forms a standard part of the Ministry of Health contract specifications for the provision of primary maternity care (Regulations to the NZ Public Health and Disability Services Act 2000, s.88). Mitchell (2003) found in a UK study that the examination is most appropriately undertaken by the ongoing caregiver, and that efficacy and quality of the assessment is improved if it is undertaken by the midwife. Wolke and colleagues (2002) found that there was no difference in maternal satisfaction levels whether the examination was undertaken by midwives or junior paediatricians. They also found that satisfaction levels were increased if information about behavioural and healthcare issues was provided at the time of the examination. Glazener and colleagues (1999) found no evidence of health gain from a policy of two examinations in hospital.

General rules for examining newborn babies

- The examination should always be undertaken with the consent of the baby's mother and in her presence. The assessment findings are communicated to the baby's mother or both parents at the time of the examination.
- The baby should be in a quiet, alert state.
- Be firm but gentle. Babies feel insecure if not handled confidently. Smooth, gentle handling will give maximum information with minimum disturbance to the baby.
- Without compromising the thoroughness of the examination, minimise the time during which the baby is unclothed, to prevent chilling and disturbance.
- *Use the same process every time* so that nothing is missed.
- Examine the baby generally in a 'top-to-toe' direction.
- Pay particular attention to symmetry. Each side should be the same—sounds, length, size, creases, muscle tone, flexion.

Exceptions to the 'top-to-toe' process:
- Observe as much as possible before the baby is fully undressed. All of the head, the baby's general muscle tone and some of the reflexes can be observed while the baby is still clothed.
- It is usual to start with examination of the baby's heart and lungs while the baby is least disturbed and less likely to cry. Nearly all babies cry when naked for any length of time, so it is sensible to listen to the heart and lungs before removing the napkin.
- Examination of the hips for developmental dysplasia is uncomfortable for the baby and should be carried out at the end of the examination. Similarly, weighing the baby should be reserved until near the end of the examination (Farrell & Sittlington 2003b; Johnston et al 2003; London et al 2003; Michaelides 2004a; Varney et al 2004).

History

Factors to take into account from the clinical record and the baby's parents include:
- the parents' appearance/stature—a small baby may merely reflect the size of the parents, for example
- genetic—any known family history
- environmental—known maternal exposure to teratogenic agents, smoking, recreational or prescription drugs etc
- social factors, maternal blood group, medical conditions
- pregnancy and intrapartum variations—such as intrauterine growth, liquor volume, fetal distress, maternal analgesia, intrapartum complications
- neonatal factors—Apgar score, birthweight (Varney et al 2004).

General measurements

The crown–heel length, head circumference and weight are assessed and used as a baseline for assessment of growth over time. Observe the whole baby for symmetry and proportion, and in particular note general length-to-leanness proportion.

Crown-to-heel length

Local policy applies as to whether calibrated measuring equipment or a tape measure is used to assess length in the first few weeks of life. When a tape measure is used at the early examinations, this assessment is only an approximation. Calibrated equipment is required for accurate and reliable length measurement. For reliability the length needs to be serially assessed by the same person (Doull et al 1995).

To use a calibrated box or mat, the baby's head and feet must be flat against either end, which is quite difficult to achieve with new babies. Whichever method is used, the mother is usually asked to assist by holding the baby's leg(s) straight while the measurement is taken.

The average crown–heel length of a term baby at birth is 50 cm. (In the New Zealand population the 3rd–97th centile range is 48–53 cm (NZMOH 2004).)

Weight

Weigh the baby toward the end of the examination. To improve reliability it is preferable to use the same set of regularly maintained scales for serial weight measurements.

Babies are generally weighed at birth, sometime towards the end of the first week, then weekly until four to six weeks old. The average birthweight of a term baby is 3500 g and the New Zealand 3rd–97th centile range is 2500–4500 g (NZMOH 2004). Healthy term babies can lose a maximum of 7–10% of their birthweight due to physiological diuresis (Blackburn 2003). In practice, 7% loss is generally regarded as the alert point at which feeding patterns need to be reviewed and intake increased. The baby should regain her or his birthweight by 10–14 days. As the baby grows older, mothers usually know if their baby is gaining weight by assessing whether the baby's clothes are fitting better or getting tighter. They also notice that the baby's face and tummy are starting to fill out. Generally term infants gain 30 g/day for the first three months (Blackburn 2003). However, the emphasis is on healthy term babies and normal urinary output—that is, babies who are feeding well and having six to eight wet napkins in 24 hours. Babies who are not term, and/or not feeding well, and/or not exhibiting normal urinary output, need to be identified and individually assessed. An appropriate plan of care needs to be implemented (see Chs 29 and 38).

Head circumference

Measurement is taken round the occipito-frontal diameter (not the ears). The average head circumference for a term baby is 35 cm. The New Zealand 3rd–97th centile range is 34–39 cm (NZNOH 2004). There may be a discrepancy between the measurement at birth and the end of first week assessment, as moulding can make an accurate initial assessment difficult.

Gestational age assessment

Gestational age is formally assessed using either the Ballard or the Dubowitz gestational assessment tools (see Ch 38). While ultrasound scanning has confirmed the gestation of most pregnancies, occasionally the scan result is incorrect; also, some women choose not to be scanned, and some women arrive at the birthing unit without prior care from that service. Midwives make a general assessment of gestational age at the time the baby is born so that unexpectedly preterm infants can be readily identified.

General assessment of gestation for healthy term neonates:

- resting posture—fully flexed extremities (see Fig 27.6)
- creases cover the whole of the sole of the foot (see Fig 27.7) (Note: this is reliable only in the first 12 hours.)
- breast tissue of 6–7 mm diameter is present
- ear cartilage and curves of the pinna are complete. The

ear promptly returns to the normal position when folded forward and released.

- genitalia well developed. Male: scrotum covered in rugae and testes usually descended. Female: labia majora completely cover the clitoris and labia minora.
- elbow does not reach the midline when the scarf sign is assessed from 40 weeks gestation onward (see Fig 27.8).

Temperature

Take and record the baby's temperature. This is especially important at the initial examination when the baby is most vulnerable to hypothermia.

Examination of specific areas

Lungs

- Count the respiratory rate, and observe the rise and fall of the chest and abdomen—they should rise and fall together.
- Babies' heart sounds can be heard in many parts of the chest, so auscultate the lungs toward the lateral side of the chest to diminish the volume of the heart sounds. Focus on the breath sounds until the heart sounds are backgrounded. Then the breath sounds can be assessed.

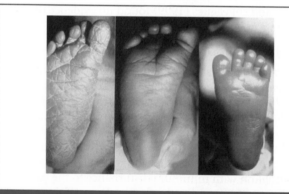

Figure 27.7 Plantar surface of the foot (Thureen et al 2005)

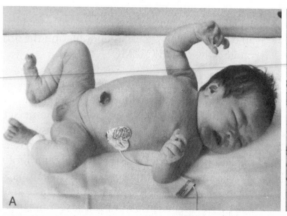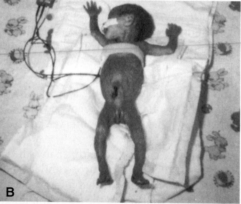

Figure 27.6 (a) Term posture (flexed) **(b)** Preterm posture (extended) (Thureen et al 2005)

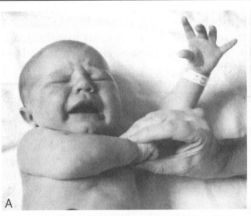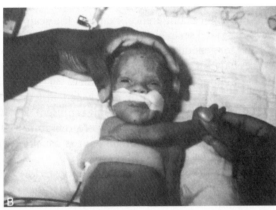

Figure 27.8 Scarf sign **(a)** Full-term infant **(b)** Preterm infant (Thureen et al 2005)

- Listen for air entry into both lungs. Note whether each side sounds similar.
- Listen for rales or rhonchi. If present, record which lung(s), volume and how it sounds (e.g. moist, rattly, dry, breezy).

Heart

The heart is examined for rate, regularity, heart sounds and the presence of murmurs. The baby is assessed for general signs that may indicate a cardiac anomaly—that is, variations in colour, raised respiratory rate, lethargy, poor feeding.

Auscultate with the stethoscope diaphragm (high pitch), then the bell (low pitch). Focus on the heart sounds, backgrounding the breath sounds. Listen carefully until the heart sounds have your full attention. The cardiac cycle can then be assessed.

- *Count*: rate and note regularity
- *Listen* to:
  - systolic (first) heart sound S_1 (lub)
  - diastolic (second) heart sound S_2 (dub)
  - the spaces in between the sounds:
        lub-space-dub-space-lub-space

Neonates sometimes have a third heart sound. Carefully assess whether there are any murmurs (other sounds in the cardiac cycle). Murmurs in newborn infants are usually flow murmurs. These can be either physiological (e.g. from a partially closed foramen ovale) or pathological (e.g. from a septal or valvular defect). Physiological flow murmurs are the most commonly heard murmurs at the initial examination. These should be reassessed in 24 hours. They have generally resolved by the examination at the end of the first week. However, until significant experience is gained, if any sound other than the normal systolic and diastolic sounds are heard, consultation with a medical practitioner is warranted.

Clinical point

Telephone consultation related to cardiac variations
Initial consultation and referral is often via the telephone and the doctor may be some distance away, so it is important to ensure that she or he can make an assessment of the urgency of the situation. The following information should be given and recorded in the clinical notes:
▶ General condition of the baby, especially colour, respiratory rate and feeding behaviour. (Major cardiac anomalies are either very soft or inaudible. These anomalies announce themselves as more general signs and symptoms.)
▶ Heart rate (normal 110–150 bpm)
▶ The extra sound(s):
  – nature—rumbling, breezy, whistling, creaking, rubbing
  – volume—soft (grade 2), easily heard (grade 3), loud (grade 4)
  – where the murmur is audible—all over the chest, in the back, a specific place on the chest or back
  – in which part of the cardiac cycle the murmur is audible (e.g. with the systolic sound)
Midwives and women need to be aware that non-specific signs and symptoms such as pallor or failure to thrive may be the only indication of a silent cardiac defect that will become apparent at a later time.

Clinical point

Auscultation of the lungs and heart
▶ Use a paediatric stethoscope. The small diaphragm makes heart sounds in particular much easier to hear. Warm the diaphragm in the hand prior to placing on the baby's chest.
▶ Use smooth, gentle actions. If the baby is disturbed and cries, the sounds will not be audible.
▶ Focus on the sound being listened to, backgrounding other sounds.

Head

After measuring the head circumference, examine the scalp for cuts and abrasions, fetal scalp electrode or blood sample sites. Assess the head for general shape, presence and shape of moulding, microcephaly, macrocephaly, caput succedaneum, cephalhaematoma, 'chignon' from vacuum delivery.

Palpate the sutures, which should be clearly felt unless overriding of the bones associated with moulding is present at the initial examination. Note width, overriding or premature fusion. Note distribution and texture of hair. Hair is usually silky and fine. Coarse-textured hair is abnormal.

Examine the anterior and posterior fontanelles. The posterior fontanelle is often not palpable as an opening from shortly after birth but does not anatomically close for 6–8 weeks. The anterior fontanelle slowly closes over by approximately 18 months. The anterior fontanelle should be flat; a sunken fontanelle is a late sign of dehydration, whereas a bulging fontanelle may indicate hydrocephalus or intracranial haemorrhage.

Plagiocephaly

Some babies always lie with their head in one position. This can lead to flattening of the occiput that becomes more noticeable after three to four weeks (Johnston et al 2003). It is important to differentiate plagiocephaly from unilateral premature closure of the coronal suture (craniosynostosis). According to Cowan (2000), Glasson, a plastic surgeon, states that there is growing evidence that plagiocephaly does not completely self-correct. In the early stages it is easily preventable and also treatable by varying the baby's head position. Mothers are encouraged to turn their baby's head to one side during the day and to the other side at night. However, Glasson goes on to state that helmet treatment may be necessary if the condition is undetected and untreated in the early stage, but that helmets are ineffective after one year.

Face

Examine for symmetry, placement of features, expression and shape.

Eyes

Examine to ensure the eyes are present, note symmetry, any discharge or swelling. The eyes should move; the baby will follow movement and gaze at the mother's face when held. The iris may be dark blue at birth but the colour may gradually change over the first three to six months. Tears are not usual for the first two months, although some babies have tears from birth.

Check for presence of subconjunctival haemorrhages (treatment not usually required), and epicanthic fold (skin fold over the medial aspect of the eye). This fold may be familial but is also seen in some congenital syndromes including Down syndrome (Hernandez & Glass 2005).

Examination for the red reflex with an ophthalmoscope confirms the clarity of the lens and the presence of the retina. The red reflex may be seen as the red pupils in photographs taken without the red eye reduction button on. If the red reflex is not assessed by the examiner, it is important to record that it has not been done in the health record so that the assessment can be undertaken at the next examination.

Nose

Check that the nostrils are patent by observing that the rate of respirations is normal and the baby is having no difficulty breathing. Note any swelling of the tear ducts. A small amount of saline drops can be used to clear the nares if the baby is 'snuffling'. Do not insert cotton buds.

Mouth

The mouth opens symmetrically but is usually held closed at rest. The lips are complete and the philtrum present. A receding jaw is sometimes associated with feeding difficulties. Elicit the rooting reflex by brushing the baby's cheek with a finger to encourage the baby's mouth to open. Use a pencil torch to view that the palate is complete, followed by palpation with a gloved finger. Assess the soft palate carefully, as small clefts can easily be missed. Check for complete gum lines and exclude premature dentition. Note the presence of tongue tie. Treatment is not required unless the tongue cannot move upward or cannot protrude over the bottom gum line.

Observe the sucking reflex (preferably when feeding). At subsequent examinations, examine the mouth for signs of *Candida* infection (thrush). Oral thrush is seen as white plaques on the gums, inside of the cheeks or a white film over the tongue. The white film left by milk is easily wiped away, whereas *Candida* plaque is not.

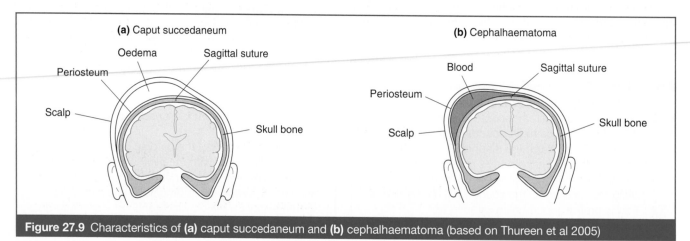

Figure 27.9 Characteristics of **(a)** caput succedaneum and **(b)** cephalhaematoma (based on Thureen et al 2005)

Ears

The auditory canals should be patent and the pinna should be flexible and cartilaginous. The upper edge of the pinna should be above or level with the outer corner of the eye. Moulding may affect these proportions at birth. Re-check at the first week examination. Low-set ears should alert for other anomalies.

Check for skin tags and spots, most commonly in front of the ear lobe but may be behind the ear. Skin tags may be benign or associated with a bone deficit under the tag and may contain meningeal tissue; they may also be associated with renal anomalies. Medical consultation is warranted when skin tags are noted. Never insert objects such as cotton buds into the auditory canal.

Hearing

A general assessment for sensitivity to noise can be made at birth, but hearing is better assessed more fully at a later date. 'Almost half of newborns with hearing impairment have no risk factors associated with this impairment' (Narrigan 2000, p 368). Routine screening for hearing using acoustic emission testing (AET) occurs in some Australian states, and trials are currently being undertaken in others and in New Zealand. Where routine AET testing is not undertaken, midwives should ask the parents if their baby is 'disturbed by loud noises—that is, jumps or blinks, stirs in sleep, looks up from sucking or stops sucking for a moment or cries' (NZMOH 2004, p 85). Note that babies can have a variable response to loud background noise in the early months.

Neck

Elicit the rooting reflex bilaterally to examine range and symmetry of movement. The head should move freely, creases should be symmetrical. Note any webbing or cystic growths, check creases for skin lesions.

Skin

Assess colour: pink, peripheral acrocyanosis at birth, jaundice, duskiness, pallor. Note the amount of vernix caseosa, lanugo and peeling. Examine creases for heat rash and pustules, the buttocks for nappy rash (bright red), or *Candida* rash (bright red, excoriated, sometimes roseate, associated with *Candida* lesions in the mouth and painful maternal nipples). Examine for common variations and birthmarks.

The full term baby's skin has few veins visible and has limited pigmentation at birth; all babies experience changes in skin pigmentation as they grow and develop. Because of the reduced pigmentation and the fact that capillaries are close to the skin surface, all healthy term neonates have a pink tinge to the skin. When the baby is first born, the skin is reddish and crinkly. The redness disappears within a few hours and the skin unfurls over the first few days. The skin is smooth and soft to the touch (Blackburn 2003; Farrell & Sittlington 2003b; London et al 2003; Michaelides 2004a; Thureen et al 2005).

The neonate's skin is thin and easily blistered or excoriated by friction, acid or alkaline substances and pressure. The epidermis is nonetheless an effective barrier preventing infection, especially as the skin pH falls from an average of 6.4 at birth to a mean of 4.9 over the first few days. Bacteriostatic capability is a feature of skin that has a pH lower than 5.0. Preterm infants are vulnerable to infection for a longer period as they take longer to form this acid mantle (Blackburn 2003; Farrell & Sittlington 2003b; London et al 2003; Michaelides 2004a; Thureen et al 2005).

There is a varying quantity of fine hair called lanugo particularly on the shoulders and upper arms. Lanugo is more noticeable over a larger area and found in greater quantities as gestation decreases. Before birth the skin is covered with varying amounts of vernix caseosa, a thick white, creamy substance that is thought to protect the skin. By term the amount has reduced so that it is primarily found in the creases of the axillae, elbows, neck and groin. Vernix does not need to be removed. If necessary it may be massaged into the skin. During the first week the skin on the hands and feet may peel, particularly if the baby is post term. Peeling requires no treatment; application of oils or creams is not necessary (Blackburn 2003; Farrell & Sittlington 2003b; London et al 2003; Michaelides 2004a; Thureen et al 2005).

Common skin variations

The following skin variations are common and clear spontaneously without treatment. Parents may need reassurance that they are normal skin variations.

- Acrocyanosis is the transitory bluish colour of the hands and feet seen in the first 2–6 hours after birth, before peripheral perfusion is fully established. Hand and foot colour is not sufficiently reliable to use for assessment of satisfactory neonatal oxygenation, and therefore assessment of the face and mucous membranes of the mouth is used to detect cyanosis.
- Superficial capillary naevi (see Fig 27.10) are pale reddish marks commonly called 'stork bites', seen on about a third of babies, on the eyelids, brows, between the nose and at the nape of the neck. They mostly disappear over the first year, although the marks at the nape of the neck sometimes persist.
- Mongolian spots (see Fig 27.10) are bluish/black or bluish/grey areas primarily seen on the buttocks or lower back, although they can be found anywhere on the body. They are more readily visible in babies with darker skins. They usually fade over the first year of life. Parents may need reassurance as the marks can look very like bruising.
- Milia are exposed sebaceous glands on the face. They look like raised white spots and can be quite profuse particularly on the nose. They disappear in the first four to six weeks after birth.
- Erythema toxicum is the term given to a transient rash that frequently comes and goes mostly on the body, in the first week of life. The baby is otherwise well. The spots are most commonly small, erythematous lesions with a white centre that look like pimples. They are not an infection; the fluid in the spots contains eosinophils,

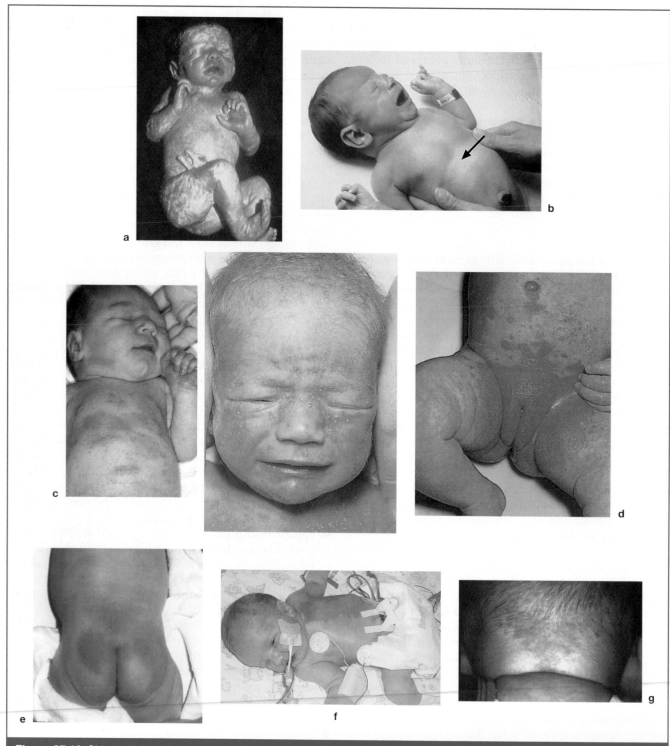

Figure 27.10 Skin variations **(a)** vernix caseosa **(b)** plethora **(c)** erythema toxicum **(d)** *Candida* dermatitis **(e)** Mongolian spots **(f)** harlequin sign **(g)** 'stork bites' (Thureen et al 2005; photograph (g) Dr AMM Oakley)

not pathogens. The rash can be quite extensive and the spots can run into each other making large blotchy red patches on the baby's skin. The rash is usually aggravated by heat. It can be unsightly and cause anxiety for parents. The rash usually clears in a few days.

- Petechiae, sometimes called traumatic cyanosis, are small, pinpoint haemorrhagic skin lesions, giving a dusky (bluish/grey) appearance to the face and head when there are multiple tiny petechiae in the skin. It is commonly seen when the head has been congested during birth, most commonly by the cord tightly wound around the neck. The mucous membranes of the mouth and the baby's body are not affected and remain pink. It disappears within 48 to 72 hours.

- Subcutaneous fat necrosis is a localised area of induration that is reddish and blotchy with a hardened area of fat underneath. Usually spontaneous, it can follow a forceps delivery when it is usually found over the zygomatic process. It gradually disappears over several months (Burden & Krafchik 1999).

- Harlequin colour change (see Fig 27.10) is an intermittent transient colour change lasting from a few minutes to half an hour more commonly seen in preterm infants. There is a clear line of demarcation between an area of redness and one of paleness. The line of demarcation may run from the head to the abdomen. It is caused by temporary imbalance in the skin vasculature. Although it may occur up to three weeks of age, it is not significant (Farrell & Sittlington 2003b; Johnston et al 2003; London et al 2003; Michaelides 2004a; Thureen et al 2005).

Birthmarks

Birthmarks need obstetric or paediatric assessment so that a treatment plan and ongoing parental support can be initiated.

Capillary haemangioma

Port wine stain (naevus flammeus) (see Fig 27.11) is a flat, dark, reddish-purple capillary haemangioma that occurs in about 1 in 3000 births. It is commonly seen on the face and may vary in shape and size. It is twice as common in girls. It does not fade or shrink over time. Parents and child will need significant support. Laser treatment and cosmetics can be used later in life to reduce the appearance. Meningeal anomalies (Sturge-Weber syndrome) should be suspected if the haemangioma follows the distribution of the trigeminal nerve (Johnston et al 2003; Thureen et al 2005).

'Strawberry mark' (naevus vasculosus) (see Fig 27.12) is a capillary haemangioma that becomes apparent during the first few weeks as a small, bright red, raised lesion that continues to enlarge over one to three months. They can be very distressing for parents and the older child as they are often on the face and can grow quite large. However, they regress spontaneously and usually disappear by five to eight years of age. Treatment is not required unless the haemangioma is in an awkward place, such as obstructing the vision (Johnston et al 2003; Thureen et al 2005).

Pigmented naevi

Pigmented naevi are rare but can be multiple, large and/or hairy. They are brown and can be flat or raised. The impact on parents can be significant. They are formed from abnormal dermal melanocytes and become malignant in approximately 30% of cases, and therefore surgical excision and skin grafting in childhood is often recommended as a preventive measure. Treatment is not usually undertaken in the neonatal period (Johnston et al 2003; Thureen et al 2005).

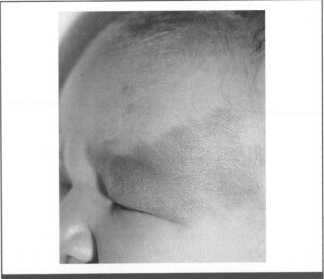

Figure 27.11 Port wine stain (Callen et al 2000)

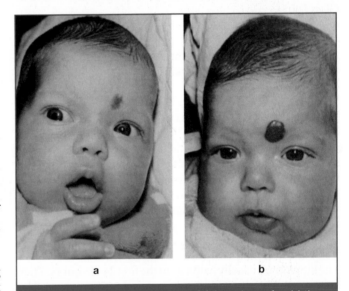

a   b

Figure 27.12 Strawberry naevus **(a)** four days after birth **(b)** six weeks after birth (Thureen et al 2005)

Chest

In a term infant the nipples should have approximately 6–7 mm of breast tissue (Leveno et al 2003). Hormonal swelling of breast tissue in both boys and girls may occur naturally and occasionally a milk-like substance may be seen. This is not an infection and will resolve naturally over one to two weeks as the level of maternal hormones decreases. Parents and health professionals alike need to be actively discouraged from squeezing the tissue, as it is easily damaged (Hernandez & Glass 2005).

Umbilicus

The cord should not be bleeding. Check that the clamp is properly fastened. Examine the cord for the presence of three vessels. A small number of babies with one umbilical artery have one or more associated congenital anomalies, usually cardiac, pulmonary or renal, especially renal agenesis (Thummala et al 1998). At birth the cord is bluish white and contains a variable amount of Wharton's Jelly. As it dries out, the cord shrinks and darkens to a yellow-brownish colour. The umbilical cord separates by dry gangrene at any time between three and seven days, most commonly at four to five days. The cord clamp remains on the cord stump for 48 hours, after which it is removed.

Serous, purulent or sanguineous drainage is abnormal and may indicate a patent urachus or omphalitis (Hernandez & Glass 2005). Observe the area at the base of the cord for redness. Redness or umbilical 'flare' is usually associated with an infection and must be medically treated *very promptly* as neonatal septicaemia can be a rapid consequence. Check for umbilical hernia. This occurs when the abdominal muscles have not completely closed around the umbilicus. Unless very large it does not usually require treatment and closes spontaneously by two to three years of age (Hernandez & Glass 2005).

Abdomen

Auscultate each quadrant of the abdomen for bowel sounds, which are present from approximately one hour after birth.

Liver

The inferior border of the liver should be palpable 1–2 cm below the costal margin in the mid-clavicular line and extends across the midline; the normal edge is 'sharp and soft' (Hernandez & Glass 2005, p 141). Start palpation at the iliac crest and work upward towards the liver to come on to the liver border. It is sometimes easier to use the edge of the thumb rather than the fingertips for this palpation. The spleen is not usually palpable.

Kidneys and bladder

The kidneys are usually palpable in the first 24–48 hours. They are moderately firm and approximately 4.5–5.0 cm long. The right kidney may not be easily palpable. The kidney is palpated by placing the hand under the baby's flank and using deep, smooth abdominal pressure over the renal area (Hernandez & Glass 2005).

The bladder becomes an abdominal organ when full and may be palpable 1–2 cm above the symphysis pubis. There should be no other masses in the abdomen. The groin should be examined for any sign of palpable hernia or undescended testicle.

Femoral pulses

Palpate the femoral pulses. Assess each pulse individually and then together. The pulses are normally present on both sides and should beat in unison when palpated together. Compare the femoral pulse with the brachial pulse. Difference between brachial and femoral pulses, absence of femoral pulse(s) or asynchronous pulsation (rate or pressure) may indicate congenital cardiovascular anomaly, in particular coarctation

---

Clinical point

Umbilical cord care

The cord stump separates by saprophytic action. Using antiseptics to clean the base of the cord interferes with this process. Umbilical cords do not require any special cleaning or treatment. There is no increase in infection when the cord is not treated with hexachlorophene powder and alcohol wipes (Dore et al 1998). Application of powders, antiseptic or alcohol wipes has been shown to delay cord separation (Barr 1984; Lawrence 1982). The cord should be washed in the bath and dried carefully. It is preferable to fold down or cut a small 'v' in the waist band of disposable napkins so that the cord is outside, where it is exposed to the air and protected from contamination by urine and faeces. If cloth nappies are used, they should be fastened so that the cord is outside the nappy. As the cord begins to separate it can become quite sticky around the base; the sticky material should be gently removed with a damp cotton bud and carefully dried. As the cord comes off there may be a *very small* amount of dark blood seen. This is normal and is only present for one or two nappy changes. Fresh blood is not normal. Occasionally the centre of the umbilicus has a small piece of raised, granulomatous flesh where the cord has separated. Occasionally this rubs on the baby's clothing and does not heal over. If this is the case, the stump can be easily and painlessly cauterised by the baby's general practitioner.

Clinical point

Palpating the abdomen

The baby's abdomen is examined in the same way as that of an adult. However, the quadrants are much smaller, so the flat surface of the fingertips is used. The palpation moves from light to deep, watching the baby's face to detect discomfort. The examiner's other hand is placed in the back of the baby to provide a firm support. The baby's hip may need to be flexed to relax the abdominal muscles during palpation.

---

of the aorta (Hernandez & Glass 2005). Any finding other than synchronous pulsation should be assessed by a medical practitioner.

Limbs

Upper limbs

Examine symmetry of length, creases, flexion and muscle tone. Check axillae and elbows for abnormalities. Open the hands to check for extra digits (polydactyly), skin tags or webbing between the fingers. Examine palms for single palmar (Simian) crease (may be associated with Down syndrome) (London et al 2003; Thureen et al 2005).

Confirm symmetry and normal range of movement in the joints. (*Do not force the joints.*) The hands are normally held as loosely clenched fists.

Lower limbs

Examine symmetry of length, creases, flexion and muscle tone. The term baby has creases over more than two-thirds of the sole of the foot (see Fig 27.7). Check for polydactyly, webbing and skin tags. Examine groin and popliteal spaces for abnormalities. Confirm symmetry and normal range of movement in the joints. Note that the knee joints often cannot be fully extended for the first few days (Johnston et al 2003).

The term baby's feet should easily dorsiflex so that the upper surface of the foot almost touches or touches the shin. (Preterm infants' feet do not fully dorsiflex.) Examine for signs of talipes equinovarus. *Do not force the foot.* If it will not naturally flex, refer the baby for paediatric or orthopaedic examination.

Spine and back

Turn baby over and examine the spine. Palpate the length of the spine to feel all the vertebral spinous processes. If there appears to be a gap, a hairy patch, or an area of thickened or differently textured skin over the spine, refer to a paediatrician for exclusion of spina bifida.

Examine the cleft in the buttocks; about 1% of babies have a dimple, usually at the top of the cleft (Johnston et al 2003). Ensure that the base of the dimple is sighted and that it is closed. The dimples are usually benign; however, very occasionally they are open to the meninges at the base, or it may be a congenital pilonidal sinus. If the base cannot be clearly seen or the dimple is deep, paediatric consultation is indicated. Dimples elsewhere on the spine should always be medically assessed (see Ch 38).

While examining the back, note the baby's posture when held in ventral suspension (see neurological section and Fig 27.13, below).

Visually check that the anus is patent and correctly positioned.

Genitalia

Female

The labia majora covers the clitoris and labia minora. The labia should be parted to examine the clitoris for appropriate size.

The hymen should be perforated, confirmed by whitish vaginal discharge. There may be a small quantity of bloodstained discharge in the first few days, which is a pseudo menstrual period caused by the withdrawal of maternal hormones at birth (Johnston et al 2003; London et al 2003; Thureen et al 2005).

Male

The foreskin should completely cover the glans penis. As it is normally adherent it should not be retracted. By three years of age, 90% are retractable (Johnston et al 2003; Thureen et al 2005). Examine the penis for hypospadias by ensuring that the urethral opening is at the end of the penis and that the tissue is intact along the full length of the inferior surface.

The scrotum should be soft and covered in rugae. Hydrocoele (collection of fluid in the scrotum) is not uncommon and should be identified. While most resolve spontaneously, consultation is appropriate (London et al 2003) as inguinal hernia should be excluded. Strangulated inguinal hernia is a surgical emergency (Thureen et al 2005).

Gently palpate the scrotum between the thumb and forefinger for the testes. They are firm, pea-like structures 1.5–2 cm long (Johnston et al 2003). The testes are sensitive to temperature and may move back up the inguinal canal when cold. It is not uncommon for one or both testes to have not descended. It they are not palpable in the scrotum, palpate the groin from the iliac crest to the external inguinal ring, where undescended testes are sometime palpable. Babies with undescended testicle(s) need medical follow-up as it can take several years for the testes to descend. Testes that fail to descend are treated surgically in childhood (Johnston et al 2003; Thureen et al 2005).

Ambiguous genitalia

Gender should not be ascribed if there is any doubt. Medical referral is required if the genitalia appear ambiguous, as it is important that gender is correctly ascribed. Chromosomal analysis may be required. Ambiguous genitalia are almost always associated with an underlying abnormality (Johnston et al 2003).

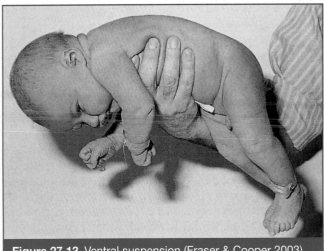

Figure 27.13 Ventral suspension (Fraser & Cooper 2003)

Elimination

Note whether the baby has passed urine or meconium.

Neurological examination

Movements and reaction to stimuli change as gestation progresses. What is normal at 34 weeks is not normal at term. When interpreting the neurological examination, the baby's gestational age and state of arousal need to be taken into account (Johnston et al 2003). The baby needs to be in a quiet alert state. The integrity and normality of the neurological system is tested by assessing the baby's posture and reflexes. Weak or absent responses may indicate immaturity or an abnormality.

Posture

- Supine—legs are semi-flexed and the head turns to one side. The arms and legs recoil readily if extended and released. The elbow should not cross the midline when the arm is drawn across the chest and up to the neck (scarf sign, see Fig 27.8).
- Prone—legs are more flexed and tucked up under the abdomen; the arms are held to the chest in a flexed position.
- Ventral suspension—when the baby is held up by the examiner's hand under the chest (see Fig 27.13), the body is semi-flexed, the head is briefly extended in line with the spine, and the limbs are momentarily flexed.
- hAll limbs move spontaneously.

Rooting, sucking and swallowing

These are easily observed when the baby commences feeding. The rooting reflex is easily stimulated by brushing the baby's cheek or upper lip with a finger. The baby will turn toward the stimulus and open the mouth ready to suck. The suck–swallow–breathe pattern is coordinated and strong enough for adequate feeding from 36 weeks.

Grasp reflexes

These can be elicited in both the hands and feet. It is strong enough in term neonates to briefly lift the baby away from the examination surface.

Traction response

When the baby is pulled forward by the hands from supine to a sitting position, the elbows, knees and ankles flex (see Fig 27.14). The head comes with the body with minimal lag. When the baby reaches the sitting position, the head falls onto the chest. The response reflects the development of flexor tone, which occurs at about 37 weeks.

Asymmetric tonic neck reflex

The head is turned to one side while the baby is supine. The limbs on the side the baby is facing extend, while the limbs on the opposite side flex (see Fig 27.15). It is strong from 30 to 36 weeks, may not be seen in the early newborn period, and returns four to six weeks after birth. A very strong response at birth needs a medical consultation (Johnston et al 2003, London et al 2003).

Moro reflex (startle reflex)

In response to a loud noise or suddenly lowering of the head into the examiner's hand, the baby extends the arms, hands and fingers outwards and the knees flex (see Fig 27.16). The arms slowly return into the chest (like a hug). The baby may cry.

Stepping response

When the baby is supported in a standing position with the soles of the feet on a firm surface, the infant will simulate walking. The presence of this reflex indicates mature extension and flexion mechanisms (Farrell & Sittlington 2003b; Johnston et al 2003; London et al 2003).

Hips

Developmental dysplasia of the hips (DDH) is a condition that has serious consequences for the child if not diagnosed and treated very soon after birth (see Ch 38 for treatment). Screening babies for this condition is non-invasive and effectively diagnoses most babies requiring orthopaedic assessment. Clinical examination using Ortolani's and

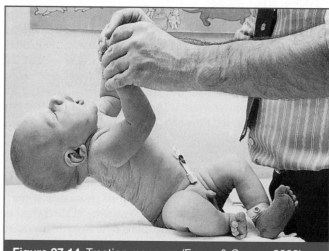

Figure 27.14 Traction response (Fraser & Cooper 2003)

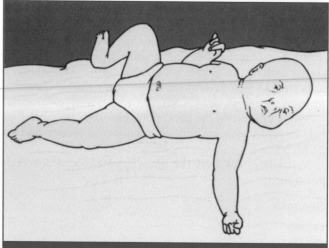

Figure 27.15 Tonic neck reflex (Thureen et al 2005)

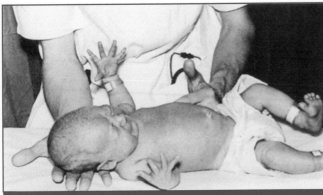

Figure 27.16 Moro reflex (Fraser & Cooper 2003)

Barlow's tests is universally used to screen newborn babies. When examiners are experienced, sensitivity is significantly improved. The tests have high specificity but a low sensitivity, resulting in a false positive rate and subsequent over-treatment and a false negative rate resulting in late detection (Eastwood 2003). Ultrasound is used for screening in some centres in Europe and Britain. Two recent reviews of the research concluded that there is as yet insufficient clear evidence for or against general ultrasound screening of neonates for DDH (Eastwood 2003; Woolacott et al 2005).

Examine the hips for:
● symmetry of thigh and buttock creases
● equal leg length
● range of abduction
● dislocation or laxity of the hip joints ('clicky hips').

Symmetry of thigh and buttock creases, leg length

The thigh and buttock creases should be symmetrical when the baby is lying prone. (Note these when examining the baby's back, to minimise handling.) The legs should be of equal length. When the baby is lying flat with knees flexed, the height of both knees should be equal. Asymmetry and/or limited range of abduction may be signs of DDH. These assessments are unreliable alone and must be accompanied by the abduction tests.

Abduction tests

Each joint should be physically assessed separately for dislocation or laxity. Two tests are normally used:
● Ortolani's test (Fig 27.18) examines for the presence of a dislocated hip.
● Barlow's test (Fig 27.17) examines the joints for laxity and the capability for the joint to dislocate with ease (see Clinical point above, for procedures).

Findings:
● Normal finding—no movement is felt in the joint.
● Joint laxity—on examination the joint feels lax or unstable (i.e. 'gives' a little) but does not clunk. It may 'click' during the examination. Joint laxity at birth is the result of the breech position in some babies or may be related to a hormonal effect on the joint capsule, especially in baby girls. In most cases the joint capsule

---

Clinical point

Examining the hips for developmental dysplasia
In all cases *be gentle*. The pressure you apply to the baby's legs should the same as you would apply in holding an egg. Excessive force is not needed. If the hip joint is unstable, it will move as the test is carried out. Normal hip joints are stable.
Preparation:
◗ consent from mother
◗ warm, relaxed baby lying flat on a warm, flat surface
◗ napkin off.
Do *not* attempt the examination if the baby is distressed.

Ortolani's test
Joints are assessed separately.
1 Stabilise the pelvis with the non-examining hand.
2 Hold each leg, place thumb on inner surface of the thigh, and the index and middle fingers over the greater trochanter of the femur.
3 Flex the knees and the hips 90 degrees.
4 Lifting the thigh slightly, abduct the leg gently, applying pressure over the trochanter with the fingers. (The aim is to slide a dislocated head of femur over the rim and back *into the acetabulum*.)
5 A positive result is a palpable clunk.

Barlow's test
Assess each hip separately.
1 Hold the knee and hip in a flexed position.
2 Gently pull the thigh upward, Adduct the thigh *slightly* and push downward toward the bed, then abduct the thigh. (The aim is to slide a dislocatable head of femur over the rim and *out of the acetabulum*.)
3 A positive result is a palpable clunk.
4 Record findings.
(Sources: Johnston et al 2003; Thureen et al 2005.)

---

tightens over several days and the laxity disappears. Persistent joint laxity is abnormal. *All* babies with joint laxity are referred for medical assessment so that the state of the joint can be monitored and treatment commenced where necessary.
● Dislocated or dislocatable hip(s)—if a distinct 'clunk' is felt and/or heard when either test is carried out, the femoral head is dislocated or dislocatable. Immediate orthopaedic referral is required so that treatment can be commenced without delay (see Ch 38).

Record of neonatal examination

Although there is no single way to record the findings from the examination, it is essential that the assessment is fully recorded. Table 27.5 shows some commonly used symbols for recording selected assessments. These records usually form

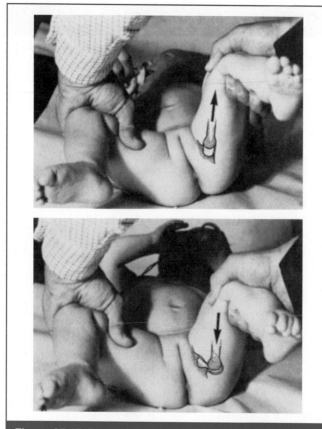

Figure 27.17 Barlow's test (Thureen et al 2005)

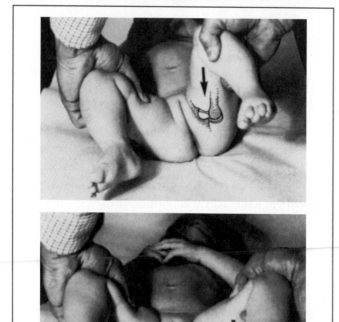

Figure 27.18 Ortolani's test (Thureen et al 2005)

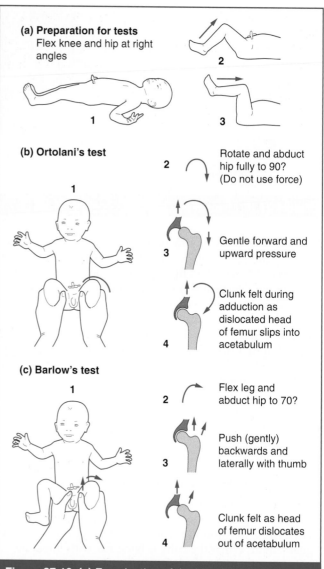

(a) Preparation for tests
Flex knee and hip at right angles

1

2

3

(b) Ortolani's test

1

2 Rotate and abduct hip fully to 90? (Do not use force)

3 Gentle forward and upward pressure

4 Clunk felt during adduction as dislocated head of femur slips into acetabulum

(c) Barlow's test

1

2 Flex leg and abduct hip to 70?

3 Push (gently) backwards and laterally with thumb

4 Clunk felt as head of femur dislocates out of acetabulum

Figure 27.19 (a) Examination of the hips **(b)** Ortolani's test **(c)** Barlow's test (based on Fraser & Cooper 2003)

part of a total record for the baby at birth and at subsequent assessment points.

Care of the newborn infant

Growth and development: birth to six weeks

Newborn infants communicate verbally by crying. Non-verbal communication is initially by reflex, such as the sucking and rooting reflexes. By the time they are four to six weeks old babies can also communicate by smiling in response to an adult and exhibit the beginnings of random 'cooing' when content. Random smiling may occur quite early but smiling socially in response to an adult does not usually appear before four weeks, and it is often closer to six weeks before it occurs.

Restlessness when hot or uncomfortable begins to be seen as the baby grows.

Initially, babies move their arms and legs and can turn their head from side to side as they seek the breast. By four to six weeks, babies can generally turn their head from side to side and raise their head from the cot when in the prone position. They have developing neck strength.

At birth, babies are usually quiet and wide-eyed, have a crinkled skin and some degree of head moulding. They lie in their mother's arms or in the bassinet generally in the same flexed position as they were in utero. They unfurl like flowers opening over the first one to two weeks of life. Head moulding disappears and the head shape becomes round. The face appears to 'open up' as the head shape changes, the crinkly reddish appearance present at birth disappears and the skin smoothes out. Their bodies also unfurl. While babies' bodies stay quite flexed while sleeping, there is a gradual straightening of the body when the baby is awake. For parents, watching this gradual unfurling is one of the precious joys of new parenthood.

Ongoing care

Everyday assessment for mothers and midwives

The thriving baby:

- *The baby should be content between feeds and have a wet nappy every feed.* In the first 24 hours the baby must pass urine, usually 2–5 times; thereafter 6–8 wet nappies every 24 hours, regular bowel motions, usually 2–3 every 24 hours (the pattern varies).
  Note: Disposable nappies are designed to pull the moisture away from the baby's skin. It is sometimes quite difficult to tell whether the baby has passed urine just by looking at the nappy. Feeling the weight of a dry, unused nappy and the one removed from the baby helps to determine this. Disposable nappies full of urine feel heavy when 'weighted' in the hand.
- *The baby should look well.* That is, the baby has a pink colour, and feels warm to the touch, including extremities. Breathing is not very noticeable (see section on normal variations in breathing, this chapter). Arms and legs are flexed and feel firm, with good muscle tone, content expression, not grimacing or frowning (although babies do have these expressions when passing a bowel motion). There should be no signs of infectious skin lesions and the umbilical cord should be clean and dry (see box, umbilical cord care, earlier).
- *When asked, the mother says the baby is well.* It is imperative that the midwife asks the baby's mother how the baby is, and *listens* to the answer. The mother has much more knowledge of the baby than the midwife. If the mother expresses concern, listen and look carefully. Babies can become seriously ill *very* quickly and do not show signs of illness in the way that adults and older children do. Signs are often subtle and/or global—

examples are: (i) a baby with a urinary tract infection will not necessarily have a high fever and cannot say where the pain or discomfort is; (ii) a baby that has been feeding well, stops feeding; (iii) significant or persistent jaundice (see Box 27.2 for danger signals).

Ongoing assessment of growth

Every baby in all Australian states and in New Zealand has an individual health record book that is maintained by all providers of healthcare during the first two to five years. The record books have a variety of local names (e.g. the Blue Book, the Plunket Book, the Well Child Health Book). The books include an ongoing record of assessments by midwives and well child healthcare providers, and information for parents about age- and stage-related issues such as making the house safe when the child begins to crawl and walk. The books also keep an ongoing record of the baby's growth and

TABLE 27.5 Recording results of neonatal examination

Clinical examination			Result*
Fontanelles	✓		
Eyes	✓	✓	Red reflex ✓ ✓
Nose/mouth	✓		Palate ✓
Ears	✓	✓	
Heart	✓		S_1✓ S_2✓ murmurs^0
Lungs	✓	✓	Air Entry =
Abdomen	✓		Soft. Liver border 1 cm ↓ costal margin
Umbilicus	✓		3 vessels
Femoral pulses	✓	✓	synchronous
Genitals	✓		N ♀
Hips	✓	✓	Stable
Back	✓		
Anus	✓		Patent
Legs/arms	✓	✓	Symmetrical
Reflexes, movements /tone	✓		Symmetrical
Skin	✓		
Signature: Date:			

*Record normal: ✓ . Record abnormal: X . Not examined: leave blank.

BOX 27.1 Decision points in the first six weeks

1st decision point (immediately post partum up to and including the first 24 hours)

Physical:

▸ full physical assessment of the baby including heart sounds, hip examination, weight and measurements

Possible tests:

▸ blood group, Rhesus factor, Direct Coombs test

Possible treatments:

▸ respect the birth plan developed with the woman in relation to administration of vitamin K, hepatitis B immunoglobulin and vaccination

▸ facilitate BCG vaccination as appropriate

Health information and education:

▸ information for baby care related to: feeding, breathing, passing urine and meconium, umbilical cord care, crying, warmth, safety

▸ national immunisation register

▸ information about developing parenting skills

▸ legal requirements

▸ birth notification.

Subsequent decision points in postnatal period

Every 24–48 hours until the woman feels confident in her home environment

Information shared:

From history:

▸ Discuss lactation and ongoing feeding.

▸ Discuss parental and baby's wellbeing.

From examination:

▸ full physical examination of the baby

Possible tests:

▸ Guthrie test; consider need for serum bilirubin estimation

Consider additional care if:

▸ feeding problems, congenital abnormalities, parenting problems

Six-week or final postnatal visit

Information shared:

From history:

▸ feeding and behaviour patterns

From examination:

▸ developmental assessment, full physical examination

Health information:

▸ immunisation

▸ community agencies and other health professionals for referral as appropriate or necessary

Well child health service:

▸ information, referral and expectations

Discuss consumer feedback and midwives' standards review process.

(Source: NZCOM 2005)

Critical thinking exercise

Baby Matt is examined at birth.

1 Plot weight, head circumference and crown–heel length on a centile chart for newborn boys.

2 Determine whether Matt is large, appropriate or small for gestational age.

3 Use a Ballard assessment score sheet to assess Matt's gestational maturity from the following features that have been observed:

 – Weight: 3000 g

 – Head circumference: 35 cm

 – Length: 50 cm

 – Skin is peeling, lanugo is in patches

 – The ears are formed, firm and show instant recoil

 – Creases cover two-thirds of the soles of the feet

 – Breast has raised areola, 3–4 mm bud

 – The scrotum is covered in rugae and contains both testes

 – Limbs are flexed at shoulders, elbows, hips and knees

 – 0° square window; arm recoil 90–100°; popliteal angle 90°; scarf sign at the midline; heel to ear scores 4 on the Ballard scale.

---

development up to two to five years of age. Weight, length and head circumference are measured regularly to assess growth.

Centile charts

Assessment of growth generally involves the use of standardised centile charts (see Fig 27.20). Consult the Well Child record book or the local area Department of Health website, as centile charts usually reflect the growth patterns of each country's population and therefore vary a little. Serial measurements of weight, length and head circumference are recorded in the clinical notes and/or on the centile charts in the baby's health record book. The centile charts provide a visual record that enables comparison of growth in the three measurement dimensions. Different centile charts are used for boys and girls. In healthy term babies, all three measurements parallel each other along the same centile curve (e.g. all following the 50th centile curve). Babies who have an initial measurement below the 3rd or above the 97th centile are carefully assessed to exclude underlying causes, as are babies with ongoing measurements that begin to fall below the initial centile curve.

Growth rate

Babies double their weight by five to six months and treble it by the end of the first year. After six months babies gain 100 g per week on average. The average length at birth is 48–52 cm. By six months, 8–10 cm is gained, and another 10 cm by the end of the first year (Sweet 2000). (See Ch 29 for feeding and weight gain.)

BOX 27.2 Child sickness danger signals

Get help from a doctor *quickly* if your baby or young child shows any of these signs.

General:

▶ Cannot be woken or is responding less than usual to what is going on around them.
▶ Has glazed eyes and is not focusing on anything.
▶ Seems more floppy, drowsy or less alert than usual.
▶ Has a convulsion or fit.
▶ Has an unusual cry for one hour or more.
▶ Has been badly injured.
▶ There is a bulge in the groin which gets bigger with crying.

Temperature:

▶ Feels too cold or too hot (temperature 38.3°C or higher).
▶ Circulation and skin colour.
▶ Body is much paler than usual or suddenly goes very white.
▶ Nails are blue or big toe is completely white, or colour does not return to toe within three seconds of a squeeze.

Breathing:

▶ Goes blue or stops breathing.
▶ Breathes more quickly than normal or grunts.
▶ Is wheezing when breathing out.
▶ In-drawing of the chest [is] visible with each breath.

Vomiting and diarrhoea:

▶ Has vomited at least half the feed after each of the last three feeds.
▶ Has green vomit.
▶ Has taken less fluid then usual.
▶ Has passed less urine then usual.
▶ Has a large amount of blood in nappy.

(Source: New Zealand Ministry of Health 2004)

Warmth and hygiene

One of the pleasures for new parents is bathing their baby. This is a time when parents can get to know their baby. Babies enjoy a deep bath, which can be a relaxing time for parents and baby. There is no 'right' way to bath a baby as long as the baby does not get cold in the process. Common-sense precautions such as warm room, towels and clothes, getting all necessary equipment ready before starting, and drying the baby thoroughly, are simple ways to prevent chilling. Soaps and shampoos should not contain strong detergents or perfumes, as the baby's skin is easily irritated.

Parents are frequently encouraged to dress their baby in many layers of clothing. Generally, it is sufficient to use one layer more than the other people in the room are wearing. Babies do not sweat very effectively and become overheated. Out of doors, especially in extreme climates, care should be taken to protect the baby's head and extremities from cold and to protect the face from cold winds (Varney et al 2003). Conversely, in hot weather keep the baby out of direct sunlight and protect the skin with light clothing.

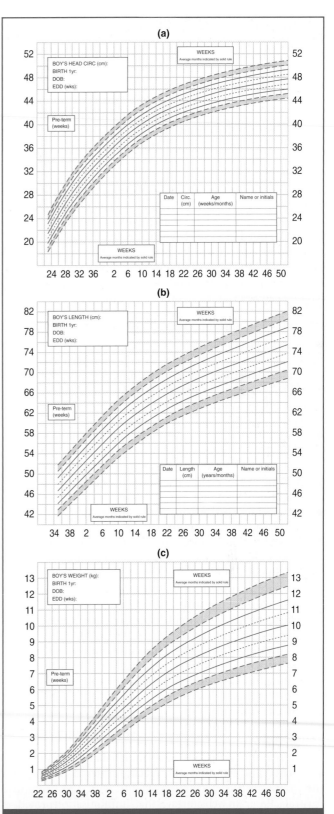

Figure 27.20 Growth charts **(a)** Head circumference from preterm (24 weeks) to one year (male). **(b)** Length from term birth to one year (male) **(c)** Weight from 23 weeks to one year (male) (adapted from Henderson & Macdonald 2004)

Prevention of injury or accident

Commonsense precautions should be observed by midwives and parents, to prevent injury. Babies should not be left unattended in cots with the sides down or on beds, chairs or tables. Pillows are not required in bassinets. Bath water should be tested before bathing the baby. Care needs to be taken with polythene bags and wrappings, and waterproof mattress covers need to be tightly fitting to avoid loose covers that may suffocate the baby (Farrell & Sittlington 2003b).

Car safety

There is evidence that death or injury in a car accident can be prevented or minimised by appropriate restraint for age. In Australia and New Zealand it is illegal for any person to be unrestrained in a car. Newborns are restrained in car seats that are the correct size for newborns. In many areas, local health authorities or well child services provide an affordable hire service. Local availability should be sourced so that women can be given the required information.

Prevention of sudden infant death syndrome (SIDS)

- Sleeping position—there is strong evidence that babies should sleep on their backs. Parents may need to be reassured that it is safe to do so. Since the introduction of the 'back to sleep' programs in Australia and New Zealand, the death rates from sudden infant death syndrome (SIDS) have fallen substantially.
- Maternal smoking—maternal smoking in pregnancy significantly increases the risk of SIDS. Ongoing smoke-change programs are working with women to reduce smoking in pregnancy. The new baby's environment should also be smoke-free.
- Bed sharing—bed sharing between a mother and her baby is a traditional and treasured practice in many places. Some situations make bed sharing less safe for young babies. The biggest risk is when there has been smoking in pregnancy. Bed sharing is also less safe when the adult is under the influence of drugs or alcohol, or is a smoker. Bed sharing should also be avoided with preterm babies (< 36 weeks gestation), low birthweight babies (< 2500 g) and babies exposed to smoking.
- Safe bedding—providing a firm sleeping surface (no soft surfaces, chairs, sofas, bean bags or waterbeds) and keeping the baby's face clear of loose bedding reduces the risk. There should be no pillows or stuffed toys in the cot while the baby is asleep (Cowan 2000).

Immunisation

Australia and New Zealand have similar standard immunisation schedules. However, the vaccines offered at birth and the timing of the vaccinations is different. The Immunise Australia Program website states that 'Immunisation providers are responsible for advising patients and parents/caregivers of available vaccine choices at the time of consultation, including those provided free under the National Immunisation Program' (DHA 2004). Each state and territory health authority has an Immunisation Infoline. The immunisation schedule and information about current vaccines are also available in *The Australian Immunisation Handbook* (DHA 2003).

The New Zealand Immunisation Schedule and information about current vaccines is available on the NZ Ministry of Health website (http://www.moh.govt.nz) or from the Immunisation Advisory Centre (http://www.immune.org.nz). The Ministry of Health also publishes a print version of the *Immunisation Handbook*. Midwives and other LMCs are required to provide parents with timely information about both the risks and benefits of immunisation and about the immunisation schedule so that an informed choice can be made. The information is usually discussed by the midwife at the four-week discharge visit, so that the parents or sometimes a child health nurse have made a decision by the six-week visit when the schedule commences.

Screening for inborn metabolic and endocrine disorders

Blood tests such as the Guthrie test are available to screen for a variety of inborn errors of metabolism and some endocrine disorders. A blood spot collection is made onto an absorbent card. For some tests the baby must have had a minimum of 48 hours of milk feeding prior to specimen collection. The conditions tested for vary in each population and with Health Department policy. They are rare conditions where very early diagnosis and treatment can prevent brain or other organ damage or prevent other serious complications.

Conditions commonly screened for can include:
- biotinidase deficiency
- congenital adrenal hyperplasia
- cystic fibrosis
- galactosaemia
- hypothyroidism
- maple syrup urine disease
- phenylketonuria
- sickle cell disease
- thalassaemia.

Population screening such as this raises ethical issues about consent, especially in relation to the addition of tests to the screen and about the long-term storage of blood samples. Murray and Clarke (2002) hold the view that 'while personal autonomy must be respected . . ., especially the need for informed consent, population screening will often be justified on the basis of benevolence' (p 447). There is no doubt that early diagnosis of hypothyroidism, for example, prevents the development of cretinism—babies treated early lead a normal life with no brain damage. However, the issue of stored blood samples has been considered by the New Zealand Privacy Commissioner (2003). The issues of explicit consent for storage, length of storage, the increasing list of items that the stored specimens can be tested for, and protection against access by other organisations or individuals, were the subject of the Commissioner's report. Storage varies between countries, from instant destruction (France), to two years (Western Australia), to indefinite (New Zealand). The information leaflet provided to New Zealand mothers prior to obtaining consent now makes the storage information explicit.

Clinical point

Bedsharing
(By Sally Baddock)

Bedsharing between babies and their mothers (and sometimes other family members) is a traditional practice in many cultures and is becoming more common again in Caucasian families (Arnestad et al 2001). Bedsharing is often chosen as a way of facilitating breastfeeding, and the majority of infants who bedshare are breastfed. However, bedsharing is not a single coherent practice. Families follow varied practices and choose to bedshare for different reasons, and this may affect the safety or otherwise of their sleeping arrangements (Baddock et al 2000).

Parents who choose to bedshare report ease of breastfeeding, reduced tiredness, emotional benefits, and having a more settled baby (Baddock et al 2004; Ball et al 1999; McKenna et al 1994). This is supported by observational studies that record increased breastfeeding, increased maternal interactions, and synchronisation of mother–baby sleep patterns during bedshare sleep. Mothers and babies are also found to sleep facing each other, in close proximity, and with the baby most often at the level of the mother's breast, facilitating breastfeeding (McKenna et al 1997; Young 1999). Fathers, if present, do not usually interact with the baby overnight.

While observational studies show that bedshare babies wake more often, their total sleep time is similar to that of cot-sleep babies, as cot sleepers tend to wake for longer at each waking (Baddock et al 2004). Waking and feeding poses less disruption in the bedsharing situation as mother and baby remain in bed, often with the mother feeding in a drowsy state. Maternal checks are sometimes prompted by infant movements, but equally the mother self-initiates many checks through the night (Young 1999). Mothers report an awareness of their babies even during sleep.

The benefits of bedsharing seem to stem from the mother–baby partnership and the facilitation of breastfeeding. As such it is a strategy incorporated into UNICEF Baby-Friendly Hospital Policies (FSID UNICEF 2003). It has been reported that non-breastfeeding mother–baby pairs do not adopt the same orientation in bed and may not derive the same benefits from bedsharing (Ball 2002). This is supported by a study of high SIDS risk, low-income families in inner-city Chicago, where bedsharing was common but breastfeeding was not (Hauck et al 2003). Bedsharing is also associated with a high rate of SIDS in cultures such as New Zealand Maori (Mitchell et al 1993), and Australian Aborigines (Panaretto et al 2002). In other cultures, however, bedsharing is common but the rate of SIDS is low—for example, Japanese (Sawaguchi & Namiki 2003), Bangladeshi infants in Wales (Gantley 1994) and infants from Pacific Island cultures (Mitchell et al 1993).

The difference in risk may be linked to high rates of maternal smoking in ethnic groups with higher SIDS rates. Bedsharing with a mother who smoked during pregnancy has consistently been identified in international studies as increasing the risk of SIDS (Carpenter et al 2004; Mitchell et al 1993). The risk from maternal smoking is greater for bedshare infants than for infants who sleep in a cot. It is possible that infants compromised by maternal smoking may not have adequate ventilatory (Campbell et al 2001) or thermal (Tuffnell et al 1995) responses to particular stresses arising in the bedsharing environment. The increased risk may be from increased head covering that inadvertently occurs during bedsharing due to the mobility of the bedding, or it may be connected with the warmer environment during bedsharing, associated with thicker adult bedding (Baddock et al 2004). The close maternal contact in bedsharing may also expose the bedsharing infant to more effects from passive smoking—for example, nicotine has been shown to accumulate on furniture surfaces and bedding, even if the mother smokes only outside the house (Matt et al 2004).

Other risk factors associated with bedsharing include recent maternal alcohol consumption or illicit drug consumption, maternal overtiredness, excessive bedding, household overcrowding, and infant age younger than eight weeks (Blair et al 1999; Carpenter et al 2004). Sleeping on a couch, chair or waterbed with a baby increases the risk of SIDS, possibly due to the likelihood of the baby becoming trapped between adult and furniture. Pillows or situations that might lead to wedging or trapping of the baby (e.g. between the bed and wall or between two mattresses) also pose a risk.

Thus the risk factors are grouped around a vulnerable baby (young age, exposure to smoking), an impaired mother (alcohol, overtired) and the physical environment (overheating, hazardous bedding). Some of these factors can be addressed, but the evidence to date suggests that a baby exposed to smoking in utero should not bedshare.

For healthy babies with mothers who are able to respond appropriately to the subtle cues of their baby, unimpaired by alcohol or overtiredness, bedsharing may offer many advantages, particularly with respect to ease of breastfeeding.

For current advice regarding safe bedsharing, check the following website: http://www.babyfriendly.org.uk/bedshare.asp

Hearing

If a universal newborn hearing screening program is not in place, the parents should be asked if they think their baby can hear before the six-week examination. Questions such as: 'Does the baby startle to loud noise?' and 'Does she turn her head in the direction of localised noise, such as the mother's voice?' are asked.

Referral to a paediatrician, otolaryngeal specialist and/or audiologist is warranted for any of the following situations:

- a close relative who has been deaf from early childhood
- rubella or contact with rubella or other congenital infection during pregnancy (e.g. cytomegalovirus (CMV))
- prematurity (< 32 weeks gestation or < 1500 g birthweight)
- malformation of head or face, or other physical findings known to be associated with deafness
- serum bilirubin levels that require exchange transfusion
- Apgar score of 0–4 at one minute or 0–6 at five minutes or more than five days ventilation
- bacterial meningitis
- received ototoxic medications (NZMOH 2004, p 76).

Vision

Before the six-week examination, parents should be asked if they think their baby can see: 'Does their baby close his/her eyes against bright light, stare at people's faces when they are up close, turn toward light, smile at the parent without being touched or spoken to' (NZMOH 2004, p 85).

Referral to an ophthalmologist or paediatrician is warranted for any of the following situations:

- close relative with an eye tumour at birth or during infancy
- close relative with a congenital eye malformation
- rubella or contact with rubella or other congenital infection during pregnancy (e.g. toxoplasmosis)
- prematurity (< 32 weeks gestation or < 1250 g birthweight)
- eye malformations (absent red reflex, bulging eye, abnormal pupil); failure to fix or follow objects/ movements; abnormal eye movements
- newborn seizures, encephalopathy, certain errors of metabolism
- trauma to the eye
- conjunctivitis that worsens or does not resolve (NZMOH 2004, p 76).

Physiological jaundice

Jaundice is a symptom that either reflects the normal breakdown of RBCs that contain HbF that is no longer required or reflects an underlying pathological process. Neonates require careful assessment in the first weeks of life to exclude hyperbilirubinaemia, particularly caused by dehydration, infection or severe physiological jaundice as kernicterus is again being reported in term infants (Bratlid 2002). Jaundice may be the only sign of bacterial infection (Garcia & Nager 2002). Hannon and colleagues (2001) showed that jaundice alarms mothers—mothers were concerned about it and perceived it as serious. In their study, Hannon and colleagues found that mothers expressed misconceptions and felt guilty, as they believed that they had caused the jaundice. However, interactions with health personnel and other mothers who had personal experience reduced their concerns. Midwives work in partnership with women to keep them informed of the baby's progress, the nature of physiological jaundice and which observed signs warrant calling the midwife.

Assessing physiological jaundice

In the community, clinical estimations of the severity of jaundice are usually made without the aid of instruments such as an icterometer or bilirubinometer, although the latter have recently made a reappearance in some hospitals. Jaundice progresses from the baby's head to the toes. The further down the body the yellow colour is, the higher the serum bilirubin level. Daily assessment of skin colour, muscle tone, alertness, feeding patterns, urinary output and sleeping behaviours assists midwives to determine whether an estimation of serum bilirubin is warranted. It is very important not to rely on skin colour alone. A dehydrated baby, for example, will exhibit the lethargy and poor urine output related to the lack of fluids while still only mildly yellow, while babies who are alert, feeding well with good muscle tone and urinary output may be quite yellow-looking and be well.

Serum bilirubin estimation in a term baby is warranted if:

- the baby is jaundiced (any degree of yellowness) and sleepy and/or feeding poorly and/or has a reduced urinary output
- the baby unexpectedly becomes jaundiced for the first time after 72 hours of age
- the baby's body is quite yellow. As rule of thumb, if the jaundice is seen in the lower abdomen or below, has spread below the mid upper arm, or the sclera are yellow, the levels are likely to be in excess of 250 mmol/L and a serum estimation is warranted.

The level of jaundice in darker-skinned babies is more difficult to assess. Blanch the baby's gums with a gloved finger. The depth of the yellow discolouration provides additional information to assist with the assessment.

Note: Assess the baby in natural light where possible; pink walls and pink or yellow clothing can affect the appearance of the skin colour.

Critical thinking exercise

At an antenatal visit, a pregnant woman asks you what sort of clothes, what size and how many she needs for her baby. She also asks you whether she should use cloth nappies. Consider your reply. Where would you access the information the woman needs in your local maternity services?

Summary

- The neonatal period lasts for 28 days. Midwives work in partnership with the baby's mother for a variable time up to six weeks of age. Midwives use professional knowledge and judgement to support new parenting, share information, and provide initial and ongoing examination and assessment of the baby's health, wellbeing and development. Timely identification, treatment and/or referral for variations from normal and appropriate transfer of care to well child services are integral to contemporary, professional midwifery care of the newborn infant.

- The transition from intrauterine to extrauterine life is characterised by physiological adaptation of many of the baby's body systems. Care of the neonate is based on supporting normal transition and early identification of variations from normal for treatment and/or referral.

- A sound understanding of neonatal anatomy, physiology and development enables midwives to support women as they learn to recognise normal behaviour and growth and development of their baby.

- Information sharing about the everyday signs that her baby is thriving, commonsense precautions to prevent heat loss and infection and common variations in baby behaviours such as sleeping and crying, assists women to develop confidence as they learn to care for their newborn infant.

- Developing the knowledge and skills to undertake a comprehensive physical examination of a newborn baby is within the scope of midwifery practice, as is ongoing monitoring of growth, development, health and wellbeing.

- Knowledge and assessment skills are required to recognise the baby who is ill, not thriving or who has a variation from normal that requires referral to another health professional.

- Good record keeping and inter-professional communication ensure that healthcare providers can continue to provide individualised and contextualised care.

Conclusion

The aims of this chapter have been to promote understanding of neonatal physiology and adaptation to extrauterine life, so that assessment skills to monitor infant health, wellbeing and development can be developed; and to promote knowledgeable and skilful midwifery practice incorporating available evidence for care that supports the newborn infant. A significant proportion of midwifery care of the newborn consists of sharing information that informs, educates and supports the baby's mother to develop confidence in her own capabilities to nurture and care for her baby and to recognise and take action when her baby is unwell.

Review questions

1   In what way do prenatal fetal breathing movements assist the assessment of post-term fetal wellbeing?

2   What would be the result if one of more of the temporary structures in the fetal circulation failed to close after birth?

3   Which babies are at higher risk of developing VKDB?

4   Are there times when vitamin K would not be administered?

5   Why can persistent jaundice be a sign of neonatal infection?

6   If you work in an area where the temperatures are extreme, what advice will you give to women about protecting their baby in very hot or very cold conditions? Find out what advice is given by midwives in your area.

7   What are the procedures in your local area if a lax hip joint is detected at birth? At one week?

8   How will you differentiate a monilial rash from nappy rash on the baby's buttocks and groin? What advice will you give the baby's mother? How will you treat the condition?

9   In your area, which conditions are tested for in the postpartum blood spot test? What is the incidence? How are they treated?

10 What action will you take if one of the blood spot tests returns a positive result?

11 In your area, what happens to the blood spot cards once the tests are completed?

Note

1 Other family members such as the baby's father, grandparents or other significant people are also part of the baby's life, and as such are included in midwifery care of the family. Nevertheless, the mother and her baby are the recipients of midwifery care and the primary interactions usually take place between the baby's mother and the midwife. This chapter refers to woman/mother and baby while respecting that others are closely involved and may also be a primary adult in the baby's life.

Online resources

Health Ministries and Departments

Australian Government, Department of Health and Ageing, http://www.health.gov.au
New Zealand Ministry of Health, http://www.moh.govt.nz
Queensland Health, http://www.health.qld.gov.au
New South Wales Health, http://www.health.nsw.gov.au
Department of Human Services, Victoria http://www.health.vic.gov.au
Department of Health, South Australia, http://www.health.sa.gov.au
Department of Health, Western Australia, http://www.health.wa.gov.au
Department of Health and Human Services, Tasmania, http://www.dhhs.tas.gov.au

Other immunisation sites

Immunise Australia Program, http://www.immunise.health.gov.au
NSW Multicultural Health Communication Service, http://www.mhcs.health.nsw.gov.au
Immunisation Advisory Centre, http://www.immune.org.nz
Immunisation Awareness Society, http://www.ias.org.nz

Other sites

Diagnostic Medlab, http://www.dml.co.nz. There is an extremely useful section for health practitioners that shows laboratory values for non-pregnant and pregnant women and for neonates, diagnostic tests, specimens required for laboratory evaluation. It is routinely updated.
The Cochrane Collaboration, http://www.cochrane.org. A major database of evaluations of the evidence for maternity care.

References

Arnestad M, Andersen M, Vege A et al 2001 Changes in the epidemiological pattern of sudden infant death syndrome in southeast Norway, 1984–1998: implications for future prevention and research. Archives of Disease in Childhood 85(2):108–115

Baddock SA, Day HF, Rimene CR 2000 Bedsharing practices of different cultural groups. Paper presented at the SIDS 2000, 6th SIDS International Conference, Auckland, New Zealand

Baddock SA, Galland BC, Beckers MGS et al 2004 Bedsharing and the infant's thermal environment in the home setting. Archives of Disease in Childhood 89:1111–1116.

Ball HL 2002 Differences in bed-sharing behaviour among breastfeeding and non-breastfeeding families. Paper presented at the Seventh SIDS International Conference, Florence, Italy

Ball HL, Hooker E, Kelly PJ 1999 Where will the baby sleep? Attitudes and practices of new and experienced parents regarding cosleeping with their newborn infants. American Anthropologist 101(1):143–151

Barclay L, Lupton D 1999 The experiences of new fatherhood: a sociocultural analysis. Journal of Advanced Nursing 29(4):1013–1020

Barr RJ 1984 The umbilical cord: to treat or not to treat? Midwives Chronicle July:224–226

Blackburn ST 2003, Maternal, Fetal, Neonatal Physiology: a clinical perspective (2nd edn) Saunders, an imprint of Elsevier Science, St Louis Missouri

Blair P, Fleming P, Smith I et al 1999 Babies sleeping with parents: case-control study of factors influencing the risk of the sudden infant death syndrome. British Medical Journal 319:1457–1462

Bliss-Holtz J 1991 Determining cold stress in full term newborns through temperature site comparisons. Scholarly Inquiry for Nursing Practice 5(2):113–123

Bratlid D 2001 Criteria for the treatment of neonatal jaundice. Journal of Perinatology 21(suppl):588–592

Brazelton TB 1984 Neonatal behavioural assessment scale (2nd edn). Heinemann, London

Brazelton TB, Nugent JK 1995 Neonatal behavioural assessment scale (3rd edn). McKeith Press, London

Burden AD, Krafchik BR 1999 Subcutaneous fat necrosis of the newborn: a review of 11 cases. Paediatric Dermatology 16:384–387

Callen JP et al 2000 Color atlas of dermatology (2nd edn). WB Saunders, Philadelphia

Campbell AJ, Galland BC, Bolton DPG et al 2001 Ventilatory responses to rebreathing in infants exposed to maternal smoking. Acta Paediatrica 90(7):793–800

Carpenter RG, Irgens LM, Blair PS et al 2004 Sudden unexplained infant death in 20 regions in Europe: case control study. Lancet 363(9404):185–191

Coad J, Dunstall M 2001 Anatomy and physiology for midwives. Mosby, St Louis

Cornelissen EAM, Kolee LAA, De Arbreu RA et al 1992 Effects of oral and intramuscular vitamin K prophylaxis on vitamin K1, PIVKA-II and clotting factors in breastfed infants. Archives of Diseases in Childhood 67:1250–1254

Cowan S 2000 Head shape, bed sharing and SIDS prevention. Education for Change. Online: http://www.efc.co.nz, accessed 20 February 2005

Department of Health and Ageing (DHA), Australian Government 2003 Australian immunisation handbook (8th edn). Online: http://www1.health.gov.au/immhandbook

Department of Health and Ageing (DHA), Australian Government 2004 Immunise Australia Program. Online: http://www.immunise.health.gov.au, accessed November 2004

Diagnostic/Medlab 2000 Blood count. In: Laboratory handbook. Online: http://www.dml.co.nz, accessed 21 August 2005

Dore S, Buchan D, Coulas S et al 1998 Alcohol versus natural drying for newborn cord care. Journal of Obstetric, Gynecological and Neonatal Nursing 27(6):621–627

Doull IJM, McCaughey ES, Bailey BJR et al 1995 Reliability of infant length measurement. Archives of Disease in Childhood 72:520–521

Eastwood D 2003 Neonatal hip screening. Lancet 361:595–597

Farrell P, Sittlington N 2003a The newborn baby: the baby at birth. Ch 38. In: D Fraser, M Cooper (Eds) Myles textbook for midwives (14th edn). Churchill Livingstone, London

Farrell P, Sittlington N 2003b The newborn baby: the baby at birth. Ch 39. In: D Fraser, M Cooper (Eds) Myles textbook for midwives (14th edn). Churchill Livingstone, London

Fleming M, Hakansson H, Svenningsen NW 1983 A disposable temperature probe for skin measurement in the newborn nursery. International Journal of Nursing Studies 10(2):89–96

Fraser DM, Cooper MA (Eds) Myles textbook for midwives (14th edn). Churchill Livingstone, Edinburgh

Fraser Garcia FJ, Nager AL 2002 Jaundice as an early diagnostic sign of urinary tract infection in infancy. Paediatrics 109(5): 846–851

FSID UNICEF 2003 Sharing a bed with your baby. FSID (Foundation for the study of infant deaths) and UNICEF UK Baby Friendly Initiative. Online: http://www.babyfriendly.org.uk/parents/sharingbed.asp, accessed 4 April 2005

Gantley M 1994 Ethnicity and the sudden infant death syndrome— anthropological perspectives. Early Human Development 38(3):203–208

Glazener CMA, Ramsay CR, Campbell MK et al 1999 Neonatal examination and screening trial (NEST): a randomised controlled switchback trial of alternative policies for low risk infants. British Medical Journal (international edition) 318(7184):627–631

Greer FR 1995 Vitamin K deficiency and haemorrhage in infancy. Clinical Perinatology 22:759

Greer FR, Marshall SP, Severson RR et al 1998 A new mixed micellar preparation of oral vitamin k prophylaxis: randomised controlled comparison with an intramuscular formulation in breast fed infants. Archives of Disease in Childhood 79(4):300–305

Golding J, Paterson M, Kirlen LJ 1990 Factors associated with childhood cancer in a national cohort study. British Journal of Cancer 62:304–308

Golding J, Greenwood R, Birmingham K et al 1992 Childhood cancer, intramuscular vitamin K and pethidine given during labour. British Medical Journal 305:341–346

Hall DMB 1999 The role of the routine neonatal examination. British Medical Journal (international edition) 318(7184):619

Hand IL, Shepard EK, Krauss AN et al 1990 Ventilation–perfusion abnormalities in the pre term infant with hyaline membrane disease: a two compartment model of the neonatal lung. Paediatric Pulmonology 9(4):206–213

Hannon PR, Willis SK, Scrimshaw SC 2001 Persistence of maternal concerns surrounding neonatal jaundice—an exploratory study. Archives of Paediatric and Adolescent Medicine 155(12):1357–1363

Hauck FR, Herman SM, Donovan M et al 2003 Sleep environment and the risk of sudden infant death syndrome in an urban population: the Chicago Infant Mortality Study. Pediatrics 111(5/2):1207–1214

Henderson C, MacDonald S 2004 Mayes midwifery (13th edn). Baillière Tindall, London

Hernandez JA, Glass SM 2005 Physical assessment of the newborn. Ch 7. In: PJ Thureen, J Deacon, JA Hernandez et al (Eds) Assessment and care of the well newborn (2nd edn). Elsevier Saunders, St Louis

Johnson R, Taylor W 2005 Skills for midwifery practice (2nd ed). Churchill Livingstone, Edinburgh

Johnston P, Flood K, Spinks K 2003 (Eds) The newborn child (9th edn). Churchill Livingstone, London

Lawrence CR 1982 Effect of two different methods of umbilical cord care on its separation. Midwives Chronicle and Nursing Notes June:204–205

Leveno KJ, Cunningham FG, Gant NF et al 2003 Williams manual of obstetrics (21st edn). McGraw-Hill, New York

Loughnan PM, Chant KM, Elliott E et al 1999 The frequency of late onset haemorrhagic disease (HD) in Australia with different methods of prophylaxis, 1993–1997. An update. Journal of Paediatrics and Child Health 38:A8

London ML, Ladewig PW, Ball JW et al (Eds) 2003 Maternal– newborn and child nursing: family centred care. Prentice Hall, London

McHugh C 2004 Newborn care: physiological transition to extrauterine life. Ch 38. In: H Varney, J Krebs, C Gegor (eds) Varney's midwifery (4th edn). Jones Bartlett, Boston

McKenna J, Mosko S, Richard C et al 1994 Experimental studies of infant-parent co-sleeping —mutual physiological and behavioral influences and their relevance to SIDS (sudden infant death syndrome). Early Human Development 38(3):187–201

McKenna JJ, Mosko SS, Richard CA 1997 Bedsharing promotes breastfeeding. Pediatrics, 100(2/1):214–219

McKinney PA, Juszczak E, Findlay E et al 1998 Case controlled study of childhood leukaemia and cancer in Scotland: findings for neonatal vitamin K. British Medical Journal 316:173

Matt GE, Quintana PJE, Hovell MF et al 2004 Households contaminated by environmental tobacco smoke: sources of infant exposures. Tobacco Control 13(1):29–37

Michaelides S 2004a The newborn baby: physiology, assessment and care. Ch 31 In: C Henderson, S MacDonald (Eds) Mayes' midwifery (13th edn). Baillière Tindall, London

Michaelides S 2004b The newborn baby: thermoregulation. Ch 32 In: C Henderson, S MacDonald (Eds) Mayes' midwifery (13th edn). Baillière Tindall, London

Mitchell M 2003 Midwives conducting neonatal examination: part 1. British Journal of Midwifery 11(1):16–21

Mitchell EA, Stewart AW, Scragg R et al 1993 Ethnic differences in mortality from sudden infant death syndrome in New Zealand. British Medical Journal 306(6869):13–16

Murray A, Clarke A 2002 The ethics of population screening. Current Paediatrics 12:447–452

Narrigan D 2000 Newborn hearing screening update for midwifery practice. Journal of Midwifery, Women's Health 45(5):368–377

New Zealand College of Midwives (NZCOM) 2001 A consensus statement: vitamin K prophylaxis in the newborn. NZCOM Journal 23.

New Zealand College of Midwives (NZCOM) 2005 Midwives handbook for practice. NZCOM, Christchurch

New Zealand Ministry of Health (NZMOH) 2004 Tamariki ora. Well child health book. Ministry of Health, Manatu Hauora, Wellington

New Zealand Privacy Commissioner 2003 Guthrie tests: a report by the Privacy Commissioner following his inquiry into the collection, retention and release of newborn metabolic screening test samples, pursuant to section 13(1)(m) of the Privacy Act 1993. Online: http://www.privacycommissioner.org.nz, accessed 17 August 2005

NHMRC 2000 Joint statement and recommendations on vitamin K administration to newborn infants to prevent vitamin K deficiencies in infancy. Commonwealth of Australia, Canberra

Novak B 2005a Adaptation to extrauterine life 1—respirations and cardiac functions. Ch 48. In: D Stables, J Rankin (Eds) Physiology in childbearing with anatomy and related sciences (2nd edn). Elsevier, London

Novak B 2005b Adaptation to extrauterine life 2—nutritional and metabolic adjustments. Ch 49. In: D Stables, J Rankin (Eds) Physiology in childbearing with anatomy and related sciences (2nd edn). Elsevier, London

Olsen JH, Hertz H, Blinkenberg K et al 1994 Vitamin K regimens and incidence of childhood cancer in Denmark. British Medical Journal 308(6933):895

Panaretto K, Whitehall J, McBride G et al 2002 Sudden infant death syndrome in Indigenous and non-Indigenous infants in north Queensland, 1990–1998. Journal of Paediatrics and Child Health 38(2):135–139

Passmore SJ, Draper G, Brownbill P et al 1998 Case controlled studies of relation between childhood cancer and neonatal vitamin K administration. British Journal of Medicine 316:178–184

Roberton NRC 1996 A manual of normal neonatal care (3rd edn). Edwin Arnold, London

Sawaguchi T, Namiki M 2003 Recent trend of the incidence of sudden infant death syndrome in Japan. Early Human Development 75(Suppl):S175–S179

Sleath K 1985 Lessons from Colombia. Nursing Mirror 160(14): 14–16

Stables D, Rankin J 2005 Physiology in childbearing. Elsevier, London

Sweet B (Ed) with Tiran D 1997 Mayes midwifery: a textbook for midwives (12th edn). Baillière Tindall, London

Thummala MR, Raju TN, Langenberg P 1998 Isolated single umbilical artery anomaly and risk for congenital malformations: a meta analysis. Journal of Paediatric Surgery 33(4):580–585

Thureen PJ, Deacon J, Hernandez JA et al (Eds) 2005 Assessment and care of the well newborn (2nd edn). Elsevier Saunders, St Louis

Tuffnell CS, Petersen SA, Wailoo MP 1995 Factors affecting rectal temperature in infancy. Archives of Disease in Childhood 73(5):443–446

Vain NE, Szyld EG, Prudent LM et al 2004 Oropharyngeal and nasopharyngeal suctioning of meconium-stained neonates before delivery of the shoulders: a multicentre randomised controlled trial. Lancet 364(9434):597–602

Varney H, Kriebs J, Gegor C 2004 (Eds) Varney's midwifery (4th edn). Jones & Bartlett, Boston

Whitelaw A, Heisterkamp G, Sleath K et al 1988 Skin to skin contact for very low birthweight infants and their mothers. Archives of Diseases in Childhood 63:1377–1381

Wells N, King J, Hedstom C et al 1995 Does tympanic temperature measure up? American Journal of Maternal Child Nursing 20:95–100

Wolke D Dave S, Hayes J et al 2002 A randomised controlled trial of maternal satisfaction with the routine examination of the newborn baby at three months post birth. Midwifery 18(2):145–154

Woolacott NF, Puhan MA, Steurer, J, Kleijen J (2005) Ultrasonography screening for developmental dysplasia of the hip in newborns: systematic review. British Medical Journal 330: 1413. Online: http://bmj.bmjjournals.com/cgi/, accessed 20 June 2005

Young J 1999 Night-time behaviour and interactions between mothers and their infants of low risk for SIDS: a longitudinal study of room-sharing and bedsharing. Unpublished PhD thesis, University of Bristol, Bristol

Zipursky A 1996 Vitamin K at birth. British Medical Journal 313:179

Zipursky A 1999 Prevention of vitamin K deficiency bleeding in newborns. British Journal of Haematology 104:430

Statutes

Regulations to the NZ *Public Health and Disability Services Act 2000*, s.88

Acknowledgement

The author wishes to thank Sally Baddock, who wrote the Clinical interest box on bedsharing.

CHAPTER 28

Supporting the breastfeeding mother

Ann Henderson and Marlene Scobbie

Key terms

ankyloglossia (tongue tie), attachment, engorgement, epidemiological research, galactopoesis, lactation, lactogenesis I, lactogenesis II, let-down reflex, mammogenesis, mastitis, positioning

Chapter overview

The purpose of this chapter is to provide an understanding of breastfeeding from both global and local perspectives. It reviews the physiology of lactation, and the benefits and properties of breast milk in establishing a natural personal and public health advantage for infants, women, families and communities. Worldwide public health initiatives that actively protect, promote and support breastfeeding provide a global context through the local application of the Baby Friendly Hospital Initiative (BFHI) and the ten steps to successful breastfeeding in healthcare services.

The chapter establishes an evidence-based framework for understanding, educating and assisting women and their families with breastfeeding. The discussion draws on research to identify benefits of breastfeeding practices and provide guidelines for midwives when working with women who are preparing, initiating and maintaining breastfeeding. Problems that may arise during breastfeeding are addressed, and evidence-based strategies for their management are discussed. Positioning and attachment are emphasised as crucial to milk production, supply and successful transfer from mother to infant. A critique of artificial feeding is presented against a background of the advantages of breast milk and breastfeeding.

Learning outcomes

Learning outcomes for this chapter are:

1 To identify the location and anatomical structures of the female breast

2 To explain the function at a cellular level of the lactating breast

3 To differentiate between mammogenesis, lactogenesis and galactopoesis

4 To identify the properties of human breast milk

5 To discuss the benefits of human breast milk

6 To discuss worldwide initiatives that promote breastfeeding

7 To identify the ten steps to successful breastfeeding

8 To describe recommended practices that assist in the preparation, initiation and maintenance of breastfeeding

9 To recognise the importance of positioning and attachment of an infant at the breast

10 To identify common problems associated with breastfeeding, and describe recommended interventions and treatments for each identified problem

12 To critically analyse artificial feeding in relation to breastfeeding.

Physiology of lactation

Breast anatomy

The mature female breast is located over the pectoralis major muscle on the chest wall, extending from the 2nd to the 6th rib and from the sternum to the axilla on each side (Stables & Rankin 2004), and is composed of glandular tissue with a branching duct structure surrounded by supportive connective and adipose tissue. Breast size, colour and shape vary from breast to breast and from woman to woman. Breast size is dependent on the amount of adipose tissue present—size is a poor indicator of breast function and breastfeeding success (Riordan 2005).

In the mature woman, each breast has 7–10 sections or lobes of glandular tissue separated by connective tissue. The gland epithelial tissue (secretory or acini cells) synthesises the breast milk, which is then stored in small clusters of sac-like spaces called alveoli. Some 10–100 clusters of alveoli cells are present in each lobe, supported by collagen sheaths (Stables & Rankin 2004). Myoepithelial (muscle) cells surround the clusters of alveoli. The breast milk passes with the aid of muscle contractions from the alveoli into small and then larger ducts as they get closer to the nipple. Several milk ducts merge close to the areola before the nipple is reached. Some 5–10 small channels or pores emerge through the nipple to the skin surface (Brodribb 2004). A diagram of the breast structure is shown in Figure 28.1.

Ultrasound technology has enabled the female breast structure and function to be more clearly visualised (Ramsay et al 2002). This research has challenged the once-familiar, well accepted and longstanding diagrams depicted in textbooks. Visualisations have indicated:

- fewer lobes (7–10, not 15–20)
- an absence of milk sinuses (reservoirs) behind the nipple and areola
- fewer openings of milk ducts at the nipple (5–10, not 15–25)
- smaller number and size of the small and larger ducts
- rapid branching of ducts close to the areola, which continue to branch and intertwine into a disorderly pattern. The assumption that there is an organised pattern of branching ducts is now obsolete.
- that the milk duct diameter increases as let-down (milk ejection) occurs
- that multiple let-downs occur during a feed.

The nipple is located in the middle of the brown pigmented area called the areola. The size and shape of both nipple and areola can vary between individuals, from large and with flat nipples and reduced or no pigmentation, to raised and small nipples with very distinctive pigmentation. Women can lactate successfully regardless of these wide variations. The nipple, which is composed of smooth muscle, becomes erect when stimulated. There are small swellings located on the areola that secrete an oily fluid that lubricates the nipple and areola surface; these are called Montgomery's tubercles. The nipple and areola also contain many nerve endings that respond to the infant's sucking at the breast and trigger the production and release of milk (Blackburn 2003).

The breast is highly vascularised via the internal mammary and lateral thoracic arteries. Arterial blood terminates in capillary networks surrounding the alveoli. Venules drain venous blood into a circular vein behind the nipple, then into the mammary and axillary veins (Stables & Rankin 2004). The lymph vessels are extensive, flowing alongside the ductal tissue and converging toward the nipple, where they form a plexus beneath the areola. Lymph glands drain into axillary nodes. The breast is innervated by the 4th, 5th and 6th intercostals, giving rise to an uneven pattern of sensation, with the areola and nipple being the most sensitive part (Riordan 2005).

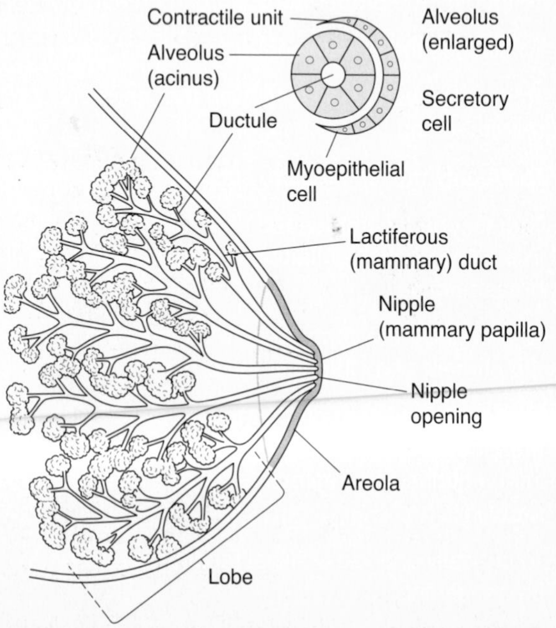

Breast physiology

The function of the breast is to synthesise and eject milk—a process called lactation. The components of milk are synthesised in the secretory cells (protein, fat and lactose) of the alveoli or extracted from the maternal plasma (minerals and vitamins) (Blackburn 2003). The secretory cells alternate between a secreting and a resting state. During infant sucking, active secretion occurs.

Breast milk production involves integration of neuronal, endocrine and autocrine processes. There are five main phases of lactation physiology.

Mammogenesis (mammary growth)

Mammary growth (mammogenesis) begins during embryonic and fetal life and accelerates at puberty under the influence of oestrogen and progesterone (Stables & Rankin 2004). Further changes occur during pregnancy and after birth, in order to

Figure 28.1 Structure of the female breast (based on Riordan 2005)

Labels: Contractile unit; Alveolus (acinus); Alveolus (enlarged); Secretory cell; Ductule; Myoepithelial cell; Lactiferous (mammary) duct; Nipple (mammary papilla); Nipple opening; Areola; Lobe

support lactation. Maturation of tissue begins shortly after conception, when there is a steady increase in breast size and weight, with a proliferation of the ducts and alveoli. Nipples become more erect, the areola pigmentation enhances and Montgomery's tubercles enlarge. Blood supply to the breast also increases, making the vessels appear more visible on the skin surface (Riordan 2005). These changes occur under the influence of oestrogen, human placental lactogen, human chorionic gonadotrophin, insulin, growth hormone, thyroid hormone, progesterone and prolactin.

Lactogenesis (initiation of milk secretion/production)

During the second half of pregnancy, the secretory cells begin milk synthesis (lactogenesis I) under the influence of prolactin, and colostrum and fat globules distend the alveoli (Blackburn 2003). Following childbirth, progesterone and oestrogen diminish in the bloodstream. Colostrum begins to change to more mature milk. At about day 2–3 up until day 8 post birth, milk production is influenced by the hormones prolactin, placental lactogen, cortisol and insulin.

When the infant sucks at the breast, mechanoreceptors (nerve endings) in the nipple stimulate the hypothalamus to suppress the prolactin-inhibiting factor and release prolactin from the anterior pituitary into the bloodstream. This initiates milk production by the acini cells in the glandular tissue (lactogenesis II). Increase in sucking and emptying the breasts leads to an increase in prolactin levels, and the prolactin receptors and milk supply increase. The breast function moves from being under initial endocrine or hormone control to autocrine or milk removal control (Riordan 2005).

The let-down (milk ejection) reflex

The let-down reflex (or milk ejection reflex) is an important process for moving milk along the system of ducts in the breast. Sucking at the breast sends messages from the nipple/areola area to the hypothalamus, which in turn releases oxytocin from the posterior pituitary gland into the bloodstream (see Fig 28.2). Myoepithelial cells around the alveoli are then stimulated to contract and push milk down the ducts toward the nipple. This same hormone stimulates uterine contractions and involution (Riordan 2005). The milk ducts increase in diameter during let-down. Multiple let-downs can occur during a breastfeed and affect the amount of milk the infant consumes (Ramsay et al 2002).

The let-down reflex can also be stimulated by the sight of an infant or the sound of an infant's cry, and inhibited by maternal pain or stress, or low milk supply. Some mothers do not notice any change in sensation during let-down but others report signs of increased thirst, a tingling sensation in the breast, a feeling of breast fullness, leaking of milk from the non-suckled breast or uterine contractions (Brodribb 2004). During let-down, the infant's sucking and swallowing pattern may also change.

Galactopoesis (maintenance of milk secretion)

The maintenance of milk production (galactopoesis) depends on active removal or non-removal of milk from the breast

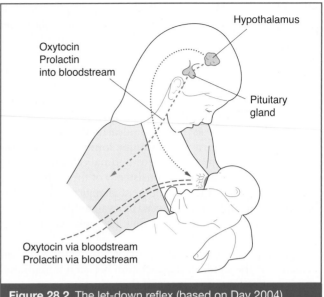

Figure 28.2 The let-down reflex (based on Day 2004)

from about day nine post birth until breastfeeding ceases. Breast function is now under the influence of a local feedback control mechanism. Production of milk depends on adequate stimulation of the breast—the more the infant sucks and the more milk is removed from the breast, the more milk is produced. The less sucking at the breast and the less milk removed, the less milk produced. As long as milk is removed from the breast regularly, the alveolar cells will continue to synthesise milk. Furthermore, the storage capacity of each breast and the quantity of milk removed at each feed influences milk synthesis between feeds (Ramsay et al 2002). The milk supply is therefore produced and influenced through the supply–demand principle as well as the functional capacity of the breast.

Weaning (involution)

If breastfeeding ceases or reduces in frequency, peptides in the milk begin to inhibit cell production and cells die, and therefore milk production decreases (Royal College of Midwives (RCM) 2002). This reduction or weaning may be infant- or mother-led. When breastfeeding ceases, involution of breast tissue occurs to the pre-pregnant state. Weaning milk begins to resemble the composition of colostrum, again with an increase in immunoglobulins, protein and sodium (Brodribb 2004).

Critical thinking exercise

Prolactin levels in the mother's blood are higher at night than during the day.
1   What are the clinical implications of this fact?
2   How would you use this fact when teaching a mother about breastfeeding?

Benefits of breastfeeding

Although instinctively known, research has clearly established the benefits of breastfeeding and the use of human milk for infants. Concomitantly, mothers, families and society can benefit from an increase in the incidence and prevalence of breastfeeding. These benefits include physiological, nutritional, health, psychological, social, economic and environmental outcomes (Bick 1999; Lutter 2000; Oddy 2002).

Physiologically, breast milk is the ideal food for infants (Bick 1999). Breast milk provides a unique fomulary of proteins, carbohydrates and fats needed for optimal cell function and growth. The breast alters the consistency of these nutrients as the infant's growth and development change over time. This balance, complexity and enhanced bioavailability of nutrients and other substances in breast milk has only recently been recognised (Brodribb 2000).

Epidemiological research has provided strong and consistent evidence of the significant association between human milk and breastfeeding of infants and the reduction in incidence and severity of acute and chronic illnesses, therefore reducing infant morbidity and mortality. Infants who receive human milk have reduced:

- gastrointestinal infections (Kramer & Kakuma 2004; Oddy 2001)
- diarrhoeal illness (Bertran et al 2001)
- necrotising enterocolitis (Bick 1999)
- otitis media (Oddy 2001)
- urinary tract infections (Bick 1999)
- respiratory infections (Bertran et al 2001).
  Breast milk also:
- protects infants from sudden infant death syndrome (McVea et al 2000)
- reduces the risk of childhood asthma
- significantly enhances cell-mediated and humoral responses to antigens (Campbell 2000)
- provides immunological protection from insulin-dependent diabetes mellitus (Bick 1999), Crohn's disease and ulcerative colitis, childhood lymphomas and those of allergic origin (Saarinen et al 2000).

Breastfed infants are less likely to develop obesity (Armstrong & Reilly 2002; von Kries et al 1999) and have lower cholesterol levels in later life (Owen et al 2002). Human milk, containing vital omega-three and omega-six fatty acids needed for brain development, also enhances cognitive development (Angelson et al 2001; Horwood et al 2001; Quinn et al 2001; Richards et al 2002) and visual acuity (Anderson et al 1999; Mortensen et al 2002).

Mothers are also likely to benefit from breastfeeding. Oxytocin, released during infant suckling at the breast, contracts the uterus and hastens involution (Riordan 2005). Breastfeeding also prolongs lactation amenorrhoea, thus reducing fertility and increasing child spacing (Kramer & Kakuma 2004). A reduction in rates of ovarian and breast cancer (Zheng et al 2000), heart disease (Owen et al 2002; Singhal et al 2001) and osteoporosis (Jones et al 2000) is revealed in mothers who breastfeed. Prolonged breastfeeding also improves the return to pre-pregnant weight. Psychologically, maternal–infant bonding is enhanced by breastfeeding, due to early contact; and maternal oxytocin levels released during a breastfeed decrease maternal anxiety, and enhance calmness and social responsiveness (Day 2004).

An increase in the prevalence of breastfeeding may provide overall medical, social and economic benefits to society. This impact may flow through to improved personal health outcomes and the possibility of healthier communities through: reduced perinatal morbidity and mortality; cost savings for parents (no need to purchase infant formula articles); fewer hospital admissions; lower healthcare costs; and less absenteeism from school or work attributable to illness (Ball & Bennett 2001). Further, global enhancements have been suggested related to reduction in world overpopulation (reduced fertility), saving on fuel and energy resources, and elimination of wastes from the production of artificial milk and its leftover containers (Biancuzzo 1999).

There is significant quality clinical and ecological evidence to support the benefits of breastfeeding and human milk consumption. Therefore the World Health Organization (WHO 2001) recommends that all babies be exclusively breastfed for the first six months to promote health and reduce illness. The WHO also recommends continued breastfeeding for a further two years. See Table 28.1 for a summary of the benefits of breastfeeding for mother and infant.

Properties of breast milk

Colostrum: the early milk

Colostrum is secreted during the last trimester of pregnancy until 10 days post partum. It is a viscous, concentrated liquid of low volume (varies from 7 mL to 123 mL in 24 hours) with an average amount of 37 mL (Riordan 2005). The newborn's kidneys are immature at birth and cannot deal with large volumes of fluid. This early fluid is high in protein, sodium, minerals and antibodies, low in carbohydrates, fats and vitamins. Colostrum facilitates the growth of gut flora, limits the growth of pathogenic bacteria and viruses, protects against illnesses and aids the excretion of meconium from the gut due to its laxative effect (Brodribb 2004).

Mature breast milk

Mature breast milk is a rich, balanced brew containing 90% water and 10% solids. Bluish in colour, it is slightly alkaline (pH 7.0–7.45), with an average calorie count of 65 kcal/100 mL, although this varies depending on fat content. It is not a uniform fluid; it varies from mother to mother and changes composition during a feed, with the time of the day and from one lactation to the next (Blackburn 2003). Breast milk has nutritional, anti-infective, immunological, bioactive and anti-allergenic properties.

TABLE 28.1 Summary of the benefits of breastfeeding for mother and infant	
Mother	**Infant**
• Hastens involution, with reduced blood loss and less anaemia. • Reduces fertility/increases child spacing. • Reduces risk of ovarian and breast cancer. • Reduces heart disease. • Reduces osteoporosis. • Possibility of improved return to pre-pregnant weight. • Enhances maternal–infant bonding. • Enhances calmness and social responsiveness. • Decreases maternal anxiety.	• Reduces gastrointestinal infections. • Reduces incidence and duration of diarrhoeal illness. • Reduces occurrence of otitis media. • Protects against respiratory infection and reduces risk of childhood asthma. • Reduces urinary tract infections. • Protects against SIDS. • Reduces the incidence of NEC. • Enhances cell-mediated and humoral responses to antigens (allergies). • Enhances cognitive development, with higher IQ scores. • Improves visual acuity • Reduces the incidence of obesity. • Protects against IDDM, Crohn's disease and ulcerative colitis. • Reduces incidence of childhood lymphomas. • Lowers cholesterol levels in later life.
(Source: WHO 2001)	

Nutritional properties

The constituents of breast milk include the following:

- Fats—fat provides half the calories of an infant's energy needs. Fats are essential for development of visual acuity, help vitamin function and form cell membranes and prostaglandins (Shinskie & Lauwers 2002). Levels vary during the feed and are higher in hindmilk than foremilk. Fat globules are small and easily absorbed, with triglycerides being broken down to free fatty acids and glycerol (Blackburn 2003).
- Carbohydrates—the carbohydrate contained in human milk is mostly lactose, being broken down slowly to glucose and galactose and providing 40–45% of an infant's energy needs. Carbohydrates enhance calcium absorption, promote the growth of lactobacilli in the intestines and reduce the growth of gut pathogens. They are also essential for central nervous system development (Shinskie & Lauwers 2002).

- Protein—human milk protein contains 40% casein (soft curds) and 60% whey (a soluble liquid), and is therefore easily digested and absorbed. The whey contains albumins, enzymes, immunoglobulins and hormones (Blackburn 2003). Infants are able to use the protein constituent efficiently. Proteins are needed for cell growth and stability, all body processes, bile salt conjugation and nerve transmission (Shinskie & Lauwers 2002).
- Vitamins—fat-soluble and water-soluble essential vitamins are available in breast milk in sufficient amounts to aid cell growth and function. Specifically, vitamins are required for blood clotting, central nervous system development and skin integrity, and to protect the retina and mediate cell function (Riordan 2005).
- Minerals—human milk contains all the essential minerals needed for electrolyte balance, and infant cell and organ function. They are highly bioavailable and suited to infant growth and development (Brodribb 2004).
- Water—water is the largest component (90%) of breast milk in which dissolved solids (10%) are carried. Water also contributes to regulation of an infant's temperature.

Other properties of milk

- Anti-infective properties—enzymes, immunoglobulin and leucocytes provide protection from infection and reduce the incidence and severity of acute and chronic illnesses (Bick 1999).
- Immunological properties—immunoglobulins are proteins produced by the plasma that block adhesion of pathogens to the infant's mucosal surfaces and produce antibodies, which in turn target microbes. B-lymphocytes help destroy antigens, macrophages engulf and absorb pathogens, neutrophils ingest microbes and T-lymphocytes kill infected cells. Lactoferrin binds iron (preventing pathogens from using it) and aids T and B cell production. The bifidus factor is an intestinal flora that promotes the growth of lactobacilli and maintains the gut pH at an acid level, which inhibits the growth of *E. coli*. Lactoperoxidase is an enzyme that, when combined with IgA, increases the ability to kill streptococcus bacteria. Oligosaccharides are simple chains of sugars that intercept bacteria and block their attachment to the gut epithelium and bind to form harmless substances (Shinskie & Lauwers 2002).
- Bioactive properties—enzymes, lysosomes, lipase, amylase, interferon and fibronectin in breast milk promote growth and development, and infection control (Riordan 2005).
- Anti-allergenic properties—breast milk facilitates early maturation of the intestinal mucosa and reduces allergic responses. There is a protective effect against skin conditions and respiratory illnesses (Bertran et al 2001; Saarinen et al 2000).

Critical thinking exercise

Draw up a table with two columns. List the components of breast milk in the left column and then add the function of each component in the right column.

Hormones and enzymes

Over 70 enzymes have been isolated from human breast milk. An insulin-like factor promotes growth, an epidermal factor aids skin growth, cortisol transports fluids and salts in the gut, thyroxine stimulates the intestine, prostaglandins aid local circulation and mucus secretion, electrolytes balance and protect the gut mucosa, and taurine is a neurotransmitter that aids brain maturation (Riordan 2005).

Worldwide initiatives to promote breastfeeding

Several worldwide primary healthcare initiatives have actively protected, promoted and supported breastfeeding and campaigned against marketing of breast milk substitutes.

World Health Organization

The World Health Organization (WHO) is a specialised agency of the United Nations with a primary responsibility for public health. Its brief extends to the role of maternity services in promoting breastfeeding (Biancuzzo 1999). A joint WHO/United Nations International Children's Emergency Fund (UNICEF) statement, launched in 1989, describes the critical role of health services and outlines steps taken to facilitate the initiation and establishment of breastfeeding (WHO/UNICEF 1989).

The WHO Global Data Bank on breastfeeding developed new breastfeeding indicators and definitions to broaden the nomenclature for describing breastfeeding behaviour and to increase the coherence, reliability and comparability of data. The 'Bank' pools information drawn from surveys and studies dealing with breastfeeding prevalence and duration. This enables comparison of representative data. National, regional and local information gathered on breastfeeding and complementary feeding practices over time provides a reliable database with which to plan promotional programs (WHO 1996).

The WHO Code

An initiative of WHO and UNICEF, the International Code of Marketing of Breastmilk Substitutes (the WHO Code), adopted in 1981, emphasises the fact that human milk and breastfeeding provides an unequalled way of providing nutrients and other biological substances necessary for the growth and development of infants. It aims to protect the wellbeing of infants through the protection and promotion of breastfeeding and ensuring that breast milk substitutes are used only when necessary. Support for and adherence to the Code is an ethical choice for countries, governments, industries, health professional organisations, educators and individuals involved in maternity and newborn care (Young 2001).

The Innocenti Declaration

In 1990 the WHO and UNICEF produced and adopted the Innocenti Declaration, which recognises the uniqueness of breastfeeding and the need to reinforce a breastfeeding culture and mobilise to stop the competition of a bottle-feeding culture. The Declaration stated that all women should be enabled to practise exclusive breastfeeding for four to six months following childbirth. It recommended that all governments implement the WHO Code and develop national breastfeeding targets and policies, and integrate them into overall health and development (Biancuzzo 1999).

In response to the recommendations, the National Health and Medical Research Council (NHMRC) developed guidelines for health workers on infant feeding (Commonwealth Department of Health and Family Services 2001). A national breastfeeding strategy was launched in the same year to provide a multifaceted primary healthcare approach to breastfeeding promotion. This was aimed at health professionals, community agencies and the general public (Commonwealth Department of Health and Aged Care 2001).

International Baby Food Action Network

Growing public and professional concern over commercial and advertising promotion of breast milk substitute foods, feeding bottles and teats encouraged development of the International Baby Food Action Network (IBFAN) (IBFAN 1993).

The network is a coalition of voluntary organisations in industrialised and developing countries working for better health through the promotion of breastfeeding and the elimination of the marketing of artificial infant foods. The IBFAN provides a written guide for health workers about the WHO Code (WHO 1993) and also monitors Code compliance. Code-breaking promotional materials and tactics are still used in systematic and blatant ways by companies that continue to undermine health in pursuit of profits (Advisory Panel in the Marketing in Australia of Baby Formula (APMAIF) 2000).

World Alliance for Breastfeeding Action

In 1990 the United Nations held a world summit for children, at which heads of state promised to work towards the rights of children, including the right to breastfeed. In 1991 groups working on maternal and child health launched the World Alliance for Breastfeeding Action (WABA). IBFAN was one founding member. The WABA group mobilised social support for the Innocenti Declaration and implemented international breastfeeding week activities on an annual basis (IBFAN 1993).

Baby Friendly Hospital Initiative

The UNICEF and the WHO jointly launched the Baby Friendly Hospital Initiative (BFHI) in 1991. This global initiative aims to provide a positive environment that promotes breastfeeding as a natural and normal primary healthcare practice and is based on the role of maternity services in protecting, promoting and supporting breastfeeding.

Ten steps to successful breastfeeding have been articulated to encompass education and counselling of new mothers, unrestricted mother–infant contact, demand and exclusive breastfeeding and maternal support in the postpartum period. Hospitals are challenged and motivated to adhere to these 10 steps when working with mothers and their families. The BFHI aims to increase the worldwide prevalence and duration of breastfeeding (Naylor 2001). The BFHI philosophy is applied universally irrespective of whether a country is developed or developing, or a society Western or traditional (WHO 1992).

The ten steps to successful breastfeeding

Hospital practices are very influential when a new mother and her family are initiating and establishing breastfeeding. Support and encouragement by informed healthcare workers, the reduced influence of artificial feeding practices, keeping mother and infant together and feeding early and frequently by infant-led demand are practices promoted by the BFHI. Successful long-term breastfeeding depends on a successful beginning. Through compliance with the 10 steps to successful breastfeeding, hospitals give mothers the best chance of establishing and maintaining breastfeeding (Philipp & Merwood 2004). The 10 steps are listed in Box 28.1.

Preparation for breastfeeding

Breastfeeding education

Successful breastfeeding depends on the mother's acquisition of basic skills and accurate information. This success is strongly influenced by the quality of help and support provided during the pregnancy, childbirth and the postpartum period. Despite the evidence of the benefits of breastfeeding, many women may choose to use artificial formula, indicating that their decision not to breastfeed may be unrelated to health factors (Earle 2000; Hodinott & Pill 1999).

The maternal decision to breastfeed is based on multiple factors, including knowledge about breastfeeding, personal attitudes and beliefs about breastfeeding, role models and support of significant others. A positive exposure to breastfeeding and observing breastfeeding as a normal event increases a commitment to and confidence in maternal ability

---

BOX 28.1   The 10 steps to successful breastfeeding

Every facility providing maternity services and care for newborn infants should:

1 Have a written policy that is routinely communicated to all healthcare staff.
2 Train all healthcare staff in the skills necessary to implement this policy.
3 Inform all pregnant women about the benefits and management of breastfeeding.
4 Help mothers initiate breastfeeding within an hour of birth.*
5 Show mothers how to breastfeed, and how to maintain lactation even if they are separated from their infants.
6 Give newborn infants no food or drink other than breast milk, unless medically indicated.
7 Practice rooming-in—allow mothers and infants to remain together—24 hours a day.
8 Encourage breastfeeding on demand.
9 Give no artificial teats or pacifiers (also called dummies or soothers) to breastfeeding infants.
10 Foster the establishment of breastfeeding support groups and refer mothers to them on discharge from hospital.

* When written in 1989, this step required breastfeeding initiation within the first half-hour. Research in the 1990s showed that the natural sequence of behaviour is for suckling to occur within the first hour. Therefore this step has been modified in some countries.

(Source: WHO/UNICEF 1989)

Critical thinking exercise

Think about breastfeeding practices that you have seen or implemented in your hospital/health facility. Compare them to the 10 steps listed above.

1   Do they support the 10 steps to successful breastfeeding?
2   How might you initiate a review of those practices?

---

to breastfeed. Decision-making is also related to a favourable attitude by significant others to breastfeeding (Hodinott & Pill 1999).

Antenatal care should include discussion on breastfeeding by the lead carer, covering aspects of attitudes to breastfeeding, expectations, knowledge and experience (family background). A positive attitude to breastfeeding by the health professional can enhance the duration of breastfeeding (Riordan 2005). Women should be informed of the benefits of breastfeeding, the disadvantages of not breastfeeding (that is, using artificial formula) and given the opportunity to discuss their feelings about their breasts and breastfeeding. Teaching mothers the practical skill of positioning and attachment can prepare new mothers and their partners for breastfeeding. (See positioning and attachment below.) The management of breastfeeding, from initiation to maintenance and weaning, infant's normal feeding cues and behaviours, and coping with problems that may arise, should also be covered. Written resources and community services that support breastfeeding are important components of any formal and/or informal breastfeeding education activities. It is also important to include partners in education, as their support and encouragement facilitates successful long-term breastfeeding (Brodribb 2004).

Positioning and attachment

Positioning and attaching a newborn at the breast is a learned and mostly manual skill that is acquired via education, observation and practice (Woolridge 1986). The mother can learn this skill by watching other breastfeeding women. However, breastfeeding is less overt in public and family environments in current times; therefore many mothers have been deprived of this experience (Biancuzzo 1999; RCM 2002). Hospital practices that provide education in and support of positioning and attachment increase the prevalence of breastfeeding (Enkin et al 2000).

Mothers can produce milk and let it flow from the breast when the infant needs it. Newborn infants are able to search for the breast, open the mouth, attach to the breast, suck, swallow and digest the milk for growth and development. The full-term healthy infant comes equipped with three specific, innate reflexes to help obtain breast milk: rooting, suckling and swallowing. The rooting or searching reflex occurs when the infant turns toward a touch on the cheek and lips. The mouth opens into a wide gape with the tongue down and forward, ready to receive the breast tissue. Suckling is the next reflex, which occurs by stimulation of the roof of the mouth with the nipple and breast tissue. The third reflex of swallowing occurs in response to breast milk coming into contact with the back of the throat and soft palate (Day 2004).

What is positioning and attachment?

Positioning refers to the position of the infant relative to the position of the mother. It is the interaction of the mother's and infant's body positions and the infant's mouth-to-breast position that allow for easy attachment. This does not mean that there is only one correct position. Any position that the mother and infant find comfortable that does not interfere with the infant being able to draw adequate breast tissue into the mouth, suck, swallow and breathe is acceptable. Principles

of correct positioning include: a relaxed and comfortable mother, so the breasts fall naturally forward; infant at level of the breast, with support behind the infant's shoulders; neck slightly extended; chest of infant turned towards the chest of mother and chin pointed towards the breast (Inch & Fisher 1999).

Attachment refers to the bringing of the infant to the breast using the rooting reflex to open the infant's mouth widely, and the drawing of the nipple and breast tissue into the mouth to the back of the soft palate. The tongue is forward over the gums but under the areola, with the chin placed on the underside of the breast (Inch & Fisher 1999) (see Fig 28.3).

The early use of cineradiographic techniques and ultrasound by Smith et al (1985) and Weber et al (1986) has helped researchers to learn about the mechanisms of infant feeding at the breast. When an infant is positioned and attached correctly at the breast, the nipple and surrounding breast tissue is drawn into an elongated teat-like shape that extends back to the junction of the hard and soft palate (see Fig 28.4).

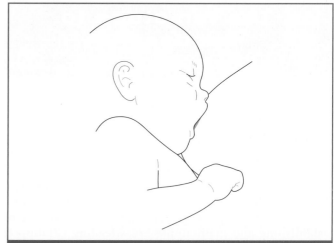

Figure 28.3 Correct attachment, external view (based on Day 2004)

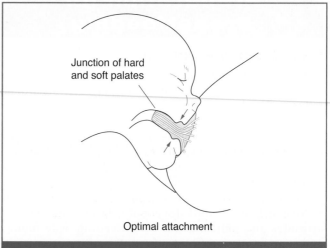

Junction of hard and soft palates

Optimal attachment

Figure 28.4 Correct attachment, internal view (based on Day 2004)

The sides of the tongue cup around the elongated 'teat', forming a central trough. A circular movement of the jaw and compression of milk sinuses milk the breast by the tongue and gums. Milk is propelled out through the nipple openings along the trough via peristaltic movement into the back of the pharynx, ready for swallowing. When the volume of milk is sufficient, swallowing is triggered. The soft palate elevates and closes the nasal area, the larynx closes over the trachea and the milk bolus moves into the oesophagus. The larynx returns to its normal position, closing off the oesophagus behind the milk, and leaves the airway open again. A fresh cycle of compression begins. When the infant is positioned and attached adequately, minimal energy is used and the breast actively ejects the milk. Suckling is free from friction, as there is little movement of the teat (Woolridge 1986).

Correct sucking technique is when the infant has a wide-open mouth, with the tongue under the areola, expressing milk from the breast by slow, deep sucks. When positioning and attachment are correct (optimal) a variation in suckling rate and pattern occurs in response to the milk flow. The first suckles are short, shallow, irregular and fast with short pauses, then the rate changes to a second stage when suckles become slower, stronger, regular and longer as the milk flows. Swallowing can be heard or seen with each or every few sucks. At this time the infant is receiving the foremilk. The third stage of suckling occurs as the feed continues when sucks are again shorter with more pauses. The infant is receiving the hindmilk at this stage. Comfort sucking occurs towards the end of the feed and the infant comes off the breast or falls asleep (Inch & Fisher 1999).

It follows that positioning and attachment plays a crucial role in the successful ejection (let-down) and transfer of milk and stimulation of milk supply. The majority of women give birth in hospital or in the home, with postpartum care provided by midwives in public, private or community settings (NHMRC 2003). Midwives can facilitate the mother's learning of correct positioning and attaching her infant at the breast through education, support and guidance. Conversely, inaccurate or inconsistent breastfeeding advice, or lack of support and guidance, may deter a new mother from breastfeeding.

Practical skills using a hands-off technique

Teaching new mothers the skill of positioning and attachment can assist in the success of breastfeeding initiation. A prevalent method involves using a hands-on technique, where midwives

---

Clinical point

With a family member, friend or colleague, assist them (using verbal interaction and a hands-off technique) to position and attach a doll/bear ready for a breastfeed.

▸ Remember the principles of positioning and attachment.
▸ Think about the language you will use in this interaction.

---

physically assist with positioning and attachment. This does not prepare the mother for confident and independent feeding. Health professionals can describe the process without using their hands. Using verbal and visual strategies (e.g. the use of dolls) to demonstrate these principles during the antenatal period and when initiating breastfeeding empowers mothers to 'do it for themselves' with autonomy and confidence, and this can have a positive effect on breastfeeding duration (Benjamin 1999; Fletcher & Harris 2000; Ingram et al 2002).

Initiation of breastfeeding

Early, frequent and correct sucking aid the physiology of lactation. Early sucking occurs as soon as possible after birth using the alert responses and reflexes of the infant and enhancing maternal feelings. Frequent sucking is maintained through continuous maternal–infant contact as well as demand and exclusive breastfeeding. Correct sucking includes the optimal positioning and attachment of the infant at the breast to aid efficient and sufficient suckling. Through correct positioning and attachment, nerve messages initiate better milk production, and sufficient suckling allows the milk ejection reflex to occur and aids milk transfer from mother to infant (Riordan 2005).

The first feed

Following birth, the infant's interest and responses are at a peak to begin breastfeeding and the mother has a heightened sense of awareness and responsiveness to her infant (Anderson et al 2003). Mother and infant should remain together and not be separated unless medically indicated, in order to maximise the alertness and responsiveness of mother and infant. Weighing, bathing and examination of the infant should be delayed until after the first feed (NHMRC 2003). However, feeding immediately after birth is not essential for successful initiation of breastfeeding. If a breastfeed does not eventuate then skin-to-skin contact at this time is reported to have a significant and positive effect on breastfeeding duration (Anderson et al 2003), although a recent systematic review does not indicate such a positive effect on timing of the first feed and highlights the need for further research (Carfoot et al 2003).

Healthy newborns placed on their mother's abdomen or chest demonstrate an ability to search for and touch the breast and nipple using their five senses. Washing the skin of the mother or infant before the first feed can interfere with these senses. Mothers should be supported to breastfeed preferably within an hour of giving birth. When infant cues of mouthing, hand–mouth movements and rooting are noted, the midwife can assist the mother to encourage her infant to the breast using the principles of correct positioning and attachment. The infant's sucking reflex is very active at this time (Lawrence 1999).

Breastfeeding will stimulate the release of oxytocin and initiate the let-down reflex, with the infant receiving colostrum. A positive experience of the first breastfeed can enhance maternal confidence (Riordan 2005). Partner presence during this time also helps establish a positive breastfeeding relationship. When the first feed is delayed (due to mother or infant needing medical attention) or if the infant is not interested in feeding due to the effect of maternal medication, the first feed should then be timed as soon as possible (Brodribb 2004).

Subsequent feeds

Following the alert period it is common for babies to be sleepy for some 24 hours as a consequence of labour and birth. Most babies begin to seek feeds frequently after their sleepy episode (NHMRC 2003). The correct principles of positioning and attachment should be reinforced at each subsequent feed, promoting the mother's confidence in her ability.

Demand feeding

Ideally, babies should be fed when they exhibit a quiet alert state of behaviour. Mothers can learn their infant's sleep–wake cycles and learn to identify the best time for feeding. It is difficult to feed an infant who is sleepy, and an infant who is crying is difficult to attach to the breast. The quiet alert state facilitates easier breastfeeding. Feeds should not be regimented by clock time, as this may not match the infant's wakefulness and may lead to reduced sucking, reduced breast stimulation and supply, and engorgement (Brodribb 2004). Demand feeding also encourages the passage of meconium and lessens the infant's weight loss (NHMRC 2003).

Unrestricted feeding

The length of a feed should be determined by the infant's needs. Variations in breast anatomy lead to variations in storage capacity and rate of milk flow. Infant-led feeding allows the infant to regulate intake according to their need (Ramsay et al 2002).

Frequency of breastfeeding for a term healthy newborn ranges from 8 to 12 feeds in a 24-hour period, with intervals varying from every hour or two during the day to a couple of times during the night. The infant will eventually develop a pattern of feeding across the day by four to six weeks of age.

Reducing sucking time or frequency of breastfeeding will reduce stimulation of milk supply and lead to engorgement (RCM 2002). Unlimited sucking at the breast also improves breastfeeding, with the infant receiving both foremilk and the higher-fat hindmilk (Shinskie & Lauwers 2002). Mothers should be encouraged to observe and interpret when their infant is satisfied. Limiting the length of a feed can result in a higher intake of foremilk and less intake of hindmilk, leading to reduced satiety and poor weight gain. It is recommended for the same reason that an infant be allowed to finish feeding on the first breast before offering the other side.

Rooming in

Keeping mother and infant continuously together from birth helps initiate breastfeeding. Mothers learn to understand their infant's cues and behaviours and how to handle the infant. This increases maternal confidence and bonding, and promotes milk supply with unrestricted access to the breast and regular stimulation (Shinskie & Lauwers 2002).

Exclusive breastfeeding

Exclusive breastfeeding ensures that the infant receives the full nutritional and protective benefits of breast milk. Full-term healthy babies do not require additional fluids. Additional fluids can interfere with sucking, and reduce the frequency of sucking at the breast, leading to reduced stimulation and inadequate initiation of breastfeeding. In addition, the mother may feel unable to provide for her infant's needs and lose confidence in her ability to breastfeed (NHMRC 2003). Infants are more likely to be weaned earlier when not exclusively breastfed. Furthermore, a Cochrane Systematic Review indicates that exclusively breastfed infants are healthier than infants who are mixed-fed, in both developing and developed countries (Kramer & Kakuma 2004).

Pacifier use

There is a strong association between daily exposure to pacifier use and breastfeeding duration (Kramer et al 2001), especially if there is frequent exposure before six weeks post partum (Howard et al 1999). Pacifier use may reduce breastfeeding episodes (frequency and duration) during a 24-hour period, therefore reducing breast stimulation and supply (Howard et al 1999). Mothers may also feel less motivated to breastfeed if a pacifier soothes a fussy baby (Bennis 2002). Pacifier use is therefore not recommended during the initiation of breastfeeding.

Maintenance of breastfeeding

Healthy newborns show signs of hunger, although the interval between feeds varies considerably. Some babies will want

---

Reflective exercise

1　Think about infant cues other than crying that may indicate readiness for a breastfeed.
2　How would you know if an infant was satisfied after a feed?

Reflective exercise

Take some time to reflect on your breastfeeding experiences/views of breastfeeding.

How do you think this affects the way you practise, especially when assisting a women with a breastfeed?

feeding every one and a half to two hours, whereas others may feed every four hours. During the early months, many babies do what is called 'cluster feeding', spacing feeds closer together at certain times of the day (typically in the evening) and going longer between feeds at other times of the day. When a baby suddenly wants to feed more often, it is called a growth spurt. These commonly occur around two or three weeks, six weeks and three months (Mohrbacher & Stock 2003).

Breast storage capacity is an important determinant of how often a baby's demand for milk is met. Women who have small breasts are still capable of producing as much milk over a 24-hour period as a woman with large breasts; however, the storage capacity is not as great and therefore her infant might need to feed more frequently (Ramsay et al 2002). If a mother is concerned about her milk supply, review the following points with her:

- How often and for how long is the baby feeding? Expect a minimum of 8–12 feeds in 24 hours and 15–20 minutes on the first breast, and 10–15 minutes on the second breast, but the baby may be satisfied after only one breast.
- The baby should have at least three bowel movements each 24 hours, and by day 4 these should be yellow, soft and of a watery consistency.
- The baby should have at least six wet napkins a day by day 4, and the urine should look clear, not dark and concentrated.
- Expect < 7% weight loss in the first week.
- Expect return to birthweight by day 14.
- Expect weight gain of 120–240 g a week until the baby's birthweight has doubled (International Lactation Consultant Association 1999, pp 21–22).

Many babies continue to have frequent bowel movements for as long as they are exclusively breastfed. However, some babies, from about six weeks of age, have bowel movements only once a week, and as long as this is plentiful in amount and remains soft in texture then this is not of concern (Mohrbacher & Stock 2003).

A breastfeeding mother should be encouraged to eat a well-balanced and varied diet. The recommended energy intake during breastfeeding is an additional 500 calories a day during the first six months and then reduced to 400 calories as milk production decreases (Lawrence 1999; Picciano 2003).

There is no scientific basis for the concern that gassy foods cause gas in the breastfed baby. The normal intestinal flora produces gas from the action on fibre in the intestinal tract; however, gas and fibre are not present in breast milk (Lawrence 1999). Extensive clinical experience does suggest that some babies do not tolerate certain foods in a mother's diet. If a mother questions the effect of a certain food on her baby, then Lawrence (1999) suggests that the mother watch the baby for colic for 24 hours post ingestion.

Some mothers are concerned that exercise might interfere with their milk supply. However, moderate exercise should not affect the milk supply or the baby's reaction to it (Riordan 2005).

> ## Critical thinking exercise
>
> Tricia is six weeks old and exclusively breastfed. Mary is concerned that she has insufficient milk supply, as Tricia is now unsettled and seems hungry all the time.
> 1   What may be happening here?
> 2   How would you help Mary?

Management of problems

With appropriate support and guidance, most common problems associated with breastfeeding can be prevented. Problems are likely to occur when the normal physiological process is interrupted, by the baby not attaching correctly to the breast, or incorrect advice, or imposed rules and regulations interrupting the normal breastfeeding process.

Early recognition and treatment of problems when they occur is required in order to preserve the breastfeeding experience for the mother and baby. For many problems, practitioners use interventions based on clinical experience rather than research; however, any interventions and treatments that are recommended should be evidence-based. Careful assessment of the situation and a plan of management should be drawn up in partnership with the mother.

Sore or damaged nipples

During the early breastfeeding experience, tenderness of the nipples is normal. As the collagen fibres are stretched in early suckling, women may feel nipple discomfort, which peaks between day 3 and day 6. Protracted nipple tenderness, or that which lasts throughout a feed, is not normal. If a mother complains of pain during breastfeeding then something is not right.

Lawrence (1999) describes common causes of nipple pain as:

- poor positioning
- nipple sucking
- nipple tipped up too much because of finger pressure above the nipple
- infant's lower lip sucked in and irritating the underside of the nipple
- taking the infant off the breast without first breaking the suction.

Riordan (2005) adds to this:

- an infant with a disorganised suck
- ankyloglossia (tongue tie)
- engorgement
- sensitivity to nipple creams
- flat or retracted nipples
- prolonged exposure to wet nipple pads
- infection or thrush.

Tait (2000) suggests that discussing latching techniques and signs of improper positioning with women during the antenatal period and again after birth may assist them in recognising the problem before damage occurs. When skilled staff are not available to assist with breastfeeding then this knowledge would be important. Breastfeeding is a two-person activity, so both mother and infant need to be considered when undertaking an assessment to identify the cause of the nipple pain.

Management will involve supporting the mother and reassuring her that this will be a self-limiting problem. Observation of a breastfeed and correcting the positioning and attachment, if necessary, may be all that is required to correct the problem. Practical suggestions may include: applying warm compresses to the breasts before feeding to stimulate the milk flow; if the breast is engorged, hand expressing some milk to make the areola softer; beginning each feed on the less sore breast; changing breast pads frequently; and expressing milk onto the nipples after a feed.

There is little evidence that nipple creams or ointments either heal or relieve soreness of nipples. Recent research suggests that the most effective treatment is warm water (Lavergne, cited in Tait 2000). However, as most applications are relatively harmless and new mothers like to use them so they feel something is being done, it may be more harmful to deny their use if a woman wishes to do so. If women choose to use cream or ointment on their nipples, they should be advised to apply it to the nipple only, as the Montgomery glands on the areola may become blocked, inhibiting the secretion of the natural oils that help maintain elasticity of the nipples.

Resting the nipple by not feeding from the breast should only be recommended if the pain of sucking is intolerable to the mother or when any bleeding or damage is worsening. Remember that while the baby is not suckling on the breast, the milk must be removed either by hand expressing or by pumping. When the baby returns to the breast, attention must be given to positioning and attachment.

Breast fullness versus engorgement

Engorgement is almost always a preventable complication of breastfeeding. Lawrence (1999) describes engorgement as having three elements:
* congestion and increased vascularity, which is the physiological response that follows removal of the placenta and does not depend on suckling
* accumulation of milk, also a physiological response
* oedema secondary to the swelling and obstruction of drainage of the lymphatic system by vascular increases and fullness of the alveoli.

Critical thinking exercise

Jemma is three weeks old and 50 grams above her birthweight. Jemma's mother Grace has a right cracked nipple and wants to wean Jemma. You observe a blister on Jemma's top lip.
How would you respond to this situation?

When this physiological process proceeds normally, it rarely lasts more than 24 hours. During this time, the mother's breasts will be full but the tissue will remain compressible, and the infant should be able to suck efficiently without trauma to the breast or nipple (Riordan 2005). If feeds are restricted, or there is poor attachment and inefficient sucking leading to incomplete removal of milk, then what was a normal process will lead to pathological engorgement. It can also occur when breastfeeding is ceased abruptly or when weaning foods are introduced.

If the milk is not removed, over-distension of the alveoli can cause the milk-secreting cells to flatten out and even rupture. The over-distension puts pressure on the surrounding tissue, exacerbating the problem by occluding the blood capillaries. This can lead to increased arterial pressure to the breasts and compression of the connective tissue, impeding drainage of the lymph fluid from the breast, which then leads to oedema (Snowden et al 2001).

When there is milk stasis, a protein called the feedback inhibitor of lactation accumulates in the breast. The accumulation of milk in the breast and the resulting engorgement are a trigger for apoptosis, or programmed cell death, which causes involution of the milk-secreting gland, milk reabsorption, collapse of the alveolar structures, and the cessation of milk production (Smith & Heads 2002).

To prevent breast engorgement there should be no delay in initiating breastfeeding, and effective positioning. Also, transfer of milk should be ensured and unrestricted breastfeeding should be promoted.

There are many suggested treatments for engorgement, including application of heat, ice packs, cabbage leaves, massage, ultrasound and frequent feeding. The Cochrane Systematic Review of treatments for breast engorgement during lactation (Snowden et al 2001) found that anti-inflammatory drugs were the most effective treatment tested. Although widely used, cabbage leaves were found to be no more effective than gel packs in relieving symptoms.

Expressing milk may be necessary to prevent the build-up of the feedback inhibitor of lactation and decrease the risk of mastitis and compromised milk production, and to give comfort to the mother.

Blocked milk ducts (plugged ducts)

There is sometimes no obvious cause of a blocked milk duct, but it may be the result of incomplete emptying of a lobe in the breast due to ineffective positioning and attachment of the baby at the breast, or an oversupply, or external pressure on the breast. This may be from finger pressure during a feed, a tight bra, sleeping prone, or straps from a baby carrier (NMAA 1999; Riordan 2005). The mother may complain of a tender lump in her breast, which may or may not be reddened, in the absence of a fever.

Assessment should include observing the mother–infant pair during a breastfeed to ensure correct positioning and attachment. The mother should be encouraged to continue to breastfeed often, applying moist heat to and massaging the affected area before and during breastfeeding. Positioning the baby so that the chin is pointing to the area of the lump will encourage better drainage from that area.

Lawrence (1999) describes improvement in women with repeated blocked ducts by limiting the mother to polyunsaturated fats and adding lecithin to her diet. If blocked ducts are left untreated, mastitis may develop.

Mastitis

Mastitis is an inflammatory condition of the breast, which may or may not be accompanied by infection. The initial cause of mastitis is an unresolved increase in the intraductal pressure, first causing a flattening of the secretory cells; a paracellular pathway then may occur between the cells, allowing the passage of some of the components in breast milk to leak into the interstitial tissue, resulting in an inflammatory response. This inflammatory response and the resultant tissue damage can be a precursor of infective mastitis (Smith & Heads 2002).

The WHO (2000) states that the two principal causes of mastitis are milk stasis and infection. Milk stasis occurs when milk is not effectively drained from the breast, as in untreated engorgement or blocked ducts, poor attachment of the baby to the breast, restriction or alteration of the frequency or duration of feeds, or an overabundant milk supply. Cracked or damaged nipples are thought to provide a portal of entry for pathogenic organisms.

The woman will present with sudden onset of flu-like symptoms, aches, chills, a fever and a red, hot, painful area on the breast, usually on the upper outer quadrant.

The WHO (2000) lists the main principles of treatment as:

- supportive counselling
- effective milk removal
- antibiotic therapy
- symptomatic treatment.

As mastitis is painful and the woman feels ill (flu-like chills and headache), she will require support and encouragement to continue to breastfeed. Reassure the woman that the breast milk is safe for her baby and that the breast will recover.

Effective removal of the milk

This is the essential part of treatment. If necessary, assist the mother to improve attachment of the baby to the breast and encourage frequent breastfeeding, as often and for as long as the infant is willing. If the woman is unable to have the baby feed from the breast, then breast milk must be expressed by hand or by pump until such time as the baby may return to the breast.

Antibiotic treatment

Staphylococcus aureus is the most common causative organism associated with mastitis. Antibiotics should be prescribed when:

- symptoms are severe from the beginning
- a nipple fissure is present, or

- symptoms do not improve after 12–24 hours of improved milk removal.

To be effective against *S. aureus* a penicillinase-resistant penicillin or a cephalosporin should be prescribed. Lawrence (1999) states that the antibiotic course should be 10–14 days, as shorter courses are associated with a high incidence of relapse.

Symptomatic treatment includes treating the pain associated with mastitis. Ibuprofen is considered to be effective as both a pain reliever and an anti-inflammatory.

Other measures to recommend are rest, increased fluids, and warm compresses on the affected breast to encourage milk flow. Delayed or inadequate treatment of mastitis can lead to abscess formation.

Flat or inverted nipples

Although the frequency of flat or inverted nipples is unknown, they can present a challenge to successful breastfeeding. Gunther (cited in Wilson-Clay & Hoover 2002) theorised that infants expect protractile nipple tissue that is sufficiently elastic to pull deeply into the oral cavity. Contact along the tongue and at a zone near where the hard and soft palate merge is necessary to stimulate the sucking reflex. In many cases the degree of inversion is such that it does not affect the ability of the baby to grasp the areola tissue and draw the nipple into the mouth, and so does not cause a problem.

Two commonly suggested antenatal interventions to stretch the nipples are Hoffmann exercises (stretching and pulling the nipple and areola) and wearing of breast shells (plastic discs with holes in the centre and a domed cover). Studies have failed to find any significant value in either of these interventions (Brodribb 2004).

The most effective intervention for treating flat or inverted nipples is to stimulate and shape the nipple just before breastfeeding. This can be done by hand massage, using the pump or a modified syringe. Select a 10 or 20 cc syringe, depending on the nipple diameter, remove the plunger and cut off the nozzle-end of the syringe barrel. Reinsert the syringe plunger into the barrel from the cut end, so it is away from the mother's nipple. The mother then applies the device to her nipple and pulls gently on the plunger to create suction (Kesaree et al 1993).

Pumping and breastfeeding will usually pull out flat or inverted nipples in a few days, a few weeks or sometimes months. If the baby remains unable to latch directly on to the breast despite efforts to evert the nipple, then consideration should be given to using a nipple shield.

Ankyloglossia (tongue-tie)

Ankyloglossia (commonly known as tongue-tie) is a congenital condition characterised by the lingual frenulum (the tissue that attaches the tongue to the floor of the mouth) being too short, too tight, or attached to the tip of the tongue, which causes the tongue to appear heart-shaped when protrusion is attempted. The forward motion of the tongue is restricted, causing it to thicken and turn downward, making it difficult to initiate the characteristic peristaltic wave that milks the ductules (Riordan 2005). It is a hereditary condition and the mother, father or another close relative of the infant may also have the same condition, which is more common in boys than girls (Messner & Lalakea 2000; O'Shea 2002).

The degree of ankyloglossia varies and although it is not always a cause for concern, the condition does represent a significant proportion of breastfeeding problems. Poor infant latch, maternal nipple pain, poor milk supply, mastitis and slow infant weight gain are frequently associated with this finding. Careful assessment, followed by frenotomy when indicated, seems to be successful in facilitating continued breastfeeding (Ballard et al 2002; O'Shea 2002). However, ankyloglossia in the newborn is the subject of ongoing controversy among various professionals as well as specialty groups (Messner & Lalakea 2000).

Is artificial feeding OK? A critique

Artificial feeding is often seen as a safe, easy alternative to breastfeeding, but there are risks. However, breast milk is a living tissue that cannot be duplicated by any other means. Infants who are artificially fed are disadvantaged due to constituents of the substitutes and also by factors associated with their manufacture (Minchin 2000; RCM 2002).

Nutrients in artificial formula can be lacking, deficient or excessive (RCM 2002). Cow's milk protein is casein-dominant, and so takes longer to digest. The fat is either butterfat or mixtures of vegetable oils with fatty acid composition very different from that of human milk. Infant formula also lacks many living cells, cholesterol, free amino acids, glycosamine, polyamines, enzymes and other bioactive substances (NHMRC 2003). Long chain polyunsaturated fatty acids are important for nervous system development, specifically in the brain and retina. They are also precursors of other substances needed for renal function, allergenic and inflammatory reactions. Breast milk contains these fatty acids and precursors needed for body processes but formula-fed babies require dietary supplements to match this component (Clandinin et al 1999; Sellmayer & Koletzko 1999). The sterilisation of formula modifies the protein structure, although allergenicity of the protein is reduced (NHMRC 2003).

Breast milk constituents change constantly throughout lactation, during a feed and during the day. The high bioavailability of micronutrients ensures that the infant receives the nutrition needed at that specific time. Infants can control their caloric intake by altering their sucking pattern. The composition of manufactured milk is homogenous and cannot change and is therefore less adaptable to the infant's needs (Shinskie & Lauwers 2002).

Although the benefits of breast milk and breastfeeding are widely recognised, the hazards of artificial feeding are less so. Randomised controlled trials involving artificial feeding are not ethically appropriate with term babies (RCM 2002). The health risks of manufactured infant milks are confirmed by epidemiological research over time, by a higher incidence and severity of illnesses and diseases and increased mortality and morbidity. Gut flora can be changed as a result of ingestion of formula sensitising the infant to cow's milk proteins and gastric-related illnesses. A reduction in personal health outcomes for both mother and infant and an increase in healthcare costs results (Ball & Bennett 2001; Bick 1999).

Safe bottle-feeding requires a safe water supply, hygienic surroundings and practices for preparation, adequate refrigeration, bottles and teats and a method of sterilising the equipment, as well as the formula itself and the ability to understand the instructions for preparation. Overheating of formula can also cause burns to the mouth and throat. Although breastfeeding is the optimal infant feeding method, when there is no alternative other than using formula, the quality and composition of manufactured milk is regulated, although potentially hazardous. The artificial formula may also be contaminated with aluminium, hydrocarbons and bacteria (NHMRC 2003).

Breast milk is a convenient, inexpensive food source posing no environmental cost. Conversely, infant formula and infant feeding bottles are costly for the family and community in terms of production and energy requirements, purchase of bottles, teats and formula and waste disposal (Biancuzzo 1999; Riordan 2005).

Breast milk may be affected by maternal medications, as most pass from the maternal plasma into the milk, although there is little evidence of harm to the infant (Hale 2002). The exceptions to this are the hepatitis B and C viruses and the human immunodeficiency virus. The WHO still recommends exclusive breastfeeding in the first months when artificial feeding is not safe, feasible, sustainable or affordable (WHO 2000). Supplementation of breastfeeding with artificial formula may interfere with the establishment of breastfeeding, although the effects of established breastfeeding mixed with infant formula are less clear (Enkin et al 2000).

Review questions

1 What are the advantages of breastfeeding?

2 What are the disadvantages of artificial feeding?

3 Where is the female breast located and what are the main structures?

4 What are three worldwide measures that promote breastfeeding?

5 What are the ten steps to successful breastfeeding?

6 What are the main components of breast milk?

7 How does the lactating breast function?

8 What is the milk ejection reflex and how does it function?

9 What strategies would you use to assist a new mother to initiate breastfeeding?

10 What hospital practices support breastfeeding initiation and continuation?

11 What common problems can be encountered during breastfeeding, and what recommended strategies would you use to manage them?

12 When do infants have growth spurts and what effect can they have?

Online resources

Australian Breastfeeding Association, http://www.breastfeeding.asn.au

Baby Friendly Hospital Initiative, http://www.bfhi.org.au

Children, Youth and Women's Health Service, 'Child and Youth Health', http://www.cyh.com.au

International Lactation Association, http://www.ilca.com

National Health and Medical Research Council Dietary Guidelines for Children and Adolescents, http://www.nhmrc.gov.au/publications/synopses/dietsyn.htm

References

Advisory Panel on the Marketing in Australia of Infant Formula (APMAIF) 2000 Annual report 1999–2000. Panther, Canberra

Anderson G, Moore E, Hepworth J et al 2003 Early skin-to-skin contact for mothers and their healthy newborn infants. Cochrane Review. Cochrane Library (3). John Wiley & Sons, Chichester

Anderson J, Johnstone B, Remley D 1999 Breastfeeding and cognitive development: a meta-analysis. American Journal of Clinical Nutrition 70:525–535

Angelsen N, Vik T, Jacobsen G et al 2001 Breast feeding and cognitive development at age 1 and 5 years. Archives of Diseases in Childhood 85(3):183–188

Armstrong J, Reilly J 2002 Breastfeeding and lowering the risk of childhood obesity. Lancet 359:2003–2004

Ball T, Bennett D 2001 The economic impact of breastfeeding. Pediatric Clinics of North America 48(1):253–265

Ballard J, Auer C, Khoury J 2002 Ankyloglossia: assessment incidence and effect of frenuloplasty on the breastfeeding dyad. Paediatrics 110(5):63–70

Benjamin M 1999 Survey of infant feeding practices in Warwickshire 1997/8. Clinical Effectiveness Department, Warwick

Bennis M 2002 Are pacifiers associated with early weaning from breastfeeding? Advances in Neonatal Care 2(5):259–266

Bertran A, Onis M, Lauer J et al 2001 Ecological study of effect of breastfeeding on infant mortality in Latin America. British Medical Journal 323(7308):303–306

Biancuzzo M 1999 Breastfeeding the newborn: clinical strategies for nurses. Mosby, St Louis

Bick D 1999 The benefits of breastfeeding. British Journal of Midwifery 7(5):312–319

Blackburn S 2003 Maternal fetal and neonatal physiology. Saunders, Philadelphia

Brodribb W 2000 Breastfeeding—the natural advantage. Nursing Mothers Association of Australia Newsletter 36(1):4–5

Brodribb W 2004 Breastfeeding management (3rd edn). Australian Breastfeeding Association (ABA), Ligare

Campbell C 2000 Childhood obesity: breastfeeding is important. British Medical Journal (letters) 320(7246):1401–1403

Carfoot S, Williamson P, Dickson R 2003 A systematic review of randomized controlled trials evaluating the effect of mother/baby skin-to-skin care on successful breastfeeding Midwifery 19:148–155

Clandinin M, van Aerde J, Parrott A et al 1999 Assessment of feeding different amounts of arachidonic and docosahexaenoic acids in preterm infant formulas on the fatty acid content of lipoprotein lipids. Acta Paediatrica 88:890–896

Commonwealth Department of Health and Aged Care 2001 National breastfeeding strategy. AGPS, Canberra

Commonwealth Department of Health and Family Services 2001 Naturally: the facts about breastfeeding. A companion document to the NHMRC infant feeding guidelines for health workers. AGPS, Canberra

Day J 2004 Breastfeeding … naturally. Australian Breastfeeding Association, East Malvern, Victoria

Earle S 2000 Why some women do not breast feed: bottle feeding and father's role. Midwifery 16(4):323–330

Enkin M, Keirse M, Neilson J et al 2000 A guide to effective pregnancy and childbirth (3rd edn). Oxford University Press, Oxford

Fletcher D, Harris H 2000 The implementation of the HOT program at the Royal Women's Hospital. Breastfeeding Review 8(1):19–22

Hale T 2002 Medications and mother's milk (10th edn). Pharmasoft, Amarillo

Hodinott P, Pill R 1999 Qualitative study of decisions about feeding among women in east end of London. British Medical Journal 318(7175):30–34

Horwood L, Darlow B, Mogridge N 2001 Breast milk feeding and cognitive ability at 7–8 years. Archives of Diseases in Childhood, Fetal and Neonatal Edition 84: F23–F27

Howard C, Howard F, Lanphear B et al 1999 The effects of early pacifier use on breastfeeding duration. Pediatrics 1033:E33

Inch S, Fisher C 1999 Breastfeeding: getting the basics right. The Practising Midwife 2(5):35–38

Ingram J, Johnson D, Greenwood R 2002 Breastfeeding in Bristol: teaching good positioning and support from fathers and families. Midwifery 18:87–101

International Baby Food Network (IFBAN) 1993 Protecting infant health. Penang, Malaysia

International Lactation Consultant Association (ILCA) 1999 Evidence-based guidelines for breastfeeding management during the first fourteen days. ILCA, USA

Jones G, Riley M, Dwyer T 2000 Breastfeeding in early life and bone mass in prepubertal children: a longitudinal study. Osteoporosis International 11:146–152

Kesaree N, Banapurmath CR, Banapurmath S et al 1993 Treatment of inverted nipples using a disposable syringe. Journal of Human Lactation 9(1):27–29

Kramer M, Barr R, Dagenais S et al 2001 Pacifier use, early weaning and cry/fuss behavior: a randomised trial. Journal of the American Medical Association 286(3):322–326

Kramer M, Kakuma R 2004 Optimal duration of exclusive breastfeeding. Cochrane Review. Cochrane Library (3). John Wiley & Sons, Chichester

Lawrence R 1999 Breastfeeding: a guide for health professionals (5th edn). Mosby, St Louis

Lutter C 2000 Breastfeeding promotion—its effectiveness supported by evidence and global changes in breastfeeding behaviors. Advances in Experimental Medicine and Biology 478:355–368

McVea K, Turner P, Peppler D 2000 The role of breastfeeding in sudden infant death syndrome. Journal of Human Lactation 16(1):13–20

Messner A, Lalakea M 2000 Ankyloglossia: controversies in management. International Journal of Otorhinolaryngology 54(2/3):123–131

Minchin M 2000 Artificial feeding and use—the last taboo. Practising Midwife 3(3):18–20

Mohrbacher N, Stock J 2003 The breastfeeding answer book (3rd edn). La Leche League International, USA

Mortensen E, Michaelsen K, Sanders S et al 2002 The association between duration of breastfeeding and adult intelligence. Journal of the American Medical Association 287:2365–2371

National Health and Medical Research Council (NHMRC) 2003 Infant feeding guidelines for health workers. Commonwealth of Australia, Canberra

Naylor A 2001 Baby-friendly Hospital Initiative. Paediatric Clinics of North America 48(2):475–483

Nursing Mothers Association of Australia (NMAA) 1999 Best practice guide to common breastfeeding problems. Commonwealth of Australia, Canberra

O'Shea M 2002 Licking the problem of tongue-tie. British Journal of Midwifery 10(2):90–92

Oddy W 2001 Breastfeeding protects against illnesses and infection in infants and children: a review of the evidence. Breastfeeding Review 9(2):11–18

Oddy W 2002 The impact of breast milk on infant and child health. Breastfeeding Review 10(3):5–18

Owen C, Whincup P, Odoki K et al 2002 Infant feeding and blood cholesterol: a study in adolescents and a systematic review. Pediatrics 110:597–608

Philipp B, Merwood A 2004 The baby-friendly way: the best breastfeeding start. Pediatric Clinics of North America 51:761–783

Picciano M 2003 Pregnancy and lactation: physiological adjustments, nutritional requirements and the role of dietary supplements. Journal of Nutrition 133(6):S1997

Quinn P, O'Callaghan M, Williams G et al 2001 The effect of breastfeeding on child development at 5 years: a cohort study. Journal of Paediatrics and Child Health 37(5):465–469

Ramsay D, Kent J, Hartman P 2002 Ultrasound imaging of the anatomy of the lactating human breast. Proceedings of the Perinatal Society of Australia and New Zealand, Christchurch, March

Richards M, Hardy R, Wadsworth M 2002 Long term effects of breastfeeding in a national birth cohort: educational attainment and midlife cognitive functioning. Public Health and Nutrition 5(5):631–635

Riordan J 2005 Breastfeeding and human lactation (3rd edn). Jones & Bartlett, Boston

Royal College of Midwives (RCM) 2002 Successful breastfeeding (3rd edn). Churchill Livingstone, London

Saarinen K, Juntunen-Backman K, Jarvenpaa L et al 2000 Breastfeeding and the development of cow's milk allergy. Advances in Experimental Medicine and Biology 478:121–130

Sellmayer A, Koletzko B 1999 Long-chain polyunsaturated fatty acids and eicoanoids in infants—physiological and pathophysiological aspects and open questions. Lipids 34:1999–2005

Shinskie D, Lauwers J 2002 Pocket guide for counseling the nursing mother. Jones & Bartlett, Boston

Singhal A, Cole T, Lucas A 2001 Early nutrition in preterm infants and later blood pressure: two cohorts after randomized trial. Lancet 357:413–419

Smith A, Heads J 2002 Breast pathology. In: M Walker (Ed) Core curriculum for lactation consultant practice. Jones and Bartlett, Sudbury, pp 175–201

Smith W, Erenburg A, Nowak A et al 1985 Physiology of sucking in the normal term infant using real time. Radiology 156(2):379–381

Snowden HM, Renfrew MJ, Woolridge MW 2001 Treatments for breast engorgement during lactation. Cochrane Review. Cochrane Library (2). John Wiley & Sons, Chichester

Stables D, Rankin J (Eds) 2004 Physiology in childbearing (2nd edn). Elsevier, Edinburgh

Tait P 2000 Nipple pain in breastfeeding women: causes, treatment and prevention strategies. Journal of Midwifery and Women's Health 45(3):212–215

von Kries R, Koletzko B, Sauerwald T et al 1999 Breast feeding and obesity: cross sectional study. British Medical Journal 319:147–150

Weber F, Woolridge M, Baum J 1986 An ultrasonographic study of the organisation of sucking and swallowing in newborn infants. Developmental Medicine and Child Neurology 28(1):19–24

Wilson-Clay B, Hoover K 2002 The breastfeeding atlas (2nd edn). Lactation News Press, Texas

Woolridge M 1986 The etiology of sore nipples. Midwifery 2(4):172–176

World Health Organization (WHO) 1993 Protecting infant health: a health worker's guide to the international code of marketing of breastmilk substitutes (7th edn). IBFAN, Malaysia

World Health Organization (WHO) 1996 WHO global data bank on breast feeding: the best start in life. Nutrition Unit, WHO, Geneva

World Health Organization (WHO) 2000 Mastitis: causes and management. WHO Department of Child and Adolescent Health and Development, Geneva

World Health Organization (WHO) 2001 The optimal duration of exclusive breastfeeding. Press Release 7. WHO, Geneva

World Health Organization(WHO)/UNICEF 1989 Protecting promoting and supporting breast-feeding: the special role of maternity services. WHO, Geneva

World Health Organization (WHO) /United Nations International Children's Emergency Fund (UNICEF) 1992 Baby friendly hospital initiative. Part II, hospital level implementation. WHO/ UNICEF guidelines. WHO/UNICEF, Geneva

Young D 2001 Violating 'The Code': breastfeeding ethics and choices. Birth 28(2):77–78

Zheng T, Duan L, Liu Y et al 2000 Prolonged lactation reduces breast cancer risk in Shandong Province, China. American Journal of Epidemiology 152(12):1129–1135

Further reading

International Lactation Consultant Association 1999 Evidence-based guidelines for breastfeeding management during the first fourteen days. ILCA, USA

La Leche League International Inc 2003 The breastfeeding answer book (3rd edn). Schaumburg, Ill.

Oddy W 2000 Breastfeeding and asthma in children: findings from a Western Australian study. Breastfeeding Review 8(1):5–11

Riordan J 2005 Breastfeeding and human lactation (3rd edn). Jones & Bartlett, Boston

Royal College of Midwives (RCM) 2002 Successful breastfeeding (3rd edn). Churchill Livingstone, London

WHO Collaborative Study Team on the Role of Breastfeeding on the Prevention of Infant Mortality 2000 Effect of breastfeeding on infant and child mortality due to infectious diseases in less developed countries: a pooled analysis. Lancet 355:451–455

CHAPTER 29

Pharmacology and prescribing

Marion Hunter and Jackie Gunn

Key terms

agonist, antagonist, bacterial resistance, bioavailability, dependent prescribing, half-life, hepatic first pass, independent prescribing, loading dose, maximum safe concentration, minimum effective concentration, NSAIDs, pharmacodynamics, pharmacokinetics, steady state, therapeutic range

Chapter overview

In this chapter, the scope of midwifery practice is discussed with respect to independent prescribing. Prescribing for women during pregnancy and lactation requires particular caution, as nearly all drugs transfer to the fetus or neonate. Pharmacological concepts are reviewed, as this understanding is essential for the administration or prescription of pharmaceuticals. Antimicrobials used during childbirth are considered in light of increasing concerns over bacterial resistance. Common conditions prescribed for in pregnancy are also discussed, and evidence-based practice is considered in order to inform the prescription of medicines. In concluding this chapter, guidelines are given for midwife prescribers and for accurate prescription writing.
Limitations of this chapter: The authors assume that readers have prior pharmacology knowledge and a comprehensive knowledge of normal and complicated childbirth. The discussion in this chapter is limited to

pharmaceutical medicines and does not cover the use of complementary or non-pharmaceutical therapies. The authors acknowledge that prescription of medicines is always evolving according to research, availability of pharmaceuticals and cost. Midwife prescribers have an obligation to maintain a current knowledge of the safety of medicines in pregnancy and lactation, and of preferred pharmaceuticals for particular conditions.

Learning outcomes

Learning outcomes for this chapter are:

1   To discuss the scope of midwifery practice in relation to prescribing medicines and the legislation associated with the prescription of medicines

2   To revise pharmacological concepts that inform the prescription of medicines and discuss the safety of drugs in pregnancy

3   To review the action and use of antimicrobials in relation to midwifery practice, in particular midwifery responsibility for minimising bacterial resistance

4   To examine the evidence in relation to accurate assessment, diagnosis and prescription of medicines related to midwifery scope of prescribing

5   To accurately prescribe appropriate medicines as part of autonomous midwifery practice.

Scope of midwifery prescribing

At the time of writing, most midwives in Australia undertake dependent prescribing (prescribing according to standing orders or protocols where authority remains with the medical practitioner), although variations might occur between states. However, it is acknowledged that midwives do initiate pharmacological substances for uncomplicated pregnancies, labour and the puerperium. A project is under way in Western Australia to consider midwifery prescribing according to a formulary (personal correspondence, K Hyde, Senior Midwifery Officer, 14 September 2004).

Midwives in New Zealand undertake dependent and independent prescribing, and the Midwifery Council of New Zealand (2004) expects all registered midwives to be able to demonstrate competence in independent prescribing. Competency 2.13 (2004) indicates that a midwife must demonstrate the ability to prescribe, supply and administer medicine, vaccines and immunoglobulins safely and appropriately within the midwife's scope of practice and the relevant legislation.

Midwives in New Zealand gained lawful prescribing rights through the passage of the *Nurses Amendment Act 1990*, which included amendments to the *Misuse of Drugs Act 1975* and the *Medicines Act 1981*. There is no defined list of medicines a midwife may prescribe, but the limits as to when a midwife can prescribe are set out in an amendment to Regulation 39 of the Medicines Regulations (1984), which states: 'No registered midwife shall prescribe any prescription medicine otherwise than for antenatal, intrapartum and postnatal care'. The Misuse of Drugs Act permits midwives to prescribe pethidine, the only controlled drug that midwives can prescribe.

Following the law changes above, the New Zealand Department of Health (1990) circulated a guide to the Nurses Act Amendment stating that midwifery prescribing would not include the treatment of underlying medical conditions such as asthma or hypertension and that 'it would also not include the prescribing of medicines such as antibiotics or oral contraceptives' (1990, p 5). However, caseloading midwives found the latter restriction untenable. It imposed additional expense on women to consult a doctor in order to obtain medicines such as the progestogen-only contraceptive pill or antibiotics for an uncomplicated urinary tract infection. The New Zealand College of Midwives (NZCOM) challenged the restrictions on prescribing, and during 1995 the New Zealand Ministry of Health agreed that there was no legal basis for restricting the prescription of antibiotics and oral contraceptives and that it may indeed be appropriate for these to be prescribed by midwives during the course of providing antenatal, intrapartum and postnatal care (personal correspondence, K Guilliland, 1998).

The NZCOM Consensus Statement on Prescribing (2002) notes that midwives can prescribe for conditions commonly associated with uncomplicated pregnancy, labour and the postnatal period, up to six weeks after the birth of the baby (Campbell 2003). Midwives need to have knowledge of the effects, side-effects and contraindications of the drugs prescribed and to prescribe within their knowledge and expertise. The NZCOM strongly discourages the use of analgesics or sedatives during labour at home. The necessity for these types of medications is an indication for transfer to hospital. If narcotics are prescribed for use in labour, these must be discussed with the woman and the midwife must have the equipment and skills necessary to cope with the effects of this medication.

In the latter half of this chapter, specific conditions are discussed in relation to midwifery prescribing. The authors do not consider that all pregnancy-related conditions warrant treatment by midwives. Women requesting medication for hyperemesis should be referred to an obstetrician, as particular caution is required during the first trimester. Obstetric doctors need to prescribe adequate postoperative analgesia for women in secondary care (e.g. women who have experienced caesarean birth). Prescribing of anti-depressants, medication for asthma or hypertension/pre-eclampsia is clearly beyond the scope of midwifery practice. It is important that midwives do not issue prescriptions for medicines outside their scope of practice. Auditing identifies the named prescriber and the types of medicines prescribed. Midwives need to insist that the obstetrician or medical practitioner fax or issue a prescription for medicines associated with underlying pathology. Midwives should not prescribe antibiotics for neonates. If an infection is present, systemic antibiotics are usually necessary for newborn babies and this is beyond the scope of midwifery prescribing. Topical eye antibiotics should be used with caution and only when chlamydial infection has been ruled out. The immaturity of the neonate liver means that prescribing paracetamol should be done by medical practitioners.

Safety of drugs during pregnancy and lactation

Thalidomide is well known as the prototype for teratogens (De Santis et al 2004). Thalidomide prescribed to pregnant women in the 1960s to relieve nausea and vomiting resulted in babies born with limb malformations, and this catastrophic effect shook the perception that the placenta provides a barrier to drugs (Gardiner 2002). Drug use during pregnancy should be restricted according to necessity, and to the use of drugs for which prior clinical evidence is available. The first trimester of pregnancy is generally considered the most critical period for teratogenic effects. After the first 11 weeks, exposure to teratogens will generally have an effect on the nervous system, gonadal tissue (due to slower development than other organs) or general growth restriction (Hansen et al 2002). Vigilance is also necessary when midwives prescribe medicines during lactation. Resources should be utilised to ascertain the safety of medicines.

Studies show that many women use drugs during pregnancy. Schirm and colleagues (2004) evaluated drug types by prescription for 7500 Danish women. The authors reported that 69% of the women used a drug during pregnancy that was not folic acid, an iron preparation or vitamins. Drugs commonly used included dermatological and gynaecological preparations, lactulose, salbutamol and paracetamol. Andrade and colleagues (2004) similarly reported that 64% of women in a study in the United States (total study $n = 98,182$) used a drug other than a vitamin or mineral supplement during pregnancy, with the most frequently used drugs being oral anti-infective medicines.

There appears to be a prevalence of drug use during pregnancy, and therefore it is important that midwives stress the safe use of medications during pregnancy, particularly with the availability of over-the-counter pharmaceuticals. The Swedish, Australian and Federal Drug Administration drug classification systems are well known for classifying drug safety and use codes (A, B, C, D, X). However, a recent evaluation showed that only 26% of drugs common to all three systems were placed in the same risk category (Schirm et al 2004). These differences in categories cause confusion for the prescriber. The Australian categorisation of drugs and safety during pregnancy provides additional narrative information to guide the prescriber with the correct choice of medicine when drug therapy is required during pregnancy. Drugs are categorised to assist the prescriber to select the 'safest' known medicine appropriate for a particular condition.

Principles of pharmacology

Some key concepts are reviewed here; for a more extensive discussion, a pharmacology text should be consulted. Pharmacokinetics is the term used to describe how drugs are absorbed, distributed, metabolised and eliminated by the body.

Absorption

In most cases, when a drug is administered to a person it has to be absorbed into the bloodstream before the molecules can be distributed around the body to the site of action. Absorption is a complex process, as age, body mass, activity and fullness of the stomach can affect both the amount and the rate at which drugs are absorbed. Decreased gastrointestinal motility can increase or decrease drug absorption during pregnancy, and vomiting could mean that the drug is not absorbed at all (Bryant et al 2003; Shargel et al 2001). Once the drug is dissolved in the gastrointestinal tract, the molecules can be absorbed. Because cell membranes primarily consist of lipid substances, drug molecules generally need to be lipophilic (having an affinity with lipids) to pass through into the capillaries (Galbraith et al 2001; Shargel et al 2001).

Distribution

Hepatic portal system

As with most other digested substances, drugs are absorbed from the intestine into the hepatic circulation via the portal vein. Therefore, before the drug molecules can reach the general circulation they must pass through the liver. This is known as the hepatic first pass. At this point, a proportion of drug molecules can be metabolised and excreted by the liver. Drugs that have a significant proportion of molecules metabolised in this way are said to have a high hepatic first pass (Galbraith et al 2001; Holland & Adams 2003).

Some of the metabolites from the liver are excreted into the small intestine via the bile duct. Bile salts are excreted in this way. The body uses intestinal bacteria to recycle bile salts. The bacteria de-conjugate the bile salts, allowing them to be reabsorbed from the small intestine so that they can be conjugated again in the liver, excreted back into the small intestine and used once again in the normal digestion process. This is known as the entero-hepatic cycle. A proportion of drug molecules metabolised in the liver on the hepatic first pass are excreted into the intestine, where they are also recycled by undergoing the process of de-conjugation, reabsorption from the gut and then passing through the hepatic circulation a second time. Oestrogen in the combined oral contraceptive pill is an example of a drug that is affected in this way (Bryant et al 2003; Galbraith et al 2001; Holland & Adams 2003).

General circulation

Once the molecules reach the general circulation, they are distributed to the site of action. Highly soluble drugs are carried in the plasma as free molecules in solution. More poorly soluble drugs are carried partially bound to serum protein molecules. Only drug molecules that are free in solution are pharmacologically active. They cannot bind to the receptor sites in the body while still bound to the serum protein. The proportion of free and protein-bound drug molecules are in equilibrium. This means that drug molecules that are bound to protein molecules are released and become active as the free molecules are used. Therefore drugs that are distributed in the body partially bound to protein molecules take longer to be released to the receptor sites. The partially bound drug is pharmacologically active for longer than a highly soluble drug that has all its molecules available to the receptor sites and all its molecules available for metabolism by the liver at the same time.

The increase in maternal plasma volume and increase in body fat during pregnancy can affect drug distribution. This does not affect drug dosing except for loading doses, where a higher dose might be required (Gardiner 2002). The increase in body fat might affect drugs that are deposited in fatty tissue, resulting in a decrease in plasma concentration. Decreased serum albumin can decrease protein binding of drugs and can be relevant for monitoring of drug concentrations such as phenytoin (Begg 2003; Bryant et al 2003; Shargel et al 2001). Phenytoin concentrations during pregnancy are extremely complicated and specialist consultation is necessary (Gardiner 2002).

Metabolism and excretion

If the drug molecules remain lipophilic they will be reabsorbed at the nephron tubules or returned to the gut from the liver. Therefore drugs are metabolised in the liver to make them water-soluble (polar) so they can be excreted from the body. Two types of enzyme are involved in metabolism of drugs. The first type (sometimes called phase I) modifies the drug by chemical processes such as oxidation, reduction or hydrolysis to make water-soluble metabolites. The cytochrome P_{450} family of enzymes found in abundance in the hepatocytes are responsible for most of these reactions. Induction or inhibition of drug metabolism during pregnancy is dependent on the specific P_{450} enzymes involved. During pregnancy, metabolism of caffeine is decreased, whereas that of phenytoin is increased (Begg 2003; Bryant et al 2003).

The second type of enzyme (phase II) conjugate either the drug molecules, or a phase I metabolite, with a polar molecule such as glucuronic acid, which renders the molecule water-soluble for excretion. Conjugation enzymes belong to the transferase family. Midwives will be familiar with the physiological process in neonates whereby excess lipophilic bilirubin molecules are conjugated to water-soluble molecules by the enzyme glucuronyl transferase in the liver (Begg 2003; Bryant et al 2003). Drugs are mainly excreted in the bile and urine. Other routes include the lungs, sweat and saliva, and breast milk in lactating women (Galbraith et al 2001). Drugs that are very water-soluble are excreted virtually unchanged into the urine. This can be helpful when treating bacterial infections of the lower urinary tract (Bryant et al 2003; Lang 2001).

Drug clearance may be increased during pregnancy due to an increase in renal and liver blood flow (Gardiner 2002).

Glomerular filtration rate increases from early pregnancy and remains elevated through the pregnancy, and therefore increased doses are used for drugs such as beta lactam antibiotics, which are eliminated through the renal system (Begg 2003; Gardiner 2002).

Bioavailability

Bioavailability is the amount of drug that is available to the receptor sites. When injected intravenously, 100% of the drug is available, but when given orally some of the drug is lost during the absorption and hepatic first pass processes. Therefore, a smaller dose is usually required when the intravenous route is used (e.g. doses of narcotics). Antibiotic therapy is the most common exception, as these drugs act directly on bacteria, not on body cells (Bryant et al 2003; Galbraith et al 2001).

Plasma concentration

The time taken after a dose of a drug to reach maximum plasma concentration is affected by absorption, distribution, metabolism and elimination rates. Drugs given orally take longer than those administered intravenously to reach peak plasma concentration. The plasma concentration is related to the therapeutic effect (Begg 2003).

Therapeutic range

In order to produce a clinical effect, a certain level of drug needs to be present in the general circulation. This level is called the minimum effective concentration (MEC). The minimum effective concentration is different for each drug. For all drugs there is also a level at which the drug will produce adverse effects on the person, known as the maximum safe concentration (MSC). The range between the MEC and the MSC that is associated with drug efficacy is known as the therapeutic range. Most drugs have a wide therapeutic range, which means that the serum levels will not normally rise to toxic levels when the usual size and frequency of dose is taken. However, a significant number of drugs, especially anti-convulsants and antibiotics from the aminoglycoside family (e.g. gentamycin) have a narrow therapeutic range. This means that it is possible for serum levels to rise to toxic levels even with normal dose and frequency regimens. People being treated with drugs that have a narrow therapeutic range have the serum levels of the drug regularly monitored so that, if necessary, the dose can be adjusted to maintain effectiveness without causing toxicity (Begg 2003; Bryant et al 2003; Galbraith et al 2001).

Half-life

The length of time for which a drug is clinically effective in the body is called its half-life. Half-life is the length of time it takes to reduce the amount of drug in the circulation by half. For example, 500 mg of a drug that has a half-life of four hours will reduce to 250 mg four hours after administration, to 125 mg after another four hours, and so on. Although there are still active molecules of the drug in the body after four hours (in this example), the clinical effectiveness of the drug has been significantly reduced. This principle is what guides recommendations for the frequency of doses. Doses are given at the half-life interval (e.g. four-hourly in the above example) (Bryant et al 2003; Galbraith et al 2001; Shargel et al 2001).

Steady state concentration

The aim of dosing regimens is to achieve a steady state concentration—that is, to maintain a constant concentration of the drug in the plasma that is consistent with a therapeutic response in the person (Fig 29.1). When a steady state is reached, the maintenance dose rate is equal to the elimination rate (i.e. it is in equilibrium) (Bryant et al 2003; Shargel et al 2001). Drugs are given at half-life intervals to reach a steady state concentration: 'In general it takes 3 to 5 half lives to reach the desired steady state' (Bryant et al 2003, p 122). To avoid the problem of delay when the half-life is long or rapid and treatment is imperative, a loading dose is often given.

While loading doses are often twice the ongoing dose, the desired plasma concentration and the apparent volume of distribution for individual drugs are taken into account (Shargel et al 2001). The initial dose is sometimes given parenterally, followed by oral administration of maintenance doses.

Pharmacodynamics

Pharmacodynamics is the term used to describe the action of a drug on the body. Nearly all drugs act on receptors in the body (antimicrobials act on microorganisms) by binding to a protein. Most drugs have some selectivity—that is, they 'see' or 'fit' particular receptors as targets. Generally, drugs act on four main types of regulatory proteins: carriers, enzymes, ion channels and receptors (Bryant et al 2003; Holland & Adams 2003). Carriers transport ions and small, poorly fat-soluble molecules across cell membranes. Examples are carriers that uptake noradrenaline and serotonin at the nerve terminals. Drugs that target carriers usually inhibit carrier-mediated uptake of such transmitters (e.g. tricyclic antidepressants) (Bryant et al 2003). *Enzymes* are biological catalysts that control cellular biochemical reactions. Drugs that interact with enzymes inhibit or alter the biochemical reaction. The sulfonamide group of drugs, which includes the drug Bactrim, are an example (Galbraith et al 2001). Ions are transported in and out of cells through specific channels in the cell membrane so that the electrochemical gradient across the cell membrane can be maintained. Drugs that interact with receptors to block the ion channels are widely used. These drugs generally have a high selectivity. Nifedipine, used for the control of hypertension, for example, is a calcium ion channel blocker that affects the arterioles but has little effect on cardiac muscle and no effect on the transport of other ions such as sodium (Bryant et al 2003; Galbraith et al 2001).

Receptors are specific proteins that span cell membranes. They are engaged in 'chemical signalling between and within cells' (Bryant et al 2003, p 95). Drug molecules bind with receptors in a 'lock and key' effect. Drugs that temporarily bind to receptors and stimulate the cell to carry out its normal biochemical actions are known as agonists, while those that bind to the receptors to temporarily block or inhibit the normal cell process are referred to as antagonists. Drugs called 'blockers' are antagonists. The beta-blocker labetalol is an example (Galbraith et al 2001; Holland & Adams 2003).

Antimicrobials

Midwives require a thorough understanding of antimicrobials, not only for prescribing and administration purposes, but also to take every opportunity to encourage health-promoting activities in childbearing families. Opportunities to reinforce information about completing courses of antibiotics, recognising adverse effects and preventing the development of resistant bacteria arise in the course of everyday midwifery practice.

Midwives do not independently prescribe for infections that require intravenous antibiotics; referral should be made

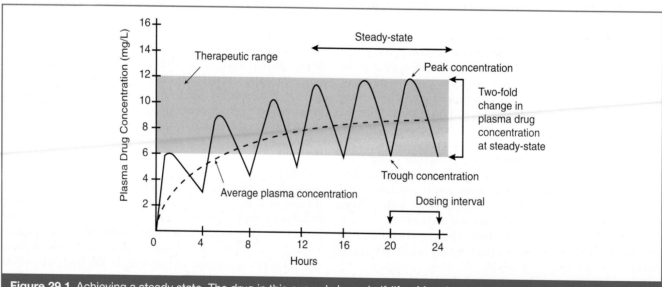

Figure 29.1 Achieving a steady state. The drug in this example has a half-life of four hours (based on Bryant et al 2003).

BOX 29.1 Barriers to distribution

Blood–brain barrier

The brain is protected from harmful substances because it has a different capillary structure from that of the rest of the body. The junctions between endothelial cells are narrower, reducing the number of pores available. Further, a web of tightly connected glial cells forms a fatty layer between the capillaries and the brain tissue. Only material that is very fat soluble or is actively transported can cross the blood–brain barrier (Bryant et al 2003; Galbraith et al 2001; Shargel et al 2001).

Placenta

Considering the size and complexity of the placenta, it is very limited barrier for many drug molecules. It does not have the selectivity of the blood–brain barrier, allowing both lipid-soluble and water-soluble drugs to cross into the fetal circulation. For example, the effect of narcotic analgesia given in labour on neonatal respiratory effort is well documented. A number of drugs can have a deleterious effect on the growing embryo or fetus (e.g. phenytoin, tetracycline).

The poor protection afforded by the placenta is the primary reason that drugs are generally contraindicated in uncomplicated pregnancies. When a pregnancy is complicated by a concurrent medical condition, medications are prescribed with caution. In these cases, the obstetrician assesses the risk/benefit of medication in each situation. Some anticonvulsants commonly used to control epilepsy in non-pregnant women pose a significant risk to the growing baby. The woman's medication may be changed to a drug that poses less risk to the baby for the duration of the pregnancy. In other medical conditions, the dose(s) of drug used to control the medical condition may need to be adjusted and plasma concentrations monitored (Bryant et al 2003).

BOX 29.2 Prescribing antimicrobials

Bryant et al (2003, p 753) list the following important principles for prescribing antibacterial drugs:

- Use an antibacterial drug only when indicated.
- Identify the infecting microorganism.
- Determine the susceptibility of the organism.
- Use a drug with the narrowest spectrum of activity for the known or likely organism.
- Use a single drug, unless combination therapy is specifically indicated to ensure efficacy or to reduce the emergence of resistance.
- Use a dose high enough to ensure efficacy (with minimal toxicity) as this reduces the likelihood of resistance.
- Use a short duration of treatment (< one week) unless evidence indicates a longer duration.

Bacterial resistance

Midwives have a responsibility not to contribute to the development of bacterial resistance and should base practice on evidence. Good prescribing and health education practices will assist in the prevention of unnecessary exposure or under-treatment with antibiotics (Foureur 2001).

Spectrum of activity

The number of types of organisms that are sensitive to the antibiotic is what determines its spectrum of activity. Antibiotics to which only a few groups of organisms are sensitive are said to have a narrow spectrum of activity, while those that are effective against a wide range of organisms are said to have a broad spectrum of activity. This does not mean that narrow-spectrum antibiotics are of no value. A well-chosen narrow-spectrum antibiotic can be very effective. An example of this is flucloxacillin, a narrow-spectrum, beta-lactamase-resistant antibiotic, effective against *Staphylococcus aureus* and *Streptococcus sp* (Miller 2002), and used for the treatment of mastitis when women are lactating (Lang 2001).

Adverse reactions

The importance of taking a careful history relating to hypersensitivity to antibiotics cannot be sufficiently emphasised. There is a world of difference between an anaphylactic reaction, fever and rash due to allergy, and adverse effects such as diarrhoea, nausea and vomiting, candidiasis or sore mouth or tongue (*New Ethicals Compendium* 2000). Clients do not always distinguish between types of adverse reaction. Women who have a history of hypersensitivity to any antibiotic should have their notes prominently marked so that it is not overlooked. In cases of hypersensitivity, drugs should be discontinued and consultation sought. 'Hypersensitivity reactions occur in 4–8% of patients. Anaphylaxis occurs in approximately 0.2% [of clients]' (Lang 2001, p 25) (see Box 29.3). Midwives need to be particularly cautious regarding

---

to an obstetrician. Midwives would not prescribe for medical conditions such as pyelonephritis or prophylactic antimicrobials for cardiac conditions. Neonates with symptoms suggestive of systemic infection should be promptly referred to the paediatric service (or a medical practitioner in areas without a paediatric service). Neonates have an immature liver enzyme system and therefore have limited ability to metabolise drugs. They can also become seriously ill very quickly.

Antimicrobials are groups of drugs that destroy or restrict the proliferation of infectious microorganisms. They work by inhibiting cell wall synthesis, disrupting cell membrane permeability, interfering with the organism's metabolic processes, or by inhibiting protein synthesis in the organism (Bryant et al 2003; Galbraith et al 2001).

Bacteriocidal antimicrobials destroy the organism and bacteriostatic drugs hinder bacterial growth, giving the body a longer period in which to mobilise its own defences. Antibiotics are used to treat bacterial infections. Other antimicrobials include antiviral, antifungal and antimycobacterial agents (Holland & Adams 2003).

BOX 29.3 Anaphylactic shock

Anaphylaxis is a potentially life-threatening, acute and severe systemic reaction that occurs after exposure to a specific antigen. Mast cells and basophils are the primary initiating cells of immunoglobulin E (IgE) mediated allergic reactions, causing severe bronchospasm, laryngospasm, angioedema, urticaria and cardiovascular collapse. Symptoms of anaphylaxis usually occur within seconds to minutes of exposure to the allergen and range from mild to very severe. Allergens include penicillins, anaesthetic drugs, some intravenous infusion liquids, and aspirin and other NSAIDs.

Signs and symptoms

▶ rapid pulse, sweating, dizziness, fainting, unconsciousness
▶ wheezing, chest tightness, difficulty breathing, coughing
▶ itchy hives, which may blend together to form larger areas of skin swelling
▶ swelling of the lips, tongue or eyes
▶ nausea, vomiting, abdominal cramps, diarrhoea
▶ paleness, bluish skin colour
▶ throat swelling, with a feeling of throat tightness, a lump in the throat, hoarseness or obstructed air flow.

Treatment

▶ Call for emergency assistance immediately.
▶ Adrenaline is the treatment of choice. The dose of adrenaline is usually 0.3 mg for an adult, to be given at the first sign of a serious reaction.
▶ Adrenaline given subcutaneously or intramuscularly will work for about 150 minutes.
▶ Following the administration of adrenaline, admit to hospital for observation for up to 24 hours, as occasionally the symptoms can return. An antihistamine or corticosteroid injection may also be administered, or given together with fluids intravenously.
▶ Oxygen may be given.

Side-effects of adrenaline

▶ Trembling, palpitations and a feeling of tension or anxiousness—these are normal effects of the adrenaline and soon wear off. Higher doses cause an extremely unpleasant feeling.

Contraindications

▶ high blood pressure or heart arrhythmias.

women with a history of penicillin allergy. A significant number of these clients will have adverse reactions or allergies to other groups of antibiotics, and hence referral to a doctor is indicated. The tetracyclines group of antibiotics cannot be used as an alternative, as they are contraindicated in pregnancy—there is risk to the fetus of teeth staining and inhibited bone growth (Lang 2001). Midwives need to be aware of local policy for reporting adverse reactions of medicines and to promptly refer women experiencing any adverse effects to a medical practitioner.

Types of antimicrobials

Beta-lactam antibiotics

These drugs are bacteriocidal substances that contain a beta-lactam ring in their molecular structure. They include the penicillins, cephalosporins, monobactams, carbapenems and beta-lactamase inhibitors (Galbraith et al 2001; Lang 2001; Miller 2002). Some bacteria have become resistant to antibiotics by developing the capacity to produce the enzyme beta-lactamase (penicillinase), which breaks the beta-lactam ring in the antibiotic molecule, rendering it ineffective (Holland & Adams 2003).

Penicillins

The penicillins are a large group of both natural and synthetic antibiotics (Miller 2002). They are grouped into several categories. Benzylpenicillin or penicillin G (parenteral) and phenoxymethylpenicillin or penicillin V (oral) are clinically comparable. They have been largely replaced by broad-spectrum penicillins such as amoxycillin, which does not need an empty stomach and is more reliably absorbed (Lang 2001). Penicillin V may be used as prophylaxis for women with a history of cardiac conditions such as bacterial endocarditis.

Narrow-spectrum penicillinase-resistant penicillins

These penicillins are beta-lactamase resistant (Bryant et al 2003; Holland & Adams 2003). Flucloxacillin and dicloxacillin are used to treat staphylococcal infections, particularly in soft tissues. They need to be taken on an empty stomach (Lang 2001).

Extended-spectrum penicillins

The spectrum of activity for amoxycillin/clavulanic acid, piperacillin/tazobactam and ticarillin/clavulanic acid is extended by the addition of the beta-lactamase inhibitors clavulanic acid or tazobactam. This makes these antibiotics effective against otherwise resistant strains of *S. aureus* and some anaerobes. Of all the penicillins, piperacillin and ticarillin have the widest range of action against Gram-negative organisms. Ticarillin is no longer available in New Zealand (Bryant et al 2003; Lang 2001).

Beta-lactamase inhibitors do not have much antibacterial activity in themselves, and reaction to clavulanic acid is extremely rare. They protect the antibiotic by binding with the beta-lactamase produced by the microorganisms (Lang 2001).

Patterns of bacterial resistance in local flora of the gut are an important prescribing consideration. For example, in some areas, amoxycillin-resistant *Staphylococcus* make an amoxycillin/clavulanic acid preparation more appropriate to prescribe if treatment needs to commence before sensitivities are known. It is important for midwives to follow up the results of bacterial culture sensitivities, to both fully treat the infection and minimise the spread of resistance.

Cephalosporins

Cephalosporins are a family of broad-spectrum antibiotics that are classified by their generation. The generation refers to the timeframe over which each group was developed, rather than increasing improvement. Each generation has specific effect on different groups of bacteria. First-generation cephalosporins are active against Gram-positive bacteria. Second-generation drugs also target Gram-negative organisms, as do third-generation drugs, which have a longer duration and target beta-lactamase-producing organisms. Fourth-generation cephalosporins have similarities with the third-generation drugs (Holland & Adams 2003). Most cephalosporins are only available for parenteral use. Therefore community prescribing is limited to the few oral preparations. Cephalosporins are judiciously prescribed, as they are valuable agents in the treatment of Gram-negative organisms and are more expensive than the penicillins.

Oral cephalosporins are alternatives to penicillins for treatment of skin and soft tissue infections of *S. aureus* and streptococcal (not enterococcal) origin (Lang 2001). Cephalosporins should not be used if a person reports a serious reaction to penicillin (Bryant et al 2003; Hansen et al 2002). Adverse effects are similar to those for penicillins but hypersensitivities are much less common. Renal toxicity has been associated with earlier-generation cephalosporins (Holland & Adams 2003).

Macrolide antibiotics

The macrolides are a group of primarily bacteriostatic antibiotics with some bacteriocidal effect that include erythromycin and azithromycin. They have a broad spectrum of activity against diverse organisms. Erythromycin is the most commonly used alternative to penicillin where there is an allergy (Holland & Adams 2003; Lang 2001). Erythromycin estolate is contradicted in pregnancy because of drug-related hepatotoxicity. Erythromycin ethylsuccinate is satisfactory for use during pregnancy.

Aminoglycosides

Prescription of aminoglycosides is outside midwives' scope of practice. However, midwives administer these drugs parenterally and monitor their effects. For example, gentamycin can be used with amoxycillin as a prophylactic regimen for women intrapartum with cardiac conditions. Gentamycin can also be used to treat sensitive bacteria causing acute pyelonephritis in pregnancy.

The aminoglycosides are a group of potent bacteriocides that act by inhibiting protein synthesis. They are generally reserved for Gram-negative infections. They are: gentamycin, neomycin, netilmycin, streptomycin and tobramycin (Bryant et al 2003; Holland & Adams 2003). Adverse reactions include serious neurological, renal and ototoxicity, and therefore careful observation for signs of adverse reactions is required. If treatment is longer than 72 hours, plasma levels and renal function are monitored to determine dose regimens (Bryant et al 2003).

Nitrofurantoin

Nitrofurantoin is a broad-spectrum bacteriocide, the mechanism of which is not fully understood. It is used for the treatment of acute urinary tract infections, as it is highly soluble. Approximately 65% of the drug is excreted in the urine unchanged. Urine alkalinisers are not recommended when women are being treated with nitrofurantoin, as it has more efficacy in an acidic environment. It should not be used when labour is imminent because of the possibility of haemolytic anaemia in the neonate due to immature erythrocyte enzyme systems (glutathione instability). Nitrofurantoin is contraindicated in women with G6PD deficiency due to potential haemolytic anaemia (Bryant et al 2003; Medsafe 2003). Antacid preparations containing magnesium trisilicate should not be used when taking nitrofurantoin, to avoid the possibility of impaired absorption.

Topical antibiotics

Topical antibiotics are used for the treatment of conjunctivitis and occasionally superficial skin/umbilical cord infections in neonates. Care must be taken to only use topical antibiotics when there is actually an infection present. A significant proportion of neonatal 'sticky eyes' in the first week of life is related to an inflamed tear duct rather than an infectious conjunctivitis. Regular cleansing (associated with gentle massage of the tear duct) is usually all that is required. If an infection is suspected, a swab should be taken for culture and sensitivities prior to starting treatment. Antibiotic therapy can mask chlamydial eye infections. Midwives need to consider this condition if the conjunctivitis does not resolve quickly.

The use of topical antibiotics for minor neonatal skin infections is controversial. A mild antiseptic wash may be just as effective. The treatment of umbilical cord stumps with topical antibiotics should rarely be necessary. Most 'sticky cords' are merely the result of saprophytic action and require hygiene measures rather than antibiotics. Umbilical cord infections can rapidly spread to become serious systemic infections. Regular observation will assist early detection; referral is indicated for babies with umbilical infections.

Antivirals: acylovir

Acyclovir is used as topical or oral preparation to increase the healing rate and to decrease the pain of genital herpes lesions

---

Critical thinking exercise

1   How do prescribers make decisions regarding which antibiotic is appropriate for treatment of a particular infection?

2   What is the rationale for prescribing more than one antibiotic in particular circumstances? For example, an obstetrician or doctor will frequently prescribe intravenous amoxicillin plus gentamycin for women with cardiac pathology (including a history of rheumatic heart disease).

3   What pregnancy-related issues need to be considered and taken into account *before* a midwife deems that it is appropriate to prescribe a pharmaceutical?

(Galbraith et al 2001). The topical preparation is widely available (OTC), as it is primarily used for the treatment of Herpes Simplex I lesions. Diagnosis of genital herpes, follow-up of partners and treatment regimens is beyond the scope of midwifery practice. Referral to a doctor is indicated.

An understanding of pharmacology and knowledge of commonly used antimicrobials is essential for safe prescribing practices. The following section refers to common conditions during pregnancy where midwives might need to consider prescription medicines in discussion with the woman.

Other drugs and conditions prescribed for

Selected other drugs commonly used, and conditions commonly prescribed for in the childbearing year, are described below.

Oxytocin

Synthetic oxytocin is used in labour to augment uterine contractions when they are absent or incoordinate, or during induction of labour (Varney 2004). Oxytocin has an immediate onset and is rapidly inactivated in the liver. As it has a half-life of 1–6 minutes, oxytocin is administered in labour via an intravenous infusion in which the dose is incrementally titrated to achieve approximately three to four contractions every 10 minutes (Bryant et al 2003). Oxytocin is also used to prevent or control haemorrhage post partum. A single-dose injection is used for the active management of the third stage of labour, while a continuous infusion is used to control postpartum haemorrhage (Varney et al 2004). When used in conjunction with prostaglandins or inhalational anaesthetics, the action of oxytocin may be enhanced. Close monitoring of both maternal and fetal wellbeing is required. Adverse reactions include nausea, vomiting, hypotension, tachycardia and irregular heart rate. Occasional fetal bradycardia, dysrhythmias or neonatal jaundice have occurred (Bryant et al 2003).

Local anaesthetic (lignocaine hydrochloride)

Lignocaine hydrochloride is used as a local anaesthetic for perineal repair. A 1% solution without adrenaline (i.e. plain) is the usual strength employed, although others can be used. The lowest dose needed to provide effective anaesthesia should be used. Injection should be made slowly with aspiration to prevent intravascular injection, as this may produce toxic effects. The amount required for individual women will depend on the size of the woman, the extent of the perineal injury and whether the infiltration is into an intact perineum prior to birth or an injured perineum after the birth. The maximum dose is 200 mg in adults (i.e. 20 mL of 1% plain solution)

(*New Ethicals Compendium* 2000). In most circumstances the dose given is significantly less than the maximum. For smaller lacerations it often does not exceed 100 mg (10 mL).

Tocolytic drugs

Tocolytic drugs have been used in the management of preterm labour to quieten uterine activity. The group of drugs most commonly used to halt uterine activity are the beta-adrenergic agonists (e.g. salbutamol). They relax smooth muscle by stimulating the beta-receptors of the autonomic nervous system. They are administered by an intravenous infusion that is titrated to achieve uterine relaxation at the minimum dose (Lindsay 2000). Common adverse effects include tachycardia, palpitations, tremor, nervousness, dizziness, malaise, nausea, vomiting, bronchospasm and hypersensitivity reactions, among others (Comerford 2003). Women receiving tocolytic drug infusions need to be carefully monitored for adverse effects. At the time of writing (2005), the calcium ion channel blocker nifedipine is used as a tocolytic agent in the management of preterm labour in some parts of New Zealand. This drug inhibits muscle contraction by interfering with the movement of calcium across the plasma membrane (Lindsay 2000).

Non-steroidal anti-inflammatory drugs

Use of non-steroidal anti-inflammatory drugs (NSAIDs) during the second and third trimester is associated with oligohydramnios and anuria. Close to term, use of these drugs is associated with premature closure of the ductus arteriosus, with subsequent pulmonary hypertension, intracranial haemorrhage and necrotising enterocolitis in the infant. During pregnancy, paracetamol is the drug of choice for analgesic, anti-inflammatory and antipyretic action (De Santis et al 2004; Gardiner 2002).

Folic acid

Supplementation with folic acid has been shown to decrease the incidence of neural tube defects (Page 2000) and is recommended for primary prevention and also for women with a previously affected baby. Stefanogiannis (2003) reported that two randomised controlled trials emphatically and rigorously confirmed that increasing the daily intake of folic acid decreases the risk of neural tube defects. The United States Public Health Service acted on this research in 1992 and recommended that women of childbearing age consume 0.04 mg of folic acid per day to reduce the risk of neural tube defects.

Other countries have adopted various approaches, such as recommending an increase in folate-rich foods, supplementation by tablets, or fortification of certain foods. The National Food Authority in Australia permitted voluntary fortification of foods with folic acid (bread, flour, breakfast cereal, pasta, yeast and fruit juices) from 1995. The Commonwealth Department of Health and Ageing recommends that women planning pregnancy take folic acid supplements of 0.5 mg per day.

TABLE 29.1 Folate recommendations for Australian and New Zealand women

Australia	New Zealand
All women planning a pregnancy should supplement their diet with 0.5 mg of folic acid/day beginning one month prior to conception until 12 weeks gestation.	All women planning a pregnancy should supplement their diet with 0.8 mg of folic acid/day beginning one month prior to conception until 12 weeks gestation.
Women with a previous neural tube defect-affected pregnancy or with close family history of neural tube defect-affected pregnancy should supplement their diet with 5 mg of folic acid/day.	
(Sources: NHMRC 1993; Ministry of Health 1997)	

Similarly in New Zealand, voluntary fortification of food has been permitted since 1996. However, evidence suggests that women still do not have a sufficient daily intake of folic acid to reduce neural tube defects (Stefanogiannis 2003). The NZ Ministry of Health recommends that folic acid 0.8 mg tablet orally be taken daily from one month pre-conception to the end of 12 weeks gestation. Women who have had a child previously affected by neural tube defect, a family history of neural tube defect, and women at risk (e.g. women on anticonvulsant medication, women with pre-existing diabetes) should take 5 mg tablet orally (Rubin 2000).

Iron supplementation (anaemia)

Iron deficiency anaemia is the most common anaemia during pregnancy; however, midwives need to be aware of other types of anaemia, including: folate, B_{12}, sickle cell, thalassemia and auto-immune anaemia. Correct diagnosis is important, to avoid inappropriate treatment regimens that might be harmful to the woman and the fetus. Iron overload can occur in women with undiagnosed haemochromatosis or ineffective erythropoiesis such as sickle-cell disease or thalassemia (Adams-Graves 2001).

Iron deficiency anaemia

Routine iron supplementation during pregnancy is not necessary in developed countries. Plasma volume increases by 40–50% during pregnancy and red cell volume increases by only 20%. Consequently, haemodilution occurs as a physiological response. The increased blood volume during pregnancy and the lower blood viscosity ensure good perfusion and oxygenation of the fetus throughout the pregnancy (McMullin et al 2003). As pregnancy progresses, there is an increase in absorption of iron from the gut. However, despite this physiological adaptation, a number of women become deficient in iron stores during the latter stages of pregnancy. It is estimated that up to a quarter of women in industrialised countries have insufficient iron in their diet to maintain sufficient intake during pregnancy (Haram et al 2001). Haem iron is the most bioavailable (absorbable) iron and is prolific in red meat. Vegetarians generally have a low intake of bioavailable iron and ingest foods with phytic acid, which decreases iron absorption (Haram et al 2001). Non-haem iron found in pulses, vegetables and fruit is not as well absorbed and can be affected by tea, coffee, excess bran and some antacids (McKay 2000). Tea is a stronger inhibitor than coffee in reducing the absorption of non-haem iron, while vitamin C can encourage the uptake of non-haem iron (Haram et al 2001).

Interpreting blood indices

It is often difficult to decide whether Hb values between 90 and 110 g/L are due to haemodilution or anaemia. Haram and colleagues (2001) considered that a 'low' Hb was 110 g/L (11.0 g/100 mL) during the first half of pregnancy and 100–105 g/L or lower after 25 weeks gestation. An Hb less than 100–110 g/L in the first and second trimester has been associated with preterm birth and low birthweight. On the other hand, a 'high' Hb (> 135 g/L) might be associated with pre-eclampsia or conditions where haemodilution has not occurred (Haram et al 2001).

When assessing a woman for anaemia, a full blood count provides initial information. Mean cellular volume increases by about 4 femtolitres in healthy pregnancy (Haram et al 2001) and is therefore not a reliable marker for diagnosing iron deficiency anaemia. Serum ferritin is the blood test of choice to determine iron stores in the body and is a reliable blood test in the first trimester of pregnancy. However, after the first trimester, serum ferritin levels will fall due to the effect of haemodilution independent of changes in iron stores. Ferritin levels can increase in response to an acute inflammatory reaction or excessive alcohol intake (the latter should not be occurring during pregnancy). A ferritin level of 15–30 μg/L indicates that iron stores are too small to cover the need for iron in pregnancy. A ferritin level of < 12–15 μg/L indicates empty stores and iron deficiency (Haram et al 2001).

How much iron supplementation is required?

Practitioners need to differentiate the woman's diagnosis to either iron deficiency anaemia or low iron stores. If the woman is iron deficient (low Hb, lower parameter mean cell volume (MCV) and almost absent ferritin) she certainly requires supplementation. If a woman has ferritin levels within the lower range, discussion needs to occur regarding increasing iron-rich foods in the diet or consideration of supplementation. Studies have shown that routine supplementation of about 60 mg iron per day *throughout* the pregnancy is sufficient to maintain iron stores during pregnancy (Haram et al 2001). The literature is less forthcoming in relation to 'need-based' supplementation. The midwife should use her discretion as to the amount of supplementation required on an individual need basis according to the blood results and the woman's diet.

Gastrointestinal side-effects might occur with iron supplementation, yet these appear to be dose dependent. Lowering the dose of iron supplement and recommending that the dose be taken at different intervals (if tablet form permits this dosing), or taken with food, should result in fewer side-effects. Taking iron supplements with fruit juice is likely to increase gastrointestinal side-effects, and vitamin C is not essential for the absorption of elemental iron.

Women are significantly more likely to take iron supplements if the midwife stresses the importance and rationale for supplementation (Wulff & Ekstrom 2003). Intake of too much iron might interfere with the absorption of trace metals such as zinc. In certain cases, iron supplementation might increase the expansion of the red blood cell mass to the extent that the increased viscosity of the blood is an additional risk factor (Haram et al 2001).

Recommended prescribing

- Obtain complete blood count and ferritin levels (iron studies include ferritin level).
- Ensure diagnosis is iron deficiency anaemia and no other pathology.
- If haemoglobin level is < 90, referral to an obstetrician is indicated.
- If ferritin is low (e.g. 12–20 µg/L), a woman might require approximately 60 mg elemental iron per day in supplement, depending on her diet and gestation.
- If ferritin is less than 12 µg/L and diet is low in haem iron, consider prescribing a higher dose of iron supplement (e.g. up to 105 mg of elemental iron supplement per day).
- Midwives need to check the amount of elemental iron in iron preparations as this can vary substantially between products. The amount of elemental iron affects the number of tablet/s prescribed.
- The amount of ferrous iron (ferrous salts: sulfate, gluconate, fumerate and succinate) absorbed is about three times greater than that of iron in the ferric form (Engstrom & Sittler 1994).
- Midwives need to consider the cost of iron supplements in partnership with the woman, provide sound education on the rationale for use and ensure safe storage from children.
- Adding vitamins to iron generally increases the cost of the supplement. One study of 371 women, undertaken by Juarez-Vazquez et al (2002) showed that iron plus folate therapy gave a better increase in Hb, particularly for women with severe anaemia.
- Assess full blood count and ferritin level within four weeks of commencing therapy.
- If the woman requires intramuscular iron therapy (due to low haemoglobin and lack of compliance with

> ### Clinical scenario
>
> Haley works in the city as a sales representative, and was having her first baby. The following were her blood results:
> *Immediately pre-conception*: Hb 120 g/L, MCV 86
> At 28 weeks: Hb 110 g/L, MCV 85, ferritin 7 µg/L
> Ferritin was ascertained with Haley's consent in view of her extreme tiredness. Haley spent a lot of time driving and tended to have quick meals. She was reluctant to eat cold meats because of concern about *Listeria* infection. Haley was advised to supplement 60 mg elemental iron per day if tolerated and try to increase haem iron intake in her diet. Note that the Hb and MCV above do not indicate any significant decrease, as Haley probably has 'latent iron deficiency'.
> *At 36 weeks*: Hb 115 g/L, MCV 84, ferritin 18 µg/L
> Haley had a caesarean birth after a long labour that was augmented with Syntocinon. Haley is a small woman and her baby weighed 4.5 kg.
> *At 41 weeks labour*: Hb 112, MCV 84, PCV .34
> *At 2/7 after LSCS*: Hb 87, MCV 84, PCV .26
> *At 3 weeks pp*: Hb 117, MCV 84, PCV .36, ferritin 30 µg/L
> The blood loss at LSCS was documented as only being 500 mL with normal postpartum bleeding, yet there is a significant decrease in the haemoglobin and packed cell volume (PCV). Haley resumed iron therapy (60 mg elemental iron daily) from a week post partum (when she felt able to tolerate iron tablets). Blood tests were taken at three weeks after the birth. The increase in Hb and PCV (haematocrit) shows that iron therapy was effective.

oral iron therapy), an obstetrician should prescribe this. Iron injections can cause staining of the skin and should be administered according to the manufacturer's instructions.

- Intravenous iron therapy requires administration in a specialist unit, where the woman is monitored for adverse reactions.

Antacids

Gastroesophageal reflux is a common occurrence during pregnancy. Reflux generally bothers up to two-thirds of pregnant women by the third trimester (Tytgat et al 2003). Reflux is aggravated by spicy or greasy foods, tomatoes, acidic products and carbonated drinks. If dietary changes do not solve reflux, calcium- or magnesium-based antacids, which neutralise stomach acids, can be used during pregnancy. High-dose aluminium-containing antacids are not generally recommended due to common side-effects of constipation and altered gastrointestinal (GI) motility (Tytgat et al 2003). Combination antacids have been formulated to reduce the risk of diarrhoea or constipation. Alginic acid forms viscous cohesive foam, preventing reflux by increasing adherence of mucus. Simethicone disperses and prevents the formation of mucous gas pockets in the GI tract, relieving flatulence (Bryant et al 2003). Antacids can bind with other medications and therefore should be taken at least an hour apart from iron preparation and other medicines. Histamine-2 receptor antagonists are also safe during pregnancy and include cimetidine and ranitidine. The latter tend to be drugs of choice prior to Caesarean birth.

Recommended prescribing

- Ensure that there is no other pathology and be aware that heartburn can mimic epigastric pain associated with pre-eclampsia. Always consider the woman's blood pressure.
- Try to encourage the woman to alter her dietary habits in the first instance before resorting to antacids.
- If reflux continues to be troublesome, advise or prescribe antacid. Recommended dose depends on which preparation is given.
- Sodium alginate: oral liquid 55 mg with sodium bicarbonate 267 mg per 10 mL (Gaviscon). Dose 10–20 mL up to four times (maximum) a day after meals and 30 minutes before bedtime.
- Simethisone: oral liquid aluminium hydroxide 200 mg with magnesium hydroxide 200 mg and activated simethicone 20 mg per 5 mL (Mylanta P).

Thrush (candidiasis or moniliasis)

Vaginal thrush is a common complaint of women and increases in prevalence during pregnancy due to changes in the vaginal flora. Predisposing factors include a recent course of antibiotics (which reduces the vaginal lactobacilli count, rendering a woman more susceptible to overgrowth of the yeast), diabetes, HIV infection, anaemia and urinary tract infection. Young and Jewell (2001) revealed that imidazole drugs (clotrimazole, miconazole) are more effective than nystatin for treating vaginal candidiasis in pregnancy. Young and Jewell also recommend treatment for a seven-day period during pregnancy (clotrimazole preparations are generally packaged for six nightly applications and this should suffice). Single-dose treatments (and four-day treatments) were shown to be less effective during pregnancy when assessed by culture and symptoms (Young & Jewell 2001). Shorter courses of antifungal therapy are stronger: 10% cream for a one-night treatment compared with 1% for the six-night course, so women are more likely to experience burning and irritation with the stronger preparations. It is possible that shorter-course treatments might contribute to non-*albicans* species such as *Candida glabrata* and *C. tropicalis*. Traditional therapy of imidazoles does not adequately treat non-*albicans* species, hence the rationale for culture of a vaginal swab (Andrist 2001). Oral antifungals are not considered safe during pregnancy (Morgan 2000). The primary mode of action of clotrimazole appears to be on the cell membrane of the fungi, damaging the permeability barrier (*New Ethicals Compendium* 2000).

There is sufficient cream in the vaginal application pack to enable women to apply cream to the vulva twice a day. Education regarding careful insertion of the applicator should be discussed, as well as hygiene to decrease the risk of re-infection. There is no evidence that treating a male sexual partner makes any difference to this episode or future episodes unless the partner already has symptoms. Douching washes out lactobacilli as well as *Candida*. Studies have shown increased pelvic infection rates after douching, so this is not a suitable treatment, particularly in pregnancy. Salt baths are helpful in reducing itching and swelling in the acute phase (Hunter & Roke 2002).

Recommended prescribing

- Treat only if the woman is symptomatic.
- While clotrimazole is classified as being safe during pregnancy, manufacturers recommend cautious use in the first trimester.
- It is advisable to confirm a suspected diagnosis with a high vaginal swab.
- Use clotrimazole or miconazole 1%. Insert applicator full of cream into vagina at bedtime for six (or seven) nights. There is sufficient cream to apply to vulva BD. Some women might prefer to use vaginal pessaries plus cream to treat the vulva.

Urinary tract infection

Urinary tract infection (UTI) is a common complication during pregnancy. Asymptomatic bacteriuria is prevalent in 5–10% of pregnant women, and almost a third of these women will develop symptomatic infection if left untreated. Acute pyelonephritis is associated with fetal morbidity and mortality (Chaliha & Stanton 2002). It is recommended that an uncontaminated mid-stream urine (MSU) be obtained from pregnant women around 12–16 weeks gestation to ascertain whether there is asymptomatic bacteriuria (Nicolle 2002). Women who have had previous UTIs often recognise the symptoms associated with a UTI and present early to their caregiver. Midwives should only prescribe for lower tract infections and refer to an obstetrician if there are any symptoms of pyelonephritis (pyrexia, loin pain) or if there are recurrent urinary infections during the pregnancy. If there are recurrent urinary infections (more than two) during the pregnancy, an obstetrician might recommend prophylactic antibiotics for the continuation of the pregnancy and/or renal investigations.

Recommended prescribing

- Diagnosis of UTI should only be made by careful assessment of symptoms and an uncontaminated MSU obtained *prior* to the commencement of any antibiotics.
- Antibiotics might need to be prescribed before laboratory results are available (if a woman is symptomatic). Microscopy of urine can occur quickly (in 1–2 hours if indicated as urgent); however, culture

of bacteria currently takes about 36 hours. If laboratory service is unavailable, urine dipstick can be done for white cells and nitrate.

- Microscopy associated with UTI generally shows a raised white count (epithelial cells should be nil or very low numbers in an uncontaminated specimen). Culture shows a high bacterial count and usually a single organism as opposed to mixed bacterial species. Consult with the local laboratory for parameters used and always consult with a microbiologist or an obstetrician if unsure how to interpret the laboratory findings (e.g. sterile pyuria).
- If a prescription for antibiotics is indicated, reassess the woman for any allergies or adverse reactions prior to prescribing.
- Consider local resistance to antibiotics and also consider microbiologist and/or obstetrician recommendations regarding first line drug of choice during pregnancy.
- Refer the woman if there are any symptoms associated with pyelonephritis or if the woman has had more than two UTIs in this pregnancy.
- Follow-up culture and sensitivity of original MSU, and alter antibiotics where indicated according to the bacteria isolated and sensitivity.
- Ensure the woman does a clean MSU 7–14 days after completing antibiotics to make certain that the infection has cleared.
- Treat women with asymptomatic bacteriuria with three-day regimen and screen monthly for UTI (Lang 2001).
- Antibiotics that can be used for UTI (not in order of preference):
  - nitrofurantoin 100 mg BD for three to five days for an uncomplicated UTI. Do not use urine alkalinisers during treatment with nitrofurantoin, as this drug requires an acidic urinary pH to work effectively. Do not use in women with G6PD deficiency or when labour is imminent. Side-effects: GI.
  - amoxycillin/clavulanic acid 625 mg TDS for three days. Side-effects: possible candidiasis.
  - cefaclor 250–500 mg q 6 hr for three days. Oral cephalosporins should not be first choice for community-acquired UTIs (Lang 2001; Nicolle 2002).

Sexually transmitted infections

New Zealand midwives are legally able to prescribe for women during the antenatal, intrapartum and postnatal period. The legislation does not allow prescribing for any partners. Hence decisions need to be made with the woman concerning screening for sexually transmitted infections (STIs) and the rationale for eradication of any infections. If a woman returns a positive *Chlamydia* or gonorrhoea swab, a discussion needs to occur regarding the importance of treatment to avoid risk of pelvic inflammatory disease, preterm labour and stillbirth (Gencay et al 2000; Say 2004). In cases of STIs, all sexual partners require simultaneous treatment. Some sexually acquired infections can be asymptomatic and might be present but undetected for a number of years. *Chlamydia* screening during pregnancy generally includes a urethral swab and a cervical swab (Say 2004). Urine screening for *Chlamydia* and self-administered swabs are still being evaluated for efficacy.

Recommended prescribing

- *Chlamydia* (partners require treatment simultaneously for all STIs):
  - Erythromycin ethylsuccinate 800 mg BD for 7–10 days.
  - Specialist doctors are currently using azithromycin 1 g orally stat. At the time of print, azithromycin is listed as Category B by the FDA.
- *Trichomoniasis*:
  - Metronidazole 200 mg TDS for seven days.
  - A longer course is more effective in pregnancy than stat doses.
- *Gonorrhoea*: current recommendations are to refer all women with gonorrhoea in pregnancy to an STI specialist in view of bacterial resistant patterns associated with treating gonorrhoea. Say (2004) recommends that all patients with gonorrhoea be treated for incubating *Chlamydia* infections at the same time.
- *Human immune-deficiency virus (HIV)*: there is currently debate as to whether HIV serology screening should be optional or routine screening during pregnancy.[1] Formal counselling prior to HIV screening is available in some areas. Treatment regimens continue to develop and antenatal therapy clearly reduces the maternal–fetal transfer of HIV. This information should be shared with women when screening is discussed.

Mastitis

The importance of good assessment skills is paramount in detecting and managing mastitis. Continuity of care and regular postnatal visits will assist the woman and the midwife to problem solve most situations related to mastitis. Complementary remedies are used by a number of women; however, these remedies lack formal evidence and are therefore at the woman's discretion. Symptoms of mastitis include 'flu-like' symptoms, sore breast with reluctance to breastfeed from that breast and possibly a firm red wedge area on the breast. Redness of the breast might not be visible until 12 or more hours after the 'flu-like' symptoms in a deep tissue breast infection. Mastitis frequently originates from a previous sore or cracked nipple. If rapid response to conservative management does not occur, treatment with antibiotics is warranted.

Recommended prescribing

- Undertake a full physical assessment of the woman, including temperature and pulse to exclude other pathology.
- Check for penicillin-related allergy.

- Flucloxacillin 500 mg QID either one-hour prior to food or two hours after food for 10–14 days (10 days is usual treatment, but 14 days might be required if recurrent mastitis).
- Rationale for flucloxacillin is to use the narrowest-spectrum antimicrobial for the pathogen. *Staphylococcus aureus* is the most common cause of mastitis, entering through a cracked or damaged nipple, and > 98% of *S. aureus* are currently susceptible to flucloxacillin. Risk factors for flucloxacillin-induced liver injury include treatment greater than 14 days, high doses, and female gender (Begg 2001).
- Dicloxacillin is an alternative to flucloxacillin (if funded) and has less risk of hepatic reaction than flucloxacillin. However, it appears to have a greater risk of interstitial nephritis.
- Amoxicillin-clavulanate and cefaclor are broader-spectrum antimicrobials and therefore have more side-effects such as diarrhoea and candidiasis. The use of these might encourage resistant organisms. First-generation cephalosporins could be used depending on restrictions such as hospital-only medicines and funding restrictions. Cefaclor is not recommended, as noted previously, because of its broader spectrum of activity and concerns about serum sickness (Begg 2001).
- If the woman is penicillin-allergic and has safely taken erythromycin previously, prescribe 400 mg erythromycin QID or 800 mg BD for 10–14 days.
- Follow up to ensure that the woman breastfeeds from the affected breast (to prevent a breast abscess). There should be notable improvement within 24 hours; if not, refer to a colleague (midwife or doctor) experienced in the management of mastitis. The woman might require intravenous antibiotics to combat severe infection, or require an incision or aspiration to remove large amounts of pus within blocked ducts.

Endometritis

Endometritis occurs more commonly after caesarean births than vaginal births. The infection may be early (two to three days post partum) or late (three to six weeks post partum) (Chaim et al 2003). This can be caused by a number of pathogens, including odourless bacteria such as Group B Streptococcus. The midwife needs to have a low threshold for consultation regarding any woman suspected of having endometritis, in view of possible systemic infection. Reporting of elevated temperature is essential and the New Zealand referral guidelines indicate consultation with an obstetrician when the woman's temperature is > 37.6°C with tachycardia.

Prescribing should be in consultation with an obstetric specialist. If fever is present, an obstetrician might prescribe intravenous antimicrobials. A cervical swab should be cultured to isolate the causative organism(s). Oral amoxicillin/clavulanic acid 625 mg TDS for five to seven days could be prescribed for women who are not pyrexic with abdominal tenderness and/or foul-smelling lochia (Chaim et al 2003). If the woman

---

> **BOX 29.4** **Prescription guidelines**
>
> To ensure accurate prescription of a pharmaceutical medicine:
>
> ▶ Use accurate physical examination and diagnostic skills.
> ▶ Consider whether a pharmaceutical is appropriate for the condition.
> ▶ Have comprehensive knowledge of 'commonly' used drugs, including action/effect, and communicate this information to the woman.
> ▶ Ensure that the treatment is regarded as safe during pregnancy or during lactation.
> ▶ Consider the evidence in relation to the clinical scenario.
> ▶ Prescribe the appropriate drug, dose, frequency and duration of treatment.
> ▶ Monitor for any adverse reactions and refer accordingly.
> ▶ Do follow-up culture and sensitivity and alter drug if necessary.
> ▶ Be able to research information about drugs used less commonly.
> ▶ Have a low threshold for consultation with an obstetrician or general medical practitioner.
>
> (Source: adapted from Banning 2004 and Lethard 2001)

is penicillin-allergic, consider erythromycin in consultation with an obstetrician.

Lower-segment caesarean section wound infection

In view of rising caesarean rates and shorter postnatal stays, midwives are increasingly monitoring women in the community for wound infections. Prescribing for wound infections should be discussed with an obstetrician, as it is outside the scope of midwifery practice. Clean the wound site prior to collecting a swab. Be vigilant at following up culture and sensitivity of the wound swab.

Postpartum contraception

Lactational amenorrhoea provides reasonable contraceptive efficacy in the first six months, provided the criteria of amenorrhoea (after 56 days post partum) and exclusive breastfeeding are met. However, many women want to add a pharmaceutical method such as the progestogen-only pill for extra protection. Lactational amenorrhoea is generally not a reliable method of family planning in Western countries (Stables & Rankin 2005).

Progestogen-only pill

The progestogen-only pill (POP) has 96–97% efficacy, depending on compliance, and is frequently chosen as an oestrogen-free contraceptive method post partum. POPs do not reduce the milk volume for lactating women (Perheentupa et al 2003) and minute amounts of the POP pass through the breast milk to the baby, according to studies done on norethisterone- and levonorgestrel-containing POPs (Guillebaud 2004). The POP, as with most other medicines, is metabolised by the liver. The most important mode of action is increased viscosity of cervical mucus, making sperm transport less favourable. Anovulation occurs in approximately 60% of women, but varies in each woman's cycle and between women, with older women more likely to experience anovulation. The variations in menstrual bleeding, from amenorrhoea to women experiencing regular menstrual cycles, are related to ovarian activity. The POP also decreases the receptivity of the endometrium and alters tubal motility (Guillebaud 2004). Perheentupa et al (2003) concluded that the POP contraceptive effect is due to local action of the POP on the endometrium and cervix, and that it is breastfeeding itself that suppresses the ovarian function.

As with any medicine, midwives should not prescribe the POP to any women with altered liver function. The POP is affected by enzyme-inducing drugs such as some anticonvulsants and rifampicin. Women taking medication should have a consultation with a medical practitioner in order to assess drug interactions and to ensure safe prescribing. Other contraindications include arterial disease (including hypertension BP > 140/90), abnormal lipids, any cancers, trophoblastic disease, pathological changes in nervous or muscle tissue, previous ectopic pregnancy, functional ovarian cysts (as these appear increasingly with use of the POP) and undiagnosed irregular menstrual bleeding (Guillebaud 2004). The World Health Organization has deemed the POP an acceptable contraceptive method for use in women with a history of venous thrombosis, pulmonary embolus, diabetes and obesity (Apgar & Greenberg 2000); however, all these conditions warrant a decision by a medical practitioner as opposed to a midwife prescriber.

Prescribing recommendations

- It is prudent to reassess the woman carefully concerning her history, and to document this discussion.
- Record the woman's blood pressure and document.
- There is increased likelihood of irregular bleeding if the POP is started before day 21 post partum. If the woman chooses, she could start the POP at six weeks post partum to lessen any exposure of the newborn to the POP (Guillebaud 2004).
- Provide sound education on the POP. A pill needs to be taken every day of the month within three hours of the same time each day (there are no inactive/sugar pills in POP packages, unlike some combined oral contraceptives).
- If a POP is 'missed'—considered as > 12 hours late if the woman is breastfeeding and has amenorrhoea (Szarewski & Guillebaud 2000), otherwise > 3 hours late—then the woman should either abstain from sexual intercourse or use a barrier method of contraception for 48 hours until viscous cervical mucus re-establishes (Apgar & Greenberg 2000).
- Antimicrobials do not affect the POP unless they are enzyme-inducing drugs (oestrogen is recycled in the entero-hepatic cycle, not progestogen) such as rifampicin for tuberculosis and griseofulvin used for fungal infections of the skin and nails (Szarewski & Guillebaud 2000).
- Counselling should be given regarding symptoms of ectopic pregnancy and functional ovarian cysts. The woman should be informed of the possibility of irregular bleeding.
- Do not write 'mini pill' on the prescription form, as the pharmacist might interpret this as a low-dose combined oral contraceptive pill.
- Brand names are acceptable on the prescription form. Check which brands are fully subsidised, to minimise cost to the woman.
- Some brands of POP include: ethynodial acetate (Femulen®); norethisterone (Noriday 28®), levonorgestrel (Microval/Microlut®).

Combined oral contraceptive

Some non-lactating women elect to use the combined oral contraceptive (COC) as their choice of contraception in the immediate postpartum period. Bryant and colleagues (2003) detail the actions of the COC containing oestrogen and progestogen. It appears that oestrogen decreases FSH release, thus impairing follicle development and reducing the likelihood of ovulation. Progestogen reduces the LH release necessary for 'triggering' ovulation, along with effects on the cervix and tubal motility. In contrast to the POP, the main action of the COC is suppression of ovulation.

COCs have been associated with venous thromboembolism (VTE) and fatal pulmonary embolism. O'Brien (1999) commented that four well-designed studies that reported an increased risk of VTE with 'third-generation' pills had been subjected to relentless criticism. O'Brien concluded that in a $3 billion world contraceptive market the stakes are high, yet on evidence the second-generation COCs should be the first choice of pill when prescribing. Factor V Leiden mutation might also contribute to VTE and is reported as the most common genetic risk factor. Vandenbrouchke and colleagues (1996) have suggested screening women who use COCs for this characteristic (referral to a doctor would be necessary).

Parkin and colleagues (2000) reviewed fatal pulmonary embolism in all New Zealand women of childbearing age from 1990 to 1998. Third-generation oral contraceptive pills containing the newer type progestogen, desogestrel and gestodene (purported to have less androgenic effects), were the most commonly used COC by the women who died. Skegg (2000) concluded that women taking third-generation (desogestrel or gestodene) COCs have about twice the risk of

Clinical point

The dose of oestrogen in the COC is kept as low as is compatible with clinical effectiveness in order to reduce the possibility of adverse effects. However, because of the high hepatic first pass, a significant percentage of molecules travel around the entero-hepatic cycle before reaching the general circulation. If a woman takes antibiotics while on the COC, the resulting lack of intestinal bacteria can reduce the amount of oestrogen that is de-conjugated in the intestine and thus available for reabsorption into the circulation. The resulting lowered blood levels can fall into the sub-therapeutic range, exposing the woman to the possibility of conceiving (Galbraith et al 2001).

Critical thinking exercise

1   How will you decide whether a woman requires antibiotics to treat mastitis or whether to consider conservative management initially?
2   Explore the research findings on the contraceptive efficacy of lactational amenorrhoea. Why do you think lactational amenorrhoea is 'under-used' by Western postpartum women?
3   Discuss how you would explain to a woman the pathophysiology of VTE in association with particular types of combined contraceptive pills.
4   Differentiate the signs and symptoms associated with each of the following vaginal infections: candidiasis, trichomoniasis, chlamydia and gonorrhoea.
5   Discuss the 'pros and cons' of injectable progestogens and the information that you would share with women who might be considering this method of contraception post partum.

VTE of women using preparations containing levonorgestrel (second-generation COC).

Prescribing recommendations

● Check thoroughly for history that would preclude midwifery prescribing of COC (e.g. past or present circulatory disease in the woman or in her family history, disease of the liver, conditions affected by sex steroids, possible pregnancy, undiagnosed genital tract bleeding, any cancers, hypertension, smokers over 35 years of age, immobilisation, use of other medication, breastfeeding, etc) (Guillebaud 2004).
● Document the investigation of risk factors and record the woman's blood pressure.
● Do not prescribe the COC prior to 21 days post partum. After 21 days post partum there is a lower risk of thrombosis, as blood-clotting factors have returned to normal levels. The earliest fertile ovulation after a full-term pregnancy was shown biochemically to be 28 days post partum in non-lactating women (Guillebaud 2004). Hence a start on day 21 post partum allows seven days to suppress follicular activity.
● Document whether or not the woman has used the COC previously and any effects related to previous use.
● Prescribe a second-generation COC with ethinyloestradiol of 30–35 µg or less, combined with levonorgestrel or norethisterone.
● It is acceptable to use a 'brand' name on the prescription. Ensure that the 'brand' selected is subsidised.
● Provide the woman with advice for taking the COC and information if a pill is 'missed' (> 12 hours late) (family planning brochures are useful).

Injectable progestogen contraceptive

The primary action of the progestogen dose given by injection is to suppress ovulation. There is a much higher dose level initially, which then declines. It is essential that the injection site is intramuscular and is *not* massaged, as this shortens the duration of action. Guillebaud (2004) recommends that postpartum women preferably receive a first injection at 5–6 weeks post partum, as earlier administration increases the likelihood of heavy and prolonged bleeding. Lactation is not inhibited by the use of injectable progestogen. There have been isolated cases of anaphylactic reactions after injection of progestogens. It is prudent practice to administer the injection in a setting where adult adrenaline and resuscitation facilities are available.

Rules for writing prescriptions

There is no formulary list for New Zealand midwives. Midwives are expected to prescribe within their scope of practice. Prescriptions must conform to the requirements of Regulation 41, Medicines Regulations 1984 (Amendment No. 3 1990):

41 – Form of prescription – Every prescription shall (a) be legibly and indelibly printed: and (b) be signed personally by the prescriber with his [her] usual signature (not being a facsimile or other stamp) and dated; and (c) set out the address of the prescriber.

Prescriptions can be made on individual client prescription form, hospital medication order charts, and women's notes for midwife administration of drugs at a home birth.

Specific rules

Individual prescription forms must include:
● *prescriber information*—name, address and contactable

telephone number, designation (i.e. registered midwife), Midwifery Council Annual Practising Certificate number, signature, date of writing prescription

- *client information*—client's title, full name (include middle name or initial), residential address (PO box number is not sufficient), date of birth (if under 13 years)
- *medication information* (use one box on the prescription form per medication)
- name of drug, strength of preparation (e.g. 250 mg), dose, frequency of dose, route of administration, instructions for administration (e.g. before food), quantity dispensed or period prescribed for. Strike out any unused medication boxes.
- *prescription codes*—codes serve an administrative function to enable batching of prescriptions and payment to pharmacists. They are altered periodically. Midwives should ensure that they use the current codes.

Only use established abbreviations that have clear meaning to pharmacists. Writing instructions in full might prevent any miscommunication.

Conclusion

In this chapter an overview of pharmacology has been provided in order to assist student midwives with revision of pharmacology and the physiological changes during pregnancy. Antimicrobials that are commonly used for conditions experienced during pregnancy and childbirth have been reviewed. Specific pregnancy-related conditions have been discussed in association with evidence-based practice in relation to assessment, diagnosis and treatment. The authors stress the need for midwives to maintain a current knowledge base of pharmacology and pharmaceuticals. Midwives need to have a low threshold for referral and to only prescribe medicines within the scope of midwifery practice and legislation. Midwives need to have particular concern for the wellbeing of the woman and baby, and consider the effects of pharmaceuticals upon the maternal–infant dyad. Midwives also have a responsibility to encourage women and families to maintain optimal lifestyles and to minimise the use of antibiotics. Finally, if midwives do undertake prescription of medicines, accuracy of the prescription and follow-up of the client are essential for best midwifery practice.

Review questions

1 How does the Australian Categorisation of Drugs and Safety during pregnancy assist midwives in safe prescribing practices?

2 What conditions (occurring during pregnancy or pre-existing conditions) might affect liver function and therefore preclude the prescription of medicines by midwives?

3 Explain the physiological changes that take place during normal pregnancy and how these might affect pharmacokinetics.

4 Explain bacterial resistance in relation to urinary tract infection and the implications this has for prescribing practice.

5 List five principles that prescribers can employ to help minimise bacterial resistance.

6 How would you decide whether to treat a pregnant woman with a suspected urinary tract infection or to wait for the availability of laboratory findings?

7 What factors would you consider in deciding (in partnership with the woman) whether or not to commence iron supplementation during pregnancy?

8 How would you respond if a pregnant woman's partner asked you to write a prescription for his/her own personal needs?

9 Review all the assessments that you would undertake prior to prescribing a postpartum woman the progestogen-only pill.

10 What sources will you need to use/access in order to maintain your current knowledge to enable safe prescribing practice as a midwife?

Note

1 In March 2006 the New Zealand Ministry of Health introduced routine antenatal screening of pregnant women for HIV. Midwives need to be aware of their responsibilities in relation to routine screening.

Online resources

American College of Obstetricians and Gynaecologists, http://www.acog.org

Australian Government, Department of Health and Ageing, Therapeutic Goods Administration, Prescribing medicines in pregnancy: an Australian categorisation of risk of drug use in pregnancy, http://www.tga.gov.au/docs/html/mip/medicine.htm

Centers for Disease Control and Prevention (search for sexually transmitted infections and pregnancy), http://www.cdc.gov

Medsafe (NZ Ministry of Health), information on medicines, http://www.medsafe.govt.nz

PHARMAC, Pharmaceutical Management Agency of New Zealand, http://www.pharmac.govt.nz (online access to New Zealand Pharmaceutical Schedule detailing which pharmaceuticals attract subsidy)

References

Adams-Graves P 2001 The clinical approach to anemia in pregnancy. Contemporary Clinical Gynecology and Obstetrics 1:309–323

Andrade S, Gurwitz M, Davis R et al 2004 Prescription drug use in pregnancy. American Journal of Obstetrics and Gynecology 191:398–407

Andrist L 2001 Vaginal health and infections. Journal of Obstetric Gynecology and Neonatal Nursing 30:306–314

Apgar B, Greenberg G 2000 Using progestins in clinical practice. American Family Physician 62(8):1839–1846

Banning M 2004 Nurse prescribing, nurse education and related research in the United Kingdom: a review of the literature. Nurse Education Today. Online: elsevierhealth.com/journals/nedt

Begg E 2001 Urinary tract infection. Premec for Midwives May 2001. National Preferred Medicines Centre Inc, Wellington

Begg EJ 2003 Instant clinical pharmacology. Blackwell, Malden, Mass.

Bryant B, Knights K, Salerno E 2003 Pharmacology for health professionals. Mosby, Sydney

Campbell N 2003 Prescribing for midwives. Midwifery News 31:14–15

Chaim W, Horowitz S, David J et al 2003 Ureaplasma urealyticum in the development of postpartum endometritis. European Journal of Obstetrics and Gynecology and Reproductive Biology 109:145–148

Chaliha C, Stanton S 2002 Urological problems in pregnancy. British Journal of Urology 89:469–477

Comerford KC (Ed) 2003 Australia New Zealand nursing drug handbook. Lippincott Williams & Wilkins, Sydney

de Santis M, Straface G, Carducci B 2004 Risk of drug-induced congenital defects. European Journal of Obstetrics and Gynecology and Reproductive Biology 117:10–19. Online: www.sciencedirect.com

Department of Health 1990 Nurses Amendment Act 1990: information for health providers. DOH, Wellington

Engstrom J, Sittler C 1994 Nurse-midwifery management of iron deficiency anaemia during pregnancy. Journal of Nurse-Midwifery 39:S20–S32

Foureur M 2001 Newsletter: midwifery prescribing and antimicrobials 2:1–2

Galbraith A, Bullock S, Manias E 2001 Fundamentals of pharmacology. A text for nurses and allied health professionals (3rd edn). Prentice Hall Health, Sydney

Gardiner S 2002 Drugs in pregnancy. New Ethicals Journal June: 61–63

Gencay M, Koskiniemi M, Ammala P et al 2000 Chlamydia trachomatis seropositivity is associated both with stillbirth and preterm delivery. Acta Pathologica, Microbiologica et Immunologica Scandinavica 108:584–588

Guillebaud J 2004 Contraception: your questions answered (4th edn). Churchill Livingstone, London

Hansen W, Peacock A, Yankowitz J 2002 Safe prescribing practices in pregnancy and lactation. Journal of Midwifery and Women's Health 47:409

Haram K, Nilsen S, Ulvik R 2001 Iron supplementation in pregnancy—evidence and controversies. Acta Obstetricica et Gynecologica Scandinavica 80:683–688

Holland LM, Adams MP 2003 Core concepts in pharmacology. Prentice Hall, New Jersey

Hunter M, Roke C 2002 Commentary on thrush and progestogen only pill. Premec. National Preferred Medicines Centre Inc, Wellington

Juarez-Vazquez J, Bonizzoni E, Scotti A 2002 Iron plus folate is more effective than iron alone in the treatment of iron deficiency anaemia in pregnancy: a randomised, double blind clinical trial. British Journal of Obstetrics and Gynaecology 109:1009–1014

Lang S (Ed) 2001 Guide to pathogens and antibiotic treatment (6th edn). Adis International, Auckland

Lethard H 2001 Understanding medicines: conceptual analysis of nurses' needs for knowledge and understanding of pharmacology part one. Nurse Education Today 21:266–271

Lindsay P 2000 Pre term labour. In: B Sweet (Ed) Mayes Midwifery (12th edn). Baillière Tindall, London

McKay K 2000 Iron deficiency anaemia. The Practising Midwife 3:25–27

McMullin M, White R, Lappin T et al 2003 Haemoglobin during pregnancy: relationship to erythropoietin and haematinic status. European Journal of Haematology 71:44–50

Medsafe 2003 New Zealand Medicines and Medical Devices Safety Authority, New Zealand Ministry of Health. Online: www.medsafe.govt.nz

Midwifery Council of New Zealand 2004 Midpoint Newsletter

Miller EL 2002 The penicillins: a review and update. Journal of Midwifery and Women's Health 47(6):69–77

Ministry of Health 1997 Code 4147 Planning for pregnancy. Folic acid and spina bifida. MOH, Wellington

Morgan J 2000 Vaginal discharge. New Ethicals Journal March: 65–69

National Health and Medical Research Council (NHMRC) 1993 Revised statement on the relationship between dietary folic acid and neural tube defects such as spina bifida. NHMRC, Canberra

New Ethicals Compendium 2000 (7th edn). Adis International, Auckland

New Zealand College of Midwives (NZCOM) 2002 Consensus statement: prescribing guidelines. Online: www.nzcom.org.nz, accessed 3 October 2004

Nicolle L 2002 Urinary tract infection: traditional pharmacological therapies. American Journal of Medicine 113:35–44

O'Brien P 1999 The third generation oral contraceptive controversy. British Medical Journal 319:795–796

Page L (Ed) 2000 The new midwifery: science and sensitivity in practice. Churchill Livingstone, Edinburgh

Parkin L, Skegg D, Wilson M et al 2000 Oral contraceptives and fatal pulmonary embolism. Lancet 355:2133–2134

Perheentupa A, Critchley H, Illingworth P et al 2003 Effect of progestin-only pill on pituitary-ovarian axis during lactation. Contraception 67:467–471

Rubin P (Ed) 2000 Prescribing in pregnancy (3rd edn). BMJ Publishing, London

Say J 2004 Management of sexually transmitted infections and related conditions for midwives. Handout for student midwives

Schirm E, Meijer M, Tobi H et al 2004 Drug use by pregnant women and comparable non-pregnant women in the Netherlands with reference to the Australian classification system. European Journal of Obstetrics and Gynecology and Reproductive Biology 114:182–188

Shargel L, Mutnick AH, Soouney PF et al (Eds) 2001 Comprehensive pharmacy review (4th edn). Lippincott Williams & Wilkins, Philadelphia

Skegg D 2000 Third generation oral contraceptives: caution is still justified. British Medical Journal 321:190–192

Stables D, Rankin J 2005 Physiology in childbearing (2nd edn). Elsevier, Edinburgh

Stefanogiannis N (Ed) 2003 Improving folate intake in New Zealand: policy implications. Ministry of Health, Auckland

Szarewski A, Guillebaud J 2000 Contraception: a user's guide (3rd edn). Oxford University Press, New York

Tytgat G, Heading R, Muller-Lissner S et al 2003 Contemporary understanding and management of reflux and constipation in the general population and pregnancy: a consensus meeting. Alimentary Pharmacology Therapy 18:291–301

Vandenbrouchke J, van der Meer F, Helmerhorst F et al 1996 Factor V Leiden: should we screen oral contraceptive users and pregnant women? British Medical Journal 313:1127–1130

Varney H, Kriebs JM, Gegor C 2004 Varney's midwifery (4th edn). Jones and Bartlett, Boston

Wulff M, Ekstrom E 2003 Iron supplementation during pregnancy in Sweden: to what extent is the national recommendation followed? Acta Obstetrica et Gynecologica Scandinavica 82: 628–635

Young G, Jewell D 2001 Topical treatment for vaginal candidiasis in pregnancy (Cochrane Review). Cochrane Library (2). John Wiley & Sons, Chichester

Statutes (NZ)

(see www.legislation.govt.nz/libraries/contents)

Medicines Act 1981

Medicines Regulations 1984

Medicines Regulations 1984 Amendment No. 3 1990

Further reading

Student midwives should access references cited in recently published journal articles and texts related to microbiology, pharmacology and prescribing practices. The following resources are useful.

Australia New Zealand Nursing Drug Handbook 2003 Lippincott Williams & Wilkins, Philadelphia

Begg E 2000 Clinical pharmacology essentials: the principles behind the prescribing process. Adis International, Auckland

Shaw JP 1994 Prescribing rights in New Zealand: a public discussion paper. Ministry of Health, Wellington

MIMS New Ethicals

New Ethicals Journal

New Zealand Pharmaceutical Schedules

CHAPTER 30

Completing the midwife–woman partnership

Rhondda Davies

Key terms

cervical screening, closure, cultural health, debrief, documentation, Edinburgh Postnatal Depression Scale, emotional health, family planning/contraception, informed choice, physical health, professional friendship, referral, sexual health, six-week development, social health, spiritual health, Standards Review, support services, vaccination, well baby, well woman

Chapter overview

This chapter outlines a model final assessment by the midwife, of the woman and her baby. This assessment ordinarily includes: modified physical assessments of both mother and baby; a final review of the mother's mental wellbeing; contraception needs/choices; cervical screening; referral to well child and well woman providers; and a final debriefing of the maternity experience and reflection on care. The chapter concludes with final documentation requirements and an indication of the role of subsequent midwifery Standards Review process.

Learning outcomes

Learning outcomes for this chapter are:

1 To explain the importance of a thorough physical, mental and social assessment of the woman and baby before transfer from the maternity carer to well woman / well child carers

2 To establish what constitutes normal six-week or four-week developments for the woman/family and for the baby

3 To identify what should be conveyed in referral notes to these carers and what may require earlier referral

4 To discuss the methods of family planning appropriate for the woman and her partner, and the provision of information and advice, and ordering/prescribing for a method within the norms and legislation of New Zealand and/or Australia, according to the woman's informed choice

5 To explain the requirements for documentation of the completion of care and safe, comfortable closure of the professional friendship with the woman and her family

6 To highlight the important aim of care in the puerperium to affirm the woman's self-esteem and confidence in independent parenting.

The woman's health

The midwife's approach to the final assessment should be a holistic one, seeking information on the woman's current health status and following up on issues that have arisen in the previous six weeks (e.g. with regard to the woman's physical health). Recent literature draws attention to the following physical symptoms at six weeks that are typically played down by postpartum women: backache; perineal pain (whether or not there is a healing wound); urinary incontinence; sexual problems; haemorrhoids; constipation; faecal incontinence; headaches; fatigue; recovery from infection (of, for example, a caesarean wound or episiotomy wound) (Glazener et al 1995, cited in Symon et al 2003; MacArthur 1999).

It is most important to attend to outstanding social issues, such as: mobility, financial restraints, access to support services and new mothers' groups (e.g. La Leche League, Australian Breastfeeding Association, Ukaiko, locally organised new mothers' groups/playgroups for older siblings). Also consider issues such as whether the woman plans to return to work, and if so, how she will continue breastfeeding.

Those who plan to return to work or study prior to their baby reaching six months may well need advice and support to continue exclusively or fully breastfeeding. Hopefully, this issue will have arisen in discussion much earlier in your care than at the discharge check. Among the information the woman will require is an explanation of why it is important to continue breastfeeding until six months, and how to inform and gain the support of her employer—for example, the advantages of a family-friendly workplace include happier workers who take less time off due to baby illness. Figure 30.1 shows some options to discuss with women who intend to work and breastfeed. It is recommended that you discuss and leave clear written instructions regarding expressing milk, storage and hygiene. The women will also require local information on organisations specialising in breastfeeding support.

Emotional health

What does the woman notice about her mood? What does her partner/family/any significant other notice? What efforts does she make to leave the house and actively seek social contact?

The Edinburgh Postnatal Depression Scale (EPNDS) questionnaire has not been universally applauded as effective (Forman et al 2000; Shakespeare et al 2003). However, Barclay

---

Clinical scenario 1

You arrive at S's basement flat. She greets you with a warm smile and welcomes you in her mid-European accent. S is a recent immigrant, resident in your country through marriage, whose husband left her during the pregnancy. She is bringing up their daughter alone with the support of her husband's family, a wide circle of friends and intermittent contact from him. She has a thriving baby girl whom she is exclusively breastfeeding. Her labour and birth were spontaneous. Her perineum sustained a second-degree tear and was sutured. A summary of her postpartum recovery includes referral to a lactation consultant for training of her daughter to breastfeed, not nipple suck, as she left hospital doing. Also her perineum continued to cause discomfort without developing an infection requiring treatment. She has, however, reported improvement over the last two weekly visits at four and five weeks.

As S's midwife, summarise your discharge visit priorities.

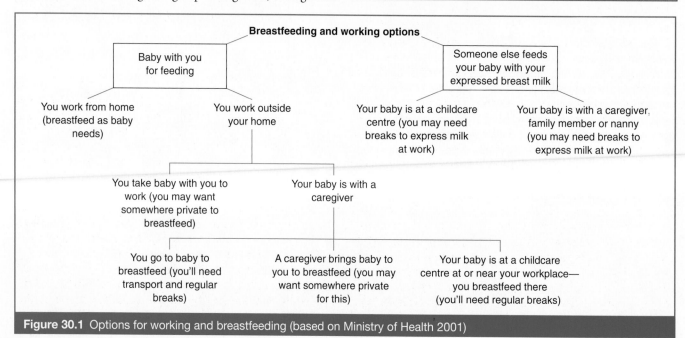

Figure 30.1 Options for working and breastfeeding (based on Ministry of Health 2001)

BOX 30.1 Support groups

Does the woman know what resources are available for support for postnatal distress? For example, the following website provides contact details of consumer mental health support groups in New Zealand: http://www.nzgg.org.nz/guidelines/0039/Appendix_8.pdf

and Lie (2004), after a chart review conducted by investigators from the University of Rochester School of Medicine in New York, reported that 'the EPNDS should be considered for use in screening for post partum depression (PPD) in the first year well-child visit setting. However, adequate quality control measures need to be in place for consistent implementation'. They also stated that 'the EPNDS results in higher rates of detection of maternal depression during the postpartum year' (Barclay & Lie 2004). This screening device is used by some New Zealand lead maternity carers to assess the need to refer with possible pathological postnatal distress/depression.

Spiritual health

Supporting the woman's spiritual needs requires a carefully accrued knowledge of the woman and her pregnancy, childbirth and early parenting journey (possible with LMC continuity of care), and actively listening to her reflections. Some women can articulate these clearly; others require gentle, persistent delving if the midwife detects spiritual pain. You might not feel qualified to support the woman in spiritual difficulty. Rather, your role might be to involve the woman's own spiritual guides through her family.

Sexual health

Many women may be reluctant to discuss sexual ill health fully with their midwife, even at six weeks. A midwife is expected to raise the topic: enquire about dyspareunia and impart the clear message (whether or not intercourse has resumed) that the woman does not need to tolerate any ongoing discomfort, and should seek help if she needs it. Sensitive questioning may help elicit other sexual health related concerns and lead to a discussion about lack of desire. Several factors such as a difficult birth, lochial discharge, tender, secreting breasts, sore nipples, altered physical appearance (some women may never have considered that their genitals would be permanently changed), or fear of becoming pregnant again, can combine to depress the woman's interest in intercourse. Breastfeeding also has an effect: 'Although there are some physiological similarities between sexual arousal and breastfeeding, erotic stimulation and/or orgasm do not usually accompany breastfeeding. The hormonal basis of breastfeeding usually causes the woman to "fall in love" with her baby, thereby ensuring that she will respond to its needs' (Auckland Homebirth Association 1993, p 139). Exhaustion, changes in libido, deterioration in general understanding and communication between the couple can

Clinical scenario 2

C is a woman who, with her second pregnancy, approached you to be her labour and birth midwife on advice from her rural midwife LMC. She chose to birth at a secondary care birth facility. Her first labour was complicated by fetal distress and she vividly remembers travelling in second stage in an ambulance from a birthing unit to a secondary care maternity facility because of concern for the baby. The resulting tension and extreme discomfort guided her choice this time, to labour and birth some 90 minutes away from home, to avoid a possible repeat of the transfer in late first stage. Her (second) labour was spontaneous and she birthed normally without fetal distress—a second daughter. However, her perineal laceration, you determined, was beyond your skills to repair, and you sought advice and assistance from a senior registrar. He speedily repaired her wound, and she returned to her local primary facility for postpartum care and six-week assessment.

Five months later, she has phoned you, seeking your help in reviewing her perineal condition. She is experiencing severe dyspareunia, to the extent that sexual intercourse is impossible, and her marriage is under strain. She very much wants a third child.

1 What steps can you take within the system of referral in your area?
2 How does any lesson learned from such a scenario guide you in your approach to sexual function assessment in future six-week discharge visits?

all develop, whether or not there is discomfort. It is beginning to be understood that such difficulties are common (Dixon et al 2000; Force 2000).

Cultural health

Like spiritual health, cultural health is largely 'glanced off' in both societies. In New Zealand the tangata whenua (people of the land) have only recently asserted the clear principle of cultural safety among the healthcare spheres of New Zealand society (Ramsden 1993). The capacity of the LMC midwife to acknowledge a culture that may be different from the dominant culture yet clearly potentially influential on the health status of her client, is to be carefully nurtured. Both countries claim multicultural communities. However, in both, the dominant ethnic group has been Anglo-Saxon. This power imbalance between the groups requires constant vigilance in order not to abuse it.

At six weeks it is late in the day to begin assessment. Ideally the midwife will already have incorporated, within her holistic approach, attention to the language, customs, culturally sensitive aspects and safety measures relevant to her client and the family. These efforts will enable her now to seek valid feedback from her client. A midwifery 'wisdom' developing in New Zealand, at least, is the appropriateness, or standard, of regarding each pregnant woman as having her own unique culture. It should be seen as one you will respect throughout the childbearing year (nine and a half to ten months) that you are alongside her.

Infant feeding

By six weeks most women have settled into the method and implementation of the feeding choice they have made for their baby. However, a small number of women may continue to have difficulty with breastfeeding and may require ongoing support. Consumer support groups such as the La Leche League can provide useful support to all breastfeeding women, whether they have experienced problems or not. It is helpful to put women in touch with such community support services. Family can also play an important role with ongoing support.

Some women will gain valuable support and advice from their well-child provider (such as a Plunket nurse or general practitioner) and it is important that your referral to this service provides appropriate information about the progress of infant feeding and any issues that may have arisen.

At the final examination it is important to find out how the woman feels the feeding is going and her reflections on the experience so far. The honest admiration you express of the thriving, smiling, healthy baby is invaluable and will leave a lasting, empowering impression on a first-time breastfeeding mother.

Physical assessment

The six-week check is so-timed as it is known that the endometrium is fully healed by six weeks (Sweet 2000; Fraser & Cooper 2001). Ideally your timing management of this physical check for the mother will ensure that this is attended to some time prior to the baby waking/being woken. Much can be discussed during this one-to-one opportunity with the woman. Wider personal and public health information can be passed on (diet, exercise, smoking, cervical screening), and final questions asked, such as:

- Does she have any concerns regarding her breasts and nipples?
- If there is a caesarean scar and if she chooses midwife discharge assessment (as opposed to returning for an obstetrician clinic appointment), how well healed is this scar?

You should find the uterus completely involuted and not palpable abdominally.

- Has her bleeding stopped? In New Zealand, funding for a scan of the uterus to detect retained products is part of the LMC budget only until six weeks. Ongoing lochial discharge, suggestive of non-involuted uterus and some retention of membrane or other placental fragment, could be assessed at five weeks and an appropriate scan ordered with consent, to avoid the woman/couple sustaining the cost. However, recent studies suggest that ongoing loss up to 42 days is not unusual (Marchant et al 2002) and a decision regarding a scan may best be held over until 8 or 10 weeks and require general practitioner (GP) referral. Obviously the budget issue does not affect Australian midwives and

---

BOX 30.2 Breastfeeding resources

Is the woman aware of all the community-based breastfeeding resources available to her, such as:

▸ La Leche League (NZ)—provide information on breastfeeding, telephone counselling, and run breastfeeding support groups.
▸ Plunket Society (NZ)
▸ hospital and community lactation consultants
▸ Australian Breastfeeding Association.

Clinical scenario 3

H and T conceived their twins by in vitro fertilisation. They live in a small town half an hour's drive out of the city. The twins were born by caesarean section at 38 weeks, as it appeared that the second twin, their son, was in distress on a routine growth scan. Both babies had good Apgars; the girl weighed 2740 g, the boy 2500 g. The girl's cord remnant swelled and oozed post partum and the boy developed mild physiological jaundice. H began by exclusively breastfeeding but the girl's failure to gain weight and show good urine output, together with H's exhaustion, meant that eventually she partially breastfed and partially bottle fed, until the twins were stronger. At home, the girl was mainly bottle fed, the boy mainly breastfed.

What are your discharge priorities and preparations for this family?

Clinical point

Continuity and perineal care
Among the continuity-of-care midwife's rarely noted but distinctive advantages in maintaining and improving good practice is the unique opportunity she has to gain insight in the way in which she looks after the woman's perineum. Such a midwife has the opportunity to follow up on the outcome of her care, and often more than once. In her recent review of midwives' approaches to care of the perineum, Wickham noted (while commenting on Lewis's study) that: 'midwives were able to reflect upon their practice in relation to the woman's experience, something which midwives working in systems without continuity of partnership are not often given the opportunity to do' (Wickham 2001, p S26). Those midwives were then able to alter their practice significantly.

Critical thinking exercise

Research and plan approaches to the following topics as part of your discharge visits:

▶ ongoing substance (including tobacco) abuse issues
▶ obesity
▶ exercise/relaxation needs.

BOX 30.3 Family violence

▶ Do you know the process of documenting your concerns and conveying them to the appropriate agency?
▶ Does your College of Midwives have Best Practice Guidelines for your response in these situations?
▶ NZ midwives can view the NZCOM Consensus Statement on family violence screening at: www.midwife.org.nz/content/documents/93/family%20violence.2002.doc

BOX 30.4 Child sickness danger signals

Is the mother aware of the list of child sickness danger signals detailed on the back cover of the *Well Child Tamariki Ora Health Book* (in New Zealand) and similar publications in Australia? (See the online resources list.)

advice by them to see the GP at the more reasonable time of eight weeks with ongoing, non-period bleeding would suffice.

● If there is bleeding, is it lochial or menstrual?

If there has been any perineal, vaginal wall or labial damage (sutured or not) the area should be assessed for degree of healing. Use a good light, and gloved hands. If she has not done so already, the woman should be encouraged to look in a mirror herself to know how differently her genital area now appears.

The question of dyspareunia is a natural one to arise now. The appropriateness of pelvic examination, cervical smear and vaginal swabbing to take place during this examination is dealt with elsewhere in this book. Do not overlook the state of the anus and the presence of haemorrhoids. Ask directly about faecal incontinence (O'Connell 1997).

Family violence screening

Family or domestic violence is a complex issue that spans all socio-economic strata. A recent study recommends that 'questions regarding abuse should be included in all clinical practices' (Hedin 2000, cited in MIDIRS 2000, p 366). New Zealand LMCs and Australian midwives who are trained to screen for family violence, screen women at booking and discharge.

Indicators of possible family violence are:

● repeated contact with health care practitioners (besides yourself) and hospitals for minor injuries or nonexistent complaints
● constant presence of partner at all your visits, who intervenes to answer your queries for the woman
● making light of bruising
● repeated non-compliance with advice or prescribed treatment.

The baby's health

As you assess baby, note her or his social development and how the mother/parents relate to the baby—that is, continue your assessment of the holistic health of the mother as you interact with the baby. You should also seek and flag any ongoing information needs, including what developments would cause the mother to seek medical attention.

Feeding and behaviour patterns

Breastfeeding

Questions to ask:

● Is breastfeeding going as well as the woman expects?
● Is the baby having yellow, paste-consistency stools?
● How many wet napkins are there in 24 hours?
● How long is the baby's longest sleep?

There might be no discernible pattern yet to the baby's sleeping and feeding behaviour. This may or may not be a concern for the mother/parents. Stress how normal it is for there to be no pattern despite popular expectations of babies quickly establishing a routine of sleeping and feeding (Gainsford 1999). Fatigue will generally be the outstanding physical symptom for the mother, and it is not too late to discuss ways in which she can manage her sleep/rest needs.

Combined breast and bottle feeding

Enquire about the balance between the two and whether the mother is satisfied. Is she aiming to achieve exclusive breastfeeding? Or is there evidence that her supply is reducing—artificial milk being used increasingly—and if so, is this of concern to her? Your goal is to enable satisfaction with her chosen method of feeding her baby; the secure emotional bond between mother and baby is a priority over the ideal of exclusive breastfeeding. Check that she has some understanding of the quantity of milk needed in 24 hours as the baby matures.

Artificial feeding

If the woman began by this method, it is important to review the amounts and the implications. If she began by breastfeeding, this is a time to touch on that experience and debrief, with her consent and readiness.

Behaviour

At six weeks many babies are typically midway through a gut maturation, which they generally achieve by 12 weeks (anecdotal evidence conforms with the author's 15-year experience; see also Viccars 1998). This manifests as distress, described by the parents as a combination of pain and tiredness, to a greater or lesser degree, usually late afternoon/evening. The parents typically report 'difficulty' with winding the baby, and a perceived reluctance by the baby to settle. This does not affect all babies. There is little a midwife can add to the resolution of this phase (ibid) but an ability to listen to the impact this has on their enjoyment of parenthood, and conveying a confidence-boosting prediction that it will normally resolve around the three-month mark. In New Zealand, a group of remedies has been suggested, but none of these, apart from removing dairy products from the maternal diet, has been researched adequately. The challenge is to distinguish, clinically, between the popular diagnoses of 'colic' and 'reflux', and the actual development of true colic and reflux. These conditions do, of course, happen, but to a far lesser extent than is reported or investigated. There is some suggestion of an ethnic basis—such 'colicky' episodes are reported less frequently by Polynesian and Aboriginal mothers/parents.

The baby's sleeping patterns may require a review of feeding or may provide some insight into the degree of the mother's postnatal distress (Greig & Sahar 1999).

Developmental assessment

The outstanding milestone at six weeks is the social smile. The majority of babies developing normally, by this age, have learned to smile directly in response to the other person smiling at them.

Full physical examination

New Zealand midwife LMCs are qualified to carry out the first three well baby checks of the eight laid down by the Department of Health, to track the child's wellbeing up until the age of five years (that is, the physical examination carried out in the baby's first 24 hours, at five to seven days of age, and at the six-week discharge visit).

Before carrying out the examination, take some care to optimise the environment. You will need to set aside an hour to 90 minutes to complete this visit unhurriedly. Ideally it will be timed as closely as possible to a loosely predictable awake time for the baby. The location should be warm and well lit. Take care to anticipate that the baby may spill, void or defecate. Assemble your equipment out of range of audience siblings, unless it has been your approach to share your less expensive, more robust items of gear with curious other children, who respond to being involved and experimenting with the instruments (and subsequently can usually be relied upon to lose interest!)—much better than when these are forbidden. Within your personal safety boundaries, at all times reinforce the discipline approach of the parents.

Engage with the baby, who ideally has had part or all of a feed, and is not unsettled or preoccupied. Note any findings if you doubt they are normal. You will develop your own style of examining; some find it useful to work methodically from 'top to toe'.

- Measure head circumference—assess contour of scalp, palpate suture lines, anterior fontanelle. Discuss this 'soft spot', how to accommodate it, and when it will close over (18 months).
- Examine the eyes with an auriscope for red reflex (both retinas).
- Observe whether the baby follows with her or his eyes as you move in front of the face. Ordinarily you will be chatting with the mother throughout the examination. Her observation of the baby 'following'—indeed, her observation of all the developments you are there to confirm—is naturally reaffirming of her unique expertise regarding her baby.
- Any pseudostrabismus? Explain, reassure, inform of regular monitoring/review.
- Examine the baby's mouth—there may be something you have overlooked in previous examinations, and you need to assess for thrush infection. Do not neglect the gums.
- Ears—ask the woman what she notices about the baby's reaction to loud noise. Any doubts about the baby's ability to hear have probably already been raised, and appropriate referral made. At this point you can remove baby's clothing down to singlet and nappy.
- Skin—as you work your way down the body of the baby, you are assessing health, integrity, colour, temperature and tone of skin and muscle. Openly inspect skin grooves and creases in the baby's body (behind the ears, neck, axillae and groin) for unavoidable moisture traps, which eventually may cause excoriations of the skin and possibly cellulitis.
- Examine the fingernails—are they healthy or is there some parenchyma?
- Auscultate the apex of the heart, preferably through a singlet. You are listening to confirm ongoing absence of murmur. Ideally any suspicion of irregularity has long ago been investigated by a paediatrician. You should also record the rate.
- Auscultate both lungs—listen just below collar bone on left and right, turn baby and listen just below the scapula bilaterally. Record respiratory rate. Remove singlet.
- Palpate the abdomen, remark on continuing breast swelling, check for obvious masses, enlarged liver, discuss benign and also reportable 'lumps' (herniations).
- Assess healing of the umbilicus—is it dry, clean, erythematous? Is there any granuloma? Polyp? Explain ongoing hygiene of the area. Remove napkin. Be aware of the contents of the napkin—comment, give assessment.
- Palpate the femoral pulses—whether or not these have been felt or believed to be felt in earlier well baby checks.
- Baby boy—assess for bilateral descent of testes. Refer to GP if feel undescended on either/both side(s). Comment on normal colour changes of scrotum. Re-check normality of location of urethral opening/meatus. Discuss current approach to hands-off cleaning beneath meatus (Johnston 1994).
- Baby girl—reaffirm, re-educate regarding hygiene and

trust of natural self-cleaning mechanism of mucous membrane, which protects vagina and interior labial walls from infection.

- If baby sufficiently relaxed, check stability of hips.
- Turn baby onto stomach and follow the backbone to the sacrum—confirm no sinus, no dimple, assess symmetry of creases of legs held extended.
- Check for reflexes—Moro or startle (elicited if you hold the baby seated and allow to fall momentarily backward, and catch), stepping reflex etc.
- Any medications due (e.g. third oral dose vitamin K)?

Appendix A shows the six-week well baby check summary documentation as used in the *Well Child Tamariki Ora* book.

Vaccinations

'The purpose of vaccination is to induce protection (immunity) from subsequent disease, similar to that of natural infection, with minimal or no systemic symptoms' (MOH 2002a, pp 1–2). Immunisation is the state of successful vaccination (passive immunity), or of having been exposed to the illness (active immunity), so that the individual is no longer susceptible to the disease.

Health department policy

Free vaccinations are provided in New Zealand and Australia for all children under 16 years of age against: diphtheria, tetanus, pertussis, hepatitis B, *Haemophilus influenzae* type b, measles, mumps, rubella, polio, tuberculosis (for high-risk individuals and groups), and group B meningococcal disease.

Tables 30.1 and 30.2 show immunisation schedules in New Zealand and Australia.

Informed choice/consent issues

An independent midwife whose philosophy includes informed choice is presented with many difficulties when discussing vaccines and informed choice. She must set aside her personal bias, in guiding new parents who may never have considered the issues. Her choices are: to educate herself intensively on all the complex arguments; or to summarise and provide couples (who are serious about choice) with avenues of research for themselves to become informed independently.

Legal provisions that the New Zealand midwife needs to be aware of include: the *Health and Disabilities Commissioner's Act 1994*, the Code of Health and Disability Services Consumers' Rights 1996; and the *Privacy Act 1991*.

TABLE 30.1 Immunisation schedule, New Zealand

	Diphtheria tetanus acellular pertussis-inactivated polio vaccine	Hib (*Haemophilus influenzae* type b) hepatitis B¹ vaccine	Hepatitis B¹ vaccine	Inactivated polio vaccine	Measles mumps rubella vaccine	DTaP/Hib vaccine	Adult type tetanus diphtheria vaccine
	DTaP-IPV	Hib-HepB	HepB	IPV	MMR²	DTaP/Hib	Td³
Route	IM	IM	IM	SC	SC	IM	IM
6 weeks	DTaP-IPV	Hib-HepB					
3 months	DTaP-IPV	Hib-HepB					
5 months	DTaP-IPV		HepB				
15 months					MMR	DTaP/Hib	
4 years	DTaP-IPV				MMR		
11 years				IPV*			Td

*For children who have not received a fourth dose of polio vaccine

IM: intramuscular. SC: subcutaneous

BCG should be offered to babies who will be living in a household or family/whanau with a person with either current TB or a past history of TB; or have one or both parents who identify as being Pacific people; or have parents or household members who have within the last five years lived for a period of six months or longer in countries where there is a high incidence of TB; or will during their first five years be living for three months or longer in a high incidence country.

1 Babies of HBsAg positive mothers need HBIG and hepatitis B vaccine (5 µg) at birth; then continue with the usual schedule at six weeks, three months and five months,. Household and sexual contacts of hepatitis B cases and carriers should be offered hepatitis B immunisation.

2 Women of childbearing age who are susceptible to rubella should be offered MMR or rubella vaccine.

3 Boosters of Td should be offered at 45 and 65 years of age, and after some injuries.

TABLE 30.2   NHMRC standard childhood vaccination schedule for Australian babies, 2005

Age	Disease	Vaccine
2 months	diphtheria, tetanus & pertussis poliomyelitis *Haemophilus influenzae* b	DTPw triple antigen OPV Sabin vaccine HibTITER
4 months	diphtheria, tetanus & pertussis poliomyelitis *Haemophilus influenzae* b	DTPw triple antigen OPV Sabin vaccine HibTITER
6 months	diphtheria, tetanus & pertussis poliomyelitis *Haemophilus influenzae* b	DTPw triple antigen OPV Sabin vaccine HibTITER
12 months	measles, mumps & rubella	MMR Measles/mumps/rubella
18 months	diphtheria, tetanus & pertussis *Haemophilus influenzae* b	DTPa Infanrix HibTITER
4–5 years	diphtheria, tetanus & pertussis poliomyelitis	DTPa Infanrix OPV Sabin vaccine
10–16 years (Year 6)	measles, mumps & rubella hepatitis B	MMR Measles/mumps/rubella Hepatitis B vaccine (3 doses)
15 years or prior to leaving school (Year 10)	diphtheria & tetanus poliomyelitis	ADT adult diphtheria & tetanus OPV Sabin vaccine

Hepatitis B vaccine should be given in a schedule of birth, one and six months for:
- infants and children up to 10 years of age where the mother is a hepatitis B carrier.
- infants and children up to 10 years of age who belong to ethnic groups in which the hepatitis B carrier rate exceeds 2%. These groups are: individuals from all countries in Asia, Africa, Oceania, central and south America, eastern Europe and the Mediterranean region, and Aboriginal and Torres Strait Islander children. Children of Aboriginal or Torres Strait Islander background should receive PedvaxHIB at two, four and 12 months rather than HibTITER.

Advice for LMCs can also be found in such governmental publications as *Principles and Guidelines for Informed Choice and Consent for all Health Care Providers and Planners* (Department of Health, Wellington, May 1991) and *Consent in Children and Youth Health: Information for Practitioners* (Ministry of Health, Wellington, December 1998). One non-governmental source is the Australian Vaccination Network (http://www.avn.org.au), which provides advice for New Zealand and Australia.

Midwife's role

The midwife's role is confined to providing balanced information and response to parents' questions regarding vaccination and immunisation schedules, diseases, reactions (and how to manage these), varying the recommended schedules, ideal timing and support of babies undergoing first immunisations, evidence-based options and alternative approaches. There are advantages in restricting the administration of vaccines to a clinic or medical centre environment: such clinics are set up to deal with reactions, including anaphylaxis; and medical centre administrations are better placed to record batch numbers and run a recall system to ensure the regimen/schedule chosen by the parent(s) is completed.

Critical thinking exercise

Research the following questions, which are typically put by parents-to-be. Try to provide a balanced response to each.
1   What is vaccination?
2   Is there a difference between vaccination and immunisation?
3   Do vaccinations work?
4   Are vaccines safe?
5   What is in a vaccine?
6   Can I alter the routine schedule?
7   What does it cost?
8   What precautions should I take if I choose vaccinations?
9   What precautions should I take if I do not choose vaccinations?
10   My baby is premature—should I delay the vaccination schedule?
11   What if my baby has a reaction?

During the woman's pregnancy you will have had occasion to discuss immunisation/vaccination information. This aspect of child health is the subject of widespread MOH advertising, and usually new parents-to-be are conscious of the government recommendations. Often a query will arise from the woman during pregnancy.

In New Zealand, Section 88 makes specific reference to the expectation that government has of LMCs. Service specification and quality requirements 4.5 (Services following birth) includes: '4.5.2 provision of Ministry of Health information on immunisation' (MOH 2002b, p 14). For the current Australian schedule of immunisation, midwives are advised to go to the NHMRC website and search for immunisation.

Contraception and sexual function

The issue of resumption of intercourse, and the need for contraception, may have arisen prior to your discharge meeting. The resumption of intercourse following childbirth has no well-defined, socially acceptable, ideal timing. The prohibition on sex until six weeks post partum is mythical but may nevertheless be a useful boundary marker for some women. Two people's needs are involved, within a wide spectrum of maturing relationships and communication skills. It could be among the first things on the woman's mind, or the very last.

It has not been established that postpartum education about contraception is effective in the long term (Hiller et al 2004). However, a midwife is uniquely placed to assess contraception needs and offer advice, towards the latter part of the postnatal care period.

You may have raised the issue; or the woman may remark that she wonders what she should do about contraception. Or she may have already asked you to provide information on a specific form of contraception. Sometimes during pregnancy the woman discusses, and enquires about, the form of future contraception she intends to try.

A caseloading midwife offering total midwifery care, or full postnatal care, will encounter the full range of contraceptive needs. These can extend from caring for a teenager pregnant from her first experience of intercourse, who has never used contraception, to a woman who has tried all known methods, knows precisely her preferred method, or has never found any to be effective. The effective outcome of your family planning counselling time will depend upon the establishment over the weeks of pregnancy of a good partnership with clear and well-established communication channels. Your intuition, professionalism and comprehensive knowledge, and her trust, will promote her assertive control over her fertility to optimise her health, both physical and sexual.

The woman may be undecided about whether she wishes to have more children. Your partnership will help you decide on the right time to offer advice and stimulate some thinking to planning beyond this baby and the sometimes all-encompassing preoccupation with this baby. It is important to spend time making the right choice for her situation. The following quote nicely summarises your message and your part in the choice: 'Choosing contraception that is right for you requires accurate information as well as negotiation and communication skills. Issues like effectiveness, safety and freedom from adverse effects need to be weighed up against convenience, cost and issues of trust and control' (Better Health Channel 2005).

In New Zealand, midwives are licensed to prescribe progesterone-only medication and condoms.

Your role as midwife encompasses the following questions and responsibilities:

- Is your information on contraceptive methods up-to-date?
- Presumably you will be aware of her sexual orientation—but this issue is mentioned to alert you to the dangers of assuming incorrectly, and the importance of thorough data collection during the establishment of the partnership.
- Do you understand and can you convey the effect that exclusively breastfeeding/partially breastfeeding/artificially feeding has on the woman's fertility?
- What impact on contraceptive choice does her birth outcome—caesarean, normal, instrumental, major perineal damage, major postpartum haemorrhage—have?
- What sensitivities are posed by her religious and/or cultural beliefs? And what by her intellectual abilities and social support deficiencies?
- Was the baby conceived by in vitro fertilisation? If so, what constitutes sensitive advice in this situation?
- Does her medical history affect her contraceptive choice?
- If she is not in a relationship, should you make any assumption about her contraceptive needs?
- Are you counselling—discharging—this woman following a miscarriage?
- How does introduction of a hormone-based contraceptive interfere with vaginal discharge—the tapering off of lochial flow as the endometrium heals and the incidental bleeding provoked by the introduction of the pill/injection and the recognition of the first real period, so a cycle can begin to be charted?

When should contraception begin again?

If the woman is not, or is partially, breastfeeding, contraception needs to begin prior to the first ovulation following birth. Menses can begin as early as day 35 to day 40 post partum. Ovulation would have happened 12–16 days prior to this. Therefore the contraception method for women who have resumed intercourse must begin by day 21. If the method is hormone-based, a 14-day period of adjustment is required before that method can be deemed reliable. Alternative methods of contraception are needed in the interim.

A detailed description of contraceptive methods is given in Chapter 31.

Well child referral

The rationale for well child referral is to provide monitoring and assessment of normality and the earliest possible documentation and follow-up care for any deviation, from birth to school age.

Well child care in New Zealand began in 1907 with the Plunket Society (originally named the Society for Promoting the Health of Women and Children). Plunket nurses were specially trained to care for babies and children (Coney 1993). But access to the Society was restricted to white middle-class mothers. The health reforms of the 1980s and the setting up of a whare Hauora concept increased access to well child care for Polynesian women. The *Plunket Book* is now called the *Well Child Tamariki Ora Health Book*. The well child system—Plunket and whare Hauora—provides:

- a free well child/Tamariki Ora service
- home or clinic visits
- key public health concepts of supportive environments, disease prevention and health promotion
- clinical assessment, core screening, surveillance, education and support entitlements.

Both organisations are staffed by registered general and obstetric nurses, or registered comprehensive nurses who have met the competencies for child health as approved by New Zealand Nursing Council. In areas not supplied by family support workers (see below), the Plunket Society also provides a home-visiting service entitled 'Plunket Additional Care Contract'. Family support is a government-funded network of organisations specifically established to address the needs of disadvantaged families. These organisations operate in conjunction with Plunket and local iwi-run, well child services.

General practitioners, sometimes through their practice nurses, simply provide the eight free well child checks or clinical assessments. This constitutes the fourth option for well child referral by LMCs.

In Australia, the equivalent well child health system varies slightly from state to state. Child health nurses are government-paid, well child care providers. Women also use their GPs. The following websites provide useful information from each state and territory regarding the child services available in each area:

ACT: http://health.act.gov.au/c/health?a=da&did=10039032

New South Wales: http://www.sch.edu.au/health/factsheets/

New South Wales Health: http://www.health.nsw.gov.au/living/child.html

NHMRC: http://www.nhmrc.gov.au/publications/subjects/childhealth.htm

Northern Territory: http://www.nt.gov.au/health/related.shtml#fam

Queensland: http://www.health.qld.gov.au/cchs/default.asp

Rural: http://www.rhef.com.au/programs/509b/509b.html

South Australia: http://www.healthysa.sa.gov.au/directory.asp?category=%27Babies%20and%20children%27

Tasmania: http://www.dhhs.tas.gov.au/services/view.php?id=5

Victoria: http://www.rch.org.au/rch/index.cfm?doc_id=1495

Western Australia: http://wchs.health.wa.gov.au/

Midwife's role

The midwife's role is to explain the local choices of well child care provider. Ordinarily this should happen during third trimester. Ideally, discussion will have begun at the fourth decision point (i.e. at the 36-week assessment) (NZCOM 2005).

Regarding the timing of referral, within your assessment of the social, emotional and education needs of woman/family/whanau, which is ongoing and dynamic, you will have assessed the level of need for well child care. Additional care needs, if present, will guide you in referral, even antenatally, to a more intensive well child support system to cultivate a relationship and understanding between woman/whanau and well child carer during the pregnancy. Otherwise, for routine well child referral, the convention in New Zealand is at four weeks. An example of a well child referral form is shown in Appendix B.

Well woman referral

Integral to a midwife's understanding of her scope is a clear recognition of normal maternity-related issues for the woman/family and how these are to be distinguished from medical issues, unrelated or only indirectly related to the pregnancy and puerperium, which are appropriately referred, with the woman's consent, to medical practitioners. The midwife recognises her limits with regard to the health of her client and her responsibility to inform the woman's usual caregiver, ordinarily the GP, with as complete, but succinct, a picture of the woman's pregnancy and birth and postpartum experience as possible.

In New Zealand the woman may have chosen not to involve her GP at any stage of her pregnancy. She may have approached her midwife from the outset to confirm her pregnancy and initiate midwifery care. Her GP may have no knowledge of this pregnancy. Alternatively, the GP may have cared for the woman until she was eligible to register with an LMC (i.e. at 14 weeks), but have had no contact since then.

Each midwife can devise her own preferred referral process. An example of a well woman referral letter template is shown in Appendix C.

Documentation: health record

The New Zealand definition of a health record is 'a record describing every aspect of the healthcare provided to an identifiable consumer/patient and may be in a single file, multiple file, hard copy (paper based) or electronic (digital, audio, video, etc.) format, and held by the consumer/patient themselves' (Standards New Zealand 2002, p 6).

Health records take a variety of forms. Institutions ordinarily devise and provide stationery that facilitates the documentation it requires to record care, communicate among caregivers, comply with legal requirements, and hold result forms. With respect to maternity information, it is likely that in the lifetime of this textbook it will become widespread practice to have minimal documentation within the institution, and that the person to whom the information belongs—the woman—will carry the bulk of the information. Care is recorded by the healthcare professional at whichever point the woman encounters this person.

Standard Four of the NZCOM Standards for Practice states that: 'The midwife maintains purposeful, on-going, updated records and makes them available to the woman and other relevant persons' (NZCOM 2005, p 11).

The main compliance requirements for documentation and structure of health records are described by Hendry in the June 2004 *Midwifery News*:

- The content must be accurate, legible, jargon-free, in chronological order and non-erasable.
- All alterations, corrections and additions must be signed and dated.
- The record must have a unique identifier that enables a correct match with a consumer.
- Alert stickers should be used to identify potential adverse reactions.
- Verbal orders and consumer information obtained from others must be dated, signed and the source identified within the health record (Hendry 2004).

Whatever format you use to document your care, you must consider its comprehensibility to the woman and provide a glossary of the abbreviations used. Any medical term must be neatly translated into lay description the first time it is used. Your language should be non-judgemental, and positively phrased where possible, and you must summarise her care as succinctly as possible without repetition. A self-evident guide to the effectiveness of your documentation is to ask yourself: 'If I was relieving this midwife, would I easily grasp the progress or current concerns of this woman/whanau and/or baby?'

The discharge visit: assessment

In New Zealand, when the midwife is concluding the discharge visit, in addition to documenting the woman's physical, mental and social state, the midwife should also ask the following questions:

- Would you like your copy of the notes sent to you/left with you?
- May I write to your GP/well woman care provider with a summary of your pregnancy experience?
- Are you aware that my practice is reviewed annually? This is an opportunity to further explain the Midwifery Standards Review and the role of the consumer feedback.

Midwifery Standards Review has been developed to provide a systematic process that enables the midwife, whatever her practice setting, to reflect on her midwifery practice with two midwifery colleagues and two consumers of midwifery services, who have been specifically educated to do this work for the New Zealand College of Midwives. The design of the process reflects the midwifery profession's partnership with women as well as the requirement for the midwife to be professionally accountable to herself, the women for whom she cares, and the profession (NZCOM 2004, p 11).

- As part of the review, may I send you the consumer feedback questionnaire?
- Would you consent to the use of your notes should yours be chosen at random by the Review Panel, just prior to Review, to check the standard of documentation?

Care of documentation

From the day you discharge the woman, you are required by law, currently (2005), to keep her records safe. 'Safe' includes protected from unauthorised access, locked securely, held in fireproof and waterproof containers. If the woman was not sent a copy then she must always know where to find her records during your guardianship of them. If you cease to practise, those records in your care must be transferred to a nominated organisation or service provider. It is even required that you nominate in your Will the appropriate transfer or disposal of these documents in the event of your demise.

An example of a summary of care assessment at discharge is shown in Appendix D. It is a useful checklist for the LMC midwife discharging a client/family at six weeks post partum.

Cervical screening

Cervical screening is a program of regular diagnostic investigation of cervical cytology among a population of women. A number of cervical cells are removed to detect cervical intraepithelial neoplasia (CIN) at the earliest possible time. These cells are taken from the squamo-columnar junction between the endocervix (columnar epithelium) and the ectocervix (squamous epithelium) in the transformation zone—the squamo-columnar junction, just at the outside end of the canal (area between internal and external os) where the canal opens into the vagina. This zone moves, depending on the stage of life and whether the woman is

Critical thinking exercise

1 If a result is not normal, what does this mean?
2 What are 'dysplasias' and CIN 1, 2 and 3?
3 How are abnormal or pre-cancerous cells treated?
4 What causes cervical cancer?
5 What are the risk factors that predispose to cervical cancer?

Clinical scenario 4

Julie is a first-time pakeha mother whose labour was augmented, as her membranes had ruptured and there was no spontaneous onset of labour within the negotiated time. Despite every effort to achieve vaginal birth, with obstetrician and midwife collaboration and planning, Julie developed a high fever and there was no acceptable progress in her labour. Her birth outcome was emergency caesarean section after 16 hours of established labour. Julie and her partner had done all they could during the pregnancy to have as natural and as 'low intervention' labour and birth experience as possible. This also is your philosophy. You choose to support women to birth relying predominantly on their own resources and the best possible information, evidence-based where possible, and emotional encouragement. You also cover the occasional discrepancy between planning for the normal and being aware of abnormal developments and intervention, based on sound obstetric rationale.

Following the birth, you debrief about the abnormal labour and outcome at as sensitive an interval as your experience clues you to do. Julie downplays the shift from dearly held expectations to the actual reality of her experience. She reports feeling well informed and able to understand the events that unfolded. She indicates that she has resolved her feelings of disappointment. She is delighted with her healthy boy. Her focus shifts to the feeding. She has some ups and downs while learning to feed but eventually achieves exclusive breastfeeding. However, the true breastfeeding commitment of such a good-sized, frequently feeding boy, and his evident need to be close, all the family and societal expectations of firmly 'disciplining' a baby from birth, as well as recovery from surgery are overwhelming and she cries most days of her postpartum time with you. You make yourself available to listen and you reinforce at every opportunity the good decisions she is making, seeking to bolster her confidence. Together you explore the source of her postnatal distress. This, you feel, is not too excessive considering what she is undergoing. She articulates many times the gap between what she expects from her partner, and what he offers. Much is attributed to fatigue and inadequate communication between the couple. During her discharge visit she admits again to crying most days.

1   How would you terminate this partnership and fulfill your role?

2   How do you yourself reflect upon and debrief this challenge so as to approach similar future cases differently?

Clinical scenario 5

Another first-time mother, Maori woman Rebekka has had a normal pregnancy, spontaneous labour and planned home birth, third-degree laceration, transferred to secondary care facility for repair, healthy baby girl, has taught herself to breastfeed, had no need to refer to any reading material you suggested. The baby is now thriving. A smear was last done three years prior, and the woman received notification that the next was due during her pregnancy. She lives with her mother. List your priorities and documentation for the six-week discharge visit for Rebekka.

breastfeeding. This is the part most likely to undergo cancerous changes.

Some midwives use the final discharge visit to offer the woman a cervical smear if it is due. Regardless of whether you plan to become a registered smear-taker and include this choice for women, the discharge visit is an appropriate time to raise the issue of screening, provide information, and address any questions the woman may have.

The rationale for routine screening is that cervical cancer is largely preventable. In 2005 the statistics showed that each year without screening, 1 in 90 women develop cervical cancer, and 1 out of 200 women will die from cervical cancer in New Zealand. Proportionally more Maori women figure in these statistics than non-Maori (cultural associations keep them away from having smears) (*Screening Matters*, Special Issue, February 2005). With screening, only 1 in 570 develop the cancer and only 1 in 1280 die from the cancer. Before symptoms develop there are changes in cervical cells that predict pathology. The success rate for adequate treatment of pre-cancers revealed by these changes is 98–100%. Any woman who has ever had sexual intercourse is at risk and would benefit from routine screening. The information you provide may ensure that the woman makes an informed decision about undergoing, or not undergoing, the screening. Explain why it is in her best interests but also how she can feel comfortable about taking the test. In your locale you should be fluent with the answers to such questions as:

● How long will the test take?
● How much will it cost?
● Who is most likely to take the smear?
● Can I have a third person present? This could be a friend, husband, partner, member of her family, practice nurse as chaperone or interpreter (if English is her second language and the smear-taker does not speak her first language).
● Any other query the woman has, until you believe that she is clear about the test.

Encourage women going for the first time to make this clear to the smear-taker. If she has never had a smear it will be necessary to explain how a smear is taken. She will be asked

Clinical scenario 6

First-time mother, Soo Lei, of Asian ethnicity, birthed by emergency caesarean section six weeks previously. You are confident that there are no ongoing issues related to that labour and birth, but Soo Lei's baby Anna had severe tongue tie. Your referral, in the postnatal ward, to a sympathetic paediatrician resulted in his recommendation to continue without frenulotomy. The baby, Anna, appeared to latch adequately and, with initial good supply, did well. Postnatal staff members were reassuring. On discharge you continued to assess the baby, however, as 'nipple' feeding. You arrange a frenulotomy with a sympathetic GP and appointment for retraining of tongue with the community lactation consultant (LC). Some improvement results (some strengthening of her untethered tongue muscle), but Anna vacillates between strong sucking and weak, tired sucking. Weight gain is just adequate and there are more visits to the LC. Any day now you expect Anna to strengthen and train herself. You continually reinforce the solid commitment and good-humoured tolerance and enthusiasm of the couple to explore every avenue to achieve exclusive breastfeeding. You arrive for the six-week visit with the feeling of a 'job not done'.

How would you vary your closure of this relationship from that of scenario 5?

Clinical scenario 7

Barbara is a 38-year-old pakeha, multiparous woman who was exposed to rubella in her mother's womb. This left her with a 40% hearing disability, and an inability to store fat reserves. She has borderline adequate nutritional status due to chronic hyperemesis throughout her 38 weeks of pregnancy; she also has cardiac and thyroid complications. She now has four children. Each of her pregnancies has resulted in labours where her hypertensive state escalated alarmingly. She has a steady relationship with this baby's father.

1 How would you advise and counsel her on her contraceptive needs?
2 What information would you accumulate before your six-week discharge visit with her?

Reflective exercise

1 What are your supervision and/or debriefing needs following on from the experiences related in these scenarios?
2 What are the major questions you need to have answered by the visit, to complete the partnership?
   If you have provided lead care or continuity of care, your 'knowing' of the woman, and every step of her maternity care experience, is an advantage to you at this visit. You can help the woman/couple/family pull the whole experience together and confront unresolved feelings that this naturally intense episode in their lives may have generated.
3 In what other ways can you evaluate satisfaction with care?

to take off her lower garments, and to lie down on her back or side. Then a warmed metal or plastic instrument called a speculum is placed in the vagina so that the cervix—she may well be familiar with this term through antenatal classes or your care of her in labour, but do not assume this—can be seen. Ordinarily the vaginal wall is collapsed like a closed umbrella, and the speculum is used to hold the walls apart, thus allowing a light source to illuminate the cervix. Once the smear-taker has positively identified the cervix, a sample of cells is gently taken with either a spatula or small brush or specially shaped 'cervi-broom', smeared onto a laboratory slide, and sprayed with cell fixative. This slide is then sent to the laboratory and the cells examined under a microscope.

If a woman is having her very first smear, and if this result is normal she is recommended to have her second test one year later. If this also is normal, then the frequency of smear tests is recommended to be three-yearly in New Zealand (www.healthywomen.org.nz) and two-yearly in Australia (DHA 2001).

Smear-taking at the six-week discharge visit

If you contemplate taking smears at the six-week discharge visit, you need to consider the following issues:

● As an LMC with an annual caseload of 40–60 women, would you do a sufficient number of smears to maintain an acceptable standard of smear-taking?
● Breastfeeding women are known to have cervical differences due to altered hormonal state when they are lactating. The crucial endocervical cells (transformation zone) retreat up the canal, are difficult to reach and, therefore, a satisfactory sample is less likely.
● If the woman is due for a smear and you do not do it within your postnatal budget module, she must then attend a clinic, or GP, at her own expense. This reduces the likelihood of compliance.
● Do you wish to return the woman to her undressed, exposed self again after she has slowly assumed her sense of privacy and dignity since the intimacies of the birth? Can you manage this return to intimate, and

possibly painful, exposure, and still end your care on the respectful, positive, uplifting note you would choose? This naturally requires good communication skills and a sensitive, professional approach.

On the other hand, the midwife is often coincidentally required to examine and assess the healing of a wound, the involution of the fundus, the appearance, or not, of a rash or a suspect discharge. Also, it can be a relief to the woman to have smear and pelvic exam complete, be reassured and then able to relax about such an exposure not being required for another three years. Often she will feel that she has done the responsible thing and attended to this aspect of her present and future health. Needless to say, you will have prepared her for the physical side of her discharge assessment and discussed with her the appropriateness of a smear being taken.

Concluding the partnership

A significant function of the discharge visit is the closure or ending of the relationship. Standard Nine of the NZCOM Standards for Practice states that: 'The midwife negotiates the completion of the midwifery partnership with the woman' (NZCOM 2005, p 21). The parting between midwife and woman/whanau is signalled at the very first introductory visit. When the woman is choosing her midwife, you explain how the partnership begins, and when it conventionally ends. Then you will have reminded the woman at least one more time, perhaps at the beginning of the postpartum period, and you signal this again as you set up the six-week assessment at four or five weeks post partum. You are explicit with each other, at that visit, regarding her readiness (or not) for discharge.

Review questions

1 Outline a holistic health assessment of the woman at six weeks post partum.

2 What key points are necessary to convey when transferring your care of baby to a well child care provider?

3 Which social and physical milestones has a baby usually achieved by six weeks of age?

4 What are a woman's choices for well child referral in your country?

5 Write a summary of the side-effects of all methods of contraception.

6 What are the legal requirements for midwifery documentation in your country?

7 Discuss the strengths and weaknesses of the support networks and resources for postpartum women in your community.

8 What is the role of Standards Review with respect to LMC midwives?

9 How would you describe the benefits of breastfeeding to a teenage mother?

10 How would you deal with the knowledge that a young unmarried woman in your care is suffering from domestic violence? Can you list the resources available to you and to her locally?

Online resources

Australian Breastfeeding Association, http://www.breastfeeding.asn.au/bfinfo/index.html

Australian Government, Health Insurance Commission (HIC), http://www.hic.gov.au

Better Health website, http://www.betterhealth.vic.gov.au/bhcv2/bhcartcles,nsf/pages/Contraception_condo accessed 25/07/04

Family Planning Australia, http://www.fpa.net.au/index.htm accessed 25/07/04.

Healthy Women website, http://www.healthywomen.org.nz

List of consumer mental health support groups in New Zealand, http://www.nzgg.org.nz/guidelines/0039/Appendix_8.pdf

World Organisation of the Ovulation Method Billings (WOOMB), http://www.woomb.org/

References

Auckland Homebirth Association 1993 Guide to Pregnancy and Childbirth, Auckland

Barclay L, Lie D 2004 Edinburgh Postnatal Depression Scale detects postpartum depression. Online: http://www.medscape.com/viewarticle/471307

Better Health Channel 2005 Victorian Government. Online: www.betterhealth.vic.gov.au, accessed 25 July 2004

Coney S 1993 Standing in the sunshine. Penguin, Auckland

Department of Health and Ageing (DHA), Australian Government 2001 Cervical cancer: the facts. Online: http://www.cervicalscreen.health.gov.au/facts/index.html. Population Health Division

Dixon M, Booth N, Powell R 2000 Sex and relationships following childbirth: a first report from general practice of 131 couples. British Journal of General Practice 50(452):223–224

Family Planning Association of New Zealand. Online: http://www.everybody.co.nz/page-18c367f0-f489-40f2-9986-406b2722b7e2.aspx

Force S 2000 The provision of community-based midwifery postnatal care in the UK—making a difference? MIDIRS Midwifery Digest 10(2):232–234

Forman DN, Videbech P, Hedegaard M et al 2000 Postpartum depression: identification of women at risk. BJOG: International Journal of Obstetrics and Gynaecology 107(10):1210–1017 (authors' abstract reprinted in MIDIRS 11(1) 2001)

Fraser D, Cooper M 2001, Myles textbook for midwives (14th edn). Churchill Livingstone, Edinburgh

Gainsford G 1999 Expectations of the normal breast fed baby. NZCOM Midwifery Newsletter 12:1–6

Greig J, Sahar M 1999 Post-natal distress survival guide (2nd edn). Post and Ante-Natal Distress Support Group, Wellington

Harvey SM, Bird ST, Branch MR 2003 A new look at an old method: the diaphragm. Perspectives on sexual and reproductive health 35(6):270–273 (reprinted in MIDIRS 14(2) 2004)

Hedin, LW 2000 Postpartum, also a risk period for domestic violence. European Journal of Obstetrics and Gynaecology and Reproductive Biology 89(1):41–45 (abstract written for MIDIRS by Price S: MIDIRS 10(3) 2000)

Hendry C 2004 MMPO Update on managing maternity notes, Midwifery News 33:24

Hiller JE, Griffith E, Jenner F 2004 Education for contraceptive use by women after childbirth (Cochrane Review). Cochrane Library (2) 2004. John Wiley & Sons, Chichester

Johnston PGB 1994 Vulliamy's the newborn child (7th edn). Churchill Livingstone, Edinburgh

MacArthur C 1999, What does postnatal care do for women's health? Lancet 353(9150):343–344 (reprinted in MIDIRS 9(2) 1999)

Marchant S, Alexander J, Garcia J 2002 Postnatal vaginal bleeding problems and general practice. Midwifery 18(1):21–24 (author abstract reprinted in MIDIRS 2002)

McCall A, Holt AK 2004 A reflective review of the progesterone-only pill and lactational amenorrhoea: do breastfeeding women really need both in the early months after birth? MIDIRS Midwifery Digest 14(1): 89–93

Ministry of Health 2001 Breastfeeding and working. MOH, Wellington

Ministry of Health 2002a Immunisation handbook 2002, MOH, Wellington

Ministry of Health 2002b Maternity services. Notice pursuant to Section 88 of the New Zealand Public Health & Disability Act 2000. MOH, Wellington

NZCOM 2004, Midwifery standards review handbook. NZCOM, Christchurch

NZCOM 2005, Midwives handbook for practice (3rd edn). NZCOM, Christchurch

O'Connell PR 1997 Post-partum bowel problems in women. Irish Medical Journal 90(8):288–289 (reprinted in MIDIRS 8(3) 1998)

Ramsden I 1993 Kawa Whakaruruhau: cultural safety in nursing education in Aotearoa New Zealand. Nursing Praxis in New Zealand 8(3):4–10

Shakespeare J, Blake F, Garcia J 2003 A qualitative study of the acceptability of routine screening of postnatal women using the Edinburgh Postnatal Depression Scale. British Journal of General Practice 53:614–619 (abstract written for MIDIRS by S Marchant, MIDIRS 14(1) 2004)

Standards New Zealand and Ministry of Health (NZ) 2002 New Zealand Standard: health records, SNZ/MOH, Wellington

Sweet BR (Ed) 2000 Mayes midwifery: a textbook for midwives (12th edn). Ballière Tindall, London

Symon A, Glazener CMA, MacDonald A et al 2003 Pilot study: quality of life assessment of postnatal fatigue and other physical morbidity. Journal of Psychosomatic Obstetrics and Gynaecology 24(4):215–219 (reprinted in MIDIRS 14(1) 2004)

Viccars A 1998 Abstract: writer's comments on effectiveness of treatments for infantile colic: systematic review, by Lucassen PLBJ et al. British Medical Journal 316(7144):1563–1569 (abstract in MIDIRS 8(3) 1998, pp 362–363)

Wickham S 2001 Perineal pampering—before, during and after birth. MIDIRS Midwifery Digest 11(suppl 1):S23–S27

APPENDIX A: Six-week well child check documentation

6 week

Well Child Tamariki Ora check

Progress:

Assessment:

Weight: ____ Head circumference: ____ Length: ____

Vision: ☐ Hearing: ☐ Development: ☐

Physical examination: yes/ok ✓ needs comment/action ✗

skin ☐	heart ☐	hips – Ortolani/Barlow ☐
fontanelle ☐	lungs ☐	– classic signs ☐
eyes – red reflex ☐	abdomen ☐	genitals ☐
nose/mouth ☐	umbilicus ☐	back ☐
ears ☐	femoral pulses ☐	anus ☐
		reflexes, movement, tone ☐

Comments/action:

Health protection (✓ if done)

Vitamin K (3rd oral) ☐   Immunisation choice made ☐

On National Immunisation Register ☐

Immunisation programme commenced Y/N ☐   record page 140

Signature: ____   Date: ____

Print name/designation: ____

6 week check

91

Source: Ministry of Health 2005 Well Child Tamariki Ora Health Book. MOH, Wellington

APPENDIX B: Example of a well child referral form

This form is used by New Zealand midwife LMCs. Note that all parties receive a copy.

Referral to Well Child Provider and Notification to GP

This form is to be sent to both the Well Child Provider and the GP in order to fulfil clauses C4.5.4 & C4.5.5

MINISTRY OF
HEALTH
MANATU HAUORA

Mother

Family name: ....

Given names: ....

Birth Date: .... NHI number: ....

Address: ....

....

....

....

Daytime phone: .... Alternative Contact: ....

Parity: ....

Baby

Family name: ....

Given names: ....

Birth Date: .... NHI number: ....

Gender: Male   Female

Baby Summary

Gestation: .... Weeks

Significant birth/postnatal event(s) (e.g. apgar score, birth weight) ....

....

Vitamin K   Guthrie test

Feeding at time of referral to Well Child Provider

Exclusive Breastfeeding   Fully Breastfeeding   Partial Breastfeeding   Artificial feeding

Comment ....

....

Summary of ongoing needs identified at time of referral (e.g. referral to Family Start, Multiple Birth Society):

....

....

Date referral/notification sent to Well Child Provider and GP:

Planned date of discharge from LMC: ....

Name of LMC: ....

LMC Contact details: ....

WHITE - **CLIENT COPY**   PINK - **WELL CHILD PROVIDER COPY**   BLUE - **GENERAL PRACTITIONER COPY**   YELLOW - **LEAD MATERNITY CARER COPY**

MOH008
REORDER NO 61287
03/03

Source: Ministry of Health, Wellington

APPENDIX C: **Example of a well woman referral letter template**

RXXXXX   DYYY   INDEPENDENT MIDWIFE... 1 VV ST
[Address]
PH: [Number]
PAGER: [Number]
[Email address]
Date:
. . . .
. . . .
. . . .

Dear . . . .

I have provided midwifery care for . . . .
. . . .
NHI:. . . . . during her pregnancy, birth and postnatal period.
The following is a summary of her experience

Gravida: Parity:
Pregnancy:

Labour and Birth:
Baby: NHI:
Birth Weight: Discharge age and weight
Where born:
Vitamin K   Audiology screen
PKU:
Vaccination:
Feeding history to date:
Six week check:
Cervical smear:
Contraception:
Follow-up by:

Yours sincerely

APPENDIX D: Checklist for the LMC midwife discharging a client/family at six weeks

postnatal care summary
MMPO

postnatal care summary (vertical, right margin)

Maternity Notes number ☐☐☐☐☐☐☐
from inside the folder

Infection
○ None ○ Breast
○ Uterine ○ Perineal ○ Wound
○ Urinary ○ Other - *specify* _____

Breastfeeding ○ Yes ○ No
If yes, did any of the following occur: ○ Engorgement ○ Nipple Trauma ○ Latching difficulty
○ Perceived over/under supply ○ Baby unable to feed ○ Social pressures ○ Blocked duct
○ Infection - treated ○ Abcess ○ Other - *specify* _____
Referral to: ○ Midwife ○ Lactation consultant ○ Other - *specify* _____

Postnatal depression / psychosis ○ Yes ○ No Referral to - *specify* _____

Postnatal complementary practices
○ Homoeopathy ○ Water ○ Massage ○ Acupuncture ○ Acupressure
○ Herbal medicine ○ Heat Packs ○ Naturopathy ○ Osteopathy ○ Positional techniques
○ Rongoa ○ Other - *specify* _____

Postnatal prescriptions given by you ○ Yes ○ No Number _____

Type: ○ Antibiotics / Antibacterials ○ Antifungals ○ Minerals *(folic acid, iron, calcium)* ○ Vitamins
○ Analgesics ○ Contraceptives - oral ○ Contraceptives - other ○ NSAIDS
○ Haemorrhoid treatment ○ Other - *specify* _____

Anti D ○ Not Applicable
○ Required ○ Yes ○ No ○ Given ○ Declined

Referral details

Date of referral *(date/month/year)*	Name of provider referred to	Specialist type *eg Obstetrician*	Hosp	Private	Reasons for referral *use referral Guidlines or Ultrasound indications List (See back page)*
☐☐/☐☐/☐☐☐☐			○	○	
☐☐/☐☐/☐☐☐☐			○	○	
☐☐/☐☐/☐☐☐☐			○	○	

Care transferred
○ Yes ○ No If yes, then date ☐☐/☐☐/☐☐☐☐ time _____
Specialist type *(eg Obstetrician)* _____ Change LMC ○ Yes ○ No
FV Screen ○

Smoking ○ Yes ○ No _____ No.at completion of care *(perday)*
Alcohol ○ Yes ○ No
Other substances ○ Yes ○ No Specify _____
Total number of postnatal visits _____
Total number of postnatal home visits _____ Readmitted Yes No
Total hospital stay *(if applicable)* _____ days _____ hours Reason _____
Care shared with ○ Not shared ○ Other Midwife ○ HHS ○ Obs ○ GP
Component of care shared ○ All ○ AN ○ L&B ○ PN *(tick as many as applicable)*
Rural travel ○ Semi-rural ○ Rural ○ Remote Rural If yes, Dornicle code _____
Physical address _____
Date of discharge *(mother and baby)* ☐☐/☐☐/☐☐☐☐ *day/month/year*
Discharge referral ○ Declined ○ GP ○ Plunket ○ Maori provider ○ Social Serv. ○ Other
Client evaluation sent ○ Yes ○ No **Copy of casenotes provided** ○ Yes ○ No

MMPO

white copy for midwife   **pink copy** post to MMPO   **blue copy** for woman

Source: Midwifery and Maternity Provider Organisation

CHAPTER 31

Contraception

Helen Calabretto

Key terms

basal body temperature, body mass index, combined oral contraceptive, emergency contraception, fertility awareness-based methods, progestogen implant, human immunodeficiency virus, intrauterine device, intrauterine system, lactational amenorrhoea method, progestogen-only injection, progestogen-only pill

Chapter overview

This chapter gives an overview of the methods of contraception used in Australia and New Zealand and will provide midwifery students with a beginning knowledge in this area. It is not within the scope of this chapter to provide complete information about each method of contraception. Rather, it should be viewed as an introduction to the methods with key points of information. Completion of a course offered at local family planning organisations and undertaking wider reading will provide additional invaluable information for midwives working with women in the antenatal and postnatal periods in particular.

Learning outcomes

Learning outcomes for this chapter are:

1   To identify contraceptive services available

2   To describe the role of the midwife in providing contraception counselling

3   To identify the factors that influence the selection of a suitable method of contraception for a woman or couple

4   To discuss the impact of culture, disability and pre-existing health problems on the choice of contraception

5   To explain the efficacy of various methods of contraception with typical and perfect use

6   To differentiate the changed patterns of contraceptive use at different times of a woman's reproductive life

7   To describe the way in which the following methods of contraception act, the reasons they may be selected as a method, and their suitability for use during lactation and the postpartum period: lactational amenorrhoea method; fertility awareness-based methods; barrier methods; intrauterine devices/systems; hormonal contraception; spermicides; vaginal douche; coitus interruptus; and sterilisation.

Introduction

Attempts to control fertility have been documented throughout history and have included methods such as the insertion of objects (e.g. stones) into the vagina or uterus, douches made of carbonated beverages, and plastic wrap to simulate the function of condoms (Varney 1997). Fortunately there are many more efficacious methods of contraception available to women. In the twentieth century, Margaret Sanger, a nurse, made an important contribution to women's quest for planning their families and the right of children to be born when they are wanted. She recognised the correlation between poverty and high birth rates, and in 1952 founded the Planned Parenthood Federation of America, which is now the International Planned Parenthood Federation (IPPF) and links national autonomous Family Planning Associations (FPAs) in over 180 countries worldwide.

In Australia and New Zealand, contraceptive services are provided in a variety of settings. These may include family planning clinics, general practice, women's health centres, community health centres, youth health centres, sexual health services and services provided within acute care hospitals. The leading organisations for contraceptive services are the Family Planning Association of Australia (with separate organisations in each state and territory), and the Family Planning Association of New Zealand. Their services encompass a broader focus than clinical services, including professional and community education, training, consultation and research. A list of the head offices is provided at the end of this chapter, as well as web addresses for other relevant organisations that provide reproductive health information (see Online resources).

Contraception counselling: the role of the midwife

Although many women plan their pregnancies, this is not the case for all women (Forrest 1994). Midwives must be cognisant of the fact that the woman's current pregnancy may not be wanted, or may be mistimed and may have resulted from contraceptive failure, error with the method or non-use of contraception. After the current pregnancy, women may wish to continue with their previous method of contraception, or may lack confidence in their previous method and want to consider a different method. Some women will want to start using contraception, and for other women a permanent method of contraception will be preferred. Midwives are therefore in a unique position to assist women during pregnancy, childbirth and the puerperium with their future contraception and safer sex needs.

Unfortunately, provision of contraceptive information is often a hasty activity included in a checklist of other topics as part of discharge education in the postnatal ward (Glasier

Critical thinking exercise

Go to the website of your local family planning organisation (see the addresses at the end of the chapter) and familiarise yourself with the services offered and location of the clinics. Compile a resource list for use in your own clinical practice.

et al 1996). A recent Cochrane Review (Hiller et al 2004) concluded that there is not enough evidence to establish that current postpartum contraception education is effective, and that research is required to examine the best timing and approaches. Until such time as this is undertaken, it would be reasonable to assume that discussion about contraception should be initiated in the antenatal period and revisited in the postnatal period. It is important that the issue is adequately discussed, and in addition to provision of verbal and written information about contraceptive methods, there needs to be referral to a primary health care provider for ongoing contraceptive needs. An up-to-date list of providers is a useful adjunct for counselling.

Advice about contraception is critical because in the absence of breastfeeding, it is possible that ovulation may occur from day 28 postnatally (Guillebaud 2004). A number of factors will influence the method of contraception selected by a woman or couple. These include:

- whether the individual or couple is seeking a permanent or temporary method of contraception
- their understanding of the effectiveness of the method (see Table 31.1)
- the perceived or actual side-effects of the method
- any previous positive or negative experience(s) of a method(s)
- the cost and convenience of the method
- the ease of use of particular methods
- the number of sexual partners
- current popularity of a particular method
- influence of the media, friends and family
- religious and/or cultural factors (WHO 2004; Varney 1997).

Choices of contraceptive method change at various times in the childbearing years, as exemplified in Tables 31.2 and 31.3. Information should be provided about the effectiveness of various methods, none of which are 100% effective (see Table 31.1), their action, potential side-effects and the benefits and risks of the method as they relate to the individual woman. The time it takes for fertility to return after cessation of the method is also important when couples want to have more children, and whether the method also affords protection from sexually transmitted infections will be important for some women. Midwives should be aware of when particular methods can be commenced in the postpartum period, and their suitability during lactation. Some women have existing health problems that affect the suitability of some methods. These are summarised in Appendix A. In the past, most women

TABLE 31.1 Percentage of women experiencing an unintended pregnancy during the first year of use and the percentage continuing use at the end of the first year, USA*

Method (1)	% of women experiencing an unintended pregnancy within the first year of use		% of women continuing use at 1 year[3] (4)
	Typical use[1] (2)	Perfect use[2] (3)	
No method[4]	85	85	42
Spermicides[5]	29	18	42
Withdrawal	27	4	51
Periodic abstinence	25		
Calendar		9	
Ovulation method		3	
Sympto-thermal[6]		2	
Post-ovulation		1	
Cap[7]			
Parous women	32	26	46
Non-parous women	16	9	57
Diaphragm	16	6	57
Condom[8]			
Female	21	5	49
Male	15	2	53
Combined pill and minipill	8	0.3	68
DMPA	3	0.3	56
IUCD			
ParaGard Copper T™	0.8	0.6	78
Multiload Cu 375® (rates not available)			
Mirena (LNG IUS)	0.1	0.1	81
LNG implants			
Implanon	0.05	0.05	84
Female sterilisation	0.5	0.5	100
Male sterilisation	0.15	0.10	100

Emergency contraceptive pills: Treatment initiated within 120 hours after unprotected intercourse reduces the risk of pregnancy by at least 75%.[9]

Lactational amenorrhoea method (LAM) is a highly effective, *temporary* method of contraception.[10]

* Equivalent data are not available from Australia and New Zealand

1. Among *typical* couples who initiate a method (not necessarily for the first time), the percentage who experience an accidental pregnancy during the first year if they do not stop use for any other reason.
2. Among couples who initiate use of a method (not necessarily for the first time) and who use it perfectly (both consistently and correctly), the % who experience an accidental pregnancy during the first year if they do not stop use for any other reason.

TABLE 31.1—cont'd.

3. Among couples attempting to avoid pregnancy, the % who continue to use a method for one year.
4. % becoming pregnant in columns (2) and (3) are based on data from populations where contraception is not used and from women who cease using contraception in order to become pregnant. Among such populations, about 89% become pregnant within one year. This estimate was lowered slightly (to 85%) to represent the percentage who would become pregnant within one year among women now relying on reversible methods of contraception if they abandoned contraception altogether.
5. Foams, creams, gels, vaginal suppositories and vaginal film. Note: vaginal suppositories and film are not available in Australia and New Zealand.
6. Cervical mucus method supplemented by calendar in the pre-ovulatory and basal body temperature in the post-ovulatory phases.
7. With spermicidal cream or jelly.
8. Without spermicides.
9. This doesn't mean a 25% pregnancy rate. If 100 women have intercourse in the middle of their cycle, approximately eight pregnancies will occur and use of the EC will reduce that number to two—a reduction of 75% (American College of Obstetricians and Gynecologists 1997)
10. However, to maintain effective protection against pregnancy, another method of contraception must be used as soon as menstruation resumes, the frequency or duration of breastfeeds is reduced, bottle feeds are introduced or the baby reaches six months of age.

(Source: adapted from Trussell 2004)

with intellectual disabilities, particularly those who were institutionalised, had induced amenorrhoea using continuous progestogens or by surgical approaches (Grover 2002). Now, their choices are the same as for non-disabled women, with infrequent use of surgical intervention.

Different cultural views about the use of contraception must also be respected by midwives when discussing ongoing contraceptive needs with women. It is not possible here to discuss each cultural group represented in Australia and New Zealand; however, it is important for midwives to be familiar with the cultural mores of the common groups of culturally and linguistically diverse (CALD) women in their care. These women (like other women in the dominant culture) may have poor knowledge of contraceptive methods from their schooling or teaching within the family, particularly where virginity is highly prized and expected until marriage. Information about contraception may be withheld as being more appropriate to be discussed at the time of marriage. Some groups of women may have had particular methods of contraception used without their informed consent and may be distrustful of all methods. Other women may be refugees or have migrated from countries where access to contraceptive services was limited or unavailable. Some women may have come from countries with pronatalist policies, and other may have come from countries where limitations are placed on family size. When discussing contraception with CALD women, traditional values must be respected and dealt with sensitively. There must also be acknowledgement that women may want to move away from traditional approaches to

TABLE 31.2 Contraceptive practices, Australia

Contraceptive method	18–24 %	25–29 %	30–34 %	35–39 %	40–44 %	45–49 %	Total %
	Age group (years)						
Use condoms[1]	35.9	30.5	25.8	20.3	12.6	9.1	22.9
Use oral contraceptives[2]	43.2	40.4	29.4	22.2	14.5	7.9	26.8
Use an IUD	0.3	0.5	1.6	2.0	1.7	1.1	1.2
Use a diaphragm	-	0.5	0.6	1.1	0.5	0.2	0.5
Use natural, rhythm or Billings method	1.4	3.1	4.9	4.8	4.0	2.0	3.3
Use withdrawal method	9.6	8.3	9.4	5.4	3.7	2.1	6.6
Had a contraceptive injection	2.0	2.5	2.6	1.2	1.9	0.7	1.9
Took the morning after pill[3]	5.4	2.2	1.7	0.3	0.1	0.4	1.8
Had a tubal ligation/tubes tied	-	1.2	4.7	10.6	15.9	20.6	8.6
Partner has been sterilised	0.4	2.3	6.7	16.9	21.6	21.3	11.2
Had a hysterectomy	-	0.2	0.9	4.0	8.6	16.1	4.7
Menopause	-	0.1	0.4	1.0	3.6	21.0	4.0
Self or partner infertile	0.3	1.6	1.9	2.0	2.4	2.5	1.7
Other	1.0	0.8	0.7	0.8	0.4	0.4	0.7
Not sexually active	16.4	8.8	6.9	8.5	8.7	9.8	10.0
None of these apply	11.3	13.0	14.9	9.0	8.0	7.8	10.7
Not stated	8.5	9.9	8.1	9.1	10.7	11.8	9.6
TOTAL[4]	100.0	100.0	100.0	100.0	100.0	100.0	100.0

1 Used for protection or contraception purposes.
2 Includes COC and POP.
3 Emergency contraception.
4 Persons may have reported more than one type of contraceptive practice and therefore components may not add to total.
(Source: adapted from ABS 2001)

contraception that may at times differ from the views of their partner and/or community.

The advice and information provided must be framed within the woman's values and beliefs. It is important that the midwives or other health professionals provide non-judgemental contraceptive advice and do not allow their own values to influence the advice they give to women. The midwife's counselling role also needs to extend beyond advice about contraception. Although the birth of a baby can strengthen a relationship and perhaps enhance sexual intimacy, resumption of sexual intercourse may take several months. Hormonal changes can result in a low libido; there can be physical discomfort from an episiotomy, perineal tear or caesarean section, and physical and emotional exhaustion from sleepless nights and the demanding role of parenting (Guillebaud 2004). Other issues include decreased lubrication from reduced oestrogen secretion; bloody lochia, which may interfere with sexual feelings; changed feelings about the erotic significance of the breasts; and adjustment of the relationship to include a new family member (Kennedy & Trussell 2004).

Reversible methods of contraception

Lactational amenorrhoea method (LAM)

Breastfeeding can provide a natural contraceptive effect and is a method that can be used when a woman is exclusively or near-exclusively breastfeeding for the first six months following a birth. Infant suckling at the breast inhibits ovulation, and although this is often attributed to high levels of prolactin, it is due to the disruption of the pulsatile release of gonadotrophic hormone (GnRH) by the hypothalamus, which in turns affects the pulsility of LH needed for follicle stimulation of the ovary. The small amounts of secreted oestrogen are insufficient to trigger the LH surge necessary to induce ovulation (Kennedy & Trussell 2004). LAM provides 98% protection against pregnancy if all of the following three criteria are met:

- The woman must breastfeed both day and night, providing a minimum of 90% of the infant's nutritional requirements.
- She must be amenorrhoeic.
- The infant must be under six months old (WHO 2004).

TABLE 31.3 **Contraceptive practices, New Zealand***

Method used	Age group (years)					
	20–24 %	25–29 %	30–34 %	35–39 %	40–44 %	45–49 %
Non-Maori women (*N* = 1292)						
Sterilisation (male + female methods)	1	8	24	42	60	72
Pill, Pill + other	47	45	29	17	11	5
Pill + condom	14	5	2	2	[0.4]	0
Condom, Condom + other	21	20	20	16	8	7
IUD or injection or diaphragm or foam	9	4	7	7	8	3
Traditional methods	2	2	3	4	3	2
No method	6	16	15	11	10	11
TOTAL %[2]	100	100	100	100	100	100
Maori women (*N* = 236)						
Sterilisation (male + female methods)	0	15	40	51	61	75
Pill, Pill + other	25	34	23	14	7	0
Pill + condom	9	0	5	0	3	0
Condom, Condom + other	16	17	16	4	3	0
IUD or injection or diaphragm or foam[3]	18	9	7	6	7	0
Traditional methods	0	4	0	0	0	0
No method	32	21	9	25	19	25
TOTAL %[2]	100	100	100	100	100	100

*Type of contraceptive method or methods used in the four weeks prior to the survey by women[1] aged < 50 years old, who were not pregnant and who had had intercourse in the previous four weeks, by age group at the time of survey and ethnicity
1 Excludes women who responded 'don't know' or 'refused'.
2 Totals may not add to 100% due to rounding.
3 Among Maori women, this category is mainly injection.
(Source: Pool et al 1995)

If supplements are given, they can only be non-milk (e.g. water and juice), given infrequently (no more than and preferably less than 5–15%), and not via a bottle (Kennedy & Trussell 2004). This ensures maximum suckling stimulation of the breast. Interestingly, in one study, higher rates of pregnancy (5.2%) were seen in working women using LAM, which indicates that even in the presence of good milk production and full breastfeeding, it is frequent suckling that is necessary to gain the maximum effect of LAM (Kennedy & Trussell 2004). In Australia, 64% of infants less than three months of age (ABS 2001) and in New Zealand, 55% of infants less than three months of age (NZ Plunket Society 2004) are fully breastfed. If women were better informed about this method, it could gain popularity and improve breastfeeding rates, although this would require good support for breastfeeding by the healthcare system, employers, and family and friends.

LAM suits women who do not want to use a hormonal method while they are exclusively breastfeeding their babies, but it is not suitable for women who plan to use supplemental feeding. However, it could be used for the time during which the woman meets the conditions described above, even if it is less than six months. Once the baby is six months old, or before that time if any of the criteria are not met, the mother should plan to use an additional method of contraception to avoid pregnancy. LAM is unsuitable for women with HIV because there is a 14–29% chance of the virus being passed through breast milk. In Australia and New Zealand, the current recommendation is to not breastfeed if the mother has HIV infection. LAM is also unsuitable if a woman has an infection or is taking particular medications that are passed in the breast milk and are harmful to the infant, or when the infant is unable to suck at the breast due to congenital abnormalities, prematurity or being small-for-dates and full breastfeeding is difficult.

Fertility awareness-based methods (FAB)

These methods, sometimes called 'natural methods' or 'natural family planning', use recognition of the changes in the woman's body at various times of the menstrual cycle. They acknowledge that the estimation of the period of fertility needs to take into account the sperm viability in the female genital tract—an average of three to four days with a theoretical possibility of up to seven days—and the fertile period of the ovum, which is estimated to be 24 hours (Guillebaud 2004).

FAB methods require cooperation and commitment within a relationship to maximise its effectiveness through agreement by the couple to abstain from intercourse or have protected intercourse using barrier methods in the potentially fertile period of the woman's menstrual cycle. The methods are suitable when religious or cultural beliefs exclude the use of contraception, and there is a preference for a method that is free of physical side-effects and one that is inexpensive once the instruction is completed. Couples are advised to learn these methods correctly from expert practitioners to maximise efficacy. Local family planning organisations (see the list at the end of this chapter) can provide information about the specialist organisations providing this education. It should also be noted that these methods may also be used to assist conception. Couples may choose one or a combination of approaches described below.

Calendar (rhythm) method

The calendar method is the least reliable of these methods (see Table 31.1). It is based on the premise that ovulation occurs in the middle of the cycle, and the fertile period lasts for six days—the five days before ovulation and the day of ovulation (Jennings et al 2004). Calendar methods are not particularly effective, and there are relatively few days in a cycle during which some women are not fertile, including the day of the cycle when they expect their next menstrual period (Wilcox et al 2000). These researchers found that only 30% of women were fertile in the currently accepted clinical guidelines as being between days 10 and 17 of the cycle. Even for women who closely study their cycles to identify shortest and longest cycle length, life events may disrupt predictions and alter the fertile period unexpectedly. Some women have less regular cycles, which makes the method even less predictable. Refer to Guillebaud (2004, p 29), who outlines the way in which the fertile period is calculated, to maximise the effectiveness of this method.

Basal body temperature (BBT)

The BBT method is based on the fact that there is a drop in the woman's body temperature 12–24 hours prior to ovulation, with a sustained rise for several days. Knowledge of temperature change is only useful in establishing when ovulation has already occurred over several cycles and thus the infertile period in which safe intercourse can occur. The temperature needs to be taken accurately each morning before the woman does *any* activity, using the same (oral, vaginal or rectal) route and charted on a temperature chart. The problem with relying on this method is that there is great individual variation in BBT, which can be affected by life events such as illness, emotional stress, irregular sleep, sedatives, use of electric blankets, alcohol intake, time of day, climate and immunisations (Varney 1997, p 77). In addition, some women have no identifiable BBT pattern (Hatcher et al 1994).

Cervical mucus charting (ovulation or Billings method)

This method originated in Australia in the 1950s (Varney 1997). In this approach, the woman is taught to recognise her fertile days by both the appearance and sensation of mucus at the vulva. She learns to recognise the difference between feelings of wetness and dryness. The fertile mucus (Spinnbarkeit mucus) assists the sperm to enter the cervix and is produced under the influence of unopposed oestrogen in the follicular phase of the cycle (Guillebaud 2004). It is likely that ovulation occurs within a day before, during or one day after the last day of abundant slippery discharge (Jennings et al 2004). The method is most effective if the fertile period is considered to begin when there is any type of mucus noted before ovulation. Following ovulation, the mucus changes under the influence of progesterone in the luteal phase, becoming impenetrable and hostile to sperm, and sticky (Guillebaud 2004). A disadvantage of this method is that some women may not secrete adequate amounts of mucus to notice cyclic changes.

Sympto-thermal method

This method incorporates cervical mucus observation and BBT as described previously and additional indicators of ovulation. These include symptoms such as the recognition of the softening and lowering of the external cervical os at the time of ovulation by the woman palpating her cervix (Guillebaud 2004). Cervical palpation each day towards the end of lactation can be a useful adjunct to assist the woman to recognise the return of fertility when using the LAM method. Additional symptoms include: mittelschmerz pain caused by follicular rupture resulting in symptoms such as dragging pain in the lower abdominal area; and rectal pain, which may occur before, during or after ovulation. Other symptoms may include increased libido, mood changes, breast tenderness and tenseness (Varney 1997).

Breastfeeding considerations

The current WHO (2004, p 3) guidelines outline the following information in relation to FAB, which may be less effective when breastfeeding.

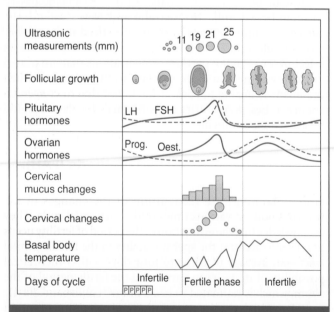

Figure 31.1 Fertility chart (based on Guillebaud 2004)

Before six weeks post partum, women who are primarily breastfeeding and are amenorrhoeic are unlikely to have sufficient ovarian function to produce fertility signs and hormonal changes during the first six months post partum. During LAM, the likelihood of resumption of fertility increases with time over the postpartum period and with substitution of breast milk by other foods.

After menses commences, when the woman notices fertility signs (particularly cervical secretions), she can use a symptoms-based method. Prior to that time, a barrier method should be offered if the woman plans to use a FAB method later.

Postpartum considerations

The current WHO (2004, p 3) guidelines outline the following information in relation to postpartum use of FAB.

Non-breastfeeding women are unlikely to have sufficient ovarian function to either require a FAB method or have detectable fertility signs or hormonal changes prior to four weeks post partum. Although the risk of pregnancy is low, a method appropriate for the postpartum period should be offered.

After four weeks, non-breastfeeding women are unlikely to have sufficient ovarian function to produce detectable fertility signs and/or hormonal changes at this time; and the likelihood increases rapidly with time post partum. Women can use a calendar-based method as soon as they have completed three postpartum menses. Methods appropriate for the postpartum period should be offered prior to that time.

Barrier methods

Barrier methods include male and female condoms, diaphragms and cervical caps. They are generally used in conjunction with spermicides and prevent spermatozoa coming in contact with the ovum. Barrier methods are used only as they are required, and in addition to their contraceptive value, prevent the transmission of some STIs.

Male condom

This is a widely available and popular male method of contraception (see Tables 31.2 and 31.3) that is readily reversible. Male condoms are one-use-only sheaths most commonly made of latex (rubber). Polyurethane (plastic) condoms are also available but are more expensive than latex condoms. They are thinner and have a higher breakage rate than latex condoms, although they provide a good alternative for individuals with allergies, sensitivities or personal preferences that might prevent the use of latex condoms (Gallo et al 2004). In some countries, 'lambskin' condoms are available, and although they are effective as contraceptives, they are not effective in preventing the transmission of infections. They are not available in Australia or New Zealand.

Condoms rarely break or slip off, and provide high contraceptive efficacy if used correctly and consistently (Walsh et al 2004). Refer to Table 31.1 for efficacy of the method. Male condoms can be used alone or with a spermicide, and can also be used as an adjunct to other methods of contraception when there is a risk of STI transmission.

Prior to use, the integrity of condoms must be confirmed by checking the expiry date, checking for the presence of a bubble when the unopened packet is squeezed gently between the thumb and forefinger, and for holes or other damage to the packet. Condoms must be stored in a cool, dry place, and therefore wallets kept in clothing pockets, and car glove boxes, are unsuitable places for storage. A new condom must be used for each act of sexual intercourse and should be put on to the erect penis before any contact is made with the female genitalia, anus or mouth. The condom is placed over the glans penis, and the air expelled from the end of the condom so that room is left for the semen after ejaculation. Failure to do this may result in the condom breaking. The condom is then rolled down to the base of the erect penis. Following ejaculation, the condom must be removed from the vagina before the penis loses its erection. The condom is held at the base of the penis during withdrawal so that it does not accidentally come off and cause spillage of semen. It is important that the used condom is removed from the woman's genital area and that the penis makes no contact with that area until the penis is cleansed.

Oils and creams can break down the latex and should not be used as lubricants with condoms. These include vaginal products used to treat *Candida albicans*, such as Nilstat™, Fungillin™, Nystatin™ and Monistat™ (Australia), and Nilstat™, Clocreme™, Clotrimaderm™, Clomazol™, Gyno-Pevaryl™ and Micreme™ (New Zealand). Oil-based lubricants like Vaseline™, baby oil, massage oils and hand and body lotions are also unsuitable. Only water-based lubricants should be used with latex condoms. Oil-based lubricants can, however, be used with polyurethane condoms. Care must be taken in the handling of all condoms to ensure that tearing does not occur at any time during their use.

Condoms come in different colours and flavours, but some of these are not safe to use. It is also important that users check that the condoms are Australian or New Zealand standards approved where pregnancy and/or STI prevention are wanted. Condoms are available from many sources including supermarkets, pharmacies, vending machines, health services and entertainment venues, and are reasonably cheap, particularly when bought in bulk. New Zealand midwives are licensed to prescribe condoms. Some manufacturers make wider and longer condoms, which suit men who find standard condoms uncomfortable. It should be noted that condoms do not afford protection against all STIs, but are effective in reducing the risk of transmission of HIV (Weller & Davis 2004), and also of herpes simplex virus 2, gonorrhoea, chlamydia and syphilis, and in protecting women against trichomoniasis (Holmes et al 2004).

Breastfeeding considerations

Male condoms do not interfere with lactation.

Postpartum considerations

Male condoms can be used when the couple are ready to resume sexual intercourse. When vaginal dryness or perineal soreness is a problem, additional water-based lubricant will make intercourse more comfortable.

Female condom (Femidom™)

The female condom is a loose polyurethane sheath (see Fig 31.2) that is inserted into the vagina. It has a 60 mm ring at one end that fits into the vaginal fornices in contact with the cervix (in much the same way as a diaphragm) and an outer ring 70 mm in diameter that is in contact with the vulva, preventing it from retracting into the vagina. Although female condoms are not a particularly popular method of contraception, they will suit women who want to control the use of a condom, because they can insert the female condom ahead of time (up to eight hours). Female condoms are pre-lubricated; however, additional lubricant can be used to assist in reducing the noise that generally accompanies their use during thrusting of the penis. As with male condoms, female condoms afford protection against several STIs (Guillebaud 2004). Because they are made of polyurethane rather than latex, they can be used with oil-based lubricants. Although it is generally recommended that female condoms are one-use only, if used for contraceptive purposes alone, they can be washed in bleach for one minute, then in soap and water and then rinsed and hung up and dried. They can be re-used up to five times (WHO 2004).

Female condoms are four times the cost of male condoms. In 2004, a decision was made to not import Femidoms™ into Australia in the future. If women want to use female condoms, they should be referred to the local family planning organisation (see contact details at the end of this chapter) for information about mail or internet ordering from another country. In New Zealand, Femidom™ is imported by the Family Planning Association and sold through clinics and by mail order.

Breastfeeding considerations

Female condoms do not interfere with lactation.

Postpartum considerations

Female condoms can be used when the couple are ready to resume sexual intercourse.

Diaphragm

A diaphragm is a soft, latex dome with a flexible metal spring encased in the rim (see Fig 31.3). It is inserted into the vagina to cover the cervix and is used in conjunction with a teaspoon of spermicide in the dome, which is in contact with the cervix

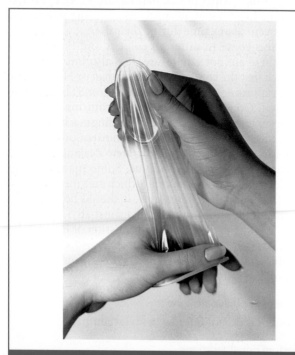

Figure 31.2 Female condom, Femidom™ (Guillebaud 2004)

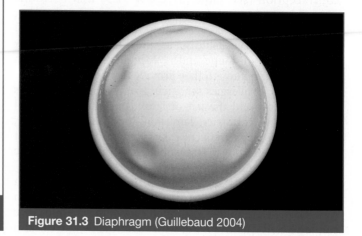

Figure 31.3 Diaphragm (Guillebaud 2004)

(Cook et al 2004a). Diaphragms come in circumferences ranging from 70 mm to 90 mm. They also come in different varieties named for the type of spring that holds the diaphragm in position: flat spring (flat band of lightweight stainless steel), coil spring (flexible circular coil), and all-flex (combination of flat and coil spring). Flat-spring diaphragms are not currently available in Australia or New Zealand. The spring in the circumference of the dome springs back into shape when the diaphragm is in place and holds in it position. There are no randomised controlled trials providing evidence that diaphragms provide protection against infection; however, it is likely that they provide protection of the cervix from infection (Cates & Stewart 2004).

Diaphragms needed to be correctly fitted by a qualified practitioner, and should be replaced after two years, after childbirth and if a woman gains or loses four or more kilograms in body weight. Failure of diaphragms is caused by poor fitting of the diaphragm, improper positioning, and inconsistent use (Guillebaud 2004). Diaphragms are not suitable for all women, in particular those with a shallow pubic ledge and women with poor vaginal and/or perineal muscle tone or with latex allergy. Women who choose this method must feel comfortable with their bodies and confident in inserting and removing the diaphragm from their vagina. They must be taught how to insert their diaphragm, check that it is in place and covering the cervix, the technique to remove the diaphragm and how to recognise when the diaphragm is no longer fitting correctly. Diaphragms can be inserted up to eight hours before intercourse and require the insertion of additional spermicide before subsequent intercourse. They need to be left in for six hours after intercourse because that is how long the spermicidal preparation takes to immobilise and kill the sperm. If intercourse takes place more than once within a six-hour period, the diaphragm should be left in place and more spermicide added using a plastic applicator. Diaphragms can be left in all the time, but must be removed every 24 hours and cleaned before replacing.

The cautions about oil-based lubricants and other products outlined earlier in the section on male condoms are the same for diaphragms. Only water-based lubricants should be used with diaphragms. Care also needs to be taken with diaphragms to prevent the latex from deteriorating. They need to be washed carefully with a mild soap, rinsed and dried well, and stored in the plastic box provided, away from light and heat. Diaphragms can be dusted with cornflour or *unscented* talcum powder before putting them in the storage box. They must also be checked regularly for holes, and the latex checked for tackiness, which indicates the need for replacement because the latex is starting to perish.

Breastfeeding considerations

Diaphragms and spermicides do not interfere with lactation.

Postpartum considerations

Diaphragms can be fitted six weeks after delivery. LAM or condoms and spermicide are suitable alternative methods that can be used in the interim.

EC alert

Women should be provided with information ahead of time about emergency contraception, so they can prevent pregnancy if they become aware that the diaphragm did not feel as though it fitted correctly, if it became dislodged, or if it was not used.

Cervical cap

The Dumas or vault cap (suitable for a woman who has a short, wide cervix) and the Prentif cavity rim cervical cap (suitable for women with a long, straight-sided cervix) are available in both Australia and New Zealand. Caps are made of latex rubber, are smaller than diaphragms and have a thick rim (see Fig 31.4). They cover the cervix and are held in place by suction. Spermicides are placed in the dome, but it is important that no spermicide gets on the rim of the cap, otherwise the suction action may be diminished (Guillebaud 2004). Fitting and care of cervical caps is the same as for diaphragms.

Breastfeeding considerations

Cervical caps and spermicides do not interfere with lactation.

Postpartum considerations

Cervical caps can be fitted six weeks after delivery. LAM or condoms and spermicide are suitable alternative methods that can be used in the interim.

EC alert

Women should be provided with information ahead of time about emergency contraception so they can prevent pregnancy if the woman becomes aware that the cap did not feel as though it fitted correctly, if it became dislodged, or if it was not used.

Intrauterine devices

The intrauterine contraceptive device (IUD or IUCD, see Fig 31.5) is a highly effective (see Table 31.1) and economical method of contraception. It is inserted into the uterus and left in situ, and when removed will provide prompt return of fertility. Because of the problems associated with the Dalkon Shield™ and subsequent litigation, the IUD has decreased

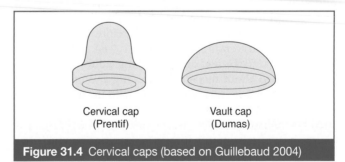

Cervical cap
(Prentif)

Vault cap
(Dumas)

Figure 31.4 Cervical caps (based on Guillebaud 2004)

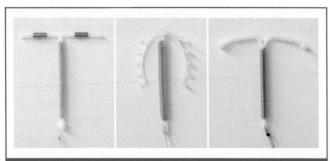

Figure 31.5 Intrauterine contraceptive devices **(a)** Copper-T 380™ **(b)** Multiload Cu 375® **(c)** Nova-T 380™ (Guillebaud 2004)

in popularity, although it is potentially a suitable method for many women. In Australia, the Copper-T 380a™ and Multiload Cu 375® are currently available and both of these are copper-bearing. The Copper-T™ can be left in place for eight years, and the Multiload for five years. In New Zealand, both the Nova T™ and Multiload Cu®375 (also copper-bearing) are available and can be left in place for three years and five years respectively. The Mirena® intra-uterine system (IUS), a levonorgestrel (LNG) releasing system, is available in both countries and has a five-year lifespan.

The IUD acts as a foreign body to change the endometrium, and also the uterine and tubal fluid. The device itself and the copper on the device act to block fertilisation and impede the transport of sperm (Guillebaud 2004). The copper on the devices is also toxic to ova and sperm. Copper IUDs can also be used for emergency contraception (see Emergency contraception section). The main disadvantage of IUDs is that they may cause a heavier menstrual flow for some women. On rare occasions they may perforate the uterine wall and occasionally migrate to the peritoneal cavity.

The end of menses through to mid-cycle is probably the best time for insertion of an IUD, because the likelihood of expulsion is minimal at that time. It is preferable for intercourse to not take place for three to four days following insertion, to minimise the risk of infection. If intercourse does take place during that time, a male or female condom should be used to counteract unexpected or unnoticed expulsion. Each month, the woman needs to check for the IUD strings, which are palpable at the cervical os.

The Mirena® IUS releases 20 µg of levonorgestrel per day. Its action is to block oestrogen and progesterone receptors, and also reduce sperm penetrability of the uterine fluid and cervical mucus. It also has an anti-implantation effect that takes time to develop (and is therefore unsuitable for emergency contraception, unlike other IUDs). IUSs are more expensive than IUDs and are better targeted to women who are concerned about menstrual bleeding and pain with an IUD. Since amenorrhoea is associated with the use of an IUS and was found to be the main reason for discontinuing the method, information about this aspect should be provided to assist women in making an informed decision about whether to use an IUS (van Vilet et al 2004).

Pelvic inflammatory disease (PID) is a complication of IUDs but is not caused by them, as was thought previously. It is possible, however, that asymptomatic cervical infection may be introduced into the uterus during the insertion process. Selective screening may be performed to exclude the presence of infection prior to insertion. A low rate of infection has been found with or without use of prophylactic antibiotics (Grimes et al 2004). IUDs do not provide protection against STIs, and so condoms should be used if there is any risk of infection.

Breastfeeding considerations

IUDs do not interfere with lactation. WHO (2004) guidelines suggest that the risk to the neonate due to exposure to steroid hormones with use of LNG-IUSs during the first six weeks post partum is the same as for other progestogen-only contraceptives.

Postpartum considerations

Although they can be inserted earlier (FFPRHC 2004), current practice is to postpone insertion of IUDs and IUSs until after six weeks post partum after a vaginal birth, and 12 weeks after a caesarean delivery. This is because the reason for postpartum bleeding will be unclear—for example, whether it is due to retained products or the IUD. LAM or condoms and spermicide are suitable alternative methods that can be used in the interim.

> **EC alert**
>
> Women should be provided with information ahead of time about emergency contraception so they can prevent pregnancy should the woman become aware that the IUD/IUS was not in situ and sexual intercourse had occurred.

Hormonal methods

Combined oral contraceptive (COC) pills

Combined oral contraception, commonly known as 'the pill', is both an effective (see Table 31.1) and popular (see Tables 31.2 and 31.3) method of contraception. COCs are a combination of synthetic oestrogen and progestogen in different amounts depending on the brand. COCs are either monophasic (all the same active pills in the packet with the same strength of oestrogen and progestogen), biphasic (two types of active pills in the packet where the oestrogen dosage and type remain constant and the type of progestin changes between the two last weeks of the active pills), or triphasic (three types of active pills in the packet where the oestrogen level may remain constant or change with the progestin component, and progestin has three different levels in the three weeks of active pills).

The action of COCs is to suppress ovulation by suppressing FSH and LH production 90–95% of the time, and also to thicken the cervical mucus, thus blocking sperm penetration. Additionally, a thinned endometrium inhibits implantation, and tubal and endometrial motility is slowed (Hatcher et al 2004a). COCs do not protect against STIs and should be used in conjunction with condoms and spermicides if the woman is at risk for STIs.

Table 31.4 shows the currently available pill brands with the combination of hormones in each formulation. Given the large number of COCs available, it is usually possible to find a formulation that suits each woman in whom this method is not contraindicated. Some pill packets have a total of 21 pills, which are all active (hormone) pills; other pill packets have a total of 28 pills—21 active pills and 7 placebo pills. Pills are taken each day at around the same time for the 21 active pills in the packet. For the remaining seven days, which is also called the 'pill-free interval' or PFI, either no pills are taken, or the placebo pills are taken. A withdrawal bleed (WTB) occurs during that time. Many women equate the WTB with a normal menstrual period. However, the normal menstrual cycle does not occur because ovulation has been suppressed; the bleeding is the result of the withdrawal of hormones resulting in endometrial shedding (Guillebaud 2004). It is important that the PFI is not extended by missing one of the active pill(s) the day before or the day after the PFI. An extension of the PFI week risks ovulation and thus the possibility of pregnancy should intercourse occur at that time. This means that every pill in the packet should be taken, and the woman needs to plan ahead so that she has a new packet ready to take at the end of the PFI.

In addition to their contraceptive effects, COCs offer other advantages. These include regular, light and less painful periods, possible reduction in premenstrual symptoms, protection from PID, and a decreased incidence of ectopic pregnancy (Fraser & Cooper 2003). Additionally, the time and frequency of menstruation can be manipulated; there is a reduction in ovarian and endometrial cancer rates, and decreased risk of death from colorectal cancer (Hatcher et al 2004a).

Complications

Some of the potential side-effects of COCs include venous thromboembolism, which is associated with the oestrogenic component. The risk is greater with 50 µg pills than with 20–35 µg pills. The risk is also higher for women with a BMI of greater than 30, those who have had a previous venous thromboembolism, and women who are immobile. In addition, women with focal migraine headaches or new onset of headaches are at greater risk of haemorrhagic stroke and should not take COCs (FFPRHC 2003; Hatcher & Nelson 2004). There is also an increased risk of acute myocardial infarction (AMI) for women over 35 years who smoke, and women with hypertension, diabetes, hyperlipidaemia or obesity. One per cent of women develop hypertension, which is reversible within 14 months of ceasing COCs. There is also a slightly increased risk for breast cancer, which declines in the first 10 years after discontinuing the Pill (Hatcher et al 2004a). Smoking potentiates most of the risks associated with COC use, such as ischaemia, and haemorrhagic stroke and AMI (Hatcher & Nelson 2004). Additional unwanted effects include headaches, breast tenderness, nausea, weight increase, depression and loss of libido. These effects often diminish over time or may improve with a change of pill.

Precautions

Some prescription medications can decrease the efficacy of COC and make it an unsuitable method for women taking these medications. Examples include rifampicin, phenytoin, primidone, carbamazepine, phenobarbitol and griseofulvin (Varney 1997). Other medications may potentiate the effect of COCs, and the efficacy of others may be reduced. Information about medication interaction is provided in the package insert, and should be highlighted to women to maximise the efficacy of COCs. St John's wort, a complementary medicine, may have a wide range of potency, and is therefore also not suitable for COC and progestogen-only pill takers. It is important that a careful prescription and non-prescription medication history is taken from women who want to commence COCs. Clearly written information about managing problems such as missed pills, vomiting, intractable diarrhoea and taking medications should be provided to women who are taking COCs. COCs should be ceased for four weeks before major surgery where the woman will be immobilised and a progestogen-only method used—otherwise thromboprophylaxis and compression stockings should be used (Guillebaud 2004; RCOG 2004). For minor surgery, COCs do not need to be discontinued.

Breastfeeding considerations

There is no consensus about when COCs should be commenced, when a woman is breastfeeding. There is a theoretical concern that the neonate may be at risk due to exposure to steroid hormones via breast milk during the first six weeks post partum, and that the duration of lactation may be decreased and therefore the growth of the infant may be affected (WHO 2004). This is, however, not supported in a recent Cochrane Review that concluded that existing randomised controlled trials were unable to establish an effect of hormonal contraception on milk quality and quantity, and the evidence inadequate to make recommendations regarding hormonal contraception for lactating women. Additionally, no adverse effects on infant growth have been documented (Truitt et al 2004). It would seem prudent, however, to advise women to postpone the commencement of COCs until lactation is well established (FFPHRC 2004). Given that there are other choices such as a combination of progestogen-only pills and LAM that provide almost 100% efficacy (Guillebaud 2004), excellent alternatives are available.

Postpartum considerations

In non-lactating women it is preferable to wait for three weeks to commence COCs. At this time, the risk of thrombosis is minimised due to the decrease of the high oestrogen levels of pregnancy. Blood coagulation and fibrinolysis are essentially normalised by this time. Additionally, ovulation will not have occurred by this time (Guillebaud 2004; WHO 2004). COCs may be used when blood pressure is back to normal levels in women who have had pregnancy-induced hypertension.

TABLE 31.4 Oral contraceptives available in Australia and New Zealand

Product	Oestrogen	Progestogen	Availability	
			Australia	New Zealand
20 µg—monophasic				
Loette®	Ethinyloestradiol	Levonorgestrel	☆	☆
Melodene™	Ethinyloestradiol	Gestodene	-	☆
Mercilon 21/28®	Ethinyloestradiol	Desogestrel	-	☆
Microgynon 20 ED®	Ethinyloestradiol	Levonorgestrel	☆	☆
30 µg—monophasic				
Femodene™	Ethinyloestradiol	Gestodene	☆	☆
Levlen ED®	Ethinyloestradiol	Levonorgestrel	☆	☆
Marvelon 21®	Ethinyloestradiol	Desogestrel	-	☆
Marvelon 28®	Ethinyloestradiol	Desogestrel	☆	☆
Microgynon 30 & 30 ED®	Ethinyloestradiol	Levonorgestrel	☆	☆
Minulet 21®	Ethinyloestradiol	Gestodene		☆
Minulet 28®	Ethinyloestradiol	Gestodene	☆	☆
Monofeme 28®	Ethinyloestradiol	Levonorgestrel	☆	☆
Nordette®	Ethinyloestradiol	Levonorgestrel	-	☆
35 µg—monophasic				
Brevinor, Brevinor 1®	Ethinyloestradiol	Norethisterone	☆	☆
Norimin®	Ethinyloestradiol	Norethisterone	☆	☆
Norimin 1®	Ethinyloestradiol	Norethisterone	☆	-
50 µg—monophasic				
Microgynon 50 & ED®	Ethinyloestradiol	Levonorgestrel	☆	☆
Nordette 50®	Ethinyloestradiol	Levonorgestrel	☆	-
Norinyl-1 21/28®	Mestranol	Norethisterone	☆	☆
Triphasic				
Improvil®	Ethinyloestradiol	Norethisterone	☆	-
Logynon®	Ethinyloestradiol	Levonorgestrel	☆	-
Synphasic 28 Day®	Ethinyloestradiol	Norethisterone	☆	☆
Trifeme 28®	Ethinyloestradiol	Levonorgestrel	☆	☆
Tri-Minulet®	Ethinyloestradiol	Gestodene	☆	-
Trioden ED®	Ethinyloestradiol	Gestodene	☆	-
Triphasil 28®	Ethinyloestradiol	Levonorgestrel	☆	☆
Triquilar & ED®	Ethinyloestradiol	Levonorgestrel	☆	☆
Biphasic				
Biphasil 28®	Ethinyloestradiol	Levonorgestrel	☆	☆
Sequilar ED®	Ethinyloestradiol	Levonorgestrel	☆	-
Progestogen only				
Femulen®		Ethynodiol	-	☆
Locilan 28®		Norethisterone	☆	-
Microlut®		Levonorgestrel	☆	☆
Micronor®		Norethisterone	☆	☆
Microval®		Levonorgestrel	☆	-
Noriday 28®		Norethisterone	☆	-

(Sources: AMH 2004; MIMS 2004)

Women who have had severe pregnancy-induced hypertension with persistent biochemical abnormalities are at greater risk of thrombosis, and if no alternative method is acceptable should wait until eight weeks to commence COCs (Fraser & Cooper 2003).

EC alert

Women should be provided with information ahead of time about emergency contraception so they can prevent pregnancy in the event that pills have been omitted (particularly those that extend the PFI), or when vomiting or intractable diarrhoea has occurred.

Progestogen-only pill

The progestogen-only pill (POP), also known as the 'mini-pill', provides the same amount of one of three progestogens (levonorgestrel, norethisterone or ethynodiol)—see Table 31.4. It is suitable for women in whom oestrogen and thus COC is contraindicated. Efficacy is listed in Table 31.1, but it should be noted that in lactating women, its efficacy is nearly 100% (Guillebaud 2004). The POP is taken every day with no PFI. Unlike the COC, which has a 12-hour leeway for the dose of active pills, POPs have to be taken within three hours of the same time each day. The action of POPs is the same as other progestogen-only contraception: blocking passage of sperm by thickening the cervical mucus, inhibiting ovulation in most women for most cycles, and decreasing endometrial receptivity. As with the other progestins, bleeding patterns may be altered during POP use, although amenorrhoea is likely during lactation (Guillebaud 2004).

Precautions

As POPs are low-dose contraceptives there is a very narrow margin of error for missed pills. If the pills are taken late, a back-up method of contraception should be used for 48 hours until the woman is back on schedule. In the event of vomiting, the usual pills should be taken and a back-up method such as condoms and spermicide should be used for 48 hours. When commencing POPs at any time other than during lactation or post partum, additional precautions are not required if it is commenced on day 1 of the cycle. Rifampicin and griseofulvin are both enzyme-inducing antibiotics, so extra precautions need to be taken during and after their use because their effect will be reduced by POPs. This does not apply to other antibiotics. As with COCs, St John's Wort is not suitable for POP users. POPs do not protect against STIs and should be used in conjunction with condoms and spermicides if the woman is at risk for STIs.

Breastfeeding considerations

The current WHO (2004) guidelines state that breastfeeding studies have shown that progestogen-only contraception did not affect breastfeeding performance and infant health and growth. However, there are no current data evaluating the effects of progestogen exposure via breast milk on brain and liver development.

Postpartum considerations

Although Fraser and Cooper (2003) state that postnatal use is associated with breakthrough bleeding, current WHO guidelines state that POPs can be started at any time during the postpartum period (WHO 2004). Some women may find the narrow timeframe in which to take POPs difficult to adhere to when they are experiencing erratic sleeping and waking patterns, so some women may prefer to commence COC instead, once breastfeeding is established.

EC alert

Women should be provided with information ahead of time about emergency contraception so they can prevent pregnancy should a dose of POP be omitted or vomited.

Injectable contraception

Depo-medroxyprogesterone acetate (DMPA), known as Depo-Provera® 150 µg, is an intramuscular contraceptive injection that is effective for three months (see Table 31.1 for efficacy). It suits women who prefer a non-coitus-dependent method of contraception, but should be used in conjunction with condoms for women who are at risk for STIs. It is suitable for women who need a method that does not include oestrogen (e.g. smoker, where there is a history of thrombosis), women who have oestrogen-related side-effects from the COCs, or who are taking medications that are contraindicated with COCs.

DMPA is administered by deep intramuscular injection into the deltoid or gluteus maximus. The woman is given the date (calculated by 12 calendar weeks) from that date for the next injection, although there is a leeway of up to 14 weeks in which it can be administered. Its action is to suppress ovulation by inhibiting the LH and FSH surge, thickening cervical mucus, thus blocking sperm entry into the upper reproductive tract, slowing tubal and endometrial motility, and causing thinning of the endometrium (Hatcher et al 2004a).

When commencing this method, the first injection should generally be administered before day 7 of the cycle, and no further precautions are required, although some clinicians advise extra precautions for a week if it is later than day 2 (Guillebaud 2004). Women currently on POP or COC and definitely not pregnant can be given the first injection at any time during the cycle with no added precautions. Some women experience irregular menstrual bleeding and spotting, particularly in the first few months of use, and with time, amenorrhoea occurs for many women (50% by one year). Importantly, fertility may take up to a year to return after ceasing DMPA, and so it is not suitable for women who want reasonably prompt reversibility of contraception. Some women experience a progressive weight gain due to increased appetite (Hatcher 2004). Headaches, dizziness, abdominal pain, or discomfort and weakness and fatigue, have been reported as other side-effects (Guillebaud 2004).

The other important issue is the greatly reduced bone mineral density in the lumbar spine and femoral neck in women who have used DMPA for at least five years, particularly after 15 years and when started before the age of 20 years (Hatcher et al 2004a). All users of DMPA should therefore be encouraged to undertake regular weight-bearing exercise. Their diet should include adequate dietary calcium, and if it does not, the need to take calcium supplements should be advised.

Breastfeeding considerations

The current WHO guidelines are that DMPA should be delayed until six weeks post partum because although breastfeeding studies have shown that progesterone-only contraception does not affect breastfeeding performance and infant health and growth, there are no data evaluating the effects of progestogen exposure via breast milk on brain and liver development (WHO 2004).

Postpartum considerations

Current guidelines are to wait until six weeks post partum, because heavy and prolonged bleeding may occur prior to that time. An alternative method must be used during that time and for seven days after the first injection. Guillebaud (2004) states that in theory, DMPA can be administered one week post partum, if the woman is not breastfeeding and might not return for the first dose.

EC alert

Women should be provided with information ahead of time about emergency contraception so they can prevent pregnancy in the event that the next DMPA injection is not given within the time limit and sexual intercourse has taken place.

Implant

Implanon® is a matchstick-sized progesterone-releasing rod, implanted under local anaesthetic, parallel to the skin on the inside upper arm (see Fig 31.6). It has a three-year lifespan and high efficacy rate (see Table 31.1) and suits women who want a non-coitus-dependent method that is 'set and forget'. The action, side-effects and precautions related to the use of Implanon® are the same as for DMPA. Implanon® contains 68 µg of etonorgestrel and releases 60 µg of progestin per day. It acts by blocking passage of sperm by thickening the cervical mucus, inhibiting ovulation, and making the endometrium atrophic (Hatcher et al 2004a). Implanon® may cause initial irregular and unexpected bleeding, which may be unacceptable to women, although supplemental hormones can be used to manage this. If at any time the method needs to be discontinued, the implant can be removed. Some women will become amenorrhoeic using this method. As with DMPA, weight gain can be a problem for some women.

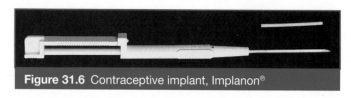

Figure 31.6 Contraceptive implant, Implanon®

Implanon® can be inserted from day 1 to 5 of the woman's cycle; however, if it is later than day 2, additional precautions should be used for seven days. If the woman is changing from COC or any other progestogen-only or uterine method, Implanon® can be inserted on any day, and the preceding method or condoms can be used for a further few days (Guillebaud 2004).

Breastfeeding considerations

The current WHO guidelines state that Implanon® should be delayed until six weeks post partum because although breastfeeding studies have shown that progesterone-only contraception does not affect breastfeeding performance and infant health and growth, there are no data evaluating the effects of progestogen exposure via breast-milk on brain and liver development (WHO 2004).

Postpartum considerations

Day 21 is recommended as the day of insertion of the implant because of the additional risk of irregular bleeding prior to that time, and to circumvent the need for additional contraceptive precautions. Another contraceptive method should be used for seven days, if the insertion takes place after day 21 (Guillebaud 2004).

Emergency contraception

Emergency contraception has been highlighted as a back-up method throughout this chapter. It is an important and under-used method of contraception that can be used for contraceptive failure (ruptured or slipped condom, dislodged diaphragm, missed pill(s) and so on), non-use of contraception, and for sexual assault. It is a method of contraception that should be included as part of counselling for most contraceptive methods as well as made more widely known about in the community (Calabretto 2004).

Hormonal emergency contraception

Hormonal emergency contraception is the main approach for emergency contraception. In the past, combined oral ethinyloestradiol and progestogen was used. In Australia this was off-label use of a COC brand, Nordiol (no longer available), and in New Zealand a dedicated product called PC4. An important multi-centre trial led to the current levonorgestrel-only method of EC (Task Force on Postovulatory Methods of Fertility Regulation: WHO 1998).

EC is sometimes erroneously thought to be an abortifacient. However, it is important to understand that EC does not interrupt an already implanted pregnancy (Calabretto & Galloway 2004). It is most likely that the main mechanism of action is to interfere with ovulation and prevent fertilisation, and there is no reliable evidence that EC interferes with implantation (Croxatto 2002). LNG is a synthetic progestin and is able to produce similar changes to the endometrium normally needed for implantation and continuation of pregnancy. This adds further support to the argument that the effect of EC is likely to be pre-ovulatory (Faundes et al 2003). Additional actions may be an effect on sperm transport, and alteration in cervical mucus (AMH 2004).

In Australia, Postinor-2® is the current levonorgestrel EC, and is available without prescription from pharmacies but requires counselling by a pharmacist prior to dispensing. It is no longer available on prescription. In New Zealand, Levonelle® is the levonorgestrel EC and can be sold with counselling, by accredited pharmacists and nurses. Postinor-2™ is a subsidised medicine available on prescription in New Zealand. EC may also available from other sources such as family planning clinics, women's health clinics, community health clinics, sexual health clinics, and youth health clinics, where it may be provided free or at a lower cost than in a pharmacy or on prescription.

The package insert states that EC must be taken as soon as possible within 72 hours of unprotected sexual intercourse, as two single doses of 750 μg, and taken 12 hours apart. In keeping with the study by Rodrigues et al (2001), current practice is now for EC to be commenced as soon as possible within 120 hours of unprotected sexual intercourse with the pills taken together as a single dose of 1500 μg. Importantly, although the extended timeframe does provide more leeway for women, the efficacy does decrease over time. In the future, it is likely that there will be a 1500 μg pill rather than the two-pill dose, and the package insert will reflect the extended timeframe.

The IUD as emergency contraception

A copper-bearing IUD (non LNG-IUS) can also be used as EC. It is inserted not more than five days after the most probable calculated date of ovulation, even if there have been multiple acts of unprotected intercourse, or five days after any single (earliest) exposure (Guillebaud 2004). Use of the IUD for the purpose of EC is most appropriate for women who want to use it as an ongoing method of contraception.

Breastfeeding considerations

EC may be safely taken during lactation (WHO 2004).

Postpartum considerations

EC may be safely taken during the postpartum period (WHO 2004).

Other contraceptive methods

Spermicides

Spermicides are chemical agents that destroy or immobilise sperm, making them incapable of fertilising an ovum. They are not recommended as a contraceptive alone (see Table 31.1 for efficacy), but are useful in increasing the efficacy of barrier methods such as diaphragms and condoms. Nonoxynol-9 is the active agent in most spermicides, and some condoms come

pre-lubricated with this spermicide. Spermicides are effective against several STIs. However, repeated and frequent use of this spermicide has been associated with increased risk of genital lesions, and may actually increase the risk of HIV (Wilkinson et al 2002). Spermicides, in the form of gels, cream or jelly, are inserted near the cervix using the applicator that comes with the product. It is important that the information provided on the package insert that comes with the particular spermicide is followed. Spermicide must be inserted prior to intercourse, and reapplied prior to subsequent episodes of intercourse.

Breastfeeding considerations

Spermicide use does not interfere with lactation.

Postpartum considerations

Spermicides can be used when the couple are ready to resume sexual intercourse.

Vaginal douche

There is an erroneous belief that vaginal douching is contraceptive by flushing sperm out of the vagina (Varney 1997). Most sperm are contained in the first few drops of ejaculate, and within 90 seconds of the deposit of semen at the cervical os, sperm have entered the cervical canal. It is simply impossible to douche in time to prevent pregnancy, and douching may also cause an increased risk of pelvic infections. It is therefore not advisable to recommend this practice (Cates & Raymond 2004).

Coitus interruptus (withdrawal)

This is a method that requires the man to withdraw his penis from the vagina before he ejaculates. The method may variously be described as 'withdrawal', 'being safe' or 'being careful' or by other euphemisms (Varney 1997). It is important to be aware of the meaning behind such descriptions when a woman discusses her contraceptive method. It has a low rate of contraceptive efficacy (see Table 31.1), although when used consistently and correctly it has the same efficacy as barrier methods and therefore should not be dismissed. It must also be appreciated that some cultural groups use coitus interruptus as their main method of contraception when spacing families and, for some people, is the only contraceptive method they will use throughout their reproductive lives. See Tables 31.2 and 31.3 for use in each age group.

Of importance to this method is the fact that sperm from a previous ejaculation may be present in the pre-ejaculate and therefore pose a pregnancy risk if intercourse occurs again within a short time. Although it has yet to be researched, it is probably advisable for the male to urinate after ejaculation to remove any sperm from his urethra, and he should also cleanse the external surface of the penis before contact with the woman's internal and external genitalia occurs (Kowal 2004). The method will fail if the man ejaculates on, or in the vicinity of, the female's external genitalia. Use of a spermicide will increase the efficacy should there be a small number of sperm in the pre-ejaculate from a previous ejaculation (Guillebaud 2004). Its advantage as a method is that it is free and always available as a method or back-up method, although it requires good communication and cooperation between the couple and excellent control by the male.

Breastfeeding considerations

Coitus interruptus does not interfere with lactation.

Postpartum considerations

Coitus interruptus can be used when the couple are ready to resume sexual intercourse.

> ### EC alert
>
> Women should be provided with information ahead of time about emergency contraception so they can prevent pregnancy should ejaculation occur in the vagina or vulva.

Permanent methods of contraception

These highly effective (see Table 31.1) surgical methods block the passage of ova in women and sperm in men. Although reversibility may be possible for some procedures, sterilisation should be considered as permanent, and it is therefore important that appropriate counselling is provided so that expectations are accurate. None of the procedures affect the hormonal levels in the body, and will not diminish and may in fact enhance sexual response because the fear of pregnancy is removed. These techniques do not provide protection against STIs, and so use of condoms and spermicides is needed for women who are at risk for STIs.

Tubal sterilisation

Female sterilisation, or tubal occlusion, is performed by a gynaecologist under conscious sedation, or general or local anaesthetic. The surgical approaches that may be used are laparoscopy, mini-laparotomy (performed after childbirth) or laparotomy. Once the fallopian tubes have been accessed, they are sealed off with clips, rings or bands applied to the tubes, or diathermy may be used to heat and seal the tubes. The method is effective immediately, and sexual intercourse may be resumed when the woman is ready to do so.

The newest method of female sterilisation—the Essure® technique—is performed using a cervical block and leaves no abdominal scars. Nickel titanium coils are inserted hysteroscopically into the ampullae of the fallopian tubes to cause scarring, and thus blockage of the tubes. At three months, a hysterosalpingogram or ultrasound is performed to confirm the presence and position of the coils (Teoh et al 2003). Until the blockage is confirmed, another method of contraception must be used. At present in Australia, the Essure® method is performed in some public hospitals

under Medicare arrangements or for a cost of $A2000 in private hospitals. In New Zealand the procedure can only be undertaken privately. Although it is the least-invasive method of female sterilisation, it is the least commonly performed procedure at present.

Breastfeeding considerations

This method does not interfere with lactation.

Postpartum considerations

The current WHO guidelines state that female sterilisation can be safely performed from immediately post partum up to seven days; however, there is an increased risk of complications from days 7–42 when the uterus has not fully involuted (WHO 2004).

A tubal ligation may be performed after a caesarean delivery. The WHO (2004) guidelines also note that women who have had pre-eclampsia or eclampsia have increased anaesthetic-related risks; and where there has been prolonged rupture of the membranes for 24 hours or more, when the woman has had puerperal sepsis, intrapartum or puerperal fever, there is an increased risk of postoperative infection. Women who have had a severe antepartum or postpartum haemorrhage may be anaemic and unable to tolerate further blood loss. If there has been severe trauma to the genital tract—cervical or vaginal tract tear at time of delivery—there may have been significant blood loss and anaemia, and the procedure may be more painful.

Prior to the procedure being done during the postnatal period, counselling needs to take place to ensure that this is a well-considered decision. It may be preferable to delay the procedure until 12 weeks post partum so that the woman will not regret a decision made at an early, more emotional time (Guillebaud 2004), unless the decision has been carefully considered in the antenatal period.

> ### EC alert
>
> Women should be provided with information ahead of time about emergency contraception so they can prevent pregnancy should intercourse take place in the first three months after the Essure® procedure.

Hysterectomy

Removal of the uterus for obstetric emergencies or gynaecological problems also confers permanent contraception.

Vasectomy

This is a male method of contraception where the vas deferens is cut and the end sutured to block the vas deferens and passage of sperm from the testes. There is local swelling and discomfort for a few days after the procedure. After vasectomy, sperm are reabsorbed. The procedure is usually performed under local anaesthesia, by a urologist, surgeon or GP. Higher rates of vasectomy success are associated with greater experience in vasectomy technique (Cook et al 2004a). Following the procedure, between 15 and 20 ejaculations are needed for the remaining sperm to be expelled from the body, so additional precautions need to be taken until a semen analysis is done to confirm the absence of sperm in the seminal fluid. After a vasectomy, the seminal fluid will not be noticeably different because only 2–5% of semen is sperm; most of the seminal fluid is composed of secretions from the seminal vesicles and prostate gland.

EC alert

Information about emergency contraception should be provided ahead of time so that pregnancy can be prevented should intercourse take place before a semen analysis has confirmed the absence of sperm.

Critical thinking exercise

Complete a table using the model below, including commencement time and compatibility with breastfeeding.

Method of contraception	When can the method be commenced during the postpartum period?	Is the method compatible with breastfeeding?
LAM		
COCs		
Condoms (female)		
Condoms (male)		
Diaphragm, cap		
EC		
Fertility awareness methods		
Implant		
Injectable		
IUD		
POPs		
Spermicides		
Tubal ligation		
Vasectomy		

Review questions

1   Are midwives adequately prepared to provide information about fertility control?

2   When is the best time to discuss fertility control with women?

3   Do you know where to refer women for contraceptive counselling and services?

4   What resources should be available in clinics or units to assist midwives to discuss contraception with women?

5   How do midwives ensure that their own negative views about a particular method(s) of contraception are not imparted to women?

6   Do you always discuss emergency contraception when you talk to women about contraceptive methods? Think about strategies to ensure that this aspect is not omitted.

7   Think about why some women or couples may be ambivalent towards the use of contraception. How might you assist them?

8   Think about the reasons that a woman might stop using a method of contraception, and how you would counsel her in this situation.

Review questions—cont'd

9 Decreased bone mineral density can be a problem for women who are long-term users of DMPA, and so these women should be taking adequate dietary calcium. How many µg of dietary calcium is adequate for a non-pregnant woman? Provide examples of common foods that would add up to this amount in a 24-hour period.

10 A woman in your care says that her partner does not want her to use any contraceptive method because of his cultural beliefs, although she would prefer to use a hormonal method, to space her family. Discuss the strategies you would use to assist your client to resolve this situation with her partner.

Online resources

American College of Obstetricians and Gynecologists, http://www.acog.org

Association of Reproductive Health Professionals, http://www.arhp.org/

Australian Sexual Health Nurses Association, http://www.ashna.com.au/

Contraceptive Technology, http://www.managingcontraception.com

Emergency Contraception Website, http://www.not-2-late.com

Faculty of Family Planning and Reproductive Health Care, http://www.ffprhc.org.uk/

Family Planning Association UK, http://www.fpa.org.uk

International Planned Parenthood Federation, http://www.ippf.org/

John Hopkins School of Public Health Information Program, http://www.jhuccp.org

Lactational Amenorrhoea Method, http://www.linkagesproject.org

Natural Fertility New Zealand, http://www.timgummerdesign.com/nf/index.htm

Ovulation Method Research and Reference Centre of Australia, http://www.billings-ovulation-method.org.au/index.shtml

Royal Australian and New Zealand College of Obstetricians and Gynaecologists, http://www.ranzcog.edu.au/

Royal College of Obstetricians and Gynaecologists, http://www.rcog.org.uk/

World Health Organization, http://www.who.int/health_topics/contraception/en/

World Organization Ovulation Method Billings (WOOMB), http://www.woomb.org/

References

American College of Obstetricians and Gynecologists 1997 ACOG Practice Patterns. Emergency oral contraception. International Journal of Gynecology and Obstetrics 56:203–210

AMH 2004 Australian medicines handbook. Australian Medicines Handbook Pty Ltd, Adelaide, SA

Australian Bureau of Statistics (ABS) 2001 National Health Survey, summary of results. Cat. No. 4364.0. ABS, Canberra

Calabretto H 2004 Emergency contraception—a qualitative study of young women's experiences. Contemporary Nurse Journal 18(1/2):152–163

Calabretto H, Galloway E 2004 Emergency contraception—issues of deregulation. Australian Pharmacist 23(1):46–52

Cates W, Raymond EG 2004 Vaginal spermicides. In: RA Hatcher, J Trussell, F Stewart et al (Eds) Contraceptive technology (18th edn). Ardent Media, NY, Ch 17

Cates W, Stewart F 2004 Vaginal barriers. In: RA Hatcher, J Trussell, F Stewart et al (Eds) Contraceptive technology (18th edn). Ardent Media, NY, Ch 18

Cook L, Nanda K, Grimes D 2004b Diaphragm versus diaphragm with spermicides for contraception (Cochrane Review). Cochrane Library (3). John Wiley & Sons, Chichester

Cook L, van Vilet H, Pun A et al 2004b Vasectomy occlusion techniques for male sterilization (Cochrane Review). Cochrane Library (3). John Wiley & Sons, Chichester

Croxatto HB 2002 Emergency contraception pills: how do they work? IPPF Bulletin 36(6):1–2

Faculty of Family Planning and Reproductive Health Care (FFPRHC) Clinical Effectiveness Unit 2004 FFPRHC guidance (July). Contraceptive choices for breast feeding women. Journal of Family Planning and Reproductive Health Care 30(3):181–189

Faculty of Family Planning and Reproductive Health Care (FFPRHC) Clinical Effectiveness Unit 2003 FFPRHC guidance (Oct). First prescription of combined oral contraception. Journal of Family Planning and Reproductive Health Care 29(4):209–223

Family Health International 2004 Chronic diseases and contraceptive use. Online: http://www.fhi.org/en/RH/Pubs/Network/v19_2/chrondiseases.htm, accessed 28 September 2004

Faundes A, Brache V, Alvarez F 2003 Emergency contraception—clinical and ethical aspects. International Journal of Gynecology and Obstetrics 82:297–305

Forrest JD 1994 Epidemiology of unintended pregnancy and contraceptive use. American Journal of Obstetrics and Gynecology 170:1485–1488

Fraser DM, Cooper MA 2003 Myles textbook for midwives (14th edn). Churchill Livingstone, Edinburgh

Gallo MF, Grimes DA, Schultz KF 2004 Non-latex versus latex male condoms for contraception (Cochrane Review). Cochrane Library (3). John Wiley & Sons, Chichester

Glasier A, Logan J, McGlew TJ 1996, Who gives advice about postpartum education? Contraception 53:217–220

Grimes D, Schultz K, van Vilet H et al 2004 Immediate postpartum insertion of intrauterine devices (Cochrane Review). Cochrane Library (3). John Wiley & Sons, Chichester

Grover S 2002 Menstrual and contraceptive management in women with an intellectual disability. Medical Journal of Australia 176:108–110

Guillebaud J 2004 Contraception. Your questions answered (4th edn). Churchill Livingstone, Edinburgh

Hatcher RA 2004 Depo-provera injections, implants and minipills. In: RA Hatcher, J Trussell, F Stewart et al (Eds) Contraceptive technology (18th edn). Ardent Media, NY, Ch 20

Hatcher RA, Nelson A 2004 Combined hormonal contraceptive methods. In: RA Hatcher, J Trussell, F Stewart et al (Eds) Contraceptive technology (18th edn). Ardent Media, NY, Ch 19

Hatcher RA, Trussell J, Stewart F et al (Eds) 1994 Contraceptive technology (16th edn). Ardent Media, NY

Hatcher RA, Zieman M, Cwiack C et al 2004a Managing contraception 2004–2005. The Bridging the Gap Foundation, Tiger Georgia

Hatcher RA, Trussell J, Stewart F et al (Eds) 2004b Contraceptive technology (18th edn). Ardent Media, NY

Hiller JE, Griffith E, Jenner F 2004, Education for contraceptive use by women after childbirth (Cochrane Review). Cochrane Library (3). John Wiley & Sons, Chichester

Holmes KK, Levine R, Weaver M 2004 Effectiveness of condoms in preventing sexually transmitted infections. Bulletin of the World Health Organization 82(6):454–461

International Medical Advisory Panel (IMAP) 1999 Statement on contraception for women with medical disorders. International Planned Parenthood Federation

Jennings VH, Arevalo M, Kowal D 2004 Fertility awareness-based methods. In: RA Hatcher, J Trussell, F Stewart et al (Eds) Contraceptive technology (18th edn). Ardent Media, NY, Ch 15

Kennedy KI, Trussell J 2004 Postpartum contraception and lactation. In: RA Hatcher, J Trussell, F Stewart et al (Eds) Contraceptive technology (18th edn). Ardent Media, NY, Ch 23

Kowal D 2004 Coitus interruptus (withdrawal). In: RA Hatcher, J Trussell, F Stewart et al (Eds) Contraceptive technology (18th edn). Ardent Media, NY, Ch 14

MIMS 2004 MIMS New ethicals catalogue (May). MediaMedia New Zealand Ltd, Auckland

New Zealand Plunket Society Inc. 2004 Breast feeding rates at 3 months of age. Online: http://www.plunket.org.nz/Other_Information_Page.htm#database

Pool I, Dickson J, Dharmalingam A et al 1995 New Zealand's contraception revolutions. Social Science Monograph Series Population Studies:47–48

Rodrigues I, Grou F, Joly J 2001 Effectiveness of emergency contraceptive pills between 72 and 120 hours after unprotected sexual intercourse. American Journal of Obstetrics and Gynecology 184(4):531–537

Royal College of Obstetricians and Gynaecologists (RCOG) 2004 RCOG Guideline No. 4. Venous thromboembolism and hormonal contraception. Online: http://www.rcog.org.uk

Sweet BR, Tiran D (Eds) 1997 Mayes' midwifery. A textbook for midwives (12th edn). Ballière Tindall, London

Task force on postovulatory methods of fertility regulation: WHO 1998 Randomised control trial of levonorgestrel versus the Yuzpe regimen of combined oral contraceptives for emergency contraception. Lancet 353:428–433

Teoh M, Meagher S, Kovacs G 2003 Ultrasound detection of the Essure permanent birth control device: a case series. Australian and New Zealand Journal of Obstetrics and Gynaecology 43:378–380

Truitt ST, Fraser AB, Grimes DA 2004 Combined hormonal versus nonhormonal versus progestin-only contraception in lactation (Cochrane Review). Cochrane Library (3). John Wiley & Sons, Chichester

Trussell J 2004 Contraceptive efficiency. In: RA Hatcher, J Trussell, F Stewart et al (Eds) 2004 Contraceptive technology (18th edn). Ardent Media, NY, Ch 31

van Vilet H, Cowan F, Mansour D et al 2004 Hormonally impregnated intrauterine systems (IUSs) versus other forms of reversible contraceptives as effective methods of preventing pregnancy (Cochrane Review). Cochrane Library (3). John Wiley & Sons, Chichester

Varney H 1997 Varney's midwifery. Jones and Bartlett, London

von Hertzen HG, Piaggio G, Ding J et al 2002 Low dose mifepristone and two regimens of levonorgestrel for emergency contraception: a WHO multicentre randomised trial. Lancet 360:1803–1810

Walsh TL, Frezieres RG, Peacock K et al 2004 Effectiveness of male latex condom: combined results for three popular condom brands used as controls in randomized clinical trials. Contraception 70:407–413

Weller S, Davis K 2004 Condom effectiveness in reducing heterosexual HIV transmission (Cochrane Review). Cochrane Library (3). John Wiley & Sons, Chichester

Wilcox AJ, Dunson D, Baird DD 2000 The timing of the 'fertile window' in the menstrual cycle: day-specific estimates from a prospective study. British Medical Journal 321:1259–1262

Wilkinson D, Ramjee G, Tholandi M et al 2002 Nonoxynol-9 for preventing vaginal acquisition of HIV infection by women from men. Cochrane Database of Systematic Reviews (3), Art No CD003936. DOI: 1O. 1002/14651858.CD003936

World Health Organization (WHO) 2004 Medical eligibility criteria for contraceptive use (3rd edn). Reproductive Health and Research, WHO, Geneva

Additional resources: family planning organisations

Useful information about clinic locations and services, and contraception, is available from the family planning organisations listed below. Also see the list of online resources, above.

AUSTRALIA

Sexual Health and Family Planning Australia
PO Box 256, Lyneham ACT 2602
email: fpa@fpa.net.au
website: http://www.fpa.net.au
ACT
Sexual Health & Family Planning ACT Inc.
Level 1, 28 University Ave (PO Box 1371), Canberra ACT 2601
Clinic : (02) 6247 3077, Education : (02) 6247 3018
email: shfpact@shfpact.org.au
website: http://www.shfpact.org.au
New South Wales
FPA Health (New South Wales)
Head Office, 328–336 Liverpool Rd, Ashfield NSW 2131
Phone: (02) 9716 6099, fax: (02) 9716 6164
email: healthline@fpahealth.org.au
website: http://www.fpahealth.org.au
Northern Territory
Family Planning Welfare Association of NT
Head Office
Unit 2, The Clock Tower, Dick Ward Drive, Trower Rd, Coconut Grove NT 0810
(PO Box 503, Nightcliffe NT 0814)
Phone: (08) 8948 0144
email: admin@fpwnt.com.au

Queensland
Family Planning Queensland
Head Office, 100 Alfred Street (PO Box 215), Fortitude Valley Qld
4006
Phone: (07) 3250 0240
Fax: (07) 3854 1277
email: enquiries@fpq.com.au
website: http://www.fpq.com.au
Victoria
Family Planning Victoria
Head Office, 901 Whitehorse Road (PO Box 1377), Box Hill Vic 3128
Phone: (03) 9257 0100
email: fpv@fpv.org.au
website: http://www.fpv.org.au
South Australia
Shine SA
17 Phillips St, Kensington SA 5068
Phone: (08) 8431 5177
Sexual health hotline: (08) 8364 0444
email: info@shinesa.org.au
website: http://www.shinesa.org.au
Tasmania
Family Planning Tasmania
Head Office, 2 Midwood St, New Town Tas 7008

Phone: (03) 6228 5244
email: info@fpt.asn.au
website: http://www.fpt.asn.au
Western Australia
FPWA (Formerly Family Planning Western Australia)
Head Office, 70 Roe St (PO Box 141), Northbridge WA 6865
Phone: (08) 9227 6177
email: sexhelp@fpwa-health.org.au
website: http://www.fpwa-health.org.au

NEW ZEALAND
Family Planning Association Inc, New Zealand
National Office, Level 6, Southmark House, 203–209 Willis St (PO
Box 11 515), Wellington
Phone: (04) 384 4349
email: national@fpanz.org.nz
website: http://www.fpanz.org.nz

Acknowledgement

New Zealand specific information was provided by Dr Christine
Roke, MB Ch B, FACSHP Cert FPRH, National Medical Adviser,
Family Planning Association Inc, Auckland, New Zealand

APPENDIX A:	Contraceptive methods for women with existing health problems	
Condition	**Unsuitable methods**	**Suitable methods**
Cardiovascular diseases		
Venous thromboembolism	COCs contraindicated. No sterilisation until condition treated and resolved.	Progestogen-only methods, IUDs.
Ischaemic heart disease or stroke	COCs contraindicated.	Progestogen-only methods when other methods are not available or acceptable.
Valvular heart disease		Progestogen-only methods. COCs if there are no complications such as pulmonary hypertension, atrial fibrillation, or history of subacute bacterial endocarditis.
Hypertension	Moderate and severe hypertension complicated with vascular disease are contraindications for COCs. Sterilisation for women increases GA risk, therefore vasectomy could be considered instead.	Low dose COC for mild hypertension and no additional risk factors (ie smoking, diabetes, obesity, or age > 35 years) when other methods unsuitable or unavailable POPs, IUDs, implants good choices, DMPA good second choice.
Diabetes	Hormonal contraception unsuitable when there are vascular complications. Female and male sterilisation can be performed but with additional precautions to anticipate hypoglycaemia or ketoacidosis and increased risk of infection. Copper IUD with screening and treatment of pre-existing infection prior to insertion, strict asepsis. Prophylactic antibiotics considered.	COCs normally contraindicated except where there is no vascular disease. POI (injectables) but only if other methods are not available or acceptable to the client. Hormonal contraception may be used if there are no vascular complications (nephropathy, neuropathy, or retinopathy). POP or Implanon can be used when there are vascular complications.
Convulsive disorders	DMPA and Copper or LNG IUD. EC—in the absence of scientific data on how drug interaction affects efficacy, the standard regimen should be used.	All methods are suitable but use of anticonvulsants— phenytoin, carbamazepine, ethosuximide, phenobarbitone & primidone—may reduce the efficacy of COCs, POPs, Implanon.
Migraine	COCs contraindicated in focal migraine. Onset or exacerbation of migraine with a new pattern which is recurrent, persistent or severe requires discontinuation of the COC and evaluation of the cause. POPS, DMPA or Implanon are usually discontinued in the presence of headache.	For focal migraine, POPs, Implanon or non-hormonal methods. POIs is last choice in the absence of hypertension. Low-dose COC for women who have simple migraine without aura.
Liver disease	COCs contraindicated in active liver disease, severe cirrhosis, or liver tumour.	Non-hormonal method should be first choice. Progestogen-only contraceptives may be used if other methods not acceptable or not available. Women who carry hepatitis viruses can use any method of contraception. Mild cirrhosis can generally use progestogen-only contraception, with COCs only as last choice.
Malignant diseases		
Breast cancer or liver neoplasms		Pregnancy should be avoided in women with a genital tract premalignant or malignant disease. With most genital tract malignancies, the treatment is such that there will be no further pregnancies. Pre-malignant conditions of the cervix—any method is suitable.

(Continued)

APPENDIX A:	Contraceptive methods for women with existing health problems—cont'd	
Condition	**Unsuitable methods**	**Suitable methods**
Breast cancer	Breast cancer: CU IUD is a good choice.	BC: COCs, POI contraindicated. POPs and LNG IUSs should not be initiated.
Endometrial, ovarian, cervical cancer		Copper IUDs should not be initiated but may be continued if cancer develops during use. Treatment usually causes sterility. If treatment is not available and contraception is needed, COCs, POPs, POI and Implanon® can be used.
Haematological disorders		
Anaemia	Copper IUCDs not suitable as they can increase blood flow.	COCs. Progestogen-releasing IUD, POI can reduce blood loss through menstruation.
Sickle cell disease		Pregnancy can be life-threatening for women with sickle-cell anaemia, therefore effective method is needed. Long-acting progestogen-only contraceptives should be first choice. COC and copper IUD are good second choices.
Thalassaemia	No methods are contraindicated.	
Infectious diseases		
Tuberculosis		Efficacy of COCs, POPs and Implanon is reduced, therefore the woman should be advised to employ a back-up method while taking Rifampicin and for two weeks after cessation of therapy.
Malaria		No contraindications to any method. No known drug interaction between antimalaria medications.
HIV infection	Spermicide used alone is not adequate.	Whatever the contraceptive choice, male condoms should also be used. The female condom is less well studied but should also reduce the risk of HIV infection when used consistently and correctly.
Psychiatric disorders	Sterilisation is not recommended for women or men with a psychiatric illness such as depression that may impair informed decision-making.	Methods that do not require strict compliance are more suitable for women with an acute or severe psychiatric disorder for whom making contraceptive choices may be difficult.
Mental disability	Careful consideration needs to be made to ensure that there is no coercion to use a particular method of contraception. Most methods are suitable and are dictated by the woman's ability to manage a particular method.	Sterilisation in the absence of informed consent by the client must involve the legal guardian and team of professionals. The decision must be guided by legislation.
(Sources: IMAP 1999; Family Health International 2004)		

CHAPTER 32

Screening and assessment

Sally K Tracy

Key terms

anaemia, asymptomatic bacterial vaginosis, asymptomatic bacteriuria, blood grouping, *Chlamydia trachomatis*, cytomegalovirus, Down syndrome, fetal anomalies, gestational diabetes mellitus, haematological conditions, hepatitis B virus, hepatitis C virus, HIV, infections, muscular dystrophies, placenta praevia, pre-eclampsia, preterm birth, red cell alloantibodies, rubella, sickle cell disorders, streptococcus group B, structural anomalies, syphilis, thalassaemia, toxoplasmosis

Chapter overview

Screening is a way of detecting a predisposition for a condition or a disease in people who are considered otherwise healthy and without any signs of the condition that is screened for. It can involve specific tests, or simple questions. It is important to note that a screening test is *not* a diagnosis or a diagnostic test. It merely brings to our attention someone or a group of women who may be at higher risk of having a disorder or disease. The next step, once a screening test has shown positive results, is for the woman to undertake further tests, which may be more expensive, invasive and time consuming. Screening usually begins early in pregnancy to check whether a woman has any conditions or infections that could affect her or her baby's health. It is important to always explain the purpose of any test that is offered, and it is of utmost importance to ascertain whether or not a woman wishes to have any

particular test. The information that tests provide may help you and the woman to consider certain pathways or treatments during the antenatal period. The test results will also invariably affect the way women make choices during their pregnancy.

This chapter builds on the information in Chapter 20. It follows on from the assessments that will have been made during the antenatal visits and discusses in depth the screening and assessment techniques currently undertaken in New Zealand and Australia. The chapter is not intended as a 'cookbook' guide on when and how to advise women about screening. You will be aware of the different screening policies at the national and area health service levels. This chapter is intended to introduce the student midwife to current debates and information appropriate to practice.

Learning outcomes

Learning outcomes for this chapter are:

1 To explain the concept of screening during pregnancy

2 To describe the test, examinations and other procedures available to women

3 To discuss the known benefits and disadvantages of screening procedures

4 To discuss the ethical, legal and social dilemmas accompanying the use of innovative medical technologies in antenatal screening.

Introduction: screening guidelines

In Australia and New Zealand there are various sets of evidence-based guidelines prepared and published to guide midwives (and others) through the maze of screening options available for women having uncomplicated pregnancies. Some of these are listed here, with brief overviews of their contents.

Three Centres Consensus Guidelines

The *Three Centres Consensus Guidelines on Antenatal Care* are available online at http://www.health.vic.gov.au/maternitycare/anteguide.pdf.

Information on the content of visits should include the rationale and timing of routine tests and investigations. Wherever possible, any reduction in the total number of visits should be accompanied by an increase in time allocated.

The evidence accumulated for the Three Centres Project suggests a baseline eight-visit antenatal schedule as follows:

- **Visits 1 and 2** are in the first trimester. From the carer's perspective, first trimester visits are primarily to assess maternal and fetal wellbeing, particularly the risk of complication, to date the pregnancy, take a comprehensive history, discuss smoking behaviour and establish care options. The visits are scheduled in order to offer screening tests recommended for asymptomatic bacteriuria, syphilis, HBV, HCV, HIV and Down syndrome.
- **Visits 3 and 4** are in the second trimester. Second trimester visits are primarily scheduled to monitor fetal growth, maternal wellbeing and signs of pre-eclampsia. If ultrasound is routinely offered, it should be included as part of a visit at 18–20 weeks. If women have glucose screening this should be part of a visit at 24–28 weeks.
- **Visits 5–8** are in the third trimester. Third trimester visits are primarily to monitor fetal growth, maternal wellbeing, signs of pre-eclampsia, and to assess and prepare women for admission, labour and going home. These visits may include bacteriological screening for GBS (at 35–37 weeks), and preparations for admission, labour and 'going home', consistent with other guidelines.

It is important to establish each person's expectations and understanding, as women may have a different perspective on the purpose and timing of antenatal visits. The option and timing of additional visits should be discussed with all women.

NICE Guidelines

The NICE (National Institute for Clinical Excellence) Guidelines are available on the RCOG website. See 'Antenatal care: routine care for the healthy pregnant woman' (http://www.rcog.org.uk/index.asp?PageID=693).

Midwives Handbook

The NZCOM's *Midwives Handbook for Practice* (NZCOM 2005) says that the first decision point in pregnancy (within the first 16 weeks of pregnancy) is timed to allow for a comprehensive assessment to be made according to the best available evidence. It is an ideal time to discuss the role that both the midwife and women will undertake in the following pregnancy and birth. It will also ensure that there is time to make appropriate decisions regarding treatment and decisions to intervene in the pregnancy if this is what eventuates following the screening procedures that may be undertaken. It is important that the midwife adequately explains to a pregnant woman what screening tests are meant to detect, how they are conducted, possible risks to her and her fetus, the type of results that will be reported (e.g. probability, risk), the likelihood of false-positive or false-negative results, and the choices she will face once results are obtained (NICE 2003).

Information shared

The first step in screening is to review the woman's history to identify any factors that may need follow-up. Midwifery factors include a discussion of what the woman and midwife understand to be the role they will play during the pregnancy. It may involve discussion of previous experiences of labour and birth; or it may include an in-depth discussion of the scope of practice of the midwife and the appropriateness of referral and consultation. In this first screening visit it is important to ascertain the support networks available and the priorities for medical consultation, if this is recommended.

Chapter 20 covered in detail how to do a booking and the regular observations that midwives attend to in the antenatal period. This chapter discusses the contemporary screening options offered to women, and discusses the appropriateness of screening for each condition.

Review of current and past maternity history

At this time you will ascertain the number of pregnancies a woman reports (gravida) and the number of births (parity). (Note: The definitions of mortality differ between Australia and New Zealand. In both Australia and New Zealand, a live birth is recorded if the fetus is 20 weeks gestation or over, and weighs 400 g or more at the time of birth (AIHW 2004). The perinatal death rate in Australia includes stillbirth (or fetal death) and death up to 28 days after birth; in New Zealand, a perinatal death is a stillbirth (fetal death) or a death up to 7 days after birth. The denominator for perinatal death rate is per 1000 births: both live and stillborn over these time periods.)

At this time it is important to ascertain whether a woman has had any spontaneous or elective abortions or whether she has experienced preterm labour and birth, or had a stillbirth or a neonatal death. This information helps to build a better picture about whether a woman might benefit from more intensive screening than the usual methods offered to most women regardless of any risk markers.

Definition of terms:

- Parity refers to the total number of pregnancies continued beyond 20 weeks gestation, regardless of the outcome (i.e. live birth or stillbirth) or the number of fetuses in the uterus (i.e. parity is not influenced by multiple births—plural pregnancies are counted as one). A nulliparous woman has never given birth to a viable infant, or, in other words has never completed a pregnancy beyond 20 weeks gestation.
- The term primiparous refers to a pregnant woman who has given birth and has had no previous pregnancy before this birth resulting in a live birth or stillbirth.
- Multipara refers to a pregnant woman who has had at least one previous pregnancy resulting in a live birth or stillbirth before this one, or, in other words, having completed at least one pregnancy beyond 20 weeks.
- Grand multipara refers to a pregnant woman who has had four or more previous pregnancies resulting in a live birth or stillbirth (i.e. this is her fifth (or more) pregnancy).

Screening tests

A good screening test should be able to discriminate clearly between those who are at high risk, and those who are not. It should be safe, have a reasonably defined cut-off level and be both valid and reliable. Although the latter two terms are often used interchangeably, they are distinct. Validity is the ability of a test to measure what it sets out to measure, usually differentiating between those with and without the disease. By contrast, reliability indicates repeatability (Grimes & Shultz 2005, p 882). It refers to a method of measurement that consistently gives the same results (NICE 2003).

However, being labelled as at 'high risk' is only useful if something can be done to alter or decrease the risk. In addition, risk factors are not things that cause an outcome —they are only markers of a particular situation, and serve to alert the midwife to the fact that diagnostic tests might be required to ascertain whether or not the woman has a certain condition. This leads us to our first ethical dilemma.

Screening differs from the traditional clinical use of tests in several important ways. When we believe there is something wrong with us, it prompts us to consult an expert (perhaps a doctor) about the complaint or problem, and this in turn prompts testing to confirm or exclude a diagnosis. By contrast, screening engages apparently healthy women who are not seeking medical help (and might prefer to be left alone). In addition, the occurrence of false-positive results and true-positive results may lead to (dangerous) interventions. Although the anxiety induced by a correct diagnosis may be overwhelming, those incorrectly thought to have a problem suffer as well. For example, although failing to diagnose sexually transmitted diseases can have important health implications, incorrectly labelling people as infected can wreck marriages and damage lives (Grimes & Schulz 2002).

Assessing the effectiveness of a test

There are four indices of the validity of a test: sensitivity, specificity, and predictive values of positive and negative (see Fig 32.1).

Sensitivity

Sensitivity is sometimes termed the 'detection rate'. It describes the ability of a test to find those with the disease (Grimes & Schulz 2002). In diagnostic testing, sensitivity refers to the chance of having a positive test result, given that you have the disease. One hundred per cent sensitivity means that all those with the disease will test positive, but this is not the same the other way around. A woman could have a positive test result but not have the disease—this is called a 'false positive'. The sensitivity of a test is also related to its 'negative predictive value' (true negatives): a test with a sensitivity of 100% means that all those who get a negative test result do not have the disease. To fully judge the accuracy of a test, its specificity must also be considered (NICE 2003, glossary).

Specificity

Specificity denotes the ability of a test to identify those without the condition (Grimes & Schulz 2002). In diagnostic testing, this refers to the chance of having a negative test result, given that you do not have the disease. One hundred per cent specificity means that all those without the disease will test negative, but this is not the same the other way around. A woman could have a negative test result, yet still have the disease—this is called a 'false negative'. The specificity of a test is also related to its 'positive predictive value' (true positives):

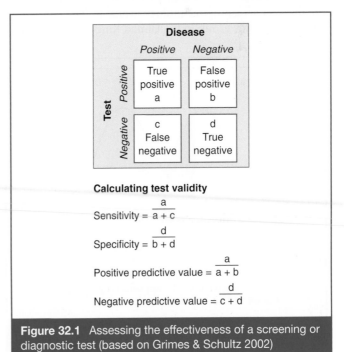

Figure 32.1 Assessing the effectiveness of a screening or diagnostic test (based on Grimes & Schultz 2002)

a test with a specificity of 100% means that all those who get a positive test result definitely have the disease. To fully judge the accuracy of a test, its sensitivity must also be considered (NICE 2003, glossary).

For the purposes of this chapter, it is important to understand these concepts broadly, so that you understand how screening works in real life. For example, the trade-off between sensitivity and specificity (see Fig 32.2) is demonstrated by the following. For any continuous outcome measurement (e.g. blood glucose), the sensitivity and specificity of a test will be inversely related. If we place the cut-off for abnormal blood glucose at a very low point, thereby producing perfect sensitivity (i.e. we manage to identify all those women with diabetes), the low cut-off identifies all those with diabetes. However, the trade-off is poor specificity—that is, those women who also have blood glucose at the level specified but are part of the 'healthy distribution' (i.e. at one end of 'normal') and are incorrectly identified as having abnormal values. Placing the cut-off higher yields the opposite result: all those who are healthy are correctly identified (perfect specificity), but the cost here is missing a proportion of women who are diabetic. Selecting a cut-off point is a compromise, mislabelling some healthy people and some people with diabetes. Where the cut-off should be depends on the implications of the test.

As in other areas of maternity care, there is healthy debate about what constitutes evidence-based screening and what does not. This has been instrumental in driving a serious attempt to outline the most reasonable path to follow with screening in pregnancy. For the purposes of this chapter, the road map for screening will be that developed by the National Institute for Clinical Excellence (NICE). The NICE Guidelines were developed in the United Kingdom and drew on the first attempt in Australia to gather evidence-based guidelines to help practitioners and women navigate their way through the maze of screening technology available. The Guidelines developed by this group in the United Kingdom represent:

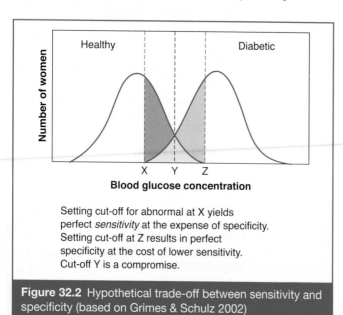

Setting cut-off for abnormal at X yields perfect *sensitivity* at the expense of specificity. Setting cut-off at Z results in perfect specificity at the cost of lower sensitivity. Cut-off Y is a compromise.

Figure 32.2 Hypothetical trade-off between sensitivity and specificity (based on Grimes & Schulz 2002)

Reflective exercise

Look closely at the references cited in the NICE Guidelines, the Three Centres Consensus Guidelines from Australia, and the New Zealand Guidelines for antenatal screening, and determine how many interventions are based on Level 1 evidence.

the view of the Institute, which was arrived at after careful consideration of the evidence available. Health professionals are expected to take it fully into account when exercising their clinical judgment. The guidance does not, however, override the individual responsibility of health professionals to make decisions appropriate to the circumstances of the individual patient, in consultation with the patient and/or guardian or carer (NICE 2003).

Appointment times for screening

The following summary of screening visits and what to do are based on the NICE Guidelines (2003, pp 10–12). Remember that these are only a guide to practice: screening is an individual thing, and many women will not necessarily find this level of surveillance a comfort or a necessity. It is therefore most important to respect women's views in these matters.

First appointment

At the first appointment:
- give information to enable informed decision-making about screening tests
- identify women who may need additional care
- check blood group and Rhesus D (RhD) status
- offer screening for anaemia, red-cell alloantibodies, hepatitis B virus, HIV, rubella susceptibility and syphilis
- offer screening for asymptomatic bacteriuria (ASB)
- offer screening for Down syndrome
- offer early ultrasound scan for gestational age assessment
- offer ultrasound screening for structural anomalies (20 weeks).

After the first (and possibly second) appointment, for women who choose to have screening, the following tests should be arranged before 16 weeks of gestation (except serum screening for Down syndrome, which may occur up to 20 weeks of gestation):
- ultrasound scan to determine gestational age using:
  - crown–rump measurement if performed at 10 to 13 weeks
  - biparietal diameter or head circumference at or beyond 14 weeks
- Down syndrome screening using:
  - nuchal translucency at 11 to 14 weeks
  - serum screening at 14 to 20 weeks.

16 weeks

The next appointment should be scheduled at 16 weeks to:
- review, discuss and record the results of all screening tests undertaken.

18 to 20 weeks

At 18 to 20 weeks, if the woman chooses, an ultrasound scan should be performed for the detection of structural anomalies. For a woman whose placenta is found to extend across the internal cervical os at this time, another scan at 36 weeks should be offered and the results of this scan reviewed at the 36-week appointment.

28 weeks

At this appointment:
- offer a second screening for anaemia and atypical red-cell alloantibodies
- investigate a haemoglobin level of less than 10.5 g/dL and consider iron supplementation, if indicated
- offer anti-D to Rhesus-negative women.

31 weeks

Review, discuss and record the results of screening tests undertaken at 28 weeks.

34 weeks

At 34 weeks, all pregnant women should be seen in order to:
- offer a second dose of anti-D to Rhesus-negative women.

36 weeks

At 36 weeks:
- for women whose babies are in the breech presentation, offer external cephalic version (ECV)
- review ultrasound scan report if placenta extended over the internal cervical os at previous scan.

Gestational age assessment

The information in this section is from the NICE Guidelines (2003, pp 7–8).

Pregnant women should be offered an early ultrasound scan to determine gestational age (in lieu of last menstrual period (LMP) for all cases) and to detect multiple pregnancies. This will ensure consistency of gestational age assessments, improve the performance of mid-trimester serum screening for Down syndrome, and reduce the need for induction of labour after 41 weeks. (The guidelines underpin this advice with a level of evidence obtained from randomised controlled trials and systematic reviews.)

Ideally, scans should be performed between 10 and 13 weeks and crown–rump length measurement used to determine gestational age. Pregnant women who present at or beyond 14 weeks gestation should be offered an ultrasound scan to estimate gestational age using head circumference or biparietal diameter. (This recommendation is based on a 'good practice point'.)

Ultrasound scans

Early in pregnancy (usually around 10 to 13 weeks), the first ultrasound scan may be offered. It is used to estimate when the baby is due and to check whether there is more than one fetus. If you don't see women this early, it is appropriate to offer the scan at the earliest time. Between 18 and 20 weeks appears to be the optimum time to offer a second scan to check for physical abnormalities in the fetus. Beyond these it is not recommended that women have any further routinely offered scans, as they have not been shown to be useful (NICE 2003).

Individual clinicians, maternity units and geographic regions have adopted widely varying strategies for combining LMP and early ultrasound (EUS) estimates of gestational age (GA). Some still use LMP, others rely exclusively on EUS, while many base GA on EUS only when the discrepancy with LMP exceeds a given limit, such as ±7, 10 or 14 days (Blondel et al 2002).

Table 32.1 shows the effect of estimating the GA in a fetus using the various methods of estimation in a study in 44,632 pregnancies in France. Note the discrepancies between postdates babies using the LMP method and the EUS method. Some authors recommend ultrasound estimation as the first choice for dating all pregnancies; others have voiced reservations about exclusive use of EUS estimates. Because of these different approaches to resolving discrepancies in LMP and EUS estimates, both among and within countries, geographic and temporal trends in preterm and post-term birth remain difficult to interpret (Blondel et al 2002).

Estimates of gestational duration based on the timing of the last normal menstrual period (LMP) are dependent on a woman's ability to recall the dates accurately, the regularity or irregularity of her menstrual cycles and variations in the interval between bleeding and anovulation. Crowther and colleagues (1999) estimate that between 11% and 42% of GA estimates from LMP are reported as inaccurate. Ultrasound measurements are based on standard growth curves, but fetal growth may deviate from the standard, even early in gestation. Fetuses that grow faster than the standard curve will be given a biased, longer gestational length, and therefore an increased probability of being classified as post-term, even when they are not (Olesen et al 2004). The opposite will be seen for slow-growing fetuses. Lower early ultrasound-based GA estimates therefore seem attributable in some cases to slower fetal growth (Olesen et al 2004). This observation was also reported by Smith et al (1998).

In a study that examined the determinants and consequences of fetal growth restriction as a function of differences in GA estimates, Morin et al (2005) found that several maternal and fetal characteristics influenced the magnitude of the discrepancy between the GA estimates. These included socio-economic differences and potential determinants of early fetal growth restriction (Morin et al 2005). Mothers with severe pre-eclampsia and short stature were more likely to have

TABLE 32.1 Rates of preterm and post-term birth, estimated from LMP or EUS, according to six algorithms for combining the two estimates (n = 44,623)

GA		Algorithm*				
	1 LMP alone	2 LMP or EUS (14-day rule)	3 LMP or EUS (10-day rule)	4 LMP or EUS (7-day rule)	5 LMP or EUS (3-day rule)	6 EUS alone
Preterm birth (%)						
< 32 weeks	1.3	1.3	1.3	1.3	1.3	1.3
< 34 weeks	2.2	2.1	2.2	2.2	2.3	2.3
< 37 weeks	7.6	7.8	8.1	8.5	9.0	9.1
Post-term birth (%)						
≥ 41 weeks	20.9	16.9	15.1	13.4	11.7	11.2
≥ 42 weeks	6.4	3.5	2.8	2.4	2.0	1.9

*EUS source if discrepancy between the two sources > 14 days (Algorithm 2), > 10 days (Algorithm 3), > 7 days (Algorithm 4), > 3 days (Algorithm 5)
(Source: Blondel et al 2002)

positive differences (higher menstrual than early ultrasound-based GA estimates), suggesting that these widely recognised determinants of fetal growth might begin to exert their effects by the early second trimester. Small differences in growth may also depend on fetal sex, maternal age, parity and smoking (Olesen et al 2004). The NICE guideline group conclude, however, that there is thought to be little variation in fetal growth rate up to mid-pregnancy and, therefore, estimates of fetal size by ultrasound scan provide estimates of GA that are not subject to the same human error as LMP (NICE 2003).

Ultrasound assessment of GA at 10–13 weeks is usually calculated by measurement of the crown–rump length. For pregnant women who present in the second trimester, GA can be assessed with ultrasound measurement of biparietal diameter or head circumference (NICE 2003). Ultrasound measurement of biparietal diameter is reported to provide a better estimate of date of delivery for term births than first day of the LMP (NICE 2003, p 51). Routine ultrasound before 24 weeks is also associated with a reduction in rates of intervention for post-term pregnancies. A 1998 Cochrane Review (Neilson 1998) found that, compared with selective ultrasonography, routine prenatal ultrasonography before 24 weeks gestation provided better GA assessment and earlier detection of multiple pregnancies and fetal malformations. This review reported, in the long-term follow-up of Norwegian and Swedish children, no adverse influence on school performance or neurobehavioral function as a consequence of antenatal exposure to ultrasound; however, fewer of the ultrasound-exposed children are right-handed (Neilson 1998). The 'Alesund' trial, which was reported in 2000 (Eik-Nes et al 2000), claimed the possible benefits of the routine use of ultrasound screening in pregnancy as a lower incidence of induced labour due to apparent post-term pregnancies—approximately 70% lower in the ultrasound-screened group. Inductions from all causes were also less frequent among ultrasound-screened women. Among the controls, three pairs of twins remained undiagnosed until the mothers were admitted to the hospital in labour at between 36 and 38 weeks gestation. The authors concluded that for women who were screened with ultrasound, obstetricians were less likely to induce labour due to apparent post-term pregnancy, than for women who were not screened (Eik-Nes et al 2000).

Accurately assessing the GA also permits optimal timing of antenatal screening for Down syndrome and fetal structural anomalies. Reliable dating is important when interpreting Down syndrome serum results, as it may reduce the number of false-positives for a given detection rate (NICE 2003).

Side-effects of ultrasound

The use of ultrasonography for evaluating the developing embryo/fetus continues to rise, although the potential risks from exposure are uncertain (Barnett et al 2000; Marinac-Dabic et al 2002; Miller et al 1998). An effect of ultrasound on intellectual performance cannot, at present, be ruled out. Researchers from Sweden who published their work in the journal *Epidemiology* in 2005 concluded that further action to evaluate possible neurotoxic effects of ultrasound should be taken, particularly because ultrasound exposure in the published studies looking at long-term effects of exposure was low compared with present levels of exposure (Kieler et al 2005).

Prenatal exposure to ionising irradiation in the second trimester has been found to affect the developing brain, resulting in intellectual impairment (Schull & Otake 1999). Whether other forms of radiation such as ultrasound have similar neurotoxic effects is not yet known (Ziskin & Barnett 2000). Ultrasound has the potential to damage tissue by

---

BOX 32.1 What is ultrasound?

The term 'ultrasound' refers to the ultra-high-frequency sound waves used for diagnostic scanning. Ultrasound waves are emitted by a transducer (the part of the machine that is put onto the body), and a picture of the underlying tissues is built up from the pattern of 'echo' waves that return. Hard surfaces such as bone will return a stronger echo than soft tissue or fluids, giving the bony skeleton a white appearance on the screen.

Ordinary scans use pulses of ultrasound that last only a fraction of a second. In contrast, Doppler techniques, which are used in specialised scans, fetal monitors and hand-held fetal stethoscopes, feature continuous waves, giving much higher levels of exposure than pulsed ultrasound.

More recently, ultrasonographers have been using vaginal ultrasound, where the transducer is placed high in the vagina, much closer to the developing baby. This is used mostly in early pregnancy, when abdominal scans can give poor pictures. However, with vaginal ultrasound, there is little intervening tissue to shield the baby, who is at a vulnerable stage of development, and exposure levels will be high. Having a vaginal ultrasound is not a pleasant procedure for the woman; the term 'diagnostic rape' was coined to describe how some women experience vaginal scans.

Another recent application for ultrasound is the nuchal translucency test, where the thickness of the skin fold at the back of the baby's head is measured at around three months; a thick 'nuch (neck) fold' indicates that the baby is more likely, statistically, to have Down syndrome. When the baby's risk is estimated to be over 1 in 250, a definitive test is recommended. This involves taking some of the baby's tissue by amniocentesis or chorionic villus sampling. Around 19 out of 20 babies diagnosed as 'high risk' by nuchal translucency will not turn out to be affected by Down syndrome, and their mothers will have experienced several weeks of unnecessary anxiety. A nuchal translucency scan does not detect all babies affected by Down syndrome.

(Source: Buckley 1998–2005)

BOX 32.2 When is ultrasound helpful?

One of the most common justifications given for routine ultrasound scanning is to detect intrauterine growth restriction (IUGR). Many clinicians insist that ultrasound is the best method for the identification of this condition. In 1986, a professional review of 83 scientific articles on ultrasound showed that 'for intrauterine growth retardation detection, ultrasound should be performed only in a high-risk population'. In other words, the hands of an experienced midwife or doctor feeling a pregnancy woman's abdomen are as accurate as the ultrasound machine for detecting IUGR. The same conclusion was reached by a study in Sweden comparing repeated measurement of the size of the uterus by a midwife with repeated ultrasonic measurements of the head size of the fetus in 581 pregnancies. The report concludes: 'Measurements of uterus size are more effective than ultrasonic measurements for the antenatal diagnosis of intrauterine growth retardation'.

If doctors continue to try to detect IUGR with ultrasound, the result will be high false-positive rates. Studies show that even under ideal conditions, such as do not exist in most settings, it is likely that over half of the time a positive IUGR screening test using ultrasound is returned, the test is false, and the pregnancy is in fact normal. The implications of this are great for producing anxiety in the woman and the likelihood of further unnecessary interventions.

There is another problem in screening for IUGR. One of the basic principles of screening is to screen only for conditions for which you can do something. At present, there is no treatment for IUGR, no way to slow or stop the process of too-slow growth of the fetus and return it to normal. So it is hard to see how screening for IUGR could be expected to improve pregnancy outcome.

We are left with the conclusion that, with IUGR, we can only prevent a small amount of it using social interventions (nutrition and substance abuse programs), are very inaccurate at diagnosing it, and have no treatment for it. If this is the present state of the art, there is no justification for clinicians using routine ultrasound during pregnancy for the management of IUGR. Its use should be limited to research on IUGR.

(Source: Proud 1997)

---

heating, cavitation or streaming, and the brain is most susceptible to environmental effects during its development (Barnett 1998; Miller et al 1998). Although epidemiological research on possible adverse effects of ultrasound is sparse, there have been published reports of an association between non-right-handedness/left-handedness in males and exposure to prenatal ultrasound. The significance of 'handedness' studies is the higher risk of an association of left-handedness in infants with lowered intellectual abilities (Kieler et al 2005). However, in a study examining the association between prenatal ultrasound exposure and intellectual performance, Kieler et al (2005) failed to demonstrate a clear association between ultrasound scanning and intellectual performance.

Screening for Down syndrome and fetal structural anomalies

The general principle guiding all screening tests is that a risk assessment is made by combining the results of the screening test with the pre-test risk, based on the woman's age and previous history.

BOX 32.3 Ultrasound past and present

Ultrasound was developed during WWII to detect enemy submarines, and was later used in the steel industry. In July 1955 Glasgow surgeon Ian Donald borrowed an industrial machine and, using beefsteaks for comparison, began to experiment with abdominal tumours that he had removed from his patients. He discovered that different tissues gave different patterns of sound wave 'echo', leading him to realise that ultrasound offered a revolutionary way to look into the previously mysterious world of the growing baby (Wagner 1999).

This new technology spread rapidly into clinical obstetrics. Commercial machines became available in 1963 (De Crepigny 1996) and by the late 1970s ultrasound had become a routine part of obstetric care (Oakley 1986). Today, ultrasound is seen as safe and effective, and scanning has become a rite of passage for pregnant women in developed countries. In Australia, it is estimated that 99% of babies are scanned at least once in pregnancy—usually as a routine prenatal ultrasound (RPU) at 4 to 5 months. In the US, where this cost is borne by the insurer or privately, around 70% of pregnant women have a scan (Martin et al 2003), and in European countries, it is estimated that 89% of pregnant women have an ultrasound, usually once in each trimester (third) of pregnancy (Levi 1998). However, there is growing concern as to its safety and usefulness. UK consumer activist Beverly Beech has called RPU 'the biggest uncontrolled experiment in history' (Beech 1993) and the Cochrane Collaborative Database—the peak scientific authority in evidence-based medicine—concludes that 'no clear benefit in terms of a substantive outcome measure like perinatal mortality [number of babies dying around the time of birth] can yet be discerned to result from the routine use of ultrasound . . . For those considering its introduction, the benefit of the

demonstrated advantages would need to be considered against the theoretical possibility that the use of ultrasound during pregnancy could be hazardous, and the need for additional resources (Neilson 1998).

The additional resources consumed by routine ultrasound are substantial. In 1997, for example, the Australian federal government paid out $39 million to subsidise pregnancy scans; an enormous expense compared to $54 million for all other obstetric Medicare costs (Senate Community Affairs Reference Group 1999), and this figure does not include the additional costs paid by the woman herself. In the US, an estimated US $1.2 billion would be spent yearly if every pregnant woman had a single routine scan.

In 1987, UK radiologist HD Meire, who had been performing pregnancy scans for 20 years, commented, 'The casual observer might be forgiven for wondering why the medical profession is now involved in the wholesale examination of pregnant patients with machines emanating vastly different powers of energy which is not proven to be harmless to obtain information which is not proven to be of any clinical value by operators who are not certified as competent to perform the operations' (Meire 1987). The situation today is unchanged, on every count.

In 1999, the Senate Committee report, 'Rocking the Cradle' recommended that the cost-benefit of routine scanning, and of current ultrasound practices, be formally assessed. Recommendations were also made to develop guidelines for the safe use of all obstetric ultrasound, as well as for the development of standards for the training of ultrasonographers . . . So far, none of these recommendations have been implemented (Senate Committee 1999).

(Source: Buckley 1998–2005)

In Australia and New Zealand

To date, there has been an 'ad hoc' approach to serum screening in Australia and New Zealand. While there have been attempts in some Australian states to make this a population-based screening program (for example, South Australia where population coverage is about 75%, and Victoria), the overall utilisation of serum screening has been low, with no more than 30% of Australian women undergoing this test. This is despite the introduction in Australia of a specific Medicare item number (MBS 66321) and rebate for the maternal serum screen. One of the reasons for this may be that antenatal care in Australian public hospitals is funded by state health departments, and only in Victoria and South Australia have public hospitals sanctioned the additional cost of introducing this test.

Recommendations for antenatal screening for Down syndrome in Australia are as follows:

Early in pregnancy, all women should receive appropriate written information concerning available screening (including potential risks and benefits, the difference between screening and diagnostic testing and possible costs to women).

The offer of screening for Down syndrome should be made available to all pregnant women, irrespective of age.

Pre-screening counselling must be given by appropriately trained staff and should be specific to the age of each woman.

If after counselling women choose to proceed with screening tests for Down syndrome:

i Screening should include accurate pregnancy dating by ultrasound, preferably in the first trimester.
ii Screening should be by either second trimester biochemistry or by nuchal translucency (alone or in combination with first or second trimester biochemistry).
iii Women should be notified of their screening result, irrespective of the risk, in a format that they understand.
iv Women who have an increased risk of Down syndrome should be offered further counselling and diagnostic testing within 72 hours or as soon as possible. (Three Centres Consensus Guidelines 2001)

In New Zealand, antenatal screening for Down syndrome has developed rapidly over the past 15 years. There is now a range of screening tests available, including:

● a first trimester blood test (not yet widely available in New Zealand), and /or

- a second trimester blood test (the Triple Test), a combination of three tests that measure quantities of various substances in the blood, usually done between 15 and 20 weeks of gestation (available but women pay $70 for this test) and/or
- an ultrasound scan at about 12 weeks for nuchal translucency (publicly funded). Women identified as 'high risk' following screening are offered invasive procedures, for example, chorionic villous sampling or amniocentesis. Both these diagnostic tests carry a small risk of fetal loss.

Development of diagnostic testing methods

When the first screening test for Down syndrome was introduced in the United Kingdom, approximately 5% of pregnant women were 35 years of age or older, and 30% of all Down syndrome births were to those women (Haddow 1998). The majority of children with Down syndrome are born to women who are younger than 35 years old. The identification of younger women with an increased risk became possible after Merkatz et al (1984) reported an association between a low alpha-fetoprotein level and fetal aneuploidy, launching an era of maternal serum screening to assess the risk of fetal Down syndrome. Subsequent studies showed that the maternal serum levels of three markers—alpha-fetoprotein (AFP), beta human chorionic gonadotrophin (β-hCG), and unconjugated oestriol (uE$_3$)—occurring between 15 and 22 weeks of gestation could be used to make adjustments to the risk based on maternal age alone (Mennuti et al 2003).

Antenatal screening for Down syndrome became possible because two components of diagnostic testing had developed to the level of clinical applicability. The first was a sampling procedure where cells were taken from the amniotic fluid (amniocentesis). Cells in amniotic fluid are fetal in origin and can be cultured for chromosome analysis. Amniocentesis was originally offered during the early second trimester and carried about a 1% risk of spontaneous fetal loss (Tabor et al 1986). The second diagnostic component that had reached clinical significance was cell culture and chromosomal analysis via karyotype. Karyotyping is still the preferred test method for most pregnancies, ascertained either through a screening program for Down syndrome or for other referral reasons. Karyotyping detects a range of numerical and structural chromosome abnormalities in addition to the common autosomal trisomies (13 (Patau's syndrome), 18 (Edwards' syndrome), and 21 (Down syndrome)) and sex chromosome abnormalities. However, since amniotic fluid and chorionic villus cells are cultured before analysis, delays of up to 14 days or longer can occur before a result is issued (Caine et al 2005). (Notwithstanding that this is currently recognised as among the most reliable diagnostic tests in clinical medicine (Haddow 1998). Culture failure is uncommon, and erroneous results from maternal cell contamination are rare (Haddow 1998).) This degree of reliability is crucial, since it forms the basis for decisions that have far-reaching consequences. During the past decade, emphasis has been placed on obtaining fetal cells earlier in gestation, by either chorionic villous sampling or earlier amniocentesis. Chromosome analysis via karyotype, however, continues to be the cornerstone of Down syndrome diagnosis (Haddow 1998).

After the landmark discovery in 1984 that AFP concentrations in maternal serum were lower in the presence of Down syndrome and could be used as a screening test (Cuckle et al 1984), screening began to be offered to pregnant women younger than age 35. The efficacy of screening with AFP was comparable to that based on maternal age (a 20–25% detection rate for a 5% false-positive rate), and since AFP was already being measured as a screening test for open spina bifida or neural tube defect, adding an interpretation for Down syndrome risk represented a negligible cost (Haddow 1998).

Further progress in screening was achieved later in the 1980s with the discoveries of hCG and uE$_3$. Measures of these markers were combined with that for AFP to produce a 'triple' test, capable of detecting 60% of Down syndrome pregnancies, at a 5% false-positive rate (Wald et al 1988). This substantial step-up in detection led many women over the age of 35 to choose serum screening rather than amniocentesis. More recently, the addition of a fourth serum marker, inhibin, has been shown to boost detection of Down syndrome to about 75% (Haddow 1998). With the advent of biochemical markers in combination with ultrasound, considerable attention was given in the 1990s to providing maternal serum screening earlier in gestation. Measurements of two markers—pregnancy-associated plasma protein A (PAPP-A) and either the free β subunit of hCG or hCG detected between 10 and 13 weeks gestation—have become nearly as efficient as the second-trimester 'triple' test (Haddow 1998). Studies in the 1990s showed an association between Down syndrome and increased nuchal translucency, a sonolucent space evident at the back of the fetus's neck in the first trimester. In 1995, Wald et al demonstrated the feasibility of first-trimester serum screening for Down syndrome (Wald et al 1995).

Screening combinations

The NICE Guidelines recommend the following screening combinations for Down syndrome:
- from 11 to 14 weeks:
  - nuchal translucency (NT)
  - 'combined' test (NT, hCG + PAPP-A)
- from 14 to 20 weeks:
  - 'double' test (hCG + AFP)

BOX 32.4 Serum markers

Abbreviations for serum markers:
▸ hCG = human chorionic gonadotrophin
▸ uE$_3$ = unconjugated oestriol
▸ AFP = alpha-fetoprotein
▸ PAPP-A = pregnancy-associated plasma protein A

- 'triple' test (hCG, SFP + uE₃)
- 'quadruple' test (hCG, AFP, uE₃ + inhibin A)
- from 11 to 14 weeks and from 14 to 20 weeks:
  - integrated test (NT, PAPP-A + hCG, AFP, uE₃, inhibin A)
  - serum integrated test (PAPP-A + hCG, AFP, uE₃, inhibin A) (NICE 2003, p 78).

The NICE Guidelines (2003) also state that:

Antenatal screening for Down syndrome can take place during the first or second trimester of pregnancy and a variety of screening tests can be used.

In the first trimester, nuchal translucency (NT), which is the measurement of the normal subcutaneous space between the skin and the cervical spine in the fetus early in pregnancy, can be used to identify women at increased risk of carrying a Down syndrome baby at around 10 to 14 weeks. Nuchal translucency may be used with or without two first-trimester maternal serum markers, human chorionic gonadotrophin (hCG) and pregnancy-associated plasma protein (PAPP-A), i.e. the combined test, or as part of the integrated test.

In the early second trimester, screening techniques include biochemical marker screening at around 15 to 16 weeks. In these tests a risk assessment for Down syndrome is made based on the differences between observed and expected levels at 15 to 18 weeks of AFP, estriol and beta-hCG.

Once a screening test is performed, the risk of Down syndrome is calculated, taking into account maternal age, gestational age and the levels of biochemical markers.

Results are 'positive' or classified as 'high risk' if the risk is equal to or greater than a locally agreed cut-off level. This is often expressed numerically to indicate the likelihood that a woman has a baby with Down syndrome when a positive screening result is returned; e.g., a 1/250 chance that a pregnant woman is carrying an affected baby. When a high-risk screening result is returned, a woman will usually be offered a diagnostic test, such as amniocentesis, which has an excess fetal loss rate of 1% (NICE Guidelines 2003, pp 74–75).

Some women undergo chorionic villous sampling during the first trimester rather than screening or amniocentesis during the second trimester. Some women, such as those carrying multiple fetuses, are not candidates for second-trimester serum screening. Others decline screening because they do not wish to undergo prenatal diagnosis or would not consider pregnancy termination on the basis of the results. The anxiety experienced by friends or relatives who had a positive screening test followed by normal findings on amniocentesis deters some women from undergoing screening. Women who are 35 years of age or older increasingly opt to undergo serum screening and ultrasonography before deciding about amniocentesis. With the emergence of alternative approaches earlier in pregnancy, decisions about screening are becoming more complex.

Summary: screening for Down syndrome

- The screening tests involved in early or first trimester pregnancy screening for Down syndrome (DS) when the fetus is between 11 and 13 weeks gestation involve a nuchal translucency (NT) screen, which takes place within the context of a detailed ultrasound scan in addition to maternal serum screening.
- DS screening in the second trimester using a variety of combinations of maternal serum markers such as the so-called 'triple test' (hCG, uE and AFP) has become an established but controversial part of antenatal care over the past decade (Vassy 2005).
- Increasingly, however, first-trimester NT screening, particularly in combination with maternal serum screening with biochemical markers, is being proposed.
- 'Nuchal translucency' refers to the subcutaneous space between the skin and the cervical spine of the fetus. An increased NT is associated with an increased risk of aneuploidy, particularly trisomies 21 (Down syndrome), 18 (Edwards' syndrome) and 13 (Patau's syndrome).
- With the advent of DS screening in the first trimester and the application of nuchal translucency measurements (NT screening) at 10–14 weeks gestation, the potential impact of combining maternal age with fetal nuchal translucency thickness and maternal serum free β-hCG and PAPP-A seems to be increasing.
- One of the latest additions to the proliferation of screening technologies is the association of increased nuchal thickness with congenital heart defects (Ray et al 2005).

Figure 32.3 illustrates the rates of use of various diagnostic tests for Down syndrome.

What to tell women

Down syndrome is caused by the presence of an extra chromosome in a baby's cells. It occurs by chance at conception and is irreversible. Women are offered screening tests to check whether their baby is likely to have Down syndrome. You must be able to spend time explaining the implications of Down syndrome, the tests you are offering and what the results may mean. Each woman has the right to choose whether to have all, some, or none, of these tests. Each woman must be aware that she is under no obligation to have any test— and that the decision to have them must be her and her family's decision. It should be explained how to 'opt out' of the screening process at any time if she wishes. Screening tests will only indicate that a baby *may* have Down syndrome. If the screening test results are positive, the woman should be offered further diagnostic tests to confirm whether her baby does in fact have Down syndrome. The time at which the woman is tested will depend on what kinds of tests are used. Screening tests for Down syndrome are not always right. They can sometimes wrongly show as positive, suggesting that the baby does have Down syndrome when in fact it does not. This type of result is known as a 'false positive'. The number of occasions on which this happens with a particular test is called its 'false-positive rate'. The screening tests available at present have a false-positive rate of less than 5 out of 100 and detect at least 60 out of 100

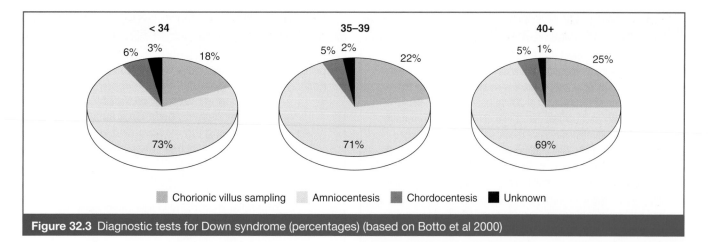

Figure 32.3 Diagnostic tests for Down syndrome (percentages) (based on Botto et al 2000)

cases of Down syndrome. The tests that meet this standard are:
- from 11 to 14 weeks:
  - nuchal translucency (an ultrasound scan)
  - combined test (an ultrasound scan and blood test)
- from 14 to 20 weeks:
  - triple test (a blood test)
  - quadruple test (a blood test)
- from 11 to 14 weeks and 14 to 20 weeks:
  - integrated test (an ultrasound scan and blood test)
  - serum integrated test (a blood test).

Use of maternal age as a primary criterion for offering amniocentesis results in very high rates of use of this invasive test and is a suboptimum use of resources. Every woman's choice to accept or reject chorionic villus sampling or amniocentesis should be based on counselling that uses the best possible estimate of her personal risk for fetal aneuploidy. Policy advisory groups in other countries should follow the UK initiative and abandon obsolete guidelines that have advocated offering amniocentesis to all women aged 35 or more, without routinely incorporating serum and ultrasound screening into their risk assessment (Benn 2003).

Birth anomalies remain a significant public health problem in Australia and are a major reason for admission to hospital during infancy and childhood. They often result in disabilities and handicaps and, in some cases, death (AIHW 2002). An estimated 5% of all Australian births and terminations of pregnancy have a major birth anomaly (Stanley et al 1995) and birth anomalies account for about 13% of the disease burden for children aged 0–14 years (AIHW 1999). Birth anomalies are also a leading cause of infant mortality in Australia, with 25% of infant deaths in 2000 caused by birth anomalies (Al-Yaman et al 2002).

Birth anomalies are caused by genetic (including chromosomal), environmental and unknown factors, or combinations of these factors. It is estimated that the cause of about 65–75% of birth anomalies is unknown. About 15–25% of birth anomalies have a genetic cause and about 10% have an environmental cause (AIHW 2004; Brent 2001).

TABLE 32.2 Expected detection rates and false-positive rates for various second-trimester protocols applied to 1999 US pregnant population

Screening protocol	Detection rate (%)	False positive rate (%)
Maternal age alone (≥ 35 years)	49	13.1
Second trimester, maternal age, plus:		
MSAFP + hCG	73	9.6
MSAFP + uE$_3$ + hCG	78	7.8
MSAFP + hCG + INH-A	82	6.9
First trimester, maternal age, plus:		
NT	74	5.1
PAPP-A + free β-hCG	75	8.6
NT + PAPP-A + free β-hCG	86	4.2
First and second trimester, maternal age, plus:		
PAPP-A + MSAFP + uE$_3$ + hCG + INH-A	87	4.9
NT + PAPP-A + MSAFP + uE$_3$ + hCG + INH-A	93	2.6
(Source: Benn 2003)		

Future fetal diagnosis

The introduction of new screening and surveillance measures continues at such a pace that it is beyond the scope of this text to inform readers of the very latest techniques. However, one of the more promising areas of screening, although still very much in the research arena, is the analysis of fetal cells and fetal DNA and RNA from the maternal circulation. It is speculated that new technologies involving sampling maternal plasma with cell-free fetal DNA may play a bigger role in

---

BOX 32.5   Screening for CHD

Congenital heart defect (CHD) is more prevalent than Down syndrome, with a reported worldwide frequency of 4–9 of every 100 births (Ray et al 2005). There is no clear consensus on the definition of CHD (Ray et al 2005); however, it is defined pragmatically as a cardiac defect that could potentially require surgical intervention, intensive medical therapy or prolonged follow-up after birth. Ray and colleagues (2005) observed that less than one-third of cases with increased nuchal translucency have chromosomal abnormality. This is an area of screening in its infancy at present. However, as more biomarkers are established and our preoccupation with reproductive perfection continues, the possibilities are unimagined.

---

non-invasive prenatal genetic diagnosis of aneuploidy by helping to identify pregnancies at sufficient risk for trisomy 21 or 18 without women having to undergo an invasive diagnostic procedure for definitive diagnosis. This new process of risk identification may avert the need for prenatal genetic diagnosis requiring invasive procedures such as amniocentesis or chorionic villous sampling. Circulating fetal DNA has also been targeted as a marker for assessing feto-maternal wellbeing. Increased fetal DNA concentrations have been reported for several pregnancy-related complications including pre-eclampsia. So far, various forms of circulating DNA in plasma have been observed: shed cells, apoptotic bodies, nucleosomes, other nucleoproteins and free DNA (Bischoff et al 2005).

Screening for genetic disorders (muscular dystrophy)

The muscular dystrophies are a group of inherited disorders characterised by progressive muscle wasting and weakness. A unifying feature of the dystrophies is the histological analysis of muscle samples, which typically includes variations in fibre size, areas of muscle necrosis and, ultimately, increased amounts of fat and connective tissue. The diagnosis therefore requires a muscle biopsy (generally a needle biopsy under local anaesthesia) and possibly electromyography (Emery 1998).

Newborn screening for genetic and other disorders is usually confined to diseases for which there is treatment—either a change of diet (as in phenylketonuria and galactosaemia) or replacement therapy (as in hypothyroidism)—or in which there is a chance of affecting morbidity or mortality early in life, as occurs in the haemoglobinopathies (particularly sickle cell disease). Screening for disorders in which the clinical course cannot be altered is generally avoided: a program of newborn screening for disorders like Duchenne muscular dystrophy could therefore create an ethical nightmare.

Ethical dilemma

Is it justifiable to offer newborn screening for a potentially untreatable genetic disorder?

For   Some would argue that newborn screening for Duchenne muscular dystrophy decreases emotional distress because it avoids delays in diagnosing the disease, and without screening two or more boys could be born with the condition before the parents realised that they were at risk of having an affected child. Accordingly, if an infant with Duchenne muscular dystrophy is identified early, the family has the option of prenatal diagnosis for future pregnancies.

Against   On the other hand, neonatal diagnosis could interfere with normal emotional growth and the child's interaction with his family.

Screening newborn infants

Duchenne muscular dystrophy is a severe X-linked inherited recessive disorder that occurs in around 1 in 3500 baby boys (Emery 1998). There may be no family history of the disorder, as the large gene responsible for it is prone to mutation, but even so, subsequent sons are at risk. It is a serious condition, with progressive muscle wasting and weakness, which causes most boys to require wheelchairs by age 12 and to die in their twenties. Up to a third of boys with Duchennetype dystrophy have some degree of intellectual impairment, and in severe cases special schooling may have to be considered. Beckertype muscular dystrophy is clinically similar but milder, with onset in the teenage years or early twenties. Loss of the ability to walk may occur later and many individuals with Beckertype dystrophy survive into middle-age and beyond (Emery 1998).

Screening of newborns for Duchenne muscular dystrophy by measurement of blood spot creatine kinase activity has

---

BOX 32.6   Muscular dystrophies

▸ At least 1 in 3000 people are affected by a serious inherited neuromuscular disorder; the muscular dystrophies make up an appreciable proportion of these.

▸ Histological examination of muscle tissue and electromyography are used in the diagnosis of muscular dystrophy to exclude other causes of muscle wasting and weakness, such as spinal muscular atrophy, myopathies, and neuropathies.

▸ On the basis of clinical and molecular genetic studies, C-linked (Duchenne) type and at least two other types of muscular dystrophy are recognised.

▸ A precise diagnosis is essential in order to provide a reliable prognosis and accurate genetic counselling.

(Source: Emery 1998)

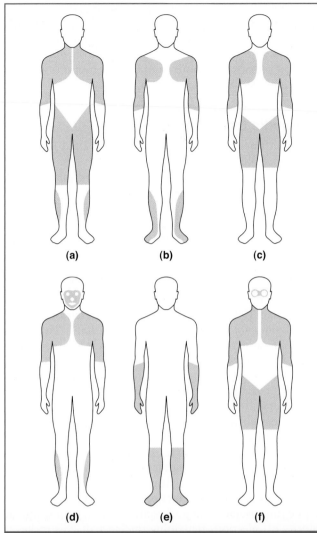

Figure 32.4 Distribution of predominant muscle weakness in different types of dystrophy: **(a)** Duchennetype and Beckertype **(b)** EmeryDreifuss **(c)** Limb girdle **(d)** Facioscapulohumeral **(e)** Distal **(f)** Oculopharyngeal (based on Emery 1998)

been technically possible since a suitable assay was devised in the mid-1970s (Bowman 1993). It is offered on a limited basis in Germany, and as a routine service in Lyons, France, and Antwerp, Belgium. Before the advent of molecular genetics, screening of newborns in the United Kingdom was generally regarded as ethically unsound because no treatment was available; it offered little advantage to the family other than the possibility of terminating all subsequent male fetuses, more than half of whom would be normal. With the isolation of the gene responsible for Duchenne muscular dystrophy it became possible to track the defective gene and to offer increasingly accurate prenatal diagnosis either by deletion analysis in many cases or by using linked markers. Consequently, although the condition was still untreatable, the neonatal identification could facilitate reproductive choice in further pregnancies in the immediate and extended family. This led to a reassessment

of the ethical issues surrounding newborn screening. The common clinical experience of diagnosing two (or occasionally more) affected boys simultaneously in a single family has to be weighed against the availability of prenatal diagnosis in future pregnancies once the first case has been identified. In addition, diagnostic delay causes considerable distress to families and may result in subsequent bitterness if the child's symptoms are not taken seriously by family or health professionals, or if a second affected boy is born. Despite such considerations, there has been concern that a neonatal diagnosis would interfere with the normal social and emotional growth and interaction of child and family (Bradley et al 1993).

Screening for infections

Asymptomatic bacteriuria

Asymptomatic bacteriuria is defined as a pure culture of at least 10^5 organisms/mL of urine. Detection of all women with asymptomatic bacteriuria is important as 25% to 30% will develop symptomatic urinary tract infection while pregnant. The sequelae of urinary tract infection in pregnancy include pyelonephritis, premature labour and preterm rupture of the membranes. In view of the potential importance of asymptomatic bacteriuria it is current best practice to send a urine sample for laboratory analysis from all women who book for antenatal care (Tincello & Richmond 1998).

According to the *Three Centres Consensus Guidelines* (2001):

> Early in pregnancy, all women should be given appropriate written information about this test and be given an opportunity to discuss it with their midwife or doctor. All pregnant women should be offered screening at booking or in early pregnancy for asymptomatic bacteriuria using either a two-step protocol or microscopy and culture of a fresh mid-stream urine sample.
>
> If using a two-step protocol, women should provide a mid-stream urine sample at the first antenatal visit that is screened for blood, protein, nitrites and leukocyte esterase using a reagent strip. If there is a positive result in any of the four categories the sample should be sent for microscopy and culture.
>
> If midwives and doctors routinely screen for asymptomatic bacteriuria using microscopy and culture then they may also need to screen women for chronic renal disease (CRD) using dipstick testing, as CRD will not be picked up by culture alone (Three Centres Consensus Guidelines 2001, p 23).

What to tell women

Asymptomatic bacteriuria is a bladder infection that has no symptoms. Identifying and treating it can reduce the risk of premature birth (NICE 2003).

Asymptomatic bacterial vaginosis

Bacterial vaginosis (BV) is characterised by a changed vaginal microflora in which the normally occurring lactobacilli yield to an overgrowth of a mixed anaerobic bacterial flora. Whether it occurs spontaneously as an ecological imbalance in the vaginal flora, and its role in both genital tract infection and in pregnancy outcome, have been the subject of study since the 1980s and still remain an enigma (Larsson et al 2005). Routine screening of all pregnant women for BV is not recommended (Kirkham et al 2005).

As BV is a possible cause of pregnancy complications as well as being socially unacceptable and disturbing for affected women, there are good reasons for finding a cure (Larsson et al 2005). The efficacy of yoghurt in treating bacterial vaginosis compared with vaginal metronidazole and vaginal placebo was tested in a trial in 1998 (Thiagarajan 1998). Although metronidazole was the most effective treatment against persistence of infection (relative risk reduction 62%, 95% CI 50–72%), yoghurt was two-thirds as effective as metronidazole when compared with the placebo group (relative risk reduction 46%, 95% CI 31–58%) (Thiagarajan 1998).

Generally speaking, treatment for BV is more effective during pregnancy because pregnant women do not menstruate and it appears that BV tends to recur during a menstrual period. Spontaneous cure among pregnant women has been noted (Larsson & Forsum 2005).

Around a dozen studies have investigated the likelihood of reducing spontaneous preterm delivery through a variety of treatments and regimens prescribed for women with BV (Larsson & Forsum 2005).

During the past 15 years there has been ongoing discussion concerning the epidemiological correlation between various complications during pregnancy and BV. Today it is clear that BV doubles the risk of spontaneous preterm birth. A meta-analysis by Leitich et al (2003) indicates that BV increases the risk of preterm delivery more than twofold (odds ratio (OR) 2.19, 95% CI 1.54–3.12). Higher risks were calculated for subgroups of studies that screened for BV at 16 weeks gestation (OR 7.55, 95% CI 1.80–31.65) or 20 weeks gestation (OR 4.20, 95% CI 2.11–8.39).

BV also significantly increases the risk of spontaneous abortion (OR 9.91, 95% CI 1.99–49.34) and maternal infection (OR 2.53, 95% CI 1.26–5.08) (Leitich et al 2003).

A recent systematic review concluded, however, that for women with bacterial vaginosis, antibiotics reduced the risk of persistent infection but did not reduce the risk of preterm birth or the incidence of associated adverse outcomes for the general population or for any subgroup analysed. For women with *Trichomonas vaginalis*, metronidazole reduced the risk of persistent infection but increased the incidence of preterm birth. Contrary to the conclusions of recent systematic reviews, there was no evidence to support the use of antibiotic treatment for bacterial vaginosis or *T. vaginalis* in pregnancy to reduce the risk of preterm birth or its associated morbidities in low- or high-risk women (Okun et al 2005)

Screening and treating healthy pregnant women (i.e. low risk for preterm birth) for asymptomatic bacterial vaginosis does not appear to lower the risk for preterm birth or other adverse reproductive outcomes. Pregnant women should not be offered routine screening for bacterial vaginosis because the evidence suggests that the identification and treatment of asymptomatic bacterial vaginosis does not lower the risk

for preterm birth and other adverse reproductive outcomes (NICE 2003, p 83).

For women with a previous preterm birth, there is some suggestion that treatment of bacterial vaginosis may reduce the risk of preterm prelabour rupture of membranes and low birthweight (McDonald et al 2003).

Chlamydia trachomatis

Chlamydia trachomatis is a sexually transmitted infection. Mother-to-child transmission can occur at the time of birth and may result in ophthalmia neonatorum or pneumonitis in the newborn (Brocklehurst & French 1998).

In Australia, notification rates for chlamydia have increased fourfold since the early 1990s, with the greatest rises seen among adolescents and young adults (Chen & Donovan 2004). In New South Wales, legislation was introduced in 1998 that made the reporting of *C. trachomatis* by laboratories mandatory. Chlamydia notifications in New South Wales increased in parallel with national rates—from 39 per 100 000 population in 1999 to 88 per 100 000 in 2002 (National Centre in HIV Epidemiology and Clinical Research 2004). The extent to which these increases in chlamydia notifications represent a true rise in chlamydia incidence is uncertain: ecological studies suggest that the higher notification rates also reflect increased chlamydia testing (Chen & Donovan 2004; Chen et al 2005; Hocking et al 2003).

The rise in chlamydia notifications could largely have been the result of increased chlamydia testing. More extensive use of nucleic acid amplification tests may also have contributed. In recent years, chlamydia testing rates have increased steadily throughout Australia, with strong correlations between the intensity of testing and detection rates for *C. trachomatis*. Despite this, overall testing rates are still low, with the great majority of infections remaining undetected. This makes it difficult to know what the true incidence and prevalence of chlamydia is in the Australian population (Chen et al 2005).

Chlamydia infection during pregnancy is associated with higher rates of preterm birth (OR 1.6, 90% CI 1.01–2.5) and intrauterine growth restriction (OR 2.5, 90% CI 1.32–4.18). Left untreated, it has also been associated with increased low birthweight and infant mortality. In a review of randomised control trials, the number of women with positive cultures for *Chlamydia* was reduced by 90% when treated with antibiotics compared with placebo (OR 0.06, 95% CI 0.03–0.12). However this did not alter the incidence of birth before 37 weeks (NICE 2003, p 83).

In industrialised countries, *C. trachomatis* is the predominant infectious agent causing pelvic inflammatory disease (PID), and as a result of damage to the fallopian tubes, accounts for up to half of all ectopic pregnancies. The substantial financial costs of genital chlamydial infections result from hospital treatment for PID, ectopic pregnancy, and infertility, which may include in vitro fertilisation.

Screening should be offered to women at increased risk for sexually transmitted infections (STIs), including those younger than 25 years. There is currently no evidence to

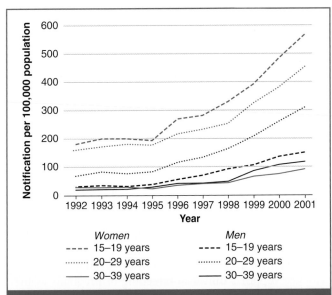

Figure 32.5 Notification rates for genital *Chlamydia trachomatis* infection in women and men by age group, Australia, 1992–2001 (based on National Centre in HIV Epidemiology and Clinical Research)

support universal screening of pregnant women for chlamydial infection. High-risk groups include women younger than 25 years; unmarried women; women with a history of STIs, new or multiple sexual partners, inconsistent use of barrier contraception; and women living in communities with high infection rates. Affected women and their partners should be treated. The optimal testing time is uncertain, but most authors recommend testing at the first prenatal visit and again in the third trimester for high-risk patients (Kirkham et al 2005).

In several remote areas in Australia, nucleic acid testing for gonorrhoea and chlamydia has been used (since 1996) and requires collection of first-void urine and an endocervical swab. Since mid-2001, self-obtained lower vaginal swabs have been available and recommended for STI screening in situations where the woman is asymptomatic, not a sexual contact of STI and does not require a Papanicolaou smear (Mak et al 2003).

Syphilis

Syphilis is a sexually acquired infection caused by *Treponema pallidum*. The body's immune response to syphilis is the production of non-specific and specific treponemal antibodies. The first notable response to infection is the production of specific anti-treponemal immunoglobulin M (IgM), which is detectable towards the end of the second week of infection. By the time symptoms appear, most people infected with syphilis have detectable levels of immunoglobulin G (IgG) and IgM.449 (NICE 2003, p 91).

Syphilis may also be asymptomatic and remain latent for many years. The availability of penicillin reduced the prevalence of syphilis significantly from 1950 onwards and

the disease is rarely seen in either New Zealand or Australia. In the United Kingdom the incidence of infectious syphilis is also low. In the United States, an 'epidemic' of congenital syphilis was reported by the Centers for Disease Control in 1994, with rates increasing from 4.3/100 000 live births in 1982 to 94.7/100 000 in 1992 (CDC 1994).

Infectious syphilis is a disease of considerable public health importance, with overwhelming health effects if not treated in pregnancy. These include adverse pregnancy outcomes, such as stillbirth and congenital syphilis. Further, concurrent infection with syphilis can facilitate transmission of HIV (Doherty et al 2002). Syphilis has disproportionate effects on vulnerable or disadvantaged populations and on people involved in high-risk activities such as illicit drug use, sex work, unprotected intercourse, and sex with multiple partners (NICE 2003). Syphilis is most infectious through sexual contact during the primary or secondary stages, but transmission can also occur during the early latent stage (Doherty et al 2002).

Syphilis is preventable, and treatable with effective and inexpensive antibiotics. The possible resurgence of infectious syphilis, a disease previously believed to be close to eradication, is a matter of increasing global concern (Doherty et al 2002).

In pregnant women with early untreated syphilis, 70% to 100% of infants will be infected and one-third will be stillborn. Mother-to-child transmission of syphilis in pregnancy is associated with neonatal death, congenital syphilis (which may cause long-term disability), stillbirth and preterm birth.

According to the Three Centres Guidelines for Australia (2001):

> Early in pregnancy all women should receive appropriate written information about antenatal syphilis testing and be given the opportunity to discuss it with their midwife or doctor. Antenatal serological screening for syphilis should be offered to all pregnant women.
>
> Screening for syphilis should be undertaken at the first antenatal visit, ideally prior to 16 weeks' gestation. Syphilis has significant long-term morbidity for mothers and can seriously complicate pregnancy, resulting in spontaneous abortion, stillbirth, nonimmune hydrops, intrauterine growth restriction, malformations and perinatal death. Congenital syphilis results in serious sequelae in live born infected children. Screening pregnant women for syphilis and treating them appropriately can eliminate complications. The evidence available indicates that screening for syphilis should be part of routine antenatal care. Universal screening programs have been shown to significantly increase the detection of pregnant women who have syphilis compared with selective screening of women considered to be a high risk (Three Centres Consensus Guidelines 2001, p 36).

What to tell women

Syphilis is a rare STI that can also be passed from a mother to her baby. Mothers and babies can be successfully treated if it is detected and treated early. A person with syphilis may show no symptoms for many years. A positive test result does not always mean you have syphilis, but your healthcare providers should have clear procedures for managing your care if you test positive (NICE 2003).

Cytomegalovirus

Cytomegalovirus (CMV) is a member of the herpes virus family. It is the most common cause of intrauterine viral infection and sensory neural deafness (Stagno & Whitley 1985). It remains latent in the host after primary infection and may become active again, particularly during times of compromised immunity.

At present, antenatal screening for this condition is thought to be inappropriate, as it is not currently possible to determine accurately which pregnancies are likely to result in the birth of an infected infant. There is no way to determine which infected infants will have serious sequelae, there are no currently available vaccines or prophylactic therapy for the prevention of transmission and no way to determine whether intrauterine transmission has occurred (NICE 2003, p 84).

In both the United States and Western Europe, CMV infection is the most common viral form of congenital infection. Intrauterine transmission of CMV takes place in approximately 40% of infections, and approximately 10% of live-born infants have symptomatic disease at the time of birth and later. Late sequelae such as sensorineural hearing loss and neurodevelopmental disorders occur in 10% to 15% of infants lacking symptoms at birth. Recurrent maternal infection contributes substantially to the rate of congenital infection (Daiminger et al 2005).

The available evidence does not support routine CMV screening in pregnant women and it should not be offered (NICE 2003, p 84).

Hepatitis B virus

The aim of screening pregnant women for hepatitis B virus (HBV) is to prevent the transmission of the virus to their children. Acute hepatitis B can cause morbidity and mortality. Perinatal infection can be prevented by prompt immunoprophylaxis at birth. The incidence of HBV is falling among infants and adults following the introduction of protocols for handling blood products, combined with immunisation and health-promotion strategies. Existing evidence supports universal screening of pregnant women for hepatitis B surface antigen by a combined prenatal and perinatal approach. This combined approach is encouraged in Australia, where antenatal hepatitis B screening is accepted practice, and the NHMRC recommends that all newborn

---

BOX 32.7 Viral transmission in pregnancy

The ability of viruses to spread from the infected mother to the fetus arises from the structure of the placenta, which anchors the fetus to the uterus. The human placenta is composed of villi that float in maternal blood and also villi within the uterine wall that anchor the placenta and attach the fetus to the mother.

The individual chorionic villus contains a connective core that contains fetal blood vessels and numerous macrophages (Hofbauer cells) that often lie under a thick basement membrane, depending on their location. In floating villi, they fuse to form a multinucleate syncytiotrophoblast covering attached at one end to the tree-like fetal portion of the placenta. The rest of the villus floats in a stream of maternal blood, which optimises the exchange of substances between the mother and fetus across the placenta. In the pathway that gives rise to anchoring villi, which attach the placenta to the uterine wall, cytotrophoblasts aggregate into cell columns of non-polarised mononuclear cells that attach to and penetrate the uterine wall. The ends of the columns terminate within the superficial endometrium, where they give rise to invasive cytotrophoblasts.

Placental cytotrophoblasts differentiate, assume an endothelial phenotype, breach uterine blood vessels and form a hybrid vasculature that amplifies the maternal blood supply for fetal development. Human cytomegalovirus (CMV), the major cause of congenital disease, infects the uterine wall and the adjacent placenta, suggesting adaptation for pathogen survival in this microenvironment.

(Source: Pereira et al 2005)

TABLE 32.3 Intrauterine viral transmission

Virus	Mode/rate of transmission
CMV	Prenatal infection affects 1–2% of live births. Virus replicates in the uterus, infects the placenta, then is transmitted to the fetus. Transmission rate approx 50% in women with primary infection.
HSV 2	Infrequent prenatal infection. Transmission occurs primarily at the time of birth (80%) and also possibly through an ascending infection after the membranes rupture.
HIV	Transmission primarily at the time of birth. Isolated cytotrophoblasts infected in vitro.
HBV	Transmission primarily perinatal. Some intrauterine infection from maternal blood (5%).
HCV	Intrauterine infection and at birth (2–12%).
Parvovirus B19	Placental infection associated with inflammatory cytokines. Complications in early gestation.
Rubella virus	Placental infection during primary maternal infection. Transmission in first trimester (80%) and second trimester (25%).
HPV	Infection via maternal genital secretions at birth.
Varicella zoster virus	Congenital infection low (2%). Transmission during primary infection in late gestation (25–50%).

(Source: Pereira et al 2005)

infants be offered immunisation (Three Centres Consensus Guidelines 2001, p 27).

Women should be offered a screening test for HBV early in pregnancy. The optimal time for screening appears to be at the first antenatal visit. There is no evidence to support repeat screening in the third trimester or that a repeat test for hepatitis B in late pregnancy will result in increased detection of hepatitis B.

Screening for active hepatitis B infection with hepatitis B surface antigen (HbsAg) is recommended at the first prenatal visit so that postnatal intervention can be offered to decrease mother-to-child transmission. Women at increased risk of acquiring hepatitis B can be vaccinated safely during pregnancy and should be screened again for surface antigen before they give birth (ACOG 2002). Women who were not screened during pregnancy and those at increased risk should be tested at the time of giving birth (Kirkham et al 2005, p 1557).

What to tell women

Hepatitis B virus is a potentially serious infection that can affect the liver. Many people have no symptoms, however. It can be passed from a mother to her baby (through blood or body fluids), but may be prevented if the baby is vaccinated at birth. The infection can be detected in the mother's blood.

Hepatitis C virus

Hepatitis C is a blood-borne viral liver infection. It is a slowly progressive disease with long-term sequelae, including cirrhosis and hepatocellular carcinoma. During 1999 the incidence of infection among pregnant Australian women was estimated at 13 per 1000. An estimated 55% of these women were diagnosed prior to pregnancy and 19% during pregnancy (Three Centres Guidelines 2001, p 30). As one of the major causes of liver cirrhosis, hepatocellular carcinoma and liver failure, hepatitis C virus (HCV) is a major public health concern. Hepatitis C antibody screening should be offered to women with risk factors (e.g. prison inmates, injection drug users, women exposed to blood or blood products, HIV-positive women, women with elevated aspartate transaminase levels, multiple sexual partners, or tattoos). Aside from the risk of vertical transmission, estimated as 6% if a woman is HCV RNA positive (Dore et al 1997), and negligible if she is HCV RNA negative, there does not appear to be an increased risk of adverse pregnancy outcomes in women infected with hepatitis C (Boucher & Gruslin 2005; Kirkham et al 2005, p 1557).

Human immunodeficiency virus (HIV)

The first recognised cases of the acquired immune deficiency syndrome (AIDS) occurred in the summer of 1981 in the United States. Reports began to appear of *Pneumocystis carinii* pneumonia and Kaposi's sarcoma in young men, who, it was subsequently realised, were both homosexual and immunocompromised. Even though the condition became known early on as AIDS, its cause and modes of transmission were not immediately obvious. The virus now known to cause AIDS in a proportion of those infected was discovered in 1983 and given various names. The internationally accepted term is now the human immunodeficiency virus (HIV). Subsequently a new variant has been isolated in patients with West African connections—HIV2 (Adler 2001, p 1226).

Infection with HIV begins with an asymptomatic stage, with gradual compromise of immune function eventually leading to AIDS. The time between HIV infection and development of AIDS ranges from a few months to as long as 17 years in untreated patients (NICE 2003, p 86).

In the absence of intervention, mother-to-child transmission (MTCT) may occur in one in four births to infected mothers in Europe or the United States, and 25% to 40% in Africa and Asia (Mohlala et al 2005). This figure may be substantially reduced following antiretroviral treatment, and a combination of interventions (i.e. combination antiretroviral therapy, caesarean section and avoidance of breastfeeding) can further reduce the risk of transmission to 1% (NICE 2003, p 86). It is estimated that up to 30% of MTCTs, with the exclusion of those due to breastfeeding, occur in utero, with the remainder occurring intrapartum (Minkoff et al 2003). The most potent predictors of perinatal HIV transmission are maternal HIV-1 load (viral load), severity of maternal disease (European Collaborative Study 1992), prolonged rupture of the amniotic membranes, and mode of delivery (Landesman et al 1996).

Several studies have demonstrated that giving birth by elective caesarean section before rupture of the amniotic membranes or the onset of labour, as well as the administration of zidovudine or nevirapine during the peripartum period, reduces MTCT significantly (Mohlala et al 2005).

The possible mechanisms responsible for vertical transmission during the peripartum period include transplacental micro transfusions of maternal blood into the fetal circulation during contractions, labour, and separation of the placenta before clamping of the umbilical cord; ascending infection from the vagina through the cervix after rupture of the amniotic membranes, which infects the amniotic fluid;

TABLE 32.4 Global transmission of AIDS	
Type of exposure	**Percentage of global total**
Blood transfusion	3–5
Perinatal	5–10
Sexual intercourse	70–80
Vaginal	60–70
Anal	5–10
Injecting drug use (sharing needles etc)	5–10
Health care (needlestick injury, etc)	< 0.01
(Source: Adler 2001)	

Clinical point

What should we say to women?

A study of all obstetricians and members of the RANZCOG in 2003 found that the percentage of respondents who always discuss the risk of transmission of hepatitis B through breastfeeding is 55.4%. The percentage of respondents who always discuss the risk with patients infected with hepatitis C is slightly higher at 67% and for HIV it is 82%.

More women are being offered hepatitis C screening than HIV despite a lack of evidence for effective interventions during labour to reduce perinatal transmission of hepatitis C.

Many women are not being asked about risk factors for exposure to these viruses. Only approximately one-third of obstetricians would alter their clinical practice and recommend caesarean section and avoid rupture of membranes in women infected with HIV despite evidence that this reduces perinatal transmission.

(Source: Giles et al 2003)

BOX 32.8 HIV in New Zealand

An estimated 56,000 women give birth in New Zealand each year. The risk of transmission from a mother with HIV to her baby can be reduced from as high as 31.5% to less than 2% if the mother uses a combination of interventions and treatment (Dorenbaum et al 2002; Duong et al 1999).

If a universal offer of antenatal screening was the policy in New Zealand then on an annual basis approximately 55,000 pregnant women would be tested for HIV (based on live births rather than total number of pregnancies). Nearly all pregnant women with HIV infection would be detected by the first test.

If all infected pregnant women were detected through antenatal screening:

▶ an additional 4–18 women would be diagnosed with HIV annually

▶ if interventions to prevent transmission were taken up by all of these women, it is estimated that on average 1–4 perinatal infections could be prevented annually (Dickson et al 2002).

The incidence of HIV is rising in New Zealand. There were 136 new cases of HIV in New Zealand in 2002, and in 2003 there were 188 new HIV cases—this was a 44% rise in the number of new infections in those two years.

HIV is increasingly affecting women. Between 1996 and 2002, 24% of newly diagnosed infections in New Zealand were in females. The women diagnosed with HIV in New Zealand are disproportionately from parts of the world where heterosexual transmission is relatively common, with 74% of HIV cases among women in New Zealand since 1996 acquired overseas—44% in Africa and 17% in Asia.

Each HIV test costs $14.70 but there are associated costs to run an effective screening program.

(Source: National Advisory Committee on Health and Disability (National Health Committee) 2004)

and absorption of the virus through the infant's immature digestive tract. Microtrauma to the fetal skin during birth, with exposure to blood and infected cervicovaginal secretions, may also be responsible for transmission of the virus. It is also possible that fetal exposure to HIV-infected amniotic fluid or to the cells that are found within amniotic fluid before rupture of the amniotic membranes could be responsible for a proportion of vertical transmission in utero (Mohlala et al 2005).

The most common way to diagnose HIV infection is by a test for antibodies against HIV-1 and HIV-2. HIV antibody is detectable in at least 95% of patients within three months of infection. Early HIV diagnosis improves outcomes for the mother and can reduce the rate of disease progression.

Pregnant women should be offered screening for HIV infection early in antenatal care because appropriate antenatal interventions can reduce MTCT of HIV infection (Kirkham et al 2005). In addition, all women should receive appropriate written information about antenatal HIV testing and be given an opportunity to discuss it with their midwife or doctor. Women at increased risk for HIV infection should be retested in the third trimester of pregnancy (Kirkham et al 2005; CDC 2002). Testing should be voluntary and done with informed consent (Kirkham et al 2005). A positive result should be verified through a second blood test. Women should be notified as soon as the result is verified and offered post-test counselling. The diagnosis should be delivered personally in a sensitive, supportive manner, allowing sufficient time for questions. Results should never be communicated by telephone, answering machine or through a receptionist. During post-test counselling, women's understanding of a positive diagnosis should be explored and further discussion

of features of the illness, diagnostic procedures and medical care may be necessary. Referrals to clinical, social and welfare services should be offered and women should know how to access support groups (Three Centres Guidelines 2001, p 33).

A system of clear referral paths should be established so that pregnant women who are diagnosed with an HIV infection are managed and treated by the appropriate specialist teams (NICE 2003, pp 86–87).

RANZCOG recommends that all women be offered HIV testing after appropriate counselling. In contrast, the Australian National Council on AIDS, HCV and Related Diseases (ANCAHRD) advocates the selective offer of testing.

In Australia it appears that approximately half of practitioners offer HIV testing to all pregnant women in their care. The vast majority of these women are tested. The other half of practitioners offer testing on the basis of exposure assessment or on request, and as a result, only a small minority of women undergo testing. The prospect of universal screening in Australia has raised concerns about cost-effectiveness, testing without informed consent, provision of pre- and post-test counselling and discrimination against women found to be positive in a population (Three Centres Guidelines 2001, p 34).

What to tell women

HIV usually causes no symptoms at first but can lead to AIDS. HIV can be passed from a mother to her baby, but this risk can be greatly reduced if the mother is diagnosed before the birth. The infection can be detected through a blood test. If the woman is pregnant and is diagnosed with HIV she should receive specialist care.

Rubella

Detection of rubella does not protect against MTCT in the current pregnancy. However, protection of subsequent pregnancies against the rubella virus will prevent future MTCT of rubella and reduce the risk of stillbirth and miscarriage due to rubella infection (NICE 2003, p 88).

Vaccination during pregnancy is contraindicated because of fears that the vaccine could be teratogenic. Screening for the rubella antibody in pregnancy helps to identify susceptible women so that rubella vaccination can be offered post partum to protect future pregnancies.

Rubella susceptibility screening should be offered early in antenatal care to identify women at risk of contracting rubella infection and to enable vaccination in the postnatal period for the protection of future pregnancies.

What to tell women

Screening for German measles (rubella) is offered so that if you are not immune you can choose to be vaccinated after you have given birth. This should usually protect you and future pregnancies. Testing you for rubella in pregnancy does not aim to identify it in the baby you are carrying (NICE 2003).

Herpes simplex virus

Both herpes simplex virus (HSV) type 1 and HSV type 2 can cause genital herpes. Because the infection is chronic, genital herpes has become the most common STI among women. The prevalence of the genital HSV infection can cause a large spectrum of disease. First-episode infections, which represent new acquisition of HSV, usually are most severe, and recurrent infections may be milder. However, as many as 75% of primary infections are unrecognised by either patient or care provider. Recurrences usually are limited to the genital area. Most women with HSV-2 do not know they have genital herpes because their recurrences are mild and infrequent. Such women may have nonspecific genital conditions and may have been receiving treatment for other genital conditions, such as recurrent yeast infections, urinary tract infections, or allergic rashes in the genital area. An important feature of HSV infection is intermittent reactivation, with or without accompanying symptoms, and resultant shedding of the virus in the genital tract. DNA from HSV can be detected in the genital tract 10–50% of the time among HSV-2 seropositive women. Women close to the time of acquisition or with severe clinical disease have a higher risk of viral shedding between symptomatic recurrences (ACOG 2004, p 1112).

It is estimated that 5% of the general population has a known history of genital herpes 1. This creates a large population of women known to be at risk for transmitting HSV to their infants during delivery, should they have a peripartum recurrence. To avoid intrapartum HSV exposure and neonatal infection, it is currently recommended that pregnant women with visible genital herpes lesions or prodromal symptoms at the time of labour have a caesarean delivery. Gravidas without visible lesions or prodromal symptoms should be allowed to continue in labour because they have a low risk of neonatal HSV transmission. Using these guidelines, it is estimated that one poor neonatal outcome from HSV infection is averted for every 1580 caesarean deliveries performed for maternal clinical HSV recurrences (at a cost of US$2.5 million) (Scott et al 2002).

It is difficult to make the diagnosis of genital herpes on clinical grounds alone. The classic presentation of a painful cluster of vesicles and ulcers occurs in a small proportion of women, and most women will have atypical lesions, such as abrasions, fissures, or itching without obvious lesions. Conversely, even in at-risk women with a presentation compatible with genital herpes, up to 20% of women will not have genital herpes. Thus, a definitive diagnosis should be confirmed by a laboratory test, even if the infection was established in the past on clinical grounds.

Traditionally, the laboratory test used most often has been viral culture because it is highly specific, widely available, and relatively inexpensive. Viral culture can be useful in women presenting with new or recurrent genital ulcer disease. However, viral culture is insensitive, even with a primary infection, with a false-negative rate up to 25%. In recurrent disease, the rate of viral isolation is less than 50%. This low rate of viral isolation results in the need for repeat visits or leaves the impression that the patient does not have genital herpes. In addition to viral detection methods, the detection of type-specific antibodies to HSV-1 and HSV-2 also can help to establish the diagnosis. The incubation period for HSV is short (approximately four days), and antibodies to HSV-2 are detected 2–12 weeks after acquisition of infection and persist indefinitely. Most women with genital HSV-1 or genital HSV-2 infection are asymptomatic. A small proportion may recall symptoms or lesions compatible with genital herpes when they receive a diagnosis of HSV-2. Because HSV is so prevalent among women, infection rates are very high among sexually active women, even if the number of sexual partners is not very high. Therefore, type-specific antibody testing is more accurate than assessment of infection based on symptoms or past sexual behavior (ACOG 2004, p 1113).

A vaginal birth is appropriate in the absence of recurrent genital herpes lesions or prodromal symptoms (Scott et al 2002). Pregnant women with a history of recurrent genital herpes might decrease their risk of clinical reactivation at the time of birth by more than 50% by using suppressive acyclovir therapy (Brocklehurst & French 1998; Scott et al 2002). The significant reduction in clinical herpes recurrences amongst women treated with acyclovir could potentially reduce the caesarean section rate (Scott et al 2002). Cost-benefit analyses performed for the use of acyclovir suppression in the last several weeks of pregnancy demonstrate that suppressive therapy would cost less, would result in decreased maternal morbidity and mortality, and would result in fewer cases of neonatal herpes than deferring acyclovir treatment and resorting to caesarean section for clinical reactivations (Randolph et al 1996).

Group B Streptococcus

Group B beta-hemolytic Streptococcus (*Streptococcus agalactiae*) (GBS or GBBS) is a Gram-positive aerobic coccobacillus that was first associated with bovine mastitis, hence the name *agalactiae,* meaning 'no milk'. Unfortunately, it is not confined just to cows, and can cause invasive disease (sepsis) of the newborn in humans. GBS disease of newborns is early-onset (occurring less than seven days after delivery, usually within 24 hours) in 80% of cases, or less frequently late-onset (occurring seven or more days after delivery) (ACOG 1996). GBS is a leading cause of sepsis, meningitis and death among newborn infants in Western countries. Early-onset infections with this organism account for approximately 80% of GBS infections in infants and are usually acquired by contact with the genital tract of the mother during labour and birth (Bergeron et al 2000, p 175). Infants who have such infections may require prolonged hospitalisation, and those who survive may have mental retardation or visual loss. Among pregnant women, the prevalence of colonisation with GBS ranges from 15% to 40%. Women who are carriers are also at risk for severe infections (Bergeron et al 2000, p 175).

Early-onset GBS infection (EOGBS) in neonates usually occurs within the first 24 hours after birth, and accounts for 80% of neonatal infections, although it is defined as that occurring within the first seven days. Late-onset GBS infection occurs from seven days until three months of age, and is less aggressive.

The bacteria ascend into the amniotic fluid (once membranes are ruptured) and enter the epithelium of the lungs, or more rarely the meninges (Feldman 2001, p 16), causing pneumonia, bacteraemia and, in approximately 15% of cases, meningitis, causing permanent neurological damage (Glantz & Kedley 1998, p 45).

Incidence

The incidence of GBS varies within and between populations. In New Zealand the most recent survey found a colonisation rate of 22% in a population of 240 women swabbed recto-vaginally at 35–37 weeks gestation (Grimwood et al 2002). Recto-vaginal colonisation rates exceed vaginal colonisation rates by > 50% (Benitz et al 1999, p 5). While ethnic, geographic and socio-economic differences in colonisation rates have

been documented, there is insufficient consistency in these factors to establish valid 'at-risk' subgroups.

An estimated 10–30% of pregnant women in Australia will have vaginal carriage of GBS. The incidence may be considerably higher in Indigenous populations. Transmission to the newborn may occur during labour, resulting in pneumonia, septicaemia and occasionally infant death. About 1–2% of infants born to GBS-colonised mothers will develop early-onset infection. In this group there is a 6% fatal outcome which is higher in pre-term infants (Three Centres Guidelines 2001, p 60).

Screening options

Either risk assessment or screening for GBS colonisation in pregnant women is recommended, to identify candidates for intrapartum prophylaxis.

- The risk-based protocol does not entail antepartum screening, but treats women with certain risk factors during labour.
- The screening-based protocol includes cultures at 35 to 37 weeks gestation, and offers intrapartum prophylaxis to all women with positive cultures. Uncultured women with risk factors are treated.

Both protocols involve high rates of intrapartum antibiotic use and both may significantly lower rates of neonatal GBS sepsis (screening-based more than risk-based for both). Figures 32.6 and 32.7 show the two management protocols.

Risk assessment is performed at the onset of labour, and the presence of fever, a prolonged interval between rupture of membranes and birth, or imminent preterm birth is considered indicative of the need for prophylaxis.

In New Zealand, the GBS Consensus Working Party provides the following guidance:

> The risk-based approach (above) should be used to identify those women at risk of giving birth to GBS-affected babies.
> Intrapartum penicillin G (1.2 g intravenously as the initial dose, then 0.6 g intravenously every 4 hours until birth) is the

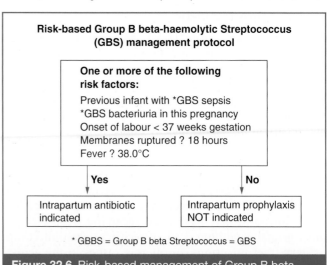

Figure 32.6 Risk-based management of Group B beta-haemolytic Streptococcus (GBS) (based on Glantz & Kedley 1998)

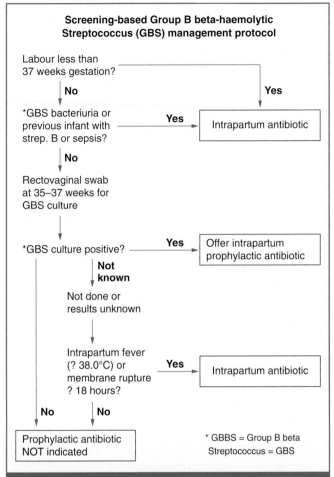

Screening-based Group B beta-haemolytic Streptococcus (GBS) management protocol

Labour less than 37 weeks gestation?

No → *GBS bacteriuria or previous infant with strep. B or sepsis? — **Yes** → Intrapartum antibiotic

No → Rectovaginal swab at 35–37 weeks for GBS culture

*GBS culture positive? — **Yes** → Offer intrapartum prophylactic antibiotic

Not known → Not done or results unknown

Intrapartum fever (? 38.0°C) or membrane rupture ? 18 hours? — **Yes** → Intrapartum antibiotic

No   **No** → Prophylactic antibiotic NOT indicated

* GBBS = Group B beta Streptococcus = GBS

Figure 32.7 Screening-based management of Group B beta-haemolytic Streptococcus (GBS) (based on Glantz & Kedley 1998)

intrapartum antibiotic of choice. Penicillin is recommended because of its narrow spectrum of activity. An alternative is amoxicillin (2 g intravenously initially, then 1 g every 4 hours until birth occurs).

As part of antenatal assessment, a history of penicillin allergy should be sought—including details of immediate (within 24 hours) hypersensitivity reactions (e.g. anaphylaxis, angioedema, laryngospasm, bronchospasm, or urticaria). Women not at high risk of anaphylaxis should receive cephazolin (2 g intravenously initially, then 1 g intravenously every 8 hours until birth). The small group of women with a definite history of immediate hypersensitivity reactions can receive vancomycin. This should be only after seeking clinical microbiology or infectious diseases advice. The recommended dose is 1 g intravenously every 12 hours until the baby is born. Neither penicillin G nor amoxicillin alone are adequate treatment for maternal chorioamnionitis (intrapartum fever with > 2 of the following signs: fetal tachycardia, uterine tenderness, offensive vaginal discharge, or maternal leucocytosis). As *E. coli*, anaerobes, and GBS can all cause chorioamnionitis, this requires immediate aggressive management with broad-spectrum antibiotics (Campbell et al 2004, p 10).

Screening consists of obtaining vaginal and anal specimens for culture at 35 to 37 weeks gestation.

Identification of GBS colonisation in pregnant women

The identification of GBS colonisation in pregnant women is fundamental to our ability to quantify the risk of infection for any infant. GBS is a 'moving target'—'both vaginal and rectal colonisation may be persistent, transient or intermittent, limiting the predictive value of screening cultures for colonisation on any future date' (Benitz et al 1999, p 5). The most accurate swabs are taken from the low vaginal-introitus area, rather than the high vaginal or cervical region (Glantz & Kedley 1998, p 46).

Yancey and colleagues (1996) found cultured vagino-rectal swabs to have a positive predictive value of at least 88% from five weeks prior to birth, but this reduced to only 43% for more than five weeks (Yancey et al 1996, p 813). They also report a negative predictive value of at least 95% in the five weeks before birth, with a still relatively high value of 80% for negative cultures taken more than five weeks before birth (Yancey et al 1996, p 813).

Benitz and colleagues (1999, p 7) report a 64.5% prevalence of vaginal colonisation among women with vagino-rectal colonisation, and that 'virtually all infants with EOGBS disease are born to mothers from whom GBS can be recovered from vaginal cultures' (Benitz et al 1999, p 7). They argue against the use of vagino-rectal cultures, asserting that it would 'not identify additional infants who are likely to become infected but would enlarge and dilute the pool of women identified as being at risk for EOGBS infection' (Benitz et al 1999, p 7).

Two issues relating to women's experience of swabbing warrant attention. First, the degree of acceptability of rectal or anal swabbing by women is uncertain. It is currently not done in New Zealand as part of GBS screening in practice, and would need to be established as necessary for women to agree either to have it done to them, or to do it themselves. The second issue is that of self-swabbing. Taylor et al (1997) found that swabs collected by women themselves were 'highly correlated with nurse-collected samples for accuracy of culture results' (p 410).

If antenatal screening is carried out, the results need to be available when the woman is in labour, to be of any value. This issue is of course secondary to the problems associated with the unreliability of swabbing as a predictive tool in relation to GBS at present.

The standard method for the diagnosis of GBS colonisation consists of culturing combined vaginal and anal secretions in a selective broth medium that inhibits the growth of other microorganisms. After collection, swabs should be placed in a suitable, non-nutritive transport medium, such as Amies, or may be directly plated at the bedside. The swab will maintain viability for up to four days at room temperature. Transport as a dry swab or in an inappropriate medium will significantly reduce detection rates. Culture is performed using selective culture media such as Lim or SBM broth (Three Centres Guidelines 2001, p 59).

Cultures may be negative in some women whose infants subsequently have GBS infections. On the other hand, the use of antibiotic prophylaxis on the basis of risk assessment leads to unnecessary treatment in many women (Bergeron et al 2000, p 175).

Intrapartum antibiotics are recommended for:
- pre-term birth < 37 weeks
- rupture of membranes > 18 hours prior to delivery
- maternal temperature = 38°C during labour
- previous GBS colonisation
- GBS bacteriuria
- previous infant with GBS.

The recommended intrapartum chemoprophylaxis for GBS is penicillin G 1.2 g (IV) load, then 0.6 g IV four-hourly throughout labour ((Three Centres Guidelines 2001, p 59) (although the Cochrane Review by Smaill (2001) reports treatment with intrapartum ampicillin 1 g intravenously every six hours during labour as the usual regimen; and alternatives included benzyl penicillin or erythromycin (Smaill 2001)).

Wherever possible, antibiotics should be commenced at least four hours prior to birth to ensure adequate prophylaxis. In the case of suspected penicillin allergy, clindamycin (600 mg IV eight-hourly) or erythromycin (500 mg IV six-hourly until delivery) may be used (Three Centres Guidelines 2001, p 59).

Risk factors for EOGBS infection

GBS colonisation

Being able to assess the colonisation of women at the time of labour is the most significant piece of information required to assess potential risks for neonates. There is a known relationship between density of colonisation in both women and neonates, and EOGBS infection—with heavier colonisation associated with 2.54 times greater odds of infection compared with lightly colonised mothers (Benitz et al 1999, p 5).

GBS bacteriuria in pregnancy

This is believed to reflect heavy colonisation in women, but the empirical evidence for this is not conclusive (Benitz et al 1999; CDC 1996).

Previous child with GBS infection

This 'risk' is also difficult to quantify (Benitz et al 1999). GBS is extremely difficult to eliminate from the GI tract and re-colonisation of the vagina is highly likely. It may be that the low incidence is a reflection of the high rates of prophylactic antibiotic use in this group, as a result of their, and/or their caregiver's, potentially high levels of anxiety to avoid a similar experience a second time.

Chorioamnionitis

This condition is clinically defined by maternal fever and 'two or more additional signs, including fetal tachycardia, uterine tenderness, foul-smelling vaginal discharge, or maternal leucocytosis, occurs in 1–3.8% of parturients and is associated with neonatal GBS attack rates ranging from 6% to 20%' (Benitz et al 1999, p 10). It is detectable, and is a condition of high risk of neonatal sepsis whatever the causative organism. It requires empirical antibiotic treatment. Further, 'chorioamnionitis is almost universally present in mothers of infants who became septic despite intrapartum prophylaxis with an appropriate IV antibiotic' (Benitz et al 1999, p 10).

This may be due to the antibiotics chosen and/or the high level of bacterial invasion prior to treatment, and/or inadequate time of treatment from diagnosis until birth.

Intrapartum fever

This is clearly related to the chorioamnionitis risk above, as fever is often the first symptom recognised, and is the point from which other investigations are instigated. Intrapartum fever is recognised as a significant risk factor for EOGBS infection, at 5–15 times the risk (Glantz & Kedley 1998, p 46). Defining fever in labour, or the level at which it is significant, is less straightforward, with differing values used by various authors: > 37.5°C (Benitz et al 1999), >37.8°C (Feldman 2001; Langley 2000) and > 38°C (Glantz & Kedley 1998; Schuchat 1999). Most do not justify the use of a particular temperature. While it is tempting to believe that the higher the temperature the higher the risk, 'there are no objective data to quantify that relationship' (Benitz et al 1999, p 10). A critical review of the literature found that 'available data do not identify specific temperature thresholds above which prophylaxis, diagnostic screening or empiric therapy are appropriate or imperative' (Benitz et al 1999, p 10).

BOX 32.8 EOGBS risk factors

Primary risk factors for EOGBS infection:
- GBS colonisation—heavier associated with increased risk
- GBS bacteriuria in pregnancy—indication of heavy colonisation, measure varies
- previous child of the woman had EOGBS infection—colonisation and bad experience
- chorioamnionitis—maternal fever and/or fetal tachycardia, offensive amniotic fluid
- maternal intrapartum fever—range in values used, > 37.5°C, > 37.8°C or even > 38°C
- rupture of membranes—prelabour or prolonged, > 18 hours before the birth
- preterm labour and birth— < 37 weeks gestation, premature and low birthweight.

Factors associated with lower or not well documented risk for EOGBS infection:
- duration of internal fetal monitoring > 12 hours
- number of vaginal examinations > 6
- young women
- lower parity
- ethnicity—varies depending on country, may well be linked to socio-economic status
- number of sexual partners—not usually defined
- frequency of sexual intercourse.

Benitz and colleagues (1999) acknowledge the influence of epidural analgesia in intrapartum fever. They note that the maternal temperature increases at 0.08–0.14°C/hour, exceeding 38.0°C in 10–15% of women, and they suggest that the use of a higher fever threshold for women who have had an epidural analgesia may be appropriate (Benitz et al 1999). Arguably, this exposes the somewhat arbitrary nature of defining maternal fever in labour.

Ruptured membranes: prolonged or prelabour

It is now generally believed that EOGBS infection occurs after membrane rupture, although there has been debate about the bacteria's ability to pass through membranes. At issue is the length of time of ruptured membranes (ROM) required for the bacteria to ascend. The full-term baby is better able to resist infection, and 18 hours has evolved as the benchmark time beyond which neonates are believed to be at increased risk, although Yancey (cited in MMWR 1996, p 3) has proposed > 6 hours, and McLaren et al (cited in Benitz et al 1999, p 9) call for > 10 hours as appropriate. The 18 hours benchmark has not been reached by any empirical methodology: rather, it is an attempt to find the optimal time to catch infections without (over) treating an unacceptable number of women, who were at no greater risk than the normal birthing population. Preterm prelabour ROMs combine two relatively high-risk groups, with these neonates reported to have attack rates of 33% to 50% (Benitz et al 1999, p 9).

Preterm birth

This is usually defined as birth before 37 weeks gestation (Feldman 2001; Langley 2000) and combines two known risk factors: prematurity and low birthweight. A gradient of increasing risk with decreasing birthweight and gestational age has been demonstrated (Schuchat 1999; Yancey et al 1996). Glantz and Kedley (1998) claim that 'preterm delivery is associated with approximately 25% of invasive disease' (p 46).

Recommendations for midwifery practice

(by Celia Grigg)

GBS presents midwives with a number of challenges when trying to keep birth normal. It is an elusive and unpredictable bacterium that may be harmless most of the time, but with the potential to become life-threatening to neonates.

A measured approach is required, to balance the harm-versus-benefit ratio. This involves establishing acceptable boundaries for risk, which is a good idea, but theory and practice are not always easily matched. Unfortunately, there are no definitive markers, only sliding scales of known risk, with numerous indices, and a significant population affected.

Midwives contracting to be with women at the hospital are, theoretically at least, bound by the hospital recommendations and policies unless clear documentation of alternative choices exists. Midwives are in the position of sharing information with women to facilitate their making decisions for themselves. It seems appropriate to provide information about GBS and the issues, risks and options, and to work with women and their families within their 'world view', accepting that some will make choices that may not fit our 'world view'.

Within the context of midwifery practice, the following are recommended:

- Avoid taking vaginal swabs during pregnancy. This helps maintain normality and avoids unnecessary anxiety for a large number of women.
- If a woman 'falls' into a risk category for EOGBS, share information about GBS and discuss options. Give written information, as the subject is complex and it is easy to not fully grasp the issues.
- See and assess a woman after prelabour ROM as soon as possible.
- Check for signs of infection in the woman and in the fetus, including chorioamnionitis. Consider taking a low vaginal swab for immediate culturing if a woman has prelabour ROM and she is likely to choose not to have prophylactic antibiotics if she doesn't give birth in the next 18–24 hours. Culture will take 24 hours, but will give very reliable information on which to base decisions at that time.
- If there are signs of chorioamnionitis, recommend IV treatment with antibiotics.
- Discuss signs of an unwell baby with all families, including temperature taking.
- Observe all neonates for sepsis in the first two to three hours.
- Carefully monitor neonates whose mothers were in an 'at-risk' category closely for six hours, but continue for 24 hours.
- If the woman is in hospital, ask midwifery staff to monitor the baby's wellbeing.
- Consider requesting specific observations, such as taking the baby's temperature four-hourly.
- If any baby has poor Apgar scores and/or respiratory distress, consider sepsis, assess the whole situation and respond quickly if concerned. EOGBS infection usually has a rapid onset and is potentially fatal.
- Do not take gastric aspirate or ear swabs from neonates at birth, even if there are risk factors.
- Unwell babies will have blood cultures taken, and GBS skin colonisation is not a useful measure.

GBS is a common but unpredictable bacterium with the potential to cause significant illness at times. It is difficult to identify its presence reliably at the time it causes most damage for neonates, during labour and birth or once women have ROM. The 24-hour timeframe for culturing swabs is usually too slow. The great majority of affected babies are symptomatic at birth, which is usually within 24 hours of ROM or the start of labour. Unfortunately, the known risk factors have poor sensitivity and specificity, and work on a poorly defined sliding scale of risk.

Intrapartum antibiotics are not a very efficient or effective way of dealing with GBS, and have several risk factors associated with them. Allergic reactions and possible resistance are well documented, but the unnecessary medicalisation of the process of labour for a significant proportion of women giving birth is of concern, when almost all of their babies are well. There is a real danger of the general public developing a misplaced expectation of antibiotics as a risk-free, fullproof prevention, when at best they will reduce the incidence of EOGBS infection and at worst make way for more serious infections resistant to available antibiotics.

EOGBS infection is very rare and can be treated effectively in most cases. Midwives need to be well informed about GBS and the management options, and work with women to maintain appropriate perspective on the minimal risks in normal labour and birth situations.

Toxoplasmosis

Caused by the parasite *Toxoplasma gondii*, primary toxoplasmosis infection is usually asymptomatic in healthy women. Once infected, a lifelong antibody response provides immunity from further infection.

Toxoplasmosis infection is acquired via four routes in humans:
- ingestion of viable tissue cysts in undercooked or uncooked meat (e.g. salami, which is cured) or tachyzoites in the milk of infected intermediate hosts
- ingestion of oocytes excreted by cats and contaminating soil or water (e.g. unwashed fruit or vegetables contaminated by cat faeces)
- transplanted organs or blood products from other humans infected with toxoplasmosis
- mother-to-child transmission when primary infection occurs during pregnancy.

Routine antenatal serological screening for toxoplasmosis should not be offered because the harms of screening may outweigh the potential benefits. Pregnant women should be informed of primary prevention measures to avoid toxoplasmosis infection, such as:
- washing hands before handling food
- thoroughly washing all fruit and vegetables, including ready-prepared salads, before eating
- thoroughly cooking raw meats and ready-prepared chilled meals
- wearing gloves and thoroughly washing hands after handling soil and gardening
- avoiding cat faeces in cat litter or in soil (NICE 2003, p 95).

Screening for clinical conditions

Blood group and Rhesus D status

You can find more information about this in the publication entitled 'Guidance on the routine use of anti-D prophylaxis for RhD negative women: information for patients', published by NICE in 2002 and available on the NICE website (see online resources list at the end of this chapter).

Anti-D

Overall a policy of anti-D administration at 28 and 34 weeks during pregnancy to all Rh (D) negative women (who have not actively formed their own anti-D) will result in a reduction of alloimmunisation from about 1% to 0.3%.

Blood must be taken for Rh antibody titre prior to administration of anti-D, which the NHMRC recommends at 28 and 34 weeks. It is reasonable to vary the timing so that this can be grouped with other tests between 28 and 38 weeks gestation.

The administration of Rh D immunoglobulin (anti-D) has been shown previously (and more recently in Cochrane Reviews) to result in a significant reduction in the incidence of Rh isoimmunisation (Crowther & Middleton 2006). In 1999 the NHMRC recommended prophylactic administration (3) of Anti-D during pregnancy (NHMRC 1999).

Only Rh (D) negative women (who have not actively formed their own anti-D) having their first baby and who have reached 28 weeks gestation should be offered anti-D prophylaxis, with a repeat dose at 34 weeks—CSL 625 IU (125 µg)

For *all* Rh (D) negative women (who have not actively formed their own anti-D):
- first trimester indications—CSL 250 IU (50 µg):
  - chorionic villus sampling
  - miscarriage
  - termination of pregnancy
  - ectopic pregnancy
- second and third trimester indications—CSL 625 IU (125 µg):
  - obstetric haemorrhage
  - amniocentesis, cordocentesis
  - external cephalic version of a breech presentation, whether successful or not
  - abdominal trauma, or any other suspected intrauterine bleeding or sensitising event
- postnatally, within 72 hours, to *all* women who give birth to an Rh (D) positive baby.

RhD immunoglobulin should not be given to women with preformed anti-D antibodies except where the preformed anti-D is due to the antenatal administration of RhD immunoglobulin. If it is unclear whether the anti-D detected in the mother's blood is passive or preformed, the treating clinician should be consulted.

If there is continuing doubt, RhD immunoglobulin should be administered.

All women should have the magnitude of potential feto-maternal haemorrhage assessed and if necessary further anti-D administered as appropriate.

Gestational diabetes mellitus

Gestational diabetes mellitus occurs in 2% to 9% of all pregnancies (NICE 2003, p 96). Although the risks associated with gestational diabetes are well recognised, there has been uncertainty about the evidence available from clinical trial data regarding whether screening and treatment to reduce maternal glucose levels reduce these risks. Given this uncertainty, professional groups have disagreed on whether to recommend routine screening, selective screening based on risk factors for gestational diabetes, or no screening. Some recommend

screening, whereas others do not. Recent evidence indicates a worrisome rise in the prevalence of gestational diabetes (Dabelea et al 2005) that is largely explained by the increase in maternal obesity. Efforts to reverse this trend are critical (Greene & Soloman 2005).

Results of the Australian Carbohydrate Intolerance Study In Pregnant Women

The recently published Australian Carbohydrate Intolerance Study in Pregnant Women (ACHOIS) trial (Crowther et al 2005) assessed whether the treatment of gestational diabetes would reduce perinatal complications, and assessed the effects of treatment on maternal outcome, mood and quality of life. The large, randomised, multicentre trial with 18 collaborating centres will give some firm evidence on which to base policy decisions for treating pregnant women considered to be at risk from gestational diabetes (Crowther et al 2005).

In the trial, pregnant women underwent a 75 g oral glucose-tolerance test between 24 and 34 weeks gestation; those with values below 7.8 mmol per litre after an overnight fast and between 7.8 and 11.0 mmol per litre at two hours were eligible for randomisation. Women were advised to follow a normal diet 48 hours before the oral glucose-tolerance test and to fast for eight hours the night before the test. Blood samples were obtained after the overnight fast and one and two hours after taking the drink of 75 g oral glucose. Women with previously treated gestational diabetes or active chronic systemic disease (except essential hypertension) were excluded (Crowther et al 2005, p 2478).

Women were told that they would be eligible for randomisation only if their blood glucose levels fell into the range specified above. If they were assigned to the intervention group, they received a slip indicating a diagnosis of glucose intolerance of pregnancy and the plan for intervention, whereas if they were assigned to routine care, they received a slip indicating that they did not have gestational diabetes. The researchers justify this approach on the following grounds:
- There remained uncertainty as to the level of glucose impairment associated with adverse perinatal outcomes.
- There was wide variation in the glucose levels used to define the need for treatment with some committees, but not others.
- There was still no clear evidence of the benefits and harms of treatment (Crowther et al 2005).

Women whose glucose levels exceeded cut-off values for eligibility were informed that they had gestational diabetes (Crowther et al 2005, p 2478).

The 490 women assigned to the intervention group were shown how to monitor their blood glucose levels (four times a day until they reached the required blood glucose levels) as well as being provided with individualised dietary counselling. They were given insulin as needed to maintain fasting and before-a-meal glucose levels below 5.5 mmol per litre and at two hours postprandial (after a meal) the levels were not to exceed 7.0 mmol per litre. This group (the intervention group) had care consistent with management approaches in which screening and treatment for gestational diabetes are routine.

The 510 women assigned to the control group received routine care that was consistent with the care provided in places in which screening for gestational diabetes is *not* standard.

In analysing the results, the researchers used an 'intention-to-treat' analysis. The results showed that among the babies born to women in the intervention group, as compared with those of women in the routine-care group, there was a significantly reduced risk of the primary outcome measures. These included one or more of the following: perinatal death, shoulder dystocia, bone fracture, and nerve palsy (1% versus 4%; adjusted relative risk, 0.33; 95% CI 0.14–0.75). There were five deaths (three stillbirths and two neonatal deaths) among the offspring of mothers in the control group, compared with none in the intervention group. Two stillbirths were unexplained intrauterine deaths at term of appropriately grown infants, and the other, at 35 weeks gestation, was associated with pre-eclampsia and IUGR. One infant had a lethal congenital anomaly, and one infant died after an asphyxial condition during labour without antepartum haemorrhage (Crowther et al 2005, p 2481).

A higher percentage of infants born to women in the intervention group than of infants born to women in the control group were admitted to the neonatal nursery (71% versus 61%, adjusted $P = 0.01$) and most babies stayed for one to two days.

Macrosomia (defined as a birthweight of 4 kg or greater) was significantly more common among the infants of mothers in the control group than among the infants of mothers in the intervention group (21% versus 10%, $p < 0.001$). There was no significant difference in the rates of shoulder dystocia between the intervention and control groups (1% and 3%, respectively). No infant in the intervention group had a bone fracture or nerve palsy, whereas in the control group, one infant had both a fractured humerus that was not related to a difficult birth and a radial-nerve palsy, one infant had Erb's palsy related to shoulder dystocia, and one infant had Erb's palsy alone.

Among the women in the study, the primary outcome measures were the rates of induction and the rates of caesarean birth. The induction of labour was significantly more common in the intervention group than in the control group (39% versus 29%; adjusted $P < 0.001$). This meant that women who were treated for gestational diabetes had a risk of 1.36 (1.15–1.62) (a third times more likely to have induction of labour after controlling for parity, maternal age and Aboriginality).

The rates of caesarean birth were similar in the two groups, as were the reasons for operative birth. More women had an elective caesarean section in the intervention group and more women had an emergency caesarean section in the control group—but these results did not reach statistical significance.

The researchers assessed the response of a subgroup of women in the trial to their perceptions of quality of life following treatment for gestational diabetes, and found no negative effect.

This trial will have major repercussions for the screening and treatment of gestational diabetes because it showed conclusively that treatment of gestational diabetes in the form of dietary advice, blood glucose monitoring, and insulin therapy to maintain control of blood glucose levels, reduces the rate of serious perinatal complications, without increasing the rate of Caesarean birth.

This trial was published just prior to this book going to press (2006). For that reason I have described the study in some detail because it will make many of the current policies redundant. See also the NICE Guidelines (2003) and the *Three Centres Consensus Guidelines* (2001).

Pre-eclampsia

Hypertensive disorders in pregnancy and pre-eclampsia remain major causes of maternal and perinatal mortality, accounting for 15% of maternal deaths and 4% of perinatal deaths. Therefore, a key aim of modern antenatal care is the timely detection and management of pre-eclampsia (Wallace & Oats 2002).

Elevated blood pressure is one of the first signs of the condition. Consequently, guidelines recommend the practice of recording blood pressure at every antenatal visit as critical in detection and management of hypertensive disorders of pregnancy. Early detection is important, as underlying conditions can progress rapidly. Current Australasian Consensus Guidelines suggest a diagnosis of hypertension when:

- systolic blood pressure is 140 mmHg
- and diastolic blood pressure is 90 mmHg,
- taken on two or more consecutive occasions over several hours,
- or an increment of 15/30.

Both diastolic and systolic pressures have been shown to be closely associated with fetal outcome. A clinical diagnosis of pre-eclampsia is usually made when hypertension occurs with one or more of proteinuria, renal insufficiency, liver disease, neurological problems, haematological disturbances or fetal growth restriction (Australian Society for the Study of Hypertension In Pregnancy 2000; Brown et al 2000; Three Centres Guidelines 2001, p 42).

Pre-eclampsia is a multisystem disorder that occurs in the second half of pregnancy and is associated with increased maternal and neonatal morbidity and mortality. The incidence of pre-eclampsia ranges from 2% to 10%, depending on the population studied and the criteria used to diagnose the disorder. Maternal symptoms of advanced pre-eclampsia may include:

- bad headache
- problems with vision, such as blurring or flashing before the eyes
- bad pain just below the ribs
- vomiting
- sudden swelling of face, hands or feet (Action on Pre-eclampsia 2004).

Although it is usually mild, it can cause serious problems for mother and baby if it is not detected and treated. It is more likely to develop in women who:

Clinical point

How to measure blood pressure in pregnancy

1 The woman should sit down with her feet supported.
2 Take measurements after the woman has been resting in this position for two to three minutes.
3 Use a standard-sized cuff for women with an arm circumference of 33 cm, a large cuff for arm circumference > 33 cm.
4 Palpate systolic blood pressure at the brachial artery and inflate the cuff to 20 mmHg above this level.
5 Deflate the cuff slowly, at approximately 2 mmHg per second.
6 Record diastolic blood pressure reading using the Korotkoff V sound. If phase V is not present, then record phase IV.

Hypertension is defined when systolic blood pressure is > 140 mmHg and/or diastolic blood pressure (Korotkoff V) is > 90 mmHg or there is an incremental rise of 30 mmHg systolic or 15 mmHg diastolic.

(Sources: Australian Society for the Study of Hypertension in Pregnancy 2000; Three Centres Consensus Guidelines 2001)

BOX 32.10 Hypertension in pregnancy

▶ Current definitions of hypertensive disorders in pregnancy:
— *pre-eclampsia*—hypertension new to pregnancy manifesting after 20 weeks of gestation that is associated with a new onset of proteinuria, which resolves after delivery
— *pregnancy-induced hypertension*—hypertension new to pregnancy that resolves after delivery but is not associated with proteinuria
— *chronic hypertension*—hypertension that predates a pregnancy or appears prior to 20 weeks gestation.
▶ Most women with hypertension in pregnancy have no clinical symptoms. Hypertension is frequently the only early sign that predates serious disease.
▶ Blood pressure measurement is routinely performed in antenatal care to allow the diagnosis and classification of hypertension in pregnancy.
▶ Pre-eclampsia is though to be caused by widespread endothelial cell damage secondary to an ischaemic placenta.
▶ Hypertension and proteinuria are two easily measured signs associated with pre-eclampsia, although they are surrogate markers indicating end-organ damage.
▶ Eclampsia is rare. It occurs in nearly 1/2000 pregnancies in the UK. It is associated with high maternal morbidity and accounts for over 50% of the maternal deaths associated with hypertensive disorders in pregnancy.
▶ Blood pressure may be of limited importance in identifying women who are going to develop eclampsia, as about one-third of first fits occur in women with normal or a mild increase in blood pressure.
▶ Oedema was originally part of the triad of signs describing pre-eclampsia but it occurs in too many pregnant women (up to 80%) to be discriminatory and has been abandoned as a marker in classification schemes.

(Source: NICE Guidelines 2003, p 99)

● have been diagnosed with pre-eclampsia in a previous pregnancy
● have not been pregnant before
● are 40 years old or more
● have a mother or sister who has had pre-eclampsia
● are overweight at the time of the first antenatal appointment
● are expecting more than one baby or already have high blood pressure or diabetes.

Urine sample

Whenever blood pressure is measured during pregnancy, a urine sample should be tested at the same time for protein (as this can be another sign of pre-clampsia). Use the same type of equipment, method and conditions each time, so that the results at different times can be compared. The diagnosis of pre-eclampsia depends on the presence of significant proteinuria as well as raised blood pressure.

Reagent strips or 'dipsticks' are commonly used to detect proteinuria. The incidence of false positive results in random urine specimens may be up to 25% in trace reactions and 6% with 1+ reactions. Therefore, dipsticks can only be a screening test and will not have much utility when not used in combination with blood pressure measurements. Due to considerable observer errors involved in dipstick urinalysis, an RCOG Study Group recommended that automated dipstick readers be employed. This can significantly improve false positive and false negative rates. An initial sample of 1+ or greater should be confirmed by a 24-hour urinary protein measurement or protein/creatinine ratio determination. Although a finding of 300 mg/24 hours or more or a protein/creatinine ratio of 30 mg/mmol of creatinine is customarily regarded as significant, a proteinuria threshold of 500 mg/24 hours has been suggested to be more predictive in relation to the likelihood of adverse outcome (NICE 2003, p 101; RCOG 2003).

Placenta praevia

Placenta praevia is a condition in which the placenta is low-lying in the womb and covers all or part of the entrance (the cervix). In most women, as the womb grows upwards, the placenta moves with it so that it is in a normal position before birth and does not cause a problem.

If an earlier ultrasound scan showed the placenta extending over the cervix, another abdominal scan should be offered at 36 weeks. If this second abdominal scan is unclear, a vaginal scan should be offered.

Non-routine tests

There are a number of screening tests that have sometimes been offered to women in the past or have been suggested for routine antenatal care. The following tests should *not* be offered as a matter of routine, because they have not been shown to improve outcomes for mothers or babies:

- cardiotocography (a record of the trace of a baby's heartbeat, which is monitored through electronic sensors placed on the mother's abdomen, called a trace or CTG)
- Doppler ultrasound (an ultrasound scan that measures the blood flow between the baby and the mother)
- vaginal examination to predict whether a baby may be born too early
- routine breast and pelvic examination
- screening for gestational diabetes mellitus (a form of diabetes triggered by pregnancy) (see Crowther et al 2005 for this update)
- daily counting and recording of the baby's movements
- screening for GBS.

Women should be asked early in pregnancy if they have had any previous psychiatric illnesses. Women who have a past history of serious psychiatric disorder should be referred for a psychiatric assessment during the antenatal period.

Pregnant women should not be offered routine screening in the antenatal period to predict the development of postnatal depression (e.g. with the Edinburgh Postnatal Depression Scale). Pregnant women should not be offered antenatal education interventions to reduce perinatal or postnatal depression, as these interventions have not been shown to be effective.

Alcohol

All pregnant women and women contemplating pregnancy should be informed of the harmful effects of alcohol on the fetus. Safe levels of alcohol consumption during pregnancy are not known; therefore, pregnant women are advised to abstain from drinking alcohol. More research into the efficacy of primary care screening and behavioural intervention for alcohol misuse among pregnant women is needed.

How many visits?

In developed countries with well-established obstetrics services, small reductions in the number of prenatal visits (equal to or less than two visits) are compatible with similar good perinatal outcomes as in the standard model. However, it can be expected that women may be disappointed with fewer visits. Two trials conducted in developing countries, in which a proportionally major reduction in the number of visits was achieved, also supports this conclusion. Therefore,

---

BOX 32.11 Family violence

Pregnancy is a particularly at-risk time for women to become victims of family violence and has been identified as a unique window of opportunity for identification and management of abused women. Currently, practitioners do not adequately identify cases of family violence, and abused women tend not to disclose it.

A pilot study by Lauti and Miller (2003) aimed to investigate the opinions of obstetricians and midwives regarding their perceived role in identification and management of family violence. Specifically, their opinions about possible barriers to identification and management were sought, and how these might be overcome.

Content analysis of focus group and semistructured interview discussions with obstetricians and midwives identified many issues:

- Time, failure of the medical model, lack of continuity of care, privacy and confidentiality issues were perceived as significant barriers to identification.
- All practitioners experienced uncertainty about appropriate management.
- Screening may pick up a woman's historical abuse, which may be inappropriate.
- Debriefing is needed after difficult cases.
- Midwives have a crucial role and can experience serious boundary issues.
- Midwives may become entangled in the power imbalance of a woman's abusive relationship.

Significant issues continue to exist in the area of domestic screening for both New Zealand and Australian midwives.

(Source: Lauti & Miller 2003)

---

attempts to provide effective interventions during pregnancy by distributing them in fewer visits than usually recommended can be attempted without risking effectiveness. Such care can be provided by staff other than the obstetrics/gynaecology specialist. In light of the available evidence, the four antenatal care visits schedule tested in the largest trials appears to be the minimum that should be offered to low-risk pregnant women (Villar et al 2004).

Effective prenatal care should integrate the best available evidence into a model of shared decision-making. Pregnant women should be counseled about the risks of smoking and alcohol and drug use. Structured educational programs to promote breastfeeding are effective. Routine fetal heart auscultation, urinalysis, and assessment of maternal weight, blood pressure, and fundal height generally are recommended, although the evidence for these interventions is variable. Women should be offered ABO and Rh blood typing and screening for anemia during the first prenatal visit. Genetic counseling and testing should be offered to couples with a family history of genetic disorders, a previously affected fetus or child, or a history of recurrent miscarriage. All women should be offered prenatal serum marker screening for neural tube defects and aneuploidy. Women at increased risk for aneuploidy should be offered amniocentesis or chorionic villus sampling. Counseling about the limitations and risks of these tests, as well as their psychologic implications, is necessary. Folic acid supplementation beginning in the preconception period reduces the incidence of neural tube defects. There is limited evidence that routine use of other dietary supplements may improve outcomes for the mother and infant (Kirkham et al 2005).

Figure 32.8 shows a summary of routine appointments during pregnancy.

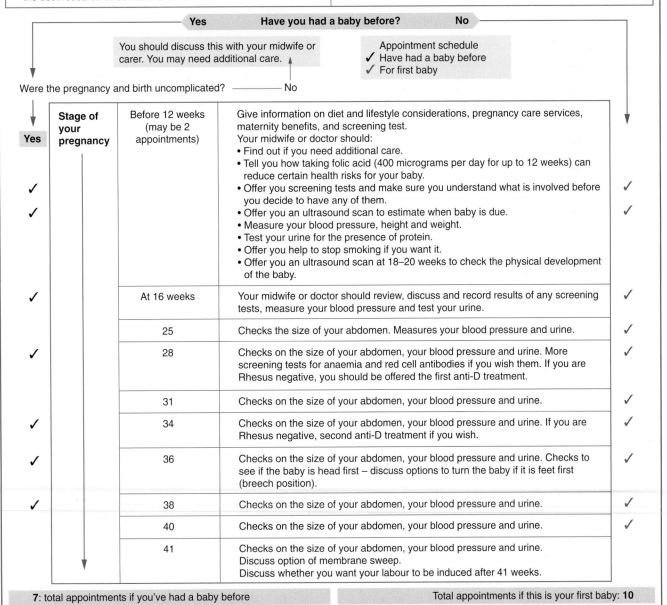

Figure 32.8 Summary of routine appointments during pregnancy (based on NICE 2003)

Review questions

1   How do you explain the importance of screening to women?

2   Describe the difference between a screening test and a diagnostic procedure.

3   What is the specificity of a screening test and how is this different from the sensitivity of a screening test?

4   How would you explain the long-term side-effects of ultrasound to a woman who is anxious about the procedure?

5   Is it justifiable to offer newborn screening for a potentially untreatable genetic disorder? Why or why not?

6   What is a serum marker? Explain the various serum markers available for screening for Down syndrome. How would you explain the notion of a false-positive result to a 40-year-old woman who is pregnant for the first time? How and when would you conclude that the test result was a false positive?

8   What is the incidence of hepatitis B in your area? What do you tell families who want to weigh up the pos and cons of hepatitis B vaccination of their baby at the time of birth? What are the long-term effects of hepatitis B? Does hepatitis B affect different populations differently?

9   Should there be a universal offer of antental screening for HIV? Do you agree with the New Zealand Ministry of Health directive? Why or why not?

10 Describe the various viral infections that may be screened for in pregnancy. What are some of the risk factors that you would describe in relation to each viral infection? How many of these viruses may be transmitted through breast milk?

Online resources

Canadian Midwives Guidelines, http://www.cmbc.bc.ca/

Consensus statement on diabetes control in preparation for pregnancy, http://www.mja.com.au/public/issues/181_06_200904/mcl196_fm.html

Guidelines on antenatal care (National Collaborating Centre for Women's and Children's Health, commissioned by the National Institute for Clinical Excellence October 2003), http://www.rcog.org.uk/index.asp?PageID=693)

National Blood Authority, http://www.nba.gov.au

National Institute on Alcohol Abuse and Alcoholism, http://www.niaaa.nih.gov/publications/instable.htm

New Zealand Ministry of Health, http://www.nzgg.org.nz/ (Go to links on this page)

NICE 2002, Guidance on the routine use of anti-D prophylaxis for RhD negative women: information for patients, http://www.nice.org.uk/pdf/Anti_d_patient_leaflet.pdf.

NZCOM consensus statements, http://www.midwife.org.nz/index.cfm/Consensus

NZCOM resource site, http://www.midwife.org.nz/index.cfm/Resources

RCOG, http://www.rcog.org.uk

References

ACOG 1996 Committee on Obstetric Practice. Prevention of early-onset group B streptococcal disease in newborns. ACOG Committee Opinion. No. 173. ACOG. Washington, DC

ACOG 2002 Practice Bulletin No. 20. Perinatal viral and parasitic infections. International Journal of Gynaecology and Obstetrics 76:95–107

ACOG 2004 Practice Bulletin. No. 57 Gynecologic herpes simplex virus infections. International Journal of Gynaecology and Obstetrics 104(5)

Action on pre-eclampsia 2004 Online: www.apec.org.uk/index.html

ADIPS 2002 Australasian Diabetes in Pregnancy Society (ADIPS) Gestational diabetes mellitus—management guidelines, updated by ADIPS December 2002

ADIPS 1998 Gestational diabetes mellitus—management guidelines (ADIPS: L Hoffman, C Nolan, JD Wilson, JJN Oats and D Simmons). Medical Journal of Australia 169:93–97. Online: http://www.mja.com.au/public/issues/jul20/hoffman/hoffman.html

Adler MW 2001 ABC of AIDS: development of the epidemic. British Medical Journal 322:1226–1229

Australian Institute of Health and Welfare (AIHW) 1999. The burden of disease and injury in Australia: the full report. AIHW, Canberra

Australian Institute of Health and Welfare (AIHW) 2002. Australia's Health 2002. AIHW Cat. No. AUS 25. AIHW, Canberra

Australian Institute of Health and Welfare (AIHW) (NPSU: Birch MR, Grayson N, Sullivan EA) 2004 Recommendations for development of a new Australian Birth Anomalies System: a review of the congenital malformations and birth defects data collection. AIHW Cat. No. PER 23. (Birth Anomalies Series 1) AIHW NPSU, Sydney

Al-Yaman F, Bryant M, Sargeant H 2002. Australia's children: their health and wellbeing 2002. AIHW Cat. No. PHE 36. AIHW, Canberra

Australian Society for the Study of Hypertension in Pregnancy 2000 The detection, investigation and management of hypertension in pregnancy: full consensus statement. Australian and New Zealand Journal of Obstetrics and Gynaecology 40:139–155

Backe B, Nakling J 1994 Term prediction in routine ultrasound practice. Acta Obstetricia et Gynecologica Scandinavica 73: 113–118

Bahado-Singh RO, Wapner R, Thom E et al 2005 First Trimester Maternal Serum Biochemistry and Fetal Nuchal Translucency Screening Study Group. Elevated first-trimester nuchal translucency increases the risk of congenital heart defects. American Journal of Obstetrics and Gynecology.192(5):1357–1361

Barnett S 1998 Can diagnostic ultrasound heat tissue and cause biological effects? In: S Barnett , G Kossoff (Eds) Safety of diagnostic ultrasound. Parthenon, Lancashire, pp 27–38

Barnett SB, Ter Haar GR, Ziskin MC et al 2000 International recommendations and guidelines for the safe use of diagnostic ultrasound in medicine. Ultrasound in Medicine and Biology 26:355–366

Beech BL 1999 Ultrasound? Unsound. A review and expansion of ultrasound research and a discussion of AIMS' concerns about the expansion of routine use in pregnancy and childbirth. Midwifery Today website. Online: http://www.midwiferytoday.com/articles/ultrasoundwagner.asp?a=1&r=1&e=1&q=ultrasound

Benitz W, Gould J, Druzin M 1999 Risk factors for early-onset Group B Streptococcal sepsis: estimation of odds ratios by critical literature review. Pediatrics 103(6)

Benn P 2003 Improved antenatal screening for Down syndrome. Lancet 361:794–795

Bergeron MG, Danbing KE, Menard C et al 2000 Rapid detection of group B streptococci in pregnant women at delivery. New England Journal of Medicine 343:175–179

Bischoff FZ, Lewis DE, Simpson JL 2005 Cell-free fetal DNA in maternal blood: kinetics, source and structure. Human Reproduction Update 11(1):59–67

Blondel B, Morin I, Platt RW et al 2002 Algorithms for combining menstrual and ultrasound estimates of gestational age: consequences for rates of preterm and post-term birth. British Journal of Obstetrics and Gynaecology 109:718–720

Botto LD, Rittler M, di Tanna GL et al 2000 Prenatal diagnosis and Down syndrome. International Clearinghouse for Birth Defects. Monitoring systems annual report on multiple congenital anomalies. Online: http://www.icbd.org/document/Ar/189_215.pdf

Boucher M, Gruslin A 2005 SOGC clinical practice guidelines: the reproductive care of women living with hepatitis C infection. Online: http://sogc.medical.org/sogcnet/sogc_docs/common/guide/pdfs/ps96.pdf

Bowman JE 1993 Editorial. British Medical Journal 306(6874):349

Bradley DM, Parsons EP, Clarke AJ 1993 Experience with screening newborns for Duchenne muscular dystrophy in Wales. British Medical Journal 306(6874):357–360

Brent RL 2001 Addressing environmentally caused human birth defects. Pediatric Review.22(5):153–165

Brocklehurst P, French R 1998 Review. The association between maternal HIV infection and perinatal outcome: a systematic review of the literature and meta-analysis. British Journal of Obstetrics and Gynaecology 105(8):836–848

Buckley S 2005 Ultrasound scans: cause for concern. In: Gentle birth, gentle mothering: the wisdom and science of gentle choices in pregnancy, birth and parenting. One Moon Press

Caine A, Maltby AE, Parkin CA et al for the UK Association of Clinical Cytogeneticists (ACC) 2005 Prenatal detection of Down syndrome by rapid aneuploidy testing for chromosomes 13, 18, and 21 by FISH or PCR without a full karyotype: a cytogenetic

risk assessment. Lancet 366(9480):123–128. Online: www.thelancet.com

Campbell N, Eddy A, Darlow B et al 2004 The prevention of early-onset neonatal group B streptococcal infection: technical report from the New Zealand GBS Consensus Working Party. New Zealand Medical Journal 117(1200). Online: http://www.nzma.org.nz/journal/117-1200/1023

Campbell S 2001 Isolated major congenital heart disease. Ultrasound in Obstetrics and Gynecology 17:370–379

Centers for Disease Control (CDC) 1994 Cigarette smoking among women of reproductive age, United States, 1987–1992. Morbidity and Mortality Weekly Report 4(43):789–91, 797

Chen MY, Donovan B 2004 Genital *Chlamydia trachomatis* infection in Australia: epidemiology and clinical implications. Sexual Health 1:189–196

Chen MY, Fairley CK, Donovan B 2005 Discordance between trends in chlamydia notifications and hospital admission rates for chlamydia-related diseases in New South Wales, Australia. Sexually Transmitted Infections 81:318–322

Crowther CA, Kornman L, O'Callaghan S et al 1999 Is an ultrasound assessment of gestational age at the first antenatal visit of value? A randomised clinical trial. British Journal of Obstetrics and Gynaecology 106:1273–1239

Crowther CA, Hiller JE, Moss JR et al 2005 Australian Carbohydrate Intolerance Study in Pregnant Women (ACHOIS) Trial Group 2005 Effect of treatment of gestational diabetes mellitus on pregnancy outcomes. New England Journal of Medicine 352(24):2477–2486

Cuckle HS, Wald NJ, Lindenbaum RH 1984 Maternal serum alphafetoprotein measurement: a screening test for Down syndrome. Lancet i:926–929

Dabelea D, Snell-Bergeon JK, Hartsfield CL et al 2005 Kaiser Permanente of Colorado GDM Screening Program. Increasing prevalence of gestational diabetes mellitus (GDM) over time and by birth cohort: Diabetes Care 3:579–584

Daiminger A, Bader U, Enders G 2005 Pre- and periconceptional primary cytomegalovirus infection: risk of vertical transmission and congenital disease. British Journal of Obstetrics and Gynaecology 112(2):166–172

Doherty DA, James IR, Newnham JP 2002. Estimation of the Doppler ultrasound umbilical maximal waveform envelope: II. Prediction of fetal distress. Ultrasound in Medicine and Biology 10:1261–1270

Dore GM, Hargreaves G, Niven BE1997 Dependent opioid users assessed for methadone treatment in Otago: patterns of drug use. New Zealand Medical Journal110(1043):162–165

Drummond LM, Veale AMO 1978 Muscular dystrophy screening. Lancet i:1258–1259

Eik-Nes SH, Salvesen KA, Økland O et al 2000 Routine ultrasound fetal examination in pregnancy: the 'Alesund' randomized controlled trial. Ultrasound in Obstetrics and Gynecology 15(6):473–478

Emery AEH 1998 The muscular dystrophies. British Medical Journal 317:991–995

Feldman R 2001 Group B Streptococcus: prevention of infection in the newborn. The Practicing Midwife 4(3):16–18

Giles M, Hellard M, Sasadeusz J et al 2003 A study investigating obstetricians' management of women infected with a blood borne virus. Australian and New Zealand Journal of Obstetrics and Gynaecology 43:398–408

Glantz JC, Kedley KE 1998 concepts and controversies in the management of Group B streptococcus during pregnancy. Birth 25(1):45–53

Greene MF, Soloman CG 2005 Gestational diabetes mellitus—time to treat. New England Journal of Medicine 352(24):2544–2546

Grimes D, Schulz K 2002 Uses and abuses of screening tests. Lancet 359:881–884

Grimwood K, Darlow BA, Gosling IA et al.2002 Early-onset neonatal group B streptococcal infections in New Zealand 1998–1999. Journal of Paediatric and Child Health 38(3):272–277

Guidelines for the use of Rh D Immunoglobulin (Anti-D) in obstetrics in Australia. Online: http://www.ranzcog.edu.au/publications/statements/C-obs6.pdf

Haddow JE 1998 Antenatal screening for Down syndrome: where are we and where next? Lancet 352(9125):336–337

Haddow JE, Palomaki GE, Knight GJ et al 1998 Screening of maternal serum for fetal Down syndrome in the first trimester. New England Journal of Medicine 338:955–961

Hocking J, Fairley C, Counahan M et al 2003 The pattern of notification and testing for genital *Chlamydia trachomatis* infection in Victoria, 1998–2000: an ecological analysis. Australian and New Zealand Journal of Public Health 7:405–408

Kieler H, Haglund B, Cnattingius S et al 2005 Does prenatal sonography affect intellectual performance? Epidemiology 3:304–310

Kirkham C, Harris S, Grzybowski S 2005 Evidence-based prenatal care: part II. Third-trimester care and prevention of infectious diseases. American Family Physician 71:1555–1560, 1561–1562

Landesman SH, Kalish LA, Burns DN et al 1996 Obstetrical factors and the transmission of human immunodeficiency virus type 1 from mother to child. The Women and Infants Transmission Study. New England Journal of Medicine 334(25):1617–1623

Langley S 2000 Group B Streptococci and early onset neonatal infection. Nursing Times 96(25)

Larsson PG, Bergström M, Forsum U et al 2005. Bacterial vaginosis transmission. Role in genital tract infection and pregnancy outcome: an enigma. Acta Pathologica, Microbiologica et Immunologica Scandinavica 113(4):233–245

Lauti M, Miller D 2003 Obstetricians' and midwives' perception of their role in the identification and management of family violence. Australian and New Zealand Journal of Obstetrics and Gynaecology 43:398–408

Leitich H, Bodner-Adler B, Brunbauer M et al 2003 Bacterial vaginosis as a risk factor for preterm delivery: a meta-analysis. American Journal of Obstetrics and Gynecology 189:139–147

Mak DB, Murray JC, Bulsara MK 2003 Antenatal screening for sexually transmitted infections in remote Australia. Australian and New Zealand Journal of Obstetrics and Gynaecology 43(6):457–462

Marinac-Dabic D, Krulewitch CJ, Moore RM Jr 2002 The safety of prenatal ultrasound exposure in human studies. Epidemiology 13:S19–S22

McDonald H, Brocklehurst P, Parsons J et al 2003 Interventions for treating bacterial vaginosis in pregnancy. Cochrane Database of Systematic Reviews (2), pp 1–30. John Wiley & Sons, Chichesters

Mennuti MT, Driscoll DA 2003 Screening for Down syndrome—too many choices? New England Journal of Medicine 349(15):1471–1473

Merkatz IR, Nitowsky HM, Macri JN et al 1984 An association between low maternal serum alpha-fetoprotein and fetal chromosome abnormalities. American Journal of Obstetrics and Gynecology 148:886–894

Miller MW, Brayman AA, Abramowicz JS 1998 Obstetric ultrasonography: a biophysical consideration of patient safety—the 'rules' have changed. American Journal of Obstetrics and Gynecology 179:241–254

Minkoff H, Hershow R, Watts DH et al 2003 The relationship of pregnancy to human immunodeficiency virus disease progression. American Journal of Obstetrics and Gynecology189(2):552–559

Morbidity and Mortality Weekly Review (MMWR) 1996 Prevention of perinatal Group B Streptococcal disease: a public health perspective. MMWR 45(RR-7): 1–24

Mohlala BK, Tucker TJ, Besser MJ et al 2005 Investigation of HIV in amniotic fluid from HIV-infected pregnant women at full term. Journal of Infectious Diseases 192(3):488–491

Morin I, Morin L, Xun Zhang et al 2005 Determinants and consequences of discrepancies in menstrual and ultrasonographic gestational age estimates. BJOG: An International Journal of Obstetrics and Gynaecology 112(2):145–152

Murray N, Homer CS, Davis GK et al 2002 The clinical utility of routine urinalysis in pregnancy: a prospective study. Medical Journal of Australia 177:477–480

National Advisory Committee on Health and Disability (National Health Committee) 2004 HIV screening in pregnancy. A report to the New Zealand Minister of Health, October 2004. Online: http://www.nhc.gov.nz

National Centre in HIV Epidemiology and Clinical Research. Annual surveillance reports. Online: www.med.unsw.edu.au/nchecr/

National Collaborating Centre for Women's and Children's Health. Antenatal care: routine care for the healthy pregnant woman. Online: http://www.rcog.org.uk/index.asp?PageID=693

National Health Committee 2004 Steering Committee of the National Public Health Initiative on Diabetes and Women's Health, Centers for Disease Control and Prevention. Report from the CDC. The National Public Health Initiative on Diabetes and Women's Health: leading the way for women with and at risk for diabetes. Journal of Women's Health13(9):962–967

Neilson JP 1998 Ultrasound for fetal assessment in early pregnancy. Cochrane Database (4)

Neilson JP 2004 Ultrasound for fetal assessment in early pregnancy. Cochrane Database (4) CD000182

NHMRC Guidelines on the prophylactic use of Rh D immunoglobulin (anti-D) in obstetrics. Online: http://www.nhmrc.gov.au/publications/synopses/wh33.htm

NICE Guidelines 2003 Antenatal care: routine care for the healthy pregnant woman. National Collaborating Centre for Women's and Children's Health Commissioned by the National Institute for Clinical Excellence. Online: http://www.rcog.org.uk/resources/Public/pdf/Antenatal_Care.pdf

Okun N, Gronau KA, Hannah ME 2005 Antibiotics for bacterial vaginosis or *Trichomonas vaginalis* in pregnancy: a systematic review. Obstetrics and Gynecology 105(4):857–868

Olesen AW, Westergaard JG, Thomsen SG et al 2004 Correlation between self-reported gestational age and ultrasound measurements Acta Obstetricia et Gynecologica Scandinavica 83(11):1039–1043

Pereira K, Maidji E, McDonagh S et al 2005 Insights into viral transmission at the uterine-placental interface. Trends in Microbiology 13(4):164–174

Proud J 1997 Understanding obstetric ultrasound (2nd edn). Books for Midwives, Hale. Excerpt on Midwifery Today website. Online: http://www.midwiferytoday.com/articles/ultrasoundwagner. asp?a=1&r=1&e=1&q=ultrasound

Randolph AG, Hartshorn RM, Washington AE 1996. Acyclovir prophylaxis in late pregnancy to prevent neonatal herpes: a cost-effectiveness analysis. Obstetrics and Gynecology 88(4/1): 603–610

RCOG Study Group 2003 Shennan AH, Waugh JJS. The measurement of blood pressure and proteinuria. In: H Critchley, AB MacLean, L PostonL et al (Eds) Pre-eclampsia. RCOG Press, London, pp 305–324

Reid MC, Fiellin DA, O'Connor PG 1999 Hazardous and harmful alcohol consumption in primary care. Archives of Internal Medicine 159(15):1681–1689

Schuchat A 1999 Group B Streptococcus. Lancet 353(9146),: 51–56

Schull WJ, Otake M 1999 Cognitive function and prenatal exposure to ionizing radiation. Teratology 59:222–226

Scott DA, Loveman E, McIntyre L et al 2002 Review. Screening for gestational diabetes: a systematic review and economic evaluation. Health Technology Assessment 6(11):1–161

Smaill F 2001 Intrapartum antibiotics for Group B streptococcal colonisation (Cochrane Review). Cochrane Library (2). Update Software, Oxford

Smith GC, Smith MF, McNay MB et al 1998 First-trimester growth and the risk of low birth weight. New England Journal of Medicine 339:1817–1822

Stagno S, Whitley RJ 1985 Review. Herpes virus infections of pregnancy. Part II: Herpes simplex virus and varicella-zoster virus infections. New England Journal of Medicine 313(21):1327–1330

Stanley F, Blair E, Rice G et al 1995 Review. The origins of cerebral palsy—a consensus statement: The Australian and New Zealand Perinatal Societies. Australian College of Midwives Inc. Journal. 8(3):19–25

Tabor A, Philip J, Madsen M et al 1986 Randomised controlled trial of genetic amniocentesis in 4606 low-risk women. Lancet i:1287–1293

Taylor M, Mercer B, Englehardt K et al 1997 Patient preference for self-collected cultures for group B streptococcus in pregnancy. Journal of Nurse-Midwifery 42(5):410–413

Thiagarajan M 1998 Evaluation of the use of yogurt in treating bacterial vaginosis in pregnancy. Journal of Clinical Epidemiology 51:22S

Three Centres Consensus Guidelines 2001 Three Centres Consensus Guidelines on Antenatal Care Project. Mercy Hospital for Women, Southern Health and Women's and Children's Health

Tincello DG, Richmond DH 1998 Evaluation of reagent strips in detecting asymptomatic bacteriuria in early pregnancy: prospective case series. British Medical Journal 316:435–437

US Preventive Services Task Force (USPSTF) 2004 Recommendation Statement. Screening and behavioral counseling interventions in primary care to reduce alcohol misuse. Online: http://www.ahrq. gov/clinic/3rduspstf/alcohol/alcomisrs.htm#ref4

Vassy C 2005 How prenatal diagnosis became acceptable in France. Trends in Biotechnology 23(5):246–249

Wald NJ, Cuckle HS, Densem JW et al. 1988 Maternal serum screening for Down syndrome in early pregnancy. British Medical Journal 297:883–888

Wallace EM, Oats JJ 2002 National guidelines for antenatal testing. Medical Journal of Australia 177(9):468

World Health Organization (WHO) 1992 The ICD-10 classification of mental and behavioural disorders: clinical descriptions and diagnostic guidelines. WHO, Geneva

Yancey M, Schuchat A, Brown L et al 1996 The accuracy of late antenatal screening cultures in predicting genital group b streptococcal colonization at delivery. Obstetrics and Gynecology 88(5):811–815

Ziskin MC, Barnett SB 2000 Ultrasound and the developing central nervous system. Ultrasound in Medicine and Biology 27:875–876

Acknowledgement

Thanks to Celia Grigg, who wrote the section on midwifery recommendations for GBS.

APPENDIX: Checklist of tests

Tests recommended at the first antenatal visit

1 **Blood group and antibody screen**
   Where the blood group has already been performed it does not need to be repeated. However, the antibody screen should be repeated at the beginning of each pregnancy.

2 **Full blood examination**

3 **Rubella antibody status**
   Although a previous high rubella antibody titre is generally used to exclude this investigation from first visit testing, there is some evidence that antibody levels may decline after rubella immunisation, especially since antibody levels are rarely boosted by exposure to wild viruses in the community.

Other tests that may be considered

1 **Cervical cytology**
   Documented normal cervical cytology within the preceding 18 months may be used to delay repeat screening if there is no clinical indication for another Papanicolaou smear.

2 **Screening for haemoglobinopathies**
   Each unit should have a defined policy for screening for haemoglobinopathies, taking into account the ethnic mix of patients screened. As a minimum, all women should be screened with MCV and MCHC. Haemoglobin electrophoresis and iron studies should be performed in the event of thresholds not being reached. Consideration should also be given to the further screening of patients with DNA analysis for alpha-thalassaemia. Testing of normal-MCV women for haemoglobinopathies may be considered if they are members of high-risk groups.

3 **Varicella**
   Consideration should be given to checking varicella antibodies at the first visit where there is no history of previous illness.

Tests after the first antenatal visit

1 **Obstetric ultrasound scan**
   All women should be offered an obstetric ultrasound before 20 weeks gestation. This will include an ultrasound for fetal morphology and placental localisation usually at 18–20 weeks gestation. Other scans may be indicated depending on individual circumstances and to assess/confirm dates.

2 **Screening for Down syndrome**
   Antenatal screening for Down syndrome and other fetal aneuploidy.

3 **Gestational diabetes**
   'Screening for GDM should be considered in all pregnant women. However, if resources are limited, screening may be reserved for those at highest risk.' (ADIPS 2002)

4 **Group B streptococcal disease**
   Swabbing for GBS

5 **Rhesus negativity blood group antibody screenings**
   Guidelines for the use of Rh-D immunoglobulin (anti-D) in obstetrics in Australia. Further screening is recommended for Rh-negative women at 28 weeks gestation. Screening of Rh-positive women is at the discretion of the clinician/managing health service.

6 **Iron deficiency**
   The haemoglobin level and platelet count should be repeated at 28 weeks gestation. If anaemia is detected, further investigation is warranted.

7 **Cytomegalovirus/toxoplasmosis**
   Screening is recommended only for those women at a substantially increased risk of acquiring an infection.

8 **Syphilis**
   Syphilis screening should be repeated at 28 weeks in high-risk populations.

9 **Late pregnancy tests of fetal wellbeing**
   Late pregnancy tests for assessment of feto-placental function should be performed when indicated on clinical grounds—either through a suspicion of placental insufficiency, a predisposing factor for placental insufficiency or through an inability to clinically ascertain fetal growth (e.g. obesity). Tests of fetal wellbeing should be considered after 41 weeks gestation. Detailed and frequent assessment of fetal wellbeing, including an assessment of liquor volume, is mandatory in pregnancies at or beyond 42 weeks gestation.

CHAPTER 33

Challenges in pregnancy

Christine Griffiths and Carol Thorogood

Key terms

chorioadenoma, choriocarcinoma, chronic hypertension, complete miscarriage, cystitis, dizygotic (binovular), endometritis, gestational diabetes, gestational hypertension, hyperemesis gravidarum, hypoglycaemia, inevitable miscarriage, ketoacidosis, ketonuria, molar pregnancy (hydatidiform mole), monozygotic (uniovular), oligohydramnios, placenta praevia, placental abruption, polyhydramnios, pre-eclampsia, pregnancy-induced hypertension, pyelonephritis, recurrent miscarriage, silent miscarriage, threatened miscarriage, thrombo-embolic disease, Type 1 diabetes, Type 2 diabetes

Chapter overview

For most women, pregnancy progresses normally and she and her unborn baby remain well. For some, however, pre-existing problems, challenges or complications that arise during the pregnancy put the woman and her baby at risk of adverse outcomes. These complications can lead to serious illness, trauma, and even the death of the woman, her baby or both. Irrespective of the final outcomes, challenges in pregnancy place tremendous stress on the family. It is essential that midwives have the knowledge and skills to recognise the physical signs that a pregnancy is not progressing as it should and can identify psycho-social and environmental stressors that create or

exacerbate complications in pregnancy. It is not enough just to recognise that all is not well. Midwives have a professional, legal and ethical responsibility to act on their findings. Irrespective of the practice setting, the woman—not clinicians or institutions or the woman's 'disease'—remains the primary focus of maternity care.

Many of the problems, challenges and complications considered in this chapter may be ones that the midwife, working in partnership with the woman, manages in a primary setting. However, when complications fall outside the scope of midwifery practice, midwives, still working in partnership with the woman, consult colleagues in a timely manner and work collaboratively with them to jointly manage secondary and tertiary levels of care.

Learning outcomes

Learning outcomes for this chapter are:

1   To describe the effects that complications in pregnancy have on the woman, her family, the pregnancy and the unborn baby

2   To discuss the pathophysiology, diagnosis, evidence for treatment of, and expected outcomes associated with, common complications in childbearing

3   To identify strategies to support women as they are challenged by and deal with the physical and psychological complications of 'high-risk' birthing.

Introduction

This chapter focuses on an exploration of the most common complications arising in pregnancy—some pre-exist pregnancy, others are exacerbated by pregnancy and a few occur de novo. All pose challenges for the parents and their unborn baby, and the clinicians' role is to ensure best practice and outcomes. This chapter cannot cover every complication, and so you are advised to use journals, the internet and others' expertise to expand on the knowledge and skills obtained from this text. This chapter builds on the philosophy, principles and actions of Chapter 20: Working with women in pregnancy, on the understanding that if a midwife is to understand the 'abnormal' she must first know the 'normal'. Chapter 20 makes the point that antenatal care consists of more than just a series of medical tests and monitoring procedures. In the same way, 'high-risk' antenatal care is not just about investigations, diagnoses, conditions and medical treatment, but is also about women from different ethnic, socio-economic and cultural backgrounds who, while pregnant, must still face common life stressors and at the same time deal with pregnancy complications and stressors, including anxiety and fear about their own and their baby's health and the wellbeing of their family. Thus midwifery care is also about supporting women as they make the uncertain journey towards birth, one sometimes complicated by obstacles that result in actual or potentially life-threatening situations. The complications discussed in this chapter include the specifics of hyperemesis gravidarum, bleeding, medical conditions, hypertension and multiple pregnancy, as well as the social and psychological variables that affect these conditions and their outcomes.

Vomiting in pregnancy

Morning sickness

Nausea and vomiting (morning sickness) is a common complication of pregnancy, occurring in approximately 80% of pregnant women. It usually begins between the fourth and seventh week and resolves by the sixteenth week of pregnancy without treatment. Between 0.05% and 2% of sufferers require hospitalisation. Morning sickness is often called a minor disorder of pregnancy, probably by clinicians who have never tried to care for small, non-toilet-trained children, cook nutritious meals and then travel to work via public transport for an efficient day at the office, while feeling very ill. Women with morning sickness are often expected to accomplish all these tasks and endure nausea and vomiting for weeks, sometimes months. It is little wonder that some women seek to end this misery by terminating the pregnancy.

Hyperemesis gravidarum

Hyperemesis gravidarum is a debilitating illness, affecting one in 200 pregnant women (Quinlan & Hill 2003), beginning at about the fourth week of pregnancy and usually improving by the twentieth week, although some women continue to have recurring periods of severe nausea and vomiting throughout the whole pregnancy. It is characterised by: persistent and intractable vomiting leading to fluid and electrolyte imbalance; marked ketonuria; and nutritional deficiency and rapid weight loss, often greater than 5%. The pathophysiology of nausea and vomiting in pregnancy and hyperemesis gravidarum is poorly understood but is likely to be multifactorial (Hyperemesis Education and Research (HER) Foundation 2004; Quinlan & Hill 2003). These are:

- elevated pregnancy hormones (e.g. human chorionic gonadotrophin (hCG), oestrogen and progesterone)—hCG levels are higher than usual in some conditions associated with hyperemesis and nausea and vomiting in pregnancy (molar pregnancy and multiple pregnancy)
- displacement of the gastrointestinal tract, delayed gastric emptying, lower oesophageal sphincter pressure and increased levels of hydrochloric acid
- autonomic nervous system disturbance related to the physiological changes in pregnancy in blood volume, temperature, heart rate and vascular resistance
- nutritional deficits (e.g. trace elements, vitamin B_6)
- liver dysfunction—however, it is possible that elevated liver function (bilirubin, aminotransferase and alkaline phosphatase) may be secondary to the condition rather than a cause of it
- lipid metabolism—a slow adaptation of the liver to the increased levels of hormones in pregnancy may cause hyperemesis gravidarum and result in abnormal levels of serum lipids and lipoproteins
- chronic infection with *Helicobacter pylori*—this may play a role in hyperemesis gravidarum (Hayakawa et al 2000)
- psychogenic factors (e.g. ambivalence or rejection of the pregnancy)
- high thyroxine levels—these may be associated with hyperemesis gravidarum.

The 5% of women who develop hyperemesis gravidarum are often offered little sympathy, let alone practical or effective solutions to a debilitating problem, one that has a major impact on their self-esteem and daily living activities and is therefore a condition of great significance to those who have it. There have been a number of explanations for this neglect, centering around clinicians' views about women, their nature and what is considered 'important'. In one study, Fairweather (1968) administered the Cornell Medical Index to 44 pregnant women with hyperemesis and 49 pregnant women without the condition. Inexplicably, the Minnesota

Critical thinking exercise

Using a physiology textbook (such as Stables & Rankin's *Physiology in Childbearing*), revise the structure and function of the 'pregnancy hormones' such as hCG, oestrogen and progesterone. Make sure you understand their relationship to hyperemesis gravidarum.

Multiphasic Personality Inventory (MMPI) was given only to the group with hyperemesis, making the findings meaningless, but saying a great deal about the researchers' beliefs about women in general and the mental health state of women with hyperemesis in particular. The results suggested that women with hyperemesis had hysteria, were overly dependent on their mothers and had infantile personalities. Despite the methodological weaknesses of studies such as this during the 1960s and 1970s, medical and midwifery students were taught that women with hyperemesis gravidarum were hysterics who were trying to eject their fetus by vomiting it out of their bodies. Forty years later, discussion with women with hyperemesis reveals that some clinicians have not moved beyond these ways of thinking.

Collaborative support for a woman with hyperemesis

When a pregnant woman contacts her midwife with a history of persistent vomiting for most of the day, is unable to tolerate fluids and voids only small amounts of concentrated urine, an immediate midwifery assessment is warranted. In severe cases the woman will be dehydrated, show signs of electrolyte imbalance, initially alkalosis from the loss of hydrochloric acid. Later, as her condition worsens, she will become acidotic and develop ketonuria, hypovolaemia, hypotension and tachycardia. Once any of these signs are observed, medical referral and hospital admission are indicated. The goals of treatment for hyperemesis gravidarum are to reverse the effects of fluid and weight loss and to provide emotional support for the woman, who must deal with the stress related to the hyperemesis.

It is important to consider and rule out other pregnancy and non-pregnancy-related causes such as pyelonephritis, drug toxicity, biliary tract and liver disease. Pregnancy-related differential diagnoses include multiple pregnancy or a hydatidiform mole. The woman needs support, understanding, and perhaps counselling, as well as education and advice about measures that can ameliorate the symptoms. Traditionally the treatment of hyperemesis has been supportive, with

---

WOMAN'S STORY

I am a successful career woman who wanted a baby very badly. After many years of infertility treatment, I became pregnant, and then the horror began. I so wanted to 'glow', like the books tell us we should. I was desperate to keep my baby safe but all I could do was stick my head in the toilet and chuck—all day, every day. I felt so helpless and out of control. There was I, a senior executive in a male-dominated, not overly sympathetic field. In the middle of meetings, I had to rush out, vomit in the loo and then come back and behave as though nothing had happened and then take up where I had left off. I needed to work, as money was very tight. I didn't want to take drugs but I knew that this persistent vomiting posed immense risks for my baby and me. A colleague, a nurse, told me that research showed that hyperemesis was all in the head and that I needed to calm down. I didn't need this! I was overwhelmed, guilty, anxious and so frustrated that I could not make myself stop vomiting—but I couldn't control it, no matter what I did. Eventually I found a doctor who believed me and, even better, acknowledged my misery, not that she could stop me vomiting. I took anti-emetics and they worked a bit but I still vomited all day, every day, week after week, month after month. I was so dehydrated that my doctor would admit me to hospital every Friday night for rehydration with IV fluids so that I could go to work on Monday. I did this for five months, and had a Caesarean section at 34 weeks. I love my baby but I can't go through that again, and so my son will have no siblings. It's sad, really. I come from a family of eight kids and I always thought that I would be like my sisters and just pop 'em out.

Critical thinking exercise

Francesca is 12 weeks pregnant. She comes to your clinic for her first antenatal check, and tells you that she vomits all day and 'can't keep anything down'.

Formulate questions for Francesca that will help you determine the severity of her nausea and vomiting, and the potential for hyperemesis gravidarum. Your questions should centre on:

▸ the frequency of vomiting
▸ risk factors
▸ pain or pyrexia
▸ tolerance of food and fluid.

Clinical point

Education for women with severe nausea and vomiting in pregnancy

▸ Eat a diet high in complex carbohydrates (such as bread, rice, potatoes) and protein, and low in fat.
▸ Drink plenty of fluids.
▸ Eat five to six small meals a day, including a late-evening snack. Low blood sugar can cause nausea and shakiness. Some women find sucking on hard sweets helpful.
▸ Try eating a small snack before getting up.
▸ Eat many small meals each day but avoid lying down immediately after eating.
▸ Get plenty of rest. Being overly tired can set off nausea.
▸ Consider taking ginger supplements.
▸ Limit stressful events.
▸ Avoid noxious odours that trigger vomiting, cigarette smoke and tastes that trigger nausea, such as coffee.
▸ Consider acupuncture or acupressure to assist in relieving nausea.

reassurance, dietary modifications and lifestyle changes, but there is no evidence of the benefits of such dietary modifications (Jewell & Young 2002).

Hospitalisation is usually required for hyperemesis gravidarum. All food and drink are stopped temporarily, to rest the digestive tract. Intravenous fluids and electrolytes are almost always needed to replace fluids and correct imbalances in electrolytes. A few women will require enteral or short-term total parenteral nutrition (TPN) via a PICC line but these should be last-resort treatments for pregnant women who continue to vomit and lose weight despite active treatment with less interventionist strategies. Both TPN and central venous access can result in significant complications, including sepsis. However, an advantage is that women can manage these therapies at home.

Since the thalidomide tragedy, anti-emetic therapy is generally reserved for those whose symptoms are so persistent and severe that they prevent daily activities and pose a threat to the safety of the mother and her unborn baby. Because of concerns about the teratogenic effects of drug treatment there have been relatively few studies on the efficacy and safety of anti-emetics used for nausea and vomiting in pregnancy.

Treatments

A Cochrane Review (Jewell & Young 2002) as well as a number of other reviews of a range of pharmaceutical and non-pharmaceutical treatments for nausea and vomiting have been published (Mazzotta & Magee 2000; Meltzer 2000; Moran & Taylor 2002; Nelson-Piercy et al 2001). In summary, these show that there is no firm evidence that the administration of pyridoxine (vitamin B_6) alone or with doxylamine has a clinically significant effect on severe vomiting in pregnancy. However, according to a Cochrane Review (Jewell & Young 2002), it may be the most effective drug with the fewest side-effects. Although steroid therapy may resolve nausea and vomiting in pregnancy, concern has been raised recently about a marginally increased risk of congenital malformations (Quinlan & Hill 2003). Anti-emetics such as promethazine are widely used and it is considered the drug of choice in pregnancy because it is the most-studied. Therapy should be stopped two weeks before birth, as withdrawal symptoms in the infant can occur. Although frequently used for the treatment of nausea and vomiting, no randomised controlled trials (RCTs) have been published to support the effectiveness of metoclopramide as a treatment for nausea and vomiting in pregnancy (Mazzotta & Magee 2000). Extrapyramidal reactions sometimes occur, particularly in young women. Similarly, no

---

Clinical point

For more in-depth information about hyperemesis gravidarum, see 'International consensus on standards for studying the efficacy of pharmacological therapies for nausea and vomiting of pregnancy' by Berkovitch et al (2001).

RCTs have investigated the effectiveness of domperidone to treat nausea and vomiting of pregnancy (Mazzotta & Magee 2000). Serotonin antagonists such as ondansetron (Zofran) have also been used to decrease stimulation to the vomiting centre in the brain, but as yet there is no evidence that this medication makes a significant difference to outcomes, although it is possible that it makes some women less sensitive to odours and movements, which are common triggers of bouts of vomiting (Mazzotta & Magee 2000).

Non-pharmaceutical treatments

Some women and clinicians doubt the safety and efficacy of pharmaceutical treatments for hyperemesis and regard complementary therapies as less toxic and more natural than synthetic remedies. It is therefore important for midwives to be knowledgeable about the evidence that supports their efficacy and, if they are to use them, are deemed competent to administer complementary therapies. Often fewer trial data exist for both safety and efficacy of complementary therapies than for drugs conventionally used to treat nausea and vomiting of pregnancy. In brief, ginger may reduce nausea and vomiting in pregnancy (Mazzotta & Magee 2000). According to Meltzer (2000) there is concern that ginger has an adverse effect on fetal brain development, and that by inhibiting thromboxane synthetase, ginger used in therapeutic quantities could increase bleeding in early pregnancy.

The acupuncture point most frequently used in traditional Chinese medicine for anti-emetic action is point 6 (P6) on the pericardium channel. Clinical trials on the use of acupressure and acupuncture including the use of Sea-Bands have not produced consistent results. A Cochrane Systematic Review (Jewell & Young 2002) showed that Neiguan point (P6) acupressure does have beneficial effects for nausea and vomiting in pregnancy. However, data from one of the largest RCTs were not included in the review, and this trial showed no benefit from acupressure (Jewell & Young 2002). Nevertheless, it has the advantage of being inexpensive and does not require consultation with the doctor or midwife.

Case reports of the efficacy of hypnosis, hypnotherapy, psychotherapy and behaviour modification on the treatment of hyperemesis have been published but as yet none have reported significant benefits (Jewell & Young 2002; Mazzotta & Magee 2000). Herbal remedies for nausea and vomiting in pregnancy, such as red raspberry or wild yam, have been used to treat hyperemesis, but again there is no evidence to support their efficacy or safety. Finally, there are no published trials regarding the efficacy of homeopathic remedies as a treatment for hyperemesis gravidarum.

Ongoing treatments

Left untreated, the woman with hyperemesis gravidarum may develop renal, neurological or hepatic damage. In severe cases, splenic avulsion, oesophageal rupture, peripheral neuropathy and pre-eclampsia as well as fetal intrauterine growth restriction and increased mortality occur (Quinlan & Hill 2003). Termination of pregnancy may be the woman's choice, especially if severe renal, neurological or hepatic

<table><tr><td>

BOX 33.1 Support for women with hyperemesis

Clinical support

Most sufferers with hyperemesis gravidarum (HG) require multiple admissions for each pregnancy. Women with HG are very miserable and deserve to be treated with great compassion. Extra measures that are beneficial, both physically and psychologically, are required to give comfort and relief. Intravenous fluids may be warmed before administration to avoid discomfort and calorie loss due to shivering. Warmed blankets will also help. If multiple IV sites are required it is important to use local anaesthetics and to use the most skilled personnel to site them, to avoid undue pain and scarring. A PICC line is useful if total parental nutrition is required.

Multiple intramuscular injections should be avoided because of muscle atrophy and general discomfort. It is important to minimise stimuli (light, noise and odours), as well as interruptions to the woman's rest. Occupational or physiotherapy consultations can be used to develop progressive exercise regimens that minimise muscle atrophy. Daily weigh-ins are unnecessary for women during extended hospital stays. Women with HG need the chance to express their feelings in an atmosphere of compassion and empathy. These feelings should be taken seriously, and the woman with HG needs to know that her midwife will do all she can to help her cope with the misery, stress and discomfort of HG.

HER Foundation

The Hyperemesis Education and Research (HER) Foundation is dedicated to those suffering from HG and those who have survived it. HER can be contacted at: http://www.hyperemesis.org.

(Source: adapted from HER 2005)

</td></tr></table>

involvement becomes apparent. If not, investigation of other associated factors causing hyperemesis gravidarum, such as multiple gestation or hydatidiform mole, are required. Social and financial assistance is often required to help the woman care for herself and her other children, especially if she cannot work until this incapacitating condition is resolved.

Bleeding in pregnancy

Any bleeding in early pregnancy—that is, the first or second trimester—is considered a threatened or an actual miscarriage (abortion) until proved otherwise. A miscarriage can be an intensely sad and frightening experience for everyone. A pregnancy that seemed normal suddenly ends, leaving the expectant parents devastated. About 20% of women with clinically diagnosed pregnancies will experience bleeding at some time in early pregnancy (Bryan 2003). Overall, up to 50% of all pregnancies end in miscarriage although many more losses occur before a woman realises she is pregnant (ACOG 2001). Of these, about 20% of recognised pregnancies end in an actual miscarriage (Bryan 2003).

Definition and classification

For most women, pregnancy loss is associated with emotions of fear, grief, guilt and sorrow, and the feeling that their body has failed them. The traditional, medical term for a miscarriage is 'spontaneous abortion', but such language should be avoided. Terminology such as 'spontaneous abortion', 'habitual abortion' and 'pregnancy failure', or 'abnormal pregnancy', may exacerbate the negative self-perceptions that women already may have—a sense of failure, even shame, guilt and insecurity. Midwives need to be aware of the language they use when talking to women and ensure that it is acceptable to both the woman and her midwife. When unsure, it is preferable to adopt the language the woman uses. The use of a common language is a step towards offering positive support for women.

There are many confusing terms and moments that accompany a miscarriage. It is best considered a process rather than an event, but for ease of understanding, the different 'types' of miscarriage are presented here as separate entities.

Threatened miscarriage (abortion)

Vaginal bleeding (spotting) before the twentieth week of pregnancy and possibly accompanied by low back or abdominal pain are usually the first signs of a threatened miscarriage. The amount of bleeding and the presence of pain have little predictive value in terms of the viability of the pregnancy (Bryan 2003). Women experiencing a threatened miscarriage have an approximately 85% chance that the pregnancy will progress to term. The bleeding is usually self-limiting, and is sometimes attributed to trophoblastic implantation within the endometrium rather than a miscarriage per se. On examination, the cervix remains closed, the uterus is soft and non-tender and of appropriate size for gestational age.

Inevitable (imminent) miscarriage

When vaginal bleeding and cramping persist and are accompanied by dilatation of the internal os or rupture of the fetal membranes, a miscarriage is inevitable. Bleeding is usually more severe than with a threatened miscarriage and is often associated with mild to moderate uterine contractions.

Complete miscarriage

In a complete miscarriage, the products of conception are expelled. Women report a history of vaginal bleeding,

<table><tr><td>

BOX 33.2 Miscarriage support

Miscarriage Support Auckland Inc. (http://www.miscarriagesupport.org.nz/support.html, www.sandsvic.org.au/services.html) is a team of volunteers who have all experienced the loss of a baby. Sharing their experience with others has assisted many women with the grieving progress and set them on the road to healing. This can be via the internet on the Bulletin Board at www.everybody.co.nz/bulletinboard.html (or via email at support@miscarriagesupport.org.nz).

</td></tr></table>

abdominal pain, and passing tissue (products of conception). Once miscarriage is completed, the bleeding and pain usually subside, the uterus contracts and the cervix closes. A completed miscarriage can be confirmed visually, by an ultrasound showing an empty uterus with close apposition of relatively thin and regular endometrial interfaces. Urine or serum β-hCG values will be falling or below the discriminatory threshold levels determined by the healthcare service.

Incomplete miscarriage

An incomplete miscarriage is more likely to occur between 6 and 14 weeks of pregnancy. Bleeding and pain may persist if the miscarriage is not completed, and this increases the risk of infection. Vaginal bleeding is usually heavy and accompanied by increasingly severe uterine contractions. The cervical os is open. The woman may say that she has passed fetal or placental fragments. Ultrasonography may reveal that some products of conception are still present in the uterus; these typically appear as echogenic material.

Silent or delayed miscarriage (missed abortion, blood mole, carneous mole or stony/fleshy mole)

Women can experience a miscarriage without knowing it. In a silent (missed) miscarriage, the fetus has died but is retained in the uterus. Uterine and breast growth cease and the woman may report vaginal 'spotting' or a brown, sometimes offensive, vaginal discharge. With widespread use of transvaginal ultrasonography, a silent miscarriage (presence of a non-viable fetus) or an anembryonic pregnancy (absent fetal echo) are now believed to reflect different aspects or stages of the same clinical process. A blighted ovum (anembryonic pregnancy) occurs when a fertilised egg implants into the uterine wall but fetal development does not begin. Often there is a gestational sac with or without a yolk sac, but there is an absence of fetal growth. Chromosomal abnormalities are a common cause of an anembryonic pregnancy. The woman may notice that her pregnancy symptoms have stopped and she may develop dark-brown vaginal bleeding. Diagnosis is confirmed by the woman's story, physical examination, laboratory tests and ultrasonography. Blood and urine tests will show a drop in β-hCG levels or a negative over-the-counter pregnancy test. An ultrasound examination shows early evidence of an intrauterine pregnancy but only an empty pregnancy sac. The miscarriage may not be completed for weeks and this may lead to fetal autolysis, which results in the release of thromboplastin and disseminated intravascular coagulation.

Molar pregnancy (gestational trophoblastic disease)

Following a silent miscarriage, a few women develop gestational trophoblastic disease. This term covers a spectrum of disorders characterised by abnormal and rapid growth of trophoblastic tissue, ranging from a molar pregnancy (hydatidiform mole) to a malignant choriocarcinoma. Trophoblastic disease is rare, occurring in 1 out of every 1000 pregnancies, but the condition varies between regions and age groups. The reasons for these geographic and age differences are unknown but may be related to poor nutrition, particularly a low intake of carotene (vitamin A precursor). The main risk factor for a molar pregnancy is advanced maternal age—women over 40 have a five- to ten-fold greater chance of a molar pregnancy. In addition, women who have had a prior molar pregnancy have a 1:100 chance of having another in a subsequent pregnancy.

Complete and partial molar pregnancies (hydatidiform moles)

Molar pregnancies are the result of a genetic error during fertilisation and comprise two distinct entities. Irrespective of whether they are complete or partial, a molar pregnancy poses a threat to the woman not only because it produces an abnormal pregnancy, but also because it may cause life-threatening complications. A complete mole differs from a partial one according to chromosomal patterns, karotype, gross and microscopic histopathology and clinical presentation. Complete moles arise from the fertilisation of an 'empty egg'—one that has lost its maternal genetic material. There is no embryo and no normal placental tissue. However, the placenta continues to grow and produces β-hCG, so the woman thinks and feels that she is pregnant. A complete mole demonstrates a characteristic vesicular pattern (resembling a bunch of grapes). However, in a partial mole, there may be some normal placental tissue and the embryo, although abnormal, begins to develop. A partial mole has duplicate paternal genetic material, although the maternal chromosomal complement is intact, so the genetic material is in triplicate. Therefore the embryo has 69 chromosomes instead of the normal 46. The fetus nearly always dies in utero.

Signs of a molar pregnancy

A molar pregnancy begins like a normal pregnancy and may entail common symptoms of pregnancy, including a missed period, positive pregnancy test and nausea. From about the 10th week of pregnancy, most women with a complete molar pregnancy experience vaginal bleeding that is dark brown in colour, and may pass vesicular tissue. These symptoms usually

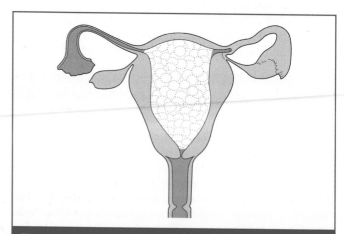

Figure 33.1 Molar pregnancy: a grapelike cluster of tissue (called a hydatidiform mole) forms around the area that normally would become the placenta, and may cause life-threatening complications.

mimic those of a miscarriage, although about 50% of women with a complete mole have uterine enlargement that is too advanced for the expected gestational age. Pre-eclampsia may develop before the 20th week of pregnancy. A few women have signs of hyperthyroidism: tachycardia, tremulousness, and feeling excessively warm.

Women with partial molar pregnancies in general have fewer symptoms and so their condition is often only confirmed following histological examination after treatment for a silent or inevitable miscarriage. They rarely have abnormally excessive uterine enlargement, hyperthyroidism or pre-eclampsia. Occasionally the fetus survives beyond 16 weeks and diagnosis is confirmed by the appearance of the placenta on ultrasound.

Medical diagnosis of a molar pregnancy

The gold standard of diagnosis remains the characteristic vesicular appearance of the placenta on ultrasound scan, typically a 'cluster of grapes' or a 'snowstorm' appearance (see Fig 33.1). Initially levels of β-hCG although not diagnostic are often higher than normal with a complete mole, but lower than normal with a partial mole.

Septic (infected) miscarriage

In a septic miscarriage, the fetus has died and the products of conception have become infected. Septic abortion was once a leading cause of maternal death across the world, and still is in countries where termination of pregnancy is illegal. The risk of death from an infected miscarriage rises with advancing gestation. If not treated, the infection may spread further into the myometrium and parametrium and cause peritonitis. The woman may develop generalised septicaemia and will require aggressive antibiotic therapy. Pelvic inflammatory disease (PID) and infertility are common long-term complications of this life-threatening disorder.

Recurrent pregnancy loss (habitual abortion)

While miscarriage is usually a one-time occurrence, about 1–2% of couples have two, three or more consecutive miscarriages (Hogge 2003). If three consecutive pregnancies end in miscarriage, the couple require referral to an obstetrician and probably a fertility specialist in an effort to determine the cause of the recurrent pregnancy loss. Possible causes for recurrent miscarriage are chromosomal or other genetic abnormality, progesterone deficiency, infection, uterine abnormality, cervical 'incompetence' or systemic disease. Any miscarriage is distressing for the parents but recurrent miscarriages are devastating, especially if it is not possible to identify a cause and therefore a 'cure'. Parents need to know that despite the battery of tests usually ordered during investigation of recurrent miscarriage, only 50% of couples will be given an answer for their inability to carry a live baby beyond two trimesters (ACOG 2001).

Implantation bleeding

It is commonly believed, even among health professionals, that as the trophoblast implants into the endometrial layer

---

BOX 33.3   Signs of infected miscarriage

Any woman of childbearing age presenting with fever, tachycardia, abdominal pain, vaginal discharge or bleeding should be evaluated for a possible septic miscarriage. Immediate referral to a medical practitioner is warranted.

Warning signs include:

- history of recent pregnancy
- pyrexia and general malaise
- abdominal pain
- vaginal discharge which may be purulent
- vaginal bleeding.

---

of the uterus, bleeding can sometimes occur and escape from the uterine cavity into the vagina—hence the term implantation bleeding (Harville et al 2003). However, Harville et al (2003) found no evidence that implantation causes vaginal bleeding. Vaginal loss is usually light and occurs a few days before menstruation would have been due and is probably a threatened miscarriage. Women may mistake this bleeding for menstruation, particularly if they normally experience minimal blood loss. It is therefore important for the midwife to take an accurate menstrual history that enables her and the woman to eliminate miscalculations in the estimated birth date.

Decidual bleeding

During pregnancy, menstruation ceases. Occasionally, however, there is a slight blood loss from the decidua in the first 10 weeks of pregnancy, usually at the time the period would be due. Decidual bleeding may be mistaken for a menstrual period and affect the accuracy of estimations of the expected birth date. Most pregnancies will proceed without further complication.

Causes of miscarriage

The causes of miscarriage are not thoroughly understood and clinicians are frequently unable to give grieving parents a precise response to questions about why the miscarriage occurred. Up to 70% of first-trimester miscarriages are caused by fetal chromosomal abnormalities (Hogge 2003). These become more common with increased maternal age, and women over the age of 35 are at much higher risk of miscarriage than younger women. There is good evidence that auto-immune diseases play a significant role in miscarriage. Autoantibodies associated with repeated miscarriage include anticardiolipin antibodies, which are associated with thrombo-embolic disorders. Studies suggest that this and related antiphospholipid antibodies cause between 3% and 15% of repeat miscarriages (ACOG 2001). In addition, a Factor V Leiden mutation, which affects blood clotting, may also play a role in repeat miscarriages (ACOG 2001).

Acute and chronic infectious diseases are well documented as causative factors in miscarriage. Bacterial vaginosis is the most common genital infection among women of reproductive age.

The US-based Centers for Disease Control (CDC) estimates that as many as 16% of pregnant women have bacterial vaginosis (CDC 2004). Although having a new sex partner or multiple partners increases the chances of infection, the exact role that sexual activity plays in the infection is unclear. A recent study found that women with bacterial vaginosis were nine times more likely to have a miscarriage than uninfected women (Leitich et al 2003). Young women of childbearing age are increasingly infected with *Chlamydia trachomatis* but as the research box below shows, the precise relationship between genital infection and early and late miscarriage is still unclear. Numerous other microbial organisms have been blamed for miscarriage, such as cytomegalovirus (CMV), herpes simplex virus (HSV), rubella, parvovirus, *Treponema pallidum* and HIV. CMV is a common viral infection of the herpes family. It is transmitted through blood, saliva, breast milk and other bodily fluids. Between 40% and 85% of people are infected with CMV during their lifetime, but most do not have any symptoms.

Chronic illnesses

Chronic illnesses, including diabetes, severe hypertension, kidney disease and auto-immune diseases, are frequent causes of miscarriage. Other postulated causative factors include low progesterone levels and thyroid dysfunction as well as anatomic defects, such as a septate or bicornuate uterus or uterine fibroids. Finally, environmental hazards (exposure to cigarette smoke, formaldehyde, pesticides), exposure to anaesthetic gases, chemotherapy and trauma are associated with miscarriage, as are maternal illness and dietary deficiencies.

Research

Association between bacterial vaginosis or chlamydial infection and miscarriage before 16 weeks gestation: prospective community-based cohort study (Oakeshott et al 2002).

The objective of this UK study was to assess whether bacterial vaginosis or chlamydial infection is associated with early miscarriage (before 16 weeks). Of the 1201 women in the study, 14.5% had bacterial vaginosis. The infection was more common in participants who: were under 25, of Afro-Caribbean or black African ethnicity, from social classes 3–5, single, and had previously used oral contraception or none, and smoked during pregnancy; and those with a history of termination of pregnancy and who had a concurrent chlamydial infection. Compared with women who were negative for bacterial vaginosis, women who were positive had a relative risk of miscarriage before 16 weeks gestation of 1.2 (0.7 to 1.9). Only 29 women had a chlamydial infection, one of whom miscarried. The authors concluded that, at least in this study, bacterial vaginosis was not strongly predictive of early miscarriage. Therefore, early screening and treatment of asymptomatic bacterial vaginosis are unlikely to improve first-trimester miscarriage rates.

In summary

Many of these factors are summarised in Box 33.4. However, in many cases there is no obvious cause of early reproductive losses. Pregnancies that proceed following a threatened miscarriage have an increased risk of complications and poor outcome compared to pregnancies where there is no bleeding (Bryan 2003).

Management of early pregnancy loss

The following summary of 'best-practice' recommendations for the collaborative management for early pregnancy loss is based on the Royal College of Obstetricians and Gynaecologists' Green Top Guidelines (RCOG 2001).

Early pregnancy assessment units

The RCOG guidelines recommend that all maternity centres provide an early pregnancy assessment service with direct access for women, midwives and medical personnel. A

BOX 33.4 Bleeding in early pregnancy

- Implantation bleeding
- Decidual bleeding
- Miscarriage
- Ectopic pregnancy
- Termination of pregnancy
- General maternal causes:
  — chronic maternal disease
  — infection (bacterial vaginosis)
  — hormonal deficiencies
  — nutritional deficiency
  — poorly controlled diabetes
  — thyroid disease
  — auto-immune disease—systemic lupus erythematosus
- Local maternal causes:
  — weakened cervix
  — abnormally shaped uterus
  — rarely a retroverted gravid uterus
  — polycystic ovary syndrome
- Other maternal causes:
  — lifestyle factors (smoking, illicit and licit drug and alcohol abuse)
  — environmental and workplace hazards
  — increased maternal age
- Hydatidiform mole
- Cervical pathology:
  — dysplasia
  — polyp
  — carcinoma
- Vaginal bleeding from non-pregnant horn of a bicornuate uterus
- Urinary tract infection
- Haemorrhoids
- Ruptured vulval varicosities

dedicated early pregnancy assessment unit (EPAU) can streamline the management of women with early pregnancy bleeding or pain and thus improve the quality of care, in the presence of a supportive, multidisciplinary team (Bigrigg & Read 1991). An effective EPAU requires:

- an efficient appointments system
- an appropriate setting (with an area for counselling)
- up-to-date ultrasound equipment (including transvaginal probes)
- easy access to laboratory facilities (for Rhesus antibody testing and selective serum β-hCG estimation)
- effective systems of communication facilitated by standardised referral and discharge letters.

Collaborative care

In many cases, and if the bleeding is not severe, women prefer to wait at home, supported by their midwife, 'to see what happens' rather than attend the local hospital or EPAU. In most cases, the woman spontaneously passes the products of conception. There are three different management options for women with an incomplete miscarriage:

- surgical evacuation
- medical therapy
- expectant treatment.

According to Bryan (2003) the choice of management options depends largely on the clinicians' and woman's preferences. However, in a partially randomised study comparing surgical and medical evacuation, 20% of women expressed a strong preference for medical management (Hinshaw 1997). The main reasons given for their choice was that they wanted to avoid general anaesthesia and felt more in control of the procedure and outcomes.

Since the 1800s, when illegal abortion was common and antibiotics were unavailable, surgical uterine evacuation (dilatation and curettage) has been the standard treatment offered to all women who have miscarried. This decision was based on the assumption that retained tissue increased the risks of infection and therefore haemorrhage and sometimes death. In recent years, with the advent of technology such as transvaginal sonography (TVS) (Bryan 2003), clinicians have questioned the need for surgical evacuation of the uterus for all women who miscarry. The consensus is that in women in whom no retained products of conception are detected by TVS, the complication rate from dilatation and curettage is higher than in women in whom no operative intervention is made and therefore a conservative approach to management is preferable (Bryan 2003). Thus a curettage is no longer considered mandatory but may be required if the woman is bleeding heavily or has an infection, or if an ultrasound examination shows that there is placental tissue remaining in the uterus.

Studies of the efficacy of the antiprogestogen mifepristone or the prostaglandin analogue misoprostol for the medical management of incomplete miscarriage (Beal & Simmonds 2002; Forna & Gulmezoglu 2004) show that these therapies are beneficial for ripening the cervix and encouraging uterine contractions and, therefore, expulsion of the pregnancy.

Clinical point

Referral to a medical centre
Most women who have an early miscarriage do not need medical treatment, although they always need supportive care. However, if vaginal bleeding is heavy, there is pyrexia, tachycardia or bradycardia and hypotension, if products of conception have been passed, or if there is severe abdominal pain, the woman must be referred for immediate gynaecological assessment. The possibility of ectopic pregnancy should always be considered if a woman in early pregnancy complains of abdominal pain or exhibits signs of peritoneal irritation.

Nevertheless, Bryan (2003) points out that misoprostol offers no advantage over either the surgical or expectant management option, mostly because of the high incidence of gastrointestinal side-effects. Expectant (conservative) management is also an accepted management alternative. Irrespective of the choice of technique used to empty the uterus, tissue obtained at the time of miscarriage should be examined histologically to confirm pregnancy and to exclude other complications such as ectopic pregnancy and gestational trophoblastic disease.

Women who miscarry should:

- be offered the opportunity to attend for follow-up care, possibly with EPAU staff or the lead carer in the community (midwife, GP or obstetrician)
- have plans for follow-up clearly recorded in the discharge letter from the EPAU to the lead carer
- be informed that they can expect a grief reaction
- be informed that lactation may need to be suppressed
- be given the contact details of their local miscarriage support group
- understand that it may take weeks to a month or more to recover physically from a miscarriage, which may be considerably longer than the time other family members think the woman needs to recover
- know that they will probably experience a menstrual period four to six weeks after the miscarriage.

Clinical point

Retained products of conception
During an incomplete miscarriage, products of conception may be caught in the cervix, causing profound vagal stimulation, bradycardia and shock. If this is suspected, the woman needs urgent hospital admission. Removal of retained products of conception will lead to rapid clinical improvement and reduction in bleeding. Any tissue passed should accompany the woman to hospital.

Clinical point

According to Weinberg (2001), approximately 4% of women who have a miscarriage will have a transplacental haemorrhage of > 0.2 mL of fetal red blood cells. Since the late 1960s, anti-D immunoglobulin has been used successfully for Rhesus prophylaxis. Non-sensitised Rhesus (Rh)-negative women should be offered anti-D immunoglobulin in the following situations: ectopic pregnancy; all threatened or diagnosed miscarriages over 12 weeks; all miscarriages; and when the uterus has been surgically evacuated. Sensitisation can occur after a transplacental haemorrhage of < 0.1 mL and so there is a potential for sensitisation in pregnancies of less than 12 weeks gestation, although research has yet to confirm this suspicion. Currently, the routine administration of anti-D immunoglobulin is not recommended in threatened miscarriages below 12 weeks gestation or if the fetus is viable. However, if the bleeding is heavy or associated with abdominal pain, Rhesus D sensitisation is more likely to occur. Weinberg's UK study (2001) shows that many women who present to emergency departments with a threatened miscarriage such that there is an increased risk of Rhesus D isoimmunisation were not offered anti-D immunoglobulin. Discharge documentation should always clearly state whether or not anti-D immunoglobulin was offered, given, and by whom.

Collaborative management of a molar pregnancy

A molar pregnancy is a very frightening experience. Not only does the woman lose a pregnancy, but she also learns that she has a risk, albeit a slight one, of developing trophoblastic disease and perhaps metastatic choriocarcinoma, a fast-growing but rare malignant growth of the chorion. In order to protect the woman, all molar tissue must be removed from the uterus. In the first trimester this is usually done with suction curettage, sometimes followed by surgical curettage, under general anaesthesia. In the second trimester, uterine stimulation with prostaglandin E_2 and oxytocin before surgical evacuation to avoid uterine perforation and severe haemorrhage are often recommended.

Occasionally, when the mole is extensive and the woman has decided against future pregnancies, she may choose a hysterectomy.

Follow-up

All women who have had a molar pregnancy are followed up regularly for the next one to two years for regular β-hCG urine tests, because molar pregnancies can recur, and to ensure that no chorionic tissue remains in the uterus because of the risk of choriocarcinoma. Follow-up consists of a baseline chest X-ray, review of the pathology specimen, and regular physical examinations of the uterus until it returns to normal size, then three-monthly check-ups for at least a year. Most importantly, to ensure no chorionic tissue remains in the uterus, the woman is advised to have weekly β-hCG levels until there are two consecutive zero results. For the next 12 months, levels are taken every month for the first six months and second-monthly for the following six months. Waiting one or two years before attempting another pregnancy is important, because a rise in β-hCG levels may indicate a normal pregnancy but may also indicate a recurrent molar pregnancy. Some physicians recommend prophylactic chemotherapy as well as or instead of the usual follow-up but this remains controversial (Khoo 2003). Chemotherapy regimens using low doses of methotrexate and folinic acid have improved survival rates.

As the pregnant woman undergoes diagnosis and treatment for a molar pregnancy, she may be concerned mainly about her own health and survival. Afterwards, she and her partner feel relief that she has come through the ordeal. Grief over the loss of the pregnancy may not become apparent for some time. As with any couple whose unborn baby has died, the family needs time to grieve and to recover emotionally. If a woman has a molar pregnancy, her outlook for a future successful pregnancy is good. It is important for women to undergo regular ultrasound in subsequent pregnancies to confirm normal fetal and placental development. The placenta is sent to the pathologist after the birth to make sure there are no abnormalities.

Emotional recovery from early pregnancy loss

The comprehensive management of pregnancy loss will be enhanced by psychological support and follow-up counselling (Boyce et al 2002). This can be provided by the woman's lead carer, who can address medical as well as psychological issues. All clinicians should be aware of the psychological sequelae associated with miscarriage and be prepared to provide support and follow-up, as well as access to a counsellor who is experienced in dealing with pregnancy loss. For some couples, a miscarriage causes both severe and protracted distress at a level not appreciated by all professionals involved.

The purpose of follow-up counselling, according to Boyce et al (2002), is to:

- allow open discussion about the loss, monitor progress and counsel the woman about future pregnancies
- provide an opportunity for her to talk about her loss and have her grieving acknowledged
- provide information about the normal grief process. This may help a woman who is masking her grief or does not believe it is legitimate.
- facilitate the grief process by enabling the woman to talk about feelings of guilt and self-blame, particularly when there is no medical explanation for her loss
- provide an opportunity for the woman and her family to discuss their dissatisfaction, if there is any, with their care, as the woman may feel angry and blame her medical practitioner for her loss.

Often women want to know how long they must wait after a miscarriage before attempting another pregnancy.

The response to this question is that the couple should not attempt another pregnancy until the woman is physically and emotionally ready and they have completed any tests recommended to determine the cause of the miscarriage. Clinicians often advise the couple to wait until the woman has had one normal menstrual cycle but it may take considerably longer before she is ready to attempt pregnancy, especially if there has been a molar pregnancy. Many women who have experienced miscarriage worry that they will miscarry again. Fortunately, the great majority of women will go on to have a subsequent successful pregnancy.

Ectopic pregnancy

An ectopic pregnancy occurs if a fertilised ovum implants at a site other than the endometrial lining of the uterus, most commonly in a fallopian tube, although ovarian, cervical and abdominal pregnancies are also possible. The incidence of ectopic pregnancy is estimated to be 1 in 200–500 pregnancies but is increasing (Tay et al 2000). The rise is greatest in women over 35 years of age. The diagnosis of ectopic pregnancy can now be made by non-invasive methods due to sensitive pregnancy tests (in urine and serum) and high-resolution TVS. Improvements and greater efficiency in diagnosis have resulted in a range of both conservative and radical treatment options. Nevertheless ectopic pregnancies are still a major cause of maternal morbidity and mortality and remain the leading cause of pregnancy-related maternal deaths in the first trimester. Most deaths result from delayed diagnosis, and inappropriate investigation and treatment.

Pathophysiology

Normally the fertilised ovum travels along the fallopian tube to the uterus via the peristaltic action of the cilia. In an ectopic pregnancy there is a delay in the passage of the ovum to the uterus, commonly due to previous tubal infection (salpingitis), which destroys the cilia that propel the blastocyst to the endometrium. Instead the blastocyst embeds in the epithelium of the fallopian tube, burrowing into blood vessels in the same way that it does in a normal implantation, and continues to develop and increase in size. This is known as a tubal pregnancy. Depending on which part of the fallopian tube the embryo has embedded in, the tube will either rupture between five and seven weeks gestation because the fallopian tube cannot stretch to accommodate the growing pregnancy, or alternatively, it is expelled from the fimbriated end of the fallopian tube into the peritoneal cavity at eight to ten weeks gestation (a tubal abortion). In both cases bleeding surrounding the embryo usually results in its demise. Rarely, transmigration of the ovum and/or sperm may occur, so that the ectopic occurs in the fallopian tube contra-laterally to the corpus luteum. Occasionally when the embryo dies it is retained within the fallopian tube surrounded by layers of blood clot, which blocks the fallopian tube, resulting in a tubal mole or haematosalpinx, similar to a uterine molar pregnancy. The 'tubal mole' may remain in the fallopian tube or be expelled as a tubal abortion.

Risks for ectopic pregnancy

Ectopics are primarily associated with an earlier tubal infection or structural abnormalities that obstruct or slow the passage of the blastocyst as it passes through the fallopian tube to the uterus where it embeds in the endometrium. Up to 50% of women with ectopic pregnancies have a medical history of salpingitis or pelvic inflammatory disease (PID). Women who have had surgery to reverse previous tubal sterilisation in order to become pregnant also have an increased risk of ectopic pregnancy when reversal is successful. In some cases, the cause is unknown. Ectopic pregnancy is more common in women with a history of:

- infertility
- endometriosis
- congenital fallopian tube abnormalities
- sexually transmitted infections (these can cause infection and scarring in the pelvis)
- previous tubal infection or surgery
- intrauterine contraceptive devices (IUCDs)
- oral contraception.

It should be remembered that the last two risks only refer to the tiny proportion of women who become pregnant while using IUCDs or when taking oral contraceptives—they do not refer to all women who have in the past used these methods and later became pregnant. Of note is that the 'morning-after pill' is associated with a ten-fold increase in ectopic pregnancy, but again this risk refers only to the proportion of women who become pregnant in spite of taking

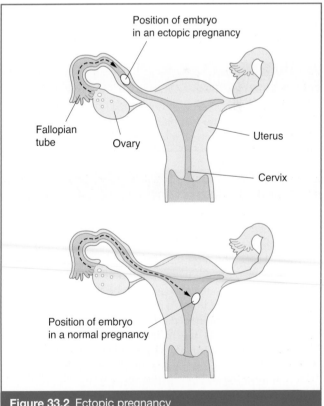

Figure 33.2 Ectopic pregnancy

the medication, rather than to women who in the past have used the drugs.

Clinical presentation

Most ectopic pregnancies are diagnosed before they rupture. Tay and colleagues (2000) state that diagnosis can be difficult and can be confused with signs of miscarriage, an ovarian cyst or PID.

In the initial stages of an ectopic pregnancy although the fertilised ovum embeds into the fallopian tube, the uterus still undergoes the normal changes of early pregnancy, and so the woman experiences the normal symptoms of pregnancy.

Tubal rupture is rarely sudden and so women who present to hospital in severe shock usually report warning signs that have been overlooked. Typically the woman presents with non-specific signs similar to those of a threatened miscarriage, but unlike miscarriage the woman complains of lower abdominal pain that precedes bleeding. On examination, abdominal pain and rigidity and rebound tenderness are palpated. These signs, especially if they are accompanied by vaginal bleeding, which may be minimal or torrential, together with signs of haemodynamic compromise/shock—hypotension, tachycardia, pallor, cold clammy skin, faintness and vomiting—should always alert the lead carer to the possibility of a ruptured ectopic pregnancy. In addition, shoulder-tip pain may be present, or pain may be referred to an iliac fossa. A mass may be felt to one side of the uterus. Any woman presenting with these signs requires immediate transfer to hospital and specialist consultation. If the clinical diagnosis is still unclear, an ultrasound scan will confirm or exclude the presence of an extrauterine gestational sac and occasionally a viable fetus.

Clinical point

Up to 9% of women with an ectopic pregnancy report no pain even if the fallopian tube is close to rupturing, and 36% lack adnexal tenderness (Tay et al 2000).

Clinical point

Always consider the possibility of ectopic pregnancy in women of childbearing age with abdominal pain. A sexually active woman with abdominal pain and vaginal bleeding after an interval of amenorrhoea has an ectopic pregnancy until proved otherwise! If there is no history of a missed period, check whether the last period was normal in duration and blood loss. The index of suspicion rises if the woman reports a history of infertility, has missed a period while using an IUCD or has been sterilised. Always ask about contraception use and remember that not all women admit to being sexually active. Others may not be aware that they are pregnant.

Incidence and rate of presenting signs of ectopic pregnancy

Tay and colleagues (2000, p 916) list the following frequencies the signs of ectopic pregnancy:

- abdominal pain (97%)
- vaginal bleeding (79%)
- abdominal tenderness (91%)
- adnexal tenderness (54%)
- history of infertility (15%)
- use of an IUCD (14%)
- previous ectopic pregnancy (11%).

Laboratory studies

Serial β-hCG levels vary in ectopic pregnancy, but compared to a uterine pregnancy the levels rise more slowly than expected and usually plateau at about six weeks gestation. Evaluating test results is complicated by the fact that at least two laboratory reporting standards are still in common use: International Reference Preparation (IRP) and the Second International Standard (2IS). IRP values are approximately twice the value of the 2IS values (Botash & Spirt 2000). Although β-hCG levels and their rate of increase may vary, a negative test result effectively excludes the diagnosis of an intra- or extrauterine pregnancy. In contrast, a positive result is highly suggestive of pregnancy. Serial testing is usually needed:

- to differentiate from a completed miscarriage
- for women in whom ultrasonography examinations are inconclusive
- to determine whether the β-hCG has reached a plateau.

A positive serum β-hCG test in combination with ultrasonographic evidence of an intrauterine pregnancy is strongly suggestive of an ectopic pregnancy or a recent miscarriage. Serum creatine kinase levels have been advocated as another marker of ectopic pregnancy but are now rejected because of their inadequate diagnostic sensitivity (Darai et al 1996).

Imaging studies

Serum β-hCG levels are most helpful if they are performed in conjunction with ultrasonography. The usefulness of ultrasound in general and TVS in particular are well documented in the assessment and diagnosis of early pregnancy complications. According to Tenore (2000), compared with abdominal ultrasonography, TVS diagnoses intrauterine pregnancies on average one week earlier because it is more sensitive and has a lower discriminatory zone. Once the β-hCG level is > 1500–2000 mIU per mL, an intrauterine pregnancy should be visible on TVS. An intrauterine pregnancy is

---

BOX 33.5 Warning signs

Warning signs of fallopian tube rupture:
- severe, sharp and sudden pain in the lower abdominal area
- feeling faint or fainting in the presence of significant bleeding
- signs of haemodynamic compromise/shock
- referred pain to the neck and shoulders.

confirmed when a gestational sac with a sonolucent centre (> 5 mm in diameter) surrounded by a thick, concentric, echogenic ring located within the endometrium and containing a fetal pole, yolk sac, or both, is visible. A probable abnormal intrauterine pregnancy is diagnosed when gestational sac > 10 mm in diameter is present without a fetal pole or when a definite fetal pole is present without cardiac activity (Tenore 2000). Finally, on ultrasound an ectopic pregnancy is characterised by the presence of a thick, brightly echogenic, ring-like structure lying outside the uterus together with a gestational sac containing an obvious fetal pole, yolk sac, or both (Tenore 2000).

Confirmation of an ectopic pregnancy

The absence of an intrauterine gestational sac on abdominal ultrasound in conjunction with a β-hCG level of greater than 6500 mIU per mL suggests the presence of an ectopic pregnancy. The ultrasound scan results combined with serial β-hCG levels > 6500 mIU per mL that do not double in 48 hours usually confirm the diagnosis.

Laparoscopy

Laparoscopy can be used for both diagnosis and treatment of ectopic gestation, although the diagnosis is missed in 2–4% of women who have very small ectopic gestations.

Collaborative management of a woman with an ectopic pregnancy

A woman presenting with classic signs of a ruptured ectopic pregnancy needs rapid transfer to an appropriate health facility with the resources to support a critically ill, shocked patient. High flow oxygen is commenced and venous access obtained before transport or en route for cross-matching of blood and to administer intravenous (IV) fluids to maintain the radial pulse and blood pressure. However, no intervention should hinder transfer to expert medical care. The receiving unit is alerted so that immediate resuscitation followed by surgery occurs on arrival.

On arrival at the medical facility, treatment consists of resuscitation followed by immediate surgery, possibly with laparoscopy, to remove the blood and blood clot and to stop the bleeding. It is often necessary to remove the fallopian tube.

Medical management of an ectopic pregnancy

Medical or expectant management with methotrexate is possible but only with haemodynamically stable women who have had minimal bleeding or pain, have no evidence of

---

tubal rupture, and have a β-hCG level below 1000 and falling (Hajenius et al 2005). Methotrexate is an antimetabolite that inhibits the synthesis of DNA and RNA, thus decreasing cell proliferation. According to Bryan (2003), medical management with methotrexate has a success rate of 75–96%, with best outcomes in small ectopic pregnancies with lower initial β-hCG levels. Gazvani and colleagues (1998) found that unruptured tubal pregnancies resolve faster in women given methotrexate in combination with mifepristone, compared to methotrexate only. Not all authors are as enthusiastic about

---

Clinical point

The ABC of all primary resuscitative efforts hold true for a woman in shock from a ruptured ectopic pregnancy. If the radial pulse is palpable, the blood pressure can be assumed to be adequate. If it is not palpable, restore circulation volume by giving IV fluids until the radial pulse is palpable again.

Research

Interventions for tubal ectopic pregnancy: a Cochrane Review (Hajenius et al 2005)

Background: The diagnosis of ectopic pregnancy is often made by non-invasive methods such as with sensitive pregnancy tests and high resolution TVS. As a consequence, various treatment options are now available: radical (salpingectomy) or conservative surgical treatment (salpingostomy); drug therapy and expectantly.

Objectives: In this review, the effects of various treatments were summarised in terms of treatment success, need for re-interventions, tubal patency and future fertility.

Main results: Laparoscopic conservative surgery is significantly less successful than the more radical approach in the elimination of tubal pregnancy due to a higher persistent trophoblast rate of laparoscopic surgery. Long-term follow-up shows similar tubal patency rates. The number of subsequent intrauterine pregnancies is comparable, but the number of repeat ectopic pregnancies is lower, although these differences are not statistically significant. Compared to laparoscopic conservative surgery, local and systemic methotrexate is significantly less successful in the elimination of tubal pregnancy. Methotrexate is not as effective in eliminating the tubal pregnancy as laparoscopic salpingostomy. Methotrexate treatment regimens are also associated with a greater impairment of health-related quality of life and are more expensive due to prolonged hospital stay and loss of productivity.

Authors' conclusions: Laparoscopic surgery is still the cornerstone of treatment in the majority of women with tubal pregnancy. If the diagnosis of tubal pregnancy can be made non-invasively, medical treatment with systemic methotrexate in a multiple-dose intramuscular regimen is an alternative treatment option but only in haemodynamically stable women with an unruptured tubal pregnancy and no signs of active bleeding presenting and with low initial serum hCG levels, after properly informing them about the risks and benefits of the available treatment options.

the efficacy of methotrexate (see the research box on the previous page). Expected management of ectopic pregnancies assumes that some of these pregnancies will resorb or resolve spontaneously (Bryan 2003).

Fertility after treatment

The prognosis for women with an ectopic pregnancy is good, provided there is early diagnosis and prompt, effective treatment. Fertility may be preserved, especially if there is early diagnosis followed by conservative management.

Local causes of vaginal bleeding

Vaginal bleeding may occur at any time in pregnancy, from benign conditions such as implantation, cervicitis or polyps, or after coitus, or from more serious conditions such as carcinoma, miscarriage, ectopic pregnancy or placenta praevia and abruption. In most non-pathological cases, treatment can be left until after the woman has had her baby.

Cervical pathology

In pregnancy the increased vascularity of the cervix may result in slight bleeding from cervical ectropian (previously called erosion). A cervical polyp may also be the cause of minimal, irregular bleeding in pregnancy. These are seen as bright red, fleshy protrusions that extend out from the cervical canal. Treatment, if required, is left until after pregnancy has been completed.

Carcinoma

Carcinoma of the cervix is a serious but rare occurrence in pregnancy, usually detected by a Papanicolau smear in pregnancy. On examination the cervix is hard and irregular and bleeds when touched. It requires immediate management. A caesarean section followed by hysterectomy is usually performed once the fetus is viable.

Cervicitis and/or vaginitis

An increased vaginal discharge is normal in pregnancy. Normal pregnancy discharge, known as leukorrhoea, is non-irritating and has no odour. Vaginal discharge may also be a symptom of genital infection. Vaginitis and cervicitis are usually due to STIs and infection with trichomoniasis or candidiasis (thrush). Microscopic examination of the discharge isolates the cause of the infection, which is then treated with antibiotics.

Bleeding from the non-pregnant horn of a bicornuate uterus

Bleeding is minimal and no treatment is required.

Haemorrhoids/vulval varicosities/urinary tract infection

While not strictly pregnancy-related bleeding, a urinary tract infection (UTI) presenting as haematuria can be the cause of a woman presenting with bleeding in pregnancy. Similarly, bleeding from haemorrhoids or vulval varicosities needs to be excluded in any assessment of bleeding in pregnancy.

Bleeding in late pregnancy: antepartum haemorrhage

Antepartum haemorrhage (APH) is defined as any bleeding into or from the genital tract after the twentieth week of pregnancy. It complicates approximately 2–5% of all pregnancies. The primary causes of APH are placental abruption (30%) and placenta praevia (20%).

Other causes of bleeding in the third trimester include: a heavy, bloody show, bleeding occurring during labour (intrapartal haemorrhage), cervical carcinoma, polyps, cervical or vaginal infection or trauma, varicosities and vasa praevia. Box 33.6 details the causes of vaginal bleeding in the third trimester.

Decisions about the management of a mild or severe APH depend on:
- whether the bleeding has settled or stopped
- whether the bleeding continues but is not life-threatening
- whether the bleeding continues and is life-threatening
- the condition of the fetus
- the gestational age of the pregnancy (Higgins 2003, p 228).

Placental abruption

A placental abruption is bleeding as a result of premature separation of a normally situated placenta from the uterine wall. Separation may be partial or complete. The aetiology is unknown but the strongest associations are trauma and hypertension. Other factors that have been associated with abruption are:
- past obstetric history of abruption
- gestational or essential hypertension
- multiple pregnancy
- increasing age
- high parity
- low socio-economic status
- renal infection
- drugs (smoking, cocaine)
- uterine anomaly or tumour
- sudden uterine decompression following rupturing membranes in polyhydramnios
- short umbilical cord
- pressure from the enlarged uterus on the inferior vena cava.

Clinical point

Placenta praevia and placental abruption can produce massive obstetric haemorrhage without any warning. With placental abruption, the clinician may not be aware of the full extent of the blood loss because a proportion of the blood may be concealed behind the placenta. Pregnant women may remain haemodynamically stable until they lose between a third and a half of their circulating blood volume.

BOX 33.6   Antepartum haemorrhage

Classification of causes of APH:

▶ bleeding from a normally situated placenta (accidental haemorrhage):
— placental abruption (concealed, revealed, combined)

▶ bleeding from an abnormally situated placenta (unavoidable or inevitable haemorrhage):
— placenta praevia
— placenta percreta/accreta/increta

▶ extraplacental/incidental causes:
— ruptured uterus/dehiscence of uterine scar (complete or incomplete)
— ruptured vasa praevia
— excessive bloody show
— cervical erosion, polyp, carcinoma
— vaginitis
— urinary tract infection
— haemorrhoids
— bleeding from the non-pregnant horn of a bicornuate uterus
— ruptured vulval varicosities.

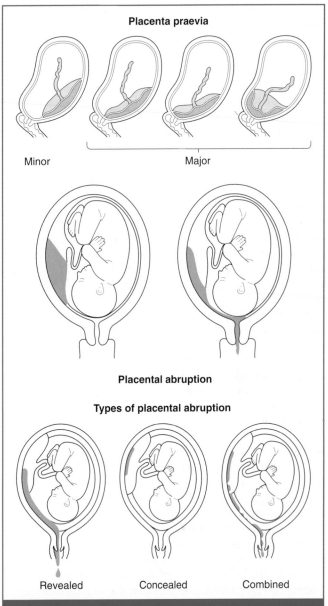

Figure 33.3 Placenta praevia and placental abruption (based on Oats & Abraham 2004)

It has been suggested also that abruption may be caused by folate deficiency, because:

● it is found more often in multiparous women with low socio-economic status

● there is an association between megaloblastic anaemia and abruption.

However:

● megaloblastic anaemia is common in developing countries but abruption is not

● folate supplements are not protective.

For most women, however, especially when bleeding is minimal, the cause is never found.

Classification of placental abruption

In placental abruption, bleeding may be:

● *central or concealed*—the separation occurs near the centre of the placenta and blood is retained between the uterine wall and the placenta as a retroplacental haematoma. In severe cases, the blood may infiltrate the myometrium until the uterus becomes swollen and engorged with blood, known as a Couvelaire uterus, increasing the woman's risk of postpartum haemorrhage (PPH) due to the inability of the uterus to contract and retract post partum.

● *revealed or marginal*—the separation occurs near the edge of the placenta and blood tracks down between the membranes and the decidua, through the cervix and into the vagina

● *partially revealed*—this is a combination of concealed and revealed bleeding, where some of the blood escapes into the vagina, the rest remaining trapped in the uterus.

Incidence

The incidence of placental abruption is 1:120 pregnancies but it accounts for 15% of perinatal mortality (Gaufberg 2001).

Clinical presentation and diagnosis

The classic manifestations of a placental abruption are dark, vaginal bleeding, and abdominal or low back pain and uterine tenderness. There may be a sudden onset of vaginal bleeding. The bleeding may be:

● *mild* with some abdominal pain, a non-tender uterus and a live fetus. The woman shows no signs of haemodynamic compromise.

● *moderate* with stronger abdominal or back pain, perhaps uterine contractions and a firm, tender uterus.

A cardiotocogram (CTG) shows a non-reassuring fetal heart rate tracing and the woman will exhibit some degree of shock.

- *profuse* with severe abdominal pain, a 'board-like', enlarging, tender uterus that fails to relax. Usually no fetal heart tones are heard on auscultation and usually real-time scan shows that the fetus is dead. The woman will be shocked, to a degree often out of proportion to the amount of visible blood loss. In severe cases significant amounts of thromboplastin are released into the circulation, making the woman at risk of disseminated intravascular coagulation (DIC).

Management

Any bleeding during pregnancy requires investigation and the pregnant woman needs to contact her lead maternity carer immediately. Should she lose more than 30 mL of blood, hospital assessment is necessary. Combined abruption is suspected if the degree of shock is out of proportion to the amount of bleeding visible. Management is dependent on the amount of bleeding, the degree of maternal haemodynamic compromise and the condition of the fetus. Careful initial assessment is required to differentiate placental abruption from placenta praevia, and to estimate the degree of maternal and fetal compromise. In contrast to placenta praevia, the fetal lie and presentation is normal.

The woman with mild bleeding may have mild abdominal pain with or without a history of precipitating factors such as some exertion, trauma or severe hypertension. Delivery of the fetus and placenta are the definitive treatments. However, if the degree of abruption is minor, and there is no fetal or maternal compromise, the pregnancy may be allowed to continue, especially if the fetus is viable but preterm.

- Venous access is obtained and blood taken for haemoglobin estimation, group and cross-matching of blood, coagulation studies and a Kleihauer Betke test.
- A careful speculum examination of the vagina may exclude other causes of bleeding. However, the clinician must be very careful to ensure that the vaginal bleeding is not from a placenta praevia.
- Tocolytic agents may be employed to stop uterine contractions.

Clinical point

During the initial assessment following an antepartum haemorrhage, look for signs of:
- ▶ cardiovascular collapse
- ▶ shock
- ▶ sepsis
- ▶ rigid abdomen
- ▶ heavy vaginal bleeding
- ▶ complications of labour
- ▶ fetal compromise.

No vaginal examinations are undertaken until the cause of the bleeding is found.

- A CTG trace of the fetal heartbeat is performed to assess fetal wellbeing.
- Depending on gestation, corticosteroids may be administered to enhance lung maturity.
- An ultrasound scan is performed to confirm placental localisation.
- Bed rest and close monitoring in hospital for at least 24 hours is recommended.
- Non-sensitised Rhesus-negative women will require anti-D immunoglobulin.
- A viable fetus near full term is often electively delivered to avoid a larger abruption later.

Every attempt should be taken to alleviate the family's anxiety and fears in honest and empathetic ways where the woman and her family feel comfortable about having their questions answered and trust that they will be given accurate, honest and up-to-date information. Diversional activities may assist the woman in dealing with the frustrations associated with prolonged bed rest and hospitalisation. Once bleeding stops and provided the maternal and fetal condition are satisfactory, the woman may go home, provided there are back-up and community resources available so that she can return to hospital if there are further signs of bleeding or if she begins labour. Assistance and support at home are often required.

The woman with moderate or profuse bleeding requires stabilisation, blood transfusion, and delivery. Resuscitation of the mother is the first objective, followed by delivery of the fetus. In many cases the fetus will be dead and vaginal delivery is preferred as the complications of serious coagulation defects are less dangerous than with a caesarean section. Provided her condition is stable, the woman's labour may be induced and a vaginal delivery attempted. There is, however, a significant danger that consumption coagulopathy (DIC) may develop with hypofibrinogenaemia. If the fetus is alive and viable, a caesarean section will be performed unless the woman is in active labour and progressing well with a reassuring fetal CTG recording. Epidural analgesia may be provided for those women, provided coagulation studies are normal and there is no evidence of hypovolaemia. Persistent haemorrhage after delivery may be due to coagulopathy or a Couvelaire uterus, or failure of the myometrium to contract once it is empty, which is a common post-delivery risk following an APH and an emergency Caesarean section. Chapter 36 discusses management of PPH in more detail.

Complications of abruption

Initial and ongoing management depends on the onset of complications, which may include:
- haemorrhagic shock
- disseminated intravascular coagulation (DIC)
- acute renal failure
- fetal compromise
- preterm labour
- intrauterine fetal death
- primary and secondary PPH
- sepsis

● anaemia.

These are dealt with in more detail later in this chapter and in Chapter 36.

Rare and ongoing complications

Sheehan's syndrome (anterior pituitary necrosis) is a rare complication following massive haemorrhage. Women with this condition demonstrate the symptoms of amenorrhoea, failure to lactate, coarsening of the hair and skin, feeling cold and, later, genital atrophy and premature sterility.

Placenta praevia: bleeding from an abnormally situated placenta

In *placenta praevia*, part of or the entire placenta is abnormally sited in the lower uterine segment (Higgins 2003). Placenta praevia may be further classified as:

● *low-lying*—lying within 2 cm but not extending to the internal cervical os
● *marginal*—extending to but not covering the internal cervical os
● *complete*—completely covering the internal cervical os.

BOX 33.7 Emergency treatment of abruption

Treat the shock

▶ Call for help and arrange escorted transfer to obstetric unit for further assessment even if bleeding seems to settle, as the fetus may still be compromised.
▶ Give oxygen via face mask at 6–8 L/min.
▶ Insert IV lines (two wide-bore cannulae).
▶ Cross-match six units of blood, coagulation profile and Kleihauer tests.
▶ Evaluate blood loss.
▶ Restore blood loss quickly with IV fluids—replace estimated losses plus 2 L of IV fluid. Give isotonic solutions followed by colloids until packed cells are available.
▶ Consider urinary catheterisation to monitor output and keep output at > 30 mL/hr.
▶ Ultrasound examination if the placenta is unsited or features suggest placenta praevia.
▶ Continuous monitoring of fetus, mother and labour.

Deliver the fetus

▶ Assess fetal maturity.
▶ Observe for the onset of labour—rupture of membranes and uterine contractions.
▶ By Caesarean section (if fetus compromised and viable).
▶ By rupturing the membranes and induction of labour (if ripe cervix or fetus nonviable).
▶ Diagnose and treat coagulopathy and disseminated intravascular coagulation (DIC).
▶ Urgent haematological consultation.
▶ Check platelet count.
▶ Transfusion—may require fresh frozen plasma and cryoprecipitate.

Maternal and fetal morbidity and mortality from placenta praevia are considerable.

The low-lying placenta

Many women in industrialised countries have one or more ultrasound scans during pregnancy and so are aware that they may be at risk of placenta praevia before the initial or sentinel bleed occurs, and have been informed about the urgent need for medical attention if they have any vaginal bleeding until the diagnosis has been confirmed. Nevertheless, in more than 98% of cases, a 'low-lying placenta' diagnosed on an early ultrasound will be found at term to have 'migrated' to the upper uterine segment. The placenta does not actually move but the growth of the uterus relative to the size of the placenta means that it appears to 'move'. Women with a low-lying placenta should have a repeat scan at about 32 weeks gestation for placental localisation.

Incidence

The incidence of placenta praevia at term is about 1% of all pregnancies. The risk increases by 1.5- to five-fold in women with a history of caesarean section. With repeated caesarean deliveries, this risk can be as great as 10%. Risks also increase with parity and there is a 4–8% recurrence of placenta praevia in subsequent pregnancies.

Causes

There is no known 'cause' of placenta praevia, but predisposing factors are well documented. Any condition that stops the blastocyst from embedding in the endometrium increases the risk of placenta praevia. The predisposing factors include:
● past history of placenta praevia
● a large placenta (e.g. with fetal erythroblastosis and multiple pregnancy)
● high parity

Clinical point

Bhide and colleagues (2003) recommend that the phrase 'placenta praevia' be restricted to diagnoses where the placental edge is equal to or less than 2 cm from the internal cervical os, as the woman will probably require a caesarean section and the risk of PPH is high. In situations where the placenta is more than 2 cm from the internal cervical os, the woman's chance of giving birth vaginally is greater than 60%, so these conditions should be defined as 'low-lying' rather than placenta praevia. The authors maintain that if a vaginal birth is to be considered, a vaginal examination is performed as a 'double set-up' and the site of the edge of the placenta is determined digitally, and a final decision reached following artificial rupture of the membranes. Once labour has commenced, or if the bleeding is severe and cannot be controlled and the maternal and/or fetal condition is compromised, a caesarean section is performed.

- an abnormally shaped uterus (e.g. fibroids, bicornuate uterus)
- previous uterine scar (myomectomy, caesarean section)
- scarring from previous uterine surgery and caesarean section
- smoking
- advancing maternal age.

Pathophysiology

As the lower uterine segment forms and the cervix begins to efface and dilate in later pregnancy (around 32 weeks gestation), there is partial separation of the inelastic placenta embedded in the lower uterine segment near or over the cervix from elastic uterine wall, and painless bleeding occurs. The closer the placenta is to the internal cervical os, and the greater the proportion of placenta covering the cervix, the earlier bleeding begins. Because these physiological changes are gradual, initial blood loss is slight and always painless and bright red in colour. Uterine contractions are rarely palpable. Bleeding may be triggered by coitus or digital examination, but usually there are no precipitating causes. It is not possible to predict when the next bleed will occur, or its severity.

Clinical presentation and diagnosis

There are two classic findings associated with placenta praevia: APH and fetal malpresentation. An APH from placenta praevia usually begins in the third trimester. It presents with recurrent, bright red, painless vaginal bleeding, although it is not uncommon for women to experience some painful uterine contractions after the bleed (Higgins 2003). The amount of blood lost is highly variable—from a few spots to several litres. The initial bleed usually ceases spontaneously as soon as the blood clots. Unlike an abruption, gentle abdominal palpation does not cause the woman pain and fetal parts are easily palpable. The presenting part usually does not engage in the pelvis and remains high, because the placenta occupies the lower uterine segment, preventing it from descending into the pelvis.

Diagnosis is confirmed by ultrasonographic imaging techniques revealing the relationship of the leading edge of the placenta to the cervical os and the leading fetal pole.

Management

The goal of management for a woman with placenta praevia is to obtain the maximum fetal maturation while minimising the risk to both fetus and mother. Management is determined by the degree of placenta praevia present, the gestational age of the fetus and the presence and amount of vaginal bleeding. Following any episode of bleeding after 20 weeks gestation, it is important that the woman be transferred to the nearest hospital for immediate assessment. In the presence of significant haemorrhage it may be necessary to summon an ambulance and initiate resuscitative measures.

On admission to hospital and depending on her haemodynamic status:

- the woman's general condition and vital signs are assessed and her records are reviewed
- an accurate history is taken that includes information about the onset of bleeding, its volume and precipitating factors
- for a diagnosis of placenta praevia to be confirmed, the location of the placenta must be determined. A transabdominal ultrasound or transvaginal ultrasound facilitates this process and should be performed as quickly as possible.
- unless bleeding is such that the woman's haemodynamic status is compromised, following a gentle abdominal palpation the fetal condition is assessed through a CTG of the fetal heart rate
- a speculum or vaginal examination must never be performed until localisation of the placenta is known.
- if the diagnosis cannot be confirmed by ultrasound, a vaginal examination using a speculum may be required. This should be performed in an operating theatre as a 'double set-up'—so the team can proceed to an immediate caesarean section should the haemorrhage become torrential.

Emergency management

Optimal outcomes depend on prompt diagnosis and appropriate, timely intervention to prevent further complications, by:

- maternal resuscitation
- continuous assessment of blood loss and maternal and fetal response to treatment;
- rapid blood-product replacement
- confirmation of the position of the placenta
- administering corticosteroids if the fetus is between 24 and 34 weeks gestation
- ruling out other causes of bleeding
- determining gestational age.
- assessing for signs of preterm labour. Tocolytic therapy may be used to inhibit labour for 48 hours.

Once the diagnosis is established, the clinical team must then decide whether the woman is a suitable candidate for expectant management, or whether in order to save the life of the mother and her baby an immediate caesarean section is needed.

Clinical point

In the presence of vaginal bleeding, do not perform a vaginal examination until placenta praevia is ruled out, as severe haemorrhage may be provoked if blood vessels lying across the os are damaged.

Clinical point

Resuscitation of the mother should always take precedence over resuscitation and delivery of the fetus.

Ongoing care

Once the initial haemorrhage is controlled, decisions about ongoing care depend on the mother's haemodynamic status, the fetal gestational age and the extent and frequency of bleeding. If the risks of preterm birth outweigh the risks of another potentially catastrophic bleed, expectant management is the preferred option because it allows more time for the fetal lungs to mature. The mother remains in hospital for at least 48 hours and an elective caesarean section is planned for about 36 weeks gestation. She is closely monitored for signs of another bleed, the onset of labour, and evidence of fetal wellbeing and/or compromise. In addition:

- blood samples for cross-match are always available at the blood bank
- an IV cannula is inserted but it may be luered
- fetal wellbeing is monitored (non-stress test and biophysical profiles)
- corticosteroids are administered if the mother is < 34 weeks pregnant
- preparations for an immediate caesarean section are always in place
- Rh D immunoglobulin (anti-D) is given to Rh D-negative women.

Measures are put in place to support the family as they deal with fear and anxiety related to the threats to the woman's life and that of her baby. These measures include:

- education about placenta praevia and treatment plans
- diversional and supportive activities to help with the boredom and anxiety associated with prolonged hospitalisation as well as the difficulties associated with being away from the family
- education about the signs of bleeding and the onset of labour.

Home versus hospital

There is little evidence of any clear advantage or disadvantage of a policy of home versus hospital care (Neilson 2004). After

---

Clinical point

When a woman presents with vaginal bleeding, the history should also include the following questions:

- When did the bleeding start, how much bleeding, and did the bleeding stop?
- Was this the first episode of bleeding?
- What was the colour of the blood (dark or bright red), were any clots present, and what was their size?
- What was the woman doing at the time of the bleed?
- Did she bleed with any of her other pregnancies?
- Does she feel the baby move?
- When did she last have sexual intercourse?
- Does she feel any contractions?
- How is her general health?
- Does she have any abdominal pain?

BOX 33.8 Mortality and morbidity

Maternal mortality (1%) and morbidity from:
- hypovolaemic shock
- postpartum haemorrhage
- invasive placenta (accreta, increta and percreta following severe haemorrhage due to major placenta praevia)
- Rhesus iso-immunisation
- disseminated coagulopathy
- anaemia
- sepsis

Perinatal mortality (4.4–67.3%) and morbidity from:
- malpresentation
- asphyxia
- prematurity and intrauterine growth restriction
- fetal anaemia from feto-maternal haemorrhage.

---

an APH the woman usually stays in hospital until there has been no further evidence of bleeding for about 72 hours. Before going home, the woman and her family are advised about the steps they can take to reduce the likelihood of another bleed (avoid sexual intercourse or any activity that may trigger labour). However, if they are to go home it is crucial that the woman always has access to transportation and can, if necessary, return to hospital within 20 minutes of the start of another episode of bleeding.

Mode of delivery

The mode of delivery needs to be planned in partnership between the woman, her family, and her care providers. Expectant management is terminated as soon as the fetus is mature, in the presence of excessive bleeding, if active labour begins or if signs of other complications such as chorioamnionitis develop.

- If the placenta praevia covers the entire os, a caesarean section is always indicated.
- If haemorrhage is life-threatening/profuse, immediate caesarean section is required.
- If the placenta is within 2 cm of the os (a low-lying placenta), a vaginal birth may be possible.
- If the fetus is dead or is not viable but there is an engaged fetal head, vaginal delivery is often attempted.

Postbirth complications

Complications include:

- coagulation disorders
- acute renal failure
- anaemia
- infection—prophylactic antibiotics should therefore be used for emergency caesarean section and considered for elective procedures
- manual removal of the placenta (often necessary)
- postpartum haemorrhage
- thromboembolism.

Research

Major placenta praevia should not preclude outpatient management (Love et al 2004)

Objective: To review current management of women with major and minor placenta praevia to assess whether outpatient care was detrimental to pregnancy outcome.

Study design: One hundred and sixty-one women with major and minor placenta praevia were separated into those who experienced an APH and those who had no bleeding during pregnancy (non-APH). Women with a major degree of praevia were not significantly more likely to experience bleeding. Women with APH were significantly more likely to be delivered early, by emergency caesarean section, of lower birthweight babies who required neonatal admission, than the non-APH group.

Conclusion: There is a place for outpatient management of women with placenta praevia. Caution is required with increasing number of bleeds but not degree of praevia.

Placenta accreta, percreta and increta, and vasa praevia

These potentially catastrophic complications are dealt with in Chapter 36.

Maternal medical conditions in pregnancy

Various medical diseases may preclude women from achieving a successful pregnancy and birth. Often, medical complications affect the mother's pregnancy, her illness and her fetus's wellbeing. It is not possible to cover all the medical disorders in a textbook of this nature, and so only the most common have been selected: diabetes, thyroid disease, heart disease, respiratory disease, renal disease, obstetric cholestasis, epilepsy, thrombo-embolic disease, genital infections, and hypertension in pregnancy.

Diabetes mellitus

Diabetes refers to a group of disorders characterised by impaired carbohydrate metabolism, all of which pose significant threats to maternal and perinatal health. Diabetes is on the rise worldwide (Amos et al 1997). The Australian Institute of Health and Welfare (2002) estimates that 940,000 Australians have diabetes but about half are unaware that they have the condition. The number of sufferers has doubled since the early 1980s and is expected to pass one million by 2010. Pregnancy presents particular challenges for women with diabetes irrespective of whether they have just been diagnosed with gestational diabetes or have been living with diabetes since childhood. Advances in medical, obstetric and intensive care of the diabetic woman have resulted in significantly better outcomes. Most women with diabetes can and do have healthy pregnancies.

Glucose homeostasis and carbohydrate metabolism are complex processes and so, before proceeding with this section, you are advised to refresh your knowledge of these topics by referring to a text such as Stables and Rankin (2004) *Physiology in Childbearing*. Briefly, energy metabolism is controlled by hormones including insulin, glucagon, epinephrine, growth hormone and the glucocorticoids. Normally the interplay

Critical thinking exercise

Why is a woman more at risk of PPH if the placenta is embedded in the lower rather than the upper uterine segment?

What is the significance of a 'low-lying' placenta?

TABLE 33.1 Comparisons between an abruption and a placenta praevia

	Abruption	Placenta praevia
Pain	Constant	Painless
Haemodynamic compromise	The actual amount of bleeding may be far in excess of observed vaginal blood loss.	Placenta praevia—the degree of shock is in proportion to amount of vaginal loss.
Uterus	Uterus is tender and tense.	Uterus is non-tender.
Fetus	Normal presentation and lie.	May have abnormal presentation and/or lie.
Fetal condition	Fetal heart trace non-reassuring/absent.	In general, fetal heart trace reassuring.
Associated problems	May be a complication of pre-eclampsia, may cause disseminated intravascular coagulation.	Small APH may occur before larger bleed.

These comparisons are generalisations and specific cases may vary in their clinical features.

between insulin and glucagon maintains blood glucose levels within a very narrow range (3–5 mmol/L). Glucagon produced by the alpha cells of the pancreas increases blood sugar levels, and insulin from the beta cells of the pancreas decreases the amount of circulating blood glucose. In contrast, insulin is required by almost all the body's cells. The stimulus for increased insulin secretion is a high blood glucose level; as blood glucose levels fall, the amount of insulin secreted by the beta cells decreases.

Glucagon is called a counter-regulatory hormone because it increases blood glucose levels: if blood glucose levels are high, glucagon is not secreted. Its most dramatic activity is its ability to initiate glycogenolysis. A reduction in circulating blood glucose stimulates the pancreas to release glucagon, which facilitates the breakdown of liver glycogen as a means of raising blood sugar levels. Glucagon also increases the transport of amino acids to the liver and stimulates their conversion, a process called gluconeogenesis.

Carbohydrate metabolism in pregnancy

Pregnant women are normally in a diabetogenic state, which ensures that the fetus has an adequate and continuous supply of glucose. It is characterised by insulin resistance with compensatory hyperinsulinaemia, beginning in the second trimester and remaining throughout the pregnancy. All pregnant women experience mild fasting hypoglycaemia and after-meal hyperglycaemia. Increased secretion of insulin between meals and during sleep enables the fetus to continue to draw glucose across the placenta from the maternal bloodstream, even during periods of maternal fasting. In the second and third trimesters, increased placental steroids and peptide hormones exacerbate tissue insulin resistance. However, if the maternal pancreatic insulin response to food intake is inadequate, first maternal and then fetal hyperglycaemia occurs.

Causes of diabetes mellitus

In diabetes mellitus there is an absolute or relative deficiency of insulin produced by the pancreas. Glucose cannot be converted to glycogen or released as energy, so it accumulates

---

BOX 33.9 Role of insulin

Insulin:
- ▶ facilitates the uptake of glucose by facilitating its movement from the blood into target cells (liver, skeletal and muscle)
- ▶ stimulates formation and storage of lipids and glycogen
- ▶ lowers circulating blood glucose.

It does this by:
- ▶ increasing glucose transport by target cells
- ▶ accelerating glucose utilisation (target cells) and enhanced ATP production
- ▶ stimulating glycogen synthesis (skeletal muscles and liver cells)
- ▶ decreasing glucogenesis.

BOX 33.10 Role of glucagon

Glucagon:
- ▶ mobilises energy reserves and promotes glucose synthesis and glycogen breakdown
- ▶ elevates blood glucose concentrations.

It does this by:
- ▶ stimulating the breakdown of glycogen in skeletal muscle and liver cells
- ▶ stimulating the breakdown of triglycerides in adipose tissues
- ▶ stimulating the production of glucose in the liver.

---

in the bloodstream, causing hyperglycaemia, some of which is excreted in the urine. Glucose is osmotically active and draws water after it, causing polyuria and thirst. Faced with a lack of glucose, the body tries to mobilise energy from fats and proteins, which leads to the production of ketones by the liver, and ketosis.

Diabetes is associated with:
- production of defective insulin
- over-production of insulin antagonists
- increased resistance to insulin (auto-immune response)
- underproduction of insulin (impaired cell function)
- inappropriate timing of insulin release.

Classification

There are three types of diabetes that affect pregnancy.
- *Type 1 diabetes* (formerly called 'insulin-dependent diabetes' (IDDM) or 'juvenile diabetes'). According to the Australian Institute of Health and Welfare (AIHW 2002), 10–15% of people diagnosed with diabetes will be Type 1. It is characterised by β cell destruction caused by an auto-immune process, usually leading to absolute insulin deficiency.
- *Type 2 diabetes mellitus* (formerly called 'non-insulin diabetes mellitus' (NIDDM), 'type II' or 'adult-onset') is the most common form of diabetes (80–90%) and is characterised by insulin resistance in peripheral tissues and an insulin secretory defect of the beta cells. Recently a new, rare form of Type 2 diabetes, known as 'maturity onset diabetes of the young' (MODY) has been identified. MODY is caused by an autosomal-dominant gene. Sufferers are usually women, of normal weight and under 25 years old. During pregnancy, women with MODY do not require insulin.
- *Gestational diabetes* (GDM) develops in pregnancy. It is characterised by carbohydrate intolerance that begins or is first recognised in pregnancy. However, most women classified with GDM have normal glucose homeostasis during the first half of the pregnancy and only develop a relative insulin deficiency (and hyperglycaemia) during the last half of the pregnancy. The hyperglycaemia resolves in most cases after birth but places them at significant risk of developing Type 2 diabetes later in life.

The following sections focus on the most common forms of diabetes affecting maternal and fetal health.

Aetiology of Type 2 diabetes

The aetiology of Type 2 diabetes mellitus is multifactorial and, like Type 1 diabetes, probably genetically based, but there are also strong behavioural components. In Australia and New Zealand, it is more common in women:

- of advancing age
- with a sedentary lifestyle
- with a family history of Type 2 diabetes
- with impaired glucose tolerance
- from low socio-economic backgrounds
- with a history of gestational diabetes
- with an 'apple-shaped figure'
- from Chinese, Indian, Maori, Pacific, Aboriginal or Torres Strait Island background.

Pathophysiology of Type 2 diabetes

People can develop Type 2 diabetes at any age—even during childhood, although usually when older. A reduced capacity for insulin secretion and insulin resistance, combined with the effects of obesity, ageing and physical inactivity, are crucial factors in determining who develops Type 2 diabetes. A relative lack of endogenous insulin plus pancreatic beta cell dysfunction reduces glucose uptake by cells, resulting in hyperglycaemia.

Diabetes, pregnancy and complications

Whatever its causation, diabetes can result in a range of complications for the mother, her baby and the progress of her disease. In women with Type 1 or 2 diabetes, glycaemic control worsens and insulin requirements change as the pregnancy progresses. Poorly controlled Type 1 diabetes causes life-threatening metabolic reactions, such as ketoacidosis and diabetic coma. In addition, hyperglycaemia is the prime determinant of the following microvascular and metabolic complications:

- diabetic ketoacidosis
- cardiovascular disease
- peripheral vascular disease
- retinopathy
- diabetic nephropathy and end-stage renal disease
- peripheral nerve disease
- cancer of the pancreas
- liver disease
- depression.

Metabolic complications

During pregnancy, lack of knowledge about the effects of pregnancy on diabetes, as well as the effects of pregnancy on glycaemic control, increases the risks of hypoglycaemic episodes as well as diabetic ketoacidosis. Women and their partners need ongoing, evidence-based information and education about the management of these conditions, including the use of glucagon to alleviate hypoglycaemia and how to recognise and prevent ketoacidosis. Midwives are

---

BOX 33.11　**Diabetes in New Zealand**

Maori and Pacific populations are among the highest-risk groups for diabetes and for cardiovascular disease and related conditions.

In New Zealand by 2011, the prevalence of diabetes is predicted to increase by 58%, 132% and 146% in European, Maori and Pacific populations respectively. This increase reflects changing demographic factors (including increased population size and changes in population age structure) and epidemiological factors (such as obesity and physical inactivity).

Effective primary prevention programs for Type 2 diabetes are largely based on programs to reduce diabetes risk factors, such as reducing overweight/obesity, stopping smoking and increasing physical activity. Such programs extend beyond the health sector, involving local government, employers, education and community groups, amongst others.

Maori and Pacific populations are among the highest-risk groups for diabetes and for cardiovascular disease and related conditions. These populations traditionally have strong community links, which are important to the success of health programs targeting the above risk factors.

(Source: New Zealand Ministry of Health, http://www.newhealth.govt.nz/toolkits/diabetes/reducing.htm)

Clinical point

Recent work suggests that an in utero environment leading to low birthweight may predispose some individuals to Type 2 diabetes mellitus in later life. Poor growth before birth may produce permanent changes in glucose metabolism. Diabetes may be linked to the so-called 'thrifty gene' that once helped hunter-gatherers survive when food was in short supply (Gautier et al 2003).

---

well placed to work with the family to develop an emergency plan that they know works and is kept in an accessible place. This plan should contain a list of local emergency contacts.

Microvascular complications

Retinal and renal disease associated with diabetes can worsen during pregnancy. Retinopathy alone is not associated with a poorer outcome for the fetus unless concurrent nephropathy is evident as well. Poor glycaemic control in the first trimester and pre-eclampsia or chronic hypertension are independently associated with the progression of retinopathy. Good glycaemic control preconceptually and during pregnancy effectively reduces the long-term risk of retinopathy.

Diabetic retinopathy may develop or worsen during pregnancy. Women are encouraged to consult an ophthalmologist before they become pregnant, and to plan further follow-up consultations during the course of the pregnancy.

Nephropathy

There is an association between pre-existing nephropathy and adverse maternal and perinatal outcomes, although not congenital malformations. As pregnancy progresses, there is an increased risk that women with diabetes will develop pre-eclampsia and experience worsening chronic hypertension. Complications associated with nephropathy and pre-eclampsia, especially if it is superimposed on chronic hypertension, are strongly associated with pre-term birth.

Effects of diabetes on the fetus

Poorly controlled diabetes may have catastrophic effects on the fetus. Temple and colleagues (2002) found a significant relationship between poor glycaemic control in early pregnancy and adverse pregnancy outcomes with Type 1 diabetes. Poor glycaemic control during fetal organogenesis is associated with increased rates of spontaneous miscarriage plus a number of congenital anomalies, such as malformations of the nervous, cardiovascular, skeletal and renal systems. In contrast, the incidence of spontaneous miscarriage for diabetic women with good glycaemic control is no different from the rate experienced by women without diabetes. Indeed, the perinatal death rate of babies born to women with diabetes is increased 1.5–2 fold compared to those without diabetes.

The main causes of perinatal death are:

- unexplained stillbirth in the third trimester
- prematurity due to a high incidence of spontaneous preterm labour and of elective premature delivery to prevent stillbirth
- low birthweight due to IUGR where the mother has diabetic nephropathy
- congenital malformations
- birth trauma due to a high incidence of macrosomic babies.

Pre-pregnancy care

Pre-pregnancy counselling should begin well before the onset of pregnancy; it is a key component of good maternity care for the woman with diabetes. Statistically, the level of risk for a woman with Type 1 or Type 2 diabetes and for the baby is determined largely by the woman's health just before conception and during the first trimester. Attendance at a pre-pregnancy clinic is associated with a reduction in the rate of spontaneous miscarriage, in risk of congenital malformations and in complications of pregnancy. Infants of mothers attending pre-pregnancy clinics have fewer problems and are kept in special care for shorter periods than infants of non-attending mothers (Kitzmiller et al 1991).

Pre-conceptional care should include consultation between an endocrinologist or physician experienced in the care of women, obstetrician, dietician, midwives and perinatologist. If glycaemic control is suboptimal, women are counselled regarding the risks of pregnancy and, in particular, the risks of fetal malformation. Contraception should be continued until glycaemic control is considered adequate.

Clinical point

Macrosomia due to poor diabetic control refers to a baby that is considerably larger than normal. The diagnosis can only be made with any certainty after birth. Fetal macrosomia has been defined in several different ways, including birthweight of 4000–4500 g or greater than the 90–95th percentile for gestational age after correcting for neonatal sex and ethnicity. Based on these definitions, macrosomia affects 1–10% of all pregnancies.

Management of Type 1 diabetes during pregnancy

The management of Type 1 and frequently Type 2 diabetes involves daily delivery of exogenous insulin by injection or an insulin pump, combined with carefully designed meal plans and exercise regimen. This, however, assumes that the insulin regimen is the guiding component of therapy. In reality the individual's typical eating pattern and lifestyle should be the key factors and the determinants of the best insulin regimen. Antenatal care for the woman with diabetes involves teamwork. Health professionals working collaboratively and in partnership with the woman plan her care during pregnancy and labour. The woman should always be referred to a consultant unit attached to a neonatal nursery. Diabetes specialist nurses and midwives have an important role in educating women about the need for home blood glucose monitoring, urine testing, intensive insulin regimens, dietary management and regular exercise.

Screening in early pregnancy

Because of the increased risk of congenital anomalies, women should be offered combined first trimester screening for aneuploidy with β-hCG and a pregnancy associated plasma protein test (PAPP-A) measured at 10 weeks gestation, followed by an ultrasound examination for dating, nuchal transparency, gross morphology and plurality at 12 weeks gestation. It is generally recommended that ultrasound be carried out at least three times in pregnancy: early or at first booking, to recognise possible early growth delay or congenital malformations as described above; later at about 28 weeks, to determine fetal size, hydramnios and further possible malformations; and finally at about 36 weeks, to identify the presence of macrosomia.

Insulin

In 1921, Frederick Banting and Charles Best discovered insulin while they were working in the laboratory of John Macleod at the University of Toronto. In 1923, Banting and Macleod were awarded the Nobel Prize for medicine. The US Food and Drug Administration first approved its use in 1939. Insulin was the first hormone to be synthesised completely in the laboratory, a feat accomplished in 1966 by Michael Katsoyannis of the United States and scientists in China. Before the advent of insulin, very few diabetic women conceived, and in those who did, perinatal mortality ranged from 40% to 60%. In the first 50 years of insulin use in diabetic pregnancy, considerable advances were made.

Insulin requirements change during pregnancy because of the effects of insulin-antagonistic placental hormones. Regimens vary but the consensus seems to be that a 'tight control' plan (Box 33.12) with frequent administration of insulin (up to four times daily) and the use of different insulin types (e.g. rapid- and long-acting insulin analogues), as well as more frequent blood glucose measurements, are better able to achieve normal blood glucose levels. Insulin therapy is usually basal-bolus with one dose of medium-acting insulin each day and short-acting insulin before each main meal.

Blood glucose monitoring

Monitoring blood glucose levels is fundamental to achieving tight diabetic metabolic control. Self-monitoring of blood glucose levels (SMBG) empowers women who have diabetes, enabling them to actively achieve their goals. In addition, the instant feedback that SMBG provides enables women to learn more about portion sizes, foods that cause hyperglycaemia, maintenance of stable temporal patterns of elevated blood glucose levels, and when exercise is most likely to help keep blood glucose in the targeted range. With this information, women are better able to make choices about their diet and activities and to see the effects of these in a timely manner. SMBG allows adjustments to be made to the meal plan/exercise/treatment regimen aimed at normalising blood glucose levels. Without SMBG these activities cannot be individualised to the different responses that many women have at any given time during their pregnancy.

Women should aim to maintain blood glucose levels as near to their non-diabetic range as possible without increasing the risk of hypoglycaemia. This usually means targeting levels between 4 and 7 mmol/L and measuring blood glucose levels four or five times a day. The glycated haemoglobin HbA_{1c} should be measured at the first visit and repeated monthly, with a target level of < 6.5%.

Laboratory tests that use plasma for measurement of blood glucose give results that are 10% higher than levels obtained from the finger prick method.

Dietary advice

Diet is another cornerstone of therapy in the management of all forms of diabetes. Expert nutritional advice should be available in all diabetic antenatal clinics in order to encourage the entire family to have a diet low in saturated fat, with high levels of complex carbohydrates, soluble fibre and vitamins. As do most women pre-pregnancy, women with Type 1 diabetes mellitus are advised to take a folic acid supplement, 4–5 mg daily, one month prior to pregnancy and for the first trimester, as the risk of neural tube defects is higher for this group of women.

Exercise

The benefits of exercise include cardiovascular fitness and psychological wellbeing. Women with Type 1 diabetes are rarely overweight but exercise is still beneficial. For women with Type 2 or gestational diabetes, the benefits of exercise also include a decrease in body fat, better weight control and improvements in insulin sensitivity. Exercise, perhaps a brisk walk for about 30 minutes a day four times a week, is an important component in establishing and maintaining 'tight' glucose control.

Maternal and fetal monitoring

Diabetic pregnancies are 'high risk' and therefore regular monitoring is appropriate. It is recommended that women with all forms of diabetes attend the antenatal clinic every two weeks. The risk is greater in women with complications of diabetes (e.g. vascular or renal disease) or hypertension in pregnancy (e.g. pre-eclampsia). A suggested minimum monitoring provision is every two weeks and then from 36 weeks weekly for clinical assessment and regular CTG. Doppler flow studies and/or biophysical profiles are recommended. The use of Doppler ultrasound in high-risk pregnancies may improve a number of perinatal care outcomes and appears promising in helping to reducing perinatal deaths (Neilson & Alfirevic 2001). Some clinicians encourage women to assess—and, if necessary, report—a perceived reduction in fetal movements during pregnancy, although there is no evidence to support the efficacy of this activity.

BOX 33.12 'Tight control' plan

Working with pregnant women with diabetes
The type of diabetes treatment program that aims to normalise blood glucose levels is referred to as a 'tight control' plan. Cornerstones of tight glycaemic control are:

▶ administering insulin and adjusting the doses, depending on results of self-monitoring of blood glucose (SMBG)
▶ frequent SMBG
▶ following an appropriate meal plan
▶ adding or maintaining an appropriate level of physical activity
▶ controlling/treating hypoglycaemia.

Clinical point

Women with diabetes should aim for near-normal glucose levels, or as close to normal as possible—ideally for three months before becoming pregnant and just as importantly for at least the first three months of pregnancy, when the fetus is developing rapidly and thus a time during which congenital malformations can occur if glucose levels are high. Studies have shown that when the glycated haemoglobin (HbA$_{1c}$) level is within 1% of normal levels, the rates of congenital deformities and spontaneous abortion are no different from those in women without diabetes. Above that, however, the incidence rises.

BOX 33.13 Type 2 diabetes support

A woman's weight influences her body image. Women with Type 2 diabetes or gestational diabetes mellitus are often overweight. Obesity makes it more difficult to maintain tight glycaemic control and this is especially true for the woman with Type 2 diabetes. In contrast, some women with Type 1 diabetes may find it very difficult to achieve their desirable weight. Women with diabetes are often advised to 'maintain a healthy weight' but this is easier said than done. It may be helpful to separate the issue of how much the woman weighs from the behaviours required for the woman to become and remain healthy. One strategy is for the woman to work with a dietician or other health professional to develop a plan of action that contains goals and strategies to meet them. In this way it is possible to focus on the plan rather than body size and weight gain or loss.

Ongoing laboratory tests

Ongoing evaluation of glycaemic control and the assessment of diabetic complications are essential components of any management plan for women with diabetes. Tests include:

- HbA_{1c}—as red blood cells are made, they combine with glucose in the blood to make HbA_{1c}. How much HbA_{1c} is produced depends on the blood glucose level at the time each red blood cell is made. Erythrocytes live for only a few months, so an HbA_{1c} test measures the average blood glucose over the previous two to three months. HbA_{1c} levels of 7% or less are associated with a reduced risk of microvascular complications, while levels > 9% are associated with increased risks. It is advisable therefore to aim for levels of 7% or less.
- serum creatinine and urinary excretion of total protein and/or albumin-to-creatinine ratio or 24-hour excretion rate—women with a protein excretion rate of > 190 mg/24 hrs are at increased risk of hypertension in pregnancy. Women with protein excretion rates > 400 mg/24 hrs are also at risk of IUGR.
- random plasma glucose and SMBG
- in the third trimester, ultrasound examination at 30 weeks for assessment of fetal growth—this should be repeated as clinically indicated, or at 36 weeks if the initial estimated fetal weight is > 80th percentile.

Self-management skills

Practical self-management skills for good glycaemic control include:

- counselling and education about the risks and prevention of congenital anomalies, maternal and perinatal complications, the effects of pregnancy on diabetes and the effects of diabetes on pregnancy, the need for effective contraception and pre-conceptual care, the importance of tight glycaemic control and its relationship to maternal and perinatal complications
- selection of appropriate anti-hyperglycaemic therapy
- development of a workable and acceptable plan to

achieve low-risk glycaemia—< 1% above the normal range
- an appropriate diet and meal plan
- self-monitoring of blood glucose levels
- self-administering of insulin and self-adjustment of insulin dose
- treatment of hypoglycaemia (woman and her family members)
- development of an emergency plan to deal with hypoglycaemia
- incorporation of daily physical activity—at least 30 minutes a day
- development of techniques to reduce stress and help cope with the condition and its potential complications.

Labour and birth

During labour, supervision by an experienced team is essential to regulate diabetic control. As yet there is no clear evidence to inform decisions about the optimal timing for birth, although common practice is that the pregnancy does not proceed past 40 weeks. The timing of birth is determined on an individual basis. If there is a risk of preterm delivery, antenatal corticosteroids are administered in line with local protocols. Even after controlling for confounding factors, women with diabetes have a high rate of caesarean section (Remsberg et al 1999). This is possibly because of clinicians' concerns about the relationship between macrosomia and shoulder dystocia. An estimated fetal weight > 4.5 kg is generally regarded as an indication for delivery by elective caesarean section, although there is no firm evidence to support the optimal fetal weight at birth. During labour and birth, evidence-based protocols for IV dextrose and insulin are necessary to maintain maternal plasma glucose between 4 and 7 mmol/L.

Post partum

Post partum, there will be a rapid reduction of insulin requirements. Usually the same meal plan used during the pregnancy is adequate to meet the needs of the breastfeeding mother with diabetes. Adjustments are made in consultation with the woman's endocrinologist and dietician. Early breastfeeding is important and adjustment of the mother's food intake to accommodate this must be recognised. There are well-documented health benefits for diabetic women in breastfeeding their babies. Six-week postpartum fasting plasma glucose levels of women with Type 1 diabetes who exclusively breastfeed have been found to be significantly lower than those who bottle feed (Ferris et al 1993). For some women with Type 1 diabetes breastfeeding may complicate their glycaemic control—they have erratic blood-glucose levels and an increase in insulin reactions. For others, it is easier to maintain tight glycaemic control; some women can eat more and take less insulin. However, others find that symptoms of hypoglycaemia are different while they are breastfeeding; perhaps these symptoms appear more quickly or without any warning. Such women may need to take extra precautions and have some form of glucose (non-diet soft drink, or glucose tablets) nearby so that they do not have to interrupt breastfeeding if a hypoglycaemic episode occurs.

Postnatal follow-up

Postnatal follow-up is a good opportunity for the team to begin pre-pregnancy care for any subsequent pregnancy, to support the woman as she works to attain good glycaemic control and to assist the family develop lifelong good health habits. The woman is advised on the necessity to make sure that the next pregnancy is planned. Effective communication between the hospital-based team, family doctor and diabetes clinic is essential. It is at this stage that a carefully documented outcome assessment for both mother and baby must take place, and this is then forwarded to the relevant clinicians responsible for the woman's ongoing care.

Management of Type 2 diabetes mellitus

Management is similar to that described for Type 1 diabetes and pregnancy.

In contrast to Type 1, Type 2 diabetes may be controlled by diet, insulin and/or medications such as metformin. Until recently it was believed that pregnant women with Type 2 diabetes who were taking oral agents such as metformin should switch to insulin as soon as their pregnancy was diagnosed, as these common medications were considered to be teratogenic and also because of concerns about the effect of transport of glucose across the placenta causing prolonged neonatal hypoglycaemia. Insulin is not associated with teratogenesis, nor does it have adverse fetal effects. In any case, many women with Type 2 diabetes require insulin during pregnancy if they are to achieve good glycaemic control.

Simmons and colleagues (2004) conducted a review of the available research and confirmed that although metformin does cross the placenta, necessitating a cautious approach to its use in pregnancy, as yet there are insufficient data to substantiate the belief that harm will always occur. They confirmed that tight glycaemic control in the pre-conceptional period and during early pregnancy is vitally important (Simmons et al 2004). If women taking metformin plan to become or are pregnant, it is crucial to ensure that the change in therapy occurs without deterioration in glycaemic control. Further, ceasing metformin may result in greater teratogenic risk by exposing the fetus to increased hyperglycaemia. Moreover, Simmons et al (2004) assert that some studies suggest that there are reduced rates of spontaneous miscarriage in women who continue taking metformin in the first trimester or throughout pregnancy. Further, there was also a reduced subsequent risk of gestational diabetes if metformin was continued during pregnancy. Simmons and colleagues (2004) conclude that it is reasonable for some women to continue metformin (e.g. if they refuse insulin therapy), or begin metformin (e.g. if they are very insulin resistant), when the likely benefits from improved glycaemic control outweigh the potential for harm.

During the postpartum period, some women will require or perhaps choose insulin as the preferred agent to maintain good glycaemic control. Metformin is not recommended if the woman breastfeeds because oral hypoglycaemic agents including metformin are passed, albeit in very small doses, into the breast milk. Some authors believe that because the quantity of the drug passing into the breast milk is so small it is safe to use in lactation. Nevertheless, others including Simmons et al (2004) assert that the safety of metformin cannot be assumed because the studies on which these conclusions were made were

---

Clinical point

Information on pregnancy and contraception should be given to all diabetic women of childbearing age. No contraceptive methods are specifically contraindicated in women with diabetes. Methods with proven high degrees of effectiveness are preferred.

BOX 33.14 Indigenous people and diabetes

Overall, compared to Europeans, Indigenous people from New Zealand and Australia as well as women from the Pacific Islands have a higher prevalence of risk factors known to be important in the development of Type 2 (non-insulin) diabetes. These include obesity, impaired glucose tolerance, hypertriglyceridaemia, hypertension and hyperinsulinaemia. Of importance also are the poor socio-economic circumstances of many Indigenous people (Colagiuri et al 1998; Simmons et al 2001a). The effect of socio-economic factors (low levels of education, unemployment, low incomes, and poor housing and related environmental conditions) are compounded through psychosocial pathways, involving stress, social support and social cohesion, social affiliations, early emotional development and social status (Marmot & Wilkinson 1999).

BOX 33.15 Reducing insulin resistance

Insulin resistance may be decreased with dietary modification, weight loss, perhaps anti-diabetic agents such as the biguanide metformin.

Clinical point

Metformin therapy should not be used routinely in women with pregnancies complicated by diabetes. The data regarding metformin use in pregnancy should be discussed with the woman before a decision is made regarding ongoing treatment. If a woman with Type 2 diabetes and taking metformin presents to the antenatal clinic already pregnant, she should be reassured that there is no evidence of teratogenesis with its use and that she should continue taking the medication until ongoing treatment options are discussed with her and clinicians in her team.

very small. Infant exposure to metformin can be minimised by breastfeeding just before taking the drug and avoiding feeding for a minimum of two to three hours after taking it.

Gestational diabetes mellitus

Gestational diabetes mellitus (GDM) affects 5% of all pregnancies and is a controversial disorder because of the uncertainties surrounding the best management. There is no consensus on the definition, management or treatment of gestational diabetes. GDM can be defined as carbohydrate intolerance of variable severity with onset or first recognition during pregnancy. This definition includes women with abnormal glucose tolerance that reverts to normal after birth as well as those with previously undiagnosed Type 1 or Type 2 diabetes, and rarely in women with maturity-onset diabetes of the young (MODY).

GDM generally resolves once the pregnancy is completed, although 50% of women will develop Type 2 diabetes in later life. The disease is usually first noticed in the last 12 weeks of pregnancy and about 50% of women diagnosed with GDM will require insulin during pregnancy. Women with GDM are more likely to experience repeated miscarriage and develop hypertensive disorders, although some of this additional risk may be associated with underlying risk factors for GDM (e.g. increased maternal age or obesity). They are also more at risk of caesarean delivery. Clinicians' fears about perceived associations between fetal macrosomia, shoulder dystocia and GDM probably account for this finding. Other potential complications for the woman include polyhydramnios, preterm labour and birth, as well as genital tract infections from *Candida albicans*, and UTIs.

Research

A New Zealand study (Simmons et al 2001b) confirms earlier findings that insulin pump therapy in Type 2 diabetes and gestational diabetes mellitus is well tolerated. Such therapy is associated with no significant hypoglycaemia, and control of hyperglycaemia is achieved to a level unlikely with large boluses of subcutaneous injections of insulin. Perinatal outcomes were comparable to those in women with less hyperglycaemia and lower insulin requirements. However, use of insulin pumps was associated with substantial weight gain and a greater likelihood of admission to the Special Care Baby Unit.

BOX 33.16 Type 2 diabetes in Australia

The likely prevalence of Type 2 diabetes among Indigenous Australians is between 10% and 30%—around two to four times that among non-Indigenous Australians. The disease also occurs at younger ages among Indigenous than non-Indigenous people (de Courten et al 1998; see also Australian Indigenous HealthInfoNet 2003).

Some studies (Turok et al 2003) assert that the fetus is at greater risk of congenital abnormalities, particularly neural tube defects. Episodes of fetal hyperglycaemia and hyperinsulinaemia may lead to fetal macrosomia, possibly traumatic birth followed by growth restriction, neonatal hypoglycaemia, hypocalcaemia, hyperbilirubinaemia, polycythaemia and intrauterine death.

Risk factors for GDM

Risk factors for GDM include obesity, family history of diabetes, being of Aboriginal or Torres Strait islander background, or of Maori, Pacific, Middle-Eastern or Asian ethnicity.

Other risk factors include previous unexplained stillbirth, poor obstetric or social history, polycystic ovarian syndrome, obesity, previous diagnosis of GDM, having a previous baby with a birth weight over 4500 g and maternal age > 25 years. In a current pregnancy, accelerated weight gain, polyhydramnios, newly detected glycosuria and multiple pregnancy are all associated with GDM.

Diagnosis of GDM

The most appropriate strategies for screening, diagnosing and managing asymptomatic GDM remain controversial (Turok et al 2003). Screening for GDM is widely practised despite a lack of evidence that it prevents adverse outcomes (Turok et al 2003). Nevertheless, many medical centres including the RANZCOG recommend a random (non-fasting) 50 g glucose challenge test as an initial screening test for GDM. If the one-hour plasma glucose is ≥ 7.8 mmol/L, women are recalled for a glucose tolerance test.

The Australasian Diabetes Society (ADIPS) (Hoffman et al 1998) has endorsed the diagnostic criteria based on modified WHO criteria. After a positive screening test, the diagnosis is confirmed with a 75 g oral glucose tolerance test (fasting) with a venous plasma glucose level at 0 hours of 5.5 mmol/L and/or at 2 hours of ≥ 8.0 mmol/L. In New Zealand, the two-hour oral glucose tolerance test (OGTT) cut-off value for a positive diagnosis is a venous plasma glucose level of 9.0 mmol/L.

Collaborative management of a woman and her fetus with GDM

The keystones of therapy—control of blood glucose levels, monitoring, diet and exercise—have already been discussed, and this section only explores material that is of direct

---

Research

New Zealand Polynesians, Maori and people from the South Pacific have a high prevalence of GDM and Type 2 diabetes, diagnosed at an increasingly young age, and obesity (Simmons et al 2001a). Compared with European women, Polynesians with GDM are older, heavier, have worse hyperglycaemia at diagnosis, are more likely to have Type 2 diabetes postnatally, and are prone to worse perinatal outcomes (Simmons et al 2000).

relevance to GDM. Women at significant risk of, or with, GDM require an interdisciplinary team approach. Ultimately the woman with GDM must become the most active member of her care team, calling on the other members for specific guidance and expertise to help her achieve her goal of a healthy pregnancy, birth and baby. If the woman has been diagnosed with GDM in earlier pregnancies, it may be possible to begin her care before conception so that she and her team can develop evidence-based strategies aimed at maintaining the maternal blood sugar levels as near to normal as possible. It is possible to stabilise the GDM by diet alone but 50% of women require insulin or a combination of both as the pregnancy progresses. Each woman requires regular antenatal assessment, including a management plan. This is usually achieved through a combination of hospital and home visits, with hospital admission if the woman's diabetes becomes unstable or if she presents with any infection or other complication such as pre-eclampsia.

After the initial visit and once she becomes pregnant (or once the condition is diagnosed), the woman is seen at four- to eight-week intervals, depending on her ability to keep to her plan of management and the presence or absence of pre-existing complications.

Insulin

Most studies involving insulin therapy in women with GDM (Turok et al 2003) have shown a reduction in the incidence of fetal macrosomia. Consequently, insulin therapy is traditionally commenced when, despite nutrition therapy and the initiation of an exercise regimen, capillary blood glucose levels exceed 5.8 mmol/L in the fasting state and 6.7 mmol/L two hours after meals (Turok et al 2003, p 1769). The combination of food diaries, SMBG records and weight changes are also used to determine whether insulin therapy is required. Women are advised to contact their lead carer if blood glucose levels exceed target goals on two or more occasions over a 1–2 week period without some obvious explanation identified in the food records, or if the blood glucose levels are consistently elevated. There is no evidence that supports the efficacy of one type of insulin regimen over another.

Dietary modification

Dietary management, with or without insulin, causes a modest but consistent reduction in neonatal birthweight. Unfortunately, the optimal distribution of calories as carbohydrates, fats and protein for women with GDM is unknown, and there is little consensus and wide variability in clinical practice. Working in partnership, the mother and midwife aim to meet the following goals for nutrition:

Reflective exercise

What would you say to a woman who says, 'My doctor says my ultrasound shows that my baby is much larger than he should be. He says he thinks this is because I have diabetes and that I will need a caesarean section.'?

BOX 33.17 Managing a GDM pregnancy

Over-zealous treatment with diet or insulin may compromise babies of mothers with GDM, especially if they are not macrosomic. Following counselling and nutritional advice, and if pre- and post-prandial glucose levels are normal and there is no evidence of excessive fetal growth, the pregnancy should be managed as a 'normal' pregnancy.

- optimal nutrition for the developing fetus
- optimal nutrition for the pregnant woman and mother
- maternal euglycaemia without distortion of dietary patterns
- good nutrition for all the family
- nutritional patterns that prevent or forestall recurrence of GDM and the onset of Type 2 diabetes mellitus in later pregnancies.

Frequency of visits

If the diabetes is well controlled, the pregnancy is treated as 'normal' and proceeds to term. It is, however, most likely to proceed to term if the woman's GDM is well controlled by diet alone. As the third trimester begins, a woman with GDM is more at risk of complications and so the schedule of antenatal visits increases—for example, for women who do not require insulin, three-weekly until 28 weeks, then two-weekly until 38 weeks, then weekly until delivery. Women receiving insulin should be seen weekly from 34 weeks. The frequency of consultations is increased if there are other complications, such as:

- pre-existing or pregnancy-induced hypertension
- fetal macrosomia

Clinical point

Community-based care

Telephone/fax/email management can be a financially and time-effective way for the midwife to maintain close contact with a woman with GDM during the intervals between face-to-face consultations with the diabetic team. Women are asked to call/fax/email records weekly. A midwife skilled in working with women with GDM can use these records to assess the woman's health and to reinforce health education, answer questions and monitor records to identify those in need of extra support. Self-maintenance of these records is empowering for the woman and also reinforces their importance. This type of monitoring also identifies the high blood glucose levels that are not necessarily brought to the attention of the diabetic team, perhaps from fear or denial of their significance. Telephone calls, rather than the more impersonal email or fax management, are probably more likely to lead to the formation of a trusting relationship between woman and midwife.

- intrauterine growth restriction
- poor glycaemic control
- inability to stop smoking.

Labour and birth

In women with good glycaemic control and no complicating factors, there is no need to induce labour before term. The chosen method of giving birth depends on choice and obstetric factors. The woman's need for exogenous insulin by itself is not an indication for earlier delivery or a caesarean section, which is often the preferred option if the estimated fetal weight at the time of delivery is > 4250 g, because of a perceived risk of shoulder dystocia. Only if there are concerns about the woman's health, her labour or the fetus is a caesarean section indicated. During labour, blood sugar levels are monitored regularly. Once the woman is in established in labour she is often commenced on an IV infusion of glucose in one line and insulin in another. The dosage required is dependent on her blood sugar levels and the unit's guidelines. The woman's condition and that of her fetus are observed and monitored as in any normal labour, although the fetal heart rate is usually continuously electronically monitored once labour commences.

Postnatal care and follow-up

Management during the early postnatal period includes frequent blood sugar estimations to detect hypoglycaemia, as the postpartum woman's insulin requirements fall rapidly after birth. If she is on insulin, the dose is reduced, depending on the blood sugar levels. Early breastfeeding is recommended and encouraged, although it does alter the woman's blood glucose levels, as it is associated with better neonatal outcomes, maternal weight loss post partum, as well as improved fasting blood glucose levels, glucose tolerance and lipid levels (Kjos et al 1993).

Before going home, the woman is counselled about family planning and advised that oral contraceptives may affect carbohydrate metabolism and hence insulin requirements. A follow-up glucose tolerance test (GTT) is recommended at six to eight weeks post partum using a standard 75 g GTT and evaluative criteria for non-pregnant women. Those with an abnormal GTT (diabetes, impaired glucose tolerance or impaired fasting glycaemia) should be reviewed by an endocrinologist. Women with a normal postnatal GTT should be advised about a healthy lifestyle, and to have a GTT every two years.

Thyroid disease

Numerous hormonal changes occur during pregnancy, resulting in complex metabolic adaptations in maternal thyroid function. Despite this, normal pregnancy is considered to be a euthyroid state. Auto-immune thyroid dysfunctions remain a common cause of both hyperthyroidism and hypothyroidism in pregnant women and these are covered briefly here. Patients with either hyper- or hypothyroidism tend to be infertile, although it is certainly possible to have these diseases and

---

> **Critical thinking exercise**
>
> What will you say to a woman with Graves' disease who says, 'I really want to breastfeed. Can I do this while taking propylthiouracil (PTU)?'

still become pregnant. Graves' disease (hyperthyroidism) accounts for more than 85% of hyperthyroid cases, while Hashimoto's thyroiditis remains the most common cause of hypothyroidism.

Hyperthyroidism

Graves' disease is an auto-immune disease characterised by hyperthyroidism due to circulating autoantibodies. If left untreated, severe thyrotoxicosis, a life-threatening thyrotoxic crisis (i.e. thyroid storm), can occur. Fortunately, pregnant women often experience temporary remission of their symptoms. Treatment of Graves' disease focuses on restoring normal thyroid function with antithyroid medication. Treatment of hyperthyroidism during pregnancy is different from that in non-pregnant women, because radioactive iodine cannot be given and surgery should not be performed because of am increased risk of miscarriage. Because of the immunosuppressive effect of pregnancy, antithyroid drugs (e.g. carbimazole) can be given in lower doses than with non-pregnant patients. Propylthiouracil is not recommended in pregnancy. Radioactive isotopes are secreted in milk and no isotope tests or isotope scans should be performed on a woman who is breastfeeding. Propylthiouracil can be used when breastfeeding, as only negligible amounts pass into the milk.

Hypothyroidism

Hypothyroidism or its associated hormonal changes are associated with anovulation, infrequent menstruation and amenorrhea. In severe cases the pituitary gland produces increased amounts of prolactin, which 'turn off' normal menstrual cycles. Thus, hypothyroidism is associated with infertility and, if pregnancy does occur, there is an increased risk of miscarriage. Very little thyroxine crosses the placental barrier so there is no contraindication to taking thyroxine in pregnancy. Many specialists increase the dose slightly during pregnancy because they feel that pregnancy increases the requirements for thyroxine and thyroid stimulating hormone levels rise. Thyroxine is also secreted in the milk, but provided the dosage in the mother is maintained in the physiological range, it appears to be quite safe for the mother on thyroxine to breastfeed. After birth, the dose of thyroxine is gradually returned to pre-pregnancy levels. The frequency of thyroid function tests is reduced and finally reviewed two months after thyroxine levels reach pre-pregnancy levels.

Heart disease

Fifty years ago, women with heart disease were advised to avoid pregnancy. Now it is not unusual for women with heart disease

WOMAN'S STORY

Type 1 Diabetes and pregnancy: one mother's story
By Kim Barwise

I was 31 years old, happily married and had no health problems despite having had Type 1 diabetes for seven years. It seemed like the right time to have a baby. But on further thought, I worried whether the risks were too high. I was aware of some of the risks to a baby caused by high blood sugars. Would my baby be okay or would he or she develop diabetes? Some of these concerns are typical to anyone with diabetes, but the fear of being responsible for the health and development of another little being was somewhat overwhelming to me. I wanted to have some guarantee that everything would turn out well.

I spoke with my endocrinologist to determine which fears were real. Statistically, the level of risk for a woman with Type 1 or Type 2 diabetes and for the baby is largely determined by the health of the woman just before conception and within the first 11 weeks of pregnancy. Women with diabetes are typically not discouraged from having a baby unless they have experienced eye complications, damage to their kidneys or have heart disease. Good blood sugar control is crucial within the first five to 11 weeks as the baby's organs are beginning to develop. If the mother's blood sugar level is high during this time period, the baby's spinal cord and heart could be affected. There are various tests offered to women at 16 weeks and at 20 weeks to determine the risk for spina bifida, Down syndrome and heart deformities.

Knowing that my blood sugar control was within a good range, and having the support of my endocrinologist and husband, I felt ready to get pregnant. It was a big disappointment. I had put a lot of effort into improving my blood sugar control, attempting to exercise, testing at least four times a day and trying to suppress my worries about my health and the baby's. Was diabetes affecting my ability to become pregnant? According to my endocrinologist, diabetes does not affect fertility. Then, as soon as I stopped worrying, I became pregnant.

Once pregnant, my motivation to manage my diabetes significantly increased. I was conscious of the grams of carbohydrate I was eating, monitored my blood sugar levels seven times a day and adjusted my insulin regularly. The blood sugar goal set by my endocrinologist was 3.5 to seven mmol/L, but this goal can vary depending on the doctor and your ability to recognise and treat hypoglycaemia. While I was able to achieve a healthy blood sugar level throughout most of my pregnancy,

I found blood sugar control difficult during the first trimester. This was probably related to the fluctuating levels of hormones that caused my blood sugar levels to become very high during my eighth week of pregnancy. Typically, women find blood sugar levels drop too low during the first trimester, but it is not uncommon for blood sugar levels to soar into the teens. The support of the endocrinologist and diabetes educators helped to calm my fears. They adjusted my insulin dose to compensate for the 'highs.'

Although I am a diabetes educator, I found it difficult at times to be objective about my health and the baby's. I had to recognise that I couldn't treat my body like a machine and expect everything to be perfect all the time. Given the psychological impact of extra monitoring and the fear of complications, it was important to discuss my concerns with both my doctor and family in order to keep my perspective. Having the opportunity to vent during the first trimester allowed me to cope with the demands of the second and third trimester.

When the third trimester arrived, I found being pregnant and having diabetes became a full-time job. The frequency of ultrasounds and visits to the obstetrician and endocrinologist increased significantly. I was also very tired at that point in my pregnancy. Once, I was caught snoozing on the floor of my office (not recommended!). The frequency of hypoglycaemia increased because the blood sugar levels were so tightly controlled. Having a knowledgeable and supportive family and work environment was crucial to coping with the demands during this trimester.

In my view, one of the few benefits of having Type 1 diabetes was the opportunity to be induced at 38 weeks instead of 40 weeks. Early induction is often recommended because diabetes may cause the placenta to mature faster. When I was at 38 weeks, the weather was hot and humid, my sense of humour was waning and I felt I couldn't possibly get any larger. I was ready to get this pregnancy over with and start being a mum.

The induction took much longer than I had expected. Yet 31 hours of labour were much more tolerable for me with an epidural. After a year and a half of planning and perseverance, the end result was a healthy, beautiful baby girl named Lindsay. All had turned out better than I had expected; it truly was a miracle!

If you are thinking about getting pregnant, my recommendation is not only 'do it' but also 'plan it'! Talk to your endocrinologist or diabetes educator a few months in advance so that the birth of your child will be as wonderful as it should be.
(Source: Barwise 2005)

---

to have a normal (albeit carefully monitored) pregnancy. It is estimated that heart disease affects 1–3% of all pregnancies. It is the leading cause of indirect maternal mortality (Slaytor et al 2004) in Australia. In their most recent report on maternal deaths in Australia, Slaytor et al (2004) report that seven of the 28 indirect maternal deaths were from cardiac-related causes.

The cause of heart disease may be congenital or related to illness, usually rheumatic heart disease. Irrespective of its causation, pre-existing or de nova heart disease is seriously complicated by pregnancy.

Congenital heart disease

The majority of pregnant women with congenital heart disease are aware of their condition and are already receiving cardiologist's care. Nevertheless, not all women are aware that they have heart disease. History taking at the first antenatal contact and questions about a past history of rheumatic fever plus auscultation of abnormal heart sounds may be the woman's first inkling that she has heart disease.

Specialist, skilled care and excellent teamwork can lead to excellent outcomes for both mother and baby. Individual counselling and ongoing care requires a multidisciplinary approach and should ideally include information regarding contraception, maternal and fetal risks of pregnancy, and expected long-term outcomes. Identification of the risks associated with pregnancy and counselling the woman with heart disease are best accomplished before conception. During counselling and information sharing, the following seven areas should be considered: the underlying cardiac lesion, maternal functional status, the possibility of further palliative or corrective surgery, additional associated risk factors, maternal life expectancy, the woman's ability to care for her child, and the possibility of an increased risk of congenital heart disease in her children.

Pregnant women with 'severe' heart disease of any causation may be at particular risk for congestive heart failure, arrhythmias, thrombosis, emboli, and adverse effects of anticoagulants. Such women should be referred to a high-risk pregnancy unit in a tertiary hospital. Ideally the woman leads a team who should meet as early as possible early in the pregnancy. With the woman and her family (unless this has

---

Clinical point

Because it is often not possible for every member of a large multidisciplinary team to attend every meeting, especially in moments of crisis, it is helpful to develop and distribute widely a readily accessible, written management plan, one that is frequently updated for foreseeable contingencies.

---

been done pre-pregnancy) and as early as possible, the team identifies the nature of the cardiac lesion, its anticipated effects on the pregnancy and the effects of the pregnancy on the disease, and explores potential problems. Women with heart disease in the 'low-risk' group can be managed with support in a Level II, community hospital setting.

Conservative medical measures designed to optimise intravascular volume and systemic loading conditions enable many women with congenital heart disease to have successful outcomes. Simple interventions such as maternal bed rest and avoidance of the supine position should not be overlooked. Whenever possible, symptomatic or severe valvular lesions should be addressed and rectified before conception and pregnancy. Pregnant women with mechanical valve prostheses have an obligate need for anticoagulation. Unfortunately, there remain significant problems and an impressive risk for both the mother and fetus from either haemorrhage or thrombosis with the use of either warfarin or heparin. Guidelines for the management of the pregnant woman with a mechanical prosthesis have been difficult to formulate due to the lack of adequate prospective randomised controlled trial data. Practice patterns vary widely and no consensus exists, as might be expected from the disparate results and claims of the retrospective and selective case series that have been reported to date.

Rheumatic heart disease

According to Northern Territory clinicians, Carapetis and Currie (1998), by the end of the twentieth century, the good news about rheumatic fever was that it was so rare that most Australian clinicians would never see a case. Since the 1930s, at least in affluent Australian populations and largely as a result of economic development and improved living conditions, with perhaps a small contribution from antibiotics and possibly altered virulence of circulating Group A streptococcal strains, there has been a dramatic decline in the incidence of rheumatic fever and its devastating complications. The authors (Carapetis & Currie 1998) then move to the bad news, that some socially and economically disadvantaged populations throughout the world, including indigenous and minority populations living in affluent countries such as Australia, still suffer high rates of rheumatic fever and rheumatic heart disease. Indeed, the highest *published* incidence of acute rheumatic fever in the world occurs in Aboriginal people living in the Top End of the Northern Territory (Carapetis et al 1996). Over a five-year study period, the authors discovered that the prevalence of rheumatic heart disease in the non-

---

Case study

A 27-year-old woman, para 0, had her antenatal care overseas. She had congenital aortic stenosis, which was managed with an aortic valve replacement. Her medication included warfarin prior to pregnancy, which was replaced by heparin. She developed gestational diabetes. At 31 weeks she was admitted to a tertiary hospital with provisional diagnosis of thrombosed prosthetic valve and infection. She was managed in the coronary care unit. Two days after admission, she developed dyspnoea, tachycardia and had a cardiac arrest one hour later, A caesarean section was carried out to deliver a stillborn infant followed by cardiac surgery. Her prosthetic valve was found to be mobile with a sub-valvular thrombus. The valve was replaced but she died shortly afterwards. Associate Professor Walters, the reviewer of this section of the report, commented that heparin is a relatively poor substitute for warfarin, and if used, low molecular heparin should be administered in an adequate dose and frequency, particularly with prosthetic aortic valves that are known to predispose to thrombosis.

(Source: Slaytor et al 2004, p 43)

Aboriginal population of the Top End was 0.014% but up to 3% of people living in remote Aboriginal communities in the Northern Territory were found to have established rheumatic heart disease. Rheumatic heart disease often leads to valvular disease such as mitral stenosis or mitral incompetence and aortic incompetence. For this reason this section is primarily focused on the effects of rheumatic heart disease, with special emphasis on the effects of valvular disease on pregnancy and its management.

Valvular heart disease

Valvular heart disease is often first recognised in pregnancy when the profound haemodynamic changes that normally occur during pregnancy put additional strain on the heart, sometimes precipitating heart failure.

Clinical presentation

Mitral stenosis is the most common rheumatic valvular lesion encountered during pregnancy. Depending on the severity and duration of the disease, pregnant women with mitral stenosis frequently present clinically with symptoms of both left-sided heart failure and right ventricular failure. However, left-sided heart failure is more common and symptoms include orthopnea, paroxysmal nocturnal dyspnoea, and dyspnoea on exertion.

Diagnostic assessment

Invasive diagnostic testing is rarely indicated in pregnant women with mitral stenosis. Echocardiography is the diagnostic test of choice because it both confirms the diagnosis and helps to determine the severity of the condition. In addition, it is used to determine pulmonary pressures, right ventricular function and mitral regurgitation.

Management in pregnancy

In addition to the measures designed to manage symptoms, rest is encouraged and dietary advice is given to aid weight control. Iron and folic acid are prescribed to prevent anaemia, and haemoglobin estimation is undertaken frequently. To prevent bacterial endocarditis (see below) a dental referral is made early in pregnancy. If the woman presents with any signs of infection, she is commenced on antibiotics. Any deterioration in the woman's condition, such as shortness of breath and a cough, requires hospital admission for ongoing observation and assessment. Rarely, some women require mitral valvotomy during pregnancy to increase the size of the narrowed mitral valve. The cardiologist on the woman's team may restrict salt and fluid intake. However, diuretics should be used with caution to avoid hypotension and increased heart rate as well as fetal compromise. Use of beta-blocking drugs to slow the heart rate can dramatically improve the woman's symptoms.

Labour and birth

In view of the increase in cardiac output during labour and after giving birth, it is important to plan management carefully. With very few exceptions, vaginal birth is preferable and possible in most women with cardiac disease including mitral stenosis. Preterm induction is rarely indicated, but planned induction of labour and delivery in high-risk situations will ensure availability of appropriate staff and equipment. Heparin anticoagulation is discontinued at least 12 hours before induction of labour, or reversed with protamine sulfate if spontaneous labour develops, and can usually be resumed 6–12 hours post partum.

Optimal management may also require invasive haemo-dynamic studies in women with moderate to severe mitral stenosis. Continuous oxygen via facial mask may be helpful to reduce pulmonary pressures and fluid restriction, and use of diuretics and epidural anaesthesia with adequate volume preloading is the technique of choice.

Labour is usually conducted with the woman lying in the left lateral decubitus position to attenuate haemodynamic fluctuations associated with contractions found if she lies in the supine position. Epidural fentanyl is particularly advantageous in women with cyanotic heart disease because it does not lower peripheral vascular resistance. Instrumental delivery with forceps or vacuum extraction will shorten the latter part of the second stage of labour and reduce the need for maternal expulsive efforts. Active management of the third stage of labour with Syntocinon—not ergometrine—can reduce the incidence of PPH and its complications.

Antibiotic prophylaxis against endocarditis

The incidence of endocarditis is no different in pregnant women with valvular heart disease than in non-pregnant women with the same condition. Streptococcal organisms (including the causative organism of rheumatic heart diseases) are the most common cause of subacute bacterial endocarditis, but acute endocarditis is usually due to more virulent organisms, such as *Staphylococcus aureus*, *Streptococcus pneumoniae* and *Neisseria gonorrhoeae*. Endocarditis prophylaxis is initiated at the onset of active labour when indicated. The American Heart Association recommendations (Bonow et al 1998) state that delivery by caesarean section and vaginal delivery in the absence of infection do not require endocarditis prophylaxis except, perhaps, in women at high risk. However, many centres with extensive experience in caring for pregnant women with heart disease use bacterial endocarditis prophylaxis routinely, as an uncomplicated birth cannot always be anticipated. However, if vaginal infection is already present, antibiotics should be started promptly. In addition, antibiotic prophylaxis seems appropriate for women in other high-risk categories. These include pregnant women who have any of the following:

- prosthetic valves
- history of bacterial endocarditis
- valvular heart disease (aortic stenosis, aortic regurgitation, mitral regurgitation or stenosis with mitral regurgitation)
- hypertrophic cardiomyopathy.

Anticoagulation therapy during pregnancy

Pregnancy involves a state of hypercoagulability caused by increased levels of various clotting factors and increased blood viscosity. Systemic anticoagulation poses major problems during pregnancy in women with prosthetic heart valves, venous or arterial thromboembolism, or atrial fibrillation with valvular heart disease. When a pregnant woman, perhaps with a mechanical heart valve, requires anticoagulation, heparin and warfarin are used but controversy continues as to which is better at different stages of pregnancy. Oral anticoagulants such as warfarin sodium cause fetal embryopathy; subcutaneous administration of heparin sodium has been reported to be ineffective in preventing thromboembolic complications (Chan et al 2000). Unfractionated heparin does not cross the placenta and has little effect on the fetus. However, long-term IV use is inconvenient and so is often unacceptable to women. Experience with low-molecular-weight heparin (LMWH) in such situations is minimal, although it appears that this drug is less effective than oral anticoagulants in preventing thromboembolism (Chan et al 2000). Moreover, LMWH is associated with low neonatal mortality and low incidences of premature delivery, spontaneous abortion, and intrauterine

fetal death. However, it can cause significant osteoporosis in pregnant women. Consequently, on the basis of the data available, most authorities (Bonow et al 1998; Chan et al 2000) recommend ceasing warfarin as early as possible in pregnancy and instead using subcutaneous heparin therapy for at least the first trimester. After this, warfarin therapy can be reinstituted.

Postnatal care and follow-up

As maternal haemodynamics do not return to baseline for many days after giving birth, the following may apply for women at intermediate or high risk:

- Provide continuous monitoring for at least 72 hours post partum.
- Rest is encouraged.
- If appropriate, antibiotic cover is continued.
- Breastfeeding is not contraindicated.

Before she goes home, family planning and contraception are discussed. The woman will be followed up at the cardiology clinic, in addition to midwife and GP follow-up.

Respiratory disease

Pregnancy induces profound changes in the mother, resulting in significant alterations in normal physiology. The anatomical and functional changes of pregnancy affect the respiratory and cardiovascular systems. Management of respiratory problems in pregnancy requires an understanding of these changes for interpretation of clinical and laboratory manifestations of respiratory diseases.

Asthma

Occurring in 4% of pregnant women and complicating up to 1.5% of pregnancies, asthma represents the most common obstructive pulmonary disease of pregnancy (Blaiss 2004). Asthma does not usually worsen during pregnancy; in fact, many women, but not all, find that their asthma improves. In their systematic review of the literature, McDonald and Burdon (1996) state that although bronchial hyper-responsiveness lessens in mid-pregnancy, studies reporting changes in asthma severity during pregnancy show widely differing results. The authors (1996) state that, overall, the

---

Critical thinking exercise

1. How will you respond to a woman with mitral valve stenosis who asks if it is safe to take warfarin in early pregnancy?

2. Women who have had valve replacements are often on oral anticoagulation therapy. Then, as the anticipated birth date draws near, this is changed to subcutaneous heparin. Why is this change of therapy necessary and what are the evidence-based advantages and disadvantages of LMWH versus unfractionated heparin in pregnancy and the postpartum period?

data indicate that the clinical severity of asthma during pregnancy improves in about 30% of women, remains stable in about 50% and worsens in about 20%. Although the specific mechanisms involved in changing the course of asthma during pregnancy have not been determined, they are likely to be multifactorial.

Avoidance and control of asthma triggers are important because poorly controlled asthma or severe asthma not only threatens the life of the mother but also threatens the fetus because of increased maternal hypoxaemia and diminution of uterine artery blood flow secondary to hypocapnic vasoconstriction. Women with poorly controlled asthma have an increased incidence of hyperemesis gravidarum, haemorrhage and pre-eclampsia. Their babies are more likely to: be low birthweight and preterm; suffer neonatal hypoxia from complications during labour; and have increased perinatal and maternal mortality (McDonald & Burdon 1996).

Unfortunately, in pregnancy asthma can still be triggered by many factors, including allergy, upper respiratory tract infection, sinusitis, exercise, aspirin, non-steroidal anti-inflammatory agents (NSAIDS), environmental toxins (e.g. tobacco smoke, chemical fumes), humidity, anxiety and emotional distress.

Asthma medications during pregnancy

Although care providers have a natural reluctance to prescribe drug therapy in pregnancy, poorly controlled asthma is potentially more dangerous for the fetus than medication. Diagnostic testing is the same for non-pregnant women and pregnant women. However, when interpreting blood gas values, it is important to remember the normal values for pregnancy. For example, the PaO_2 is higher in pregnant women than in non-pregnant women, ranging from 102 mmHg to 116 mmHg. In addition, the normal physiological increase in minute ventilation results in a lower $PaCO_2$ range of 28 mmHg to 30 mmHg. Therefore, a low PaO_2 or a high $PaCO_2$ associated with an acute episode of asthma may represent significantly more severe respiratory compromise than similar blood gas values in a non-pregnant woman. Nevertheless, mild changes in pulmonary function are usually reversible and tolerated in healthy pregnant women. However, in some circumstances an increased basal metabolic rate, increased oxygen consumption, decreased carbon monoxide-diffusing capacity, decreased buffers and alterations in lung volumes increase the woman's susceptibility to the detrimental effects of hypoxia caused by asthma. Women should therefore be advised to continue with their pre-pregnancy medication in consultation with specialist care providers.

Management of asthma

As with non-pregnant women, beta-2 agonists are used for symptomatic benefit during acute asthma. Inhaled corticosteroids remain the mainstay of therapy for asthma control. Long-acting adrenergic agonists might be used in symptomatic patients on adequate corticosteroid therapy. Generally a stepwise approach to management is preferred,

---

BOX 33.18 Asthma management

Environmental control, pharmacological treatment and specific allergen immunotherapy are the cornerstones of asthma management for all patients. Of these, institution of environmental control measures to lessen exposure to triggers is even more vital during pregnancy, Helping women to learn how to watch for and avoid these triggers will probably improve symptom control, and may possibly result in pregnant women needing less medication. Gastroesophageal reflux is a common problem in late pregnancy and is a documented asthma trigger. Advising the woman to eat small meals and to raise the head of her bed by several centimetres may help alleviate this problem. Some women may require antacids or H_2-receptor-blocking medications.

Clinical point

Medications for asthma have been shown to be safe for both the mother and the developing baby. It is more dangerous to have untreated asthma during pregnancy than to continue with prescribed asthma therapy. Asthma reduces the amount of oxygen available to the fetus. To maintain optimum control of their asthma it is important for women to follow an individualised asthma action plan very carefully.

BOX 33.19 Asthma update

The National Heart, Lung and Blood Institute (NHBLI) website (see below) has updates on the *Report of the Working Group on Asthma and Pregnancy*, published by the National Asthma Education and Prevention Program (NAEPP): *Managing Asthma During Pregnancy: Recommendations for Pharmacologic Treatment—Update 2004*. It also has the *Expert Panel Report: Guidelines for the Diagnosis and Management of Asthma* (1997) available for download. The new guidelines offer recommendations regarding the use of allergy medications in pregnancy based on recent studies of these medications. Information about the expert panel and its financial disclosures are included in the full report.

National Heart, Lung and Blood Institute (NHLBI) http://www.nhlbi.nih.gov/health/prof/lung/asthma/astpreg.htm

---

one that gradually increases the number of medications used and their doses. Occasionally corticosteroids are necessary but should be used only for short periods. An increased risk of cleft palate and placental abnormalities is reported in animals given oral steroids in first trimester, but not humans. Nonetheless, the benefits of oral steroids may outweigh the risks if they are used to manage severe asthma or during life-threatening exacerbations because the steroidoral cleft palate relationship is irrelevant after the first trimester.

Breastfeeding

Breastfeeding should be encouraged in women with asthma, as breast milk confers some immunity to infection to the baby, especially to respiratory and gastrointestinal infections. Breast milk contains very small amounts of the usual medications used to prevent and treat asthma, but there is no evidence that this is harmful to the infant. However, the manufacturers of budesonide have recommended discontinuation of this drug during lactation because of an absence of information regarding its transmission into breast milk. The decision to alter a successful medication regimen that is controlling the mother's asthma must be weighed against any potential detrimental effects to the infant from continuation of the drug.

Consequently, women should be reassured that although asthma medications do enter breast milk, their concentrations are extremely small and do not have any adverse effects on their babies.

Acute asthma exacerbation

Acute exacerbations that necessitate emergency department visits typically require a course of systemic corticosteroids. In addition, oxygen therapy is used to maintain oxygen saturation levels at or above 95% to ensure both maternal and fetal wellbeing. There is no evidence of teratogenic effects associated with bronchospasm relaxants such as the beta-2 agonists (category A)—salbutamol, terbutaline and fenoterol. Although IV salbutamol is used to delay the onset of preterm labour, these affects do not occur with bronchodilators administered by metered-dose inhaler or wet nebulisation.

Tuberculosis

Tuberculosis (TB) is an infection caused by *Mycobactrium tuberculosis*. Its inflammatory process causes destruction of lung tissue, increased production of sputum and coughing. If a woman receiving medication for active TB becomes pregnant, she continues with her medications. If the disease is diagnosed for the first time during pregnancy, anti-tuberculoid medication is still commenced and this protects the fetus from the disease. Labour is managed normally and, in the presence of active disease, an elective vacuum extraction or forceps delivery may be recommended to shorten the second stage of labour.

The disease may reactivate in the postnatal period. Breastfeeding is contraindicated if the woman has active TB while treatment is established. However, anti-tuberculoid medications cross into the breast milk. Vaccination is always recommended in high-risk groups, such as people from Asian or Pacific backgrounds and Indigenous Australians, or if other members of the household have or have had a history of pulmonary TB or if they are likely to come in contact with people at high risk of infection. In Australia and New Zealand, parents are encouraged to immunise their babies with BCG (bacille Calmette-Guerin) vaccine.

Renal disease

The renal system undergoes monumental physiological and anatomical changes during a normal pregnancy. An understanding of these changes is necessary in order to understand how they may lead to or worsen pre-existing or new renal disease. Only the most common conditions are dealt with in this section. Others such as glomerular nephritis, chronic renal disease and renal transplantation are not included here and the reader should refer to the appropriate specialist texts.

Urinary tract infection

Urinary tract infections (UTIs), especially asymptomatic bacteriuria and cystitis, are common pregnancy complications. Pyelonephritis is less common but has the potential to cause significant morbidity and adverse outcomes. Early identification and treatment of UTIs in pregnancy and post partum are crucial because of their close association with maternal hypertension, anaemia and preterm labour, making the fetus at risk of all the complications associated with low birthweight. The fetus is also at risk of IUGR. It seems that the bacterium that causes the UTI has the potential to infect fetal membranes, leading to chorioamnionitis. Finally, inadequately treated UTIs and upper tract infections such as pyelonephritis have a high incidence of later chronic renal pathology.

Traditionally, screening pregnant women's urine for glucose, ketones and protein at every antenatal visit has been a common practice. The gold standard for screening for asymptomatic bacteriuria is growing bacterial cultures of urine samples from women in early pregnancy. Contrary to popular belief, non-culture methods such as dipsticks are not generally reliable for the identification of bacteriuria in asymptomatic

---

Revision

Normal anatomical and physiological changes in pregnancy

The normal anatomical and physiological changes in pregnancy predispose the pregnant woman to UTIs and the reader may need to refresh their pre-existing knowledge by revising an appropriate textbook. In brief, starting in the first weeks of pregnancy, most pregnant women develop hydronephrosis of pregnancy. Under the influence of pregnancy hormones, increased bladder volume and decreased bladder tone, along with decreased ureteral tone, contribute to increased urinary stasis and ureterovesical reflux. This urine becomes a good growth medium for bacteria. Also, an increase in the plasma volume during pregnancy decreases urine concentration. More than two-thirds of pregnant women develop glycosuria, which encourages bacterial growth in the urine. Increases in urinary progestins and oestrogens reduce the ability of the lower urinary tract to resist pathogens.

populations, including pregnant women. Routine urinalysis is imprecise for identification of pyuria. Pyuria-based methods, particularly leucocyte-esterase dipstick, are subject to false negatives in bacteriuria without pyuria and false-positives with contamination from vaginal secretions. Nevertheless, many maternity centres require urinalysis at every antenatal consultation. If this is the case, women may prefer to test and interpret their own urine specimens for the presence of protein and nitrites or other evidence of infection. In addition to laboratory screening tests, it is important that the midwife gathers data about the woman's history of infections and existing renal pathology, renal function studies and family or personal history of renal disease, hypertension or connective tissue disorders.

Asymptomatic bacteriuria and cystitis

As many as 11% of pregnant women will develop asymptomatic bacteriuria and, as the name suggests, have no symptoms of a UTI. The prevalence is higher among women from lower socio-economic backgrounds and those with a history of asymptomatic urinary infection. Increased frequency of screening during pregnancy identifies more cases. Approximately 1–2% of women who are not bacteriuric at initial screening early in pregnancy will develop bacteriuria later in the pregnancy. Asymptomatic bacteriuria is significant if there are 10^5 organisms per mL of cultured urine. The usual organism responsible is *Escherichia coli* (over 90%). Other possible organisms include *Proteus mirabilis*, *Klebsiella pneumoniae*, *Staphylococcus saprophyticus*, *Pseudomonas aeruginosa* and the alpha-haemolytic or beta-haemolytic *Streptococcus*.

The choice of antibiotic should address the most common infecting organisms (i.e. Gram-negative gastrointestinal organisms such as *E. coli*). Historically, ampicillin has been the drug of choice, but in recent years *E. coli* has become increasingly resistant to ampicillin. Other antibiotics include nitrofurantoin, the cephalosporins, cefaclor or amoxicillin-clavulanate. Fosfomycin (Monurol) is taken as a single dose. Sulfonamides can be taken during the first and second trimesters, but during the third trimester their use carries a risk of kernicterus of the newborn, especially preterm infants. Tetracyclines are contraindicated for use in pregnancy because of rare maternal acute fatty liver necrosis. In addition, they cause permanent staining of the fetal dentition. A five- to 10-day course of antibiotic treatment is usually sufficient to eradicate the infecting organism(s). Some authorities have advocated shorter courses of treatment—even single-day therapy.

Symptomatic cystitis

A woman with symptomatic cystitis often complains of urgency and frequency of micturition and dysuria. She may have some lower abdominal discomfort and a slightly raised temperature and pulse rate. In general, treatment is initiated before the results of the culture are available. A midstream urine sample (MSU) is sent to the laboratory for a bacterial count, the leucocyte (pus) cell count and the identification

---

Research

A study of various tests to detect asymptomatic urinary tract infections in an obstetric population (Bachman et al 1993)

Bachman and colleagues compared the efficacy of faster, and usually less expensive, screening methods (e.g. dipstick, nitrite dipstick, urinalysis and urine Gram staining) with urine culture and found that although it was quicker and more cost-effective to screen for bacteriuria with dipsticks, less than half of the women with bacteriuria were identified compared with screening by urine culture. Further, the increased rate of false-negatives and the relatively poor predictive value of positive tests made the faster, albeit cheaper, methods less efficacious. The authors recommended that a urine culture be routinely used to screen for bacteriuria at the first antenatal visit and again in the third trimester.

BOX 33.20 Preventing UTIs

Midwives are ideally placed to work with women to prevent the initial occurrence of UTIs and ongoing problems. Measures include the following:

▶ Drink 6–8 glasses of water each day, to flush out bacteria. Unsweetened cranberry juice may prevent UTIs.
▶ Avoid refined foods, fruit juices, caffeine, alcohol and sugar.
▶ Develop a habit of urinating as soon as the need is felt, emptying the bladder completely.
▶ Wipe the perineum from front to back after voiding or defecation.
▶ Avoid using strong soaps, douches, antiseptic creams, feminine hygiene sprays and powder.
▶ Urinate before and after intercourse.
▶ Wear cotton underwear and avoid tight-fitting pants.
▶ Use lubricating jelly if needed during sexual intercourse.
▶ Report early signs of UTI or genital infection.
▶ Always complete a course of antibiotics.

---

of the organisms present and their sensitivity to several antibiotics. If the bacterial count is over 10^5 organisms per mL of urine, the woman is commenced on a broad-spectrum antibiotic (see above). Usually the infection is due to *E. coli*. Antibiotic choice, as in asymptomatic bacteriuria, should focus on coverage of the common pathogens and can be changed after the organism is identified and sensitivities are determined.

An increased intake (3000 mL) of oral fluids is encouraged. The woman is observed for any signs of the onset of labour, and fetal wellbeing assessed through CTG recording of the fetal heart rate. A repeat MSU should be obtained one to two weeks later and a further course of antibiotics prescribed if infection is still present. Women who present with more than three UTIs in the antenatal period require a renal physician consult and further investigation, and may be commenced on an antibiotic such as nitrofurantoin for the remainder of the pregnancy in addition to regular assessment.

Pyelonephritis

Acute pyelonephritis during pregnancy is a serious systemic illness that can progress to maternal sepsis, preterm labour and birth. It is defined as inflammation of one or both kidneys. Pyelonephritis occurs in 2% of pregnant women; almost a quarter of these have another episode of the disease in the same pregnancy. Infected urine is forced up through the ureters and infects the renal pelves and the kidney substance, causing pyleonephritis. The diagnosis is made when the presence of bacteriuria is accompanied by systemic symptoms or signs such as fever, chills, nausea, and vomiting and flank pain. The woman feels most unwell, has a high temperature, rapid pulse and shivering, and rigors may occur. Headaches, nausea and vomiting may also be present. Symptoms of lower tract infection (i.e. frequency and dysuria) may or may not be present.

Collaborative management

Early, aggressive treatment is important in preventing complications from pyelonephritis. Hospitalisation is not always necessary, although it is indicated for women who are exhibiting signs of sepsis, who are vomiting, perhaps dehydrated and who may be having uterine contractions. Intravenous antibiotic therapy (and IV fluids, if hospitalisation is required) may be initiated before obtaining the results of urine culture and sensitivity. Several antibiotic regimens may be used. The woman's vital signs are recorded four-hourly and she is observed for signs of the onset of labour. Fetal wellbeing is assessed through CTG recording of the fetal heart rate. Follow-up and repeat MSUs are undertaken to ensure the infection has been adequately treated. Other diagnostic tests may include renal ultrasonography or, if indicated, an abbreviated IV pyelogram. Even the low-dose radiation involved in an IV pyelogram may be dangerous to the fetus and therefore such tests should be avoided during pregnancy whenever possible. However, in the presence of recurrent pyelonephritis, an IV pyelogram may be necessary.

There are a number of non-pharmacological, 'natural' remedies for the prevention and treatment of UTIs:

- Urinary antiseptics are antimicrobial: uva ursi (*Arctostaphylos uva ursi*), buchu (*Agathosma betulina*), thyme leaf (*Thymus vulgaris*), pipissewa (*Chimaphila umbellata*).
- Urinary astringents tone and heal the urinary tract: horsetail (*Equisetum arvense*), plantain (*Plantago major*).
- Urinary demulcents soothe the inflamed urinary tract: corn silk (*Zea mays*), couch grass (*Agropyron repens*).

> ### Clinical point
>
> The most common reason for treatment failure in pyelonephritis is antibiotic resistance.

There has been little research and no well-controlled studies examining the effectiveness of homeopathic remedies in the treatment of UTIs. Qualified homeopaths, however, may recommend a range of treatments for UTI, based on their expertise and clinical experience. Before prescribing a remedy, homeopaths take into account the woman's constitutional type—physical, emotional, and intellectual make-up—before deciding on the most appropriate remedy for a particular individual.

- *Apis mellifica* or *Berberis*—for dysuria
- *Aconitum*—for early symptoms of UTI
- *Cantharis*—this is the most common and considered the most effective homeopathic remedy for UTI.
- *Mercurius* and *Nux vomica*—urgency and dysuria
- *Pulsatilla*—for bladder inflammation
- *Staphysagria*—for UTIs usually associated with sexual intercourse or sexual abuse.

Obstetric cholestasis (intrahepatic cholestasis)

Obstetric cholestasis is a rare liver disease characterised by itching and abnormal liver function tests (Coombes 2000). The itching initially is in the palms of the hands and the soles of the feet and there is no rash. It commences in the last 12 weeks of pregnancy and increases in severity, spreading and becoming more centralised and more distressing as the pregnancy progresses, especially at night (Coombes 2000). Other symptoms may be dark urine, pale stools and/or jaundice. The term 'cholestasis' refers to the diminished secretion of bile formed by the liver to the intestines. Bile accumulates in the bloodstream and may cause itching. The cause is unknown but it is thought that the high levels of circulating oestrogen in pregnancy may cause the reduction in the flow of bile (Turner 2000). Fat-soluble vitamins such as vitamin K are not absorbed, resulting in increased risk of PPH and fetal intracranial haemorrhage. In addition the fetus of a woman with cholestasis is at risk of premature birth, meconium aspiration, intrauterine death, stillbirth and non-reassuring fetal heart tracings.

Diagnosis is made by a history of itching in the presence of abnormal bile acid (salts) test results. Liver function tests may be normal. The woman with obstetric cholestasis requires close monitoring of herself and her fetus. This includes regular CTG recordings, fortnightly ultrasound assessment for growth, weekly liquor and Doppler placental function scans and weekly blood tests. Rest and a good diet are encouraged. Associated UTIs are common. For her comfort the woman is advised to have frequent cool baths, to use skin lotions to soothe the itch and to wear loose-fitting cotton clothing. Ursodeoxycholic acid (Urso) improves the itching and normalises biochemistry. Dexamethasone and vitamin K administration are also helpful. Labour is induced at about 37 weeks to avoid an increased risk of stillbirth (Kenyon et al 2002). Itching resolves during in the first two postnatal weeks (Turner 2000). The woman should be warned that oral contraceptives can cause a similar condition and that obstetric cholestasis is likely to recur in subsequent pregnancies.

Epilepsy

While most women with seizure disorders find that pregnancy has no effect on their disease, about one-third will have an increase in seizure activity. Epilepsy is a disease of the central nervous system resulting in convulsive seizures accompanied by paroxysmal cerebral dysrhythmia, followed by a period of unconsciousness. Women of childbearing age who have epilepsy have many concerns about how their epilepsy will affect their chances of having a baby. They want to know how anti-convulsive medications will affect them in pregnancy and their unborn child. Epilepsy imposes special risks for pregnancy and the woman and the clinicians who support her should be aware of these. Ideally, planning for a baby begins well before conception, so the woman and her clinical team can work together to keep the mother healthy and give her a very good chance of delivering a normal, healthy baby.

Risks to pregnancy

During pregnancy, the number of seizures may increase or decrease or remain unchanged. About 50% of pregnant women have no change in the number of seizures during pregnancy. Many women experience an increase in seizure frequency because they have changed or reduced the amount of anti-convulsive medication they take. Therefore, whenever possible, the anticonvulsant medication the woman has been prescribed prior to becoming pregnant should be maintained, though the dosage may require adjusting later in the pregnancy. Nevertheless, anti-epileptic medications pose significant risks for the fetus.

Risks to the mother and fetus

Reports of congenital malformations associated with anti-epileptic drugs (AEDs) are well documented. Unique malformations are associated with many of the commonly prescribed AEDs: phenytoin, phenobarbitone, primidone, valproate, carbamazepine and trimethadione. Children born to women with epilepsy are, on average, smaller in size and weight than those children born to women who do not have epilepsy. The reasons for this discrepancy are not clear. However, there is some evidence that the increased incidence of growth disparities and congenital malformations in babies of mothers with epilepsy occurs even without AED use.

Types of fetal malformation when the mother has epilepsy include microcephaly, slowed growth and impaired intellect. Certain other abnormalities, such as cleft lip, cleft palate, heart abnormalities and spina bifida, are seen more frequently in children born to mothers on AEDs. Less serious fetal abnormalities include ptosis, decreased muscle tone, hernias and talipes.

The mother's seizures represent the single largest risk to the fetus because it is deprived of oxygen during the seizure. Rarely, the fetus may be injured if the mother falls, is involved in a motor vehicle accident or injures herself during a seizure. Therefore the goal during pregnancy should be to prevent all seizures. There is still considerable controversy about the use of AEDs in pregnancy, which drugs to use and the associated risks to the fetus. In general, since the risk from the drugs is very small, having a seizure during pregnancy is much more dangerous to the fetus than the dangers associated with anti-epileptic medications. Therefore, if the risk for recurrent seizures is high then medication should still be used. However, in women at low risk of seizure, before becoming pregnant it may be possible for the woman to decrease pharmacotherapy or to taper the dosages of AEDs. Though it might appear that the ideal situation would be to stop AEDs, for most women this is not a realistic option. In the twenty-first century, the potential disruption of the woman's lifestyle by seizures, such as the risk of loss of driver's licence, makes elimination of AEDs impractical. Just as importantly, maternal seizures increase the risk of injury, miscarriage, epilepsy in the offspring and children's developmental delay.

Collaborative management

All women diagnosed with epilepsy or other neurological disorders causing seizures and wanting to have a baby require an expert, multidisciplinary team who work collaboratively with the woman to provide her and the baby with quality care.

Preconceptual care

The woman should be supported in ways that ensure that her pregnancies are planned, and so it is crucial that she has access to and uses effective contraception. Combined pill regimens are required by women on enzyme-inducing anticonvulsants (carbamazepine, phenytoin, primidone, phenobartitone) because these drugs reduce the effectiveness of oral contraceptives. All women should be offered genetic counselling. Pre-pregnancy discussions should include information about the risks to mother and fetus as well as the need for modification of her AED regimen to reduce the number of drugs and total dose. Anticonvulsant drugs may result in folic acid deficiency, so the woman is advised to take oral folic acid 5 mg daily for the first three months of pregnancy.

The following is a checklist for preconceptual discussion:
● Find out what the woman knows and fill in the gaps.
● Discuss the diagnosis and its implications for childbearing.
● Review seizure frequency and severity.

Clinical point

More than 95% of pregnant women with epilepsy give birth to normal, healthy babies. Women should be reassured that the risk of fetal malformations associated with epilepsy and associated medications is very small. Other serious diseases represent a much higher risk for fetal deformity than epilepsy. For example, diabetic women deliver, on average, 92 healthy babies out of 100.

- Consider use of a seizure diary.
- Discuss drugs—benefits, disadvantages, modifications and side-effects.
- Discuss the impact of pregnancy on the woman and her family's lifestyle.
- Provide addresses of support organisations.
- Discuss contraception and pregnancy with the woman.
- Agree on a timetable for follow-up support.

Pregnancy

The woman is offered serum screening at 16 weeks and at least one detailed ultrasound (by an appropriately skilled sonographer) at 11–13 weeks and then again between 18 and 22 weeks. It may be necessary to adjust the anticonvulsant regimen. For women on enzyme-inducing anticonvulsants, the risk to the baby of haemorrhagic disease of the newborn is increased, so vitamin K 10–20 mg daily may be administered to the woman from 36 weeks until delivery. Excessive weight gain due to fluid retention during pregnancy may exacerbate seizure activity and so the woman will need advice about how to manage her weight gain.

Intrapartum care

The usual anticonvulsant regimen is maintained during labour. The same range of analgesia (including epidural) available to other mothers should be available. Early recourse to caesarean section under general anaesthesia may be necessary if it is not possible to control seizures, which often occur during labour. Where possible, a paediatrician should review the baby to exclude the possibility of rare congenital malformations secondary to the teratogenic effects of anticonvulsants.

Postpartum care

Anticonvulsant drugs also cross the placenta and the neonate may develop withdrawal symptoms. As the risk to the baby of haemorrhagic disease of the newborn is increased, vitamin K is administered to the infant immediately after birth. Midwives should support and encourage breastfeeding, and provide advice about safe and suitable settings for feeding, bathing, and so on. Before discharge it is important to review AEDs and contraceptive regimens and to reiterate the need for pre-conceptual care for future pregnancies.

Management of seizures

In the community or in hospital, for patients with generalised tonic-clonic seizures, the following general guidelines should be followed:

- Secure the airway.
- Call for help—midwives, anaesthesiologists, obstetrician, physician and paediatrician.
- Give oxygen.
- Assess cardiac and respiratory function.
- Secure IV access in large veins.
- Manage seizures acutely with IV benzodiazepines (10 mg of diazepam or lorazepam 4 mg IV), then load phenytoin (1 g loaded over one hour). If there is a delay in gaining IV access, give diazepam 10–20 mg rectally.

- Assess the fetal heart rate or fetal status.
- Rule out eclampsia.
  On admission to hospital, care may include the following:
- Collect blood for full blood count, urea and electrolyte, liver function tests, calcium, glucose, clotting, AED levels and storage for later analysis.
- Check fetal status. A non-reassuring heart rate trace may indicate an emergency caesarean section.
- Measure blood gases to assess extent of acidosis.
- Establish aetiology. Give 50 mL 50% glucose IV if there is any suggestion of hypoglycaemia and IV thiamine (given as Pabrinex two pairs of ampoules) if there is any suggestion of alcohol abuse or impaired nutritional status.
  If the seizures persist (status epilepticus), the woman is:
- admitted to an intensive care unit (ICU) and administered general anaesthesia
- monitored using EEG to assess seizure control
- referred for specialist advice.

Thromboembolic disease

Venous thromboembolic (VTE) disease causing deep vein thrombosis and pulmonary embolism is a major cause of maternal mortality in Australia, the United Kingdom and the United States, occurring at a rate of approximately one death per 100 000 maternities (Obstetric Medicine Group of Australasia 2001). The rate is much higher in older women. In the United Kingdom, women aged over 39 years had a mortality rate of one death per 3300 pregnancies (Obstetric Medicine Group of Australasia 2001). Pulmonary thromboembolism (PTE) is also a leading cause of maternal mortality in Australia (Slaytor et al 2004). There were six deaths out of a total of 90 mortalities in the 1997–1999 triumvirate in which PTE was judged to be the principal cause of death. All six were classified as Direct Maternal Deaths. In their report, Slaytor et al (2004, p 26) comment that based on a preliminary analysis of hospital discharge data from 1997–1999 it is likely that there were 500–600 cases of pulmonary embolism associated with pregnancy and the post partum.

Pathology

The development of venous thromboembolism (VTE) requires the compounding effect of three factors, often referred to as Virchow's triad, after the scientist who first described these aetiological associations in relation to VTE 150 years ago. The basis of the triad is stasis, vessel trauma, and hypercoagulability. Progesterone-mediated changes in the blood vessels causes stasis of the venous blood flow, resulting in pooling of blood. Compression of the pelvic blood vessels compounds this physiological change. Damaged endothelium may be caused by direct trauma, such as during birth via caesarean section, infections of surrounding soft tissue, IV catheters or prolonged use of them. The trauma releases platelet-activating factors, initiating the coagulation cascade, which results in platelet adhesion to the blood vessel wall and the beginning of thrombus formation. Thirdly, clotting

WOMAN'S STORY

From Living with Epilepsy, by Julie Dennison

Here is one of the many talks I have given on my personal experiences with epilepsy. This was to the staff at the Epilepsy Centre of the National Society for Epilepsy.

So you want children! What a wonderful way to seal a relationship. Is it always possible to do this? Not in all cases. There are many illnesses where pregnancy is thought to be too dangerous and very unwise. So what about epilepsy?

Is it possible to give birth? And do you pass on the gene that says: 'You will have epilepsy and have the same problems as your parents'? Perhaps, perhaps not. No-one can be sure. Epilepsy is not always hereditary. Just in some cases. I was lucky.

Despite family members trying to get me to adopt children, I went ahead and had children of my own. As there was no history of epilepsy in my family—I was just unlucky to be born with it—the doctors seemed to think that all would be well. So we went ahead.

All medication had to be stopped on the doctor's advice. I put on a lot of weight. . . . The seizures were occurring so frequently that everything became difficult. I was lucky, though, as friends and local children were a great help. The local shop was only just down the road, a mere few minutes away, but that walk became a major trip. People would walk with one on either side of me.

. . . So let's get to the practical side of things. Before cooking, I prepared most of the food in the dining room, rather than the kitchen. If I did have a fall, it would be onto a carpet rather than a concrete floor. This would be safer for me as well as my unborn child.

Getting upstairs? Well, I would walk upstairs sideways and slide downstairs, step by step, on my bottom. This was the safest way to travel.

The side door of the house was always left open in the summer. This was so that my neighbours could hear the noise I would make when a seizure took place. . . . I was even having seizures in my sleep. There seemed to be no escape. Most of my life was lived indoors whilst I was pregnant. . . .

The next stage was the birth. Once again it was hard work. . . . Then an eight pound, twelve ounce baby boy was born, measuring twenty-three and a half inches long. He was beautiful, and within less than a few months he had been declared free of epilepsy. All that stuff I had been told about my children being less than perfect was just sheer and utter rubbish. My baby was fine: No illness, no disease no nothing.

[At home] the rules, regulations and just simple common sense had to apply. I had a life in my hands. So how did I cope? When the babies (we had another boy 18 months later) were small, night feeds were always done by my husband. He knew that to get through the day safely I had to have rest, so he had a day job then had to come home to a not very restful night! One thing about a relationship is that it's a partnership. . . .

We had an electric bottle warmer . . . so I didn't have to go near a gas stove. [We bought a microwave to heat the baby feeds.] . . . Feeding time was difficult. It was too dangerous to put my baby in my arms and feed him. I had no warning of my seizures so anything could happen. So I used to feed my son in his buggy. I would kneel beside the buggy and lean backwards with my arm outstretched as far as possible. If I did have a fall I would fall backwards, and not on my young child. . . .

Bathing my baby could only be done with someone else in the house. . . . I always took part in the little things, and these meant so much to me. Changing my baby was very similar to feeding; kneeling down on the floor beside my baby, and if possible leaning away from him. . . .

As the babies got older they wanted to crawl. But I couldn't let them crawl freely. I used to put them in a playpen with their favourite toys. My absences were occurring at a rate of about 20 to 30 every day. They didn't last long, but each was long enough to cause a tragedy. . . . I regret I could never take my boys to playschool or primary school. It was too dangerous, so someone would take them for me and I would watch from the window. Every detail of our lives had to be discussed and thought out very carefully.

The children were told at a very young age about their Mum's problems. They had to be, so they would be prepared. I think we told them in simple terms that Mum would fall down from time to time, or she would blank out and may not hear what they were saying. It was difficult to explain to them without putting them in a panic, but the best way is simple honesty. Children accept things far easier than many people think.

From a very early age, they were able to get help. They were too small to do first aid, but by getting help they were on the right track. . . . Once I burnt myself with an iron. I have had many falls on concrete floors resulting in broken and cracked ribs, cuts, bruising and sprains. . . .

My children, who are now 16 and 18 respectively, still care and each is there like a coiled spring every time I make an involuntary movement. They tell their friends, and none of them seem to worry. They take me for what I am and, like myself, they raise a smile when a blackout occurs. It is the only way to cope.

(Source: Dennison 2004)

factors alter during pregnancy. There are increased levels of Factor V and VIII and fibrinogen, acquired resistance to activated protein C (an endogenous anticoagulant) and a reduction of its co-factor, protein S. Increased inhibitors of plasminogen activator result in impaired fibrinolysis. In addition, hypercoagulability of blood may be caused by other haematological conditions such as anaemia or infectious disease (pneumonia) or as a secondary complication to renal disease, hypercoagulable medications and oral contraceptives. Drife (2003) makes the very important point that compared to the non-pregnant population, there is a twelve-fold increased risk of thromboembolism in pregnant women. In contrast, oral contraceptives increase the risk of thromboembolism three-fold. However, the risk of thromboembolism associated with the Pill is better known than the risks associated with pregnancy. Drife (2003) argues that it is regrettable that such misconceptions are helping to restrict the availability of oral contraceptives to women in developing countries, where deaths from repeated unplanned childbirths are a more significant cause of maternal mortality.

Risks for venous thromboembolism

Pregnancy is a risk factor for VTE and has a ten-fold increase in risk in comparison to non-pregnant women (RCOG 2004). The risk is even higher if delivery is by caesarean section, especially if it is an emergency procedure. Although it is associated with high degrees of morbidity and mortality, VTE during pregnancy and the immediate postnatal period is rare. A Cochrane Review identified the best estimate of incidence as 0.13%; however, other estimates varying from 0.06% to 0.11% have been published. Women particularly at risk of thromboembolic disease include those over 35 years of age, women who have undergone an operative delivery including unplanned caesarean section, immobility, maternal weight over 80 kg, women with significant medical disorders such as heart disease or previous thromboembolic disorders, women with infection, high parity and women with a diagnosis of pre-eclampsia. Recently a number of congenital thrombophilias have been discovered; the most common abnormality underlying VTE is Factor V Leiden (activated protein C resistance) and thrombophilias also associated with deficiencies in protein C and protein S. Antithrombin III deficiency is the rarest but carries the highest thrombogenic risk. Pregnant women with these thrombophilias are at significant risk of VTE.

Diagnosis

Diagnosis depends first and foremost on an awareness of the condition. Successive reports for the United Kingdom (*Ministry of Health Confidential Enquiries: Why Mothers Die*) have included case studies of women whose care providers failed to recognise the classic symptoms even when risk factors such as obesity or a family history of VTE are present.

Prophylaxis

The Obstetric Medicine Group of Australasia (2001) stresses that VTE can occur at any time during pregnancy; its prevalence is approximately equally distributed between the three trimesters. Although two-thirds occur during pregnancy, the day-by-day risk is greatest in the first weeks after birth. Major known risk factors for VTE in pregnancy have been identified. These risk factors often coexist and reinforce each

---

Research

Prophylaxis for venous thromboembolic disease in pregnancy and the early postnatal period (Cochrane Review) (Gates et al 2005)

Background: Venous thromboembolic disease, although very rare, is a major cause of maternal mortality and morbidity, hence methods of prophylaxis are often used for women at risk. This may include women delivered by caesarean section, those with a personal or family history of VTE and women with inherited or acquired thrombophilias. Many methods of prophylaxis carry a risk of side-effects, and as the risk of thromboembolic disease is low, it is possible that the benefits of thromboprophylaxis may be outweighed by harm. Current guidelines for clinical practice are based on expert opinion only, rather than high-quality evidence from randomised trials.

Objectives: To determine the effects of thromboprophylaxis in association with pregnancy in women who are pregnant or have recently delivered on the incidence of venous thromboembolic disease and side-effects.

Main results: Eight trials involving 649 women were included in the review. Four compared methods of antenatal prophylaxis; low molecular weight versus unfractionated heparin (two studies), aspirin plus heparin versus aspirin alone (one study), and unfractionated heparin versus no treatment (one study). Four studies assessed postnatal prophylaxis after caesarean section; one compared hydroxyethyl starch with unfractionated heparin, two compared heparin with placebo (one low molecular weight heparin, one unfractionated heparin) and the other compared unfractionated heparin with low molecular weight heparin. It was not possible to assess the effects of any of these interventions on most outcomes, especially rare outcomes such as death, thromboembolic disease and osteoporosis, because of small sample sizes and the small number of trials making the same comparisons.

Authors' conclusions: There is not enough evidence to show which are the best ways to prevent DVT around pregnancy, after a caesarean or in the early postnatal period. Large-scale randomised trials of currently used interventions should be conducted.

---

other (Obstetric Medicine Group of Australasia 2001). The Royal College of Obstetricians and Gynaecologists (2004) recommends that although the efficacy or benefit of the following recommendations is unknown, no high-grade evidence is available:

- all 'at-risk' women should be monitored for symptoms and signs of VTE during the first week post partum

- hydration should be maintained and early mobilisation encouraged
- graduated compression stockings with or without calf stimulation should be used during and after Caesarean section in women at moderate risk (one or two risk factors)
- in women at high risk (three or more risk factors), LMWH or unfractionated heparin prophylaxis should be used and continued for at least five days.

Deep vein thrombosis

Deep vein thrombosis (DVT) or thrombophlebitis/phlebo-thrombosis is seen more frequently in women with a history of venous thrombosis. In more than 70% of cases the thrombosis is in the iliofemoral veins, which are more likely to embolise (Greer 1999). There is clot formation in the deep veins of the leg, typically the calf or femoral veins, or occasionally the iliac veins. With a DVT the woman usually complains of pain or swelling (usually the left leg). Features such as immobilisation, asymmetric calf swelling (> 3 cm difference in calf circumference measured 10 cm below the tibial tuberosity) or swelling of the entire leg are the most reliable signs. At worst, the entire affected leg may be white, cold and oedematous. This rare condition is known as *phlegmasia alba dolens*. DVT can occur at any time during pregnancy. Diagnosis can be difficult. A positive Homans' sign (pain on dorsiflexion of the foot) is not a reliable diagnostic sign.

The gold standard for diagnosis of DVT has been contrast venography but this is invasive. Doppler ultrasonography is now the most widely used modality for evaluating patients with suspected DVT. When used in combination with a clinical prediction 'rule', ultrasound examination is accurate in predicting the need for anticoagulation therapy. However, a normal ultrasound study in a 'high-risk' woman requires additional investigation before DVT can be ruled out. Colour duplex ultrasonography allows direct visualisation of the deep veins and detection of venous flow. It is non-invasive, safe and readily repeatable. Ultrasound assessment has several limitations: its accuracy depends on the operator; it cannot distinguish between old and new thrombi; and it is not accurate in detecting DVT in the pelvic veins or the small vessels of the calf, or in the presence of morbid obesity or significant oedema. Diagnosis of DVT is based on:

- failure of the vein to compress
- presence of a thrombus

Critical thinking exercise

Barbara (G4P3), aged 40 years, had an emergency caesarean section for prolonged labour two days ago. As she walks to the nursery to see her baby for the first time, you notice that she is limping. Barbara laughs and tells you she is sore all over but her left leg is really sore.

What will you do? And what will you say to Barbara?

Clinical point

Midwives are well placed to support women requiring management of DVT at home. All aspects of the management plan must be clearly defined for the woman, her family, and her caregivers, including the family's GP. Ideally, the plan should be individualised from a standardised protocol and written in consultation with the woman and her team of medical and midwifery professionals experienced in the treatment of DVT. Each medical facility will need a protocol that fits its own practice patterns as well as the unique needs of the woman, who may be pregnant or have a newborn baby to care for as well. It is important that hospital-based and community-based team members (including the woman) work together to adopt the management plan so that it ensures consistent, seamless transition from acute care to the home-care setting. The guidelines should include criteria for anticoagulant therapy, patient and caregiver education, and type and frequency of monitoring.

Multidisciplinary teamwork is essential and follow-up care is crucial. Monitoring community-based treatment of DVT should include tracking for compliance, subcutaneous injection technique, local adverse effects from the injections, signs of bleeding, signs of recurrent thrombosis, and initiation and monitoring of warfarin therapy. Much of this can be done on an outpatient basis by midwives or nurses specialised in anticoagulation therapy. Initially they will need to visit the woman daily for the first weeks of treatment.

- absence of venous flow augmentation during compression of the calf.
- non-compressibility of the vein—this is the most sensitive and specific feature of proximal DVT (> 95%).

Magnetic resonance venography (MRI) is a relatively new technique with a sensitivity and specificity > 90% for DVT. It is not a routine test, as it is expensive and not widely available. Nevertheless, it is potentially useful in diagnosing DVT involving the pelvis, abdomen and upper extremities. MRI appears to be at least as sensitive as ultrasonography in detecting calf and pelvic DVTs because these thromboses are so difficult to compress with ultrasonography and hard to visualise with venography.

Management

Once a diagnosis is made, the woman is commenced on heparin to prevent further clotting. During labour, heparin should be given in a thromboprophylactic dose, returning to a therapeutic dose after the birth. Heparin dosage is based on estimations of the APTT, international normalised ratio (INR) and prothrombin times (Jilma et al 2003). LMWH is preferred because it is simpler to administer and the woman can be taught how to self-inject. Warfarin may be commenced after birth in combination for about three months. The woman wears anti-embolic stockings and is usually on bed rest until the swelling has reduced and the anticoagulant therapy is beginning to take effect. She often requires analgesics and will need physiotherapy.

Pulmonary thromboembolism

Pulmonary thromboembolism (PTE) is more common in the postnatal period than in pregnancy. The signs and symptoms of PTE are non-specific and so the clinical recognition of PTE is notoriously inaccurate. The lack of sensitivity of the clinical diagnosis of PTE is evident from postmortem studies demonstrating that most cases of PTE detected post mortem were not diagnosed (or treated) prior to death. Shortness of breath and rapid respirations accompanied by leg or chest pain with cyanosis are the most common symptoms, although a cardiac arrest may also be the first indication. Frothy, bloodstained sputum may also be apparent. To confirm the diagnosis, the woman requires blood gases, a chest X-ray, electrocardiogram and a ventilation-perfusion (V/Q) scan of the lungs. If the V/Q scan shows low or intermediate probability of a PTE, a pulmonary angiography is indicated.

Any woman with a suspected PTE requires hospitalisation, anticoagulation and supportive care in consultation with an obstetrician and a physician. Supplemental oxygen should be provided to reverse hypoxia and maintain a PaO_2 of more than 60 mmHg. Intubation may be required to maintain adequate fetal oxygenation (i.e. PaO_2 of < 60 mmHg) or for uncontrolled rising maternal $PaCO_2$. Fluid resuscitation and pressors such as dopamine may be used to maintain adequate blood pressure (systolic pressure > 80 mmHg), but there is a significant risk that uterine blood flow may be compromised. Narcotic analgesics should not be withheld. Only women with life-threatening manifestations of PTE should be treated with a fibrinolytic agent such as tissue plasminogen activator, since as yet there are currently no data on the risk of placental abruption or potential injury to the fetus. These agents are contraindicated post partum. Emergency thoracotomy and embolectomy may be beneficial as a last-ditch effort for critically ill patients.

Once the woman's condition has been stabilised, anticoagulation treatment to prevent further clot formation is commenced with heparin (Jilma et al 2003). Dosage is based on regular estimation of APTT, INR and prothrombin times. Medication is later changed to warfarin with regular prothrombin times taken, and continued for at least three months (Jilma et al 2003).

Infections

Like every other person in society, pregnant women are at risk of viral and bacterial infections. Infections are a particular concern during pregnancy because some infections increase the chance that problems will occur in the fetus or newborn, or are more severe in pregnant women. Of specific interest in this chapter are genital infections that complicate pregnancy. Other common infections are described briefly in the following sections but we place most of our focus on the diseases caused by Group B Streptococcus (GBS) in part because of its potentially catastrophic effects on the fetus but also because of the controversies surrounding the issue of screening for GBS infection.

Listeriosis

Listeriosis is a notifiable disease and a form of food poisoning caused by the bacterium *Listeria monocytogenes*, a Gram-positive, aerobic, motile bacillus with aerobic and facultative anaerobic characteristics. The organism is found in soil and water and can be carried by animals that do not appear ill, leading to contamination of food of animal origin such as meat and dairy products. Unpasteurised raw milks or foods are also sources of *Listeria* organisms.

Pregnant women are about 20 times more likely than other healthy adults to get listeriosis. The real incidence is not known, as listeriosis is an uncommonly diagnosed infection (FSANZ 1999). In Australia the number of cases of listeriosis reported averages about 50 to 70 per year (FSANZ 1999). While there have been many reported outbreaks of this disease overseas, there have been few reported in Australia and New Zealand. In Western Australia in 1990 there were six stillbirths reported in a cluster of nine cases. The implicated food was a particular brand of pâté. In New Zealand in 1992, the perinatal death of twins was linked to the mother consuming contaminated smoked mussels during her pregnancy (FSANZ 1999).

Listeriosis is difficult to diagnose. Pregnant women with listeriosis are often asymptomatic, or they may have a febrile illness similar to influenza with symptoms of fever, muscle aches and, sometimes, nausea or diarrhoea during the

---

Case study

Pulmonary embolism with bilateral DVT

A 29-year-old woman (para 0) weighing 79 kg had a spontaneous onset of labour at 41 weeks gestation. An emergency Caesarean was performed for non-progression of labour, despite oxytocin augmentation and an epidural. There were no operative difficulties. On day two, she suddenly collapsed with dyspnoea and rapidly deteriorated. Resuscitation was not successful. There were no other apparent risk factors for thromboembolism.

(Source: Slaytor et al 2004, pp 25–26)

Critical thinking exercise

How would you answer the following question? 'Should I get a flu shot now that I am pregnant, or should I wait until the pregnancy is a bit more advanced?'

bacteraemic phase of the disease. Although the symptoms may be mild, listeriosis can still lead to preterm birth, neonatal sepsis or even stillbirth. In neonates, the mortality rate is approximately 50%.

Prevention

According to the FSANZ (1999), it is not possible to prevent raw food from becoming contaminated with *Listeria*. However, it is easy to make food safe to eat. Freshly prepared food is safe, as the bacteria have not had a chance to grow in the food. However, raw fruit and vegetables should be washed thoroughly before eating. Listeria is also destroyed during normal cooking, so freshly cooked food is safe. If it has been more than 12 hours since a perishable food such as salad or meat has been prepared, it should not be eaten, as *Listeria* can grow on these foods, even in the refrigerator.

It is vital that pregnant women eat healthily during pregnancy, choosing from a wide variety of foods including vegetables, fruit, dairy foods, bread, cereals, pasta, lean meat, fish, eggs and nuts. To guard against listeriosis, pregnant women should avoid eating:

- certain refrigerated ready-to-eat food that has not been freshly cooked or prepared. This includes cold meats, salads, soft cheeses and pâté.
- raw meats, raw seafood and unpasteurised milk.

Treatment

Treatment is usually with antibiotics—penicillin or amoxyl/ampicillin either alone or in combination with trimethoprim and sulfamethoxazole. For penicillin-sensitive women, trimethoprim and sulfamethoxazole may be used alone.

Sexually transmitted infections

There are more than 50 sexually transmitted infections (STIs) and numerous other genitourinary infections that have the potential to affect the health and wellbeing of the woman, her partner and the unborn baby. Some STIs, such as genital herpes, chlamydia and bacterial vaginosis, are quite common in pregnant women. In Australia and New Zealand, other STIs, notably HIV and syphilis, are much less common. However, in some areas such as the Kimberley of northern Australia, syphilis is increasingly common. Early diagnosis and treatment are extremely important for preventing the effects of the disease on pregnant women and their infants.

Genital herpes

Infection with genital herpes simplex virus Type 2 (HSV-2) is a major reproductive health problem. Transmission occurs through direct, intimate, oral–genital or genital–genital contact. The first episode is called the initial or primary infection, and it is at this stage that some virus retreats to the nerve ganglia. Subsequent episodes, known as recurrences, occur if and when the virus replicates in the ganglion, releasing virus particles that travel along the nerve back to the site of the initial infection. Typically, lesions appear 2–14 days after exposure. Without antiviral therapy, the lesions usually last for 20 days. For most people, the first indication of infection starts 2–12 days after exposure to the virus. The development of symptoms may take longer or be less severe in some people, especially those who have previously developed partial immunity to the virus, perhaps having a Type-1 infection (e.g. cold sores). Antibody response occurs three to four weeks after the infection and is lifelong. However, unlike protective antibodies to other viruses, antibodies to HSV-2 do not prevent local recurrence(s) and so HSV-2 becomes a chronic infection characterised by periods of remission and exacerbation. The symptoms associated with local recurrences tend to be milder than those occurring with the primary disease.

Symptoms associated with primary infections are both local and systemic, although more than 75% of people with a primary HSV-2 infection are asymptomatic and these are responsible for many neonatal HSV infections. Local symptoms include intense pain, dysuria, occasional itching, vaginal discharge and, commonly, lymphadenopathy. Systemic

---

BOX 33.21 Information on STIs

- Centers for Disease Control and Prevention 2002 Sexually Transmitted Diseases Treatment Guidelines 2002. *Morbidity and Mortality Weekly Report 51* (RR06):1–80. Online: http://www.cdc.gov/std/treatment/default.htm
- *Australian Medicines Handbook* (5th edn) 2004 Adelaide: Australian Medical Handbook Pty Ltd
- Brown K 2000 *Management Guidelines for Women's Health Nurse Practitioners*. FA Davis, Philadelphia
- Brocklehurst P, Rooney G 2003 Interventions for treating genital *Chlamydia trachomatis* infection in pregnancy (Cochrane Review). Cochrane Library (4). John Wiley & Sons, Chichester
- Campos-Outcalt D 2003 Sexually transmitted disease: earlier screening tests, single dose therapies. *Journal of Family Practice* 52(12):965–969
- Centers for Disease Control and Prevention 2002 Sexually transmitted disease treatment guidelines. *Morbidity and Mortality Weekly Report* 51(RR-6):32–36
- Denham I, Meese P, Bradford D et al (Eds) 2002 *National Management Guidelines for Sexually Transmissible Diseases and Genital Infections* (6th edn). Venereology Society of Victoria, Commonwealth Department of Health and Family Services

---

Clinical point

Listeria infection is usually asymptomatic. Accurate clinical diagnosis is difficult in most cases. Minor illnesses in pregnancy do not warrant speculative treatment with antibiotics because of concern over listeriosis. The main protection against *Listeria* infection is through careful attention to food preparation and storage and to personal hygiene.

symptoms are due to viraemia and include fever, headache, nausea, malaise and myalgia. Women particularly often experience pain on urinating, and when this happens, it is important to avoid problems of urinary retention by drinking plenty of fluids to dilute the urine and thereby reduce pain and stinging. Some women may also notice vaginal discharge. Not everyone experiences symptomatic recurrences but of those that do, recurrences are usually shorter and less severe than the initial episode.

Diagnosis

In order to confirm a diagnosis of genital herpes simplex virus (HSV) infection, it is necessary to prove the presence of HSV. Detection of HSV antibodies in the bloodstream is not sufficient because this cannot define the site of HSV infection. Laboratory analysis is usually made either by virus culture (where the virus is grown in material known as a culture medium) or by antigen detection, where components of the virus are specifically identified.

Pregnancy and HSV-2

Women with HSV-2 can experience a safe pregnancy and normal vaginal childbirth. This is especially so when the diagnosis is made prior to becoming pregnant. If she already has a history of genital herpes, the woman's antibodies will protect the fetus from an infection during pregnancy and the neonatal period. Recurrent genital herpes presents only a minimal risk in pregnancy, though it may interfere with the woman's enjoyment of pregnancy. However, the fetus may be at risk when the woman has:

- a severe primary infective episode during the first trimester, which can lead to miscarriage. This is a very uncommon complication and it is important to reassure the woman that this hazard is also present with a number of other viral infections, including the flu.
- a primary episode of HSV-2 in the last trimester of pregnancy, because there are large amounts of circulating virus present and insufficient time for the mother to produce enough antibodies to protect the fetus. Transmission of virus to the fetus causes neonatal herpes, a potentially fatal but rare condition. Careful monitoring, judicious use of antiviral therapy and/or caesarean delivery in the presence of an active lesion can reduce the risk to the baby.

Care during pregnancy

It is important that a pregnant woman informs her lead carer if either she or her partner has genital herpes. In the third trimester, regular checks should be made and the woman and her caregiver can discuss the best option for giving birth, including a caesarean section or the use of antiviral drugs. Other than this, the pregnant woman should simply observe the normal guidelines for healthy pregnancy as closely as possible. Good nutrition and rest are even more important at this time.

Acyclovir treatment of HSV-2 can significantly reduce morbidity in the mother and potentially in the infant. It is, however, not recommended in pregnancy, although there is no evidence of adverse fetal effects. Its use should be considered when it is judged that its benefits outweigh the risks. After birth, specimens for viral culture should be collected from the baby for early identification of infection. If cultures are positive, acyclovir treatment of the neonate is advised. Parents should be advised to report early signs of perinatal HSV-2 infection (lethargy, fever, poor feeding or lesions). Breastfeeding is recommended unless the mother has lesions around the nipples. Acyclovir is excreted in breast milk but its use is not contraindicated as it does not appear to harm the infant.

Chlamydia

Chlamydia is the most common STI in Australia and New Zealand, especially among young people. In Australia, chlamydial notifications have increased four-fold over the past decade (Chen et al 2003). However, as most infections are asymptomatic, the 26,000 cases reported in 2002 probably represent only a fraction of the true incidence and prevalence (Chen et al 2003). Infection with *Chlamydia trachomatis* has become a major public health problem because of the long-term consequences of infection experienced predominantly by women. These include chronic pelvic pain, ectopic pregnancy and infertility. Rarely, males may also become infertile.

Chlamydia trachomatis is an obligate intracellular parasite. Once considered a virus, it is now classified as a bacterium, based on its sensitivity to antibiotics and its reproduction cycle. According to Chen et al (2003), although chlamydia can easily be treated and cured, it can have dire consequences if left untreated: 40% will develop pelvic inflammatory disease (PID). Of these women, 20% will become infertile; 18% will develop chronic pelvic pain, and 9% will have potentially life-threatening tubal pregnancy. More than two-thirds of women with chlamydia are asymptomatic.

Screening

Consensus has not been reached on the optimal time for screening for chlamydia or even whether it should be a 'routine' screening test. Screening early in pregnancy increases the opportunity to improve the pregnancy outcome, whereas screening in the third trimester prevents transmission to the infant. Testing women at high risk of chlamydial infection is, however, recommended. High-risk individuals include those with a clinical presentation suggestive of chlamydial infection, individuals attending GPs for testing of STI, those attending STI and family planning clinics, gay men's health centres and the partners of those already diagnosed with an STI.

Laboratory investigations currently available are:

- cell culture (only in specialised laboratories)
- antigen assays, including direct immunofluorescence or enzyme immunoassay
- hybridisation assays such as the DNA probe
- amplification assays including polymerase chain reaction (PCR) and ligase chain reaction (LCR).

Treatment

In asymptomatic women with positive culture findings and in symptomatic women, erythromycin, amoxicillin, clindamycin and azithromycin are all used to treat chlamydia.

Research

A systematic review, published in 2005, investigating 'Antibiotics for bacterial vaginosis or *Trichomonas vaginalis* in pregnancy' concluded that there was no evidence that treatment of bacterial vaginosis reduced perinatal or serious bacterial morbidity.

Okun N, Gronau KA, Hannah ME 2005 Antibiotics for bacterial vaginosis or *Trichomonas vaginalis* in pregnancy: a systematic review. American College of Obstetrics and Gynecology 105(4):857–867

Bacterial vaginosis

With bacterial vaginosis, the population of normal lactobacilli is decreased, with resultant overgrowth of other organisms, including *Gardnerella vaginalis*, *Mobiluncus* and anaerobes. The dominant commensal found in the vagina is *Lactobacillus*, and the constitution of vaginal flora is altered by the pH of the vagina. Bacterial vaginosis is associated with an increased risk of several pathological conditions, including postoperative infection and PID.

In pregnant women, bacterial vaginosis is associated with preterm rupture of the membranes and preterm labour and birth. The microbes found in bacterial vaginosis are also often found in the amniotic fluid of women with chorioamnionitis. The presence of atypical cells on Papanicolaou smear is also more common in women with bacterial vaginosis.

Diagnosis

Bacterial vaginosis is diagnosed by the presence of clinical and microscopic findings. Women with bacterial vaginosis report an abnormal vaginal discharge and may complain of an unpleasant, fishlike vaginal odour, especially after sexual intercourse. The discharge is generally white or grey, and women may have burning during urination or itching around the vagina, although the colour and amount of discharge varies greatly from woman to woman. The normal pH of vaginal secretions is less than 4.5. In women with bacterial vaginosis, the pH is usually greater than 4.5. The organisms responsible for causing bacterial vaginosis depend mainly on the pH of the vagina. With a pH of more than 4.5, *Gardnerella vaginalis* and anaerobes become the most likely causative organism.

Laboratory tests include:
- *wet mount*—a sample of vaginal discharge is examined to identify the bacteria present, to look for white blood cells that indicate an infection, and to look for unusual cells called clue cells. The presence of 'clue cells' is the most reliable indicator of bacterial vaginosis.
- *culture*—a culture of vaginal discharge may show heavy growth of microbes associated with bacterial vaginosis
- Gram stain
- *oligonucleotide probes*—to detect the genetic material (DNA) of the bacteria causing the infection.

Treatment

The drugs of choice for bacterial vaginosis are metronidazole (Flagyl™), which reports a cure rate of 84–96%, or oral clindamycin (Cleocin™) with a cure rate of 94%. When prescribing metronidazole, the lead carer should stress the importance of abstaining from all forms of alcohol, as a disulfiram-type reaction can occur. In addition, metronidazole may interfere with the metabolism of warfarin (Coumadin™) and anticonvulsants; consequently, dosages of these medications may need to be altered. Women taking barbiturates may require a higher dosage of metronidazole. In contrast, although clindamycin is also an effective treatment for bacterial vaginosis it is much more expensive and is associated with gastrointestinal irritation such as diarrhoea and, rarely, colitis.

Syphilis

In some parts of Australia such as the Northern Territory and certain locations in New Zealand, syphilis has again become a major cause of stillbirth, and babies with congenital syphilis are increasingly common. In other locations the prevalence of syphilis is so low that clinicians are now questioning the benefits of screening for the disease (Public Health Laboratory Service Syphilis Working Group 1998).

Early diagnosis and treatment are extremely important if the effects that syphilis has on pregnant women and their infants are to be prevented. Untreated primary or secondary syphilis in pregnant women can lead to congenital syphilis in 40–50% of cases. A lack of or inadequate antenatal care and failure to properly diagnose and treat maternal syphilis are the most important factors leading to congenital syphilis, and so adequate screening of high-risk populations and treatment should be the focus of widespread public health strategies aimed at prevention, early diagnosis and treatment. Syphilis, a notifiable disease, is caused by *Treponema pallidum*, a helical, tightly coiled, motile spirochete. The disease is characterised by: a primary lesion; a secondary eruption involving skin and mucous membranes; and long periods of latency culminating with late lesions of skin, bone, viscera, cardiovascular and central nervous systems. The stage of maternal disease during which the fetus is exposed to infection determines the degree and type of morbidity; the earlier the disease stage, the higher the morbidity. Untreated primary or secondary syphilis in pregnancy causes almost a 100% rate of infection in the fetus. The disease can cause stillbirth, neonatal death or congenital syphilis.

Screening

Even when syphilis is considered unlikely, routine antenatal screening is probably warranted for prevention and surveillance, especially since the tests are relatively easy to administer and inexpensive. The earlier in pregnancy the treatment, the more efficacious it is. Therefore, serological tests should be performed at the initial prenatal visit. If the woman is considered to be at high risk, it may be necessary to perform a re-test at about 28 weeks gestation and again after birth.

Diagnosis

Diagnosis of syphilis is made in the same manner as for a non-pregnant woman. In primary syphilis, the diagnosis is confirmed by identifying *T. pallidum* in dark-field examination of material taken from a lesion. However, because most pregnant women do not have visible lesions, serological screening is the primary means of establishing the diagnosis. Traditionally, screening strategies used an initial non-treponemal test (e.g. rapid plasma reagin (RPR) or Venereal Disease Research Laboratory (VDRL)). Because these tests are highly sensitive but non-specific, pregnancy often causes false-positive results; therefore, positive findings are followed up with specific anti-treponemal antibody tests such as the microhaemagglutination assay-T pallidum and the fluorescent treponemal antibody absorption test. However, many laboratories now screen with an automated enzyme immunoassay (EIA) test for anti-treponemal IgG. Unless treatment is instituted in the very early stages of infection, the EIA usually remains positive for life, unlike the non-treponemal tests, which show falling levels (or may become non-reactive) after treatment or occur spontaneously over time.

Treatment

Treatment is the same as for non-pregnant women, with a single dose of 2.4 million units of benzathine penicillin for both primary and secondary syphilis, although some experts recommend another dose a week after the initial one, especially in the third trimester or in the case of secondary syphilis. For latent syphilis, treatment consists of three doses of benzathine penicillin. In pregnancy, penicillin is the only drug that can be used to treat syphilis because the accepted alternatives to treatment are erythromycin and tetracycline and both of these are teratogenic; in any case, erythromycin may not prevent congenital syphilis.

Gonorrhoea

Gonorrhoea is caused by *Neisseria gonorrhoeae*, a Gram-negative diplococcus, and is transmitted by close sexual contact. Although many women are asymptomatic there are some reports of women presenting with endocervicitis, premature rupture of membranes, chorioamnionitis, septic miscarriage, IUGR, prematurity, and postpartum sepsis leading to PID. Proctitis is diagnosed in up to 50% of women with gonorrhoea and may be the only site colonised with *N. gonorrhoeae* thus warranting testing of rectal specimens for the disease. Similarly, individuals with gonococcal pharyngitis are frequently asymptomatic, and again the pharynx may be the only site colonised. Gonorrhoea is transmitted vertically during the birth process but there is no evidence to suggest placental transmission. Therefore newborns are exposed to the disease only during vaginal birth. The babies are at risk of an acute conjunctivitis known as ophthalmia neonatorum.

Screening

Gonococcal infections cause no symptoms in approximately 50% of women and therefore testing for gonorrhoea is one of the recommended routine, universal screening tests in pregnancy. However, some centres recommend screening only high-risk pregnant women at the first antenatal visit and again in the third trimester.

Diagnosis

The laboratory diagnosis of gonorrhoea depends on the demonstration of *N. gonorrhoeae*, or detection of its DNA in samples from the endocervix, pharynx, rectum and urethra.

Treatment

The treatment of choice is an antibiotic such as ciprofloxacin or ofloxacin, but ciprofloxacin is contraindicated in pregnancy. Unfortunately there is increasing evidence that some strains of *N. gonorrhoeae* are resistant to antibiotics. All patients treated for gonococcal infection should also be empirically treated for chlamydial infection.

Group B Streptococcus

Group B Streptococcus (GBS) is a naturally occurring Gram-positive bacterium found in the rectovaginal flora of up to 30% of healthy women. GBS colonisation is rarely life-threatening but it has the potential to cause infection and ongoing complications for the pregnant woman, the fetus and baby during pregnancy, labour and the postpartum period.

Intra-amniotic infections are often polymicrobial and occur more frequently in women with marked GBS colonisation. The time-honoured clinical signs and symptoms of chorioamnionitis include the following:
- pyrexia (an intrapartum temperature > 37.8°C)
- significant maternal tachycardia (> 120 bpm)
- occasional chills, malaise
- fetal tachycardia (> 160 bpm)
- purulent or offensive amniotic fluid or vaginal discharge
- varying levels of uterine tenderness
- maternal leucocytosis (total blood leucocyte count 15,000–18,000 cells/mm^3).

Of the criteria listed in above, intrapartum maternal pyrexia appears to be the most frequent, and other findings, such as fetal tachycardia, may be less important in the absence of maternal fever. While GBS may cause clinical urinary tract infections in pregnant women, many will have no symptoms of genital tract colonisation. UTIs caused by GBS complicate up to 4% of pregnancies. Women can contract amnionitis, endometritis, sepsis or meningitis antenatally from GBS, but associated maternal mortality is rare (Schrag et al 2002). Fetal and neonatal GBS infection is mostly preventable, provided it is identified early and managed appropriately. Antibiotics such as penicillin or ampicillin are used prophylactically or in the treatment of maternal infection and to prevent fetal infection or early-onset neonatal disease associated with maternal urogenital colonisation by GBS. Penicillin is the agent of choice for intrapartum antibiotic prophylaxis. Ampicillin is an acceptable alternative, but penicillin is preferred because of its narrower spectrum of antimicrobial activity. Intravenous administration is the only route of administration recommended for preventing GBS disease in the intrapartum period because of the higher intra-amniotic concentrations achieved with this method.

James (2001) warns of the potential adverse and unintended effects of using antibiotics prophylactically or to treat active GBS infections such as: allergic or anaphylactic reactions to the drugs used for intrapartum antibiotic prophylaxis, the emergence of strains of GBS resistant to standard therapies and, increasingly, serious antibiotic-resistant neonatal infections caused by agents other than GBS. Nevertheless, when it is transmitted to the fetus or the neonate, GBS is a common and significant cause of neonatal mortality and morbidity (Gilbert et al 2002). While only a small proportion of the babies of women known to be carriers of GBS are actually infected, up to 80% of the mothers of infected babies have one or more identifiable risk factors in labour (Gilbert et al 2002).

Before the onset of labour, ascending infection spread from the maternal gastrointestinal tract or vagina may cause fetal infection in utero. Grimwood and colleagues (2001) comment that after the introduction of intrapartum IV antibiotic therapy, the incidence of GBS infection in New Zealand fell to 0.5 per 1000 live births. Moreover, the fetus may become infected with GBS if it aspirates infected amniotic fluid. Nevertheless, GBS infections frequently result in stillbirth, neonatal pneumonia or sepsis. If the fetus does not contract the infection until it begins its passage through the birth canal, despite becoming colonised it will probably remain asymptomatic (Schrag et al 2002). Babies with late-onset GBS (after one week of age) usually present with meningitis.

Screening for GBS

(For additional information, see Ch 32.) Because of the potentially catastrophic outcomes following perinatal GBS infection, most centres advocate screening all pregnant women for GBS. Currently there are two schools of thought. In the culture-based screening method (Schrag et al 2002), universal antenatal screening for vaginal and rectal GBS colonisation of all pregnant women is performed at 35–37 weeks gestation to identify GBS carriers. These women are offered IV antibiotic cover in labour. In addition, women diagnosed with GBS bacteriuria during their current pregnancy and those who have previously given birth to a baby with early-onset GBS infection are also offered intrapartum antibiotics. Proponents of the risk-based method screen only those deemed to be at risk of a GBS infection once they are in labour. Critics of this approach argue that although attempts have been made to identify risk factors that influence GBS infections, such as ethnicity, smoking, maternal age, and number of partners, colonisation rates are so inconsistent that targeting only high-risk women for selective screening is not an effective strategy.

Women whose culture results are unknown at the onset of labour are managed according to a risk-based approach. These risk factors include labour < 37 weeks gestation, ruptured membranes for over 18 hours, and/or maternal pyrexia of 38.0°C or above. Women with negative vaginal and rectal GBS screening cultures within five weeks of delivery do not require intrapartum antibiotic cover even if they later develop these risk factors (Schrag et al 2002).

The recommended intrapartum regimen is five million units of penicillin G intravenously followed by 2.5 million units every four hours until birth. Penicillin G is preferred because of its narrow spectrum profile, although ampicillin,

---

Clinical point

Possible effects of Group B streptococcal colonisation
Asymptomatic bacteriuria
Intra-amniotic infection
Endometritis
Stillbirth
Premature rupture of membranes
Urinary tract infection
Wound infections
Preterm labour/preterm birth
Spontaneous miscarriage
Sepsis
(Source: James 2001, p 660)

Research

Group B streptococcal disease in the era of intrapartum antibiotic prophylaxis (Schrag et al 2000)
A comparison between the risk-based and culture-based approaches to screening for GBS colonisation in 5144 births demonstrated that the culture-based screening approach was 50% more effective than the risk-based strategy in preventing neonatal GBS disease. Although the risk-factor approach was the least expensive option, universal screening at 35 to 37 weeks of gestation followed by treatment of all colonised women during labour was the most effective option.

cefazolin, clindamycin, erythromycin and amoxycillin are acceptable alternatives if penicillin G is unavailable or if the woman is allergic to penicillin.

Early-onset neonatal GBS infection

Unless neonatal GBS infections are diagnosed early and treated with antibiotics and supportive therapy, morbidity and mortality are high. Symptoms of early-onset GBS in newborn babies often begin before the baby leaves the birthing room (Gomella et al 1999). They include: respiratory grunting, lethargy, irritability, poor feeding, tachycardia or bradycardia, pyrexia or low temperature, rapid or slowed respirations and hypotension. There are raised white cell count and cell-reactive protein (CRP) levels. Blood, urine or cerebral spinal fluid cultures confirm that the baby has a GBS infection.

Hypertension in pregnancy

Hypertension is the most common medical problem encountered during pregnancy, complicating 2–3% of pregnancies. This chapter uses the classificatory system used by the Australasian Society for the Study of Hypertension in Pregnancy (ASSHP). The ASSHP define the following types of hypertension in pregnancy:

● *hypertension*—systolic blood pressure (BP) greater than or equal to 140 mmHg, or diastolic BP greater than or equal to 90 mmHg when repeated over several hours (Korotkoff V)

● *chronic (pre-existing) hypertension*—hypertension diagnosed before pregnancy or in the first 20 weeks of gestation in the absence of any underlying cause. Hypertension that is diagnosed for the first time during pregnancy and does not resolve post partum is also classified as chronic hypertension. There may be proteinuria. In contrast, chronic hypertension that is primary or secondary to an underlying condition, such as renal disease, renovascular disease, pheochromocytoma or Cushing syndrome, is known as essential hypertension.

● *gestational hypertension* (pregnancy-induced hypertension (PIH))—hypertension detected for the first time after 20 weeks gestation without proteinuria. It usually resolves by three months post partum without any other signs of pre-eclampsia.

● *pre-eclampsia (PE)*—a multisystem disorder associated with hypertension and proteinuria, which rarely presents before 20 weeks gestation. The pathological changes are primarily ischaemic, affecting the placenta, kidney, liver, brain and other organs. The exact cause of pre-eclampsia is unknown, although abnormal placental implantation, endothelial dysfunction, and/or abnormal immune responses have all been suggested as possible factors.

● *pre-eclampsia superimposed upon chronic hypertension*—pre-eclampsia that occurs in women who are already hypertensive; in such cases, the outlook is much worse than for either condition alone.

● *eclampsia*—one or more seizures that occur in association with pre-eclampsia. Eclampsia is an obstetric emergency (see Ch 36).

Chronic (pre-existing) and gestational hypertension

The incidence of chronic hypertension in pregnancy is 1–5%. Management aims to achieve a diastolic blood pressure of less than 90 mmHg. In contrast to chronic hypertension, gestational hypertension is a provisional diagnosis: some women may go on to develop proteinuria (pre-eclampsia), whilst others may have pre-existing hypertension that has been masked by the physiological drop in blood pressure in the early part of pregnancy. A diagnosis of gestational hypertension is confirmed if pre-eclampsia does not develop and the blood pressure returns to normal by 12 weeks post partum.

Appropriate baseline assessment in women with chronic hypertension includes an evaluation of pre-existing target organ damage including cardiomegaly, renal insufficiency and retinopathy, preferably made prior to pregnancy. These are important for diagnosis and ongoing management. Renal function is assessed with a 24-hour urine protein and creatinine excretion, and/or a serum creatinine or a spot urine protein/creatinine ratio. An electrocardiogram will detect left ventricular hypertrophy. Baseline ultrasounds for dating the pregnancy are useful, as are follow-up scans, to detect fetal growth restriction—these usually begin at 28 weeks gestation and are repeated every four weeks until birth.

Women with chronic hypertension often continue taking their antihypertensive medication, although it may be necessary to switch to a different medication during pregnancy (Magee et al 1999). There is, however, no evidence that anti-hypertensive therapy improves perinatal outcomes, and some studies show an increase in fetal growth restriction in women taking these medications (Magee et al 1999). This is especially true for the beta-blockers, with the exception of labetalol. Methyldopa and hydralazine have the best 'track records' and are the preferred agents. However, the ACE inhibitors have been implicated in fetal renal damage and are therefore contraindicated in the first trimester. There is little data on calcium channel blockers such as nifedipine, but what does exist shows neither deleterious nor advantageous effects.

There is no evidence to demonstrate that bed rest is an effective therapy. Similarly, weekly non-stress tests (NSTs) after 32 weeks gestation may be prudent, but there is little objective evidence of benefit. If fetal growth restriction, oligo-hydramnios or superimposed pre-eclampsia are diagnosed, twice-weekly NSTs beginning at 32 weeks gestation are commenced. Doppler flow studies and biophysical profiles are useful adjuncts to NSTs and ultrasounds in assessing fetal wellbeing. Complications of chronic hypertension are: an exacerbation of maternal hypertension, superimposed pre-eclampsia and uteroplacental insufficiency, IUGR and placental abruption. Provided these complications do not arise and hypertension does not worsen, the woman can be delivered at term.

Pre-eclampsia

Pre-eclampsia (PE) complicates about 8% of pregnancies and is a multiorgan disease associated with abnormalities of the coagulation system, disturbed liver function, renal failure, cerebral ischaemia and fetal growth restriction. PE is always characterised by hypertension and proteinuria with or without oedema (Brown et al 2000). The exact mechanisms that lead to PE are still unclear. What is known is that some women have predisposing factors and are more at risk of the disease than others. PE is more common in: primigravidas, those aged over 40, women with a new partner, women with a previous history or family history of PE, multiple pregnancies, hydrops fetalis, women with other medical conditions such as diabetes or renal disease, obesity and women who have used some reproductive technologies (Brown et al 2000). In addition, PE is more common in women with large placentas, those whose sisters or mothers had PE and in women with auto-immune (collagen vascular) diseases.

Pathophysiology

Postulated mechanisms underlying the pathophysiology of PE are complex and beyond the brief of this text, and the reader should combine this account of PE with an appropriate anatomy and physiology text as well as literature from journals. It is likely that the primary trigger in PE is poor placental perfusion due to abnormal placental trophoblastic infiltration of the uterine spiral arteries (Lew & Klonis 2003), a process that occurs many weeks before the signs of PE become apparent, resulting in a high impedance circulation instead of a low-pressure system necesary if the fetus is to be adequately oxygenated.

The secondary pathology in PE is probably related to reduced blood flow to the woman's major organs, which causes endothelial damage. This causes a cyclic pathological process. Decreased blood flow to the placenta causes inadequate

placental perfusion. In response, vasoactive substances are released by the hypo-perfused placenta, which in turn leads to further widespread endothelial damage and profound vasospasm, with a consequent reduction in plasma volume. Endothelial damage activates the coagulation cascade; platelets adhere to the sites of endothelial damage. Prostaglandin metabolism is also altered, with an increase in thromboxane and a decrease in prostacyclin concentration contributing to further platelet dysfunction and vasoconstriction. Because these pathological changes occur so near the beginning of pregnancy, the fetus is compromised very early in the pregnancy. Table 33.2 lists the effects of PE and the primary body systems affected.

Diagnosis

According to the ASSHP (Brown et al 2000), for PE to be diagnosed there must be:

- hypertension after the 20th week of gestation, and rarely earlier, perhaps when there are extensive hydatidiform changes in the chorionic villi
- a diastolic blood pressure of at least 90 mmHg and a systolic blood pressure of at least 140 mmHg. These blood pressures must be manifested on at least two occasions six hours or more apart.
- proteinuria (presence of 300 mg or more of protein in a 24-hour urine collection or a protein concentration of 1 g/L or more. This level of proteinuria should produce a 2+ reaction on a standard urine dipstick in at least two random urine specimens collected six hours or more apart; and possibly evidence of:
  - renal insufficiency
  - liver disease
  - neurological problems
  - haematological disturbances
  - fetal growth restriction.
- oedema is now considered to be of little clinical importance as it occurs equally in women experiencing normal pregnancy and in PE. However, the rapid onset of oedema is usually abnormal (Brown et al 2000). Pathological oedema is defined as a generalised accumulation of fluid of greater than 1+, pitting oedema after 12 hours of bed rest or weight gain of 2 kg or more in 1 week, or both.

In addition, many women with PE will have abnormal liver function tests:

- aspartate aminotransferase (SGOT) level higher than 72 IU/L, and LDH levels > 600 IU/L
- alanine transaminase (ALT) levels > 40 IU/L
- alkaline phosphatase levels > 60 IU/L in first trimester, > 80 IU/L second trimester and > 140 IU/L in third trimester
- total albumin level 34 g/L decreases to 28 g/L at term. There is a strong relationship between low serum albumin levels and adverse maternal and fetal outcomes.
- total bilirubin levels > 17 μmol/L.

Although transaminase levels rise as a result of hepato-cellular necrosis, prothrombin time remains within the

---

Critical thinking exercise

You find that a woman who books into your antenatal clinic for the first time at 25 weeks pregnant has a blood pressure of 150/95. There is no proteinuria. What is the most likely cause of her hypertension and what are you going to do about it?

TABLE 33.2	Effects of pre-eclampsia
System	**Effects**
Maternal	
CVS	Widespread vasoconstriction
	Normal or increased systemic vascular resistance
	Left ventricular failure
	Increased vascular permeability and oedema
	Decreased circulating blood volume
CNS	Headaches
	Visual disturbance
	Hyper-reflexia
	Cerebral haemorrhage
	Convulsions
Renal	Reduced glomerular filtration rate
	Reduced urea clearance and increased uric acid concentration
	Proteinuria and hypoproteinaemia
	Oliguria
	Acute renal failure
Respiratory	Pulmonary oedema
	Facial and laryngeal oedema
	Adult respiratory distress syndrome
Liver	Abnormal liver function tests
	Subcapsular hemorrhage and epigastric pain
	Liver rupture
Coagulation	Increased turnover of fibrinogen, fibrin and platelets
	Thrombocytopaenia
	Impaired platelet function
	Disseminated intravascular coagulation
	HELLP syndrome
Fetal	
	Decreased placental circulation
	Placental ischaemia and infarction
	Intrauterine growth restriction
	Placenta abruption
	Preterm labour
(Source: Hart & Coley 2003, p 39)	

reference range. As PE worsens there may be evidence of haematological abnormalities: haemolysis (haemoglobin < 110 g/L, with reticulocytosis) or thrombocytopaenia ($< 150 \times 10^9$ g/L platelets).

Renal function tests (plasma creatinine, creatinine clearance, blood urea and total urea protein and uric acid) are often abnormal. However, a total urinary protein of > 500 mg/L in 24 hours is associated with severe PE . A serum creatinine level ≥ 0.10 mmol/L also indicates significant renal

impairment. In women with PE, serum uric acid levels are slightly increased but levels > 0.35 mmol/L are associated with poor fetal outcomes, although women with normal serum uric acid levels and clinical signs of PE may still develop complications.

Classification

The ASSHP classifies PE as mild or severe (Brown et al 2000).
Criteria for mild pre-eclampsia:
- hypertension as defined above but not meeting the criteria for severe pre-eclampsia (below).
- proteinuria > 300 mg/24 hours.
- urine output > 500 mL/24 hours.
Criteria for severe pre-eclampsia:
- BP of > 160/110 on two occasions at least six hours apart.
- The presence of an elevated blood pressure and any of the systemic symptoms noted below categorises the patient as having severe PE regardless of the blood pressure:
  - proteinuria > 500 mg/24 hours or 3+ or 4+ on urine dipstick
  - massive oedema
  - oliguria < 400 mL/24 hours
  - systemic symptoms including pulmonary oedema, headaches, visual changes, right upper quadrant pain, elevated liver enzymes, or thrombocytopaenia
  - signs and symptoms of imminent eclampsia; at least two of hyperreflexia with clonus, visual disturbances and severe headaches.
- intrauterine growth restriction.
Severe PE and eclampsia are dealt with in Chapter 36.

Management

Because PE is a multiorgan disease that compromises maternal and fetal health, any woman with hypertension must be referred to a medical practitioner, and will need to birth in hospital. Management of PE depends on several factors:
- gestational age of the pregnancy
- severity of the disease
- presence of complicating factors
- evidence of maternal or fetal compromise.

The definitive treatment for PE is delivery of the fetus and placenta. This is a reasonable choice for viable fetuses or when the mother's health is significantly compromised. Examples of these risks include signs of: impending eclampsia, pulmonary oedema, compromised renal function, placental abruption, a platelet count < 100,000/μL, a ratio of serum alanine aminotransferase to serum aspartate aminotransferase that is twice the reference range with concomitant epigastric and right upper quadrant tenderness, persistent severe headache or visual changes, and uncontrolled severe hypertension.

Expectant management

In the past, pregnant women with hypertension were admitted to hospital. Admission to hospital is always stressful and, for many women, emotionally and financially costly. In many

Research

Prevention of PE

Currently there are no well-established therapies to prevent PE (Duley 2003). However, it seems that low-dose aspirin therapy (100 mg per day or less) probably reduces the incidence of PE and eclampsia in women who have an abnormal uterine artery function on Doppler ultrasound examination performed in the second trimester. The results of studies supporting its use should be discussed with women known to be at risk of PE.

Small trials have studied the efficacy of daily calcium supplementation as a preventive measure (Atallah et al 2004). As with aspirin therapy, calcium supplementation may produce modest blood pressure reductions in pregnant women who are at above-average risk for PE and in pregnant women with existing low dietary calcium intake, but the optimum calcium dosage has not been established (Atallah et al 2004).

For decades, women have been advised to make a range of changes to their lifestyles and implement numerous dietary modifications in an effort to prevent or manage PE (Brown et al 2000). None of these have been shown to be effective. Research on the use of antioxidants (high doses of vitamins C and E) in the prevention of PE is promising (Duley 2003). However, further large studies are needed to confirm these early findings, and so as yet antioxidant therapy is not recommended.

cases, hospitals are not restful places. This intervention would be justified if there were clear benefits but as yet there is no evidence that hospitalisation for mild PE improves maternal and fetal outcomes (Duley 2003). Women with mild PE without significant proteinuria often prefer to be an 'outpatient' and remain at home or be admitted as a 'day case' for assessment and evaluation. Expectant management at home (or in hospital) requires reduced activity and careful checking and daily recording of:

● fetal activity
● blood pressure
● urine protein.

A daily log of symptoms and assessments is combined with frequent (at least twice-weekly) checks by the lead carer. The woman may be advised to stop employment, reduce her activity level and, if possible, spend a considerable amount of time in bed. However, although bed rest is considered a reasonable and logical treatment for PE, its ability to improve outcomes has not been proved—in fact, it may be harmful (Duley 2003). Strict bed rest for three days or more significantly increases the risk of thromboembolic disease in either the legs or lungs (from 1 in 1000 to 16 in 1000) when it is used to prevent preterm labour (Kovacevich et al 2000).

Collaborative management

The goals of management are twofold: first, to recognise PE early; and second, to monitor the mother for evidence of disease progression that would mandate either delivery or more intensive fetal surveillance. Baseline laboratory evaluations should be performed early in pregnancy for all women known to be at high risk of PE. All women should have their blood pressure recorded at each antenatal consultation and more frequently in women at high risk of PE. Although increases above the baseline (> 30 mmHg systolic or > 15 mmHg diastolic) are no longer considered a criterion for the diagnosis of PE, rapid increases warrant closer observation. Fundal height should be measured at each visit because a fundal height less than expected for the estimated gestation may indicate IUGR or oligohydramnios, both of which are associated with PE. In addition, evidence suggestive of IUGR and/or oliguria may be apparent long before the diagnostic criteria for PE are apparent. Further assessment of rapidly increasing, generalised oedema or maternal facial and periorbital oedema combined with rapid weight gain is warranted because marked fluid retention may be associated with the onset of severe PE.

Once hypertension is documented during the second half of pregnancy or if the onset of PE is suspected, laboratory tests to confirm the diagnosis and to track its progression include hepatic enzyme levels, platelet counts, serum creatinine levels and a 12- to 24-hour urine collection (or spot creatinine tests) for total protein measurement. Blood tests include a full blood count, urea and electrolytes and coagulation profiles (APTT, PT, fibrinogen). Antepartum surveillance (NSTs) two or three times a week and/or biophysical profiles and/or Doppler flow studies are used to monitor fetal growth and to ascertain the most appropriate and safest time for delivery.

Education for the family begins as soon as the diagnosis is confirmed and should include information about the disease process, signs and symptoms of worsening disease, proposed course of treatment, including physical and laboratory assessment, medications, potential complications for the woman and her baby and the plan for birthing.

Hospital management

Hospital admission may become necessary if the woman feels 'safer' in hospital, if her hypertension worsens, in the presence of proteinuria, if there are signs of end organ involvement, or if there are concerns about fetal wellbeing. The laboratory tests and assessments described above are used to monitor the progress of the disease. It is crucial that an accurate fluid balance chart is maintained and reviewed daily to ensure that renal impairment is detected quickly. Table 33.3 lists the systemic complications of mild and severe PE.

Antihypertensive therapy

Antihypertensive therapy for PE is indicated once the BP is persistently > 160/100 mmHg, with the aim of achieving a diastolic BP of 90 to 100 mmHg. This is to avoid 'overcorrection' and the risk of exacerbating placental hypoperfusion. Antihypertensive drugs used to control hypertension include methyldopa, atenolol and labetalol. Angiotensin-converting enzyme (ACE) inhibitors are contraindicated in pregnancy.

TABLE 33.3 Systemic complications of eclampsia/pre-eclampsia

System	Complication
Cardiovascular	Cardiogenic and non-cardiogenic pulmonary oedema
Neurological	Cerebral oedema Cerebral haemorrhage, a direct consequence of hypertension Convulsions, coma
Hepatic	Subcapsular haematoma (epigastric or right upper quadrant pain) Hepatic rupture
Renal	Renal failure Proteinuria
Haematological	Thrombocytopaenia Disseminated intravascular coagulopathy (DIC) Haemolysis
Fetal	Fetal growth restriction Placental abruption

(Source: Lew & Klonis 2003, p 362)

Timing of delivery

Delivery is the only 'cure' for clinically diagnosed PE and should be accomplished as soon as the fetus is mature, or earlier if the mother's condition deteriorates or if there is evidence of significant fetal compromise. The timing and management of delivery requires close collaboration between the woman and her obstetric, midwifery, paediatric and anaesthetic team members. If the fetus is between 24 and 34 weeks gestation and urgent delivery is required, corticosteroids are administered to the mother to stimulate fetal lung maturation and the production of surfactant. Vaginal birth is preferable and epidural analgesia is the preferred choice of analgesia for labour. Epidurals reduce the maternal stress response and release of catecholamines, which occur in labour when pain cannot be controlled. Epidural analgesia and anaesthesia are contradicated if there is evidence of coagulopathy (platelet count < 50 000 × 10^9/L).

Indications for immediate delivery

Fetal indications:
- IUGR
- non-reassuring NST
- oligohydramnios.

Critical thinking exercise

Why are ACE inhibitors contraindicated in pregnancy?

Maternal indications:
- progressive deterioration of liver function
- progressive deterioration of renal function
- suspected placental abruption
- persistent severe headache or visual changes
- persistent severe epigastric pain, nausea or vomiting.

Pre-eclampsia superimposed on chronic hypertension

PE superimposed on chronic hypertension is characterised by new-onset proteinuria (or by a sudden increase in the protein level if proteinuria is already present), a rapid increase in blood pressure (assuming hypertension already exists), or development of the HELLP (haemolysis, elevated liver enzymes, low platelet count) syndrome. Recognising PE superimposed on chronic hypertension can be very challenging. The condition should be suspected when any one of the following is present: BP > 160/110 mmHg; heavy proteinuria (more than 2 g per day), or existing proteinuria that abruptly worsens; BP suddenly increases after a period of good control; or serum creatinine levels rise to more than 110 mmol/L. Immediate management is similar to that described for PE. Once the baby is born, further assessment and treatment of ongoing hypertension is required.

Postpartum management of hypertensive disease

Although birth is the only 'cure' for PE, the condition often deteriorates immediately after delivery, and up to 30% of cases of PE are only diagnosed post partum when the mother develops eclamptic seizures. Most maternal deaths occur after delivery. It is therefore important that in the first 72 hours after birth, clinicians continue to monitor the mother's blood pressure, continue therapy and ensure that she is not 'overloaded' with fluid. If she has been diagnosed with severe PE it is crucial that a meticulous fluid balance chart is still maintained and carefully reviewed. Good analgesia cover is also important after operative delivery to reduce the stress response associated with uncontrolled pain. In women with PE, antihypertensive medication may be required post partum for three or four weeks. Little information is available on the effects of antihypertensive medication during lactation, although as yet there is no evidence that antihypertensive drugs have a detrimental effect on the baby. Hypertension and other signs of PE should remit by six to 12 weeks post partum. At a follow-up consultation, the woman should be informed of her risk of PE and its consequences in subsequent pregnancies. Women with PE do not appear to have an increased risk of future hypertension or cardiovascular disease, although women with transient hypertension or chronic hypertension do.

Clinical point

Up to 40% of eclamptic seizures occur before delivery; approximately 16% occur more than 48 hours after birth.

Multiple pregnancy

Twin birth occurs in approximately 1 in 80 pregnancies and triplets once in 80 × 80 (6400) pregnancies. Multiple gestations have a higher incidence of complications than singletons from conception until the birth of the second twin. The complications associated with multiple pregnancies have resulted in a significant increase in the proportion of preterm births and the number of babies admitted to neonatal intensive care units.

Incidence of multiple births

According to the Australian Bureau of Statistics' *Year Book Australia* (ABS 2002), birth registrations over the past 20 years indicate that while the number of pregnancies (births) resulting in a live birth has been declining, the number of multiple births has increased (see Fig 33.4). This is primarily attributed to the increased use of assisted conception technologies and the increasing number of births to older women. While the actual number of multiple births remains relatively low, there has been a steady increase in Australia and New Zealand since the 1970s.

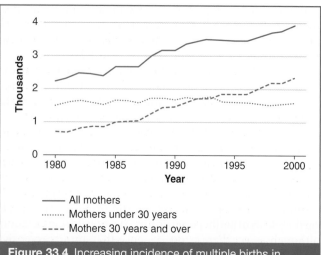

Figure 33.4 Increasing incidence of multiple births in Australia (based on ABS 2002)

Classification

There are two major types of twin gestations: dizygotic (DZ) and monozygotic (MZ). MZ twins (uniovular and identical) occur sporadically. In contrast, the incidence of DZ (binovular and fraternal) increases with advancing maternal age and parity. In some families, DZ twinning is probably inherited. DZ twins are more common than MZ twins (see Fig 33.5). In Caucasians about 30% of twin pregnancies are MZ and about 70% DZ.

DZ twins develop from two ova fertilised by different spermatozoa. They have separate gestational sacs with separate placentas, chorion, amnion and umbilical cords. The developing fetuses may be of the same or different sex and are no more alike than siblings. In contrast, MZ twins develop from a single ovum, which splits within a few days of embryogenesis into two identical halves, each developing into one twin with a separate amnion and umbilical cord but usually sharing one placenta and chorion. These babies are of the same sex, have the same blood group and share very similar physical and psychological characteristics.

Chorionicity

Zygosity refers to the type of conception, whereas chorionicity refers to the type of placentation. Twin placentas are classified into two categories according to the number of layers in the septum between the two amniotic sacs. Depending on the stage of embryogenesis at which the zygote splits, four different types of twins may result. All dizygotic twins have DC (dichorionic/diamniotic) placentas. The placentas may be fused or separate, but when examined after birth blood vessel anastamoses between the two vascular beds are seldom discovered.

In MZ twins, if the zygote splits early (within 72 hours after fertilisation) each twin will lie in its own sac and the placentas have separate chorions and amnions (dichorionic/diamniotic). However, in about 70% of MZ twins, division does not occur until the blastocyst stage between four and eight days after conception. In this case each twin will have its own amniotic sac but the placenta will only have one chorion but two amnions. An even smaller number (< 1%) of MZ twins will have monochorionic-monoamniotic placentas, so the twins share the same amniotic sac. There is no intervening membrane and so the fetuses and their umbilical cords can freely intermingle and entwine. Monoamniotic placentation

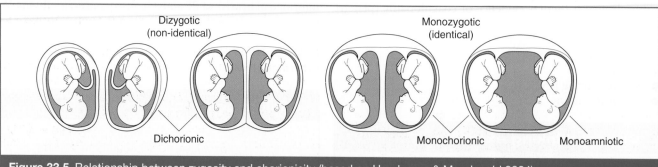

Figure 33.5 Relationship between zygosity and chorionicity (based on Henderson & Macdonald 2004)

occurs when division takes place between days 7 and 11—that is, after the amnion has differentiated. Conjoined twins are an even rarer subtype of monozygotic twinning and occur because splitting of the embryo does not take place until after the primitive streak has differentiated. Triplets can be MZ, DZ or trizygotic.

Mortality/morbidity

Multiple pregnancies are considered to be 'high risk' because the mortality rate is about four times that for singletons. Evidence suggests that about 75% of one or both twins are miscarried (Sebire et al 2000; Sutcliffe et al 2001). In many cases this is due to congenital abnormalities, which are more common in MZ and monochorionic twins. In the so-called 'vanishing twin' syndrome, the 'lost' twin is reabsorbed into the mother's body or miscarried with few or no symptoms. Occasionally one fetus dies early in the pregnancy and is retained in the uterus until term, becoming flattened and mummified. This is known as a *fetus papyraceus* ('paper-like'). Depending on local regulations, the fetus may require birth and death certificates.

Higher-order multiple births have even higher mortality and morbidity rates compared to twins and singletons. This is mostly due to the increased proportion of infants with low birthweight and preterm delivery and the complications associated with these. Several authors dispute this, however, arguing that regular fetal surveillance and appropriate steroid administration is necessary for good perinatal outcomes in monoamniotic twin gestations (Allen et al 2001; Sebire et al 2000; Sutcliffe et al 2001). Twin-to-twin transfusion syndrome, in which blood from one twin is transfused to the other twin via blood vessels in their shared placenta, is a rare but serious and potentially life-threatening condition affecting 15% of MC twins (Sutcliffe et al 2001).

Other complications include:
- preterm labour and birth
- low birthweight
- placenta praevia
- placental abruption
- intrauterine growth restriction
- pre-eclampsia
- increased frequency of birth asphyxia
- malpresentation
- pre-labour and preterm rupture of the membranes and GBS infection
- umbilical cord accidents
- operative delivery
- postpartum haemorrhage.

Goals of management

Care of the woman and her muti-fetal pregnancy should be designed to prevent and/or treat the complications that may occur in order to optimise physical and psychosocial outcomes for the mother, baby and family. Supporting the parents of twins is not just about obstetric management of the pregnancy;

it is also about helping the woman and her family to adapt to a rapid increase in their family, to prepare for parenting multiples and supporting them to make informed decisions about the management of their 'high-risk' pregnancy. Maternal adaptations to pregnancy are exaggerated with twins. Plasma volume increases an additional 10–20% in twin over singleton pregnancies. Nutritional requirements rise, carbohydrate metabolism may differ, but the most marked changes arise because of the increase in maternal blood volume and consequently maternal cardiac output. Red blood cell mass increases to a lesser degree than plasma volume and so there is a relative anaemia because of this haemodilution. Both iron and folate requirements are higher in twin pregnancies. Because of the complications associated with multiple pregnancy, most women are referred to a medical practitioner and prepare for hospital births and, increasingly often, an operative birth. However, many of the complications associated with multiple pregnancy occur irrespective of the place of birth and, indeed, hospitalisation cannot prevent their occurrence.

Diagnosis of multiple pregnancy

Generally, the diagnosis of twins is not difficult for the astute midwife. By the end of the first trimester, uterine size is larger than expected for gestational age by last menstrual period and/or earlier examinations. The woman may report excessive nausea and vomiting or that she 'feels as if she is having twins'. In the second trimester, abdominal palpation of multiple fetal parts may suggest the presence of more than a single fetus, and occasionally, two sets of fetal heart rates may be detected. Ultrasound early in the first trimester usually confirms any suspicion the woman has that she is having twins. During abdominal ultrasonography, two gestational sacs can be visualised after six weeks gestation; vaginal ultrasound allows for an even earlier diagnosis. If the initial diagnosis is made very early in pregnancy, a repeat ultrasound several weeks later will confirm the presence of twins, rule out anomalies and determine chorionicity. Because of the increased rate of congenital abnormalities, women should be offered both biochemical genetic and nuchal translucency tests. Many practitioners recommend serial scans every four to six weeks to evaluate fetal growth and for concordance, especially if the twins are MZ. Non-stress tests, Doppler flow studies and biophysical profiles all play an important role in the ongoing assessment of fetal wellbeing, especially IUGR and growth discrepancies. The NST is reasonably reliable in assessing fetal wellbeing in multiple gestations. A problem arises when the NST results are discordant for the two fetuses. If only one NST is non-reactive, another test such as the biophysical profile should be performed on both fetuses. If this suggests fetal compromise, delivery or hospitalisation may be indicated. These decisions are based on gestational age, degree of compromise, and assessment of fetal maturity.

Sometimes one of the twins dies. Grieving for the dead baby while at the same time celebrating the life of the second child is very difficult for the parents.

WOMAN'S STORY

We were thrilled to find that at last I was having twins, after so many unsuccessful cycles of IVF. And then one day they told me one of my precious babies had died. Knowing that I was carrying a dead baby and a live one was very strange. Every time I went for a scan I was terrified that they would tell me that the second baby was going to die. I used to wonder if the one who was left knew that her sister was dead. I wanted to grieve for my dead baby and I felt guilty if I felt happy for the one who was still alive, but I was. When Linda was born, so beautiful and so healthy, we were so grateful and wanted to celebrate her birth, but I mourned for my second baby girl all over again. I wasn't sure what I was supposed to feel and I alternated between relief, guilt, sorrow and intense joy. Linda is too young to talk about it yet but I often wonder if she misses her identical sister. One day we will talk about it, but not today.

BOX 33.22 Symptoms of preterm labour

▶ All women should be aware of the symptoms of preterm labour, primarily after 20 weeks gestation. These include cramps, contractions, menstrual pains, increasing pelvic or vaginal pressure, increasing low back pain, heavy vaginal discharge, vaginal spotting or bleeding, rectal pressure.

▶ There is no evidence that bed rest improves fetal outcomes but it may improve the woman's sense of wellbeing

▶ Adequate hydration, 6–8 glasses of liquid per day, is helpful.

▶ Recognise whenever an activity is associated with the above symptoms, and then stop or reduce that particular activity.

▶ For any pattern of symptoms suggestive of preterm labour that does not resolve within one hour of bed rest, contact the lead carer.

Collaborative management in pregnancy

Care of the woman with a twin pregnancy is designed to support the parents as they prepare for parenting and to prevent, identify and treat the complications that may arise. These have been dealt with earlier in the chapter. Consequently, many clinicians recommend: more frequent consultations with the obstetric team; more ultrasounds and tests for fetal wellbeing and to predict preterm labour; iron and calcium supplements; and sometimes restrictions and limitations on the woman's activities.

Preparation for birth

The mechanisms involved in vaginal birth of the first twin are similar to those for singleton pregnancies; however, malpresentation, fetal compromise, maternal and placental bleeding and the need for abdominal delivery are increased in twin pregnancies. Therefore, intensive and continuous monitoring of maternal and fetal wellbeing and the progress of labour are essential. Induction of labour and augmentation with Syntocinon and artificial rupture of membranes for one or both babies are used if necessary. Blood is cross-matched and IV access obtained because of the increased risk of PPH. Epidural analgesia is recommended if there is hypertension or if the labour is preterm or complicated by the possibility that there will be malpresentation of the second twin.

Equipment is prepared for the births of two babies, keeping in mind that the babies may be small for dates or preterm and that the birth of the second twin may be complicated. Each twin is monitored simultaneously. Immediate availability of two paediatricians and an anaesthetist is recommended.

Once Twin A is born and the umbilical cord is clamped, blood should not be collected until after delivery of the second twin. There are two reasons for this:

• There may be vascular connections between the placentas, such that blood from Twin B escapes from the cord of Twin A.

• Removal of blood from the placenta may hasten its separation from the uterine wall, leading to placental abruption.

A section of umbilical cord can safely be ligated and removed for blood gases if this is hospital protocol.

Delivery of the second twin

Route of delivery of the second twin engenders significant controversy in the intrapartum management of twins. There is general agreement that vaginal delivery is safe in twins who both present as vertex, and caesarean delivery is indicated only in the presence of the usual obstetric and fetal indications. Management of vertex–nonvertex twins is perhaps the most controversial. The options are caesarean delivery, external cephalic version (ECV), and assisted vaginal breech delivery or breech extraction. An important factor in this decision is the skill and experience of the personnel available. If the decision is made to proceed with a vaginal birth, as long as the fetal heartbeat of the second twin is reassuring, the time interval until the baby's birth is not critical. What is critical, however, is that the labour is progressing. As soon as the first baby is born, the second baby's heart tones are monitored continuously, and the baby's position, lie and presentation determined by palpation and vaginal examination or, as is increasingly common, with real-time ultrasound. If the lie is longitudinal, whether the vertex or the breech is presenting, the membranes are artificially ruptured and a short period of time left to elapse to see if contractions establish. If they do not, augmentation with oxytocin is warranted. The delivery of the second twin usually occurs quite quickly as the cervix has already been fully dilated. Because of the risk of PPH, the third stage is managed actively. Syntocinon® is given only after the birth of the second baby and after confirming that there is not a third baby waiting to be born. Many clinicians recommend that an IV infusion of Hartmann's solution or normal saline containing 40 mIU of Syntocinon® is commenced to ensure the uterus remains well-contracted in the immediate postnatal period, thereby avoiding a PPH. The placenta and membranes are examined to determine that they are complete and whether the twins are MZ or DZ, although this is confirmed by placental histology.

Care of the woman in the puerperium proceeds as for a singleton pregnancy, though the woman may require extra practical support and assistance to establish feeding and organise the care of two babies. Contact with local support groups such as the local multiple birth association is encouraged from early in pregnancy.

Conclusion

For the woman experiencing a complicated pregnancy, many associated issues arise. The woman's level of anxiety increases as the pregnancy progresses. The woman needs assistance and support if she is to be away from her normal place of residence for a period of time, including possible transfer to a regional tertiary unit and the associated dislocation from her close family and friendship network. Adequate childcare for other children may need to be organised. The cost in time and dollars of attending specialist appointments needs to be addressed. The emotional toll of a complicated pregnancy is ongoing and may not necessarily be resolved with delivery of the baby. The compromised fetus often results in the birth of a baby requiring specialist paediatric services for a period of time. At the same time, the new mother needs time to recover both physically and emotionally from a complicated pregnancy. The midwife's involvement in each woman's pregnancy is fundamental to ensuring that the woman receives appropriate care that is not compromised by exposure to unnecessary risk.

Review questions

1. At 10 weeks pregnant, Neve is unable to eat any food without vomiting and feels nauseated all day. What actions will you take?

2. Beth is eight weeks pregnant and rings you to say she has had some fresh vaginal bleeding. What advice will you give her?

3. Lydia is 32 weeks pregnant. She tells you as she has had some fresh vaginal bleeding. What are possible causes for the bleeding? What information will you need to help you make a diagnosis? Describe the advice you will give Lydia.

4. Victoria is 22 weeks pregnant. She comes to your clinic complaining of feeling unwell and with lower abdominal crampy pain. What other information do you require? What will you do?

6. Isabella's first pregnancy has progressed normally. However at her 36 week antenatal check, Isabella has a blood pressure recording of 140/98 mmHg and + protein on dipstick. What actions do you take?

7. At 32 weeks pregnant, Joanna rings you, saying that her skin feels very itchy, especially on her palms. She tells you that she has no rash. What do you advise?

8. RE results of Kelly's 28-week gestational diabetes challenge test (50 g glucose polymer load) at one hour post glucose dose is 9 mmol/L. The normal range is < 7.9 mmol/L. What are your obligations as the midwife providing Kelly's care?

9. Portia has a fundal height of 15 weeks at her 12-week antenatal visit. A subsequent USS confirms a twin pregnancy. Portia is very keen for you to continue to provide midwifery care for the remainder of her pregnancy. Under what conditions could this be provided? What plan for care and ongoing management will you negotiate with Portia?

10. Rae is 37 weeks pregnant with her first baby. She rings you at 2 am and says she has heartburn, can't stop vomiting and 'feels most unwell'. Her pregnancy has proceeded normally so far. What will you suggest?

Online resources

Australian Herpes Management Forum, http://esvc000204.wic009u.server-web.com/

Australian Indigenous HealthInfoNet 2003 Frequently asked questions: what do we know about diabetes among Indigenous people? http://www.healthinfonet.ecu.edu.au/html/html_keyfacts/faq/faq_specific_health/diabetes.htm

Centers for Disease Control, http://www.cdc.gov

Hyperemesis Education and Research (HER) Foundation, http://www.hyperemesis.org

Miscarriage Support Auckland, http://www.miscarriagesupport.org.nz/support.html

New Zealand Herpes Foundation, http://www.herpes.org.nz/pregnancy.html

Statistics New Zealand (2006) Demographic trends 2005, http://www.stats.govt.nz

References

Allen VM, Windrin R, Barrett J et al 2001 Management of monoamniotic twin pregnancies: a case series and systematic review of the litereature. British Journal of Obstetrics and Gynaecology 108:932–936

American College of Obstetricians and Gynaecologists 2001 Management of recurrent early pregnancy loss. ACOG Practice Bulletin 24

Amos A, McCarty D, Zimmet P 1997 The rising global burden of diabetes and its complications: estimates and projections to the year 2010. Diabetes Medicine 14(suppl. 5):S1–S85

Atallah A, Hofmeyr G, Duly L 2004 Calcium supplementation during pregnancy for preventing hypertensive disorders and related problems. Cochrane Database of Systematic Reviews (2): CD001059

Australasian Society for the Study of Hypertension in Pregnancy (ASSHP) 2000 Consensus Statement of the ASSHP. In: MA Brown, WM Hae, J Higgins et al, Australian and New Zealand Journal of Obstetrics and Gynaecology 46:139–154

Australian Bureau of Statistics (ABS) 2002 Yearbook Australia. ABS, Canberra

Australian Indigenous HealthInfoNet 2003. Online: http://www. healthinfonet.ecu.edu.au

Australian Institute of Health and Welfare 2002 Diabetes: Australian facts 2002. ACNCDS No 3. AIHW, Canberra

Bachman J, Heise R, Naessens J et al 1993 A study of various tests to detect asymptomatic urinary tract infections in an obstetric population. Journal of the American Medical Association 270:1971–1974

Barwise K 2005 Type 1 diabetes and pregnancy: one mother's story. Canadian Diabetes Association. Online: http://www.diabetes.ca/ Section_About/type1preg.asp, accessed 15 August 2005

Beal M, Simmonds K 2002 Clinical uses of mifepristone: an update for women's health practitioners. Journal of Midwifery and Women's Health 47(6):451–460

Berkovitch M, Briggs G, Chin R et al 2001 International consensus on standards for studying the efficacy of pharmacological therapies for nausea and vomiting of pregnancy. Online: http: www.nvp-volumes.org/consensu.htm

Bhide A, Prefumo F, Moore J et al 2003 Placental edge to internal os distance in the late third trimester and mode of delivery in placenta praevia. British Journal of Obstetrics and Gynaecology 110:860–868

Bigrigg M, Read M 1991 Management of women referred to early pregnancy assessment unit: care and cost effectiveness. British Medical Journal 302(6776):577–579

Blaiss M 2004 Managing asthma during pregnancy: the whys and hows of aggressive control. Postgraduate Medicine 115(5): 55–64

Bonow R, Carabello B, de Leon A Jr et al 1998 Guidelines for the management of patients with valvular heart disease: executive summary. A report of the American College of Cardiology/ American Heart Association task force on practice guidelines (committee on management of patients with valvular heart disease). Circulation 98:1949–1984

Botash R, Spirt B 2000 Ectopic pregnancy: review and update. Applied Radiology:7–12

Boyce P, Condon J, Ellwood D 2002 Pregnancy loss: a major life event affecting emotional health and well-being. Medical Journal of Australia 176(6):250–251

Brown M, Hague W, Higgens J et al 2000 The detection, investigation and management of hypertension in pregnancy: full consensus statement. Australian and New Zealand Journal of Obstetrics and Gynaecology 40(2):139–155

Bryan S 2003 Current challenges in the assessment and management of patients with bleeding in early pregnancy. Emergency Medicine 15(3):219–222

Carapetis J, Currie B 1998 Preventing rheumatic heart disease in Australia. A coordinated approach is needed, together with improved living conditions in affected indigenous communities. Medical Journal of Australia 168:428–429

Carapetis J, Wolff D, Currie B 1996 Acute rheumatic fever and rheumatic heart disease in the Top End of Australia's Northern Territory. Medical Journal of Australia 164:146–149

Centers for Disease Control (CDC) 2004 Bacterial vaginosis: fact sheet. Online: http://www.cdc.gov/std/bv/STDFact-Bacterial-Vaginosis.htm. Last reviewed May 2004.

Chan W, Anand S, Ginsberg J 2000 Anticoagulation of pregnant women with mechanical heart valves. A systematic review of the literature. Archives of Internal Medicine 160:191–196

Chen M, Donovan B 2003 Screening for genital *Chlamydia trachomatis* infection: are men the forgotten reservoir?' Medical Journal of Australia 79(3):124–125

Colagiuri S, Colagiuri R, Ward J 1998 National diabetes strategy and implementation plan. Diabetes Australia, Commonwealth Department of Health and Family Services, Canberra

Coombes J 2000 Cholestasis in pregnancy: a challenging disorder. British Journal of Midwifery 8(9):565–570

Darai E, Vlastos G, Benifla J et al 1996 Is maternal serum creatinine kinase actually a marker for early diagnosis of ectopic pregnancy? European Journal of Obstetrics and Gynaecology Reproductive Biology 68:25–27

de Courten M, Hodge A, Dowse G et al 1998 Review of the epidemiology, aetiology, pathogenesis and preventability of diabetes in Aboriginal and Torres Strait Islander populations. Commonwealth Department of Health and Family Services, Canberra

Dennison J 2004. Weathering the storms. Living with epilepsy. Emdee Publishing, UK. Extract from website: Julie Dennison–living with epilepsy. A personal guide, http://apersonalguide.co.uk/ livingwithepilepsy/talks/talk-preg.htm

Department of Health (2004) Why Mothers Die 2000–2002. Report on confidential enquiries into maternal deaths in the United Kingdom. RCOG Press, London

Drife J 2003 Thromboembolism. British Medical Bulletin 67:177–190

Duley L 2003 Pre-eclampsia and the hypertensive disorders of pregnancy. British Medical Bulletin 67:161–176

Fairweather D 1968 Nausea and vomiting in pregnancy. American Journal of Obstetrics and Gynecology 102:135–175

Ferris A, Neubauer S, Bendel R et al 1993 Perinatal lactation protocol and outcome in mothers with and without IDDM. American Journal of Clinical Nutrition 58:43–48

Food Standards Australia New Zealand (FSANZ) 1999 Listeria and pregnancy. Online: http://www.foodstandards.gov.au/mediareleas espublications/factsheets/factsheets1999/listeriaandpregnancy.cfm

Forna F, Gulmezoglu A 2004 Surgical procedures to evacuate incomplete abortion. Cochrane Database of Systematic Reviews (2). John Wiley & Sons, Chichester

Gates S, Brocklehurst P, Davis LJ 2005 Prophylaxis for venous thromboembolic disease in pregnancy and the early postnatal period (Cochrane Review) Cochrane Library (3). John Wiley & Sons, Chichester

Gaufberg S 2001 Abruptio placentae. EMedicine 2(3). Online: http://www.emedicine.com

Gautier G-F et al 2003 Effect of a diabetic environment in utero on predisposition to type 2 diabetes. Lancet 361(9372):1839–1840

Gazvani M, Baruah D, Alfirevic Z et al 1998 Mifepristone in combination with methotrexate for the medical treatment of tubal pregnancy: a randomised controlled trial. Human Reproduction 13(7):1987–1990

Gilbert G, Hewett M, Turner C et al 2002 Epidemiology and predictive values of risk factors for neonatal group B streptococcal sepsis. Australian and New Zealand Journal of Obstetrics and Gynaecology 42(5):497–503

Gomella T, Cunningham M, Eyal F et al 1999 Neonatology: management, problems, on-call problems, diseases and drugs. Appleton & Lange, Conn.

Greer L 1999 Thrombosis in pregnancy: maternal and fetal issues. Lancet 353:1258–1265

Grimwood K, Darlow B, Gosling I et al 2001 Early onset neonatal Group B Streptococcal infections in New Zealand 1998–99. Unpublished, Wellington.

Hajenius P, Mol B et al 2005 Interventions for tubal ectopic pregnancy (Cochrane Review). Cochrane Library (2). CD000324. DOI: 10.1002/14651858.CD000324. John Wiley & Sons, Chichester

Hart E, Coley S 2003 The diagnosis and management of pre-eclampsia. British Journal of Anaesthesia 3(2):38–42

Harville E, Wilcox WA, Baird D et al 2003 Vaginal bleeding in very early pregnancy. Human Reproduction 18(9):1944–1947

Hayakawa S, Nakajima N, Karasaki-Suzuki M et al 2000 Frequent presence of *Helicobacter pylori* genome in the saliva of patients with hyperemesis gravidarum. American Journal of Perinatology 17:243–247

Henderson C, Macdonald S 2004 Mayes' midwifery (13th edn). Ballière Tindall, London

Higgins S 2003 Obstetric haemorrhage. Emergency Medicine 15:227–231

Hinshaw H 1997 Medical management of miscarriage. In: J Grudzinskas, PMS O'Brien (Eds) Problems in early pregnancy: advances in diagnosis and management. RCOG Press, London, pp 284–295

Hoffman L, Nolan C, Wilson JD et al 1998 Gestational diabetes mellitus—management guidelines. Medical Journal of Australia 169:93–97

Hogge W 2003 The clinical use of karyotyping spontaneous abortions. American Journal of Obstetrics and Gynaecology 189(2):397–402

Hyperemesis Education and Research (HER) Foundation 2004 Diagnosis and assessment tools. Online: http://www.helpher.org/health-professionals/diagnosis-assessment/index.php

Hyperemesis Education and Research (HER) Foundation 2005 Patient comfort measures. Online: http://www.helpher.org/health-professionals/patient-comfort-measures.php, accessed 26 June 2005

James D 2001 Maternal screening and treatment for Group B streptococcus. Journal of Obstetric, Gynecologic and Neonatal Nursing 30(6): 659–666

Jewell D, Young G 2002 Interventions for nausea and vomiting in early pregnancy. Cochrane Database of Systematic Reviews (1): CD000145

Jilma B, Kamath S, Lip GY 2003 Antithrombotic therapy in special circumstances. 1. Pregnancy and cancer. British Medical Journal 326:37–40

Kenyon A, Piercy C, Girling J 2002 Obstetric cholestasis, outcome with active management: a series of 70 cases. British Journal of Obstetrics and Gynaecology 109:282–288

Khoo S 2003 Clinical aspects of gestational trophoblastic disease: a review based partly on 25 year experience of a statewide registry. Australian and New Zealand Journal of Obstetrics and Gynaecology 43:280–289

Kitzmiller J, Gavin L, Gin G et al 1991 Preconception care of diabetes. Glycaemic control prevents congenital anomalies. Journal of the American Medical Association 265:731–736

Kjos S, Henry O, Lee R et al 1993 The effect of lactation on glucose and lipid metabolism in women with recent gestational diabetes. Obstetrics and Gynaecology 82:451–455

Kovacevich G, Laich S, Lavin J et al 2000 The prevalence of thromboembolic events among women with extended bed rest prescribed as part of the treatment for premature labour or preterm rupture of membranes. American Journal of Obstetrics and Gynaecology 182(5):1089–1092

Leitich H, Bodner-Adler B, Brunbauer M et al 2003 Bacterial vaginosis as a risk factor for preterm delivery: a meta-analysis. American Journal of Obstetrics and Gynecology 189(1):139–147

Lew M, Klonis E 2003 Emergency management of eclampsia and pre-eclampsia. Emergency Medicine 15:361–368

Love C, Fernando K, Sargent L et al 2004 Major placenta praevia should not preclude out-patient management. European Journal of Obstetrics, Gynaecology and Reproductive Biology 117(1): 24–29

Magee L, Ornstein M, von Dadelszen P 1999 Management of hypertension in pregnancy. British Medical Journal 318:1332–1336

Marmot M, Wilkinson R (Eds) 1999 Putting the picture together: prosperity, redistribution, health and welfare. Social determinants of health. Oxford University Press, Oxford

Mazzotta P, Magee L 2000 A risk-benefit assessment of pharmacological and nonpharmacological treatments for nausea and vomiting of pregnancy. Drugs 59:781–800

McDonald C, Burdon J 1996 Asthma in pregnancy and lactation. A position paper for the Thoracic Society of Australia. Medical Journal of Australia 165:165

Meltzer D 2000 Selections from current literature. Complementary therapies for nausea and vomiting in early pregnancy. Family Practice 17(6):570–573

Moran P, Taylor R 2002 Management of hyperemesis gravidarum: the importance of weight loss as a criterion for steroid therapy. Quarterly Journal of Medicine 958:153–158

Neilson J, Alfirevic Z 2001 Doppler ultrasound for fetal assessment in high risk pregnancies (Cochrane Review). Cochrane Library (3). Update Software, Oxford

Neilson J 2004 Interventions for suspected placenta praevia. Cochrane Library (1). ID#CD001998. Update Software, Oxford

Nelson-Piercy C, Fayers P, de Swiet M 2001 Randomised, double-blind, placebo-controlled trial of corticosteroids for the treatment of hyperemesis gravidarum. British Journal of Obstetrics and Gynaecology 108:9–15

Oakeshott P, Hay P, Hay S et al 2002 Association between bacterial vaginosis or chlamydial infection and miscarriage before 16 weeks' gestation: prospective community based cohort study. British Medical Journal 325:1334

Oats J, Abraham S 2004 Llewellyn-Jones fundamentals of obstetrics and gynaecology (8th edn). Elsevier, Sydney

Obstetric Medicine Group of Australasia 2001 Position paper: anticoagulation in pregnancy and the puerperium. Medical Journal of Australia 175:258–263

Public Health Laboratory Service Syphilis Working Group 1998 Antenatal syphilis screening in the UK: a systematic review and national options appraisal with recommendations. Online: http://www.phls.org.uk/publications/syphil~1.pdf, accessed September 2001

Quinlan J, Hill D 2003 Nausea and vomiting in pregnancy. American Family Physician 68(1):121–128

Remsberg K, McKeown R et al 1999 Diabetes in pregnancy and Caesarean delivery. Diabetes Care 22:1561–1567

Royal College of Obstetricians and Gynaecologists (RCOG) 2001 Clinical Green Top Guidelines. The Management of Early Pregnancy Loss (25). Online: http://www.rcog.org.uk/index.asp?PageID=515

Royal College of Obstetricians and Gynaecologists (RCOG) 2004 Evidence-based clinical guidelines 7. RCOG, London. Online: http://www.rcog.org.uk

Schrag SJ, Zywicki S, Farley MM et al 2000 Group B streptococcal disease in the era of intrapartum antibiotic prophylaxis. New England Journal of Medicine 342:15–20

Schrag S, Gorwitz T, Fultz-Butts K et al 2002 Prevention of perinatal Group B streptococcal disease: revised guidelines from CDC. Morbidity and Mortality Weekly Report 51:1–24

Sebire N, Souka A, Skentou H et al 2000 First trimester diagnosis of monoamniotic twin pregnancy. Ultrasound in Obstetrics and Gynaecology 16(3):223–225

Simmons D, Thompson C, Conroy C 2000 Incidence and risk factors for neonatal hypoglycaemia among women with gestational diabetes in South Auckland. Diabetes Medicine 17:830–834

Simmons D, Thompson C, Voaklander D 2001a Polynesians prone to obesity and type 2 diabetes but not hyperinsulinaemia. Diabetic Medicine 18:1–6

Simmons D, Thompson C, Conroy C et al 2001b Use of insulin pumps in pregnancies complicated by type 2 diabetes and gestational diabetes in a multiethnic community. Diabetes Care 24:2078–2082

Simmons D, Walters B, Rowan J et al 2004 Metformin therapy and diabetes in pregnancy. Medical Journal of Australia 180(9): 462–464

Slaytor E, Sullivan E, King J 2004 Maternal deaths in Australia 1997–1999. AIHW Cat. No. PER 24. Maternal Deaths Series No. 1. Australian Institute of Health and Welfare, National Perinatal Statistics Unit, Sydney

Stables D, Rankin J 2004 Physiology in childbearing. With anatomy and related biosciences. Baillière Tindall, London

Sutcliffe A, Sebire N, Pigott A et al 2001 Outcome for children born after inutero laser ablation therapy for severe twin-to-twin transfusion syndrome. British Journal of Obstetrics and Gynaecology 108:1246–1250

Tay J, Moore J, Walker J 2000 Clinical review: ectopic pregnancy. British Medical Journal 320:916–919

Temple R, Aldridge V, Greenwood R et al 2002 Association between outcome of pregnancy and glycaemic control in early pregnancy in Type 1 diabetes: Population based study. British Medical Journal 325:1275–1276

Tenore J 2000 Ectopic pregnancy. American Family Physician 61(4):1080–1088

Turner A 2000 Obstetric cholestasis: symptoms, causes and treatments. British Journal of Midwifery 8:530

Turok D, Ratcliffe S, Baxley E et al 2003 Management of gestational diabetes. American Family Physician 68(9): 1767–1772

Weinberg L 2001 Use of anti-D immunoglobulin in the treatment of threatened miscarriage in the accident and emergency department. Emergency Medicine 18:444–447

CHAPTER 34

Disturbances in the rhythm of labour

Carol Thorogood and Catherine Donaldson

Key terms

cephalo-pelvic disproportion, dystocia, Friedman's curve, hypertonic uterine action, hypotonic uterine action, incoordinate uterine action, malposition, malpresentation, partogram, prolonged labour, 'trial' of caesarean scar, 'trial' of labour, VBAC

Chapter overview

Maternity care in most developed countries including Australia and, until recently, New Zealand is dominated by a medicalised, technologically orientated, interventionist model of maternity service provision. Soaring intervention rates suggest two things: that Western women's bodies are no longer able to cope with labour and birth without medical intervention; and that intervention is occurring in many 'normal' labours and births. Whatever the cause, increased intervention in birth, including inductions of labour, caesarean sections, the use of regional anaesthesia and analgesia, and operative deliveries, has not made substantial differences in improving maternal and neonatal outcomes for women living in resource-rich nations.

Despite the very best of care and support, not all labours proceed as planned and an exploration of the causes, associations and management of these deviations from the usual birthing journey is the overall aim of this chapter. First, however, the authors reconsider what a 'normal' journey is and what it is not. The chapter then describes the factors that disturb the rhythms of labour, leading to what is commonly called dystocia (difficult labour), such as prolonged labour, malpresentations and positions, and preterm labour, as well as the interventions used to manage these, such as augmentation and induction of labour, and operative delivery (caesarean section, forceps and Ventouse extractions). The authors draw on woman-focused and empowering language—disturbance in the rhythms of birth—to describe some of the causes of dystocia, rather than mechanistic and disempowering idiom, such as the oft-used but ill-defined 'failure to progress' or 'trial of labour' and 'trial of scar', because the former is more women-centred and does not ascribe notions of failure and inadequacy or blame to the birthing woman. However, because the latter terms are part of the everyday language found in the literature and in most delivery wards, they are included here as well.

The anatomical structures, physiology and biosciences underpinning disturbances in the rhythms of labour are covered only briefly in this chapter. Therefore it is important that students who may be unfamiliar with these concepts refer to a specialised text to enable them to apply this material to the content of this chapter.

Learning outcomes

Learning outcomes for this chapter are:

1 To analyse the causes, identification, effects and management of disturbances in the rhythms of labour and birth

2 To critically discuss the evidence that supports common medical interventions in birth

3 To describe the ways in which midwives work to keep birth culturally, emotionally and physically safe when disturbances in the rhythms of labour occur.

Introduction

Many midwives do not subscribe to an interventionist model of care for all women. For example, in New Zealand, the Midwifery Council's (2004) Scope of Practice clearly places emphasis on the midwife supporting the physiological processes of normal birthing, and this is evident throughout the Council's Competencies for Registration as a midwife. As Powell-Kennedy and Shannon (2004) discovered in a qualitative study, the support of normalcy is fundamental to a midwifery model of care, one that is prefaced by a view that birth for most women should be a normal process even though some labours are more difficult than others. Participants in the study commented that women's bodies are physiologically prepared for labour and birth (Powell-Kennedy & Shannon 2004). The midwives described how they reassured birthing women that even though their labour might be long and painful, it was still normal (ibid). Moreover, they 'embraced a tolerance for wide variations in normal labour and for sustaining as much normalcy as possible, even when pathology had been identified'(Powell-Kennedy & Shannon 2004, p 256). These midwives believe, as does the WHO (1997), that there should always be a valid reason for intervention in the natural process of birth.

A review of the literature concerned with labour and birth reveals that since the seventeenth century, clinicians have endeavoured to differentiate between a 'normal' and an 'abnormal' labour and birth. Certainly, the history of midwifery and obstetrics suggests that across time and place, clinicians have created, eliminated and re-worked descriptions of 'normal' labour. Many of these are still in use, although they are not supported by scientific or research-based evidence, and more often than not have been created according to the authors' hunches, opinions, cultural beliefs or convenience rather than evidence. Gross and colleagues (2005) comment on the difficulties associated with determining the precise onset of labour and the duration of each of its phases and stages. There are still large gaps in our knowledge and understandings about birth. As yet there is no consensus about the appropriate length of each stage of labour or how to differentiate between a 'normal' and an 'abnormal' labour and the risk factors associated with it. For instance, despite a paucity of evidence, an unengaged fetal head in a nullipara at the beginning of labour has long been held to be a risk factor for cephalo-pelvic disproportion (CPD) and therefore is cited as an indication for a 'trial' of labour or caesarean section. This is despite research by authors such as Takahashi and Suzuki (1982), and Diegmann et al (1995), who found no significant differences in labour outcomes between nulliparas with an engaged fetal head at the beginning of labour and those with an unengaged fetal head. Similarly, medical and midwifery students are often introduced to notions of specific time intervals expected from each phase of labour, and this knowledge is reinforced by what they see in the hospital environment even though these are arbitrarily timed.

The Greek word for 'difficult' or abnormal labour is 'dystocia' and this topic is the focus of this chapter. Every midwife will

Reflective exercise

If they are to provide quality midwifery care, midwives need to consider how knowledge is generated, where it comes from and how their own value and belief systems affect their understanding of 'normal' birth, its duration, the role of pain in labour and complications such as cephalo-pelvic disproportion. As you work through this chapter, reflect on the 'facts', especially those taken for granted, by asking the kinds of questions posed by Walsh (2003):

▶ Whose purpose does knowledge serve?
▶ Where does knowledge come from?
▶ Who created it and why?
▶ Who benefits?
▶ How has knowledge of birth been influenced by a technological-mechanistic view of birth that is readily apparent in twenty-first century popular and medical culture?

at some time be confronted with complications in labour or deviations from a normal labour. The midwife must know how to recognise these variations and take appropriate action until they are resolved, or make a referral and transfer care to a specialist lead carer. Irrespective of the place of birth, the composition of the healthcare team or planned interventions, midwives always work in partnership with each woman to create a space for birth that is culturally, emotionally and physically safe (Powell-Kennedy & Shannon 2004).

Midwives who are evidence-informed and reflective practitioners often find that obstetric interventions such as the induction of labour, especially if there are no accepted medical indications for the procedure, pose ethical and professional dilemmas that need to be addressed. The benefits of a clearly defined midwifery philosophy (Clarke 2002) along with the relevant Standards for Practice and Codes of Ethics, enable midwives to determine their own boundaries in regards to decision-making about their participation in interventions in the labour and birth processes.

Rhythms of labour

Midwives' and women's perceptions of the expected length of labour have been seriously undermined by dominant medical hegemony (Bates 2004). This has culminated in the overuse of protocols such as the 'active management of labour'. According to Thornton (1996) there is scant evidence to support this practice but it is still used in many maternity units.

Understanding the physiology and the mechanisms or cardinal movements of labour, including how the shape of the maternal pelvis influences the passage of the fetus through the birth canal, aids recognition of deviations from the usual pattern and rhythm of labour.

In the late 1970s and early 1980s, two Irish clinicians, O'Driscoll and Meagher (1980), introduced to maternity units in Dublin a 'package' of care that they termed 'active management', which, they argued, resulted in a reduced incidence of prolonged labour and a caesarean section rate of less than 7%. The package included: antenatal education; one-to-one midwifery care; precise criteria for the diagnosis of the onset of labour; two-hourly timed vaginal examinations, and early use of high doses of Syntocinon that achieved a rate of cervical dilatation of at least 1 cm/hr. Across the world this model of care was welcomed and widely accepted. Even today, few randomised studies have evaluated the efficacy of 'the active management of labour package'. Frigoletto and colleagues (1995) found no significant differences between the 'active management' group and a 'usual-care' control group in the rate of caesarean section. However, the median duration of labour was shorter in the 'active management' group by 2.7 hours. Nevertheless, the authors concluded that there was no justification for the universal recommendation of 'active management of labour'. Moreover, beginning in the mid-1980s, research confirmed what midwives intuitively knew—that constant social support during labour is associated with shorter labours, higher rates of vaginal births, and a reduction in the amount of pharmaceutical analgesia used in labour (Klaus et al 1986; Hodnett 2003). In other words, the same outcomes may have been achieved by midwifery one-to-one support without the other arms of the 'package'.

Critical thinking exercise

The following list identifies the assessments a midwife makes and records in every labour:

▶ *fetal heart rate*—by intermittent auscultation, or continuous electronic fetal heart rate monitoring
▶ *cervicogram*—rate of cervical dilatation and descent of the fetus through the pelvis
▶ *uterine contractions*—quantification of frequency, duration and strength
▶ *amniotic fluid* (if the membranes have broken)—state of fluid; presence of meconium
▶ *maternal urine production*—assessed for the presence of ketones and protein
▶ *maternal adaptation to labour*—blood pressure, pulse rate and temperature
▶ *hydration and nutrition*—fluid and dietary intake and output
▶ *maternal wellbeing*—behaviour and response to labour, levels of fatigue, pain and coping ability
▶ *family support*—level, type and effect.

Using the above headings as a guide, determine how frequently various clinicians (medical practitioners, midwives working in the community, birth centres or in tertiary hospitals) assess these variables and the range they use to establish whether labour is progressing normally.

Slower than expected progress in labour and midwifery support

The first clinician to provide a definitive instrument for the assessment of individual labours was a US obstetrician, Emanuel Friedman (1954). It remains the standard for defining the normal progress of labour. Friedman's initial predictions about the normal progress of labour were based on the evaluation of the labour progress of 100 women. The rate of cervical dilatation was determined by frequent rectal examinations. No exclusions were made for malpresentations, malpositions or multiple pregnancies. Work by Albers (1999) and Zhang et al (2001) have challenged Friedman's work on the duration of labour. Friedman set the normal progress of labour as a cervical dilatation rate of 1.2 cm/hr for primigravidas and 1.5 cm/hr for multigravidas (Friedman 1954). He depicted labour as a sigmoid curve, with the first stage of labour divided two distinct phases: *latent* and *active* (Fig 34.1). The active stage begins at 3–4 cm of cervical dilatation and can be further subdivided into three sequential phases: acceleration, maximum slope and deceleration.

In an attempt to improve maternity services in Rhodesia, Philpott and Castle (1972) refined Friedman's work. They described the active phase of labour as progressing in a straight line and at a cervical dilatation rate of 1 cm/hr, with no distinction for parity. In an 'advance' of Friedman's

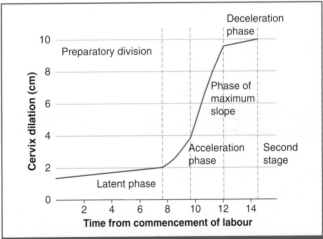

Figure 34.1 The Friedman curve (based on Friedman 1954)

work, they placed an alert line on the cervicograph (Fig 34.2). The alert line, unlike the sigmoid curve described by Friedman, was a straight line and calculated on a rate of cervical dilatation of 1 cm/hr irrespective of parity. A second parallel line, known as the action line, was later drawn on the cervicograph (partogram), four hours to the right of the alert line. The latter was an arbitrarily chosen time that was considered to allow sufficient time for a woman to be transferred from a local maternity unit in Rhodesia (now Zimbabwe) to a tertiary hospital in Harare (then Salisbury).

Cervicographs with warning and action lines are now in general use in many Western countries, and clinicians are expected to plot the rate of cervical dilatation and descent of the fetal head on a cervicograph, an important component of intrapartum assessment. Many clinicians intervene in labours as soon as they extend beyond predetermined intervals, even if there are no indications that maternal or fetal wellbeing is jeopardised.

The majority of trials testing the efficacy of the partogram have taken place in hospital settings. To date no trial has demonstrated that the partograph has lowered the rate of maternal mortality. Moreover, work by Albers et al (1996; Albers 1999) shows clearly that normal labour can and does last much longer than is commonly believed. These labours are not inevitably associated with increased morbidity in mothers or infants. Indeed, the complications often linked to prolonged labours may be caused as much by interventions (repeated vaginal examinations, augmentation of labour, epidural analgesia, operative delivery) than a lengthy labour itself.

Slow progress in the latent phase of labour

During the latent phase, the contractions become more regular and increase in intensity; there is slow but gradual cervical dilatation. Its precise duration is difficult to determine and probably the best option is to ask the woman when her labour began, and believe her. Women empowered to take control of their birth experience will alert the midwife of changes in their labour and are best placed to determine whether they are 'in' or 'not in' labour. Walsh (2003) makes the point that in a partnership of reciprocal respect and trust, women's fear of intervention during the usual ebb-and-flow patterns of labour can be minimised. According to current medical thinking, a prolonged latent phase of labour (from beginning of labour to the onset of active labour and cervical dilatation of 3–4 cm) is defined as one lasting more than 20 hours, with a mean of 8.6 hours.

Slow progress in this phase of labour is not necessarily indicative of dystocia or CPD. Further, active interventions to accelerate labour in the latent phase are not always associated with improvements in outcomes and may actually be harmful because of the increased risk of intrauterine infection and umbilical cord prolapse. The treatment of choice for a lengthy early labour is rest and sleep.

Slow progress in the active phase of labour

According to medical dictum, the active phase of labour is characterised by increasing frequency and intensity of contractions, progressive descent of the presenting part and dilatation of the cervix of 1 cm/hr. It covers the period from the end of the latent phase (3–4 cm of cervical dilatation) to complete dilatation of the cervix (10 cm of cervical dilatation). Figure 34.2 uses a partogram to plot the expected progress of labour and the typical pattern of prolonged labour based on Friedman's 'ideal' of normal labour. Alternatively, using Alber's work (1999) as a guide, the usual rate of cervical dilatation

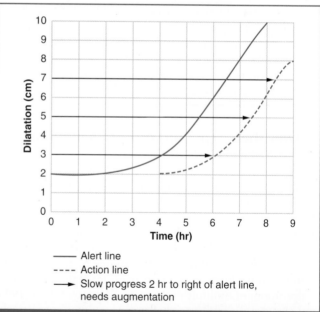

--- Alert line
---- Action line
→ Slow progress 2 hr to right of alert line, needs augmentation

Figure 34.2 Partogram plotting the alert and action lines (based on Stables & Rankin 2004)

Critical thinking exercise

Friedman described three stages in the active phase of labour: acceleration, maximal slope and deceleration. Make your own partogram and draw the typical curve. As you support women in labour, plot their labours on a 'personal' partogram. Later, reflect on how many 'normal' labours actually fitted this pattern but still had positive outcomes.

in this stage for nulliparas is 0.5 cm/hr in the absence of complicating factors, and the mean duration of active labour is 7.7 hours. For the duration of labour, the upper limit (mean + 2 standard deviations, i.e. the variance around the average) is 17.5 hours. In multiparas the mean duration is 5.6 hours and the upper duration 13.8 hours. Thus there are wide variations in the duration of women's labours, and these do not fit the expected Friedman pattern.

A misdiagnosis of slower than expected labour in the active phase can lead to unnecessary obstetric intervention, such as augmentation of labour using oxytocic drugs and artificial rupture of the membranes (ARM). Empowered, knowledgeable women will alert the midwife to an apparent slowing down in the pattern of contractions once labour has established. Non-invasive evaluation of contraction patterns occurs by gentle abdominal palpation, which tracks the descent of the fetus through the birth passage, and by careful assessment of the strength, regularity and duration of contractions. This assessment is subjective and should always be considered along with the patterns of the woman's behaviour and reactions to each contraction. Findings are confirmed by vaginal examination. A change in an established pattern of labour may indicate that there are potential complications that require investigation and possible intervention (Enkin et al 2000). The pattern of contractions can be altered by other factors including fear and anxiety. Transfer to hospital will often slow labour down. Similarly, labour often slows just before the second stage of labour begins, probably to give the mother a much needed rest before the work of second stage begins.

Although a longer than expected, albeit normal, duration of labour is not uncommon in primigravidas, there are other potentially problematic reasons for observed changes in contraction rhythms and these are now explored. They are:

- maternal dehydration or ketosis
- anxiety and fear
- ineffective pattern of contractions
- malposition (an occipitoposterior position)
- malpresentation
- cephalo-pelvic disproportion.

Maternal dehydration, ketosis and the progress of labour

Labour is hard work, and the body needs energy to work effectively. However, in industrialised countries, the effect of restricting fluids and food in labour is controversial. Restricting women's intake to fluids or ice chips during labour is a widely accepted obstetric tradition, which began about 50 years ago, when women frequently gave birth under general anaesthesia and were therefore at risk of aspiration pneumonia. However, modern anaesthesia techniques have improved, and in any case general anaesthesia is rare in modern obstetrics. Moreover, no period of fasting guarantees an empty stomach, and clear liquids leave the stomach almost immediately. Other clinicians have argued, with scant evidence to support this hypothesis, that fasting causes ketosis and dehydration, which leads to more painful contractions, slower labour and fatigue. Moreover, according to Enkin et al (2000), withholding food and drink from women in labour is unlikely to be beneficial. For these reasons, many healthcare providers no longer restrict eating and drinking during a normal labour.

Anxiety and fear

The relationships between continuous support in labour, fear, anxiety and the progress of labour are described elsewhere in this text. In brief, anxiety, excessive pain and fear are known to increase the amount of catecholamines ('fight-or-flight' hormones) released into the maternal circulation, and these influence the effectiveness of uterine contractions. For centuries, midwives and women have known that uncontrollable anxiety and fear increase the pain of labour and inhibit its progress. There is now qualitative and quantitative evidence to support this ancient knowledge. Moreover, we now know that women who feel in control of their bodies, their labour and what is happening to them are less likely to experience uncontrollable pain (Hunter 2002). Women who experienced sexual abuse in childhood or have had prior traumatic birth experiences, or have strong 'control' issues, may sometimes have difficulty surrendering to the power of their labour (Hofberg & Brockington 2000; Sjogren & Thomassen 1997). Indeed, maternal fear of childbirth is the most common reason for nulliparous women's request for caesarean delivery (Hildingson et al 2002). Women with extreme fear of labour (tocophobia) may develop post-traumatic stress disorder if they feel 'forced' to go through vaginal birth, but may benefit from counselling or psychiatric consultation (Hofberg & Brockington 2000).

Ineffective contraction patterns

Dystocia encompasses various complications in labour, the most common being incoordinate uterine contractions that result in an extremely painful and prolonged labour. Other contraction patterns include coordinate hypotonic and hypertonic uterine activity.

Incoordinate uterine action

Incoordinate uterine action is characterised by asynchronous, hypotonic or hypertonic uterine contractions, which, because they do not begin in the uterine fundus and do not pass in a wave downwards to the cervix, result in ineffective contractions. It is associated with frequent, painful contractions often combined with constant backache and pain that persists well after the contraction has finished. There is a loss of fundal polarity, and

---

> ### Clinical point
>
> Strategies to prevent, or support women in dealing with, anxiety and fear in labour are:
> - one-to-one midwifery care in which a trusting relationship has been established
> - eating and drinking to avoid fatigue and dehydration, which may slow labour
> - massage, acupressure and warm tub baths or showers to ease pain and induce relaxation, which may enhance progress
> - warm water immersion, which has been called the 'midwives' epidural'
> - talk, which provides comfort, reassurance and encouragement, and aims to relieve anxiety and explore the psychological or emotional issues or adverse environmental elements that might be causing the 'slow' labour.

---

in hypertonic incoordinate uterine action there is an increased uterine resting tone. Consequently, placental blood flow is reduced and fetal compromise may occur (Liu et al 2003). Two variations of hypertonic incoordinate uterine activity are the so-called 'colicky uterus' and 'constriction ring dystocia'. In the former, various parts of the uterus contract independently and this is combined with generalised and severe pain. An extreme form of incoordinate uterine action occurs with a localised spasm of one part of the uterus. However, constriction ring dystocia is rarely seen in developed countries. In association with ineffectual uterine contractions it occurs when an annular spasm arises at the junction between the upper and lower uterine segment, usually in late first stage or early in the second stage of labour. Unlike Bandl's pathological retraction ring, constriction rings are not associated with obstructed labour and cannot be palpated abdominally. Often, constriction rings arise from injudicious use of oxytocin or during intrauterine manipulation such as an internal podalic version. Relaxants including inhalation of amyl nitrate, or deep anaesthesia with a drug such as halothane, may eliminate the localised myometrial spasms, but as a last resort caesarean section with a vertical incision may be required.

Hypotonic uterine contractions

Ineffective contractions are commonly associated with a poorly fitting presenting part on the cervix. Hypotonic uterine action (contractions are short in duration and of weak intensity) result in a slower than expected rate of cervical dilatation and prolonged labour. The pattern may occur in early labour (primary) or later after a normal contraction pattern has been established (secondary). Typically this pattern is observed after the administration of epidural or narcotic analgesia but is frequently associated with some degree of cephalo-pelvic disproportion. There is also evidence that women are genetically predisposed to hypotonic uterine action (Dizon-Townson & Ward 1997). Once the presence of factors that preclude the use of oxytocics are eliminated, many clinicians advocate augmentation of labour with an artificial rupture of membranes (ARM) and Syntocinon infusion. However, studies of the effectiveness of amniotomy have not demonstrated that it significantly improves outcomes, although the duration of labour is shortened slightly.

Hypertonic uterine contractions

A precipitated labour is defined as one with total duration of less than two hours. For some women this may be their normal pattern, but the most common cause of hypertonic uterine action is the injudicious use of oxytocic drugs. Fetal welfare may be compromised when the intensity of uterine contractions is increased, resting intervals are shortened and duration of the contraction is increased. Hypertonic contractions may also cause maternal trauma—including uterine rupture or perineal damage. A combination of excessively forceful uterine contractions and minimal soft tissue resistance can give rise to precipitate labour, fetal anoxia and cerebral trauma, maternal lacerations, and postpartum haemorrhage caused by uterine atony. Early recognition of the problem, timely preparation for birth under controlled conditions, and properly administered analgesia or anaesthesia may minimise these risks.

Working with women experiencing ineffective contraction patterns

The woman and her support people should be active participants in all decision-making. Encouragement from the midwife and support persons in labour often improves outcomes in slower labours, reducing the need for augmentation of labour (Enkin et al 2000). A longer than expected labour can affect the woman's ability to cope, leading to an increased release of catecholamines (stress hormones), which cause the labour to slow down. The midwife will need to use all her skills in supporting women in a long labour, in particular taking care to avoid maternal dehydration and ketosis, which is best determined by measuring urine output and urinalysis. It is important to avoid a full bladder because this may inhibit descent of the presenting part in the pelvis and delay the second stage of labour. Regular assessment of and documenting maternal and fetal wellbeing as well as the progress of labour are useful to detect the onset of complications and guide the selection of strategies to treat them. According to Enkin et al (2000), research suggests that simple measures such as encouraging the woman to ambulate assists the birth process, as gravity facilitates the descent of the presenting part. Research by authors such as Cluett et al (2004) indicates that labouring in water may alleviate the effects of dystocia. Indeed, Enkin et al (2000) state that ambulation and ensuring women eat and drink as they wish may be as effective as augmentation of labour with oxytocin for a significant number of women. However, because of the hypothetical risk of aspiration of gastric contents during general anaesthesia, many hospitals have a policy of 'fluids only' in labour for *all* women. Indeed, restriction of all food in labour, ketosis and dehydration may exacerbate ineffective contraction patterns and dysfunctional labour (Newton & Raynor 2000). Moreover, fasting, enforced bed rest, intravenous therapy and continuous electronic fetal monitoring imply notions of loss of control, sickness and helplessness, which may also interfere with the progress of labour and necessitate intervention such as augmentation of labour, epidural analgesia and operative delivery (Broach & Newton 1988).

Women experiencing ineffective contraction patterns and prolonged labour are more at risk of postpartum haemorrhage (PPH). Therefore, a discussion of the management of the third stage of labour should occur early enough for the woman to be able to make informed decisions about the need for an active management of the third stage of labour.

Collaborative interventions

The primary goal of all clinicians working with women as they labour is to provide the safest outcome for both mother and infant. It is crucial that midwives have the skills and knowledge required to detect labour and contraction patterns that pose risks for the mother and fetus. Once dystocia is recognised, it is important to identify its cause and, if possible, correct it

> ### Reflective exercise
>
> How will you, as the midwife, support a woman's choice to refuse medical advice that she have her labour augmented or other interventions such as an operative delivery?

or minimise the harmful effects it may have on the mother and her baby and treat the causes of the dystocia. Frequently this can be relieved by simple measures such as alleviating intolerable pain or fear. In most cases this will include transferring primary care to a multidisciplinary team. The lead midwife should avail herself of support from her back-up midwife in primary settings or support from the midwifery staff in secondary/tertiary hospitals so that the lead carer can take regular breaks and have adequate rest while continuing to provide continuity of care in partnership with the woman (NZCOM 2005).

Augmentation of labour with an amniotomy (ARM)

There is no need to artificially rupture membranes with an amniotomy if labour progresses normally. Nevertheless, early amniotomy has been advocated as a component of the active management of labour, especially if there is slower than expected progress in the active phase of labour (Fraser et al 1999). It is often used to accelerate the progress of labour by increasing the frequency and quality of contractions, and performed prior to inducing or augmenting the labour. It may also be performed to obtain access to the fetus for a scalp pH assessment, to attach a fetal scalp electrode or to assess the liquor.

An ARM requires the woman's consent. According to a Cochrane Review (Fraser et al 2000), amniotomy is associated with risks as well as benefits and should only be performed in the presence of abnormal labour progress. Benefits include a reduction in labour duration and a possible reduction in abnormal five-minute Apgar scores. The reviewers (Fraser et al 1999) found no support for the hypothesis that routine early amniotomy reduces the risk of caesarean delivery. Indeed, there was a trend (non-significant) toward an increase in caesarean section. An association between early amniotomy and caesarean delivery for fetal distress was observed in one large trial. As soon as the membranes are ruptured there is an increased risk of umbilical cord prolapse, fetal compromise and chorioamnionitis. Once an ARM has been performed, birth should occur within 24 hours. Many Australian clinicians now advocate the administration of intravenous antibiotics if the membranes are ruptured for more than 12 hours; this is not yet common practice in New Zealand hospitals. Nevertheless, if the baby is at risk of infection from Group B Streptococcus (NZCOM 2004), intravenous antibiotics are recommended after rupture of membranes for more than 18 hours.

The amniotic sac and its liquor protect the fetal head; once the membranes break, this effect is removed. Compression of the fetal head leads to increased moulding and changes in the fetal heart rate—variable decelerations are often apparent on the electronic fetal heart rate trace because the fetal head is no longer cushioned by the amniotic fluid. Below are listed some of the potential consequences of an amniotomy that may require emergency intervention:

- maternal risk factors:
  - prolapse of the umbilical cord
  - chorioamnionitis
  - sepsis
  - significant umbilical cord compression
  - rupture of a vasa previa
- fetal risk factors:
  - preterm birth
  - infection
  - cord prolapse
  - malpresentation.

Indications for amniotomy

- to augment or stimulate labour
- to look for the presence of meconium in the liquor
- placement of a fetal spiral electrode (Boston 2004).

Contraindications for amniotomy

- presentation unknown or unstable
- cervix dilated less than 3 cm
- fetal head not engaged
- non-vertex position of the fetal head
- woman refuses the procedure
- HIV-positive
- active genital herpes simplex virus.

Clinical point

Before performing an ARM, the midwife:

▶ ensures the woman has consented to the procedure

▶ ensures that there is indication for the intervention and no contraindications

▶ performs an abdominal palpation and vaginal examination to determine the stage of labour, presentation, position, cervical dilatation and position of the fetal head relative to the ischial spines

▶ during a vaginal examination, assesses the progress of labour by cervical dilatation. Unless the fetal head is well engaged in the pelvis, ARM is not advocated.

▶ introduces the amniohook through the cervix and makes a small tear in the membranes lying in front of the fetal head

After the procedure, the midwife:

▶ checks and records the colour, odour and quantity of the liquor and the fetal heart rate

▶ ensures that the woman is dry and comfortable, and informs her of findings.

Critical thinking exercise

You are the midwife for Maria, a primigravida who has been in labour for 15 hours. Maria's mother Henrietta asks you to 'break the waters—my midwife broke mine'. What will you say and do?

BOX 34.2 ARM terminology

ARM = amniotomy or artificial rupture of membranes
SROM = spontaneous rupture of membranes
PROM = prelabour or premature rupture of membranes
PPROM = preterm, prelabour rupture of membranes

Augmentation of labour with Syntocinon

Before intravenous oxytocics are administered, cephalo-pelvic disproportion needs to be excluded by careful abdominal palpation and vaginal examination. The most frequent complications of oxytocin-augmented labours are uterine hyperstimulation causing excessive maternal pain, fetal compromise, cord compression and, more rarely, uterine rupture. Consequently, most hospitals have a policy of continuous electronic fetal monitoring once augmentation or induction of labour with oxytocin begins. After birth, PPH from uterine atony is a significant risk.

Malposition

There is only one malposition—an occipitoposterior (OP) position of the fetus (Fig 34.3). In about 10% to 25% of pregnancies, the fetal head enters the maternal pelvis with the occiput lying in the posterior segments of the pelvis. In most cases the architecture of the pelvis is normal, but in others the pelvic diameters may be reduced. OP positions are more common in the presence of long, narrow pelvic walls (oval-shaped pelvis) or with convergent pelvic side walls and prominent ischial spines. For the baby lying in a right occipitoposterior (ROP) position to rotate to a right occipitoanterior (ROA), the head must rotate 135° from an ROP to a right occipitolateral (ROL), to ROA and then, as the head begins to birth, a direct OA (DOA). Thus, prolonged labour is a frequent complication associated with an OP position. In more than two-thirds of cases, the fetal head achieves this rotation. However, in about 15% of cases the fetal attitude is one of deflexion, and the sinciput becomes the denominator. If this happens, the sinciput, not the occiput, rotates to the front of the pelvis so that the fetal head completes a short rotation of 45° and the head is born 'face-to-pubes'. With a deflexed fetal head, the presenting diameter is 12.5 cm—much larger than the 9.5 cm of the suboccipitobregmatic diameter of the well-flexed head, and so as the head births there is a much higher chance of perineal lacerations. In 20% of cases the fetal head attempts the 'long rotation' but

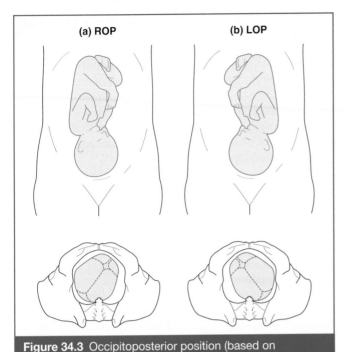

Figure 34.3 Occipitoposterior position (based on Henderson & Macdonald 2004)

arrests at the level of the ischial spines—known as deep transverse arrest.

Working with a woman experiencing an OP labour

The woman usually experiences a long, discouraging and trying labour with intense pain in the small of her back. Others will have an uncontrollable urge to push before the cervix is completely dilated. Many require pharmaceutical analgesia, including epidurals, to cope with intolerable pain and exhaustion. However, encouraging the woman to ambulate, assume positions such as the all-fours position and squatting in the first and second stage, as well as offering massage or labouring in water helps the pain and may aid the fetus to rotate anteriorly. Although there is no evidence that assuming an all-fours position and pelvic rocking (Kariminia et al 2004) achieves fetal rotation in the last weeks of pregnancy, anecdotal evidence indicates that once they are in labour many women find this activity and positioning more comfortable than assuming a supine or semi-recumbent position in bed.

Diagnosis

On abdominal palpation, the fetal back is often felt on the mother's flanks, there is a sensation of 'limbs everywhere', and the fetal head (Fig 34.3) is deflexed and slow to engage in the pelvis. A saucer-shaped depression is often seen at or just below the umbilicus because the shoulder is lying posteriorly. On vaginal examination, the anterior fontanelle can be felt in the anterior quadrant of the mother's pelvis and the posterior fontanelle at the back. Deep transverse arrest must always be considered if, during second stage on vaginal examination:

- the sagittal suture remains in the transverse diameter of the pelvis
- in a primigravida the uterine contractions become hypotonic
- there is increasing and extensive moulding of the fetal head
- there is increasing caput succedaneum
- the fetal head does not descend past the ischial spines.

It is possible to manually rotate the fetal head to an OA position once the cervix is completely dilated. As in all instances of dystocia with an OP position there is a higher incidence of early rupture of membranes, chorioamnionitis, fetal infection, fetal compromise and asphyxia. Infection occurs because the membranes are ruptured for a longer period of time and from multiple vaginal examinations. Operative intervention—episiotomy, ventouse, forceps or caesarean section—is more common in OP positions. Operative delivery carries with it the inherent risks of major surgery: infection, haemorrhage, wound infection, urinary retention and infection, pulmonary embolism and anaesthesia-related complications.

Malpresentations

Malpresentations are defined in the tenth edition of *Baillière's Midwives' Dictionary* (Tiran 2003) as 'any presentation of the fetus other than vertex. It may be a breech, face, brow, or shoulder presentation'. Many medical texts assert that failure to recognise malpresentations and manage them appropriately—that is, with immediate medical intervention—often leads to catastrophic complications, including uterine rupture, obstructed labour, and maternal and fetal death. Such language sets 'high-risk' alarm bells ringing. All midwives must be competent to recognise and deal with emergencies as they arise (Midwifery Council of New Zealand 2004). Operative intervention is not always the best way to deal with malpresentations, and skilled practitioners can often achieve good outcomes with a less interventionist approach. However, in an era of 'defensive medicine' this mode of care is becoming increasingly difficult to support because of the pressure to resort to immediate obstetric intervention as the first line of management.

A good example of how some research fails to support a non-interventionist model of care is the Canadian Term Breech Trial. Since its publication (Hannah et al 2000), debate has raged about how best to safely birth a baby presenting by the breech. Despite its findings and recommendations, a few clinicians still argue that the recommended practice of delivering breech babies by elective caesarean section has more to do with clinicians' personal fears and prejudices, often caused by lack of personal experience and competence, conflicting research evidence, policies and guidelines for both midwives and women, than evidence (Crabtree 2004; Hall & Taylor 2004). Nevertheless, the Term Breech Trial (TBT), a large multi-centre randomised controlled trial (Hannah et al 2000), supports earlier and well-substantiated findings that all babies presenting by the breech, regardless of the mode of birth, are significantly more at risk of perinatal mortality and morbidity even if these babies are at term and have no congenital anomalies. Secondly, during the TBT, which involved 2088 women with a singleton fetus in a breech presentation at term where women were allocated to either planned caesarean or a planned vaginal birth group, the authors discovered that the risk of perinatal or neonatal death or serious neonatal morbidity was significantly lower in the planned caesarean group, without a significant increase in the risk of maternal death or serious maternal morbidity (Hannah et al 2000). There have been several published critiques of the trial, for example by Halmesmäki (2001), which have argued that factors other than the mode of delivery confounded the findings. There is no doubt, however, that since the publication of the results of the TBT, at least in industrialised countries, few babies presenting by the breech are born vaginally. This means that midwifery and medical practitioners do not have the opportunity to birth breech babies, yet some women still want vaginal breech births. Despite modern technology some breech babies are undiagnosed and if women labour quickly, clinicians have little option but to assist in the vaginal birth of a breech baby.

The New Zealand Guidelines Group (October 2004), a multidisciplinary team, has produced clinical guidelines for clinicians that, while recognising the potential complications of vaginal breech birth in terms of fetal mortality and morbidity, recommends that women be given evidence-based information about the risks and benefits of both vaginal breech birth and caesarean section *prior to* (our emphasis) birth so that they can make informed decisions and choices about their care. This gives rise to the debate over what actually constitutes the provision of informed choice and the use of evidence-based information. As research by Stapleton et al (2004) into the culture of informed choice demonstrated, fear of litigation was a major factor influencing the way in which choices were presented to or withheld from women. Such fears prevent the development of a trusting relationship between the woman and her midwife.

The New Zealand Guidelines group authors stress that maintaining skills for facilitating vaginal breech birth remains important for all clinicians. While these guidelines have been developed specifically for the care of women undergoing a breech birth, they hold true for all women with a malpresentation, or indeed any complication in labour.

Breech presentation

Midwives sharing practice stories will often relate tales of how they diagnosed breech babies in labour and that these women went on to have successful uncomplicated vaginal births. Others talk about the detrimental effects of obstetric interventions such as epidurals, unnecessary ARM or making women birth in bed in the lithotomy position. Anecdotes from midwives experienced in vaginal breech birth show how they defend maternal choice for a standing vaginal breech birth, and how they coped with coercive behaviour from midwife colleagues and obstetricians who insist on a caesarean delivery rather than adopting a watching, observing and supportive approach to breech birthing.

Authors such as Crabtree (2004) maintain that women with a breech baby are now opting to birth at home or arrive in advanced labour at the hospital to avoid an operative delivery. As this chapter has already pointed out, babies presenting by the breech are at greater risk of complications than babies presenting by the vertex (Hofmeyr & Hannah 2002). Consequently, most hospitals bound by strict protocols and guidelines (Stapleton et al 2004) insist that all babies presenting as a breech be delivered by caesarean.

In most developed countries, less than 1% of all breech babies are born vaginally. Emphasis is now being placed on testing the efficacy of external cephalic version (ECV) in late pregnancy to reduce the incidence of breech presentation at the onset of labour (Hofmeyr 2002; Hofmeyr & Hannah 2002; New Zealand Guidelines Group 2004).

Sometimes a breech presentation is diagnosed late in labour. The lead midwife who finds a breech presentation should inform the woman of her findings and, as far as possible given the stage of labour, provide an evidence-informed, objective description of all possible outcomes, and follow guidelines/protocols concerned with consultation and referral. A breech presentation in labour presents a challenge for all midwives, especially those unfamiliar with vaginal breech birth. An emergency vaginal breech birth should not result from lack of care or expertise in diagnosis of the presentation in pregnancy and in labour.

Diagnosis

In late pregnancy or during labour, the breech baby may often be well 'engaged' in the pelvis and the fetal head positioned 'under the diaphragm' so that it is very difficult to identify on abdominal palpation. Real-time ultrasonography confirms the diagnosis and rules out hyper-extension of the head, hydrocephalus or footling or kneeling breech, all of which pose unacceptably high risks for a vaginal breech birth.

Types of breech presentation

There are three types of breech: legs extended at the knee (frank), 65%; both legs flexed at the hips and knees (complete), 10%; and a single or double footling breech—one or both feet are tucked underneath the buttocks, 25% (Fig 34.4).

Mechanisms of labour

The mechanisms of a right sacroanterior (RSA) position are as follows:

- The lie is longitudinal.
- The attitude is complete flexion.
- The presentation is breech.
- The position is RSA.
- The denominator is the sacrum.
- The presenting part is the right buttock.
- The bitrochanteric diameter of 10 cm enters the pelvis in the right oblique diameter of the pelvic brim.
- The sacrum points to the right iliopectineal eminence.

Descent occurs with increasing impaction of the buttocks. The right buttock reaches the pelvic floor and rotates forward into the pelvis one-eighth of a circle; internal rotation of

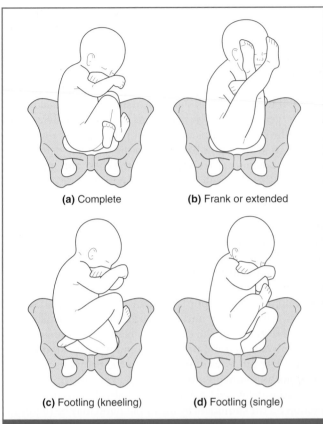

(a) Complete

(b) Frank or extended

(c) Footling (kneeling)

(d) Footling (single)

Figure 34.4 Breech presentations (based on Henderson & Macdonald 2004)

the buttocks occurs. The leading buttock escapes under the symphysis pubis; the posterior buttock sweeps the perineum and the buttocks are born by lateral flexion. Restitution of the buttocks now takes place. The anterior shoulder enters the pelvis in the same oblique diameter as the buttocks and rotates forwards one-eighth of a circle, escaping under the symphysis pubis. The posterior shoulder now sweeps the perineum and the shoulders are born. The head enters the pelvic brim in the transverse diameter; the occiput rotates forwards along the right side of the pelvis; at the same time external rotation of the body occurs so the back remains uppermost. The chin, face and sinciput sweep the perineum and the head is born in a flexed attitude.

Birthing a breech baby

Breech presentation is the most common malpresentation, occurring in about 4% of all births. The incidence is directly related to the gestational age of the fetus. Prematurity is the most common cause of breech presentation. At about 25 weeks gestation, more than 25% of babies present by the breech. By 34 weeks the incidence has decreased to 6% and by term to 3%. Other causes include: chance, parity, multiple births, uterine anomalies, placenta praevia; fetal anomalies (polyhydramnios, hydrocephalus, fetal neuromuscular disorders, macrosomia). The main causes of perinatal morbidity and mortality are: cord prolapse, intracranial

haemorrhage, low Apgar scores, asphyxia, cervical spine injury, fractures of the long bones (humerus and femur), and fracture of the clavicle. Of note is that in the seventh *CESDI Report* (CESDI 2000), the single most important and avoidable factor in causing stillbirth and death in breech births was suboptimal care in labour. While it is true that a few babies presenting by the breech are born at home, it is generally accepted that because a breech is a malpresentation and therefore birthing a breech baby is outside the scope of midwifery practice except in an emergency situation, all babies diagnosed as a breech should be referred to a medical consultant for collaborative care in a hospital with facilities for caesarean section and ready access to a team of midwives, obstetrician, paediatrician and anaesthetist.

According to Varney (2004), before birthing a breech baby vaginally, nine criteria should be met:

- careful abdominal examination or sonography to rule out hyperextension of the fetal head, hydrocephalus or a footling breech
- complete cervical dilatation
- elimination of any doubts about the adequacy of the size of the pelvis
- emptying of the bladder
- consideration of whether or not to cut an episiotomy
- determination of effective pushing efforts
- preparation in place for a full-scale newborn resuscitation
- positioning of the woman so that there is plenty of room for lateral flexion and downward traction of the body, shoulders and finally the head
- consultation with an obstetrician, who should either be present or immediately available.

Labour and breech birth

Vaginal examination must be performed when a breech presentation is suspected, not only to establish that labour has commenced but to exclude a cord presentation, cord prolapse once the membranes rupture, as well as a foot, knee or compound presentation. When labour is well established, asking the woman to remain upright and mobile will greatly aid descent of the buttocks and dilatation of the cervix. Midwifery support and care during labour is no different from that for a cephalic presentation. Intermittent fetal monitoring is important and usually adequate, although many hospital institutions have protocols in place for continuous fetal monitoring. The membranes should be left intact; if they spontaneously rupture, then meconium is often seen and should not be considered a sign of fetal distress but a positive sign of descent of the buttocks. A vaginal examination is recommended before maternal pushing commences, as the buttocks may descend without the cervix being completely dilated, especially if the baby is small. Banks (1998), a midwife experienced in breech births, writes that 'the premature urge to push before full dilatation that is often mentioned to women as being problematic in breech births is unlikely to be noticeable in a term infant who will have a hip size in a flexed or extended legs position equal to head size' (p 70).

An upright position will aid descent of the baby once pushing begins in second stage but this should not commence until the buttocks distend the vulva. At this time the membranes should be ruptured if this has not already occurred, to reduce contact of meconium with the baby's after-coming head. As the buttocks are born it is possible to see the buttocks move 'up and down' just before crowning—this is known as 'rumping'.

Physiological birth of a breech baby

The midwifery adage, 'hands off the breech' and 'keep the back uppermost', holds true today. This is easier to achieve if the woman is in an upright position. If the baby's legs are extended they will not be released until the chest is born. Watchful patience will usually see the extended legs birth on their own but the midwife can bring the leg down if necessary by placing a thumb on the popliteal fossa with two fingers of the same hand over the baby's shin to bring down the leg. When the baby's head enters the pelvis, the fetal heart rate may drop as the umbilical cord is compressed between the mother's bony pelvis and the baby's head. Once this happens the baby needs to be birthed within six minutes and continuous pushing may be required to facilitate a timely birth. As the cord is now visible, the baby's heart rate can be checked by gently feeling its pulsations or the chest felt once that appears. The baby's head should be born slowly to avoid a tentorial tear. Wrapping a warm towel around the baby's bottom and gently supporting the body helps to stop the head from extending. Once the nape of the baby's neck is visible, the woman is asked to lean forward from the waist and this tilts her pelvis to aid clearance of the baby's nose and mouth from the perineum while the rest of the head is born slowly.

Various techniques can be used to deal with assisting the breech baby birth should this be necessary. These are rarely required if the woman maintains an upright standing or squatting position with patient birth supporters. Practising these manoeuvres using a doll and pelvis or mannequin can reduce fear of having to perform them in an emergency. For example, a flexed fetal arm can be bought down across the chest by use of the index and middle fingers splinting the baby's arm and bringing the arm down across its face 'like a cat washing its face' Banks (1998, p 88).

Delivering the after-coming head of a breech baby

Most vaginal birth breech babies born in hospital take place with the mother lying in a semi-recumbent position, often with an epidural in situ. According to the Canadian Consensus Statement (Society of Obstetricians and Gynaecologists of Canada (SOGC) 1994), there is no evidence that epidural analgesia is an essential component of vaginal breech birth. Induction or augmentation of labour are also justified (SOGC 1994). However, because of the increased risk of prolapsed umbilical cord if the membranes rupture and the presenting part does not fit snugly in the pelvis, so that the cord prolapses, hospital protocols often state that the woman should be encouraged to remain in bed, frequently with an electronic fetal monitor attached to her body. Similarly,

because of the increased risks associated with breech births, the woman is often fasted and prepared for an immediate operative delivery.

As the baby begins to birth, it is crucial not to apply traction on the baby because this may deflex or extend the head, causing entrapment. The baby is allowed to 'hang'—hands off the breech! If the baby's back starts to rotate so that it is facing up, it can be gently rotated by two hands around the pelvic girdle so that the back remains uppermost (Fig 34.5). At this point the baby is again left to hang. When the scapulae deliver, the arms can be optionally swept across the chest and out of the birth canal, or they will birth spontaneously.

Mauriceau-Smellie-Veit

Delivery of the head should be by flexion, which ensures the same favourable diameters to delivery as with a cephalic presentation. A modified Mauriceau-Smellie-Veit (MSV, Fig 34.6) manoeuvre is used to flex the head. It is best to do this from a position below the baby, probably kneeling. One hand and forearm supports the baby's body, which straddles the arm, with the ring and index finger on the maxillae, the middle finger under the chin (not the mouth). An assistant may apply suprapubic pressure to maintain flexion of the occiput. The other hand is placed on the baby's back with a finger pushing down on the occiput to keep the head flexed. The head is delivered by drawing the baby downwards. Some traction on the shoulders by the upper hand may be required. As the head is delivered very slowly, the baby's body is kept in a neutral position in respect to the head and then gently raised in a large arc so that the child rests on the mother's abdomen.

Lovset manoeuvre

The Lovset manoeuvre (Fig 34.7) is particularly useful in the delivery of shoulders when the arms are extended, or in the presence of a nuchal arm. It involves a series of rotations combined with downward traction. Lateral flexion of the fetus is exaggerated to enable descent of the posterior shoulder below the sacral promontory. The midwife or obstetrician rotates the body 180°, always keeping the back uppermost—the posterior shoulder rotates anteriorly, and then lies beneath the symphysis pubis. The midwife then

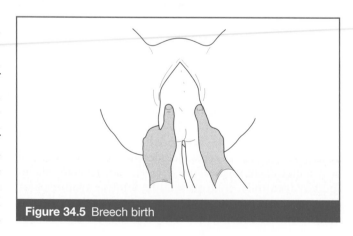

Figure 34.5 Breech birth

brings the arm downwards, then rotates the body back 180° in the opposite direction to deliver the second shoulder anteriorly once it too rotates to below the symphysis pubis. The other arm can now be delivered in the same way.

Complications of a breech birth

Complications of a breech birth are identified as cord prolapse, premature separation of the placenta, fetal hypoxia and an impacted breech when the baby is too large for the pelvis (Coates 2004). The breech baby is at risk of complications from mismanagement by the operator, such as Erb's palsy from damage to the brachial plexus when the neck is twisted, fractures of the clavicle, humerus or femur, or dislocation of hips or shoulders. Internal trauma can occur to the adrenal glands or rupture of the spleen or liver, again by grasping the baby's abdomen tightly. Some degree of bruising is to be expected, especially of the male genitalia, and so the parents should be reassured about this before the birth.

External cephalic version

Version or turning of the breech is a technique used to change a fetal presentation by abdominal or intrauterine manipulation. The latter, usually an 'internal podalic version', is rarely performed. It is used to convert the second twin from a transverse lie to a cephalic or breech presentation. In contrast, the procedure of external cephalic version (ECV) is becoming increasingly common. This section focuses on the use of ECV to turn a breech presentation to cephalic. Spontaneous version of a breech presentation occurs in about 20% of cases. In the remainder, an ECV is a useful technique to 'turn a breech', and has been practised since the time of Hippocrates. The efficacy of ECV has been rigorously appraised in six randomised controlled trials. There is a significant reduction in caesarean section in women where there is an intention to undertake ECV (Hofmeyr and Kulier 2000). Consequently, it is recommended that all women with an uncomplicated breech presentation be offered an ECV between 37 and 42 weeks of pregnancy (New

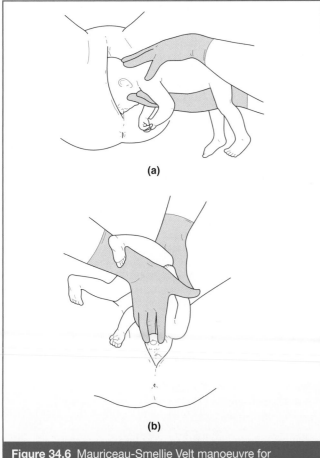

Figure 34.6 Mauriceau-Smellie Velt manoeuvre for delivering the after-coming head of breech presentation **(a)** The hands are in position before the body is lifted. **(b)** Extraction of the head

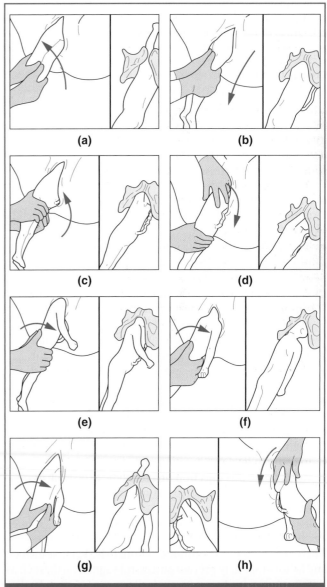

Figure 34.7 Lovset manoeuvre for delivery of extended arms (based on Fraser & Cooper 2003)

Zealand Guidelines Group 2004). Most versions are performed at about 37 weeks because at this stage most babies still in a breech position will not spontaneously revert to a cephalic presentation. In addition, if complications occur as a result of the ECV, the risk of preterm birth is eliminated.

Factors associated with a successful ECV

ECV is best carried out with the woman awake and facilities for emergency caesarean birth nearby. Lau and colleagues (1997) list nine factors that are good predictors of successful ECV:

- multiparity
- maternal weight
- placental site
- type of breech or presentation
- position of fetal spine
- adequate amniotic fluid volume
- engagement
- station of the breech at the pelvic brim
- estimated fetal weight.

Criteria for ECV

According to Hofmeyr and Kulier (2000), before an ECV is attempted, the following criteria should be met:

- The fetus must be a singleton.
- The breech must not be engaged.
- There must be adequate amniotic liquor.
- A reactive non-stress test (NST) should be obtained prior to the procedure.
- The fetus must be 36–37 weeks or more gestation.

Other authors such as Edelestone (2000) make the following recommendations:

- The woman should give informed consent for the procedure. She should be informed of the benefits and risks of ECV—failed version, reversion (2%), fetal stress related to cord entanglement or abruption, ruptured uterus and abruptio and unexplained fetal death. Benefits of a successful ECV (more than 50%) include decreased caesarean section rate. The woman and her support people also need information about alternatives to an ECV—postural exercises, moxibustion, visualisation.
- The ECV should only be performed in a maternity unit that can proceed to an immediate caesarean section.
- A real-time ultrasound should be performed prior to beginning the procedure to rule out placenta praevia and to confirm fetal presentation and position.
- A subcutaneous injection of a tocolytic drug such as terbutaline is administered to achieve uterine relaxation.

Contraindications for ECV

There are few absolute contraindications to ECV. These include any factors that may prevent successful vaginal birth, such as IUGR, multiple gestation, previous caesarean section, fetal or maternal compromise, placenta praevia and oligohydramnios and, of course, maternal refusal.

ECV procedure

The woman is admitted to a day-only unit or delivery suite in case an immediate caesarean section is necessary. Before the procedure begins, the obstetrician checks that the woman has given consent for the version and demonstrates that she understands the risks and benefits of the version and has all her questions answered. An ultrasound confirms that the baby is still in a breech position and that there is no evidence of congenital anomalies that preclude vaginal birth. An NST is performed for 20 minutes or until it is reactive. Maternal and fetal vital signs are recorded and documented. A tocolytic is sometimes administered according to the unit's protocols. The woman is placed in a supine position (with a wedge under her buttocks). Once she is relaxed, the obstetrician gently turns the baby by pushing the presenting part upwards, and the fetal head is pushed in the opposite direction towards the pelvis. This procedure should not be painful. After the version has been completed the CTG is reconnected and the FHR observed for signs of fetal compromise. If the woman is Rh-negative she will require one dose of immunoglobulin. Before she goes home, the woman should be asked to contact her lead

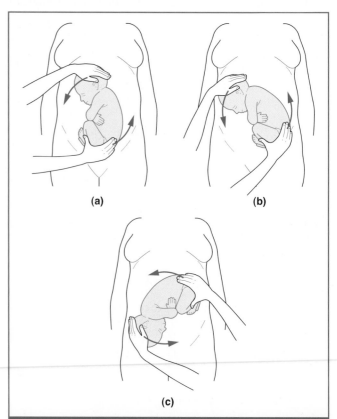

(a)   **(b)**

(c)

Figure 34.8 External cephalic version **(a)** The right hand lifts the breech out of the pelvis. The left hand makes the head follow the nose. Flexion of head and back is maintained throughout. **(b)** Flexion is continued. The left hand brings the head downwards. The right hand pushes the breech upwards. **(c)** Pressure is exerted on head and breech simultaneously until the head is lying at the pelvic brim (based on Fraser & Cooper 2003).

Recommended readings

▶ Articles on breech birth, evaluation of the term breech trial, http://www.birthspirit.co.nz/
▶ Assisted breech birth pictures, http://www.birthdiaries.com/diary/47vbirth.htm
▶ Midwives' tales of breech births, http://www.radmid.demon.co.uk/breech.htm

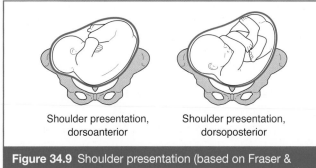

Shoulder presentation, dorsoanterior   Shoulder presentation, dorsoposterior

Figure 34.9 Shoulder presentation (based on Fraser & Cooper 2003)

carer if there are signs of vaginal bleeding, if the membranes rupture, contractions begin or if she is worried about her own or the baby's wellbeing. Women are sometimes asked to complete a kick chart for 24 hours after the version. If the ECV is unsuccessful or if the fetus reverts to a breech, the version may be repeated in one week.

Alternative techniques to reduce the incidence of breech presentation

There is no evidence that postural management—'breech exercises'—are effective in converting a breech into a cephalic presentation (Hofmeyr & Kulier 2000). Similarly, although there is anecdotal evidence that moxibustion is effective in converting a breech into a cephalic presentation, there is as yet no firm evidence to support its use. On the other hand, there is no evidence that moxibustion is harmful. Moxibustion involves the application of a heated mixture made from the dried leaves of a herb, mugwort (*Artemis vulgaris*), directly to the designated meridian point (BL67), located beside the outer corner of the fifth toenail. Treatment may take from two to seven weeks. Alternatively, the heat from a burning moxa stick is used to warm acupuncture needles that have already been inserted in the appropriate meridian point. The heat and aroma of the mugwort is believed to stimulate the meridian point, so that energy moves through it, increasing fetal activity and encouraging the fetus to move to a cephalic presentation.

Shoulder presentation

This rare complication is associated with a transverse or oblique lie, where the long axis of the fetus lies transversely across the long axis of the mother's uterus (Fig 34.9). Causative factors include placenta praevia, fetal anomaly, lax multiparous uterus, polyhydramnios and uterine malformation. An abdominal palpation will reveal that the presenting part is the shoulder (in a compound presentation, the shoulder is presenting but a hand extends down into the vagina). The firm, ballottable fetal head is found near one iliac fossa and a softer mass on the other. It is important not to perform a vaginal examination until placenta previa has been excluded as the cause of the shoulder presentation. It is not possible to deliver a baby presenting by the shoulder vaginally and so the lead carer needs to inform the woman and her support persons of the diagnosis and, if necessary, arrange a referral for transfer to hospital for collaborative care.

An experienced obstetrician may choose to perform a cephalic version so that the fetal head lies over the pelvis, sometimes followed by an induction of labour with Syntocinon and an ARM. The fetal head is then pressed down into the pelvis as the liquor escapes. If the woman has commenced labour before the version can take place, an immediate emergency caesarean section is indicated.

Face and brow presentations

Face presentation

A face (mentum) presentation is also rare, occurring once in every 500 births (Parker & Napolitano 2005). The fetal head is in an attitude of extension rather than flexion; the denominator is the mentum (Fig 34.10). If the chin (mentum) is lying in the anterior quadrant of the pelvis (left mentoanterior (LMA) or right mentoanterior (RMA)), labour usually proceeds as with a normal vertex labour and vaginal birth is possible. This is because the widest diameter of the presenting part, the face, is similar (submental bregmatic, 9.5 cm) to the presenting diameter of an OA position (suboccipitobregmatic, 9.5 cm) and the neck easily glides around the symphysis pubis. A face presentation is rarely diagnosed before labour begins. Babies lying in a mentum posterior position, unless they rotate anteriorly, rarely achieve spontaneous vaginal birth because the chin wedges on the anterior surface of the sacrum. If the posterior position persists, an emergency caesarean section is necessary.

It is not possible to detect a face presentation by abdominal palpation but a vaginal examination will reveal the contours of the face, and often a mouth will suck incoming fingers. The midwife should be careful to lessen risks of facial and eye bruising during the examination and to take care that she excludes a breech presentation, because a soft breech and a face can often be confused.

Clinical point

On vaginal examination how would a midwife differentiate between a face and a frank breech presentation?

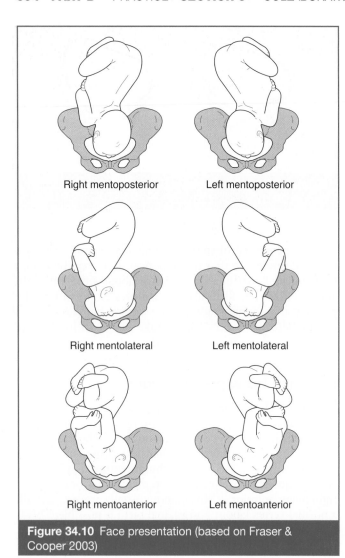

Right mentoposterior   Left mentoposterior

Right mentolateral   Left mentolateral

Right mentoanterior   Left mentoanterior

Figure 34.10 Face presentation (based on Fraser & Cooper 2003)

Understanding the 'mechanisms' of labour will help both midwife and mother deal with a face presentation.

The mechanism of labour for an RMA position is as follows:

● The lie is longitudinal.
● The attitude is one of extension of the head and back.
● The presentation is face.
● The position is right mentoanterior.
● The denominator is the mentum.

Descent occurs with increasing extension and the mentum becomes the leading part. Internal rotation of the head occurs as the chin meets the pelvic floor and rotates forward one-eighth of a circle, escaping under the symphysis pubis. Flexion occurs and the sinciput, vertex and occiput sweep the perineum and the head is born. Restitution takes place and the baby's chin faces the mother's right side. Internal rotation of the shoulders occurs as they enter the pelvis in the right oblique diameter; the anterior shoulder touches the pelvic floor and it too rotates forwards one-eighth of a circle along the left side of the pelvis. External rotation of the head

MIDWIFE'S STORY

I was supporting a woman in spontaneous labour with her third baby; labour was progressing well and abdominal palpation indicated a longitudinal lie and cephalic presentation. The baby's head was engaged and after the membranes ruptured physiologically and at the mother's request, I performed a vaginal examination to exclude a cord prolapse and to assess progress of labour. I had already examined her in early labour at home, again at her request, as she had been having the typical 'stop-start' labour with third babies so I knew it was a cephalic presentation. I had felt the bony head, and knew it was poorly applied to the 3 cm dilated cervix.

Now, five hours later and in hospital, the cervix was 8–9 cm dilated and I was very surprised to feel a nose and mouth. My first thought was, 'It's a breech', then, 'Don't be silly, it's a face'. I asked for midwife colleague support as I had not seen a face presentation birth before. Very shortly afterwards, the woman began to push strongly and the face birthed easily but she was very bruised as her 'lips came first'. The perineum was intact but the baby was quite small. We all reflected afterwards on how midwifery challenges us with variations of normal birth.

takes place at the same time, with the chin rotating another one-eighth of a circle to the right. Lastly, the anterior shoulder escapes under the pelvic arch and the rest of the baby is born by lateral flexion.

Before birth, the parents need to be warned that their baby's head may remain in an extended position (head falls back) for a little while and that facial oedema and distortion of facial features, petechiae and ecchymoses will subside after 24 hours and completely disappear in a few days. If the mother consents, an injection of vitamin K for the baby is indicated.

Brow presentation

A brow presentation (Fig 34.11) occurs in only 1 in 1500 births (Parker & Napolitano 2005). The fetal head presents in a position midway between flexion and extension. The forehead (more precisely the glabella) is the presenting part. This means that the fetal head enters the pelvis with the widest diameter of the head (occipitomental, 13.5 cm) leading. Possible causative factors include multiparity, placenta praevia, uterine anomaly, hydramnios, prematurity, multiple births and macrosomia. It cannot reliably be detected before labour begins. Abdominal palpation may reveal a high fetal head that does not descend into the pelvis despite effective contractions and progressive dilatation of the cervix. Diagnosis is confirmed by vaginal examination; on vaginal examination, the midwife may detect the sagittal suture in a transverse or oblique position; the anterior fontanelle feels very large and orbital ridges are palpable. The mouth and chin are not palpable. These indicators are not easy to detect if a large caput succedaneum

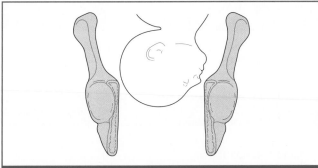

Figure 34.11 Brow presentation (based on Fraser & Cooper 2003)

BOX 34.3   Pelvic contracture

Clues to contracture of the maternal pelvis are:
▶ diagonal conjugate < 11.5 cm (contracture of inlet), outlet < 8 cm (contracture of the outlet)
▶ unengaged fetal head in early labour in primigravidas (consider contracture of inlet, malpresentation or malposition)
▶ hypotonic uterine contraction pattern (consider contracted pelvis)
▶ deflexion of fetal head (fetal head not flexed on fetal chest; may be associated with occipitoposterior)
▶ uncontrollable pushing prior to complete dilatation of cervix (may be associated with occipitoposterior)
▶ failure of fetal descent (consider contracture of the inlet, midpelvis or outlet)
▶ oedema of anterior portion (lip) of cervix (consider obstructed labour at the inlet).

(Source: Olds et al 2004)

---

has formed. There is no mechanism of labour for a brow presentation, unless the fetus is very small or it converts to a vertex or face presentation, and a caesarean section is often required.

Cephalo-pelvic disproportion

Cephalo-pelvic disproportion (CPD) is a disproportion between the size of the fetus and the size of the maternal pelvis—that is, the pelvis is not large enough to accommodate the passage of the fetus through the birth canal. CPD is usually relative because a pelvis that is adequate for a fetus weighing 2500 g may not be adequate for one weighing 3500 g. On the other hand, a healthy young woman in strong labour and effective contractions, who is not dehydrated and is coping well, may have a pelvis that accommodates a 4500 g fetus presenting as an LOA. In a second labour the same woman may be diagnosed with CPD because she has a malpresentation, an ineffective uterine action pattern, prolonged labour and is exhausted and disillusioned. This time her pelvis cannot accommodate a fetus weighing 3000 g. Therefore the adequacy of the pelvis must be re-evaluated with each pregnancy and birth.

In contrast, absolute CPD means that this fetus will never pass through the brim of the pelvis. In developed countries, it is most unusual to find a pelvis so severely contracted that labour is absolutely contraindicated. If this is the case, a caesarean section is the only option. Increasingly, midwives report that women tell them that they were told they needed an elective caesarean section because they had a 'big baby' and CPD. Clinical and ultrasound estimation of fetal size is often inaccurate, especially at the higher ranges of fetal weight. There is good evidence to suggest that estimation of fetal weight with ultrasound is no more accurate than estimations via abdominal palpation (American College of Obstetricians and Gynaecologists (ACOG) 2000a). Studies have shown that clinical estimation of fetal weight can be in error by a mean of 300 g (Zamorski & Biggs 2001). In most cases the only true test for relative CPD is labour—the so called 'trial of labour', a

term that brings with it connotations of failure and inadequacy and should be avoided.

Care of the woman at risk of CPD

Absolute CPD in developed countries is rare and therefore all women should be encouraged to labour provided there are effective uterine contractions, the labour progresses, there is descent of the presenting part and progressive dilatation of the cervix, and both mother and baby are coping with the labour. If there are no signs of absolute CPD, but the uterine contractions are inefficient (fewer than three contractions in 10 minutes) augmentation with an ARM followed by an intravenous infusion of Syntocinon® may improve the effectiveness of the contractions and facilitate descent of the fetal head. Positioning (ambulation, standing, squatting) may help to maximise pelvic space and descent of the fetus through the pelvis. Avoiding the onset of exhaustion, judicious use of measures for pain relief, perhaps epidural analgesia, and prevention of dehydration and ketosis encourage effective uterine action. Careful assessment of the progress of labour, abdominal palpation to track descent of the presenting part (vaginal examination: presentation, position, attitude, dilatation, effacement, moulding and the presence of caput succedaneum), assessment of the contraction pattern and assessment of maternal and fetal wellbeing are essential components of midwifery support of the woman suspected of CPD. Ineffective contraction patterns, failure of the labour to progress, a poorly flexed head, oedematous cervix, increased fetal head moulding, asynclitism and slow or absent cervical dilatation are all signs that labour is obstructing and that an operative delivery is warranted unless it is managed appropriately.

According to Varney (2004), dysfunctional labour caused by CPD may result in the following tragedies:
● fetal damage (e.g. brain damage)

BOX 34.4 Cervical dilatation and CPD
Slow cervical dilatation may be an early warning of CPD in primigravidas, but may not be so in multiparas.

BOX 34.5 CPD or obstruction?
There is no sharp, easily discernable line between CPD and the onset of obstruction.

- fetal or neonatal death
- intrauterine infection
- uterine rupture
- maternal death.

The goal of all maternity care providers is birth to a healthy mother who is psychologically and emotionally ready to mother her well newborn infant, not a damaged baby and a severely traumatised mother. As Varney (2004) puts it: 'there are times when obstetric heroics with forceps or a vacuum extraction to satisfy the goal of a vaginal birth is not worth the price paid. Midwives should be just as well known for calling for a caesarean section when it is truly indicated as we are for promoting and facilitating vaginal birth'.

Obstructed labour

The term 'obstructed labour' indicates a failure of the labour to progress because of mechanical problems—there is a barrier to descent of the presenting part despite an effective contraction pattern. Most of the following causes of an obstructed labour are dealt with in earlier sections of this chapter. They are:

- deep transverse arrest
- cephalo-pelvic disproportion
- pelvic mass
- fetal abnormalities
- malpresentation.

Obstructed labour increases the risk of maternal and perinatal mortality and morbidity but is rare in developed nations, due to improved antenatal and labour support from qualified health professionals with access to well-equipped health services. In developed countries, more often than not an obstructed labour is the end result of a poorly managed labour, where clinicians have failed to detect absolute CPD or a malpresentation.

Uterine rupture after a previous caesarean section

Considerable attention has been given to assessing the risk of uterine rupture in subsequent pregnancies after a previous caesarean section. In 1916, Edward Craigin (1916) made his now famous statement: 'Once a caesarean always a caesarean', a dictum that still dominates obstetrics even though there is scant evidence to support it. His advice was probably influenced by the high rate of uterine rupture known to occur with the 'classic' or vertical uterine incision used at that time (Toppenberg & Block 2002). The introduction of

Clinical point

The midwife should be aware of the late signs that a labour is obstructing:

- no descent of the presenting part
- no further dilatation of the cervix, oedema of the cervix, poorly fitting presenting part
- severe moulding
- fetal compromise (caused by moulding, meconium-stained liquor, or offensive-smelling liquor)
- abnormal contraction pattern (weak, absent or hypertonic with very little resting phase). In primigravidas, uterine contractions will often cease, leading to 'secondary arrest'. In contrast, in multigravidas the uterine contractions try to overcome the obstruction and push the fetus through the pelvis. With each contraction, the myometrial fibres shorten (retraction) and the upper uterine segment becomes thicker and the lower segment progressively thinner. The junction between the two segments is known as a Bandl's pathological retraction ring (Fig 34.12). It is observed as a ridge of tissue lying obliquely across the abdomen and may be confused with a full bladder. General signs: maternal pyrexia, exhaustion, rapid pulse rate, anxiety.
- maternal abdominal tenderness over a Bandl's ring
- abdominal distension
- distended bladder, oliguria, bloodstained urine.

a lower, non-contractile uterine segment caesarean section (LUSCS), improvements in maternity care and more reliable electronic fetal monitoring have made Craigin's dictum largely redundant.

Over the past 20 years in developed countries, the incidence of caesarean section has escalated from about 6% to 25% per year. Until recently, labour has been discouraged for women who have had a previous caesarean delivery (Guise et al 2004). There is still, however, a slightly increased risk of uterine rupture in subsequent births in a 'scarred uterus' irrespective of planned mode of delivery. Initial enthusiasm for VBAC (vaginal birth after caesarean section) has been tempered by reports of poor maternal and perinatal outcomes following attempts at a VBAC. Thus the proportion of women who attempt a VBAC after a prior caesarean delivery is again decreasing, largely because of alarm about issues of safety in general and uterine rupture in particular.

Landon and colleagues (2004) state that the absolute and relative risks associated with a trial of labour in women with a history of caesarean delivery, compared with elective repeated caesarean delivery without labour, are uncertain. The authors (Landon et al 2004) conducted a large, prospective four-year observational study of all women with a singleton pregnancy and a prior caesarean delivery at 19 teaching hospitals. Maternal and perinatal outcomes were compared between women who underwent a *trial of labour* (authors' emphasis) and women who had an elective repeated caesarean section prior to the onset of labour. The authors found that symptomatic uterine rupture occurred in 124 women who underwent a trial of labour (0.7%). Hypoxic–ischaemic encephalopathy occurred in none of the infants whose mothers underwent elective repeated caesarean delivery and in 12 infants born at term whose mothers underwent a trial of labour ($P < 0.001$). Of these 12, seven babies developed hypoxic–ischaemic encephalopathy after uterine rupture and there were two neonatal deaths. In addition, the rate of endometritis was somewhat higher in women undergoing a trial of labour than in women undergoing repeated elective caesarean delivery (2.9% vs 1.8%), as was the rate of blood transfusion (1.7% vs 1.0%). Neither the frequency of hysterectomy nor the rate of maternal death differed significantly between the groups (0.2% vs 0.3%, and 0.02% vs 0.04%, respectively). Given these results, the authors concluded that a trial of labour after prior caesarean delivery is associated with a greater perinatal risk than is elective repeated caesarean delivery without labour, although absolute risks were low.

In contrast, a systematic review of 568 articles concerned with the incidence and consequences of uterine rupture in women with previous caesarean section conducted by Guise et al (2004) concluded that although the literature on uterine rupture following an earlier caesarean section was imprecise and inconsistent, 7142 elective repeat caesarean section would need to be performed to prevent one rupture-related perinatal death, and 370 elective caesarean deliveries to prevent one symptomatic uterine rupture. In this review no maternal deaths were related to uterine rupture. In statistical terms, for women attempting a vaginal birth, the additional risk of perinatal death from rupture of a uterine scar was 1.4 per 10,000 births and the additional risk of hysterectomy following rupture was 3.4 per 10,000. The authors made the important point that most studies focus on the risk of uterine

rupture in the VBAC group, assuming that a repeat caesarean section eliminates the risk of uterine rupture. However, elective caesarean section does not protect the woman from uterine rupture; the rates of asymptomatic uterine rupture do not differ significantly between VBAC and repeat caesarean section births.

Guise and colleagues (2004) comment that in two of the studies they reviewed, induction of labour with oxytocin was associated with a two- to four-fold increase of uterine rupture, although in the other reviewed studies the use of oxytocin or prostaglandins was not associated with a higher risk of uterine rupture. They make several other important points that women making choices about subsequent births after a caesarean section should reflect on. Indeed, all women considering an elective caesarean section should understand that any uterine scar increases the risk of uterine rupture irrespective of the mode of delivery; as many as a third of these ruptures will occur in pregnancy before labour begins (Toppenberg & Block 2002). However, a woman choosing VBAC faces an additional risk of uterine rupture of 0.27%. Thirdly, even if the rupture does occur, serious maternal and perinatal morbidity and mortality are rare. Therefore clinicians and women may wish to base their decisions on the likelihood of significant mortality or morbidity for the mother and baby rather than the uterine rupture itself (Guise et al 2004). Other causes of morbidity and mortality include risks from anaesthesia, inadvertent damage to the bladder and bowel, wound and uterine infection, haemorrhage, deep vein thrombosis and pulmonary oedema,

---

BOX 34.6 Uterine rupture

Conditions associated with uterine rupture:

▶ uterine scars
▶ prior caesarean section
▶ prior rupture
▶ trauma
▶ injury from instrumentation during an abortion
▶ significant myomectomy
▶ any cause of uterine perforation
▶ uterine anomalies (i.e. undeveloped uterine horn)
▶ prior invasive molar pregnancy
▶ history of placenta percreta or increta
▶ difficult forceps delivery
▶ malpresentation
▶ fetal anomaly
▶ obstructed labour
▶ induction of labour (suspected association)
▶ excessive uterine stimulation
▶ prostaglandins E_1 (misoprostol (Cytotec®))
▶ prostaglandins E_2 (dinaprostone (Cervidil®))
▶ oxytocin (pitocin), especially high infusion rates
▶ alkaloid/crack cocaine abuse.

(Source: Toppenberg & Block 2002)

as well as neonatal problems such as respiratory distress syndrome.

Detection and management

Timely detection and management are keys to the prevention and management of uterine rupture in labour.

In the past, clinicians were taught to look for classic signs of uterine rupture: the appearance of a Bandl's ring (an indication that the uterus may rupture at any time; Fig 34.12); sensation of sudden tearing uterine pain, abdominal or shoulder tip pain; cessation of uterine contractions, maternal shock, haemorrhage, andf regression of the fetus, signs of severe fetal compromise and fetal death (Toppenberg & Block 2002). It is now recognised that, apart from signs of fetal distress, these signs are unreliable and often absent, especially with the increased use of epidurals for VBAC births.

Because the presenting signs of uterine rupture are often non-specific (Toppenberg & Block 2002), management is often the same as for any other cause of severe fetal compromise. Delay in delivery may be catastrophic and both mother and baby may die. The woman is prepared for an immediate emergency caesarean section.

Before transport, resuscitation measures are put in place—adequate intravenous access, blood is taken for cross-match, and the emergency team (obstetricians, midwives, anaesthetist and paediatrician) is summoned.

In developed countries, maternal death is rare but the mother may die following a ruptured uterus from haemorrhage, infection and peritonitis. Perinatal outcomes depend on the speed with which the surgery can take place. The fetus may die from asphyxia, infection or irreversible brain damage. If they survive, most will require transfer to a neonatal nursery.

Neglected obstruction of labour and its aftermath

Many women, especially those living in developing countries, do not have access to health services that have the human and

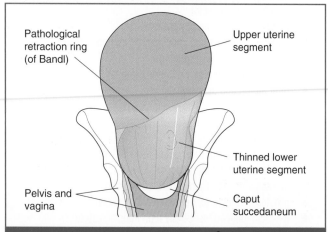

Figure 34.12 Bandl's pathological retraction ring (based on Oats & Abraham 2004)

Labels in figure:
- Pathological retraction ring (of Bandl)
- Upper uterine segment
- Thinned lower uterine segment
- Pelvis and vagina
- Caput succedaneum

> ### Clinical point
>
> Two types of uterine rupture may occur in a scarred uterus:
> - *Catastrophic (symptomatic)*—the old scar separates along its length, the amniotic sac ruptures and the fetus is extruded into the abdominal cavity. There is significant bleeding and shock.
> - *Asymptomatic*—more commonly, the scar dehisces part-way along its length, the amniotic membranes do not rupture, and so the fetus remains within the uterus. Bleeding and shock are minimal, and the fetus usually survives. This form of rupture may not be detected until subsequent births.
>
> It is important to remember that rupture of a lower segment uterine scar, although a serious complication, is generally not catastrophic.

> ### Clinical point
>
> Prolonged late or variable fetal heart rate decelerations and bradycardia seen on an electronic fetal heart rate trace are the most common—and often the only—manifestation of uterine rupture (Toppenberg & Block 2002).

physical resources to perform an immediate caesarean section for an obstructed labour and impending uterine rupture. In Australia and New Zealand, clinicians do not see the effects of a neglected shoulder presentation, obstructed labour and uterine rupture, but these are common occurrences in many developing countries.

The prevalence of obstructed labour is more common in developing countries because of a lack of adequate health care services, poor nutrition and poverty (Konje & Ladipo 2000). In these countries, obstructed labour remains a frequent cause of maternal morbidity and death. If she survives, a primigravida may develop a vesico-vaginal fistula (between the bladder and vagina) or recto-vaginal fistula (between the rectum and vagina). In the famous fistula hospital in Ethiopia, 97% of vesico-vaginal fistulas occurred after obstructed labour; 65% of women were aged less than 25 years of age; and 63% were primigravida at the time of the labour (Kelly & Kwast 1993).

According to Konje and Ladipo (2000), prevention of this dreadful scourge can be achieved in the short term by identifying women at risk of obstructed labour and transferring them to centres with the resources to deal with obstruction of labour. In the long term, efforts need to centre on improving the health and nutrition of children and young women by detecting and treating diseases that lead to growth retardation. Early motherhood should be discouraged and strategies to improve nutrition during infancy, childhood and early adulthood, and in pregnancy, put in place. Improving access to and promoting the use of reproductive and contraceptive services, including the prevention of HIV infections, will also help reduce the prevalence of this complication.

Induction of labour

Induction of labour is the artificial initiation of labour before its spontaneous onset, for the purpose of birthing the baby. The rate of induction varies between countries and between centres, and ranges from 10% to 30%. Enkin and colleagues (2000, p 375) make the point that 'the decision to bring pregnancy to an end before the spontaneous onset of labour is one of the most drastic ways of intervening in the natural history of pregnancy and childbirth'.

There are two forms of labour stimulation. The first, augmentation, has been discussed earlier in this chapter. It involves the stimulation of uterine contraction in a labour that has already begun. If the rhythms of labour are ineffective, contractions may be stimulated by augmenting labour with an ARM alone or in combination with an infusion of an oxytocic drug such as Syntocinon. It should only be used once non-invasive strategies, such as positioning and ambulation, emptying the bladder, relief of unbearable pain and anxiety (perhaps with hydrotherapy), and correcting dehydration and ketosis with fluid and nutrition, have been tried. In contrast, induction of labour refers to the artificial induction of labour with or without rupturing the amniotic sac before the spontaneous onset of labour for the purpose of accomplishing birth.

Indications for induction

Induction of labour should only be performed if the health of both mother and baby would be compromised if pregnancy

---

Clinical point

In an editorial in the *American Family Physician*, Elizabeth Baxley (2003) comments that induction of labour (social induction) is a common phenomenon in labour wards. Many women and their lead carers have valid reasons for wanting the 'labour to be brought on', including mutual convenience, logistic issues such as child care and transportation, and to ensure that a known and trusted caregiver will be present for the birth. As Baxley points out, since most induced births occur between the hours of 10.00 am and 8.00 pm, it is reasonable to presume that the obstetrician and staff will be alert and better able to respond to an emergency. However, she warns that elective induction is not without potential risks, including iatrogenic prematurity, uterine hyperstimulation, non-reassuring fetal heart rate tracing, and greater likelihood of operative delivery, shoulder dystocia and PPH. While these complications are rare in multiparous women, nulliparous women have significantly higher rates of caesarean delivery, instrumented delivery, epidural analgesia, and neonatal intensive care unit admission. Baxley concludes that because the risk of caesarean delivery with elective induction is potentially as high as 2.8 times that for spontaneous labour, it is difficult to advocate elective induction in a nulliparous woman.

---

continues; that is, the benefits of imminent delivery outweigh the risks associated with the induction of labour. Table 34.1 summarises the indications for the induction of labour. Women are informed of the risks and benefits of an induction of labour as well as the difficulties associated with accurate determination of gestational age.

TABLE 34.1   Indications for induction of labour

Maternal	Fetal	Both
Prolonged pregnancy past 41 weeks	Severe congenital abnormalities	Placental abruption
Medical conditions, e.g. Type 1 diabetes, cardiac disease, reduced renal function, central nervous system disorders, pulmonary disease, antiphospholipid syndrome, chronic hypertension	Severe Rhesus isoimmunisation	Unstable lie
Prolonged and/or spontaneous rupture of membranes. Suspected or diagnosed chorioamnionitis	Fetal death	Complications of pregnancy, e.g. pre-eclampsia
Previous obstetric & reproductive history, e.g. previous stillborn baby, precipitate labour, cervical dystocia	Potential fetal compromise (significant growth restriction, oligohydramnios and placental insufficiency) Non-reassuring fetal surveillance	
Maternal request for social reasons, or logistic reasons		

Two indications for induction of labour have resulted in significant debate and controversy, and are discussed in more detail here.

Induction and post-date pregnancies

The most frequent indication for an induction of labour and the most difficult to assess is the so-called post-dates pregnancy. There is considerable confusion about the definitions of a term and a post-term pregnancy. Commonly accepted midwifery and obstetric language used to describe the indication for induction of labour from 37 completed weeks to 43 weeks gestation, include: 'term pregnancy', 'prolonged', 'post-mature', 'post-dates' and 'post-term', which many assume are synonymous albeit vague terms that differentiate between the 'normal' and 'abnormal' range of pregnancy. This terminology contributes to the confusion about options for optimum best care at this time.

Determining the woman's actual expected date of birth may not be easy. Records of the actual date of the first day of the last normal period, an appreciation of differing lengths of menstrual cycles and an accurate early scan dating may assist in this process. Two systematic reviews (Crowley 2003; Sanchez-Ramos et al 2003) report that routine ultrasonography in early pregnancy (even in 'low-risk' ones) reduced the number of women who needed their labours induced for apparent post-dates pregnancies. As the woman approaches 41 weeks of pregnancy, midwives need to have a conversation with her about the length of her pregnancy and the indications for induction of labour after 41 weeks. To aid informed choice and consent, full disclosure of potential risks associated with induction of labour needs to take place.

Despite evidence that actual benefits for the fetus from induction occur only after 41 completed weeks of pregnancy (Crowley 2003), inducing labour at term—38 weeks of gestation—is a commonly cited reason for inducing labour (Downe & McCourt 2004). A Cochrane Review by Crowley (2003) of 19 randomised controlled trials (RCTs) found that compared to a policy of expectant management, routine labour induction at 41 weeks gestation resulted in a decrease in perinatal deaths but similar caesarean section rates. Approximately 500 women needed to have their labours induced to prevent one perinatal death. Meconium-stained fluid was more common in the expectant management group, but rates of neonatal meconium aspiration syndrome and other similar morbidities were not significantly different between the two groups. In a more recent meta-analysis (Sanchez-Ramos et al 2003) of 16 RCTs comparing induction of labour at 41 weeks of pregnancy with a policy of expectant management, the women in the induction group were less likely to require a caesarean section. There was also a non-significant reduction in perinatal mortality in the induction group. The authors concluded that about 16,000 women would need to have their labours induced to detect a 50% reduction in perinatal mortality.

However, neither review (Crowley 2003; Sanchez-Ramos et al 2003) reported any adverse perinatal complications from labour induction of pregnancies greater than 40 weeks. Of significant interest for this chapter is that both reviews found that the results were consistent irrespective of the Bishop's score. An 'unfavourable' cervix at the time of the induction did not increase the number of caesarean sections or other adverse outcomes (Crowley 2003; Sanchez-Ramos et al 2003).

'Social' induction

Labour is sometimes induced for 'social' or 'geographic' reasons without a medical or obstetric indication. There have been no RCTs evaluating induction of labour for these reasons since 1983 (Crowley 2003). The induction of labour is not an isolated intervention. It frequently results in a cascade of interventions (see Box 34.7) that have the potential to negatively affect the childbirth process and its outcomes (Alexander et al 2000).

Contraindications for induction

All contraindications to spontaneous onset of labour and vaginal birth are also contraindications for the induction of labour. These include:

- maternal refusal
- any maternal or fetal condition that precludes vaginal birth
- malpresentation—transverse or oblique lie, compound or shoulder presentation
- previous major uterine surgery—'classical' caesarean section
- absolute cephalo-pelvic disproportion
- cord prolapse
- active genital herpes
- placenta previa
- invasive carcinoma of the cervix

BOX 34.7 Cascade of intervention

The cascade of intervention following induction of labour includes:

- intravenous lines
- enforced bed rest
- continuous electronic fetal heart rate monitoring
- amniotomy
- increased pain and discomfort
- epidural analgesia
- operative delivery
- prolonged hospital stay.

Clinical point

There is compelling evidence that elective induction of labour significantly increases the risk of caesarean section, especially for nulliparous women (ACOG 2000b).

- a severely compromised fetus.
Relative contraindications include:
- non-reassuring fetal heart rate trace
- breech presentation
- unknown fetal presentation
- multiple pregnancy
- polyhydramnios
- presenting part above the pelvic brim
- severe maternal hypertension
- maternal heart disease.

Risks of induction

Induction of labour is perceived by many midwives as the first step in an often irreversible cascade of interventions that ultimately culminates in an increased need for epidural analgesia, operative delivery and caesarean section, particularly among primigravid women. For example, in 2002 the New Zealand Maternal and Newborn Information System recorded a national induction rate of 19.7% (New Zealand Ministry of Health 2004) and a caesarean section rate of 22.7%. There were considerably more inductions for European women than for Maori, Pacific Island and Asian women. When induction of labour was combined with the use of epidural analgesia, only 44.4% had a normal vaginal birth and 31.2% required a caesarean section. However, for those women who did not require an epidural, the spontaneous birth rate increased to 77.6% and only 16.7% needed a caesarean section.

Prerequisites for induction

Induction of labour is associated with potential complications and so it should only be undertaken if there is a medical indication to do so and only after the woman has had the opportunity to make an informed decision about whether or not she wishes her labour to be induced and understands the risks and benefits of the procedure. The mother must be given full disclosure of the procedure, its risks and benefits, as well as information about the limitations of the birthing unit—for example, perhaps there is no 24-hour epidural service, or if she requires a caesarean section 'out of hours' she will have to be transferred to another hospital with these facilities. In addition, the following criteria should be met:

- There is documented evidence that the procedure has been discussed with the woman, that the risks and benefits of induction of her labour have been discussed and that she has given her consent for the procedure.
- There is a documented indication for the induction of labour as well as the presence of any contraindications.
- Parity is confirmed.
- The gestational age is confirmed.
- There is documented assessment of cervical favourability, fetal position and presentation and relationship of the fetal head to the pelvic brim.
- Membrane status has been assessed—intact or ruptured.
- The adequacy of the pelvis has been ascertained.
- The presence of uterine activity is known.
- The fetal heart rate has been recorded (NST).

Midwifery support prior to induction

Induction of labour may result in maternal feelings of loss of control, and loss of continuity of midwifery care if the maternity unit is some distance from the woman's place of residence, as well as other physical complications. Discussion about the indications for an induction of labour during pregnancy aids informed decision-making at a time when a woman who is already compromised in her ability to cope with the physical discomforts of late pregnancy is more vulnerable than usual to others' coercive decision-making.

The process of induction

There are various 'natural' methods for non-invasive induction of labour (Adair 2000; Kavanagh et al 2002; Kelly et al 2002; Smith & Crowther 2002). These include: cod liver oil; herbal remedies such as blue and black cohosh; acupuncture; nipple stimulation; sex (because semen has natural prostaglandins); and the use of raspberry leaf tea during the latter stages

---

MIDWIFE'S STORY

As a core midwife working in a tertiary maternity unit on the delivery suite, I was allocated a woman who was coming in from an outlying area at 0800 for an induction of labour. This was the first time I or the doctor on duty in the labour ward had met her. It was the woman's first baby and she was exactly 39 weeks gestation by sure dates. I welcomed her into the birthing room and completed her baseline observations, an abdominal palpation and assessment. Her uterine fundus was equal to dates; the baby was felt to be about 3500 g and on palpation I found a cephalic presentation with a right occipitolateral position, and a well-engaged flexed head deep in the pelvis. The baby's heart rate ranged from 120 to 140 bpm. Her baby had been moving well and there did not appear to be any medical indication for an induction of labour. I asked her what she understood was the reason for the induction and what she had been told about the procedure. She told me that her midwife, who was not in attendance due to distance, had made her a hospital appointment after seeing her at 40 weeks one week ago and she had been booked for induction today after seeing a doctor in another antenatal clinic three days before. She said that 'it was necessary to bring the labour on because she was overdue'. The woman gave no indication that she was aware she had alternative choices and options, or that she wanted to know about them. Nor did the woman seem to have much understanding about what was going to happen today or the risks and benefits of an induction of labour.

Reflection

Consider the above story and reflect on your responsibilities and subsequent actions, taking into consideration your philosophy of practice, research findings, hospital guidelines, Standards for Practice and Codes of Ethics. You might like to consider the ethical principle of 'best interests'.

of pregnancy. The risks and benefits of these methods are unknown because the quality of evidence is based on a long tradition of use and on anecdotal case reports rather than quality research. The only conclusion that can be drawn at this time is that the efficacy of all these interventions is still uncertain.

Both the New Zealand and Australian Colleges of Midwifery recommend that before using these therapies, the woman should seek advice from a registered therapist unless her midwife has undertaken a recognised education program that entitles her to use these treatments.

Bishop's score

Before induction takes place, assessment of the cervix to determine readiness for labour is essential, and is done using the Bishop's score (Bishop 1964). A Bishop's score (Table 34.2) is ascertained by assigning points to the parameters of cervical readiness (ripeness) for labour. The higher the Bishop's score, the greater the likelihood of a successful induction of labour. Although this is an attempt at objectivity, the care provider still makes a subjective assessment of the cervix. That is, she is still making a judgement that differs from that of another practitioner. Induction should not be attempted unless a mother has a favourable Bishop's score. If the cervix is unfavourable (Bishop's score is ≤ 6), cervical ripening prior to the induction with misoprostol (Cytotec®) or endogenous prostaglandin (PGE_2) to help ripen the cervix and improve the score is warranted, because if the cervix does not readily dilate then a long labour ending in a caesarean section with resulting potential complications is more likely (Enkin et al 2000). A score of eight or nine would indicate that the cervix was very ripe and induction has a high probability of success.

Pharmacological cervical ripening

Synthetic forms of prostaglandins—PGE_2 either as a gel or pessaries (dinaprostone: Prepidil®, Cervidil®, Prostin®)—are marketed for cervical ripening. Prostaglandins facilitate cervical ripening (softening and effacing the cervix) via a number of different mechanisms. The pre-labour production of PGE_2 by the amnion causes dissolution of the cervical collagen bundles and increases the activity of collagenase in the cervix, as well as the levels of elastin, glycosaminoglycan, dermatan sulphate and hyaluronic acid, thereby facilitating water absorption by the cervix, leading to a softer, more stretchable cervix. Relaxation of smooth muscle fibres facilitates cervical dilatation and may produce uterine contractions.

Types of PGE_2

Midwives should be aware of the clinical implications of each of the pharmacological agents used for cervical ripening. The types of exogenous PGE_2 are:
- intravaginal insert containing dinoprostone
- intracervical dinaprostone gels
- hospital compounded intravaginal gels.

A reactive NST should be obtained prior to the insertion of PGE_2 and the CTG trace is continued for at least half an hour after its insertion. Prostaglandins (PGE_2) as Prostin® comes as a 1 mg or 2 mg gel and is administered vaginally into the posterior fornix. The prescribed dose is determined by parity and the obstetrician's preferences, but the gel may be reapplied every 6–12 hours if necessary. The manufacturers recommend an initial dose of 1 mg followed by a second 1 mg or 2 mg dose six hours later if necessary, up to a maximum of three doses. The woman remains in a semi-recumbent position for several hours.

Cervidil® comes as a 10 mg controlled-release (over 10 hours) vaginal insert, which has a removable cord for easy removal if necessary. After administration, the woman must remain semi-recumbent for two hours before ambulating.

Misoprostol (Cytotec®) is a synthetic PGE_1 analogue. Although it has been suggested as a useful agent for pre-induction cervical ripening and labour induction, it has not been approved for use and should only be used in the context of clinical trials until it is approved by the appropriate authorities.

Complications

There have been no randomised trials evaluating the level or duration of fetal heart rate and uterine activity monitoring

---

TABLE 34.2 Bishop's score: pre-induction assessment of cervical ripening

Examination findings	Score			
	0	**1**	**2**	**3**
Dilatation (cm)	Closed	1–2	3–4	> 5
Effacement (%)	0-30	40–50	60–70	> 80
Station	3	2	1 or 0	+1, +2
Consistency	Firm	Medium	Soft	–
Position of cervix	Posterior	Midposition	Anterior	–
(Source: Bishop 1964)				

post insertion of the gel. Uterine contractions usually start one hour after insertion and peak in the first four hours (Miller et al 1991). Uterine hyperstimulation with or without a non-reassuring fetal heart rate patterns occurs in a very small number of women. Other complications include gastrointestinal effects (nausea and diarrhoea), back pain, a warm feeling in the vagina and pyrexia. Treatment of uterine hyperstimulation includes: removing the gel, positioning the woman in the left lateral position and administering oxygen 6 L/min. A tocolytic drug such as a sub-cutaneous injection of 250 µg of terbutaline may be indicated.

Mechanical ways to ripen the cervix

Mechanical methods of cervical ripening share a similar mechanism of action: namely, local mechanical pressure stimulates the release of prostaglandins. They include Foley catheter (with or without extra-amniotic saline infusion), natural dilators (laminaria) and synthetic dilators. The risks associated with these methods include infection (endometritis and neonatal sepsis associated with natural osmotic dilators) (Kazzi et al 1982), antepartum bleeding and pre-labour membrane rupture.

Several RCTs have compared the use of a balloon device with administration of an extra-amniotic saline infusion, or prostaglandin E$_2$ (PGE$_2$). Results from these trials indicate that each of these methods is an effective means of cervical ripening with an unfavourable cervix and each has comparable caesarean-section delivery rates in women (Guinn et al 2000; Sherman et al 2001).

Membrane stripping/sweeping

This practice has long been advocated as a relatively non-invasive, albeit uncomfortable, means to induce labour. The amniotic fetal membrane is separated from the decidua of the lower uterine segment. It is believed that this process increases the release of F$_2\alpha$ prostaglandin production from the decidua and adjacent fetal membrane, thereby stimulating the onset of 'spontaneous' labour. According to the Cochrane Database (Boulvaine et al 2005), a review of 27 research trials demonstrates that this procedure does not appear to demonstrate clinically improved benefits when used to induce labour.

Induction of labour with oxytocin

Several options are available for labour induction. The ones considered here are amniotomy and oxytocin. Amniotomy is considered earlier in this chapter in the section on augmentation of labour. Intravenous oxytocin has been widely used to induce and augment labour for more than 50 years. Once the cervix is ripe, oxytocin is still the favoured pharmacological agent for inducing labour. Endogenous oxytocin, an octapeptide hormone, is secreted in the hypothalamus and transported to the posterior pituitary gland, where it is stored. It is chemically related to vasopressin (antidiuretic hormone, ADH). Its effects are enhanced by high levels of oestrogen—the highest levels occur just prior to term. Released in a pulsatile fashion, oxytocin stimulates both the frequency and strength of uterine contractions and has antidiuretic properties. Synthetic oxytocin—Syntocinon®—maintains these properties.

Low- and high-dose protocols for Syntocinon®

Oxytocin has been used for decades for induction of labour at term. It has a short biological half-life (10–12 minutes), making dosing easier than concomitant dosing with the PGE$_2$ dinaprostone (Cervidil®). Oxytocin has few adverse side-effects and therefore has been approved for use in the induction of labour at term. It should always be administered via an infusion pump and 'piggy-backed' to the main IV line and as close to the IV puncture site as possible.

There are a number of protocols for administering Syntocinon®. Studies indicate a wide range of effective dosages and change intervals, and no protocol has been shown to be clearly superior. The two commonly used protocols for dosage of oxytocin are the active or high-dose labour management protocol, and a low-dose one. There are variations between hospitals and so the ones provided here are examples of a 'typical protocol'.

The active management of labour (high-dose) protocol for Syntocinon® has been derived from the work of O'Driscoll and Meagher (1980). In rapid increments an oxytocin infusion is begun at 5–6 mU/min and increased by 5–6 mU/min to a maximum of 40 mU/min. A significant drawback to the protocol for active management of labour is the incidence of uterine hyperstimulation seen with rapid incremental dosing of oxytocin. Darwood (1995) noted that most women achieve adequate uterine activity with 12 mU/min of Syntocinon®.

The low-dose protocol for oxytocin was first advocated by Seitchik and Castillo (1982), who studied uterine hyperstimulation using both the active management of labour and low-dose oxytocin protocols. In a typical 'low-dose' approach, an infusion is prepared by placing 10 units of Syntocinon® in 1 L of an isotonic intravenous solution such as Hartmann's to achieve a concentration of 10 mU/mL. Because severe maternal hypotension or fetal compromise can occur with rapid bolus doses, the drug is 'piggy-backed' into the main IV line, and a controlled infusion pump *must* be used to determine its rate. The infusion is begun at 0.5–1 mU/min and increased every 30 to 60 minutes by 1 mU/min until adequate uterine contractions are established or until the infusion reaches 40 mU/min. The dose is always titrated according to the maternal–fetal response to the labour. The lowest dose possible to achieve adequate progress of labour is recommended. An effect is noted within three to five minutes, and a steady state is achieved within 15 to 30 minutes. Once the cervix is 6 cm dilated, often the oxytocin infusion can be reduced in similar decrements.

Contractions should not be closer than every two minutes. Low-dose protocol resulted in less uterine hyperstimulation and an overall decrease in induction to delivery time over a high-dose active labour management protocol. The disadvantage in the low-dose oxytocin protocol was the amount of time required to complete successful induction in nulliparous women with an 'unfavourable cervix'.

Complications

Oxytocin has a short half-life and is generally well tolerated by mother and baby, although induction of labour is never without some risk.

Hyperstimulation of the uterus, resulting in hypertonic uterine contractions, may occur (see Clinical point below). If this complication is not managed appropriately, the uterus may rupture. Because synthetic oxytocin is close to vasopressin in structure, it has an antidiuretic effect when given in high dosages (40 mU/min), and therefore water intoxication is a possibility in prolonged inductions—a strict input and output chart needs to be maintained.

When the uterine resting tone remains above 20 mmHg, uteroplacental insufficiency and fetal hypoxia can result. This complication underscores the importance of close FHR monitoring. There have as yet been no randomised trials of the level of fetal heart rate monitoring required for women whose labours are being induced. However, the need for close assessment of uterine activity and maternal and fetal wellbeing necessitates one-to-one midwifery care.

If fetal compromise is suspected, the oxytocin dosage can usually be lowered rather than stopped completely. This allows the fetus to recover without unnecessarily slowing the entire labour. Other steps include changing the mother's position, assessing maternal blood pressure, administering oxygen and increasing intravenous fluid administration. In emergency situations, the infusion is discontinued. A vaginal examination is performed to assess the progress of labour and rule out umbilical cord prolapse.

The intensity of uterine activity and the rapid and early onset of contractions, often from the start of labour, often means that the pain relief method of choice is frequently an epidural, and this too increases the likelihood of further interventions (Gilbert & Harmon 2003). An actively managed third stage of labour is recommended due to the increased risk of PPH.

Uterine hyperstimulation

Uterine hyperstimulation from the use of intravenous oxytocin or the administration of prostaglandins occurs in 1–5% of women (Kelly et al 2001). Other potential risks include an increased rate of operative delivery (Crowley 1995), caesarean birth (Seyb et al 1999), non-reassuring fetal heart rate patterns (Kelly et al 2001), uterine rupture (Flanelly et al 1993), delivery of preterm infant due to incorrect estimation of fetal maturity, and possible umbilical cord prolapse following an ARM when the fetal head is still above the pelvic brim.

Midwifery assessments for induction of labour

Before induction

Pre-induction assessments:
- Ensure that the woman has given informed consent for the labour to be induced.
- Identify indications for, contraindications to, or risk factors for the procedure.
- Determine lie, presentation of the fetus and the relationship of the fetal head to the pelvis.

> ### Clinical point
>
> **Uterine hyperstimulation**
> Uterine hyperstimulation (five or more contractions in 10 minutes or lasting more than 90 seconds) results in decelerations in the fetal heart rate and/or other signs of fetal compromise.
>
> If hyperstimulation occurs with signs of fetal compromise:
> - Discontinue oxytocin infusion.
> - Position the woman on her left side.
> - Administer oxygen 10 L/min.
> - Consider increasing infusion rate in the main line.
> - Notify the lead carer.
> - Prepare for possible caesarean section if the fetal heart rate does not return to normal.
> - Consider tocolysis: IV nitroglycerine 50–200 mg, or 1–2 metered doses of a sub-lingual spray (400–800 mg); terbutaline 250 µg subcutaneously.
> - If intrauterine resuscitation is successful, re-start oxytocin infusion at half the last dose.
>
> Should hyperstimulation occur without fetal compromise, decrease infusion rate and reassess its effects on the uterine contraction pattern and the fetal heart rate. It may be possible to increase the infusion rate once the contraction pattern returns to its normal state.

- Ensure that the Bishop's score has been calculated.
- Assess amniotic membrane status.
- Obtain a baseline CTG if hospital policy requires this, and analyse it for non-reassuring features.
- Obtain baseline assessments of mother's blood pressure, pulse rate, temperature and respiratory rate.
- Assess for the onset of labour.

During induction

Midwives often question the feasibility of documenting maternal and fetal status every 15 minutes during an induction of the first stage of labour and every five minutes during the second stage. Automated devices are sometimes used to record the maternal blood pressure and pulse rate. The inaccuracies of these devices are well documented (Marx et al 1993). One study (Marx et al 1993) assessed the concordance of recording the blood pressure with an automated blood pressure device and those obtained with the auscultatory method. The authors concluded that in labouring women there is a discrepancy between systolic and diastolic pressures obtained by the auscultatory versus the oscillatory method of measurement, although mean pressures are not significantly different. They therefore recommended that during labour the diagnoses of hypertension and hypotension be based on the mean rather than the systolic or diastolic pressure.

Preterm labour

Preterm labour, or, as it is often referred to, premature labour (PTL), is defined as one that begins after 20 weeks but before 37 completed weeks of pregnancy (259 days). Most mortality and morbidity occurs in babies born before 34 weeks. Despite new diagnostic and therapeutic modalities, efforts to prevent the onset of PTL have largely been ineffective and it remains the leading cause of neonatal mortality and morbidity (Norwitz & Robinson 2001).

Epidemiology of preterm labour

Approximately 5–10% of all births are preterm. For example, the 2004 New Zealand Ministry of Health report of the Maternal and Newborn Information Services from 2002 showed a 7.4% rate of premature births, a slight increase from 7.2% in 1999 (NZMOH 2004). Preterm birth was the most common cause of death for babies in New Zealand in 2002. A similar pattern is apparent in other industrialised nations including Australia—the frequency has not decreased for more than 20 years; indeed, there is some evidence that it may be increasing (Challis 2001). The increased use of reproductive technologies and the escalating frequency of multiple births are the primary causes of this increase (Gilbert & Harmon 2003).

McNamara (2003, p 79) makes the important point that PTL is 'not a disease but an event, which may result from single or multiple, independent or interdependent pathways. Preterm labour is often the final step in a multifactorial process'. Although the actual cause of PTL is unknown, there are a number of identified risk factors and these can be divided into four main areas: reproductive history; biological/medical factors; current pregnancy; and socioeconomic, behavioural and stress-related factors. According to Haram et al (2003, p 690), the two strongest risk factors for idiopathic PTL are low socio-economic status and previous preterm birth. Approximately 85% of women with one previous preterm birth between 20 and 36 weeks of gestation will birth at term next time. After two preterm births, only 70% of women will deliver their next baby at term, although about 20% of preterm births are iatrogenic.

McNamara (2003, p 80) comments that the relationships between genetics, infection and preterm labour are continually under investigation because scientists believe that these may shed further light on the precise aetiology of preterm labour, either independently or in combination. In terms of other variables, such as socio-economic status, social behaviour and stress-related issues, research will need to re-examine whether these so-called 'social' issues are causal, or have confounding or modifying effects on other causal factors. These interrelationships seem to be the key to understanding the multiple interrelated aetiologies of preterm labour.

Prevention, identification and management

The identification of women at risk of PTL, and its prevention and management, have been widely studied and are important challenges in reducing the number of preterm births and improving outcomes for mothers and babies. Maternal health is not usually adversely influenced by preterm labour, although psychosocial morbidities are high and include increased levels of anxiety and the potential for feelings of failure unless there

---

BOX 34.8 Risk factors for premature delivery

Risk factors for premature delivery are:

▶ anaemia (haemoglobin <11 and S-ferritin 12–15 µg/L)
▶ abnormal uterine anatomy
▶ abruptio placentae
▶ cervix insufficiency
▶ drug use (heroin and cocaine)
▶ fetal anomalies
▶ iatrogenic
▶ infections (UTIs, infections caused by GBS, intrauterine infections, bacterial vaginosis)
▶ low maternal weight
▶ low social status
▶ multiple gestations
▶ placenta praevia
▶ polyhydramnios
▶ premature rupture of membranes
▶ previous preterm birth
▶ smoking
▶ stressful lifestyle
▶ young mother (< 15–19 years)
▶ domestic violence.

(Source: Haram et al 2003, p 689)

Research

Effects of domestic violence on preterm birth and low birthweight (Neggers et al 2004)
Background: Domestic violence is increasingly recognised as a potentially modifiable risk factor for adverse pregnancy outcomes. This study evaluated the relationship between abuse during pregnancy or within the last year and low birthweight and preterm birth.
Methods: From 1997 to 2001, 3149 low-income, relatively low-risk pregnant women (82% African-American) participated in this prospective study. The Abuse Assessment Screen, which assesses emotional, physical or sexual abuse, injuries due to physical abuse and physical abuse in the index pregnancy, was completed by 3103 women.
Results: Of the women screened, 26.6% reported emotional abuse, 18.7% reported physical abuse in the past year and 10.3% women reported being beaten, bruised and threatened with a weapon or being permanently injured. Abuse during pregnancy was reported by 5.9% of the women. Low birthweight and preterm birth occurred in 10.9% and 10.2% of the pregnant women, respectively. Logistic regression analyses indicated that injury due to physical abuse within the past year was significantly associated with both low birthweight and preterm birth. The mean birthweight of infants born to women who were injured due to physical assault was significantly lower than the mean birthweight of infants of women who were not physically injured.

---

are medical and or obstetric indications such as pre-eclampsia or cardiac disease. The baby's ability to cope with extrauterine life depends greatly on the gestation at birth and significantly affects mortality and morbidity (Enkin et al 2000; Gilbert & Harmon 2003). Perinatal survival rates have improved substantially in recent years because of developments in neonatal technology, facilities and appropriately trained staff.

Assessing risk of PTL in pregnancy

Assessing a woman's risk of PTL and birth is part of the midwife's standard care in pregnancy. Beginning with an extensive booking history early in pregnancy, the midwife assesses for and documents risk factors for preterm labour and birth, making an appropriate early referral in consultation and with consent from the women to a specialist if necessary. Nevertheless, in 60% of cases PTL will occur in women with no risk factors. The midwife should inform the woman that if, at any time, signs of labour are apparent before 37 weeks she should contact the midwife immediately. This is of particular importance for women residing in rural areas with limited access to secondary or tertiary maternity and paediatric services, as TPL may mean a transfer of considerable distance to an appropriate facility.

Later, as her relationship with the woman grows, the midwife gathers information about the woman's past and present birthing, her physical and social histories including stressors (such as housing and food availability), social support, cultural safety, financial stressors, history of family violence, the presence of infections or the earlier diagnosis

---

Clinical point

Many pregnant women experience symptoms that suggest preterm labour. These may include uterine contractions, changes in vaginal discharge, backaches, pelvic pressure, cramping and cervical dilatation. Not all symptomatic women will actually have a preterm birth.

---

of antiphospholipid syndrome, anticardiolipin antibodies and lupus anticoagulant antibodies as well as the presence of structural abnormalities.

Tests for preterm labour

No risk assessment tool has proved effective in lowering the incidence of PTL. The most common clinical tests used to determine the risk of PTL are transvaginal ultrasonography (TVS) to measure the length of the endocervix (the shorter the cervix the greater the risk of PTL and birth), and the cervicovaginal fibronectin (fFn) test. Among women with *symptoms* of PTL, cervicovaginal fibronectin appears to be the most effective predictor of PTL (Haram et al 2003). In early pregnancy, fibronectin is normally found in cervicovaginal fluid but after 22 weeks it can no longer be found in normal vaginal secretions. It reappears two weeks before the onset of either preterm or term labour. Unfortunately, neither the fFn test nor TVS has proved its clinical usefulness as a *predictor* of PTL. Although there does not seem to be a role for either of these two procedures as routine screening tests for PTL, both have high negative predictive values and are useful in that they may help to prevent unnecessary intervention and family stress. A negative fFn means that there is a 95% probability that a woman will not begin labour for the next 7–10 days. This finding may provide the woman and her caregivers with the confidence to stay in her community and support for a decision not to commence immediate tocolytic therapy or administer corticosteroids to mature fetal lungs.

Signs of preterm labour

Accurate diagnosis of PTL is difficult. McNamara (2003, p 80) makes the point that 50% of women diagnosed with PTL do not go on to have a preterm birth. In the past this has been attributed to 'false' labour or an 'incorrect' diagnosis but this may not be the case. An alternative explanation is that 50% of PTLs do not result in preterm birth, which, as McNamara (2003) says, is a completely different issue.

Many of the early signs of PTL are common in normal pregnancy. They include:

● abdominal pain or increased painful or painless uterine contractions
● dull, low back pain
● painful menstrual-like cramps
● vaginal bleeding
● change in character of or increased vaginal discharge
● supra-pubic and pelvic pressure with a sensation of 'heaviness'
● urinary frequency
● diarrhoea.

Collaborative support

When a woman who has not completed 37 weeks of pregnancy reports any of the above signs, she needs to be referred to a hospital-based specialist medical team who will decide whether she is in 'true' labour. The diagnosis of PTL is usually made in the presence of four uterine contractions in 20 minutes plus the presence of cervical changes—dilatation and effacement. A sterile speculum examination is performed to estimate cervical length and dilatation, look for signs of bleeding or amniotic liquor and obtain endocervical swabs for microbiological examination. If possible, digital vaginal examination is avoided. A CTG trace is useful to identify the presence of uterine contractions, and to assess fetal wellbeing. Fetal tachycardia and reduced baseline variability are often the first signs of maternal and fetal infection, such as chorioamnionitis. Nevertheless, interpretation of a CTG trace at early gestation is difficult. Diagnostic data that can be used to guide management decisions are:

● complete blood cell count with differential and platelet counts
● urinalysis for microscopy and sensitivity to rule out urinary tract infection
● cervical, high vaginal and ano-rectal swabs for bacterial vaginosis, gonorrheae, chlamydia and *Trichomonas vaginalis*, to rule out infection
● fetal surveillance studies to determine signs of fetal compromise
● ultrasonography to determine biometry, fetal size, presentation, amniotic fluid volume, fetal anomalies, placentography
● Doppler studies of the umbilical artery
● fibronectin evaluation
● transvaginal ultrasound to determine cervical length.

Ongoing care and support in preterm labour takes place in collaboration with midwifery, obstetric and paediatric secondary/tertiary services. Management depends on gestation, the availability of neonatal intensive care unit (NICU), stage of labour, and evidence of complicating factors such as: cause of the preterm labour, viability of the fetus, presence of infection, state of the membranes, or maternal illness. Thus, if there is evidence of maternal or fetal infection, management centres on treating the infection and, if necessary, the administration of corticosteroids and tocolysis to inhibit labour so that the woman can be transferred to a Level III hospital with a NICU.

McNamara (2003, p 82) describes some of the critical issues concerned with PTL and maternal transport. She contends that the critical issue is the clarification of which team is 'sending' or 'receiving', and is responsible for the woman while she is in transit. McNamara (2003) makes the crucial point that the best location for a preterm birth is in a tertiary referral centre and the worst is in a transport vehicle en route to the hospital. The following factors influence decisions about when to transfer, how it will take place and where the woman will be transferred to:

- availability of NICU beds/neonatal care
- length of time before birth
- transfer time
- availability of space for the mother at a tertiary centre/ perinatal care facility
- fetal weight
- gestational age
- availability of two qualified transporting staff—one for the mother and one for the baby—should complicated delivery take place en route
- cervical dilatation—reassess immediately prior to transport; if the cervix is > 6 cm dilated, transport is generally not advised (McNamara 2003, p 82).

Inhibition of preterm labour

In up to 50% of women, uterine contractions will stop spontaneously and the pregnancy will continue to term without any medical treatment. Clinicians need to discern those in whom drug therapy (tocolysis) is warranted and whether it is the drug of choice. Tocolytic therapy can successfully, albeit temporarily, inhibit labour. Its main function is to delay labour for 24–48 hours to enable the woman and her fetus to be transferred to a suitable facility and to allow maximal effect of corticosteroids used to induce pulmonary surfactant in the fetal lungs. Generally, if the pregnancy is between 24 and 34 weeks gestation, and the baby has an estimated weight of > 2500 g, it is not recommended that uterine action be suppressed with drug therapies. After 34 weeks it is reasonable to let labour continue.

A wide variety of drugs are used to inhibit uterine activity in TPL, and some have significant side-effects. These drugs should be used if the fetus is not viable, or if fetal wellbeing is in jeopardy, or if maternal health is severely compromised, such as with an abruption.

β-adrenergic receptor agents

The most common β-adrenergic receptor agents are ritodrine hydrochloride, salbutamol and terbutaline sulfate. These

Scenario

It is afternoon, you are recently qualified and the only midwife on duty in a rural health centre about 40 minutes from the nearest maternity unit. A woman arrives at the front door exhibiting signs of advanced labour. It is her third baby and she says she is 32 weeks pregnant. You take baseline observations, and assess the strength, length and regularity of her contractions, which appear to be two to three minutes apart, becoming expulsive and strong. Abdominal palpation reveals a breech presentation, deeply engaged, with a fetal heart rate of 140–160 bpm. There are no signs of bleeding and the membranes are intact.

You inform the woman and her support persons of your findings and what you plan to do, also taking into account her birth plan, which is rather sketchy at this stage. You resist the urge to panic, ask an enrolled nurse to quickly telephone the maternity unit and a medical practitioner for consultation. He suggests that you perform a vaginal examination to determine the degree of cervical dilatation and, depending on these findings, transfer the woman to the referral centre. The hospital contacts the referral team for you. Vaginal examination reveals that the woman's cervix is 8–9 cm dilated with a well-flexed breech presentation at the ischial spines. Shortly afterwards she begins to push, shouting loudly, 'I can't stop!' even though you advise her not to. Quickly you prepare for birth, heating the room and checking resuscitation equipment.

She stands up, the membranes rupture and the baby births, with you gently supporting the buttocks once they come out, to prevent sudden birth of the head and the added risk of a tentorial tear. The baby is born with Apgar scores of eight at one minute and nine at five minutes; the baby is carefully wrapped, and nestled close to mum's skin to keep warm. A physiological third stage occurs after five minutes, with minimal blood loss, then you carefully examine the baby, noting indicators for gestational age and signs of respiratory distress.

The paediatric retrieval team phones to tell you it is ten minutes away. Documentation is completed and you accompany the family to the hospital.

Reflection

On reflection, what would you have done differently? In this situation, what are your legal and professional responsibilities? Are there particular learning points for you in this story?

Clinical point

Tocolytics are only of value in about a quarter of preterm labours.

drugs are well known for their side-effects: tachycardia and pulmonary oedema, palpitations, headache, skin flushing, hyperkalaemia, hypotension, rarely right-sided heart failure, hyperglycaemia, fetal tachycardia, hypoglycaemia and hyperinsulinism.

Calcium channel blockers

Calcium channel blockers prevent the entry of calcium through cell membranes, which inhibits contractions of the smooth muscle of the uterus. Nifedipine (Adalat®) in slow release is an effective oral tocolytic agent and increasingly popular tocolytic. Side-effects are less distressing than those occurring with the β-adrenergic receptor agents. Maternal tachycardia, headache and dizziness are the most common. One regimen involves an initial dose of 10 mg sublingually every 20 minutes for three doses and then 10–30 mg every six hours orally.

Magnesium sulfate

Magnesium sulfate ($MgSO_4$) acts as a uterine muscle relaxant, by substituting for calcium. It is as effective as the β-adrenergic receptor agents but without many of their distressing side-effects and is the first line of choice in the United States. A loading dose of 4–6 g is given intravenously, followed by a maintenance dose of 2–6 g/hr until uterine contractions cease or signs of toxicity appear. Signs of toxicity include respiratory depression, absence of deep tendon reflexes, severe hypotension and eventually respiratory and cardiac arrest. $MgSO_4$ crosses the placenta, leading to reduced baseline variability and making interpretation of a CTG difficult.

Oxytocin antagonists

Atosiban (Tractocile®) has recently been developed to avoid the side-effects of some of the other tocolytic drugs but it is more expensive than the β-adrenergic receptor agents. It acts as an oxytocin antagonist. Its clinical efficacy is yet to be determined. A typical regimen is: IV bolus 6.75 mg then 300 µg/min IV for three hours, followed by 100 µg/min IV for up to 18–48 hours. Side-effects are nausea and vomiting, headache, chest pain and dysgeusia.

Antimicrobial therapy

The relationship between infection (chorioamnionitis, bacterial vaginosis, Group B streptococcal infections as well as urinary tract infection) and PTL is well documented. Consequently the use of therapeutic and prophylactic broad-spectrum antibiotics has become popular in some centres. Randomised studies and two meta-analyses have demonstrated that in the presence of ruptured membranes, especially in mothers who have Group B streptococcal infections, antibiotic therapy prolongs pregnancy and reduces the incidence of chorioamnionitis, and postpartum and neonatal sepsis. In a review of the literature, Kenyon et al (2004) concluded that the administration of antibiotics after pre-labour rupture of the membranes (PROM) is associated with a delay in delivery and a reduction in maternal and neonatal morbidity. The findings are not so clear in the presence of intact membranes (King &

Flenady 2002). A review by King and Flenady for the Cochrane Database (2002) failed to demonstrate a clear overall benefit from prophylactic antibiotic treatment for preterm labour

Research activity

Coping with the stress of premature labour (Lowenkron 1999)

Preterm birth, the leading cause of perinatal morbidity and mortality in the United States, affects between 8% and 12% of all live births. Approximately 80% of preterm births are preceded by preterm labour. Significant progress has been made in the physical treatment of preterm labour; however, the psychological cost to women being treated needs further study. This study assessed the stress experienced by women treated at home for premature labour and to examine methods they used to cope. The theoretical framework was provided by Lazarus's model of Stress, Coping, and Emotion. A total of 50 women participated. Twenty responded to a questionnaire that included the Perceived Stress Scale (PSS) and the Ways of Coping Questionnaire only, 10 were interviewed only, and 20 completed the questionnaire and the interview.

Results: The women reported experiencing a moderate amount of stress. Their mean stress score was 26.75, just below the mean for the instrument (M = 28) and slightly less than the stress score of 27.52 reported by women experiencing a 'normal' pregnancy. Appraisal was assessed by analysing the data from the interviews. The women appraised their situation as both threatening and challenging. They described their emotional response most frequently as frustration because of fear concerning the pregnancy outcome, loss of control over their life, and inability to perform their usual roles of mother, wife and worker. The women reported on the Ways of Coping Questionnaire that they used strategies from three subscales to cope with the premature labour. Those subscales were Seeking Social Support, Planful Problem-Solving, and Positive Reappraisal.

Questions

After reading the abstract above, respond to the questions below as if you were explaining the study's findings to women attending childbirth parenting classes.

1   What is this study about?
2   How was the study done?
3   What were the results of the study?
4   What are its strengths and weaknesses?

When you have done that, ask yourself the next two questions:

5   What additional information do I need?
6   How can I use this study in my work?

with intact membranes on neonatal outcomes, and raised concerns about increased neonatal mortality in those infants who received antibiotics.

Midwifery support

The midwife's role in supporting women at risk of or in PTL is to administer the prescribed treatments according to local protocols, make ongoing regular assessments of maternal and fetal wellbeing, provide psychological and emotional support, and take appropriate action if labour continues, ensuring that the documentation is up to date. If labour does proceed, tocolysis will be discontinued and the labouring woman will be offered labour support, and pain relief if required, although narcotic drugs are not recommended because of the respiratory suppressant effect upon the preterm baby. Midwives need to take the time to provide psychological as well as physical support and education on the processes of labour, especially if, as is often the case, no childbirth preparation sessions have been accessed.

Continuous CTG is usually recommended to monitor fetal wellbeing during labour to detect fetal compromise, as the premature baby has less tolerance to stress and has an increased risk of hypoxia at birth. The midwife should carefully observe and assess the woman in PTL as the progress of labour may vary from that expected of a term baby, and specialist help including a paediatrician should be present at the birth. Timely preparations for receiving and transfer to the newborn unit after immediate resuscitation is required. Preterm contractions are not as easily palpated as those at term and the CTG monitor will not accurately indicate the strength of contractions, which depend upon maternal position. There is no evidence to support IV hydration unless the woman is already dehydrated. Nor is there any evidence to support bed rest either in hospital or at home if labour 'stops'.

There is still controversy over the type of birth recommended for preterm babies. Caesarean section is often advocated, to decrease fetal trauma associated with vaginal birth, but these assumptions have never been substantiated (Atalla et al 2000). Moreover, an elective caesarean does not reduce fetal mortality or morbidity if the presentation is cephalic and the delivery may lead to additional complications. Labour debriefing is advised following preterm birth for mother and family/whanau to reduce the likelihood of post-traumatic stress disorder and other potential postnatal psychological complications.

Operative birth

An operative or instrumental delivery is performed if it is necessary to expedite the birth of the baby. Chamberlain and Steer (1999) subdivide operative deliveries into abdominal methods (caesarean section) and vaginal assisted births (forceps deliveries and vacuum extractions). This section focuses on vaginal assisted deliveries. At present, both forceps and the vacuum extractor are in widespread use, although

there is some evidence that, as the rate of caesarean section continues to rise, the incidence of forceps deliveries declines (Patel & Murphy 2004). Controversy continues concerning whether and when to conduct operative vaginal deliveries and which instruments are best. Currently as many as 25% of women in industrialised countries have a vaginal assisted birth. Both forceps and vacuum extractors (Ventouse) are acceptable and safe instruments for operative vaginal delivery. While the procedures fall outside the scope of midwifery practice, it is important that all clinicians understand the indications for an assisted vaginal delivery, the risks and benefits associated with both, and the principles of management.

Forceps

The history of obstetric forceps is long and colourful. Sanskrit writings from approximately 1500 BC contain evidence of single and paired instruments. These were designed to deliver the baby only after it had died. The credit for the invention of the precursor of the modern forceps used on live infants goes to Peter Chamberlen (1575–1628), an English man-midwife. The family kept his invention a secret for more than 100 years and only his sons were privy to their design and use. Even when the design became public knowledge, their use was restricted to man-midwives (the forerunner of today's obstetrician) and were used primarily as a measure to save the life of the mother once the fetus was dead. In 1845, Sir James Simpson developed a forceps that was designed to appropriately fit both cephalic and pelvic curves. According to Patel and Murphy (2004, p 1302), there are more than 700 types of obstetric forceps. Three of the most common are Wrigley's, Simpson's and Kielland's, used for rotational deliveries (Fig 34.13 (b) to (d)). Each of the three main types (outlet, mid-cavity or rotational) is designed for specific clinical situations and requires different levels of expertise (Fig 34.13 (a)). The criteria for an outlet forceps delivery are that the vertex (the bony skull) is visible at the introitus and the sagittal suture is in the anteroposterior position of the pelvis. For a low (outlet) forceps application, the vertex must be at station +2 or more below the ischial spines but on the pelvic floor. The fetus must be lying in an occipitoanterior position. In a mid-cavity delivery, which often requires rotation of the fetal head, the head must be engaged in the pelvis and the vertex positioned at station +1 or +2. There is no place for a 'high forceps'—the biparietal diameter of the fetal head is above the pelvic inlet—in modern obstetrics.

Structure of forceps

Forceps have four major components (Fig 34.13 (b)):
- *blades*—this is the portion of the instrument that fits around the fetal head (each blade is curved so that it fits around the head)
- *shanks*—these connect the blades to the handles and are either parallel or crossing
- *lock*—this is the articulation between the shanks
- *handles*—these are for the accoucheur to hold when applying traction to the fetal head.

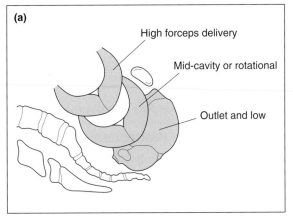

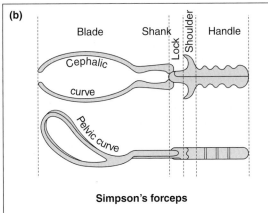

Simpson's forceps

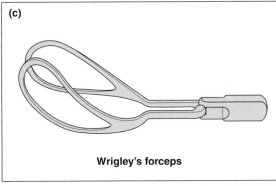

Wrigley's forceps

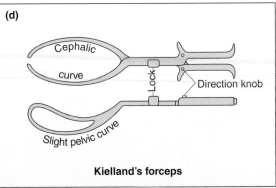

Kielland's forceps

Figure 34.13 Obstetric forceps. Top panel shows the station of the head when the forceps is applied (based on Oats & Abraham 2004)

Indications for forceps delivery

Indications for the use of forceps include the presence of any condition that threatens the wellbeing of the mother or fetus if she proceeds to a spontaneous vaginal birth. Absolute and relative conditions that put the woman at risk include:

- maternal:
  - need for prophylactic shortening of the second stage of labour (cardiovascular disease and hypertension, including severe pre-eclampsia)
  - pulmonary oedema
  - infection
  - neurological disease (spinal cord injury, myasthenia gravis)
- obstetric:
  - maternal distress and exhaustion
  - malposition of the fetus
  - forceps to the after-coming head in a breech birth
  - controlled delivery of the head in a caesarean section
  - cord prolapse in the second stage of labour
  - lack of advance of the fetal head in the second stage of labour
  - dense epidural block (ineffective pushing efforts in second stage)
- fetal:
  - signs of fetal compromise (non-reassuring fetal heart rate)
  - placental abruption in the second stage.

Contraindications

Contraindications for forceps delivery include:

- incompletely dilated cervix
- unknown fetal position
- station higher than +1 or > 1/5 palpable abdominally
- inexperienced accoucheur
- evidence of absolute CPD.

Prerequisites

Prerequisites for forceps delivery include the following:

- As with any invasive procedure, the woman must consent to the procedure.
- Adequate anaesthesia must be administered.
- The head must be engaged in the pelvis.
- The station, presentation and position of the head must be known.
- The cervix must be fully dilated.
- The amniotic membranes must be ruptured.
- The bladder should be empty.
- There should be no evidence of absolute CPD.
- Episiotomy may be performed.
- Adequate facilities and supportive elements should be available.
- The accoucheur should be competent in the use of the instruments and the recognition and management of potential complications.
- The accoucheur should be prepared to stop (i.e. to not 'force the issue').

Complications

The medical literature contains considerable information about the risks and complications of forceps delivery. Reports of maternal and fetal complications vary depending on the skill and judgement of the accoucheur. The most common are associated with increased perineal and vaginal trauma (Patel & Murphy 2004). Other maternal complications associated with forceps-assisted vaginal deliveries are:

● postpartum haemorrhage (third stage should be actively managed)
● intrapartum rupture of the unscarred uterus
● late complications, which are mainly related to injury to the pelvic support tissues and organs, often leading to faecal and urinary incontinence.

Evidence evaluating neonatal morbidity is inconsistent (Patel & Murphy 2004). Neonatal complications include:

● transient facial forceps marks, bruising, lacerations and cephalohaematoma
● facial nerve palsy (cranial nerve VII)
● skull fractures, intracranial haemorrhage with falx, or tentorial lacerations
● an increased incidence of shoulder dystocia.

Vacuum extraction (Ventouse)

A vacuum extraction is an obstetric procedure used to facilitate the birth of the fetus by applying suction to the fetal head (Fig 34.14). The indications for its use are mostly the same as for a forceps delivery. However, it is contraindicated in preterm births and malpresentations including a face presentation. Cups are available in various sizes. Some (Bird) are metal and the newer ones consist of a plastic or silastic cup connected to silastic tubing, which in turn is attached to a hand- or foot-controlled pump or wall-connected device that produces the negative pressure necessary to create a vacuum (approximately 60–80 kPa or 600–800 cmH_2O). The suction creates an artificial caput or 'chignon' as the scalp is pulled into the cup (Fig 34.15). It is important that the accoucheur ensures that no

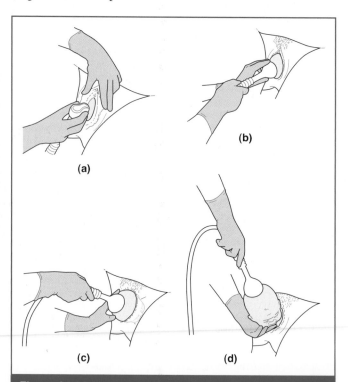

Figure 34.14 Ventouse extraction. **(a)** Application of the vacuum cup so that the centre of the cup is placed over the flexion point of the fetal skull (1 cm anterior to the posterior fontanelle) **(b)** to **(d)** With each contraction, traction is applied in a line perpendicular to the plane of the cup's ring. The fetal head is slowly lifted out of the vagina. Only two or three pulls should be required for the fetal head to birth. (based on Henderson & Macdonald 2004)

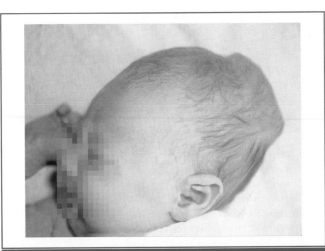

Figure 34.15 Baby with chignon (Henderson & Macdonald 2004)

vaginal tissue (if the cervix is not completely dilated) is caught by the cup. With maternal expulsive aid during contraction, the accoucheur applies traction to the fetal head. If there is no evidence of bony descent after three pulls, or if the baby is not born after 20 minutes, the procedure is stopped. Compared with forceps delivery, the vacuum extractor is associated with an increased incidence of neonatal cephalohaematoma, retinal haemorrhages and jaundice. Midwives should always remember that when the natural process and movements of birthing are disrupted, as with an instrumental delivery, there is always a higher risk of shoulder dystocia.

Mothers' perspectives on operative delivery

Most women anticipate a spontaneous vaginal birth in a joyous atmosphere, and so unexpected outcomes can often lead to disappointment and regret. Women's experience of birth determines their attitudes and feelings towards subsequent ones, and affects what they tell their daughters, friends and relatives. Murphy and colleagues (2003) (see Research box earlier) explored women's experiences of operative delivery in the second stage of labour. They explored how prepared the women felt for operative delivery, the perceived usefulness of their birth plan, their understanding of why operative delivery was needed, their views on debriefing after delivery, and their preferences for future pregnancy and delivery. Of significant interest to midwives is that while the vast majority had a good knowledge of the apparatus used for assisted birth, in more than 50% of cases this information was gathered from non-professional sources, such as magazines, books, friends, family and television. Most study participants made birth plans but these were poorly predictive of obstetric outcomes and, importantly, maternal satisfaction with their birth. The challenge is for midwives to ensure that in pregnancy, women are empowered to make informed choices about their care and that they have an opportunity to create realistic birth plans. Moreover, all women should be given the chance to discuss the events leading up to, during and after the birth. As one of the women in Murphy et al's (2003) study said, 'I'd like to have sat down and talked it through, but yes there are things that are left unanswered' (p 1134). Another said, 'The consultants came round but they never actually came and seen me' (Murphy et al 2003, p 1134).

Web activities

1 Use a search engine such as Google, PubMed or Ovid to research a specific complication discussed in this chapter.

2 Use the information you gain from these sites to help you create teaching–learning activities for the women you work in partnership with during pregnancy and birthing.

4 How might midwives help women view external cephalic version positively?

5 Describe the impact of selected interventions in labour on the childbearing woman and her support team.

6 How might a midwife support a woman dealing with a slower than expected labour?

7 Should women be offered fluids during labour? Provide arguments for and against. If a woman asks your advice on this issue, what will you tell her?

Review questions

1 How is the diagnosis of preterm labour made?

2 Discuss the advantages and disadvantages of forceps deliveries and vacuum extraction, including indications, procedures, complications and related midwifery support.

3 Discuss the advantages and disadvantages of amniotomy during a 'normal' labour.

8 What are the risks and benefits of vaginal birth following caesarean section (VBAC)? What information will you provide to a woman and her partner when asked about this procedure?

9 How do you describe the progress of labour? As an exercise, ask 10 of your colleagues how they recognise progress during labour.

Review questions—cont'd

10 You are asked to give a talk to a group of pregnant women about what to expect in terms of the progress or natural rhythm of labour.

Outline the main points you would cover and provide references to back up the points you make.

Online resources

American Family Physician, http://www.aafp.org/about.xml
Association of Radical Midwives, http://www.radmid.demon.co.uk
Australian College of Midwives, http://www.acmi.org.au/
Breech birth, evaluation of the term breech trial, http://www.
birthspirit.co.nz/
CESDI publications, http://www.cesdi.org.uk/CESDIpublications.htm
Confidential Enquiry into Maternal and Child Health (CEMACH),
http://www.cemach.org.uk/
Medical Journal of Australia, http://www.mja.com.au
New Zealand College of Midwives, http://www.midwife.org.au

References

Adair C 2000 Nonpharmacologic approaches to cervical priming and labour induction. Clinics in Obstetrics and Gynaecology 43:447–454

Albers L 1999 The duration of labour in healthy women. Journal of Perinatology 19(2):114–119

Albers L, Schiff M, Gorwoda J 1996 The length of active labour in normal pregnancies. Obstetrics and Gynecology 87(3):355–359

Alexander J, McIntire D, Leveno K 2000 Forty weeks and beyond: pregnancy outcomes by week of gestation. Obstetrics and Gynecology 96(2):291–294

American College of Obstetricians and Gynaecologists (ACOG) 2000a Evaluation of Caesarean delivery. ACOG, Washington DC

American College of Obstetricians and Gynaecologists (ACOG) 2000b Operative vaginal delivery ACOG Practice Bulletin No. 17. ACOG, Washington, DC

Atalla R, Kean L et al 2000 Preterm labour and prelabour rupture of the fetal membranes. In: L Kean (Ed) Best practice in labour ward management. WB Saunders, Sydney

Banks M 1998 Breech birth woman wise. Birthspirit Books, Hamilton

Bates C (Ed) 2004 Midwifery practice: ways of working in pregnancy, birth and maternity care. Feminist perspectives. Books for Midwives, London

Baxley E 2003 Editorial: Elective labour induction: a decade for change. American Family Physician 67(10). Online: http://www.
aafp.org/afp/20030515/editorials.html

Bishop E 1964 Pelvic scoring for elective induction. Obstetrics and Gynecology 24(2):267

Boulvain M, Stan C, Irion O 2005 Membrane sweeping for induction of labour. Cocharane Database of Systematic Reviews (1). CD000451

Broach J, Newton M 1988 Food and beverages in labour II: the effects of cessation of oral intake during labour. Birth 15(2):88

Cesario J 2004 Reevaluation of Friedman's labour curve: a pilot study. Journal of Obstetric, Gynaecologic and Neonatal Nursing 333:713–722. Online: http://www.jognn.awhonn.org

CESDI 2000 CESDI 7th Annual report: confidential inquiry into stillbirths and deaths in infancy. Maternal and Child Health Research Consortium, London

Challis J 2001 Understanding preterm birth. Clinical Investigations in Medicine 24:60–67

Chamberlain G, Steer P 1999 ABC of labour care: operative delivery. British Medical Journal 318:1260–1264

Clarke IJ 2002 Two decades of measuring GnRH secretion. Reproduction 59(suppl): 1–13

Cluett ER, Pickering RM, Getliffe K et al 2004 Randomised controlled trial of labouring in water compared with standard of augmentation for management of dystocia in first stage of labour. British Medical Journal 328(7435):314

Coates J, Smith K 2004 Reform of ACC Medical Misadventure. New Zealand Medical Journal 117(1201):U1050

Crabtree S 2004 Midwives constructing 'normal birth'. In: S Down (Ed) Normal childbirth, evidence and debate. Churchill Livingstone, London

Craigin E 1916 Conservation in obstetrics. New York Medical Journal 104:1–3

Crowley P 1995 Elective induction of labour < 41 weeks gestation. Cochrane Pregnancy and Childbirth Database (2). Update Software, Oxford

Crowley P 2003 Interventions for preventing or improving the outcome of delivery at or beyond term (Cochrane Review). Update Software, Oxford

Darwood M 1995 Pharmacologic stimulation of uterine contractions. Seminars in Perinatology 19:73–83

Diegmann E, Chez R, Danclair W 1995 Station in early labour in nulliparous women at term. Journal of Nurse Midwifery 40(4):382–385

Dizon-Townson D, Ward K 1997 The genetics of labour. Clinical Obstetrics and Gynaecology 40:479–484

Downe S, McCourt C 2004 From being to becoming: reconstructing childbirth knowledge. In: S Downe (Ed) Normal childbirth, evidence and debate. Churchill Livingstone, London

Edelestone D (Ed) 2000 Breech presentation. Best practice in labour ward management. Saunders, Philadelphia

Enkin M, Keirse M, Neilson J et al 2000 A guide to effective care in pregnancy and childbirth. Oxford University Press, New York

Flannelly G, Turner M, Rassmussen M et al 1993 Rupture of the uterus in Dublin. Journal of Obstetrics and Gynaecology 13:440–443

Fraser D, Cooper M 2003 Myles textbook for midwives (14th edn). Churchill Livingstone, London

Fraser W, Turcot L, Kraus I et al 1999 Amniotomy for shortening spontaneous labour. Cochrane Database of Systematic Reviews (4). Art. No.: CD000015. DOI:10.1002/14651858.CD000015

Friedman E 1954 Graphic analysis of labour. American Journal of Obstetrics and Gynecology 68:1568–1575

Frigoletto F, Lieberman E, Lang J et al 1995 A clinical trial of the active management of labour. New England Journal of Medicine 33:745–750

Gilbert E, Harmon S 2003 Manual of high risk pregnancy and birth. Mosby, St Louis

Gross M, Drobnic S, Keirse M et al 2005 Influence of fixed and time-dependent factors on duration of normal first stage labour. Birth 32(1):27–33

Guinn D, Goepfert A, Christine M et al 2000 Extra-amniotic saline, laminaria, or prostaglandin E_2 gel for labour induction with unfavourable cervix: a randomised controlled trial. Obstetrics and Gynecology 96:106–112

Guise J, McDonagh M, Osterweil P et al 2004 Systematic review of the incidence and consequences of uterine rupture on women with previous Caesarean section. British Medical Journal 329:1–7

Hall J, Taylor M 2004 Birth and spirituality. In: S Downe (Ed) Normal childbirth: evidence and debate. Churchill Livingstone, London

Halmesmäki E 2001 Vaginal term breech delivery: a time for reappraisal? Acta Obstetrica et Gynecologica Scandinavica 80(3):180

Hannah M, Hannah W, Hewson S et al 2000 Planned Caesarean section versus planned vaginal birth for breech presentation at term: a randomised multicentre trial. Term Breech Collaborative Group. Lancet 367:1375–1383

Haram K, Helge-Mortensen J, Wollen A 2003 Preterm delivery: an overview. Acta Obstetrica et Gynecologica Scandinavica 82:687–704

Henderson C, Macdonald S 2004 Mayes' midwifery (13th edn). Baillière Tindall, London

Hildingson I, Radestad I, Rubertson C et al 2002 Few women wish to be delivered by Caesarean section. British Journal of Obstetrics and Gynaecology 109:618–623

Hodnett E 2003 Is the hospital culture a major risk factor for abnormal labour and birth? Key note address. First Normal Birth Conference, Lancashire, England, October 2003

Hofberg K, Brockington I 2000 Tokophobia: an unreasoning dread of childbirth. A series of 26 cases. British Journal of Psychiatry 176:83–85

Hofmeyr G 2002 External cephalic version for breech presentation before term (Cochrane Review). Update Software, Oxford

Hofmeyr G, Hannah M 2002 Planned Caesarean section for term breech delivery (Cochrane Review). Update Software, Oxford

Hofmeyr G, Kulier R 2000 External cephalic version for breech presentation. Cochrane Database of Systematic Reviews (4). Update Software, Oxford

Hunter J 2002 Being with woman: a guiding concept for the care of labouring women. Journal of Obstetric Gynaecology and Neonatal Nursing 31:650–657

Kariminia A, Chamberlain M, Keogh J et al 2004 Randomised controlled trial of effect of hands and knees posturing on incidence of occiput posterior position at birth. British Medical Journal 328(7438):490. Online: http://bmj.bmjjournals.com/cgi/content/full/328/7438/490

Kavanagh J, Kelly A, Thomas J 2002 Sexual intercourse for cervical ripening and induction of labour. Cochrane Database of Systematic Review (2) CD003093

Kazzi G, Bottoms S, Rosen M 1982 Efficacy and safety of Laminaria digitata for preinduction ripening of the cervix. Obstetrics and Gynecology 60(4):440–443

Kelly A, Kavanagh J, Thomas J 2001 Vaginal prostaglandin (PGE$_2$ and PGF$_2$) for induction of labour at term (Cochrane Review).

Cochrane Database of Systematic Reviews (2). Update Software, Oxford

Kelly A, Kavanagh J, Thomas J 2002 Castor oil, bath and/or enema for cervical priming and induction of labour. Cochrane Database of Systematic Reviews (2). CD003099

Kelly K, Kwast B 1993 Epidemiologic study of vesico vaginal fistulas in Ethiopia. International Urogynaecological Journal 4:278–281

Kenyon S, Boulvain M, Neilson J 2004 Antibiotics for preterm rupture of the membranes: a systematic review. Obstetrics and Gynecology 104:1051–1057

King J, Flenady V 2002 Prophylactic antibiotics for inhibiting preterm labour with intact membranes (Cochrane Review). Cochrane Database of Systematic Reviews (4). CD000246. DOI: 10.1002/14651858

Klaus M, Kennell J, Robertson S et al 1986 Effects of social support during parturition in maternal and infant morbidity. British Medical Journal 2930:586–587

Konje J, Ladipo L 2000 Nutrition and obstructed labour. American Journal of Clinical Nutrition 72(suppl):S291–S297

Landon M, Hauth J, Leveno K et al 2004 Maternal and perinatal outcomes associated with a trial of labour after prior caesarean delivery. New England Journal of Medicine 351(25):2581–2589

Lau T, Lo L, Rogers M 1997 Pregnancy outcomes after successful external cephalic version for breech presentation at term. American Journal of Obstetrics and Gynecology 176:218–223

Liu D, Mukhopadhyay S, Arulkumaran S (Eds) 2003 Induction and augmentation of labour. Labour ward manual. Churchill Livingstone, London

Lowenkron A 1999 Coping with the stress of premature labour. Health Care of Women International 20:547–562

Marx G, Schwalbe S, Cho E et al 1993 Automated blood pressure measurements in labouring women: are they reliable? American Journal of Obstetrics and Gynecology 168(3 Pt 1):796–798

McNamara H 2003 Problems and challenges in the management of preterm labour. British Journal of Obstetrics and Gynaecology 110(suppl. 20):79–85

Midwifery Council of New Zealand 2004 Scope of practice. Online: http://www.midwiferycouncil.org.nz/main/Scope

Miller A, Rayburn W, Smith C 1991 Patterns of uterine activity after intravaginal prostaglandins E$_2$ during preinduction cervical ripening. American Journal of Obstetrics and Gynecology 165:1006–1009

Murphy D, Pope C, Frost J et al 2003 Women's views on the impact of operative delivery in the second stage of labour: qualitative interview study. British Medical Journal 327:1132–1135

Neggers Y, Goldenberg R, Clivers S et al 2004 Effects of domestic violence on preterm birth and low birth weight. Acta Obstetrica et Gynecologica Scandinavica 83(5):455

NZCOM 2004 New Zealand College of Midwives. Online: http://www.midwife.org.nz

NZCOM 2005 New Zealand College of Midwives. Online: http://www.midwife.org.nz

New Zealand Guidelines Group 2004 Care of women with breech presentation or previous Caesarean birth. NZGG, October 2004

New Zealand Ministry of Health 2004 Report of maternity, maternal and newborn information system 2002. Ministry of Health, Wellington

Newton C, Raynor M (Eds) 2000 Routine intrapartum care. Best practice in labour ward care. WB Saunders, Philadelphia

Norwitz E, Robinson J 2001 A systematic approach to the

management of preterm labour. Seminars in Perinatology 25:223–235

Oats J, Abraham S 2004 Llewellyn-Jones fundamentals of obstetrics and gynaecology (8th edn). Elsevier, Sydney

O'Driscoll K, Meagher D 1980 The active management of labour. WB Saunders, London

Olds S, London M, Ladewig P 2004 Maternal–newborn nursing and women's health care. Prentice Hall, New Jersey

Parker J, Napolitano P 2005 Brow presentation. eMedicine Journal. Online: http://www.emedicine.com/med/topic3274.htm, accessed 7 July 2005

Patel R, Murphy D 2004 Forceps delivery in modern obstetric practice. British Medical Journal 328:1302–1305

Philpott R, Castle W 1972 Cervicographs in the management of labour in primigravidae. The alert line for detecting abnormal labour. British Journal of Obstetrics and Gynaecology 79:592–598

Powell-Kennedy H, Shannon M 2004 Keeping birth normal: research findings on midwifery care during childbirth. Journal of Obstetric, Gynecologic and Neonatal Nursing 33:554–560

Sanchez-Ramos L, Olivier F, Delke I et al 2003 Labour induction versus expectant management for post-term pregnancies: A systematic review with meta-analysis. Obstetrics and Gynecology 101:1312–1328

Seitchik J, Castillo M 1982 Oxytocin augmentation of dysfunctional labour: clinical data. American Journal of Obstetrics and Gynecology 144:899–905

Seyb S, Berka R, Socol M et al 1999 Risk of Caesarean delivery elective induction of labour in nulliparous women. Obstetrics and Gynecology 94:600–607

Sherman D, Frenkel E, Pansky M et al 2001 Balloon cervical ripening with extra-amniotic infusion of saline or prostaglandin E_2: a double-blind, randomised controlled study. Obstetrics and Gynecology 97:375–80

Sjogren B, Thomassen P 1997 Obstetric outcome in 100 women with severe anxiety over childbirth. Acta Obstetrica et Gynaecologica Scandinavica 76:948–952

Smith C, Crowther C 2002 Acupuncture for induction of labour. Cochrane Database of Systematic Reviews (2) CD002962

Society of Obstetricians and Gynaecologists of Canada 1994 Policy statement: Canadian consensus on breech management at term. Journal of the Society of Obstetricians and Gynaecologists 16:1839–1858

Stables D, Rankin J 2004 Physiology in childbearing. Baillière Tindall, London

Stapleton H, Kirkham M, Thomas G 2002 Qualitative study of evidence-based leaflets in maternity care. British Medical Journal 324:639–643

Takahashi K, Suzuki K 1982 Incidence and significance of the unengaged fetal head in nulliparas in early labour. International Journal of Biological Research in Pregnancy 3(1):8–9

Thornton J 1996 Active management of labour. British Medical Journal 313:378

Tiran D 2003 Baillière's midwives' dictionary. Baillière Tindall, London

Toppenberg K, Block W 2002 Uterine rupture: what every family physician needs to know. American Family Physician 66(5):823–828

Tranmer J, Hodnett E, Hannah M et al 2005 The effect of unrestricted oral carbohydrate intake on labour progress. Journal of Obstetrics, Gynecology and Neonatal Nursing 34(3):319–328

Varney H 2004 Varney's midwifery. Jones and Bartlett, New York

Walsh D 2003 We should go with the rhythm of labour. British Journal of Midwifery 11(11):656

World Health Organization (WHO) 1997 Care in normal birth: report of a technical working group. WHO, Order No. 19301104. WHO, Geneva

Zamorski M, Biggs W 2001 Management of suspected fetal macrosomia. American Family Physician 63(2):302–306

Zhang J, Troendle J, Yancey M 2001 Reassessing the labour curve. American Journal of Obstetrics and Gynecology 15(suppl. 6):71–72

CHAPTER 35

Interventions in pregnancy, labour and birth

Sally K Tracy

Key terms

dural tap, post dural puncture headache, acupuncture, admission trace, antenatal fetal surveillance, biophysical profile, birth asphyxia, blood patch, caesarean section (C section), cascade of intervention, caulophyllum, combined spinal and epidural block, electronic fetal monitoring, epidural analgesia and anaesthesia, fetal blood sampling, induction of labour, intermittent auscultation, intrathecal injection, intravascular injection, antenatal cardiotocograph, non-stress tests, non-reassuring trace, opioids, patient-controlled epidural analgesia, post-neonatal cerebral palsy, spinal block, subdural injection, umbilical artery Doppler velocimetry, unfavourable cervix, vaginal birth after caesarean section

Chapter overview

In both New Zealand and Australia, only about two-thirds of all childbearing women have spontaneous vaginal births. Even though we live in an age of evidence-informed practice, offering women many interventions for which the evidence is either nonexistent or very weak has become almost routine. The difficulty for student midwives is in separating practices based on sound evidence from those driven by opinion, authority, dogma, market or business principles, or other needs. This chapter will discuss common interventions in pregnancy, labour and birth in the light of findings from recently published research.

Learning outcomes

Learning outcomes for this chapter are:

1 To describe interventions in birth in relation to the normal physiology of birth

2 To explore the cascade of intervention in pregnancy, labour and birth, including the known benefits and harms of each intervention

3 To outline the aetiology of cerebral palsy

4 To explore how various interventions contribute to antenatal surveillance in pregnancy

5 To explore the use of electronic fetal monitoring and the cardiotocograph in labour, including indications and contraindications in relation to current evidence and best practice

6 To discuss the reasons for induction of labour in relation to the current evidence and best practice models, and to identify the outcomes associated with induction of labour

7 To outline the use of augmentation of labour

8 To describe the implications of epidurals and combined spinal epidurals for labour and birth

9 To explore indications and outcomes of caesarean section deliveries.

Introduction

Routine use of interventions during pregnancy, labour and childbirth is common in both Australia and New Zealand. These interventions include electronic fetal monitoring, epidurals, oxytocin, episiotomies, instrumental birth with either forceps or vacuum, and caesarean section.

Evidence is available to guide practice on a number of interventions during pregnancy, labour and childbirth, such as: restricting the use of episiotomy; promotion or discontinuation of active management of the third stage of labour; routine use of 10 units of oxytocin; routine amniotomy; continuous electronic fetal heart rate (FHR) monitoring; epidural analgesia; and use of oxytocin–ergometrine to prevent postpartum haemorrhage. However, there is no evidence for the routine use of many interventions and technologies such as electronic fetal monitoring, epidurals, oxytocin or episiotomies in women who have normal, uncomplicated pregnancies. Evidence does exist for alternatives such as intermittent auscultation of the fetal heart, non-pharmacological measures for pain relief, low-technology strategies such as walking and baths for comfort and stimulation in labour. Further evidence is required on how women cope emotionally with the consequences of labour interventions.

As confusing as this may seem, there are several other factors worth considering. Physiologists claim that a woman should not be removed from her safe environment for labour because this will invariably result in inhibition of uterine contractions. We are advised that the safest way to help labouring women is to 'respect nature and not to interfere with spontaneous events unless there is clear evidence that to do so would be beneficial' (Naaktgeboren 1989). However, there is an opposing view that labour might be best avoided altogether and women delivered routinely by abdominal operation (Hannah 2004).

Avoiding unnecessary intervention

There are two golden rules for midwives faced with the plethora of routine interventions found in most hospitals in New Zealand and Australia today:

● There must be a good reason for intervening in a woman's labour. This means that you must be able to describe and support with good evidence the 'clinical indications' that require you to do anything that would interfere with the normal physiological process of labour and birth. Then you must weigh up the evidence to show that the intervention you are about to undertake will not cause more harm than good.

● By supporting a woman fully with appropriate and adequate information, you will find that many unnecessary interventions can be avoided.

Much of the intervention that is routinely used in hospitals today evolved from the use of technology to 'save' mothers or babies when they were in distress during birth. 'Distress'

itself is a subjective term and now there are parameters—or measurements—that enable us to see whether or not a woman may need medical intervention. Figure 35.1 shows an 'intervention clock', which was presented in the journal *Birth* in 1991. Even though it is over 20 years old, it still resonates for many of us. Twenty years ago, Iain Chalmers described the need to intervene in pregnancy and childbirth in terms of a 'decision to intervene' clock: 'As you go around the clock … from unambiguous 'need' at 1 o'clock to 'commercial interests' at 11 o'clock, the factors that influence the decision to intervene become less and less defensible' (Chalmers 1991, p 137). Several published studies demonstrate that there is still a need to question the effect of non-clinical factors on the rates of operative intervention during childbirth (Carey 1990; Roberts et al 2000; Shorten and Shorten 1999).

There are two other influences that must be considered when addressing the rates and role of intervention in childbirth: the 'seductive' nature of technology, and the belief that all forms of intervention will avert or prevent an adverse outcome such as brain damage or cerebral palsy. Our technocratic society places great value on intervention and the use of machines and monitors, and as a result, midwives and obstetricians are confronted with an ever-expanding array of technologies, both reproductive and information-based, that have a significant impact on the level and nature of care provided.

Cerebral palsy

A major influence on the use of intervention was the belief until very recently that intervention in birth would be effective in preventing cerebral palsy (Blair & Stanley 1997). In some cases this may be so, but the birth prevalence of cerebral palsy

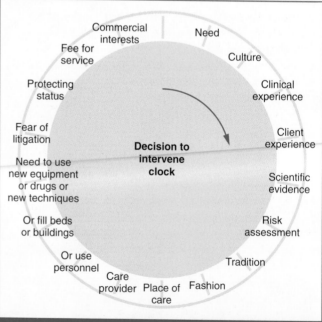

Figure 35.1 The 'decision to intervene' clock (based on Chalmers 1991)

in the developed world has not declined since the mid-1950s, in contrast to perinatal mortality. In developed countries, the majority of aetiological paths are likely to commence before labour and birth. Approximately 10% of cases are believed to now be causally associated with adverse intrapartum events. This is less than the proportion traditionally assumed to be due to intrapartum damage, and less than the proportion caused post-neonatally (after the baby is born) (Blair & Stanley 1997).

Cerebral palsy (CP) is a term of convenience applied to a group of motor disorders or motor impairment, stemming from a malfunction of the brain (rather than spinal cord or muscles). CP refers to brain malfunction that is non-progressive and manifests early in life. It is not a diagnosis, because it infers nothing about pathology, aetiology or prognosis. It is an umbrella term covering a wide range of cerebral disorders that result in childhood motor impairment (Badawi et al 1998).

In a study that reviewed data from the Western Australian Cerebral Palsy Register, three major areas were examined, to see:

- if the prevalence of cerebral palsy has fallen with increasing use of obstetric and neonatal interventions aimed at reducing birth asphyxia
- if there is any evidence that cerebral palsy is caused by birth asphyxia
- if there is any evidence that intrapartum fetal monitoring or caesarean section reduces the prevalence of cerebral palsy.

The study found that that:

- cerebral palsy proportions are not falling in spite of significant increases in obstetric and neonatal interventions aimed at reducing asphyxia
- cerebral palsy proportions in low birthweight infants are rising in most developed countries, coincident with increases in the neonatal survival of low birthweight babies
- few cases of cerebral palsy seem to be caused by birth asphyxia, and those that are may not have been preventable by obstetric care.

The study concluded that parents will continue to sue if obstetricians keep promising perfection from obstetric care in the face of 2.0–2.5 cases of cerebral palsy per 1000 children born (Stanley & Blair 1991).

In pregnancy, the risk of cerebral palsy is inversely associated with birthweight ratio (Blair & Stanley 1997; Palmer et al 1995). Researchers agree, however, that it is not low birthweight alone that increases the risk of cerebral palsy, but rather, birthweight in association with intrauterine growth restriction (Blair & Stanley 1997).

Primary antenatal causes of cerebral palsy are thought to be:

- intrauterine viral infections (Stanley et al 1986)
- iodine deficiency (Pharoah et al 1971)
- exposure to methyl mercury during pregnancy (Amin-Zaki et al 1979; Murakami 1972).
- maternal thyroid abnormalities (Blair & Stanley 1993).

More recent suggestions support a causal role for chorioamnionitis (Leviton 1993).

Some causes of poor growth may inte development, or it may be that a previousl fetus moves and grows less well (Blair Multiple birth is also strongly associated and the risk increases with the number of fetuses. Th cerebral palsy in twins of > 2500 g birthweight is about four times that of singletons of > 2500 g birthweight, suggesting aetiological factors specific to multiple gestation (Blair & Stanley 1997).

Intrapartum factors

Intrapartum factors producing hypoxia and/or trauma have traditionally been assumed to be the principal cause of cerebral palsy. This has, no doubt, contributed to the increasing use of obstetric intervention and is responsible for malpractice suits being brought against perinatal caregivers (Tito 1995).

Birth asphyxia is a poorly defined term relating to an exposure–response–outcome sequence initiated by hypoxia (Blair & Stanley 1993). Hypoxia is normal during vaginal delivery. For hypoxia to constitute asphyxia, it must have pathological effects. There is no definitive test for asphyxia (Blair & Stanley 1997). Recent studies suggest that:

- birth asphyxia may not be as important a cause of cerebral palsy as previously assumed; it may sometimes constitute one step of a multifactorial cause
- neonatal signs associated with birth asphyxia may be early manifestations of cerebral palsy from a variety of causes, of which birth asphyxia is only one
- most pathways to cerebral palsy commence before birth
- infants with evidence of damaging birth asphyxia may not have fared better with alternative obstetric care (Blair & Stanley 1997; Stanley & Blair 1991).

The risk of developing cerebral palsy appears to be elevated in infants:

- with Apgar scores 0–3 at 5 min
- with pH in the umbilical artery < 7.00
- with a base deficit in the umbilical artery < –16
- who develop hypoxic ischaemic encephalopathy (HIE) in the immediate neonatal period (MacLennan 1999; van Geijn 2005).

BOX 35.1   Birth asphyxia

Birth asphyxia is evident in a newborn baby who has had significant reduction in oxygenation or perfusion in utero and prior to birth. The clinical features are described in the clinical syndrome of hypoxic ischaemic encephalopathy (HIE). The measurement of hypoxic stress at birth includes:

- an umbilical blood gas of pH < 7.0 or a base excess of ≥ 12 mmol/L
- an umbilical arterial lactate of > 6 mmol/L
- a five-minute Apgar score of < 7.

The baby may have seizures or be in a coma together with multi-system organ failure (e.g. cardiovascular, renal, haematological, pulmonary).

Clinical point

Risk factors
Risk factors cannot be assumed to be causes, even when they do have a causal potential. Risk factors are markers that we interpret as needing further intervention or assistance.

BOX 35.2 Anti-D and cerebral palsy

A success story in the prevention of cerebral palsy
Anti-D immunoglobulin is now administered to Rh-negative women at risk of an Rh-positive feto-maternal haemorrhage. This prevents the possibility of maternal Rh isoimmunisation producing maternal Rh antibodies, which can cause kernicterus and choreoathetosis with deafness in a subsequent Rh-positive fetus. This anti-D injection has almost eliminated choreoathetosis with deafness in developed countries.
(Source: Blair & Stanley 1993)

Post-neonatal cerebral palsy

After birth, the causes of cerebral palsy (CP) are known to be infective, anoxic or traumatic, with septicaemia and meningitis accounting for the majority, particularly in developing countries. In developed countries, there is a greater variety of post-neonatal aetiology, with trauma accounting for up to 24% (including motor vehicle accidents and non-accidental injury), and cerebrovascular accident and postoperative causes accounting for up to another 25%. Because these are the most aetiologically obvious, they may also be the most preventable (Blair & Stanley 1997).

Interventions in pregnancy

Assessing the wellbeing of the fetus

Interventions to assess the wellbeing of the baby while it is in utero are intended to provide obstetricians and mothers with the best information about the optimum time for birth. Intrauterine growth restriction (IUGR) affects approximately 10% of pregnancies and is associated with significant adverse perinatal outcomes. Severe IUGR results from multiple causes, such as genetic syndromes, aneuploidy or congenital infections, and is thought to be the result of a 'compromised' placenta. When a placenta is not functioning optimally, there is a risk that the fetus will suffer from a lack of oxygen (known as 'placental respiratory failure' or 'fetal hypoxemia'). Obstetricians believe that the inherent risks of delaying delivery of the severely growth-restricted fetus include those of worsening hypoxia, long-term neurodevelopmental complications and even perinatal death. Antenatal tests of fetal wellbeing are performed with the intention of identifying severely growth-restricted fetuses with early signs of compensatory failure and fetuses who are most at risk for adverse outcomes. However, the optimal antenatal test to guide obstetricians about the timing of delivery for the preterm fetus with severe IUGR remains uncertain.

Fetal movements

Fetal movements (FM) are one of the first signs of fetal life and are an indirect measure of central nervous system integrity and function. Because of this, FM are regarded as an expression of fetal wellbeing (Olesen & Svare 2004). Pregnant women usually sense FM from 18 to 20 weeks of gestation in a first pregnancy, and at about 16 weeks of gestation in the second or subsequent pregnancy. As pregnancy proceeds, the weekly number of FM increases, peaking between 29 and 38 weeks of gestation (Olesen & Svare 2004). The movements are related to neuromuscular development and a normal metabolic state of the central nervous system of the fetus (Olesen & Svare 2004). A gradual decline in the total number of FM during the last trimester is suggested to be due to improved coordination and reduced amniotic fluid volume coupled with the increased fetal size (Rayburn 1990). On average, the fetus is active between 9% and 18% of the time in late pregnancy (Olesen & Svare 2004), or has movements of about 4 to 100 an hour (Mangesi & Hofmeyr 2004).

On ultrasound it can be observed that babies display chest wall movements that appear to be 'breathing' movements. During the last couple of months in a normal pregnancy, these 'breathing' movements may become irregular and have a frequency between 10 and 200 breaths/min (Adelson et al 1999). The complete absence of breathing is observed in some normal fetuses for up to 122 min (fetal apnoea), which indicates that monitoring of respiratory movements may require long observation time (Adelson et al 1999, Rayburn 1990). Women often report fetal hiccup movements that can be very intense, but there is no known pathology associated with this.

During the past decades, new methods for fetal assessment in various clinical settings have been introduced. Antenatal

---

BOX 35.3 Count to 10 method

Fetal movements in a day
In the 'count to 10' method of counting fetal movements, the woman is asked to count 10 movements from a specific time each day. She is advised to report whether the fetus takes longer than usual to achieve the 10 movements, or whether there are fewer than 10 movements in 12 hours. This is taken as a warning sign that the fetus may be becoming compromised.

When counting fetal movements at rest, a woman may be asked to empty her bladder, lie on her side, relax, put her hand on her abdomen and count the fetal movements over the period specified for the method used. Fetal movements may also be counted during normal activity.
(Sources: Bennet & Brown 1999; Mangesi & Hofmeyr 2004)

tests currently used to evaluate fetal wellbeing include the non-stress test (NST) or antenatal cardiotocogram (CTG), Doppler velocimetry (DV) and fetal biophysical profile (BPP). Earlier methods of detecting fetal wellbeing depended largely on the mother recognising fetal movements.

Methods of antenatal fetal surveillance

For each admission to hospital for birth in Australia, there are about 15–20 antenatal admissions (Adelson et al 1999). During these admissions, women very often undergo one or other of the following tests to ascertain fetal wellbeing.

Non-stress test (antenatal cardiotocography)

In the 1960s and 1970s, before the introduction of antenatal CTG, biochemical tests of placental or feto-placental function were widely used in high-risk pregnancies to try to predict, and thus avoid, adverse fetal outcome. Because the placenta provides nourishment for the baby in the uterus during pregnancy, it had been thought that testing women's hormone levels during pregnancy might show how well the placenta was functioning and whether the baby was growing as would be expected. A review of trials in the Cochrane Database found evidence that measuring oestriol levels in high-risk pregnancies did not affect the outcome of the pregnancy (Neilson 2003). Trials of antenatal CTG or non-stress tests were conducted in the early 1980s when the antenatal CTG was being introduced and at a time when biochemical tests were the benchmark of fetal monitoring.

The Cochrane Reviewers stated that:

> It is not possible to judge whether the CTGs would have been interpreted and acted upon as they would today. There have been no trials in recent years despite the CTG being used extensively in modern practice ... For high risk patients: A considerably larger study would be necessary to address the question of the effect of the antenatal CTG on perinatal mortality. Such a study is unlikely in the current environment, where the CTG has become an integral part of modern antenatal care (Pattison & McCowan 2003).

Antenatal CTG (or non-stress test, NST) has become widely accepted as the primary method of antenatal fetal monitoring in conjunction with ultrasound imaging and Doppler measurements. It has been used routinely to monitor post-term pregnancies, reduced FM, hypertensive disease, growth restriction and bleeding in pregnancy since its introduction in the 1980s. There is no doubt that clinicians and women are reassured by the findings of antenatal CTGs. They are able to record movements that the mother may not have felt. However, like many other interventions in pregnancy and labour, there is no definitive evidence for their efficacy. The Cochrane reviewers conclude that:

> on the basis of the information presented in this review the antenatal CTG has no significant effect on perinatal outcome or interventions such as early elective delivery. The suggested effect on reduced antenatal intervention is the main reason for the widespread current use of the CTG. The content of this review

neither adds to nor detracts from current practice where the CTG is used extensively to monitor the high risk pregnancy (Pattison & McCowan 2003, p 3).

Fetal biophysical profile

Although there have been no trials of antenatal fetal surveillance, and antenatal fetal surveillance has not definitively demonstrated improved perinatal outcome, the indications for antenatal testing should be considered somewhat relative. Conditions in which testing is usually advised include the following:

- maternal conditions:
  - antiphospholipid syndrome
  - poorly controlled hyperthyroidism
  - haemoglobinopathies such as thalassemia
  - cyanotic heart disease
  - systemic lupus erythematosus
  - chronic renal disease
  - Type 1 diabetes mellitus
  - hypertensive disorders.
- pregnancy-related conditions:
  - pregnancy-induced hypertension
  - decreased fetal movement
  - oligohydramnios
  - polyhydramnios
  - intrauterine growth restriction
  - post-term pregnancy
  - moderate to severe isoimmunisation
  - previous fetal demise (unexplained or recurrent risk)

BOX 35.4 The antenatal CTG

The antenatal CTG or NST is a continuous record of the FHR obtained via an ultrasound transducer placed on the maternal abdomen. The FHR, including variability, accelerations and decelerations, if any occur, is recorded electronically on a paper trace. Interpretation of the FHR pattern can be difficult.

A reactive (normal) CTG is deemed by two accelerations exceeding 15 bpm, sustained for at least 15 seconds in a 20-minute period (Pattison et al 2005).

Or

The NST is considered reactive, or normal, if there are two or more FHR accelerations within a 20-minute period, with or without FM discernible by the woman (ACOG 2000).

Reduced variability and the presence of decelerations are abnormal.

Various scoring systems have been devised to classify the CTG. Initial observational studies have showed a strong correlation between the abnormal CTG and poor fetal outcome (Freeman 1982; Phelan 1981).

Introduction of this test followed rapidly without supportive evidence of benefit from randomised trials.

(Sources: ACOG 2000; Freeman et al 1982; Pattison & McCowan 2003; Phelan 1981)

● multiple gestation with significant growth discrepancy.

The biophysical profile (BPP) usually includes ultrasound monitoring of fetal movements, fetal tone and fetal breathing, ultrasound assessment of amniotic fluid volume and assessment of FHR by electronic monitoring.

The BPP method of fetal assessment was derived, as a concept, from the Apgar score, which is used to assess the condition of a baby at birth. The method was introduced in the 1980s, again without substantial evidence from randomised controlled trials. However, substantial and extensive observational literature over the years suggests a link between low biophysical scores and poor pregnancy outcome. This has resulted in wide clinical use of BPP in the United States, Canada, Australia and New Zealand.

Preboth (2000) explains the BPP as follows:

> The biophysical profile consists of a non-stress test plus four observations made by real-time ultrasonography. The five components of the biophysical profile are as follows:
> 1 non-stress test
> 2 fetal breathing movements (one or more episodes of rhythmic fetal breathing movements of 30 seconds or more within 30 minutes);
> 3 fetal movement (three or more discrete body or limb movements within 30 minutes);
> 4 fetal tone (one or more episodes of extension of a fetal extremity with return to flexion, or opening or closing of a hand); and
> 5 determination of the amniotic fluid volume (a single vertical pocket of amniotic fluid exceeding 2 cm is considered evidence of adequate amniotic fluid).

Each of the components is given a score of 2 (normal or present as defined previously) or 0 (abnormal, absent or insufficient). A composite score of 8 or 10 is normal, a score of 6 is equivocal and a score of 4 or less is abnormal. In the presence of oligohydramnios, further evaluation is warranted regardless of the composite score.

During the late second or third trimester, the amniotic fluid reflects fetal urine production. Placental dysfunction may cause diminished fetal renal perfusion, which can lead to oligohydramnios. Therefore, assessment of amniotic fluid volume can be used to evaluate long-term uteroplacental function. The modified biophysical profile combines the nonstress test with the amniotic fluid index, which is the sum of measurements of the deepest cord-free amniotic fluid pocket in each of the abdominal quadrants, as an indicator of long-term function of the placenta. An amniotic fluid index of more than 5 cm is thought to be an adequate volume of amniotic fluid. The modified biophysical profile is considered normal if the non-stress test is reactive and the amniotic fluid index is greater than 5 cm and abnormal if the non-stress test is non-reactive or the amniotic fluid index is 5 cm or less (Preboth 2000, p 2).

Umbilical artery Doppler velocimetry

Doppler ultrasonography is used to assess the flow velocity waveforms in the fetal umbilical artery. Some clinicians also observe the maternal vessels supplying the placental intervillous space and (especially since the development of colour-flow imaging) other fetal vessels, including aorta and cerebral arteries (Alfirevic et al 1995). The study of the

---

TABLE 35.1 Components of the biophysical profile

Biophysical variable*	Normal score (score = 2)	Abnormal score (score = 0)
Fetal breathing movements	At least one episode of fetal breathing of ≥ 30 s duration	Absent fetal breathing, or no episode of ≥ 30 s duration
Gross fetal body movement	At least one episode of active extension with return to flexion of fetal limbs or trunk. Includes opening or closing of the hand.	Slow extension with return to partial flexion or limb movement without flexion or absent fetal movement
Fetal heart rate		
< 26 weeks	At least two episodes of ≥ 10 beat accelerations of ≥ 10 s duration	
26–36 weeks	At least two episodes of ≥ 10 beat accelerations of ≥ 15 s duration	Fewer than two episodes of accelerations and durations as specified
> 36 weeks	At least two accelerations of ≥ 20 beat accelerations of ≥ 20 s duration	
Amniotic fluid volume	At least one amniotic fluid pocket of 2 × 2 cm in perpendicular plane	No amniotic fluid pocket of 2 × 2 cm in perpendicular plane

*All parameters are examined in a 30-minute monitoring interval.
(Sources: Manning 1999; Preboth 2000)

umbilical artery has remained the most widely used approach, however, because less experienced operators can achieve highly reproducible results with simple, inexpensive continuous-wave equipment. Umbilical artery Doppler flow velocimetry has been adapted as a fetal surveillance technique because it is believed that flow velocity waveforms in the umbilical artery of fetuses with normal growth differ from those of fetuses with growth restriction. The umbilical flow velocity waveform of a normally growing fetus has high-velocity diastolic flow, while in cases of intrauterine growth restriction (IUGR), the umbilical artery diastolic flow is diminished. With extreme IUGR, the flow may be absent or even reversed. There is a high perinatal mortality rate among such pregnancies. It became clear from observational data that many of the fetuses with extremely abnormal waveforms had a poor outcome (Bricker & Neilson 2000). A meta-analysis published in 1995 (Alfirevic et al 1995) shows that assessment of umbilical artery waveforms by Doppler ultrasonography in high-risk pregnancies reduces the odds of perinatal death by 38% (CI 15–55%) (Alfirevic et al 1995).

A Cochrane Review of routine Doppler in pregnancy concluded that 'Abnormal waveforms from Doppler ultrasound may indicate poor fetal prognosis. The use of Doppler ultrasound in high-risk pregnancies appears to improve a number of obstetric care outcomes and appears promising in helping to reducing perinatal deaths' (Bricker & Neilson 2000). The review concludes, however, that although the study of umbilical artery waveforms helps identify the compromised fetus in 'high-risk' pregnancies, based on existing evidence, routine Doppler ultrasound in low-risk or unselected populations does not confer benefit on mother or baby. Future research should be powerful enough to address small changes in perinatal outcome, and should include evaluation of maternal psychological effects, long-term outcomes such as neurodevelopment, and issues of safety. Doppler ultrasound uses sound waves to detect the movement of blood. It is used in pregnancy to study blood circulation in the baby, uterus and placenta. Using it in high-risk pregnancies where there is concern about the baby's condition reduces the risk of the baby dying and the need for interventions around birth, such as caesarean section. However, its value as a screening tool in all pregnancies is limited by the rarity of complications, and the greater possibility of unnecessary intervention and adverse effects. A review of trials of routine Doppler ultrasound in pregnancy found that it does not improve the health of either the woman or the baby, and may do some harm (Bricker & Neilson 2000).

The techniques discussed here are the most commonly used interventions to monitor and study the growth and development of the fetus while is it is still in utero. Women whose babies appear to be at risk are often advised to have their labour induced in order to give birth to their babies early. Depending on how preterm or how growth restricted these infants are, they may stay for days or weeks in the neonatal intensive care unit (NICU) until they are strong enough to go home.

Interventions in labour

Electronic fetal monitoring

Electronic fetal monitoring (EFM) is defined as 'the use of electronic fetal heart-rate monitoring for the evaluation of fetal wellbeing in labour' (NICE 2003).

EFM was introduced with the aim of reducing perinatal mortality and cerebral palsy; however, systematic reviews of randomised controlled trials (RCTs) have not demonstrated their effectiveness to date (NICE 2003), and an increase in maternal intervention rates has been shown (NICE 2003).

Both the admission CTG and continuous EFM are the subject of widespread concern in midwifery. The student must discern, in collaboration with the woman she is caring for, what to do in practice.

This section will address the specific objective of reducing inappropriate or inadequate intrapartum fetal surveillance and reducing adverse perinatal outcomes, with special reference to:

- decisions relating to the use of admission CTG
- decisions relating to the use of EFM (both continuous and intermittent) or intermittent auscultation.

Admission CTG

The following statement is reprinted from the Royal Australian and New Zealand College of Obstetricians and Gynaecologists recommendations for the admission CTG (RANZCOG 2004).

> The admission cardiotocogram is a short, usually 20 minute, recording of the fetal heart rate immediately after admission to the labour ward. The most commonly heard rationale or routine justification for the admission cardiotocography is that the uterine contractions of labour put stress on the placental circulation and therefore an abnormal tracing might indicate a deficiency and hence identify potential fetal compromise at an early enough stage to allow intervention. Furthermore, a normal admission cardiotocogram offers reassurance. However, the incidence of intrapartum fetal compromise is low in pregnancies that have been uncomplicated before the onset of labour. Thus, labour admission cardiotocography may represent unnecessary intervention. In such low risk cases, confirmation of a normal fetal heart rate by Doppler auscultation should be sufficient (RANZCOG 2004).

The most important finding from a recent RCT of admission CTG by Mires et al (2001) is the increased rate of operative delivery in women who had admission CTG. Among women who were low-risk at admission, there was an absolute increase of 5.5% in operative delivery and 1.5% increase in caesarean sections. The increased use of continuous monitoring of FHR in labour in women who had admission CTG in this study is likely to be a contributing factor. This study has confirmed that among women with low-risk features at the onset of labour, the admission CTG is no better than Doppler auscultation of the fetal heart in identifying a potentially compromised fetus. Admission CTG was associated with increased obstetric intervention, including higher rates of operative delivery.

Although caution is needed in generalising conclusions to the whole population, the results point to potential problems with admission CTG. These problems are likely to persist while difficulties remain in interpreting CTGs.

The student is advised to watch very carefully for evidence to support the use of the routine admission trace for women with no other risk markers. There appears to be no substantial evidence for its use.

Continuous EFM

The assessment of fetal wellbeing is only one component of intrapartum care. It is an important area where due consideration must be given to maternal preference and priorities in the light of potential risk factors to both mother and baby, i.e. one that strikes the right balance between the objective of maximising the detection of potentially compromised babies and the objective of minimising the number of unnecessary maternal interventions. The provision of accurate information in these circumstances is essential to allow each woman to make the right decision for her (NICE 2001, p 35).

In the last century some asphyxiated babies were noted to have abnormally fast—or slow—heart rates, and auscultation evolved as a component of intrapartum care. The human ear is insensitive to subtle changes in rate, so electronic methods of recording were developed. These generate paper traces that show features not obvious on auscultation, including the degree of variation of the heart rate and the shape of accelerations and decelerations in rate. But more information is not necessarily more instructive, or we should judge textbooks simply by their size (Neilson 1993, p 347).

The use of continuous EFM for intrapartum fetal surveillance has now become entrenched in obstetric practice without robust RCT evidence to support it. The RCTs that have been undertaken confirm that the use of continuous EFM significantly increases the rate of operative delivery. To a certain extent, this can be minimised with the concomitant use of fetal blood sampling. No statistically significant improvements in long-term neonatal outcomes such as cerebral palsy have been demonstrated in these RCTs. Not surprisingly, concerns about maternal hazards and small or absent perinatal benefit have led some authorities to advise against the routine use of continuous EFM for low-risk labours (RANZCOG 2004, p 10). The NICE guidelines from the United Kingdom recommend that continuous EFM be offered and recommended for high-risk pregnancies where there is an increased risk of perinatal death, cerebral palsy or neonatal encephalopathy. They also recommend that continuous EFM be used where oxytocin is being used for induction or augmentation of labour.

Fetal heat rate monitoring is a highly complex task, often undertaken in a stressful working environment. It requires:
- a sound understanding of fetal physiological responses to hypoxia
- good pattern-recognition skills
- the ability to integrate this knowledge with each clinical situation.

In a review assessing the efficacy and safety of EFM, Thacker et al (2003) included nine trials of 18,561 pregnant women and their 18,695 infants in both high- and low-risk pregnancies from seven clinical centres in the United States, Europe and Australia. Overall, a statistically significant decrease was associated with routine EFM for neonatal seizures (relative risk (RR) 0.51, 95% CI 0.32–0.82). The protective effect for neonatal seizures was only evident in studies with high-quality scores. No significant differences were observed in one-minute Apgar scores below four or seven, rate of admissions to NICUs, perinatal deaths or cerebral palsy. An increase associated with the use of EFM was observed in the rate of caesarean delivery (RR 1.41, 95% CI 1.23–1.61) and operative vaginal delivery (RR 1.20, 95% CI 1.11–1.30). The authors concluded that the only clinically significant benefit from the use of routine continuous EFM was in the reduction of neonatal seizures. In view of the increase in caesarean and operative vaginal deliveries, the long-term benefit of this reduction must be evaluated in the decision reached jointly by the pregnant woman and her clinician to use continuous EFM or intermittent auscultation during labour (Thacker et al 2003). In the rare instances in which long-term outcomes of childbirth are measured, the findings are sometimes unexpected. Continuous electronic FHR monitoring in labour was associated with reduced neonatal convulsions, yet long-term follow-up in two studies showed a trend to increased cerebral palsy compared with the intermittent auscultation group (RR 1.66, 95% CI 0.92–3.0) (Hofmeyr 2004; Thacker et al 2004).

Following this review, Banta and Thacker (2002) concluded that:

> Our findings of insufficient evidence of efficacy and concerns about safety have been confirmed by subsequent research. Still, despite findings and recommendations of prominent professional and governmental bodies, EFM continues in widespread use in the United States and Europe and is spreading into developing countries around the world. Aggressive attacks on our assessment as well as our skills and integrity have been mirrored in recent years by criticism of other researchers in health technology assessment. The case of EFM points to the limitations of assessment without other actions to assure the implementation of results. Health technologies that are accepted by the majority of clinicians in a particular field may require extraordinary efforts to assure appropriate use of technology assessments (Banta & Thacker 2002, p 762).

EFM is a complex technology applied to monitor the fetus during labour and delivery. Introduced in the 1960s as an alternative to the traditional auscultation by stethoscope or fetoscope, it involves monitoring the FHR by either internal or external methods. The external method uses Doppler ultrasound. The internal method uses electrocardiographic leads attached directly to the fetus after rupture of the amniotic sac. Sampling of the fetal scalp blood during labour and delivery and testing it for pH (a measure of acid–base balance) complements the external and internal methods. EFM diffused rapidly into practice in the 1970s; it was used in the majority of deliveries in the United States by 1975. By 1976, when assessment of EFM began, it was already becoming controversial, but no systematic assessment had been carried out.

BOX 35.5 Monitoring a 'normal' pregnancy

Appropriate monitoring in an uncomplicated 'normal' pregnancy
Intermittent auscultation
For a woman who is healthy and has had an otherwise uncomplicated pregnancy, intermitten auscultation should be offered and recommended in labour to monitor fetal wellbeing.

In the active stages of labour, intermittent auscultation should occur after a contraction, for a minimum of 60 seconds, and at least:
- every 15 mins in the first stage
- every 5 mins in the second stage.

Continuous EFM
Continuous EFM should be offered and recommended in pregnancies previously monitored with intermittent auscultation:
- if there is evidence on auscultation of a baseline less than 110 or greater than 160 bpm
- if there is evidence on auscultation of any decelerations
- if any intrapartum risk factors develop.

Admission CTG
Current evidence does not support the use of the admission CTG in low-risk pregnancy and it is therefore not recommended.

(Source: NICE 2003)

BOX 35.6 EFM policy

Before any form of fetal monitoring is undertaken, it is always wise to palpate the maternal pulse simultaneously with FHR auscultation in order to differentiate between maternal and fetal heart rates.
- The date and time clocks on the EFM machine should be correctly set.
- Traces should be labelled with the mother's name, date and hospital ID number.
- Any intrapartum events that may affect the FHR should be noted when they happen on the EFM trace, signed and the date and time noted (e.g. vaginal examination, fetal blood sample, insertion of an epidural).
- Any member of staff who is asked to provide an opinion on a trace should note their findings on both the trace and the maternal case notes, along with date, time and signature.
- Following the birth, it is good policy for the midwife to sign and note the date, time and mode of birth on the EFM trace.
- The EFM trace should be stored securely with the maternal notes at the end of the monitoring prcess.

(Source: NICE 2003)

BOX 35.7 CTG settings

It is recommended that settings on cardiotocographs in institutions in Australia and New Zealand show:
- paper speed of 1 cm/min
- sensitivity displays of 20 bpm/cm
- FHR range displays of 50–210 bpm.

(Source: RANZCOG 2004)

TABLE 35.2 Categorisation of fetal heart traces

Category	Definition
Normal	A CTG where all four features fall into the reassuring category (see Table 35.3).
Suspicious	A CTG where features fall into one of the non-reassuring categories and the remainder of the features are reassuring (see Table 35.3).
Pathological	A CTG whose features fall into two or more non-reassuring categories or one or more abnormal categories (see Table 35.3).

(Source: NICE 2001)

Intermittent auscultation

In a pregnancy where there are no identified risk markers, the preferred method for assessing the wellbeing of babies is intermittent auscultation. This should be carried out in the following way:
- The FHR should be auscultated at specified intervals (usually every 15 minutes in the first stage and every five minutes in the second stage. This of course depends on whether the woman is comfortable with this arrangement.).
- Any intrapartum events that may affect the FHR should be noted, at the time that they happen, in the mother's notes and signed, and the time noted as usual.

Measuring lactate through fetal blood sample

The pH analysis is the standard technique of determining metabolic acidosis in the fetus during labour. However, it may be time consuming and there are difficulties in getting adequate samples, as a minimum of 35–50 mL is needed for most machines for automated analysis. Fetal blood analysis using lactate levels is comparable to pH in fetal scalp blood in predicting fetal compromise. The procedure for measuring

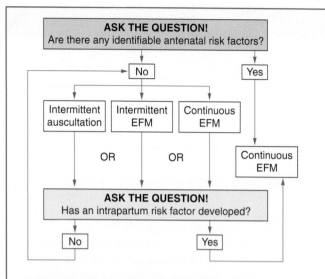

ASK THE QUESTION!
Are there any identifiable antenatal risk factors?

No   Yes

Intermittent | Intermittent | Continuous
auscultation | EFM | EFM

OR   OR   Continuous
                                    EFM

ASK THE QUESTION!
Has an intrapartum risk factor developed?

No   Yes

ANTENATAL RISK FACTORS

Evidence of fetal compromise, including:
- Abnormal Doppler artery velocimetry
- Abnormal antenatal CTG
- Suspected intrauterine growth restriction
- Oligohydramnios
- Prolonged pregnancy > 42°
- Multiple pregnancy
- Breech presentation
- Antepartum haemorrhage (significant)
- Prolonged rupture of membranes (> 24 hours)
- Known fetal abnormality which requires monitoring
- Prior uterine scar/caesarean section
- Pre-eclampsia (current pregnancy)
- Diabetes on insulin or poorly controlled
- Other medical conditions which constitute a significant risk of fetal compromise

INTRAPARTUM RISK FACTORS

- Induction of labour with prostaglandin/syntocinon
- Abnormal admission CTG (if performed)
- Oxytocin augmentation
- Epidural analgesia
- Excessive vaginal bleeding in labour
- Maternal pyrexia > 38°C
- Meconium or blood-stained liquor
- Oligohydramnios at amniotomy
- Active first stage labour > 12 hours (ie regular uterine activity, cervix > / = 4cm dilated)
- Active second stage (ie pushing) > 1 hour
- Abnormal auscultation

DISCLAIMER: *This algorithm is for general guidance only and is subject to a clinician's expert judgement. The algorithm should not be relied upon as a substitute for clinical advice.*

Figure 35.2 The Australian and New Zealand College of Obstetricians and Gynaecologists algorithm for fetal surveillance in labour (based on RANZCOG 2002)

lactate has been shown to be more successful than that for pH because the sample volume needed for this bedside analysis is 5 mL. Lactate analysis as an alternative for detecting acidosis is preferred in some centres because less blood is required and can usually be obtained with a single scalp incision and sampling attempt (Okosun & Arulkumaran 2005; Pennell & Tracy 1999).

Induction of labour

Induction of labour is one of the fastest-growing obstetric interventions in modern maternity care. In New Zealand in 2002, the rate of induction was 19.7% of all births recorded by the Ministry of Health (MOHNZ 2002). In the United States, the rate of labour induction has increased from 9.0% to 20.6%, for all births between 1989 and 2002 (a 129% increase since 1989). Australia has higher rates of induction than New Zealand and the United States (Martin et al 2002). In Australia in 2002, labour was induced in 26.6% of women and augmented in 19.2% of all births (Laws & Sullivan 2004). There is evidence that induction of labour may be efficacious where a pregnancy is well overdue and the woman is feeling anxious about being post term, or where the mother or infant is sufficiently ill to make continuation of the pregnancy hazardous. However, the recent rapid increase in induction, and particularly the doubling of the induction rate for preterm pregnancies in the United States (from 6.7% in 1989 to 13.4% in 1998), is cause for concern (MacDorman et al 2002).

In the Netherlands, the labour induction rates remained fairly constant at about 15% between 1993 and 2002, although large differences have been demonstrated in the frequencies of labour induction rates in Dutch hospitals even after adjustment for population differences (Elferink-Stinkens et al 1996; Rayburn & Zhang 2002).

Reasons for these differences relate to the widespread availability of cervical ripening agents, pressure from patients, convenience for physicians, logistic factors, psychosocial reasons and litigious constraint (Rayburn & Zhang 2002).

Indications for induction of labour are not absolute. Examples of maternal or fetal conditions that may be indications include:

- placental abruption, where the mother and baby are in danger if the pregnancy continues
- premature rupture of membranes, where the baby or mother are in danger of complications due to infection
- post-term pregnancy, when the mother or baby appear to be at risk
- medical conditions that are threatening the health of the mother or baby
- fetal compromise
- pre-eclampsia/eclampsia.

Better detection has identified pregnancies at risk. For example, borderline hypertensive disorders or an abnormally low volume of amniotic fluid are common indications for induced labour (Zhang et al 2002). It is difficult to precisely measure the effect of induction of labour in terms of cost, psychological effects and intrapartum procedures such as epidural analgesia, instrumental delivery or caesarean delivery. Research undertaken in New South Wales demonstrated the effect of a cascade of intervention associated with the

TABLE 35.3 Categorisation of fetal heart rate features

Feature	Baseline (bpm)	Variability (bpm)	Decelerations	Accelerations
Reassuring	110–160	≥ 5	None	Present
Non-reassuring	100–109 161–180	< 5 for more than 40 and less than 90 minutes	Early deceleration Variable deceleration Single prolonged deceleration up to 3 mins	The absence of accelerations with an otherwise normal CTG is of uncertain significance
Abnormal	< 100 > 180 Sinusoidal pattern ≥ 10 mins	< 5 for greater than or equal to 90 mins	Atypical variable decelerations Late decelerations Single prolonged Single prolonged deceleration > 3 mins	The absence of accelerations with an otherwise normal CTG is of uncertain significance

(Source: NICE 2001)

BOX 35.8 FBS guidelines

Classification of fetal blood sample (FBS) results

▶ pH > 7.25   FBS should be repeated if the FHR abnormality persists.

▶ ph 7.21–7.24 Repeat FBS within 30 minutes or consider operative delivery if rapid fall since last sample

▶ pH < 7.20   Operative delivery is indicated.

Note: All scalp pH estimations should be interpreted taking into account the previous pH measurement, the rate of progress in labour and the clinical fetaures of the mother and baby.

Contraindications to FBS

Contraindications include:

▶ maternal infection (e.g. HIV, hepatitis viruses and HSV virus)
▶ fetal bleeding disorders (e.g. haemophilia)
▶ prematurity (< 34 weeks).

Prolonged use of maternal facial oxygen therapy may be harmful to the fetus and should be avoided. There is no research evidence evaluating the benefits or risks associated with the short-term use of maternal facial oxygen theapy in cases of suspected fetal compromise.

During episodes of abnormal FHR patterns when the mother is lying supine, the mother should adopt the left-lateral position.

In cases of uterine hypercontractility in association with oxytocin infusion and with a suspicious or pathological CTG, the oxytocin infusion should be decreased or discontinued.

(Source: NICE 2001)

---

little is known about how women view the experience of being induced (Grant 2001). Responses to labour induction have varied from dissatisfaction with the entire birthing experience (Bramadat 1994) and mainly negative views (Out et al 1985; Salmon & Drew 1992; Salmon et al 1990) to a response where 80% of women reported that they would accept induction in any subsequent pregnancy (Nautila 1999).

What the Cochrane says

A Cochrane Systematic Review assessing the effects of interventions aimed at either reducing the incidence or improving the outcome of post-term pregnancy (pregnancies of more than 42 weeks that were otherwise 'low risk') (Crowley 1997) concluded that:

In health systems in which reliable early pregnancy ultrasound is available at an acceptable cost, it should be performed routinely and the expected date of delivery should be revised, to avoid unnecessary induction of labour for a mistaken diagnosis of post term pregnancy.

In health systems in which induction of labour is a safe and acceptable option, the question of induction of labour should be discussed with women after 41 weeks' gestation. They should be informed that about 500 inductions of labour may be necessary to prevent one perinatal death, and that there is no evidence that induction either increases or reduces the likelihood of delivery by caesarean section.

If the woman opts for induction of labour, the choice of method of induction should be based on evidence from randomized trials comparing the available methods.

Women or obstetricians who opt for conservative management should be aware of the lack of evidence to support the effectiveness of any particular method of antenatal fetal surveillance.

The implications for practice in developing countries are likely to be different. Access to early pregnancy ultrasound is unlikely, the cost of induction of labour with vaginal prostaglandins is likely to be unacceptable and any reduction in perinatal mortality must be viewed in the context of overall perinatal and maternal risks locally (Crowley 1997, p 2).

introduction of induction or augmentation (Roberts et al 2000) and further research demonstrated the incremental cost as interventions are introduced (Tracy & Tracy 2003).

Much emphasis has been placed on looking at clinical outcomes and the cost of different methods of induction. Very

Outcomes vary for women when they undergo 'cervical ripening' with pharmacological agents. Vahratian and colleagues (2005) found that women who had an elective induction with cervical ripening, indicating an unfavourable cervix, had a significantly longer latent and early active phase and a two- to three-fold increased risk of caesarean delivery compared with those with a spontaneous onset of labour. After controlling for potential confounders, women who had an elective induction with cervical ripening had 3.5 times the risk of caesarean delivery during the first stage of labour (95% CI 2.7–4.5), compared with those admitted in spontaneous labour. Elective induction without cervical ripening, on the other hand, was associated with a faster labour progression from 4 cm to 10 cm (266 mins compared with 358 mins, $P < 0.01$) and did not increase the risk of caesarean delivery, compared with those in spontaneous labour (Vahratian et al 2005).

The Cochrane Library also records the effectiveness (according to RCT evidence) of complementary therapies. In a review of acupuncture for induction of labour, the authors report:

> Acupuncture involves the insertion of very fine needles into specific points of the body. The limited observational studies to date suggest acupuncture for induction of labour appears safe, has no known teratogenic effects, and may be effective. The evidence regarding the clinical effectiveness of this technique is limited (Smith & Crowther 2004).

The effectiveness (measured by RCTs) of homeopathic methods is also reported in the following way:

> There is insufficient evidence to recommend the use of homoeopathy as a method of induction. It is likely that the demand for complementary medicine will continue and women will continue to consult a homoeopath during their pregnancy. Although caulophyllum is a commonly used homoeopathic therapy to induce labour, the treatment strategy used in the one trial in which it was evaluated may not reflect routine homoeopathy practice. Rigorous evaluations of individualised homeopathic therapies for induction of labour are needed (Smith 2003).

Epidural analgesia and anaesthesia

The popularity of epidural anaesthesia for childbirth is a relatively recent phenomenon. It blocks pain without rendering the mother unconscious. No other current drug or technique has that degree of selectivity. Epidural anaesthesia is also adaptable to the wide variety of pain patterns encountered during the course of a normal labour (Caton 2002). The character and neurological basis of childbirth pain change during the course of labour. During the first stage, the primary nerves mediating pain are small fibres of the sympathetic division of the autonomic nervous system. This pain is also known as visceral pain, mediated by the nerve fibres from T10 to L1 of the spine (Eltzschig et al 2003). Women typically perceive this pain as diffuse abdominal cramps, in phase with each uterine contraction. In contrast, pain of the second stage of labour is more continuous than rhythmic, sharper in character, and sensed in the perineum rather than in the abdomen or back. It is mediated by larger, somatic sensory fibres from sacral portions of the spinal cord (Caton 2002) mediated by fibres from S1 to S4 of the spinal cord (Eltzschig et al 2003).

Other types of pain may superimpose on the basic patterns described above. For example, when the head of the fetus is pushed hard against a large nerve against the posterior wall of the pelvis, the woman may experience intense pain in the lower back or in a discrete area of a hip or leg. If this pressure is prolonged or severe, it may result in temporary or even permanent nerve damage. A full, distended bladder may cause continuous suprapubic pain that may be confused with the pain of labour. Other patterns of pain may be caused by placental abruption or a ruptured uterus. An experienced midwife may easily evaluate the distribution and character of labour pain, but judging its severity may be far more difficult. Individuals respond to pain differently according to personal, familial and cultural factors (Caton 2002).

In Australia each year, about 125,000 women—51% of all women who give birth—experience either an epidural or a spinal block during labour (Tracy et al 2006). In the United States approximately 60% of women, or 2.4 million each year, choose epidural or combined spinal–epidural analgesia for pain relief during labour (Eltzschig et al 2003). In New Zealand each year, approximately 13,500 women, nearly 25% of all women giving birth, have an epidural (MOHNZ 2004)

Current popularity of epidurals

A study of women's attitudes to analgesia in labour between 1995 and 2001 found that the preference for epidural analgesia rose from 57% in 1995 to 66.5% in 2001, and the preference for opioids decreased from 31.5% in 1995 to 18.5% in 2001 ($P < 0.001$). The rate of epidural use in a previous birth rose accordingly, from 26% to 63%. The rates of satisfaction with the method used in previous births were similar in 1995 and 2001—about 30% not satisfied, 50% satisfied, and 20% very satisfied. The study found that in 1995, none of the women questioned opted for avoiding all kinds of analgesia, whereas in 2001, 8% did so. The research showed that women's attitudes to analgesia during labour changed during the six years of the study. Epidural block has become very popular, while

---

BOX 35.9 150 years on

One and a half centuries since Scottish obstetrician James Simpson expressed concern about the possible adverse effects of anaesthesia in 1847, saying, 'It will be necessary to ascertain anaesthesia's precise effect, both upon the action of the uterus and on the assistant abdominal muscles; its influence, if any, upon the child; whether it has a tendency to haemorrhage or other complications', it has become increasingly clear that potentially unwanted effects of analgesia for women in labour and their children cannot be determined easily.

(Source: Eltzschig et al 2003)

opioids lost popularity, and the number of women who prefer to avoid all analgesia during labour has increased (Horowitz et al 2004).

Mechanism of epidural and spinal anaesthesia

Labour pain is transmitted through lower thoracic, lumbar and sacral nerve roots, which are amenable to epidural blockade (Eltzschig et al 2003). Epidural analgesia is achieved by placement of a catheter into the lumbar epidural space or the space between the dura mater and the ligamentum flavum at spinal cord levels C7 to C10. The space is filled with loose adipose tissue lymphatics and blood vessels, and the solution tends to remain localised at the level where injected. The solution does not contact the spinal cord or the cerebrospinal fluid, so there is less risk of central nervous dystem infection than with a spinal injection. Postoperative urinary retention is common, as parasympathetic nerves are blocked (Bryant et al 2003, p 229). Solutions of a local anaesthetic, opioid or both can then be administered as intermittent rapid doses or as a continuous infusion. In the alternative technique of combined spinal–epidural analgesia, a single bolus of an opioid, sometimes in combination with local anaesthetic, is injected into the subarachnoid space, in addition to the placement of an epidural catheter (Eltzschig et al 2003, p 319).

In spinal anaesthesia, the local anaesthetic is injected into the cerebrospinal fluid in the subarachnoid space below the level of termination of the spinal cord—at about the level of L3–4 or L4–5. The needle and solution come into contact with the cerebrospinal fluid, necessitating strict aseptic techniques in order to prevent infections such as meningitis occurring (Bryant et al 2003, p 229).

The use of a subarachnoid bolus of opioids results in the rapid onset of regional anaesthesia with virtually no motor blockade. In contrast to epidural local anaesthetics, spinal opioids do not cause impairment of balance, giving the labouring woman the option to continue moving around (Eltzschig et al 2003). Some studies have suggested that there may be an increase in the frequency of non-reassuring patterns in the FHR, particularly bradycardia, with combined spinal–epidural analgesia, and such patterns may necessitate emergency caesarean delivery (Clark et al 1994; Eltzschig et al 2003; Gambling et al 1998). Other studies have demonstrated that regional analgesia during labour, compared with other methods of pharmacological pain relief, does not necessarily increase the risk of caesarean delivery (Sharma et al 2004; Segal et al 2000). Although there are insufficient data to establish whether there is a causal association, there are no studies that suggest that combined spinal–epidural analgesia is associated with an increase in adverse outcomes for the fetus (Eltzschig et al 2003, p 321).

For many years there has been debate about the efficacy of an epidural offered early in labour. There is a widely held opinion that having an epidural early in labour—before about 4–5 cm dilatation—increases the risk of operative intervention. However, in the United States, a recent large RCT of 750 women at term having their first baby who had a cervical dilatation of less than 4.0 cm were randomly assigned to receive epidural or systemic opioids at the first request for analgesia. The researchers showed that women who were assigned to 'early' regional analgesia had the combined spinal–epidural analgesia administered truly early in labour, in most cases at or near a cervical dilatation of 2.0 cm, whereas most of the women assigned to receive regional analgesia after a delay had a cervical dilatation at or near 5.0 cm when it was initiated. The primary outcome was caesarean section and the results show no significant difference between the two groups in the rates of caesarean delivery and instrumental vaginal delivery (Wong et al 2005). One of the alarming things revealed by the study is the rate of infusion of oxytocin. More than 90% of women in both arms of the study experienced augmentation or induction of labour (Wong et al 2005). The results of a French study undertaken at this time demonstrate that the placement of epidural analgesia when cephalic presentation is still 'high' is associated with a higher percentage of occiput posterior and transverse positions during labour, independently of other risk factors studied (Le Ray et al 2005). Lieberman and colleagues (2005), in studying the position changes of the fetus during labour, concluded that the consistently higher rate of instrumental vaginal delivery associated with epidural analgesia in randomised trials (Lieberman et al 2002) could result from an increase in abnormal fetal position complicating delivery. Use of epidural analgesia for pain relief has been consistently associated with a lower rate of spontaneous vaginal delivery (Howell et al 2001; Lieberman et al 2002; Roberts et al 2000, 2002). Almost all randomised studies have reported an increased rate of instrumental vaginal delivery, and a meta-analysis of randomised trials has estimated a two-fold increase (Leighton & Halpern 2002). The association of epidural analgesia with caesarean section is less clear and may vary across providers and institutions (Lieberman et al 2002; Roberts et al 2000, 2002). The reason for the lower rate of spontaneous vaginal delivery is not clear. It has been hypothesised that women who receive epidural analgesia are unable to push as effectively during the second stage of labour (Lieberman et al 2005). A large prospective cohort study undertaken by Lieberman et al (2005) found that epidural analgesia may contribute to an increase in the occurrence of occiput posterior position, representing a mechanism by which epidural analgesia may decrease spontaneous vaginal deliveries (Lieberman et al 2005).

Managing an epidural

Midwives will be guided in their management of the epidural by the policies and procedures of each institution. There are no hard and fast rules about epidurals—it is another area of practice that has evolved through expert opinion and received wisdom. As far as research-based evidence goes, there is very little to guide midwives in the best way to look after a woman who has requested an epidural.

This section outlines for the student some of the most commonly observed side-effects and the most commonly used techniques for managing epidurals. Figures 35.3 and 35.4 show the mechanism and the pathways affected by the epidural and spinal anaesthesia.

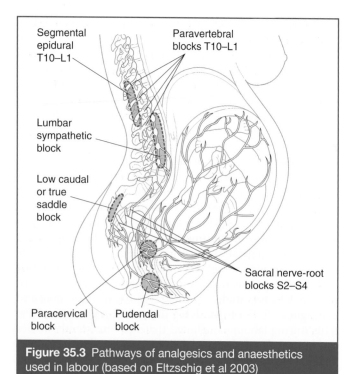

Segmental
epidural
T10–L1

Paravertebral
blocks T10–L1

Lumbar
sympathetic
block

Low caudal
or true
saddle
block

Sacral nerve-root
blocks S2–S4

Paracervical
block

Pudendal
block

Figure 35.3 Pathways of analgesics and anaesthetics used in labour (based on Eltzschig et al 2003)

Eltzschig et al (2003) describe the pathways of labour pain and its blockage as follows:

Labour pain has a visceral component and a somatic component. Uterine contractions may result in myometrial ischemia, causing the release of potassium, bradykinin, histamine, and serotonin. In addition, stretching and distension of the lower segments of the uterus and the cervix stimulate mechanoreceptors. These painful impulses follow sensory-nerve fibres that accompany sympathetic nerve endings, travelling through the paracervical region and the pelvic and hypogastric plexus to enter the lumbar sympathetic chain. Through the white rami communicants of the T10, T11, T12, and L1 spinal nerves, they enter the dorsal horn of the spinal cord. These pathways could be mapped successfully by a demonstration that blockade at different levels along this path (sacral nerve-root blocks S2 through S4, pudendal block, paracervical block, low caudal or true saddle block, lumbar sympathetic block, segmental epidural blocks T10 through L1, and paravertebral blocks T10 through L1) can alleviate the visceral component of labour pain (Eltzschig et al 2003, p 320).

Epidural analgesia [Fig 35.4 (a)] is achieved by placement of a catheter into the lumbar epidural space (1). After the desired intervertebral space (e.g., between L3 and L4) has been identified and infiltrated with local anaesthetic, a hollow epidural needle is placed in the intervertebral ligaments. These ligaments are characterized by a high degree of resistance to penetration. A syringe connected to the epidural needle allows the anaesthetist to confirm the resistance of these ligaments. In contrast, the epidural space has a low degree of resistance. When the anaesthetist slowly advances the needle while feeling for resistance, he or she recognizes the epidural space by a sudden loss of resistance as the epidural needle enters the epidural space (2). Next, an epidural catheter is advanced into the space. Solutions of a local anaesthetic, opioids, or a combination of the two can now be administered through the catheter. For combined spinal–epidural analgesia

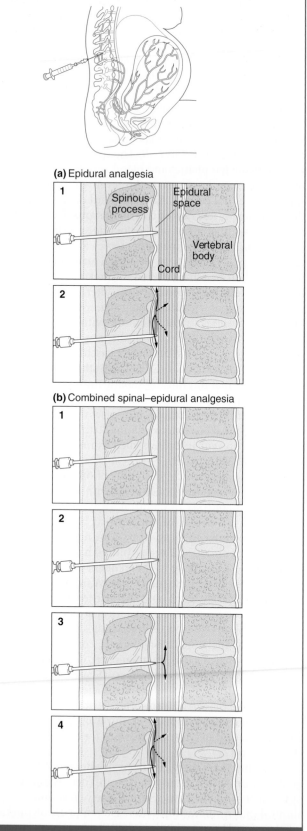

(a) Epidural analgesia

1 Spinous process   Epidural space   Vertebral body   Cord

2

(b) Combined spinal–epidural analgesia

1

2

3

4

Figure 35.4 Epidural and combined spinal–epidural anaesthesia (based on Eltzschig et al 2003)

[Fig 35.4 (b)], the lumbar epidural space is also identified with an epidural needle (1). Next, a very thin spinal needle is introduced through the epidural needle into the subarachnoid space (2). Correct placement can be confirmed by free flow of cerebrospinal fluid. A single bolus of local anaesthetic, opioid, or a combination of the two is injected through this needle into the subarachnoid space (3). Subsequently, the needle is removed, and a catheter is advanced into the epidural space through the epidural needle (4). When the single-shot spinal analgesic wears off, the epidural catheter can be used for the continuation of pain relief (Eltzschig et al 2003, p 322).

Siting an epidural or a spinal block

The method for siting an epidural or spinal block differs according to the practice of each anaesthetist. Women will be given instructions by the anaesthetist and the midwife is primarily called on to help position and attend to the comfort of the woman as she tries to position herself as directed by the anaesthetist. Depending on the stage of labour and the level of distress the woman is feeling, this could be a gruelling procedure for all concerned.

Additional interventions before placement of the epidural catheter

- Intravenous fluids are commenced prior to the introduction of spinal or epidural anaesthetics. This is to prevent the onset and effects of maternal hypotension. The most commonly used solutions include warmed (37.8°C) Ringer lactate solution IV before the induction of anaesthesia. The Cochrane recommendation for IV fluids (pre-load) is that 500–1000 mL of a non-glucose balanced sodium chloride solution may be administered 15 to 30 minutes before the procedure, to minimise the effect of hypotension. Glucose solutions are contraindicated because of the risk of fetal hyperglycaemia and rebound hypoglycaemia in the infant. A Cochrane Review of studies designed to assess the effect of prophylactic IV fluid preloading before epidural analgesia concluded that there may be beneficial fetal and maternal effects of this approach to minimising maternal hypotension (Hofmeyr 2000).
- If the woman is having an elective caesarean section, she may be prescribed an antibiotic prophylactic—this is not routine, although most hospitals have local policy and guidelines for these matters. The antibiotic most commonly prescribed is metoclopramide 10 mg and 10 mL/kg in the IV fluid. (Cochrane Reviews advise that the reduction of endometritis by two-thirds to three-quarters and a decrease in wound infections justifies a policy of recommending prophylactic antibiotics to women undergoing elective or non-elective caesarean section (Smaill & Hofmeyr 2002).)
- A urinary catheter is inserted. Before initiating an epidural, women should be encouraged to void because the sensation of a full bladder will not be felt after the introduction of intrathecal anaesthetic. Catheterisation ensures an empty bladder, preventing concerns about a full bladder impeding uterine contractility and the risk

of bladder trauma during surgery. There may be a lack of postpartum bladder tone, and therefore it is most important to keep an eye on this following birth or post caesarean section where a woman has had an epidural or combined epidural/spinal block. Urinary catheterisation poses an additional risk for the development of subsequent postpartum infection (Mayberry & Clemmens 2002).

- Some hospitals routinely offer oxygen, 6 L/min, administered through a transparent face mask.
- An electrocardiogram is attached to monitor the FHR continuously.
- A blood pressure cuff is placed (in a permanent position) so that the maternal blood pressure can be measured at two-minute intervals (using an automatic cycling device, if the hospital has one) and following insertion of the block; the maternal blood pressure is measured every five minutes.
- An oxygen saturation monitor may be attached to the woman (if the hospital has one) to measure the heart rate and peripheral oxygen saturation continuously.

Combined spinal and epidural block

The anaesthetist will perform a lumbar puncture at the L2–3 or L3–4 interspace with the woman in a sitting position. The dural puncture is usually made with a 27 G (may use a 29 G) pencil-point needle after the introduction of a Tuohy needle and identification of the epidural space. Once correct placement of the spinal needle has been confirmed by the aspiration of cerebrospinal fluid, 1.5–1.8 mL of 0.5% hyperbaric bupivacaine is given (varying with each woman's height: 1.5 mL for women under 1.65 m tall; 1.8 mL for those 1.65 m tall or taller and over 30 s). A 20 G epidural catheter is inserted 3–4 cm into the epidural space and secured in place with adhesive tape after withdrawal of the spinal needle, and the woman is positioned supine with a 15 degree left lateral tilt achieved by placing a wedge under her right hip. Uterine displacement by either lateral tilt positioning or wedging the right hip minimises the maternal–fetal effects of compression of the aorta or inferior vena cava. (Compression of the aorta or inferior vena cava decreases the blood return to the right side of the heart, which in turn contributes to maternal hypotension, which in turn contributes to a decrease in uteroplacental perfusion (Conklin & Backus 1999; Poole 2003).) If the block does not reach the T4 level after about 10 minutes, 10 mL of 0.25% plain bupivacaine plus 50 mg fentanyl (top-up) may be given epidurally in addition. The aim of this technique is to raise the level of spinal block to T8–9 by using low doses of local anaesthetic and to cause it to reach the T4 level by means of a low epidural top-up dose given in the next 10 minutes. There is not as yet any consensus about the nature of the mechanism by which the epidural top-up dose works (Karaman et al 2005).

It takes about 10 minutes to achieve a block using the combined method. If the woman is having an elective caesarean section, it may be about 15 minutes before surgery begins.

This description is one way of inserting a spinal epidural block. There are many variations—different anaesthetists will use different-sized needles and catheters, and different cocktails of anaesthetic.

Epidural block

The woman is placed in the sitting position and a lumbar puncture is made with an 18 G Tuohy needle at the L2–3 or L3–4 interspace. An epidural catheter is introduced, and 3 mL 2% lignocaine may be injected as a test dose. The epidural solution may consist of 16 mL 0.5% bupivacaine mixed with 100 mg Fentanyl. After an initial dose, an additional 2 mL 0.5% bupivacaine per unblocked segment may be given until a sensory block extending to the T4 level is achieved. It takes about 20 minutes to achieve a good block using the epidural (without added spinal) method, and for women having a caesarean section it may be about 25 minutes before surgery begins.

Once again, this is a description of one way of inserting an epidural block. Different anaesthetists and different hospitals will have different policies and protocols for anaesthetics and procedures. The midwifery student will always be instructed on what to do in assisting in this procedure. *Always* ask if you are in any doubt about any part of these procedures. Anaesthetics is a very complicated and potentially life-threatening business, and midwives are not permitted or expected to make any *autonomous* decisions concerning the insertion or safe maintenance of an anaesthetic. The midwife will always follow an anaesthetic policy or guideline on these matters. The midwife is always expected to safely monitor, report and document anything that she feels calls for consultation and advice.

Advantages of combined spinal and epidural blocks

Combined spinal and epidural blocks have become popular because they combine the rapid onset and intensity of a subarachnoid block with the facility of having an epidural catheter in place for follow-up intraoperative extension of anaesthesia, if necessary, and post-caesarean epidural analgesia. A spinal lumbar block requires a smaller amount of local anaesthetic to produce an effective block with complete muscle relaxation (Karaman et al 2005). The use of combined spinal–epidural analgesia (which involves the injection of minimal doses of medications directly into the spinal, rather than the epidural, space) has facilitated profound analgesia without concomitant motor block; moreover, the ability of women to ambulate while receiving this method of pain relief has added even greater flexibility to analgesic options (Camann 2005). The disadvantages of spinal lumbar anaesthesia, such as the risk of an extensive block, the fixed duration of anaesthesia, hypotension, and the risk of post-dural puncture headache (PDPH), have given rise to the use of epidural anaesthesia as an alternative method (Thoren et al 1994). In placing an epidural, the anaesthetist is able to target the exact level the block will extend to and maintain the block with supplementary doses. The catheter can remain in place for surgical anaesthesia and subsequently for postoperative pain relief. However, epidural

anaesthesia is more time consuming and involves a higher incidence of insufficient or superficial block, especially of the motor roots, despite the use of larger doses of local anaesthetic agent (Karaman et al 2005). The use of epidural anaesthesia for caesarean sections has been criticised because of the 25–38% rate of ineffective anaesthesia. It is difficult to obtain complete anaesthesia during this operation in pregnant women, because of the anatomical changes in the epidural space (Choi et al 2000). This is why fentanyl, epinephrine and $NaHCO_3$, with proven effects of potentiating the effects of local anaesthetics, are used to increase the efficacy of epidural analgesia (Choi et al 2000; Davies et al 1997; Karaman et al 2005).

Patient-controlled epidural analgesia

Patient-controlled epidural analgesia (PCEA) is becoming a more popular method for the administration of epidural anaesthetic because it allows the woman to control the rate of anaesthetic drug according to her needs rather than having to call someone to 'top up' the epidural. It differs from continuous epidural infusions in reducing the dose of local anaesthetic used. PCEA provides equivalent analgesia with lower anaesthetic usage, lower rates of supplementation, and higher patient satisfaction. Currently, there is no consensus on the most appropriate PCEA solutions, basal infusion rates, lockout intervals and demand dosing (Poole 2003). Threats to maternal safety, including hypotension, catheter misplacement, high blocks and respiratory depression, appear to be lessened with PCEA. Hypotension is more common following the initial placement of the epidural with the initial sympathetic blockade. PCEA maintains a more stable maternal haemodynamic status, and hypotension is rare, even after self-administered boluses (Paech 2000; Poole 2003).

Positions during labour with an epidural

After the insertion of an epidural, depending on the type, some women may be advised to move cautiously during labour (walking epidural). Other women may find the trailing leads of IV fluids, catheter bags and CTG leads too cumbersome to contemplate moving from a stationary position for the duration of the labour. A controversial area of management of epidurals in labour has to do with how long a woman remains in 'second stage' without pushing the baby out. Soo Downe and colleagues (2003) used an RCT to study the different positions women might best use for the second stage of labour with an epidural. Women are normally encouraged to sit up, to maximise the use of gravity in encouraging descent of the fetus (Downe et al 2003). However, the women randomised to the lateral position had a greater chance of a spontaneous birth, and of avoiding an episiotomy, than those randomised to the sitting position. The number-needed-to-treat calculation indicates that, for every five women using the lateral position (as opposed to the sitting position), one more experienced a normal birth, and one less an episiotomy. However, the 95% upper limit of 1.01 for the relative risk ratio implies that, for the population as a whole, there may be no advantage in the use of the lateral position in the context of epidural analgesia in labour (Downe et al 2003).

BOX 35.10 Common terms

Commonly used terms in analgesia/anaesthesia:

▸ *analgesia*—the use of medication to decrease or alter the normal sensation of pain

▸ *anaesthesia*—the use of medication to provide partial or complete loss of sensation with or without the loss of consciousness

▸ *combined spinal/epidural*—the simultaneous combination of both spinal and epidural anaesthesia

▸ *local anaesthetic agent*—a pharmacological agent capable of producing a loss of sensation in an area of the body

▸ *epidural (lumbar or peridural) block*—injection of an anaesthetic again with or without added opioid and/or epinephrine into the epidural space (lumbar spinous interspace between L4 and L5) as intermittent boluses or a continuous infusion

▸ *neuraxial analgesia*—administration of analgesic agents (local anaesthetic or opioids) either continuously or intermittently into the epidural or intrathecal space to relieve visceral pain

▸ *patient-controlled epidural*—a technique that allows the woman to self-administer a dose of epidural medication

▸ *regional (as opposed to general) anaesthetic*—the use of local anaesthetic agents to induce anaesthesia through the effect onto the spinal cord and nerve roots. Techniques include epidural, spinal, combined epidural and spinal. Obstetric regional generally refers to a partial or complete loss of sensation below the T8 to T10 level.

▸ *spinal anaesthesia (saddle block)*—an injection of an anaesthetic agent with or without added opioid and/or adrenaline into the subarachnoid space (lumbar spinous interspace between L4 and L5) as single-dose intermittent boluses or as a continuous infusion.

(Sources: Poole 2003a,b)

BOX 35.11 Commonly used drugs

Opioids

▸ *morphine*—crosses placenta rapidly; fetal effects dose and GA dependent; decreased FHR variability; maternal and neonatal CNS depression; inhibits oxytocin release and decreases uterine contractions

▸ *fentanyl*—potent respiratory depressant; cumulative effect with large dose over time; crosses placenta rapidly; excreted in breast milk

Analgesia/anaesthesia

▸ *provocaine/novocaine*—slow onset with short duration; one of the first ester local anaesthetics; poor spreading and penetrating properties; has been used for spinals but because of short duration is generally combined with another agent for labour

▸ *lignocaine/xylocaine*—relatively fast onset with intermediate duration; produces profound motor blockade; generally used for surgical block; 5% hyperbaric lignocaine may produce transient neurological symptoms involving lower back and extremities when used for spinal injections; crosses placenta rapidly; fetus and newborn can metabolise; elimination half-life in newborns is approx. 3 hrs; may produce CNS depression in newborn; small amounts excreted into breast milk but considered compatible with breastfeeding

▸ *ropivacaine*—moderate onset with long duration; less potent than bupivacaine; similar blocking properties to bupivacaine; intensity and duration of motor blockade shorter than that of bupivacaine when used for caesarean.

▸ *bupivacaine/marcaine or sensorcaine*—moderate onset and long duration; used for subarachnoid blockade for caesarean birth; duration and extent of blockade is dose-related; approx. four times as potent as lignocaine; duration is enhanced if adrenaline is added; accidental IV administration can cause acute cardiovascular collapse.

(Sources: Poole 2003a,b)

Side-effects of epidural and spinal anaesthesia

Side-effects of epidural and spinal anaesthetic in childbirth range from moderately mild to catastrophic. Lumbar epidural block provides safe obstetric analgesia and anaesthesia, but inadvertent intravascular, intrathecal or subdural injection are potentially life-threatening. There were four maternal deaths due to high spinal block reported in the Confidential Enquiries into Maternal Deaths in the United Kingdom, between 1982 and 1999 (Jenkins 2004).

The signs of catastrophic side-effects are described by Jenkins et al (2004) as follows:

● *Intravascular injection* is diagnosed when the woman complains of perioral paraesthesia, visual disturbance or tinnitus, usually following the test dose or an incremental dose of low concentration local anaesthetic. Intravascular injection of local anaesthetic may lead to convulsions, loss of consciousness and cardiac arrest.

However, these symptoms are frequently preceded by premonitory signs, such as minor auditory or visual symptoms and complaints of a metallic taste. Incidence 1 in 5000 epidurals.

● *Intrathecal injection* is diagnosed when injection of local anaesthetic, usually the test dose or an incremental dose of low concentration local anaesthetic, leads to a rapid onset of dense sensory and motor block with sacral involvement. Incidence 1 in 2900 epidurals.

● *Subdural injection* is diagnosed when injection of local anaesthetic leads to an unexpectedly high block, often asymmetric and involving the arms and face nerve roots. Subdural block is slower in onset than subarachnoid block, taking 15 to 30 minutes, and motor block and hypotension may be minimal or absent. However, it can also lead to life-threatening collapse with hypotension and apnoea. Incidence 1 in 4200 epidurals.

● *High or total spinal block* due to subarachnoid or subdural injection of local anaesthetic is diagnosed in the presence of a rapidly progressing motor and sensory block followed by respiratory paralysis requiring intubation, hypotension and loss of consciousness occurring within seconds to 20 minutes. High spinal block may occur after an apparently normal test dose. Incidence 1 in 16,200 epidurals.

Headache caused by 'dural tap'

A common and very unpleasant side-effect of an epidural is known as a 'dural tap'. Insertion of an epidural needle for obstetric epidural analgesia or anaesthesia is complicated by accidental dural puncture in 1 in 50–250 cases (Paech et al 2001), or a 1.5% risk of accidental dural puncture, with the rate among maternity units in the United Kingdom ranging from 0.19% to 3.6% (Baraz & Collis 2005). Accidental dural puncture is the most common major complication of epidural pain relief, and the headache following this complication can be very distressing and extremely disabling to the mother who is trying to nurse her newborn in the postnatal period. Following a dural tap, postdural puncture headache (PDPH) develops in at least 80% of women. Although serious, morbidity is rare, severe and prolonged headache is common, and the health care costs are enormous. According to Paech et al (2001), the Australian Patient Safety Foundation calculated that, based on an estimated 180,000 deliveries with a 33% epidural rate, a 1% incidence of dural puncture, inpatient costs of A\$500 per day and an additional hospital stay of three days, the penalty imposed on the national health budget exceeds A\$1 million per year.

As the use of epidurals is burgeoning, and the incidence of dural tap has not improved much, this poses a real cost to women and the health system. PDPH has implications for the mental and physical health of the mother. It often lasts several days, prolongs hospitalisation, and may be associated with auditory and visual disturbances, nausea and vomiting, and cranial nerve palsy.

The early or immediate headache that follows puncture with an epidural needle is attributed to the effects of rapid caesarean section and accidental subarachnoid injection of air (Paech et al 2001). PDPH usually presents within 24 hours. Despite a variety of definitions, most women report that PDPH after accidental dural puncture is severe. Many symptomatic therapies have been tried during expectant management, including systemic opioids, NSAIDs and cerebral vasoconstrictors such as caffeine. Epidural or systemic morphine appears to relieve established PDPH. Caffeine has been advocated, but has a weak and transient effect, is occasionally associated with postpartum seizures and is not widely used. Untreated PDPH after dural puncture is said to last six to eight days, but many patients remain symptomatic for weeks if untreated (Paech et al 2001). After several days of persistent PDPH, closure of the dural hole by a blood patch is advisable, to avoid not only chronic headache but also serious complications such as subdural haematoma or durocutaneous fistula (Paech et al 2001).

Inserting a blood patch

Contraindications to blood patch are fever and risk of bleeding.

The woman is usually placed in the left lateral position and the procedure carried out under strict aseptic conditions, including skin preparation and the wearing of mask, gloves and gown when identifying the epidural space, and mask and gloves when performing venipuncture.

Autologous blood is collected by the second anaesthetist and handed to the first, who injects slowly into the epidural space until 15–20 mL is delivered or a feeling of intense pressure or pain is reported by the woman. Women are advised to remain recumbent for two hours (Banks et al 2001). All patients are reviewed after the blood patch and discharged within a few hours. Patients are routinely informed that they should report back to the hospital if they have any concerns following discharge (Banks 2001).

Serious complications associated with epidural blood patch include lumbovertebral syndrome, arachnoiditis (thought to be due to injection of blood into the subarachnoid space via an intrathecally placed catheter), acute meningeal irritation, deterioration of mental status and seizures, subdural haematoma, acute exacerbation of PDPH and transient bradycardia (Banks et al 2001). The incidence of these events is unknown, but case reports are sporadic and infrequent. Nevertheless, because they may have serious consequences for the patient, such complications should be discussed when obtaining informed consent for a blood patch (Banks et al 2001).

Hypotension associated with epidural or spinal blocks

The incidence of hypotension among women having an epidural is between 0% and 50%, and hypotension is described as a maternal systolic arterial blood pressure either below 90–100 mmHg or a 20–30% decrease below baseline (Mayberry & Clemmens 2002). Blood pressure is carefully monitored in all patients receiving epidurals regardless of the technique or drug combination/dosage regimen. Maternal blood pressure should be assessed frequently (as often as every five minutes during the first 30 minutes and every 15 minutes thereafter with stabilisation, and then continued frequently throughout the remainder of labour). Each hospital will have a local policy for the management of fluids for women having epidurals. It is important for the student to be aware of local guidelines and standard procedures. A drop in blood pressure usually happens soon after the introduction of an epidural, but it is wise to continue monitoring during labour. The development of orthostatic hypotension when women move to an upright position or get out of the labour bed is also a potential risk for women receiving epidurals. Appropriate positioning to relieve potential aortal and inferior vena caval compression is necessary to minimise the risk of hypotension and the reduction of blood return to the heart, lowering of cardiac output and reduction of placental perfusion associated with recumbent positions in labour (Mayberry & Clemmens 2002). The lateral position is preferable to a supine position if there are problems with hypotension. If the hypotension persists and is not alleviated with positional changes after administration of an epidural, sometimes vasopressors may be required.

Overuse of electronic FHR monitoring has been an issue in obstetric care for at least the past five years, but the increased epidural rate is likely to be a primary reason for its continued use. Standard hospital protocols require that women be monitored using electronic FHR monitors throughout the duration of labour. One reason is that potential FHR changes in response to a decrease in uterine blood flow is a risk associated with maternal hypotension (Mayberry & Clemmens 2002).

Standard management of epidurals requires the woman to have IV fluid administration and regular monitoring. Blood pressure changes occurring with an epidural are associated with the blocked sympathetic outflow resulting in vascular vasodilatation.

Shivering

Shivering occurs in at least 20% of women during labour without neuraxial analgesia, and about 35% with epidural analgesia. Shivering can be distressing for women and can interfere with monitoring. Its impact can be minimised by warming IV fluids; and administering epidural fentanyl can reduce its incidence and severity (Karaman et al 2005).

It is curious that shivering is observed so often, because increased energy expenditure during labour presumably requires heat dissipation rather than heat production.

Physiologists believe that the shivering in labour is largely nonthermoregulatory, and the causes of these responses remain unknown (Panzer et al 1999).

Pruritus associated with epidural and spinal blocks

Epidural morphine is used widely for pain relief because it has a prolonged analgesic effect but it produces many side-effects such as pruritus, nausea, vomiting, respiratory depression and difficulty in micturition. Epidural morphine produces better analgesia than IV morphine, but more severe pruritus. The exact mechanism of pruritus is not clear; medullary dorsal horn activation may be related (Jeon et al 2004). The treatment of opioid-induced side-effects remains a challenge. From a systematic review of the side-effects of epidurals, Mayberry et al (2002) found that the incidence of pruritus among women who were given drug combinations containing one or the other opioids (with or without anaesthetics) ranged between 8% and 100%, with an average of 62%. The highest incidences were noted in study groups in which the highest doses of narcotics were administered. The incidence of pruritus within studies in which women were not given a drug combination including either fentanyl or sufentanil was 0% to 4%. The average length of discomfort was not specified in the studies, but most investigators reported symptoms of pruritus that were not considered severe enough to require treatment. Women who have 'fentanyl-only' epidurals experienced more widespread body distribution of pruritus than the other groups, in which only facial symptoms predominated.

Treatments for pruritus may consist of IV administered opioid antagonist or diphenhydramine. Effectiveness in terms of the extent of relief (i.e. complete or not) and how long the medications took to work are not known.

Nausea and vomiting

The risk of nausea and vomiting in caesarean sections performed under local anaesthesia depends on the technique used, the severity of hypotension, surgical stimulus, the woman's position, and any medications given. The incidence varies from about 30% to 35% of women who have an epidural (Davies et al 1997; Karaman et al 2005) and between 20% and 25% of women who have a combined spinal and epidural block (Davies et al 1997; Karaman et al 2005). The occurrence of this side-effect is lower when women have a block not followed by caesarean section. The average incidence of nausea alone is about 7.3% (Mayberry & Clemmens 2002) and the average incidence of nausea accompanied by vomiting is about 5%, with a range of 0% to 13% (Mayberry & Clemmens 2002). Severe nausea accompanied by vomiting may be an added risk for hypoglycaemia associated with prolonged fasting, particularly for women who have spent a lengthy period in the labour and delivery ward without food (Mayberry & Clemmens 2002).

Maternal and neonatal outcomes

Randomised studies show that compared with other forms of analgesia, epidurals are associated with increased length

TABLE 35.4   Explaining epidural anaesthetic risks to women

		Epidural complication
1 in 1	Something happens every time	
1 in 10	Something happening to one person in a family	Progress to instrumental birth
		Difficulty moving legs
		Itching
		Difficulty passing urine
1 in 100	Something happening to someone in your street	Headache
		'Failure' of epidural
1 in 1000	Death from smoking > 10 a day	Severe fall in blood pressure
	Death in car accident in your lifetime	Neurological injury from spinal
		Neurological injury from epidural
1 in 5000		Intrathecal injection
		Intravescular injection of local anaesthetic
1 in 10,000		Total spinal block
		Meningitis
		Nerve damage
1 in 15,000		
1 in 100,000	Being murdered	Spinal haematoma after spinal
		Spinal haematoma afer epidural
		Paralysis
1 in 1,000,000	Death due to the Pill	
1 in 10,000,000	Struck by lightning	Maternal death from anaesthesia
1 in 100,000,000	Something happening to someone in Europe	
1 in 1,000,000,000	Something happening to one person in the world	

(Source: adapted from Adams & Smith 2001 and Bethune et al 2004)

of labour, oxytocin augmentation, instrumental deliveries, perineal trauma and maternal fever/neonatal sepsis evaluation (Leighton & Halpern 2002). There is little evidence from randomised trials specifically about labour management among women with epidurals (Lieberman & O'Donoghue 2002). In 2005 research was undertaken in Australia to determine the association between epidurals and other interventions in labour and birth (Tracy et al 2006). The cascade of interventions that follows the introduction of an epidural indicates that interventions such as epidurals during labour and birth should have been evaluated more thoroughly before their 'wholesale' introduction into maternity practices. Women are very often given no indication of the rate of risk associated with having an epidural for pain relief in labour. Figures 35.5 and 35.6 illustrate the association between interventions such as oxytocic induction of labour with or without an epidural for labour, and the resulting use of forceps or vacuum instrumental birth or caesarean section. The data were derived from a population of women who had no risk markers for obstetric complications such as gestational hypertension or gestational diabetes, or pre-medical problems such as hypertension or diabetes noted during pregnancy. They represent the average healthy woman in Australia or New Zealand who is about to give birth, or has given birth in the past five years. The graphs show that when an epidural is used during labour, the rate of spontaneous vaginal birth falls, for first-time mothers and for mothers having a subsequent baby.

Side-effects for the baby

A recent meta-analysis (Reynolds & Seed 2005) showed that spinal anaesthesia for caesarean section is associated with a greater degree of fetal metabolic acidosis than is either general or epidural anaesthesia. The study concluded that although the limited evidence from randomised studies is a reason for caution, it is entirely consistent with that from non-randomised studies.

Many factors may influence neonatal acid–base balance at caesarean section, such as a direct effect resulting from placental drug transfer, or an indirect effect resulting from maternal physiological or biochemical changes. There are numerous aspects of management that may affect the baby indirectly, including IV fluid loading, the use of vasopressors, maternal position or uterine displacement, the presence and extent of sympathetic blockade, inspired oxygen concentration, skin incision and uterine incision, delivery intervals and previous use of sedative drugs (Reynolds & Seed 2005). The normal umbilical artery pH has been taken as ≥ 7.2 and the base excess as -10 to 0 mEq/L (Reynolds & Seed 2005); consequently, fetal acidosis is defined as umbilical arterial blood pH < 7.20 (Kansal et al 2005). Metabolic acidosis is a marker of anaerobic metabolism and hypoxia, but it does not identify, by itself,

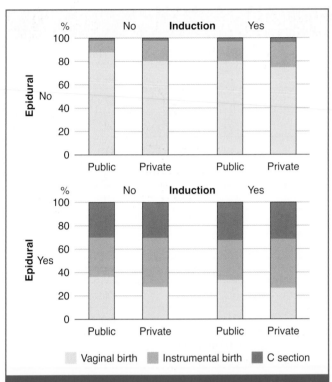

Figure 35.5 The cascade of labour interventions followed by birth interventions for primiparous women with medically uncomplicated pregnancies in Australia, 1999–2002, showing rates for women in public hospitals and women who had private health insurance. Interventions in labour are strongly associated with a falling rate of spontaneous vaginal birth and a rising rate of instrumental birth and caesarean birth (based on Tracy et al 2006)

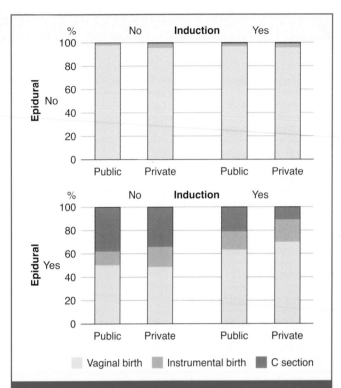

Figure 35.6 The cascade of labour and birth interventions for multiparous women with medically uncomplicated pregnancies in Australia, 1999–2002, showing rates for women in public hospitals and women who had private health insurance. As more interventions were introduced in labour, the rate of spontaneous vaginal birth fell and the rate of instrumental birth and caesarean birth rose (based on Tracy et al 2006)

newborn infants with a risk of long-term sequelae. Base excess measures or quantifies metabolic (non-respiratory) acid–base status (Reynolds & Seed 2005).

It is remarkable that spinal anaesthesia can induce a significant increase in fetal metabolic acidosis over the normally short time interval between administration of anaesthesia and delivery of the baby by caesarean section. Maternal blood pressure cannot be used as a surrogate for fetal outcome, as the changes may be too short-lived. Moreover, placental intervillous blood flow is dependent not solely on maternal blood pressure but also on maternal cardiac output and its distribution. It has been shown that spinal but not epidural anaesthesia is associated with a reduction in cardiac output even in the presence of a normal blood pressure (Reynolds & Seed 2005).

Breastfeeding

A dose–response relationship between fentanyl and artificial feeding was recently reported. When well-established determinants of infant feeding are accounted for, intrapartum fentanyl may impede establishment of breastfeeding, particularly at higher doses (Jordan et al 2005)

General anaesthesia

General anaesthesia is most likely to be used for a caesarean birth when there are no obstetric anaesthetists available to administer a spinal or epidural anaesthetic, or during an emergency, or if the woman has a contraindication to the use of regional anaesthesia. Pregnant women respond differently than non-pregnant women to the pharmacological agents used for general anaesthesia. Cricoid pressure may be called for to reduce the risk of aspiration of gastric contents. To reduce gastric acidity, an H_2-receptor antagonist, proton pump inhibitor, and/or metoclopramide and/or a clear antacid administered orally may be given (Poole 2003). Although maternal mortality from anaesthesia-related causes has declined since the mid-1980s (Poole 2003), anaesthetic-related deaths in Australia are still more likely to be related to general anaesthetic than to epidural or spinal anaesthetic (see Table 35.5).

Caesarean birth

There is a possible physiological explanation for the fact that epidural analgesia increases the likelihood of caesarean

TABLE 35.5   Leading principal causes of direct maternal deaths, Australia, 1973–1996

Direct cause of death	1973–1984		1985–1996		1973–1996	
	No.	MMR*	No.	MMR*	No.	MMR*
Pulmonary embolism	35	1.2	32	1.1	67	1.2
Hypertensive disorders**	36	1.3	23	0.8	59	1.0
Amniotic fluid embolism	22	0.8	19	0.6	41	0.7
Postpartum haemorrhage	18	0.6	11	0.4	29	0.5
Ectopic pregnancy	16	0.6	12	0.4	28	0.5
Infections	18	0.6	8	0.3	26	0.4
Anaesthetic complications	13	0.6	8	0.3	21	0.4
Ruptured uterus	14	0.5	4	0.1	18	0.3
All other causes of direct death	45	–	29	–	74	–
Total no. direct deaths	217	7.7	146	4.8	363	6.2

*Maternal mortality ratio per 100,000 confinements. **Includes pre-eclampsia, eclampsia and pregnancy-induced hypertension.
(Source: Sullivan et al 2004)

section. Lower-body muscle weakness resulting from epidural analgesia may inhibit normal fetal rotation and descent and maternal expulsive efforts, particularly when the epidural agent is administered in early labour (Camann 2005). Some retrospective observational studies have shown a higher incidence of fetal malpresentations among women who received an epidural analgesic during labour; particularly early labour (Eltzschig et al 2003). However, Wong et al (2005) report the results of an RCT of 750 primiparous women who had a spontaneous onset of labour and were offered opioids by a combined spinal–epidural 'early' in labour (at about 2.0 cm) compared with a control group who were administered analgesia at cervical dilatation of about 5.0 cm. The results

showed that there were no significant differences observed between the two groups in the rates of caesarean delivery and instrumental vaginal delivery (Wong et al 2005). Even so, the caesarean rate was 17.8% (65/366) in the intervention group and 20.7% (75/362) in the control group. In addition, the instrumental rate was 19.6% and 16% respectively, with over 90% of all women in the trial being augmented with an oxytocin infusion (Wong et al 2005).

Why caesarean delivery?

The rates of caesarean delivery continue to rise in Australia, New Zealand and the rest of the industrialised world. There is evidence that elective caesarean delivery is increasingly chosen by healthcare professionals and women. The rise in proportion of deliveries by caesarean does not seem to be explained by a change or increase in obstetric complications (Bell et al 2001). It is therefore of public health importance that the short- and long-term consequences of caesarean delivery are well understood and available to inform choice (Black et al 2005). There were 67,806 caesarean sections performed in Australia in 2002 (Laws & Sullivan 2004), representing 27% of all births in Australia for that year; and 22.7% or 12,053 of the 53,039 mothers who gave birth in hospital in New Zealand were by caesarean section (MOHNZ 2004). Collectively this means that, each year, more than 80,000 women are having major surgery when they give birth to a baby in our two countries. This represents a very large rate of morbidity in an otherwise healthy and strong cohort of women. In fact, for the year 2002 in Australia, less than 2% of all women had risk markers for a medical condition during pregnancy, and less than 10% had a previous obstetric complication such as gestational

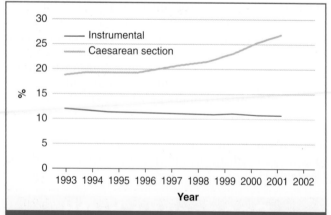

Figure 35.7 Rates of caesarean and instrumental births for women in Australia, 1993–2002 (based on Laws & Sullivan 2004)

diabetes or gestational hypertension (Tracy et al 2006). This means that less than 12% of Australian childbearing women have risk markers that suggest an intervention may be required. Why, then, has the rate of caesarean delivery climbed so dramatically in the past 25 years?

The explanations include a lower tolerance for taking risks; fear of malpractice litigation; increased use of epidural anaesthesia; increased use of EFM, which has a high false-positive rate for the detection of fetal hypoxia or acidosis; and physicians' convenience. It can be quicker to do a caesarean delivery than a vaginal delivery during a difficult labour. A couple's expectation of a perfect baby, as well as a woman's previous experience of a difficult labour undoubtedly play a part in the decision to perform a caesarean delivery. Epidural anaesthesia has afforded women relatively effective and safe analgesia during labour, but it may increase the risk of dystocia and therefore the frequency of caesarean delivery in primiparous women. In the absence of previous caesarean delivery, the reasons for selecting caesarean delivery as the method of delivery are complex and are influenced by factors affecting women, obstetricians and midwives. The literature describes a diverse range of factors influencing this decision, from fear of childbirth, potential for perineal injury, incontinence, sexual dysfunction and fear of fetal injury, to convenience and control (Wax et al 2004).

The evidence to support the relative safety of different surgical modes of delivery is complex, often controversial, and remains conflicting. Other than one trial of vaginal compared with caesarean delivery for term breech presentation, little evidence from RCTs exists to compare the safety of caesarean with vaginal delivery (Bell et al 2001). With the growing trend toward 'patient choice' or 'purely elective' caesarean deliveries, there is a need for better understanding of the risks of all forms of delivery, to enable informed consent (Black et al 2005). In countries where the age of first-time motherhood has increased—in countries such as New Zealand and Australia—caesarean section rates have increased with maternal age. In New Zealand in 2002, 36.1% (640/1774) of women over 40 years had a caesarean section, whereas only 13.1% (467/3568) of women in the 16–19 years age group had a caesarean section.

A similar phenomenon has occurred in Australia, where older first-time mothers are much more likely to have intervention in labour and birth (including caesarean section) than first-time mothers between the ages of 25 and 29 years (Tracy et al 2006). Women having their first baby between the ages of 35 and 39 years are three times more likely to have an elective caesarean section, and women aged between 40 and 44 years and having their first baby are eight times more likely to have an elective caesarean section than women aged between 25 and 29 years (Tracy et al 2006).

Although caesarean section rates have increased over the past 10 to 15 years, the major clinical determinants of the caesarean section rate have not changed (NICE 2004).

Lowering caesarean rates

In Australia, caesarean rates rose from the rate of 18.0% in 1991 (Lancaster & Pedisich 1994) to 23.3% in 2000, and 27% in 2004. This is similar to the rate in the United States, 26.1%, the highest level ever reported in that country (Martin et al 2004). Similar alarming rates are reported in the United Kingdom.

New Zealand has a significantly lower national caesarean section rate than Australia, and in particular the primary units (where women are attended mainly by midwives) in both New Zealand and Australia are showing extraordinary gains in lowering the caesarean section rate. This is also noted worldwide, and the NICE guidelines (2004) have an entire section on the lowering of caesarean section rates through birth in primary units, birth centres or outside hospital with midwives at home.

TABLE 35.6 Type of birth among New Zealand women, 2002

| Age group (years) | Normal birth (%) | Caesarean section | | | Operative vaginal birth | | | | Total (%) |
		Total (%)	Actue (%)	Elective (%)	Total (%)	Breech (%)	Forceps (%)	Vacuum (%)	
Under 16	77.5	11.6	10.9	0.8	10.9	0.8	3.1	7.0	100.0
16–19	78.0	13.1	11.2	1.9	8.9	0.6	3.4	4.9	100.0
20–24	76.6	15.0	11.2	3.7	8.5	0.6	3.2	4.7	100.0
25–29	69.8	20.4	13.7	6.6	9.8	0.6	3.8	5.5	100.0
30–34	63.8	25.4	15.5	10.0	10.8	0.6	4.5	5.7	100.0
35–39	59.8	31.4	17.0	14.5	8.7	0.7	3.7	4.4	100.0
40+	56.4	36.1	18.2	17.9	7.5	1.1	2.7	3.7	100.0
Total	67.7	22.7	14.3	8.4	9.6	0.6	3.8	5.1	100.0

(Source: MOH 2004)

Indications for caesarean section

The main indications for a caesarean delivery are:

- a prior caesarean delivery (accounting for 35% of all caesarean deliveries)
- dystocia or cephalo-pelvic disproportion (30%)
- breech presentation (12%)
- 'non-reassuring' fetal heart rate tracings (9%) (Black et al 2005).

The fifth most common reason given for performing a caesarean section has changed and is now reported to be 'maternal request' (7%) (NICE 2004).

Caesarean birth is the delivery of the infant through an abdominal and uterine incision. The method originated as a salvage procedure to rescue a child from a dying or dead mother. Technological and medical advancements have altered society's attitude towards caesarean birth from considering it a 'procedure of last resort' to an 'alternative birth method'. Nevertheless, it is a traumatic and often difficult decision for all concerned, and the risks and benefits of surgical birth should always be thoroughly discussed with each woman.

Shoe size, maternal height and estimations of fetal size (ultrasound or clinical examination) do not accurately predict CPD and should not be used to predict 'failure to progress' during labour. Although there are insufficient data on the morbidity of the mother and the baby to fully support the benefit of caesarean section over vaginal birth, the following reasons are usually given:

- Breech presentation—following the publication of the results of the term breech trial of Hannah et al (2000) in *The Lancet*, the rate of caesarean delivery for breech presentations has increased in all countries where this surgical option is available.
- Fetal distress—at some point during the progress of labour, a decision may be made to surgically intervene and deliver the baby to prevent the development of asphyxia.

Caesarean section 'on demand'

Michel Odent makes the observation, in his booklet on caesarean sections (Odent 2004, p 7), that at the end of the twentieth century, we were wondering whether it is ethical for women to 'demand' to have a caesarean section on request (without known medical indicators), and at the beginning of the twenty-first century, we are wondering whether all women should give birth by caesarean section! The phenomenon of elective caesarean section on demand began in Italy and in the largest Latin American cities (Behague et al 2002; Belizan et al 1999; Potter et al 2001) before the rest of the world (Odent 2004). There has been vigorous debate about the ethical and biological 'need' for women to have an elective caesarean section on demand. In Australia, several factors have influenced the prevalence of elective caesarean birth. These include the belief that caesarean section is protective of urinary and fecal incontinence, that elective caesarean section is safe, and that women's autonomy around birth translates into their right to choose an elective caesarean section regardless of clinical indication. (For further discussion of the concept of a woman's right to choose caesarean section, you are advised to read Bewley & Cockburn 2002, Clement 1995, O'Neill 2002 and Odent 2004.)

The following dot point summaries will give you an idea of how contentious the subject is:

- In 1998, Professor Philip Steer argued that as a race we are still evolving, and as our brains and (therefore craniums) are expected to become larger, there will be a time when the baby's head may no longer be able to squeeze out of the birth canal in the conventional way (Steer 1998).
- The American College of Obstetricians and Gynaecologists released a statement in 2003 that it considered elective caesarean section to be 'ethical' (ACOG 2003). It qualified this statement by saying that in the absence of a specific patient request for elective caesarean, the lack of hard data favouring this procedure does not obligate the obstetrician to initiate discussion regarding relative risks and benefits versus vaginal delivery. However, if a patient requesting a caesarean continues this request after informed counselling, and the physician believes that caesarean will promote the overall health of the patient and fetus more than vaginal delivery, then elective caesarean is ethically justified (ACOG 2003).

- The National Institute of Clinical Excellence (NICE) stated at the same time that in its considered opinion, doctors should not refuse a woman the right to have an elective caesarean section, but that the reasons for the request should be sought, recorded and discussed in depth (NICE 2004, p 38).

- The International Federation of Gynaecology and Obstetrics (FIGO) stated that it is unethical to perform a caesarean section without a medical reason because of inadequate evidence to support a net benefit (Schenker & Cain 1999).

To maintain objective decision-making in the face of a barrage of medico-legal, media and emotional concerns is difficult, and it would be easy for women and doctors to slip into a short-term approach of doing caesarean section as the easy way out: 'the belief that a caesarean delivery is the easy way does not appear to come from facts about caesarean birth itself but rather from deeply rooted fears about vaginal childbirth' (Clement 1995). Is it fear, or simply that obstetricians are rightly more relaxed about the dangers of caesarean section and focusing more on the recently and incompletely researched complications of vaginal delivery? (Bump 1998, cited in Bewley & Cockburn 2002).

The Canadian Association of Midwives (CAM) argued that presenting interventions such as caesarean section as 'options'

BOX 35.13 Lack of information for women

Even if doctors genuinely believe in fulfilling informed choices regardless of other ethical considerations, there is presently inadequate unbiased literature to help women. There are no standard evidence-based, or even uncertainly-based, leaflets (such as the MIDIRS Informed Choice leaflets) to help women make any postulated choice. Who knows what properly informed and assessed womean prefer?

Caesarean section rates, especially for request, are very variable, suggesting that currently women are not given fully unbiased information and so remain susceptible to cultural, media and medical fashion.

(Source: Bewley & Cockburn 2002)

BOX 35.15 CAM statement on caesarean section

Extract from statement by the Canadian Association of Midwives Board of Directors, June 2004

The debate around c-section on demand raises deep concerns for midwives about the persistent increase in obstetrical interventions and surveillance technologies used for pregnancy and birth. In many cases the increase is occurring without regard for substantiating data and despite efforts by professional organizations and consumer groups to curb rates of intervention which are not supported by evidence. This trend both reflects and serves to construct a mechanical and fragmented vision of the body and birth and also of the pregnant woman and her unborn baby. It is a product of our society's 'culture of fear' around childbirth and demonstrates the extent to which the 'epidemic of risk' is reflected in maternity care.

Presenting interventions such as c-section as 'options' puts maternity care providers and women in a consumerist relationship, and treats childbirth as a problem to be solved rather than a process to be respected. The importance of the social and cultural aspects of birth is supported by a broad humanistic discourse in the scholarly and public literature. Moreover, strong scientific evidence supports a low intervention approach. Vaginal birth is not 'an option'. It is a complex, highly developed physiologic process that deserves our fundamental respect. It is the role of midwifery and medicine to understand, promote and facilitate physiologic processes, and to intervene only when necessary.

The benefits of caesarean section and certain obstetrical interventions for specific problem situations are irrefutable. However, widespread use of intervention and technology creates fear and doubt about the adequacy of the female body, and reinforces distrust about the reproductive powers of women. When women request interventions that are not medically indicated, and when professionals offer unnecessary technology rather than support and reassurance, it may simply be an expression of those doubts. These requests can also be seen as a reflection of a system greatly in need of improving its ability to provide sensitive, supportive care in childbirth. The research on caesarean section by request clearly shows that anxiety and fear play a major role and that these factors can be addressed by more effective means than by surgery. Offering all women the choice of caesarean section is not safe and not ethical.

Midwives work in a model of care that supports the development of relationship. The potential for empowerment through 'informed choice' is much more than a neutral offer of choice. Midwifery care involves mutual trust, dialogue and acknowledgement of the fundamental uncertainty and complexity of pregnancy and birth. In that sense, empowerment comes through a process of shared decision making, not through a 'menu' of choices.

For women, families, midwives and for many other maternity care providers, childbirth is a deeply meaningful event. As a multidimensional life experience, its significance and symbolism touch the core of every society and every culture. Embedded in a historical and socio-cultural context, childbirth is far more than a medical event. As professionals, midwives consider the individual woman within her life context, and take into account factors that affect her overall health. Health policy must also take into account the societal implications affecting health as a common good. To build maternity care that is truly women-centred will require beginning with the fundamentals: trust in women and supporting their ability to trust themselves, their bodies and the birth process.

(Canadian Association of Midwives 2004)

BOX 35.14 Elective caesarean

We conclude that beneficence-based, justice-based, and autonomy-based considerations do not support routinely recommending or even offering elective caesarean delivery.

The physician should respond to questions with a thorough informed consent process and a suggestion that the woman reconsider her request in order to ensure that her autonomy is being meaningfully exercised.

In these cases, implementing her request is ethically permissible. The physician should beware of the potentially insidious influence of economic and other forms of conflict of interest. Acting on self-interest in increased income or convenience distorts clinical judgement and undermines the physician's fiduciary obligations to patients.

However, by neither dismissing a patient's informed desire regarding caesarean delivery, nor automatically acquiescing to it, the physician maintains both a responsibility to professional integrity and a respect for the patient's autonomy.

(Statement made by a group of physicians, obstetricians and medical ethicists in the United States and published by the ACOG (Minkoff et al 2004))

---

puts maternity care providers and women in a consumerist relationship, and treats childbirth as a problem to be solved rather than a process to be respected (CAM 2004). From an anonymous survey sent to all gynaecologists and registrars in the Netherlands in 1999, the researchers concluded that 'in The Netherlands, a woman can always find a gynaecologist willing to perform a caesarean section for non-medical reasons. This willingness increases with the age of the doctor. There is a need for guidelines when handling these cases' (Kwee et al 2004).

Preventing urinary incontinence

Many caesarean sections are performed in the belief that avoiding vaginal birth is a means of avoiding future urinary incontinence. However, the finding that prevalence of urinary incontinence in postmenopausal nuns who had never been pregnant is similar to rates reported in parous, postmenopausal women appears to be contrary to the conventional wisdom that nulliparity protects against stress urinary incontinence (Buchsbaum et al 2002). It is clear that our understanding of factors leading to pelvic floor disruption over a woman's lifetime is limited, and that the topic is extremely complex. Pregnancy itself, tissue rigidity, trauma, birth interventions, and mode of birth all probably influence the integrity of the pelvic floor (McFarlin 2004). Childbearing is an established risk factor for urinary incontinence among young and middle-aged women. It has been suggested that vaginal delivery is the main contributing factor, possibly because of damage to important muscle tissue or nerves.

However, pregnancy itself may predispose to mechanical changes, hormonal changes, or both, that can lead to urinary incontinence (Rortveit et al 2003). Studies showing the association between the mode of delivery and incontinence have so far been inconclusive. The mechanical strain during labour may add to the risk associated with pregnancy itself. In the EPINCONT study undertaken in Norway between 1995 and 1997, among 15,307 women aged between 20 years and 65 years, the prevalence of any incontinence was 10.1% in the women who had never had a pregnancy. Age-standardised prevalences were 15.9% in the caesarean-section group and 21.0% in the vaginal birth group (Rortveit et al 2003). The absolute difference of 5.7% in the prevalence between women who had never been pregnant and women who had had caesarean sections was significant. The researchers concluded that if 15% of women had caesarean sections, the population attributable risk, that is, the proportion of incontinence in the population that is attributable to vaginal birth, would be 30% for any incontinence and 41% for moderate or severe incontinence. These figures imply that attempts to prevent both any incontinence and moderate or severe incontinence in the population by encouraging the use of caesarean section would have limited effect, unless a very large proportion of women were to give birth by caesarean section only (Rortveit et al 2003). The individual woman's risk of moderate or severe incontinence would be decreased from about 10% to about 5% if she gave birth to all of her children by caesarean section, and this decrease would apply only until 50 years of age, since there was no association of incontinence with mode of birth in older age groups (Rortveit et al 2003). This study did not attempt to assess the greater risk of incontinence where women had an assisted instrumental birth. In addition, a previous report from the EPINCONT study (Rortveit et al 2001) did not show an association between parity and incontinence after 65 years of age. That study implies that the mode of birth is of minimal importance in elderly women, who have the highest prevalence of both any incontinence and moderate or severe incontinence. The EPINCONT researchers recommended that the risk of other conditions, the risk of death, or economic costs associated with the mode of birth should be considered in any policy decisions (Rortveit et al 2003).

A study comparing 184 first-time mothers who had caesarean sections with 100 controls who had a non-instrumental vaginal birth to determine incidence and severity of anal incontinence found that severe anal incontinence followed elective and pre-labour emergency caesarean, and that the risk after elective caesarean is comparable to that after non-instrumental vaginal delivery with an intact perineum (Lal et al 2003). Similar findings were reported from a large study undertaken in Australia (MacLennan et al 2000). In this study of 1546 women, in whom pelvic floor morbidity, including anal incontinence, occurred after caesarean delivery with a prevalence comparable to that after non-instrumental vaginal birth, the investigators concluded that pregnancy, not childbirth (unless compounded by instrumental vaginal birth), was responsible for the frequency of pelvic floor dysfunction. In an editorial on these Australian findings, the editor of the *British Journal of Obstetrics and Gynaecology* remarked on the fact that it is pregnancy itself, not childbirth that has the greater effect on the frequency of pelvic floor dysfunction in the population (Grant 2000). One in eight women who have never been pregnant had some form of pelvic floor dysfunction, compared with one-half of the women who had a caesarean section or a spontaneous vaginal delivery and two-thirds of the women who underwent an instrumental vaginal delivery (Grant 2000). Meanwhile, in the United States, Diony Young, editor of *Birth*, lamented: 'What is a woman's chance of having a caesarean delivery? Certainly these days she's at high risk if she's too big or too small; too early or too late; too old or too fearful; too tired of being pregnant or too tired of being in labour; if she's having twins, if she's breech, if she's previously had a caesarean; or if she's due and so is the weekend, Christmas ...' (Young 2003).

Breech presentation at term

Breech presentation is now one of the major contributing factors to the rate of caesarean section in Australia. In 2002, 4.5% of Australian babies presented by the breech (Laws & Sullivan 2004). This means that among singleton pregnancies (and the first of twins), 1 in every 22 babies (11,309 babies) is breech. Breech presentation is now a primary indication for caesarean section.

External cephalic version

Interventions to promote cephalic version of babies in the breech position include external cephalic version (ECV), moxibustion and postural management. ECV involves applying pressure to the mother's abdomen to turn the fetus in either a forward or backward 'somersault' to achieve a vertex presentation. Recognised complications of ECV attributable to the procedure (and incidence) include:

- FHR abnormalities, the most commonest being transient bradycardia (1.1% to 16%)
- placental abruption (0.4% to 1%)
- painless vaginal bleeding (1.1%)
- admission for induction of labour (3%) (NICE 2004).

Maternal morbidity following caesarean section

In a study of all first-time mothers in Washington State 1987–1996, to determine the association between method of birth and maternal rehospitalisation within 60 days of birth, women who gave birth via caesarean or instrumental vaginal birth were twice as likely to be readmitted to hospital than those who gave birth spontaneously. Reasons for readmission were: uterine infection, gallbladder disease, genitourinary conditions, obstetric surgical wound complications, cardiopulmonary disorders, thromboembolic phenomena or appendicitis (Lydon Rochelle et al 2000). The study found an 80% increased risk among primiparous women who had a caesarean section and a 30% increased risk of hospitalisation at two months post partum for women who had an instrumental birth. The rates of admission to hospital for infection represented a 30-fold increase in surgical wound infection amont the primiparous women who had had a caesarean section. After caesarean, women were less likely to be readmitted for pelvic injury. Those women who had a forceps or vacuum birth were at increased risk for rehospitalisation

for PPH, genitourinary conditions, obstetric surgical wound complications or pelvic injury compared with those having a spontaneous normal birth. Overall readmission rates were 17 per 1000 for caesarean, 12 per 1000 for operative vaginal, and 10 per 1000 for spontaneous vaginal birth (Lydon Rochelle et al 2000).

Abnormalities of placentation

Following a first caesarean section, women having their second or subsequent birth are at an increased risk of placental abruption and placenta praevia in their next pregnancy, compared with first-time mothers who give birth vaginally (Lydon-Rochelle et al 2001). The abruption risks in these groups are 13.7 per 1000 versus 10.9 per 1000 (relative risk (RR), 1.3; 95% CI 1.1–1.5) and the praevia risks are 6.9 per 1000 versus 4.7 per 1000 (RR 1.4; 95% CI 1.1–1.6), respectively (Lydon-Rochelle et al 2001). The risks appear to be a function of both parity and previous caesarean sections (Wax et al 2004). The rising caesarean section rate over the past 20 years has been accompanied by a 10-fold rise in the incidence of placenta accreta. The incidence is reported as anywhere between 1 per 1667 and 1 per 2510 births (Gilliam et al 2002; Hemminki & Merilainen 1996; Kastner et al 2002; Miller et al 1997; Wax 2004). The occurrence of abnormally implanted placentas appears to be directly related to the number of prior caesareans, mother's age either over 35 years or less than 35 years, and placental implantation over the prior uterine incision site. As early as 1997, researchers reported that a total of 3.7% of women less than 35 years of age with one prior caesarean and a placenta implanted away from the scar site had an accreta, in contrast to 38.1% of women over 35 with more than two previous caesareans and a placenta implanted over the previous uterine incision (Miller et al 1997). With the increased incidence of primary caesarean section worldwide, we can expect to see peripartum hysterectomy becoming a major morbidity among women who have had previous caesarean sections.

Neonatal outcomes

Neonatal outcomes following caesarean section vary in seriousness and long-term morbidity. Although birth asphyxia is the most worrying outcome both initially and because of the long-term sequelae (see cerebral palsy, above), serious morbidity is experienced in other forms of birth trauma. Serious trauma has been defined as subdural or cerebral haemorrhage, fractured clavicle, other injuries to skeleton, injury to spine or spinal cord, facial nerve palsy, brachial plexus injury, subarachnoid haemorrhage, convulsions, other and unspecified cerebral irritation, or cerebral depression/coma. Minor trauma may be defined as injuries to the scalp, other cranial or peripheral nerve injuries, other specified birth trauma, and birth trauma that is not otherwise specified (Baillit et al 2002). A study undertaken in Washington State from 1995 to 1996 evaluated the outcomes for all 158,177 births with no major anomalies (Baillit et al 2002) to determine the optimal caesarean delivery rate to balance quality care for

---

BOX 35.16   Abnormal placentation

Abnormal placental implantation with myometrial penetration can be a potentially life-threatening condition. Placenta accreta, increta and percreta represent a continuum under the broader category of placental implantation disorders. The mildest form of these is placenta accreta, which involves myometrial invasion. Placenta increta involves deep myometrial invasion. Placenta percreta is the most severe form of implantation anomaly and is defined as invasion through the serosal layer of the uterus with potential invasion of adjacent organs. Abnormal implantation of the placenta in or through the uterine wall can precipitate profuse haemorrhage, often at the time of delivery. The most common treatment for this is a hysterectomy performed immediately following birth. The incidence of emergency hysterectomy after childbirth is reported to range from 1.55 per 1000 deliveries in the United States to 0.2 per 1000 deliveries in Norway.

(Source: Engelsen et al 2001)

---

pregnant women and neonates. The researchers wanted to find out how low the caesarean birth rate could be before it would adversely affect babies. The study didn't set a number for caesarean sections per year but found that in hospitals where the caesarean section rate was above the average for the state, the neonatal outcomes were worse. This was also the case where the caesarean section rate was lower than the average (Baillit et al 2002). This finding suggests that the caesarean section rate can in fact become too high and cause more harm than good to babies.

The incidence of respiratory distress syndrome (RDS) and transient tachypnoea of the newborn (TTN) differs according to the method of birth of babies, whether by elective caesarean, caesarean following labour, or labour followed by vaginal birth. Studies in the United Kingdom undertaken by Morrison et al (1995) found that among term babies, the risk of neonatal respiratory distress necessitating oxygen therapy is higher if delivery is by caesarean (35.5 with pre-labour caesarean, vs 12.2 with caesarean during labour, vs 5.3 with vaginal delivery, per 1000 live births). This relationship is maintained week by week up to 40 weeks gestation, after which respiratory morbidity is statistically similar regardless of the birth delivery mode (Morrison et al 1995). Furthermore, after 35 weeks, infants delivered by elective caesarean exhibit a markedly increased risk of RDS, TTN and pulmonary hypertension relative to vaginally delivered neonates (Levine et al 2001; Wax et al 2004). The most recent study demonstrating risk associated with caesarean section found that delivery by caesarean section in the first pregnancy could increase the risk of unexplained stillbirth in the second (Smith et al 2003). In women with one previous caesarean delivery, the risk of unexplained antepartum stillbirth at or after 39 weeks gestation is about double the risk of stillbirth or neonatal death from intrapartum uterine rupture. Risk was not attenuated

by adjustment for maternal characteristics or outcome of the first pregnancy (2.74, CI 1.74–4.30). The absolute risk of unexplained stillbirth at or after 39 weeks gestation was 1.1 per 1000 women who had had a previous caesarean section and 0.5 per 1000 in those who had not. The difference was due mostly to an excess of unexplained stillbirths among women previously delivered by caesarean section after 34 weeks (Smith et al 2003).

Prophylaxis for caesarean section

Both ampicillin and first-generation cephalosporins have similar efficacy in reducing postoperative endometritis. There does not appear to be added benefit in using a broad-spectrum agent or a multiple-dose regimen. There is need for an appropriately designed randomised trial to test the optimal timing of administration (immediately after the cord is clamped versus preoperative).

Preparing the woman for a caesarean section

These issues are discussed in full in the section above, on fluids and surveillance for epidural and spinal blocks. When the decision to move to caesarean section is made, there may not be much time to lose; however, it is of paramount importance that you are aware not only that the birth has become a major surgical procedure, but also that it is the beginning of a special relationship between a woman and her baby. As the midwife you will facilitate a discussion of the options surrounding caesarean section between the obstetrician and the woman, and the anaesthetist and the woman. It is important that the partner or husband is also included in the discussion and information-sharing session. Often you will be called upon to recount the events leading up to and including the caesarean birth of a baby. This is often crucial to the reconciliation of the fact that a caesarean section has had to be performed where the mother and her significant others were not planning for an emergency. Many women feel a sense of loss and grief when they have had a caesarean section. Some women feel guilty that they were unable to experience a normal, natural vaginal birth. For whatever reason women have a caesarean section, it is important to remember that this is a special event in a woman's life. There are ways of making it memorable for her, without succumbing to the depersonalising effect of technology.

Procedure for caesarean section

The procedure for an elective or emergency caesarean section is as follows:

1   Check that the woman has not had anything to eat or

Reflective exercise

What is the average number of caesarean sections in your country or state? What does the WHO recommend? Can you think of 10 ways to lower the caesarean section rate in your maternity unit or in your own practice?

BOX 35.17 Caesarean theatre staff

Theatre staff present for a caesarean include:
▶ obstetrician
▶ obstetrician's assistant (may be a student obstetric registrar or resident)
▶ anaesthetist
▶ anaesthetist's assistant (optional)
▶ 'scrub nurse/midwife'—the midwife or nurse who takes the sterile instruments and passes them to and from the obstetraicn who is operating. She wears full theatre dress—sterile gown and gloves. The scrub nurse/midwife is responsible for the instrument and swab count at the end of surgery. She also documents the blood loss and records the observations regarding the placenta.
▶ paediatrician (optional)—if there is an emergency Caesarean section and fears are held for the health of the baby, a paediatrician should be present
▶ 'scout nurse/midwife'—the midwife or nurse who assists the others and runs errands out of the theatre if necessary. She will not be scrubbed or gowned and gloved.
▶ midwife—the midwife is not scrubbed or gowned and gloved. She remains with the woman and her partner at the head of the theatre table, to attend to the woman undergoing surgery. She will also help the women put the baby to the breast in theatre or in recovery immediately after theatre.

---

drink (not even water) for six hours prior to elective surgery.

2 On admission, follow the preoperative guidelines for your unit.

3 Maternal vital signs will be checked (BP, pulse and temperature).

4 An IV line for fluids is inserted (see above for epidural/ spinal block).

5 Any hair on the incision site is removed.

6 A urinary catheter is inserted to keep the bladder empty during surgery.

7 Spend some time 'walking' the woman through the procedures that are about to take place. Inform her of the people who will be present in the theatre when the caesarean section is performed.

8 Make sure that her partner is either present at the bedside in theatre or is made comfortable outside the theatre

9 Anaesthetic guidelines concerning blood products and cross-matching will need to be adhered to.

10 The theatre should be prepared, instruments laid out and the wraps for the baby should be warmed.

11 Record all relevant details contemporaneously.

12 At the conclusion of the surgery, you may need to be vigilant in making sure the mother and baby are reunited as soon as possible, and that the baby is offered the mother's breast as soon as can be achieved.

There is often no reason why babies cannot be tucked up with their mothers immediately after a caesarean birth as they would be after a vaginal birth, including in recovery rooms. Because the baby will not have had the added benefit of being squeezed through the pelvic canal of its mother, you may need to be vigilant for signs of respiratory effort. Sometimes babies born via caesarean section have 'wet lungs' that have not had the benefit of being 'squished' dry though the normal process of birth. (In fetal lambs it was observed that 75% of the fluid in their lungs at birth is squeezed out during the birth process (Berger et al 1998).)

13 Be aware that drugs such as fentanyl are very quick to cross the placenta and if they have been administered too close to birth, the baby may need to be observed for signs of respiratory arrest.

Caesarean section following previous C section

When caring for women who are attempting a vaginal birth after a caesarean section, the strongest indicator that all is not well is an abnormality in FHR. This is the most common sign of rupture, occurring in 55–87% of uterine rupture events (Guise et al 2004). Other signs may be vaginal bleeding, pain, and disturbances of uterine contractions.

Most of the information concerning the success or failure rate of vaginal birth after a caesarean (VBAC) has been forthcoming from tertiary institutions in the developed world. The set standards of practice that have resulted from these reports may well be out of reach of and irrelevant to non-academic institutions, especially in the developing world.

Of major concern is the possible maternal morbidity and mortality (mainly the risk of uterine rupture) resulting from a trial of labour after caesarean birth. In a study of births recorded in the population-based data from the Scottish birth registry, the risk of uterine rupture was a rare event, occurring in 3.5 per 1000 trials of labour (Smith et al 2004). This showed a higher rate of rupture than a systematic review of available studies, where the rate was reported to be 2.7/1000 trials of labour (Guise et al 2004). In the Scottish study, women who gave birth in a hospital with fewer than 3000 births per annum did not experience a significantly increased rate of uterine rupture; however, the risk of perinatal death following uterine rupture was increased threefold. The perinatal mortality rate was one per 1300 births in hospitals with fewer than 3000 births a year, and one per 4700 births in hospitals with more than 3000 births a year (Smith et al 2004).

There is mounting evidence that vaginal birth and uterine rupture are less likely for women with prior vaginal birth than for women without.

The risk of perinatal death due to uterine rupture was also higher in women who had not previously given birth vaginally and in women who had been induced with prostaglandins but not with other methods of induction (Smith et al 2004, p 376).

Among women who had not previously given birth vaginally,

the risk of uterine rupture without induction of labour with prostaglandin was one in 210 and with induction of labour with prostaglandin was one in 71. Among women with a previous vaginal birth, the risk of uterine rupture without induction of labour with prostaglandin was one in 514 and with induction of labour with prostaglandin was one in 175 (Smith et al 2004, p 377).

Clearly the induction of labour is an intervention *not* without serious implications and risks. A large study from Washington State also found that use of prostaglandin was associated with uterine rupture (Lydon-Rochelle et al 2001a).

Guise and colleagues (2004), in their systematic review, set out to address the practice policy question: what additional risks does a woman who has had a caesarean birth assume if she chooses to attempt vaginal birth rather than have a repeat caesarean section? (Guise et al 2004). Most of the literature focuses on the risk of uterine rupture in those attempting a vaginal birth following caesarean section, with an implicit assumption that this risk would be eliminated by elective repeat caesarean birth. If this assumption were true, it would take 263 elective repeat caesareans to prevent one uterine rupture due to trial of labour (Guise et al 2004). However, elective repeat caesarean birth is not guaranteed to prevent uterine rupture. Studies to date have reported an additional risk posed by attempting a vaginal birth after caesarean birth up to 2.7 per 1000 births (McMahon et al 1996). This means that it would take 370 (213 to 1370) elective repeat caesareans to prevent one symptomatic uterine rupture due to trial of labour (Guise et al 2004).

Ideally, women should be informed of all the morbidity associated with caesarean sections and repeat caesarean sections, and this of course includes not only the rare event of a uterine rupture, but also the risk of the baby dying if such an event should happen; and also the risk of hysterectomy in a subsequent pregnancy following a first caesarean section. In the systematic review of studies to date, Guise et al (2004) report that about 5% of symptomatic uterine ruptures were associated with perinatal mortality and 13% with hysterectomy.

This translates to 7142 elective repeat caesareans to prevent one rupture-related perinatal death and 2941 to prevent one rupture-related hysterectomy. The authors of the systematic review urge caution with these results, stating that 'it would take only one misclassified case of symptomatic uterine rupture in the smaller study and five in the largest to entirely negate the observed difference in symptomatic uterine rupture between groups' (Guise et al 2004). Serious morbidity or mortality due to uterine rupture is rare, making it difficult to study. As a result, studies have focused on the occurrence of uterine rupture rather than how often bad outcomes result from it. The existing evidence is sufficient to conclude that there is an increased risk of symptomatic uterine rupture for trial of labour over elective repeat caesarean and that caesarean delivery is not completely protective. However, most uterine ruptures do not have serious consequences, and patients and clinicians may wish to base decisions on the likelihood of significant morbidity or mortality for the mother and baby rather than on the occurrence of uterine rupture itself. For every 10,000 women attempting trial of labour there would be 27 additional symptomatic uterine ruptures, 1.4 perinatal deaths related to rupture, and 3.4 hysterectomies related to rupture (Guise et al 2004, p 6).

A study released in December 2004 in the *New England Journal of Medicine*—the largest to date, involving almost 34,000 births at 19 academic hospitals from 2000 to 2003—confirms the VBAC's minimal risk. The study included 17,898 women who attempted to give birth vaginally and 15,801 women who elected a repeat caesarean (Landon et al 2004). Of note is the increased risk of uterine rupture associated with induction of labour or augmentation with both prostaglandin and Syntocinon. The risk was increased by two- to three-fold. Of those women who attempted a vaginal birth there were two perinatal deaths due to uterine rupture. There were 12 cases of hypoxic–ischaemic encephalopathy among the infants of the women attempting labour, and none among the women undergoing elective repeated caesarean birth. Combining these cases with cases of hypoxemic–ischaemic encephalopathy and neonatal deaths to represent 'poor perinatal outcomes' associated with the chosen method of delivery, there would need to be 588 elective repeated caesarean births to prevent one poor perinatal outcome. The corrected rates of perinatal death (after the exclusion of deaths associated with congenital malformations) were 4.0 per 10,000 in women undergoing a trial of labour and 1.4 per 10,000 in women undergoing elective repeated caesarean delivery. Demographic and perinatal characteristics of women and infants in the two groups show that, compared with women who underwent elective repeated caesarean delivery, women who underwent a trial of labour were more likely to be less than 30 years of age, black, unmarried, non-obese, and in receipt of government assistance (Medicaid or Medicare), and to have a preterm delivery (delivery before 37 weeks of gestation) or a delivery at 41 or more weeks of gestation. The elective caesarean following a previous caesarean group, meanwhile, saw twice as many maternal deaths (seven versus three). The three maternal deaths among women who underwent a trial of labour were due to severe pre-eclampsia with hepatic failure, sickle cell crisis with cardiac arrest, and postpartum haemorrhage. Of the seven maternal deaths among the women who had elective repeated caesarean delivery, two could be attributed to caesarean section (one resulted from haemorrhage and the other from anaesthetic complications). Of the five remaining deaths, four were caused by suspected amniotic-fluid embolism and one by aortic dissection.

Reflective exercise

What are the known risk factors that predispose women to the risk of uterine rupture? Where should these women give birth? Can we establish definitive risk criteria for women wanting to give birth vaginally following a previous caesarean section?

Overall, the data suggest a risk of an adverse perinatal outcome at term among women with a previous caesarean delivery of approximately 1 in 2000 trials of labour (0.46 per 1000), a risk that is quantitatively small but greater than that associated with elective repeated caesarean delivery (Landon et al 2004). Remaining issues of concern are the increased risks of placenta previa and placenta accreta for pregnancies subsequent to elective repeated caesarean delivery.

Summary: caesarean section

Caesarean section has become one of the most common surgical procedures in both Australia and New Zealand. (For current rates see the mothers and babies yearly report for your country—Australia's Institute of Health and Welfare and the New Zealand Ministry of Health publish yearly rates.) Decisions to deliver by caesarean can be made before the onset of labour (elective caesarean) or after the onset of labour (emergency caesarean). Delivery by caesarean may be appropriate in a range of circumstances related to the clinical characteristics of women where a vaginal birth is not possible. Some of the reasons for this may include breech or transverse presentation, cephalo-pelvic disproportion, placenta praevia, placental insufficiency, a prolapsed cord, multiple pregnancy, dangerously high blood pressure in the mother, and older women having a first baby. However, studies across the world have shown that non-clinical factors also contribute to the rising rates of caesarean section. These include women's requests for delivery by elective caesarean section when they perceive that the benefits of a planned elective caesarean outweigh the risks, elective induction of labour (with no obvious clinical indication), the different practice patterns of individual doctors, and the private health insurance status of women.

The escalation in the total caesarean rate is fuelled by both the rise in the primary caesarean rate and the steep decline in the rate of vaginal birth after caesarean (VBAC) delivery. In the United States, the primary rate rose 7% in 2002, and the rate of VBAC delivery plunged 23% (Martin et al 2003). In Australia, the rates have increased in both public and private hospitals, although they remain consistently higher in the private sector. Higher rates of electronic fetal monitoring, induction and epidural analgesia have been implicated in the rise in caesareans, but other factors are also contributing. Studies have shown that induction (including elective induction) may increase the risk of caesarean delivery in nulliparous women (Seyb et al 1999).

Randomised controlled trials and some multicentre trials (Hannah et al 1992, 2000) concluded that professional management guidelines should promote caesarean section for breech birth, and the latest data on birth following a previous caesarean section advises in favour of a repeat elective caesarean section (Landon et al 2004) in terms of perinatal risk. Greater access to private hospitals and changes in practice responding to the medical indemnity crisis have also contributed to rising rates (Laws & Sullivan 2004). Of the 21 OECD countries that reported caesarean section rates

for 1999, Italy had the highest (32.4%), and the Netherlands had the lowest rate (11.3%). The median was Iceland (17.3%). Six countries were below 15%. Australia's rate of 21.7% of all live births was 25% higher than the OECD median and fourth-highest of the 21 OECD countries that reported that year (OECD 2002).

Implications

What are the risks of caesarean delivery? One of the most significant risks is the need for a subsequent caesarean birth (Bernstein 2002). Yet there is steady growth in the research evidence that illustrates the seriousness of the rising caesarean section phenomenon in terms of maternal and infant complications, and the importance of the debate about the appropriateness of caesarean delivery in maternity care.

Studies investigating whether caesarean section may prevent injury of the pelvic floor and the genesis of stress urinary incontinence are scarce and controversial. Contrary to popular belief, MacLennan et al (2000), in an Australian study, found that pregnancy, not childbirth (unless compounded by instrumental vaginal delivery), was responsible for the frequency of pelvic floor dysfunction. Grant (2000) added to the debate by noting that what is remarkable is the frequency of pelvic floor dysfunction in the population. One in eight women who have never been pregnant had some form of pelvic floor dysfunction, compared with one-half of the women who had a caesarean section or a spontaneous vaginal delivery and two-thirds of the women who underwent an instrumental vaginal delivery. However, Groutz et al (2004) in a urodynamic study of 300 women of similar maternal age, weight, and height, found that the prevalence of postpartum stress urinary incontinence was similar after spontaneous vaginal delivery (10.3%) and caesarean section performed for obstructed labour (12%), but stress urinary incontinence was

---

BOX 35.18 Framing risk

How should we frame risk in conditions of uncertainty?
In their Nobel Prize winning work, Tversky and Kahneman discovered that framing of outcomes, choices and contingencies influences decision-making (Kahneman & Tversky 1979; Tversky & Kahneman 1981). The reference points and language chosen by providers and policy-making organisations influence public perceptions, policy formulation, and the climate for practice and research. Whether discussions highlight benefits or risks and whether the portrayal is relative or absolute can affect perceptions. Society often behaves as if the risk threshold is set at perfection and no risk is acceptable. Modern technology and superior medical care cannot remove all risk completely. Therefore, to decide on thresholds for risk for vaginal birth and repeat Caesarean section we need to look at rates for harms such as uterine rupture and benefits, and also to ensure consistency with other issues when we interpret the thresholds (Guise et al 2004).

significantly less common following elective caesarean section with no trial of labour (3.4%, $P < 0.05$) (Groutz et al 2004).

With regard to life-threatening risks of caesarean sections, Hall et al (1999) in their analysis of the maternal mortality report for 1994–96 in the United Kingdom found that the fatality rate for all caesarean sections was six times that for vaginal birth, and even for elective caesarean section the rate was almost three times as great. These differences are highly significant. The maternal mortality was higher than that associated with vaginal birth (5.9 for elective caesarean delivery versus 18.2 for emergency caesarean versus 2.1 for vaginal birth, per 100 000 completed pregnancies in the United Kingdom during 1994–96). In the absence of other evidence (e.g. from RCTs of different modes of birth), any decision to undertake major surgery with an associated mortality should be taken very seriously by all concerned (Hall et al 1999). Maternal mortality reports from both the United Kingdom and Australia consistently report death from direct causes related to surgical procedures.

Other morbidities associated with caesarean section include an increase in subsequent problems in placentation, including placenta praevia (Ananth et al 1997), placental abruption and ectopic pregnancies (Rasmussen et al 1999). In 2001, Lydon-Rochelle et al (2001b) found that there may be an increased risk of major bleeding in a subsequent pregnancy because of placenta praevia (5.2 per 1000 live births) and placental abruption (11.5 per 1000 live births). As yet, there are no significant studies demonstrating the risk of peripartum hysterectomy following a life-threatening postpartum haemorrhage from placenta accreta in pregnancies subsequent

---

BOX 35.19 Definitions: infant and maternal mortalities

1 WHO definitions

The World Health Organization (WHO) definition of fetal death is the absence of evidence of life after birth of babies of at least 500 grams birthweight or, if birthweight is not available, whose gestational age is at least 22 weeks.

WHO recommendations differ from the Australian Bureau of Statistics (ABS) standard for neonatal death and include only early neonatal deaths occurring in the first seven days, not all neonatal deaths up to 28 days, as reported by the ABS.

The WHO has also recommended that, for international comparisons, countries should report data based on lower limits of 1000 grams or, when birth weight is not available, a gestational age of at least 28 weeks, excluding births and fetal and neonatal deaths that do not meet these criteria.

2 Mortality rates / death rates (Australia and New Zealand)

▶ *Stillbirth rate (fetal death rate)*—the number of fetal deaths in 1000 total births.

▶ *Neonatal death rate*—the number of neonatal deaths in 1000 live births.

▶ *Perinatal death rate* (Australia)—the sum of fetal and early and late neonatal deaths in 1000 total births (both live and stillborn).

▶ *Perinatal death rate* (New Zealand)—the sum of fetal and early neonatal deaths in 1000 total births (both live and stillborn).

▶ *Infant mortality rate*—the number of infant deaths in a calendar year per 1000 live births in that year.

3 Births, perinatal and infant mortality (Australia and New Zealand)

▶ *Stillbirth* (fetal death)—death prior to the complete expulsion and extraction from its mother of the products of conception of 20 or more completed weeks of gestation or 400 grams or more birthweight: the death is indicated by the fact that after such separation the fetus does not breathe or show any other signs of life, such as heartbeat, pulsation of the umbilical cord or definite movement of voluntary muscles.

▶ *Neonatal death*—death of a live-born infant within 28 days of birth.

▶ *Early neonatal death*—death of a live-born infant within seven completed days after birth.

▶ *Late neonatal death*—death of a live-born infant after seven completed days and before 28 completed days after birth.

▶ *Post neonatal death*—death of a liveborn infant after the first completed 28 days after birth and before the end of the first year of birth.

▶ *Perinatal death* (Australia)—includes fetal and early and late neonatal deaths.

▶ *Perinatal death* (New Zealand)—includes fetal and early neonatal deaths

▶ *Infant death*—the death of a live infant born in the first year of life. This includes neonatal deaths, early and late, but does NOT include stillbirths (fetal deaths).

4 Maternal mortality (Australia)

The Australian definition of *maternal mortality* based on the WHO ICD-10 definition of a maternal death is the death of a woman who is pregnant or who dies within 42 days of a pregnancy being delivered or terminated. Maternal deaths are then classified as *direct*, *indirect* or *incidental*. These are defined as follows:

▶ *Direct deaths* arise from obstetric complications of the pregnancy state (pregnancy, labour and puerperium), from interventions, omissions or incorrect treatment from a chain of events resulting from any of the above.

▶ *Indirect deaths* result from pre-existing disease or disease that developed during pregnancy and was not due to direct obstetric causes, but which might have been aggravated by the physiological effects of pregnancy.

▶ *Incidental deaths* are those due to conditions occurring during pregnancy, where the pregnancy is unlikely to have contributed significantly to the death.

(Sources: 1,2, 3, above: Laws & Sullivan 2005; 4 above: Sullivan et al 2004)

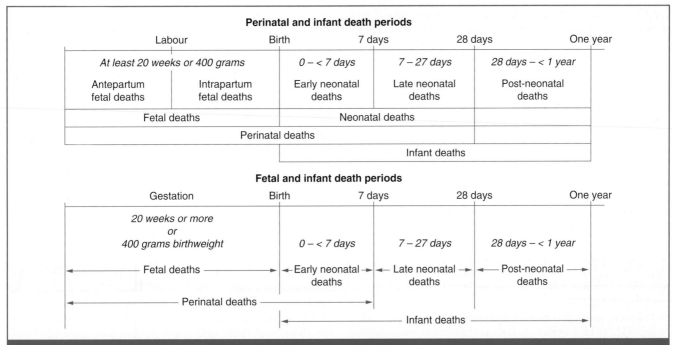

Figure 35.8 Perinatal and infant death periods, Australia (top) and fetal and infant death periods, New Zealand (bottom) (based on Laws & Sullivan 2004 and NZHIS 2004)

to a previous caesarean section. However, according to the American College of Obstetricians and Gynaecologists, the incidence of placenta accreta has increased ten-fold in the past 50 years and now occurs with a frequency of one per 2500 deliveries. Women who have had two or more caesarean deliveries with anterior or central placenta praevia have nearly a 40% risk of developing placenta accreta (ACOG 2002). Factors suggested as being associated with a higher incidence of placenta accreta include scarred uterus, multiparity and previous uterine surgery. Maternal complications in cases of placenta accreta usually occur in the third stage of labour and, rarely, in cases of placenta percreta during the pregnancy period. Women may present with a severe life-threatening hemorrhage requiring extensive surgical interventions, such as major pelvic vessel ligation and/or hysterectomy (Gielchinsky et al 2004).

Caesarean section also requires a longer recovery time, and operative complications such as lacerations and bleeding may occur, at rates varying from 6% for elective caesarean to 15% for emergency caesarean (Bergholt et al 2003; Hannah et al 2000). Babies are also implicated in risks associated with caesarean sections. Studies in the United Kingdom undertaken by Morrison et al (1995) found that among term babies, the risk of neonatal respiratory distress necessitating oxygen therapy is higher if birth is by caesarean (35.5 with a pre-labour caesarean vs 12.2 with a caesarean during labour vs 5.3 with vaginal delivery, per 1000 live births). Of potentially greater concern is data from a recent case-control study in Scotland. Over 120,000 second births from 1980 to 1998 were evaluated using linked maternal and stillbirth records. The investigators noted a 2.2-fold increased risk of unexplained stillbirth after

34 weeks gestation in association with a prior caesarean. This relationship was maintained weekly thereafter, including a risk of unexplained stillbirth after 39 weeks of 1.1 per 1000 versus 0.5 per 1000 for prior caesarean versus prior vaginal delivery (Smith et al 2003; Wax 2004). Pooled data from Sweden, Australia, Canada, Scotland, Denmark, England, the United States, Norway and Ireland reveal rising caesarean rates from the 1970s to the mid-1980s, after which rates remain stable or slightly increase.

Despite the marked increase in caesarean rate, cerebral palsy rates remained stable or slightly decreased. Therefore, caesarean is not neuroprotective for the fetus (Clark & Hankins 2003; Scheller & Nelson 1994; Wax 2004).

The Nordic countries remain lowest on the list for infant mortality rates reported by the CIA (2005). Australia, New Zealand and the United States, regardless of the rising intervention levels, remain woefully low on the rankings for resource-rich countries, especially compared to the Nordic countries and Europe (CIA 2005) (see Table 35.8).

Conclusion

Routine use of multiple childbirth procedures—that is, the over-treatment of normal childbirth—is not fiscally or medically defensible. Each procedure adds more costs to intrapartum care (Tracy & Tracy 2003), has potential adverse health effects for mother and baby, and necessitates use of still more technical care measures (Tracy et al 2006). No evidence supports routine use of electronic fetal monitoring, epidurals, oxytocin or episiotomies in low-risk women (Albers 2005).

TABLE 35.8 Infant mortality rates	
Country	**No. deaths / 1000 live births**
United States	6.5
New Zealand	5.85
Australia	4.69
Denmark	4.56
Norway	3.7
Finland	3.57
Iceland	3.31
Sweden	2.77
(Source: CIA 2005)	

In fact, the available evidence favours alternatives (Enkin et al 2000; WHO 1996) such as intermittent auscultation of the fetal heart, non-pharmacological measures for pain relief, low-technology strategies (ambulation, hydration) for labour stimulation, and no routine episiotomy. These care measures are both more pleasant for labouring women and feasible in the context of individualised care and intensive labour support. The short-sighted idea that a 'safe birth' is the only appropriate goal of maternity care fails to challenge the prevailing norm of over-treatment in hospital settings.

Ideally, a safe birth and optimal health of the new mother are both necessary goals, for which spontaneous vaginal birth and an intact genital tract are key elements. Such a mother will have the best postnatal health, including fewer hospital readmissions for post-delivery morbidity, less perineal pain and a stronger pelvic floor, better sexual function, and better overall physical functioning (Thompson et al 2002; Lydon-Rochelle 2001c). The mother's optimal health should be a high priority of caregivers, because newborn wellbeing depends so greatly on her health and functional status, which help equip her to undertake the complex and demanding task of mothering an infant with confidence (Albers 2005, p 68).

Common obstetric interventions are often for 'convenience' rather than for clinical indications. Before proceeding, it should be clear who the beneficiary of the convenience is. The midwife must make every effort to make sure that women and their partners have a full understanding of what is known about the associated risks, benefits and alternative approaches of the proposed intervention. Thorough and accurate information allows women to choose what is best for them and their infant on the basis of the individual clinical situation. Ideally, this discussion takes place during the antenatal time when there is ample opportunity to ask questions, reflect on the potential implications, and confer with partners and family members. While the interventions outlined above often are medically indicated for the wellbeing of mothers and infants, the evidence supporting their benefits when used electively may not be based on rigorous research and in many cases remains controversial.

Review questions

1   What are two points that midwives must consider when considering the use of interventions as routine practice?

2   What factors are associated with cerebral palsy in the antenatal period, during labour and in the postpartum period?

3   What is the evidence for the use of CTG assessment of fetal wellbeing in pregnancy?

4   What is the evidence for the use of routine CTG assessment on admission in labour?

5   What is the most appropriate form of fetal monitoring in an uncomplicated labour?

6   List six practices that should be performed whenever a CTG assessment is being undertaken.

7   List four characteristics of a non-reassuring CTG tracing.

8   What is the evidence in relation to the timing of induction of labour?

9   What interventions in labour are associated with the use of epidural anaesthesia?

10 List six possible reasons for the increasing caesarean section rate in Western health systems.

Online resources

Central Intelligence Agency 2005 The world factbook. Rank order—infant mortality rate, http://www.odci.gov/cia/publications/factbook/fields/2091.html

Ultrasound: causes for concern, by Sarah Buckley, MD, http://www.birthlove.com/free/ultrasound.html

Ultrasound: more harm than good? by Marsden Wagner, MD, http://www.midwiferytoday.com/articles/default.asp?a=1&r=1&e=1&q=ultrasound

Ultrasound: weighing the propaganda against the facts by Beverley Lawrence Beech. http://www.midwiferytoday.com/articles/default.asp?t=ultrasound

References

Adams AM, Smith AF 2001 Risk perception and communication: recent developments and implications for anaesthesia. Anaesthesia 56:745–755

Adelson PL, Child AG, Giles WB et al 1999 Antenatal hospitalisations in New South Wales, 1995–96. Medical Journal of Australia 170:211–215

Albers L 2005 Overtreatment of normal childbirth in US hospitals. Birth 32(1):67–68

Alfirevic Z, Neilson JP 2003 Biophysical profile for fetal assessment in high risk pregnancies (Cochrane Review). Cochrane Library (4). John Wiley & Sons, Chichester

Alfirevic Z, Neilson JP 1995 Doppler ultrasonography in high-risk pregnancies: systematic review with meta-analysis. American Journal of Obstetrics and Gynecology 172(5):1379–1387

American College of Obstetricians and Gynecologists (ACOG) 2000 Guidelines on antepartum fetal surveillance. American Family Physician 62(5):1184, 1187–1188

American College of Obstetricians and Gynecologists (ACOG) 2002 ACOG committee opinion. Placenta accreta. Committee on Obstetric Practice. International Journal of Gynaecology and Obstetrics 1:77–78

American College of Obstetricians and Gynecologists (ACOG) 2003 Surgery and patient choice: the ethics of decision making. ACOG Committee Opinion No. 289. Obstetrics and Gynecology 102:1101–1106

American College of Obstetricians and Gynecologists (ACOG) 2004 ACOG Committee Opinion No. 303. ACOG, Washington, DC

Amin-Zaki L, Majeed MA, Elhassani SB et al 1979 Prenatal methylmercury poisoning. Clinical observations over five years. American Journal of Diseases in Childhood 133(2):172–177

Ananth CV, Smulian JC, Vintzileos AM 1997 The association of placenta previa with history of Caesarean delivery and abortion: a meta-analysis. American Journal of Obstetrics and Gynecology 177:1071–1078

Association of Canadian Midwives. Online: http://www.canadianmidwives.org/

Badawi N, Watson L, Petterson B et al 1998 What constitutes cerebral palsy? Developmental Medicine and Child Neurology 40(8):520–527

Bailit JL, Garrett JM, Miller WC et al 2002 Hospital primary cesarean delivery rates and the risk of poor neonatal outcomes American Journal of Obstetrics and Gynecol 187:721–727

Banks S, Paech M, Gurrin L 2001 An audit of epidural blood patch after accidental dural puncture with a Tuohy needle in obstetric patients. International Journal of Obstetric Anesthesia 10:172–176

Banta HD, Thacker SB 2002 Electronic fetal monitoring: lessons from a formative case of health technology assessment. International Journal of Technology Assessment in Health Care 18:762–770

Baraz R, Collis RE 2005 The management of accidental dural puncture during labour epidural analgesia: a survey of UK practice. Anaesthesia 60(7):673–679

Behague DP, Victora CG, Barros FC 2002 Consumer demand for Caesarean sections in Brazil: informed decision making, patient choice, or social inequality? A population based birth cohort study linking ethnographic and epidemiological methods. British Medical Journal 324:942–945

Belizan JM, Althabe R, Barros FC et al 1999 Rates and implications of Caesarean sections in Latin America: ecological study. British Medical Journal 319:1397–1400

Bell JS, Campbell DM, Graham WJ et al 2001 Do obstetric complications explain high Caesarean section rates among women over 30? A retrospective analysis. British Medical Journal 322:894–895

Bennet VR, Brown LK 1999 Myles textbook for midwives. Churchill Livingstone, Edinburgh

Berger PJ, Kyriakides MA, Smolich JJ et al 1998 Massive decline in lung liquid before vaginal delivery at term in the fetal lamb. American Journal of Obstetrics and Gynecology 178:223–227

Bergholt T, Stenderup JK, Vedsted-Jakobsen A 2003 Intraoperative surgical complication during Caesarean section: an observational study of the incidence and risk factors. Acta Obstetrica et Gynecologica Scandinavica 82(3):251–256

Bernstein PS 2002 Elective Caesarean section: an acceptable alternative to vaginal delivery? Medscape Obstetrics, Gynecology and Women's Health 7(2). Online: http://www.medscape.com/viewarticle/441201

Bethune L, Harper N , Lucas DN et al 2004 Complications of obstetric regional analgesia: how much information is enough? International Journal of Obstetric Anesthesia 13(1):30–34

Bewley S, Cockburn JI 2002 The unethics of 'request' Caesarean section. British Journal of Obstetrics and Gynaecology109:593–596

Black C, Kaye JA, Jick H 2005 Caesarean delivery in the United Kingdom. Time trends in the general practice research database. Obstetrics and Gynecology 106:151–155

Blair E, Stanley F 1993 Aetiological pathways to spastic cerebral palsy. Paediatric and Perinatal Epidemiology 7:302–317

Blair E, Stanley F 1997 Issues in the classification and epidemiology of cerebral palsy. Mental Retardation and Developmental Disabilities Research Reviews 3:184–193

Bramadat IJ 1994 Induction of labour: an integrated review. Health Care Women International 15:135–148

Bricker L, Neilson JP 2000 Routine Doppler ultrasound in pregnancy (Cochrane Review). Cochrane Library (4). John Wiley & Sons, Chichester

Bryant SA 2003 Making culture visible: an examination of birthplace and health status. Health Care for Women International 24(2):103–114

Buchsbaum GM, Chin M, Glantz C et al 2002 Prevalence of urinary incontinence and associated risk factors in a cohort of nuns. Obstetrics and Gynecology 100:226–229

Camann W 2005 Pain relief during labor. New England Journal of Medicine. 352(7):718–720

Canadian Association of Midwives 2004 Statement on caesarean section by Board of Directors, June 2004. Birth Matters 8.3:14. Online: www.maternitycoalition.org.au/journal/Birth_Matters_Vol_8.3_Sept_04.pdf

Cary AJ 1990 Intervention rates in spontaneous term labour in low-risk nulliparous women. Australian and New Zealand Journal of Obstetrics and Gynaecology 30(1):46–51

Caton D, Frölich MA, Euliano TY 2002 Anesthesia for childbirth: controversy and change. American Journal of Obstetrics and Gynecology186:S25–S30

Central Intelligence Agency (CIA) 2005 The world factbook. Rank order—infant mortality rate. Online: http://www.odci.gov/cia/publications/factbook/fields/2091.html

Chalmers I 1991 Factors that influence the decision to intervene during pregnancy, childbirth, or the puerperium. Birth 18(3):137–141

Choi DH, Kim JA, Chung S 2000 Comparison of combined spinal epidural anesthesia and epidural anesthesia for Caesarean section. Acta Anaesthesiologica Scandinavica 44:214–219

Clark SL, Hankins GDV 2003 Temporal and demographic trends in cerebral palsy—fact and fiction. American Journal of Obstetrics and Gynecology 188:628–633

Clarke VT, Smiley RM, Finster M 1994 Uterine hyperactivity after intrathecal injection of fentanyl for analgesia during labour: a cause of fetal bradycardia? Anesthesiology 81:1083

Clement S 1995 The Caesarean experience. Pandora, London

Conklin K, Backus A 1999. In: D Chestnut (Ed) Physiologic changes in pregnancy, obstetric anesthesia: principles and practice (2nd edn). Mosby, St Louis, pp 17–42

Crowley P 1997 Interventions for preventing or improving the outcome of delivery at or beyond term. Cochrane Database of Systematic Reviews (1)

Davies SJ, Paech MJ, Welch H et al 1997 Maternal experience during epidural or combined spinal-epidural anesthesia for Caesarean section: a prospective, randomized trial. Anesthesia and Analgesia 85:607–613

Downe S, Gerrett D, Renfrew MJ 2004 A prospective randomised trial on the effect of position in the passive second stage of labour on birth outcome in nulliparous women using epidural analgesia. Midwifery. (2):157–168

Elferink-Stinkens PM, Brand R, le Cessie S et al 1996 Large differences in obstetrical intervention rates among Dutch hospitals, even after adjustment for population differences. European Journal of Obstetrics, Gynecology and Reproductive Biology 68:97–103

Eltzschig HK, Lieberman ES, Camann WR 2003 Regional anesthesia and analgesia for labour and delivery. New England Journal of Medicine 348(4):319–332

Engelsen IB, Albrechtsen S, Iversen OE 2001 Peripartum hysterectomy—incidence and maternal morbidity. Acta Obstetrica Gynecologica Scandinavica 80(5):409–412

Enkin M, Keirse MJ, Neilson J et al 2000 A guide to effective care in pregnancy and childbirth (3rd edn). Oxford University Press, Oxford

Expert Advisory Group on Caesarean Section in Scotland 2001 Report and recommendations to the Chief Medical Officer. May 2001. Online: http://www.show.scot.nhs.uk/crag/topics/reprod/EAG1.htm

Freeman RK, Anderson G, Dorchester W 1982 A prospective multi-institutional study of antepartum fetal heart rate monitoring. I. Risk of perinatal mortality and morbidity according to antepartum fetal heart rate test results. American Journal of Obstetrics and Gynecology 143:771

Gambling DR, Sharma SK, Ramin SM et al 1998 A randomized study of combined spinal–epidural analgesia versus intravenous meperidine during labour: impact on Caesarean delivery rate. Anesthesiology 89:1336–1344

Gielchinsky Y, Mankuta D, Rojansky N et al 2004 Perinatal outcome of pregnancies complicated by placenta accreta. Obstetrics and Gynecology 104:527–530

Gilliam M, Rosenberg D, Davis F 2002 The likelihood of placenta previa with greater number of cesarean deliveries and higher parity. Obstetrics and Gynecology 99:976–980

Grant JM 2000 Editorial. Pregnancy, not childbirth, causes pelvic floor dysfunction. British Journal of Obstetrics and Gynaecology 107:viii

Grant JM 2001 Qualitative and quantitative research in women's health. Editor's choice. British Journal of Obstetrics and Gynaecology 108:231–232

Groutz A, Rimon E, Peled S et al 2004 Caesarean section: does it really prevent the development of postpartum stress urinary incontinence? A prospective study of 363 women one year after their first delivery. Neurourology and Urodynamics 23(1):2–6

Guise JM 2004 Vaginal delivery after Caesarean section. British Medical Journal 329:359–360

Guise JM, McDonagh MS, Osterweil P et al 2004 Systematic review of the incidence and consequences of uterine rupture in women with previous Caesarean section. British Medical Journal 329:19–25

Hall MH, Bewley S 1999 Report on Why Mothers Die. Report on confidential enquiries into maternal deaths in the United Kingdom 1994–96. London: Stationery Office, 1998. Lancet 354:776

Hannah ME 2004 Planned elective Caesarean section: a reasonable choice for some women? Canadian Medical Association Journal 170:813

Hannah ME, Hannah WJ, Hellman J et al and the Canadian Multicenter Post-Term Pregnancy Trial Group 1992 Induction of labour as compared with serial antenatal monitoring in postterm pregnancy: a randomized controlled trial. New England Journal of Medicine 326:1587–1592 (published correction appears in 327:368)

Hannah ME, Hannah WJ, Hewson SA et al for the Term Breech Trial Collaborative Group 2000 Planned Caesarean section versus planned vaginal birth for breech presentation at term: a randomised multicentre trial. Lancet 356:1375–1383

Hemminki E, Merilainen J 1996 Long-term effects of cesarean sections: ectopic pregnancies and placental problems. American Journal of Obstetrics and Gynecology 174:1569–1574

Hofmeyr G 2000 Prophylactic intravenous preloading for regional analgesia in labour (Cochrane Review). Cochrane Library (3). Update Software, Oxford

Hofmeyr GJ 2004 Evidence-based intrapartum care. Best Practice Research in Clinical Obstetrics and Gynaecology 19(1):103–115

Horowitz JA, Goodman JA 2004 Longitudinal study of maternal postpartum depression symptoms. Research and Theory in Nursing Practice 18(2/3):149–163

Howell CJ, Kidd C, Roberts W et al 2001 A randomised controlled trial of epidural compared with non-epidural analgesia in labour. British Journal of Obstetrics and Gynaecology 108:27–33

Jenkins JG 2004 Some immediate serious complications of obstetric epidural analgesia and anaesthesia: a prospective study of 145 550 epidurals. International Journal of Obstetric Anesthesia 14:37–42

Jeon Y, Hwang J, Kang J 2004 Effects of epidural naloxone on pruritus induced by epidural morphine: a randomized controlled trial. International Journal of Obstetrics and Anesthesia 14:22–25

Jordan S, Emery S, Bradshaw C 2005 The impact of intrapartum analgesia on infant feeding. British Journal of Obstetrics and Gynaecology 112(7):927–928

Kahneman D, Tversky A 1979 Prospect theory: an analysis of decision under risk. Econometrica 47:263–291

Kansal A, Mohta M, Sethi AK 2005 Randomised trial of intravenous infusion of ephedrine or mephentermine for management of hypotension during spinal anaesthesia for Caesarean section. Anaesthesia 60:28

Karaman S, Akercan F, Akarsu T et al 2005 Comparison of the maternal and neonatal effects of epidural block and of combined spinal-epidural block for Caesarean section. European Journal of Obstetrics and Gynecology 121(1):18–23

Kastner ES, Figueroa R, Garry D et al 2002 Emergency peripartum hysterectomy: experience at a community teaching hospital. Obstetrics and Gynecology 99:971–975

Kwee A, Cohlen BJ, Kanhai HH et al 2004 Caesarean section on request: a survey in The Netherlands. European Journal of Obstetrics, Gynecology and Reproductive Biology 113:186–190

Lal M, Mann CH, Callender R et al 2003 Does cesarean delivery prevent anal incontinence? Obstetrics and Gynecology 101:305–312

Lancaster P, Pedisich E 1994 Caesarean births in Australia, 1985–1990 AIHW, Perinatal Statistics Unit. Online: http://www.npsu.unsw.edu.au/Publications.htm#PS

Landon MB, Hauth JC, Leveno K et al 2004 Maternal and perinatal outcomes associated with a trial of labour after prior Caesarean delivery. New England Journal of Medicine 351:2581–2589

Laws PJ, Sullivan EA 2004 Australia's mothers and babies 2002. AIHW Cat. No. PER 28, AIHW National Perinatal Statistics Unit (Perinatal Statistics Series No. 15), Sydney

Laws PJ, Sullivan EA 2005 Australia's mothers and babies 2003. AIHW Cat. No. PER 29. Perinatal Statistics Series No. 16. Australian Institute of Health and Welfare, Canberra

Le Ray C, Carayol M, Jaquemin S et al. 2005 Is epidural analgesia a risk factor for occiput posterior or transverse positions during labour? European Journal of Obstetrics, Gynecology and Reproductive Biology123(1):22–26

Leighton BL, Halpern SH 2002 The effects of epidural analgesia on labour, maternal, and neonatal outcomes: a systematic review. American Journal of Obstetrics and Gynecology 186(suppl):S69–S77

Levine EM, Ghai V, Barton JJ et al 2001 Mode of delivery and risk of respiratory diseases in newborns. Obstetrics and Gynecology 97:439–442

Leviton A 1993 Review. Preterm birth and cerebral palsy: is tumor necrosis factor the missing link? Developmental Medicine and Child Neurology.35(6):553–558

Lieberman E, O'Donoghue C 2002 Unintended effects of epidural analgesia during labor: a systematic review. American Journal of Obstetrics and Gynecology 186(suppl):S31–S68

Lieberman E, Davidson K, Lee-Parritz A 2005 Changes in fetal position during labor and their association with epidural analgesia. Obstetrics and Gynecology 105:974–982

Liston RM, Bloom K, Zimmer P 1994 The psychological effects of counting fetal movements. Birth 21:135–140

Lydon-Rochelle M, Holt VL, Martin DP 2000 Association between method of delivery and maternal rehospitalization. Journal of the American Medical Association 283:2411–2416

Lydon-Rochelle M, Holt VL, Easterling TR 2001a Risk of uterine rupture during labour among women with a prior Caesarean delivery. New England Journal of Medicine 345(1):3–8

Lydon-Rochelle M, Holt VL, Easterling TR 2001b First-birth Caesarean and placental abruption or previa at second birth. Obstetrics and Gynecology 97(5 pt 1):765–769

Lydon-Rochelle MT, Holt VL, Martin DP 2001c Delivery method and self–reported postpartum general health status among primiparous women. Paediatrics and Perinatal Epidemiology 15:232–240

MacDorman MF, Mathews TJ, Martin JA 2002 Trends and characteristics of induced labour in the United States, 1989–98.Paediatric and Perinatal Epidemiology 16(3):263–273

MacLennan A 1999 for the International Cerebral Palsy Task Force 1999 A template for defining a causal relation between acute intrapartum events and cerebral palsy: international consensus statement. British Medical Journal 319:1054–1059

MacLennan AH, Taylor AW, Wilson DH et al 2000 The prevalence of pelvic floor disorders and their relationship to gender, age, parity and mode of delivery. British Journal of Obstetrics and Gynaecology 107:1460–1470

Mangesi L, Hofmeyr GJ 2004 Fetal movement counting for assessment of fetal well-being. (Protocol). Cochrane Database of Systematic Reviews (2)

Manning FA 1999 Fetal biophysical profile. Obstetric and Gynecological Clinics of North America 26:557–577

Martin JA, Hamilton BE, Ventura SJ et al 2002 Births: final data for 2001. National Vital Statistics Report 51(2):1–103

Martin JA, Hamilton BE, Sutton PD et al 2003 Births: final data for 2002. National Vital Statistics Report 52(10):1–113

Martin JA, Hamilton BE, Sutton PD; Centers for Disease Control and Prevention, National Center for Health Statistics. 2004 Births: preliminary data for 2003. National Vital Statistics in Reproduction 53(9):1–17

Mayberry LJ, Clemmens D, De A 2002 Epidural analgesia side effects, co-interventions, and care of women during childbirth: a systematic review. American Journal of Obstetrics and Gynecology 186(5 Suppl Nature):S81–S93

McFarlin BL 2004 Review. Elective cesarean birth: issues and ethics of an informed decision. Journal of Midwifery Women's Health. 49(5):421–429

McMahon MJ, Luther ER, Bowes WA 1996 Comparison of a trial of labor with an elective second cesarean section. New England Journal of Medicine 335:689–695

Miller DA, Chollet JA, Goodwin TM 1997 Clinical risk factors for placenta previa and placenta accreta. American Journal of Obstetrics and Gynecology 177:210–214

Ministry of Health NZ 2002 Section 88 Maternity Notice. Online: http://www.moh.govt.nz/moh.nsf

Minkoff H, Chervenak FA 2003 Elective primary cesarean delivery. New England Journal of Medicine 348:946–950

Minkoff H, Powderly KR, Chervenak F 2004 Ethical dimensions of elective primary cesarean delivery. Review. Obstetrics and Gynecology103(2):387–392

Mires G, Williams F, Howie P 2001 Randomised controlled trial of cardiotocography versus Doppler auscultation of fetal heart at admission in labour in low risk obstetric population. British Medical Journal 322(7300):1457–1460; discussion 1460–1462

Morrison JJ, Rennie JM, Milton PJ 1995 Neonatal respiratory morbidity and mode of delivery at term: influence of timing of elective Caesarean section. British Journal of Obstetrics and Gynaecology 102(2):101–106

Naaktgeboren C 1989 The biology of childbirth. In: I Chalmers, M Enkin, MJ Keirse (Eds) Effective care in pregnancy and childbirth. Oxford University Press, Oxford, pp 795–804

National Institute for Clinical Excellence 2003 Clinical Guideline C. The use of electronic fetal monitoring: the use and interpretation of cardiotocography in intrapartum fetal surveillance. Online: http://www.nice.org.uk/pdf/efmguidelinercog.pdf

Nautila M, Halmesmaki E, Hiilesmaa V et al 1999 Women's anticipations of experiences with induction of labour. Acta Obstetrica et Gynaecologica Scandinavica 78:704–709

Neilson JP 1993 Editorial. Cardiotocography during labour. An unsatisfactory technique but nothing better yet. British Medical Journal 306(6874):347–348

Neilson JP 2003 Interventions for treating placental abruption. Cochrane Database of Systematic Reviews (1). Update Software, Oxford

New Zealand Health Information Service (NZHIS) 2004 Report on Maternity 2002. Online: http://www.moh.govt.nz/moh.nsf

NICE 2001 The use of electronic fetal monitoring: the use and interpretation of cardiotocography in intrapartum fetal surveillance. Evidence-based Clinical Guideline Number 8. RCOG Press, London. Online: http://www.rcog.org.uk/resources/public/pdf/efm_guideline_final_2may2001.pdf

NICE 2003 Antenatal care. Routine care for the healthy pregnant woman. Clinical Guideline 6. NICE, UK. Online: www.nice.org.uk/pdf/CG6_ANC_NICEguideline.pdf

NICE 2004 National Collaborating Centre for Women's and Children's Health. Caesarean section. Online: http://www.nice.org.uk/pdf/CG013fullguideline.pdf

O'Neill O 2002 Autonomy and trust in bioethics. Cambridge University Press, Cambridge

Odent M 2004 Are caesareans the future? RCM Midwives Journal 7(7):276

Okosun H, Arulkumaran S 2005 Intrapartum fetal surveillance. Current Obstetrics and Gynaecology 15(1):18–24

Olesen AG, Svare JA 2004 Decreased fetal movements: background, assessment, and clinical management. Acta Obstetrica et Gynecologica Scandinavica 83:818–826

Out JJ, Veirhout ME, Verhage F et al 1985 Elective induction of labour: a prospective clinical study. II. Psychological effects. Journal of Perinatal Medicine 13:163–170

Paech MJ 1991 The King Edward Memorial Hospital 1,000 mother survey of methods of pain relief in labour. Anaesthesia and Intensive Care 19:393–399

Paech M 2001 The use of combined spinal epidural anaesthesia for elective caesarean section is a waste of time and money. International Journal of Obstetric Anesthesia 10(1):32–35

Paech MJ, Gurrin LC 1999 A survey of parturients using epidural analgesia during labour. Considerations relevant to antenatal educators. Australian and New Zealand Journal of Obstetrics and Gynaecology 39(1):21–25

Paech M, Banks S, Gurrin L 2001 An audit of accidental dural puncture during epidural insertion of a Tuohy needle in obstetric patients. International Journal of Obstetrics and Anesthesia 10(3):162–167

Palmer L, Blair E, Petterson B et al 1995 Antenatal antecedents of moderate and severe cerebral palsy. Paediatric and Perinatal Epidemiology 9:171–184

Panzer O, Ghazanfari N, Sessier D et al 1999 Shivering and shivering-like tremor during labour with and without epidural analgesia. Anesthesiology 90:1609–1616

Pattison N, McCowan L 2003 Cardiotocography for antepartum fetal assessment (Cochrane Review). Cochrane Library (4). John Wiley & Sons, Chichester

Pennell CE, Tracy MB 1999 A new method for rapid measurement of lactate in fetal and neonatal blood. Australian and New Zealand Journal of Obstetrics and Gynaecology 39(2):227–233

Pharoah PO, Buttfield IH, Hetzel BS 1971 Neurological damage to the fetus resulting from severe iodine deficiency during pregnancy. Lancet 1(7694):308–310

Phelan JP 1981 The nonstress test: a review of 3000 tests. American Journal of Obstetrics and Gynecology 139:7–10

Poole J 2003a Neuraxial analgesia for labour and birth: implications for mother and fetus. Journal of Perinatal and Neonatal Nursing 17(4):252–267

Poole J 2003b Analgesia and anesthesia during labour and birth: implications for mother and fetus. Journal of Obstetric Gynecologic and Neonatal Nursing 32(6):780–794

Potter JE, Berquo E, Perpetuo IH et al 2001 Unwanted Caesarean sections among public and private patients in Brazil: prospective study. British Medical Journal 323:1155–1158

Preboth M 2000 ACOG Guidelines on antepartum fetal surveillance. American Family Physician 62(5):1187–1188

Rasmussen S, Irgens LM, Dalaker K 1999 A history of placental dysfunction and risk of placental abruption. Paediatric and Perinatal Epidemiology 13:9–21

Rayburn WF 1990 Fetal body movement monitoring. Obstetrics and Gynecology Clinics of North America 17:95–110

Rayburn WF, Zhang J 2002 Rising rates of labour induction: present concerns and future strategies. Obstetrics and Gynecology 100:164–167

Reynolds F, Seed PT 2005 Anaesthesia for Caesarean section and neonatal acid-base status: a meta-analysis. Anaesthesia 60:636–653

Roberts CL, Tracy S, Peat B 2000 Rates for obstetric intervention among private and public patients in Australia: population based descriptive study. British Medical Journal 321(7254):137–141

Roberts CL, Algert C, Peat B et al 2002 Trends in labour and birth interventions among low-risk women in an Australian population. Australian and New Zealand Journal of Gynaecology 42(2):176–181

Roberts CL, Raynes-Greenow CH, Upton A et al 2003 The management of labour among women with epidural analgesia. Australian and New Zealand Journal of Obstetrics and Gynaecology 43:78–81

Rortveit G, Hannestad YS, Daltveit AK et al 2001 Age- and type-dependent effects of parity on urinary incontinence: the Norwegian EPINCONT study. Obstetrics and Gynecology 98:1004–1010

Rortveit G, Daltveit AK, Hannestad YS et al 2003 for the Norwegian EPINCONT Study. Urinary incontinence after vaginal delivery or cesarean section. New England Journal of Medicine 348:900–907

Royal Australian and New Zealand College of Obstetricians and Gynaecologists 2002 (rev. 2004) Intrapartum fetal surveillance. Guidelines commissioned by RANZCOG.

Royal Australian and New Zealand College of Obstetricians and Gynaecologists (RANZCOG) 2004 Standards for epidural/spinal anaesthesia in obstetric practice. Online: http://www.ranzcog.edu.au/publications/statements/C-obs9.pdf

Salmon P, Drew NC 1992 Multidimensional assessment of the women's experience of childbirth: relationship to obstetric procedure, antenatal preparation and obstetric history. Journal of Psychosomatic Research 36:317–327

Salmon P, Miller R, Drew NC 1990 Women's anticipation and experience of childbirth: the independence of fulfillment, unpleasantness and pain. British Journal of Medical Psychology 63:255–259

Scheller JM, Nelson KB 1994 Does cesarean delivery prevent cerebral palsy or other neurologic problems of childhood? Obstetrics and Gynecology 83:624–630

Schenker JG, Cain JM 1999 FIGO Committee report. FIGO Committee for the Ethical Aspects of Human Reproduction and Women's Health. International Federation of Gynecology and Obstetrics. International Journal of Obstetrics and Gynaecology 64:317–322

Segal S, Su M, Gilbert P 2000 The effect of a rapid change in availability of epidural analgesia on the Caesarean delivery rate: a meta-analysis. American Journal of Obstetrics and Gynecology 183:974–978

Seyb ST, Berka RJ, Socol ML et al 1999 Risk of Caesarean delivery with elective induction of labour at term in nulliparous women. Obstetrics and Gynecology 94(4):600–607

Sharma SK, McIntire DD, Wiley J et al 2004 Labour analgesia and Caesarean delivery: an individual patient meta-analysis of nulliparous women. Anesthesiology 100:142–148

Shorten A, Shorten B 1999 Episiotomy in NSW hospitals 1993–1996: towards understanding variations between public and private hospitals. Australian Health Review 22(1):18–32

Smaill F, Hofmeyr GJ 2002 Antibiotic prophylaxis for Caesarean section. Cochrane Database of Systematic Reviews (3)

Smith CA 2003 Homoeopathy for induction of labour. Cochrane Database of Systematic Reviews (4)

Smith CA, Crowther CA 2004 Acupuncture for induction of labour. Cochrane Database of Systematic Reviews (1)

Smith GC, Pell JP, Dobbie R 2003 Caesarean section and risk of unexplained stillbirth in subsequent pregnancy. Lancet 362(9398):1179–1184

Smith GC, Pell JP, Pasupathy D et al 2004 Factors predisposing to perinatal death related to uterine rupture during attempted vaginal birth after Caesarean section: retrospective cohort study. British Medical Journal 329:375–380

Stanley FJ, English DR 1986 Prevalence of and risk factors for cerebral palsy in a total population cohort of low-birthweight (less than 2000 g) infants. Developmental Medicine and Child Neurology 28(5):559–568

Stanley FJ, Blair E 1991 Why have we failed to reduce the frequency of cerebral palsy? Medical Journal of Australia 154(9):623–626

Steer PJ 1998 Caesarean section: an evolving procedure? British Journal of Obstetrics and Gynecology 105(10):1052–1055

Sullivan EA, Ford JB, Chambers G et al 2004 Maternal mortality in Australia, 1973–1996. Australian and New Zealand Journal of Obstetrics and Gynaecology 44:452–457

Thacker SB, Stroup DF. 2003 Revisiting the use of the electronic fetal monitor. Lancet. 361(9356):445–446

Thacker SB, Stroup D, Chang M 2001 Continuous electronic heart rate monitoring for fetal assessment during labour (Cochrane Review). Cochrane Library (2). Update Software, Oxford

Thacker SB, Stroup D, Chang M 2004 Continuous electronic heart rate monitoring for fetal assessment during labour (Cochrane Review). Cochrane Library (1). Update Software, Oxford

Thompson JF, Roberts CL, Currie M et al 2002 Prevalence and persistence of health problems after childbirth: associations with parity and method of birth. Birth 29:83–94

Thoren T, Holmstrom B, Rawal N et al 1994 Sequential combined spinal epidural block versus spinal block for Caesarean section: effects on maternal hypotension and neurobehavioral function of the newborn. Anesthesia and Analgesia 78:1087–1092

Tito F 1995 Review of professional indemnity arrangements for health care professionals:compensation and professional indemnity in health care: report. AGPS, Canberra

Tracy SK, Tracy M 2003 Costing the cascade: estimating the cost of increased obstetric intervention in childbirth using population data. British Journal of Obstetrics and Gynaecology 110: 717–724

Tracy SK, Sullivan ES, Wang YA et al 2006 The cascade of obstetric interventions in childbirth in Australia, unpublished paper

Tversky A, Kahneman D 1981 The framing of decisions and the psychology of choice. Science 211:453–458

Vahratian A, Zhang J, Troendle JF et al 2005 Labour progression and risk of Caesarean delivery in electively induced nulliparas. Obstetrics and Gynecology 105(4):698–704

van Geijn HP 2005 Intrapartum fetal heart rate monitoring. International Congress Series, 1279:332–337

Wax JR, Cartin A, Pinette MG et al 2004 Patient choice. Caesarean: an evidence-based review. Obstetrics and Gynecology Survey 59:601–616

Wong CA, Scavone BM, Peaceman AM et al 2005 The risk of Caesarean delivery with neuraxial analgesia given early versus late in labour. New England Journal of Medicine 352: 655–665

World Health Organization (WHO) 1996 Maternal and Newborn Health/Safe Motherhood Unit. Family and reproductive health. Care in normal birth: a practical guide. WHO, Geneva

Young D 2003 Editorial. The push against vaginal birth. Birth 30(3):149–152

Zhang J, Yancey MK, Henderson CE 2002 National trends in labour induction, 1989–1998. Journal of Reproductive Medicine 47:120–124

CHAPTER 36

Life-threatening emergencies

Carol Thorogood and Sue Hendy

Key terms

amniotic fluid embolism, artificial rupture of the membranes, decision-time to delivery, diagnostic peritoneal lavage, disseminated intravascular coagulation, eclampsia, external cephalic version, fetomaternal haemorrhage, fire drills, HELLP syndrome, inotropes, Kleihauer Betke, magnesium sulphate, placenta praevia, postpartum haemorrhage, seizures, severe pre-eclampsia, shoulder dystocia, symphysiotomy, tocolysis, umbilical cord (funic) presentation, umbilical cord prolapse, uterine inversion, vasa praevia

Chapter overview

For most women, childbirth is a healthy event. However, some women may develop complications requiring complex levels of medical and technological intervention, and it is these complications that are the focus of this chapter. Healthcare practitioners ensure that their practice is current, skilled and based on the best available evidence. This chapter is concerned with the most frequent life-threatening complications, which often transpire with little or no warning. It does not provide a definitive guide to the management of obstetric emergencies—this belongs to experts in obstetrics, midwifery or medicine, or trauma specialists. A thorough understanding of the biosciences and pathophysiology underpinning emergency conditions in obstetrics is crucial to best practice. Therefore, readers will need to supplement the information they gain from this chapter with other texts.

Learning outcomes

Learning outcomes for this chapter are:

1 To identify factors that indicate the potential for emergency situations for mother and baby in pregnancy, birth and the puerperium

2 To describe the aetiology and management of a range of emergency situations in pregnancy, birth and the puerperium

3 To apply best available evidence in the identification, assessment and collaborative management of: umbilical cord presentation and prolapsed cord; shoulder dystocia; postpartum haemorrhage; eclampsia; amniotic fluid embolism; uterine inversion; maternal trauma; stabilisation; cardiopulmonary resuscitation and transport; and neonatal resuscitation.

Introduction

Researchers have developed a number of screening tools to help clinicians make accurate predictions about which women are most at risk of complications in pregnancy and birth, with limited success. Birth is never 100% predictable, and hence the rationale underpinning the policy that there should be a skilled attendant at every birth. Worldwide, between 9% and 15% of all birthing women will experience potentially life-threatening complications, and at least 1–2% will need a major intervention to survive (Maine et al 1992). Midwifery is grounded by a primary health model of practice. For birth to be satisfying and safe, midwives have a statutory responsibility to adhere to the principles outlined by their professional and regulatory authorities. These are grounded in a primary health model of practice that is influenced by particular sociocultural, spiritual and politico-economic environments. The midwife 'respects and supports the needs of women and their families/whanau to be self-determining in promoting their own health and well-being' (NZMC 2004, p 1.7). The midwife 'accepts accountability and responsibility for her actions, whilst recognising her own knowledge base and scope of practice. She is able to identify complications with appropriate and timely consultation and referral as needed. She delegates when necessary, always providing the appropriate supervision' (ANMC 2006, p 2) and 'collaborates with other health care providers when care is outside the scope of practice' (ANMC 2006, p 2.1). While some complications can be prevented, and others predicted in time, the majority of severe complications can be neither prevented nor predicted. When these do occur it is crucial that the midwife consults the most appropriate care provider. The *Australian College of Midwives' National Guidelines for Consultation and Referral* (2004) provide an evidence-based framework for consultation and transfer of care between midwives and doctors. These guidelines inform decision-making by midwives about the care, consultation and referral of women at booking, during the antenatal period, throughout labour and birth, and in the postnatal period. They help the midwife and woman determine the most appropriate place of birth, and who should be the lead care provider.

Because some complications occur with little or no warning, it is crucial that midwives are able to recognise and then manage a range of obstetric emergencies until help comes or until the woman is transferred to an appropriate facility. When complications arise, a multidisciplinary approach is usually required and so there must be a system in place for access to consultation and referral to medical facilities, personnel and emergency transport. Effective communication is pivotal to best practice in maternity care but never more so than when emergencies occur.

Fire drills

Because an obstetric emergency is unpredictable, it is imperative for all midwives, including those in an out-of-hospital setting, to have 'crash' protocols or 'fire drills' in place to facilitate effective management of emergencies such as umbilical cord prolapse. The aims of these 'fire drills' (scenario-based training in emergencies) are to test local systems and protocols for responding to emergencies, and to facilitate interdisciplinary teamwork and the development of individual skills and knowledge. 'Fire drills' should include: the procedures to be taken in the event of activation, calls for help, first-level management, staff responses, and home/birth centre/labour ward/operating logistics.

Every maternity setting should have protocols in place for the management of obstetric emergencies such as postpartum haemorrhage, shoulder dystocia and eclampsia. They also need to ensure that the fire drills are feasible and reflect best practice. All members of staff, including those working in blood banks and laboratory services (e.g. to ensure that adequate quantities of cross-matched blood and blood products are available) and orderlies must know exactly what to do, how to do it and when it is to be done. In the hospital setting, the activation of such a fire drill is usually through the hospital main switchboard, which preferably has a dedicated 'hotline' and code for this purpose. Activation of an emergency fire drill should not compromise the level of care to the woman, as the most experienced person in each 'crash' team is directly responsible for the conduct of the emergency. This extends to the woman's right to be involved in decisions about her care. It is crucial that, as soon as possible, the woman and her family are provided with an explanation of the circumstances surrounding the emergency and the need for urgent action.

Decision to delivery

In an emergency, the time from the decision to deliver by caesarean section and the actual delivery of a baby is known as the 'decision to delivery' (D-D) interval. The accepted interval of 30 minutes was recommended in a Canadian consensus statement in 1986 (Hannah et al 1986) with little evidence to support it. Since then, several studies examining the association between D-D interval and maternal and baby outcomes have found little difference between babies born with a D-D interval of 15 mins and those with a D-D interval between 16 and 75 mins (Thomas et al 2004). Other researches found that 'fewer than 40% of intrapartum deliveries by caesarean section for fetal distress were achieved within 30 minutes of the decision' and 'no evidence to indicate that overall an interval up to 120 minutes was detrimental to the neonate unless the delivery was a "crash" caesarean section' (MacKenzie & Cook 2001, p 498). Although the D-D interval remains an important measure of quality of maternity care, very short D-D intervals have been associated with poorer baby outcomes and may harm the mother as a result of surgery or factors such as general anesthesia (RCOG 2001).

Cord presentation and prolapse

Umbilical cord prolapse constitutes an obstetric emergency with potential for fetal death. With up to a 50% perinatal mortality rate, umbilical cord prolapse is one of the most catastrophic events in the intrapartum period (Curran 2003). It occurs in about 1 in 1000 births and is associated with significant perinatal morbidity and mortality. In many cases it is iatrogenic and thus a preventable condition. The risks increase whenever the presenting part does not fit snugly into the pelvis. Although a prolapsed cord poses no immediate physical threat for the woman, interventions to save the fetus, such as an emergency operative birth, will threaten her safety and wellbeing. An unexpected emergency situation combined with fear for the wellbeing of her child causes immense stress for the woman and her family.

Umbilical cord presentation

An umbilical cord presentation (Fig 36.1) is a condition in which the umbilical cord is interposed between the leading part of the fetus and the internal os of the uterine cervix but the amniotic membranes remain intact. Once the membranes break, the risk that the cord will prolapse through the cervix into the vagina increases significantly. In an occult cord presentation, a loop of cord lies alongside, instead of in front of, the presenting part and may not be felt on vaginal examination. A non-reassuring fetal heart rate (FHR) trace with deep, early decelerations may be an early sign of this complication. As labour establishes, umbilical cord compression associated with contractions causes variable FHR decelerations. If the umbilical cord prolapses through the cervix when the membranes break, it is compressed with every contraction and so severe variable FHR decelerations and/or profound fetal bradycardia may become apparent. If an umbilical cord presentation is diagnosed before the cervix is completely dilated, perhaps during ultrasonography, an obstetrician may, after obtaining informed consent from the woman, choose to perform a

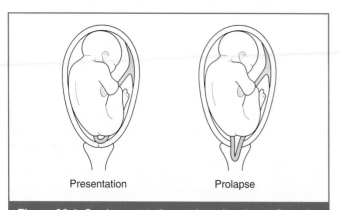

Figure 36.1 Cord presentation and cord prolapse (based on Henderson & MacDonald 2004)

'controlled' artificial rupture of the membranes (ARM) and at the same time push the cord away from the presenting part. Alternatively, once the cervix is fully dilated but before the fetal head reaches the pelvic floor, it is often possible to gently lift the fetal head up and push the umbilical cord upwards and away from it. If this is unsuccessful or if the umbilical cord prolapses, an immediate emergency Caesarean section is often necessary.

Umbilical cord prolapse

Prolapse of the umbilical cord is a rare obstetric emergency requiring immediate, skilled action on the part of the clinician who first recognises the problem. In many cases this is the midwife. An umbilical cord that, in the presence of ruptured membranes, lies in front of or beside the presenting part is said to be prolapsed (Fig 36.1). It occurs when the cord falls or is washed down through the cervix into the vagina when the membranes break and becomes trapped between the presenting part and the maternal pelvis. Thus, it is most likely to occur if the pelvic inlet is not completely filled by the presenting part.

Much more is known about umbilical cord prolapse than cord presentation, because the former is dramatically apparent and the latter is usually diagnosed by sonography or during a 'routine' vaginal examination of a clinically asymptomatic woman. If the umbilical cord prolapses through the cervix or even lies between the presenting part and the pelvis, during uterine contractions the umbilical cord will be exposed to intermittent compression, which compromises the fetal circulation. Depending on its duration and the degree of compression fetal hypoxia, brain damage and fetal death may occur. Dramatic changes in the fetal heart rate are often the first signs of a cord prolapse.

Risk factors

The risks of umbilical cord presentation and prolapse increase in frequency with malpresentations and with poorly fitting presenting parts such as in a transverse lie, shoulder and breech presentation. A flexed or footling breech poses the most risk for cord prolapse due to the increased space through which the umbilical cord can fall into the vagina. Prematurity also increases the risk of cord prolapse because these babies are more likely to present as a malpresentation and their small size in relation to the pelvis means there is more room for loops of cord to escape through the cervix. There is also more liquor volume in relation to fetal size than for a term infant.

Any structural abnormalities of the placenta, uterus or pelvis may also stop the presenting part from fitting snugly into the pelvis and thus increase the risk of prolapse (e.g. succenturiate placental lobe or contracted pelvis). A low-lying placenta (placenta praevia) can prevent the presenting part from entering the brim of the pelvis and it too increases the risk of cord prolapse. Repeated pregnancies interfere with the integrity of the abdominal musculature, which means that some multiparous woman may have lax abdominal muscles, which also increases the likelihood of an ill-fitting presenting

Clinical diagnosis of umbilical cord presentation and prolapse

▶ *Cord presentation*—loops of cord are palpated through the membranes. The presence of umbilical cord lying in front of the presenting part can also be visualised using colour Doppler studies.

▶ *Cord prolapse*—diagnosis is made by visual inspection or palpation of a pulsing umbilical cord during a vaginal examination. The umbilical cord is felt below or beside the presenting part.

▶ *Occult prolapsed cord*—is rarely felt on vaginal examination and the only indication may be FHR changes.

▶ *Overt prolapse*—the umbilical cord can be seen protruding from the introitus or loops of cord palpated within the vaginal canal.

part at term. Finally, the use of external cephalic version (ECV) to prevent breech presentation at birth is occasionally associated with cord prolapse, so it must be conducted in an environment where fetal wellbeing can be assessed and resources available to proceed to an emergency Caesarean section.

Whenever the presenting part is not engaged, an amniotomy—especially in the presence of polyhydramnios—poses a real risk of an iatrogenic cord prolapse. Of course, spontaneous rupture of the membranes can also trigger cord prolapse and so it is important for the midwife to auscultate the fetal heart prior to amniotomy and immediately after spontaneous or artificial breaking of the membranes.

Incidence

Gabbe and colleagues (2002) state that the rate of umbilical cord prolapse is much lower in fetuses presenting by the vertex than in fetuses with breech presentation or transverse lie.

The precise incidence of occult cord prolapse is unknown, but half of electronically monitored labours show fetal heart

TABLE 36.1 Incidence of cord prolapse	
Overall risk in vertex presentation	0.2–0.5%
Overall risk in breech presentations	3.5%
Complete breech	2–5%
Footling breech	15%
Transverse lie	20%
Multiple pregnancies	4%
Preterm labours and birth	5–10%
(Source: Gabbe et al 2002)	

rate (FHR) changes suggestive of umbilical cord compression, which is usually transitory and relieved by changing the maternal position. Approximately 50% of prolapsed cords occur in the second stage of labour. An additional 47% result from some obstetric intervention such as amniotomy or ECV (Usta et al 1999).

The presence of repetitive, early FHR decelerations may be indicative of umbilical cord compression or occult cord presentation, especially in the presence of oligohydramnios. This occurs because the umbilical vein is thinner than the arterial walls and therefore more susceptible to compression. Usually these apparently dramatic heart rate decelerations resolve rapidly after the contraction is finished. Unresolved cord compression will result in further fetal hypoxia, an increase in the severity of the decelerations and, eventually, prolonged fetal bradycardia. Cord prolapse is usually associated with profound fetal bradycardia.

If the cord is presenting and the amniotic membranes are still intact, during a vaginal examination the midwife may palpate a pulsating membrane, at the same rhythm and rate as the fetal heart. It is important to differentiate this rate from the maternal pulse, which may also be felt through the vaginal fornices. When the umbilical cord has prolapsed through the cervix or vagina, the midwife may palpate a 'rope-like pulsing, soft structure' in the vagina. Sometimes the cord is visible at the introitus. The midwife may also diagnose vasa praevia during a vaginal examination. This is a very rare condition where the umbilical cord vessels covered only by chorion and amnion lie across the cervical os and ahead of the fetus. This means that the cord has very little protection and the vessels often tear as the membranes break, causing asphyxia, exsanguination and death.

Management

Cord presentation

If the midwife suspects a cord presentation she must immediately and gently withdraw her fingers from the vagina to reduce the risk of rupturing the membranes. Medical assistance is summoned immediately. The aim is to relieve pressure on the cord to ensure an adequate oxygen supply to the fetus. A full explanation is given to the woman, and she is placed in an exaggerated Sim's position (left lateral, right knee to chest, resting on bed in front of left, hips supported by wedges/pillows or turned over face down with knees to nipples (see Fig 36.2).

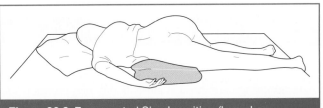

Figure 36.2 Exaggerated Sims' position (based on Henderson & MacDonald 2004)

Changing maternal position may resolve a cord presentation by enabling the presenting part to engage in the pelvis after the cord has moved away. Administering oxygen at 6–8 L/min may help to prevent fetal hypoxia. Unless the cord can be pushed away from the fetal head during an ARM, an emergency caesarean section is warranted.

Cord prolapse

As already noted, if the umbilical cord prolapses through the cervix or even lies between the presenting part and the pelvis, during uterine contractions the umbilical cord will be exposed to intermittent compression, compromising the fetal circulation. Exposure of the umbilical cord to air in an overt prolapse causes irritation and cooling of the cord, which produces vasospasm of the cord vessels. Delays in recognition and management are associated with significant perinatal morbidity and mortality. Therefore, cord prolapse requires urgent intervention and assistance.

In brief, if the fetus is alive and the cervix is not completely dilated, prompt delivery via caesarean section offers the best chance for a favourable fetal outcome. However, effective elevation of the presenting part, and tocolysis where necessary, removes the urgency of immediate caesarean section. Even with a prolapsed cord, a vaginal birth may still be possible if the birth is imminent—that is, the cervix is completely dilated, the presenting part is well down and there are no contraindications that will slow immediate delivery. If the fetus is not viable, labour should proceed to a vaginal birth.

First-level strategies (until help arrives)

Strategies to improve oxygen delivery to the fetus include:
- changing the mother's position
- techniques to stop compression of the cord against the fetal head and the pelvis
- administering oxygen.

If the fetus is viable and birth is not imminent, the woman is asked to assume an exaggerated Sim's position (her hips can

> ## Clinical point
>
> Prolapse of the umbilical cord is an obstetric emergency demanding immediate attention. Delay in management is associated with significant perinatal morbidity and mortality, due mainly to complications associated with preterm birth and birth asphyxia.

> ## Clinical point
>
> Faced with a cord prolapse, the main aims of management are: prevention, early diagnosis and temporising care through alleviation of compression on the prolapsed cord until emergency delivery of the baby can be effected.

> ## Clinical point
>
> Repetitive variable decelerations (see Fig 36.3) suggest umbilical cord compression, especially in the presence of oligohydramnios or amniotomy.

be elevated on pillows) and the midwife inserts two fingers into the vagina to push the presenting part up and away from the cord to relieve compression during contractions. This manoeuvre is maintained until help arrives or the baby is born. If the cord is visible at the introitus it is carefully replaced in the vagina, to minimise chilling and vasospasm. The midwife then makes a rapid assessment to determine the degree of cervical dilatation, fetal position and descent of the presenting part, as management now depends on the viability of the fetus, the stage of labour and whether or not birth is imminent. This assessment guides strategies for the ongoing management of this emergency.

Second-level strategies

Before moving on to the next steps in the management of cord prolapse, it is vital to assess fetal wellbeing. Fetal demise is a complication of cord prolapse and should be excluded before proceeding to operative delivery. Continuous electronic FHR monitoring is a useful adjunct in assessing fetal wellbeing and if the techniques to eliminate cord compression are successful. Maternal oxygen therapy at 6–8 L/min may have a positive impact on fetal blood arterial levels but only in the presence of a functioning gaseous interchange between the maternal and fetal circulation. This is why it is critical that the midwife's first action must be to minimise compression of the umbilical cord.

Umbilical cord compression may also be relieved by first pushing the fetal head out of the pelvis and then inserting a Foleys catheter into the maternal bladder and filling it with 500–700 mL of normal saline (Griese & Prickett 1993; Runnebaum & Katz 1999). This procedure is of most use if

> ## Critical thinking exercise
>
> Given that cord prolapse often has catastrophic consequences, think of strategies that you as a midwife can use to prevent or minimise this complication. You may like to consider:
> - how to identify risk factors for umbilical cord prolapse
> - how to recognise a cord presentation in a timely way
> - why an ARM should not be performed without a clinical indication
> - what you can do if a clinician tells you he or she wishes to perform an amniotomy when the fetal head is still 4/5 above the brim of the pelvis.

the woman needs to be transferred from an outlying facility without operative delivery capabilities to hospital, and a D-D interval of more than one hour is expected.

If vaginal birth is not possible, it is important to inhibit uterine contractions. Syntocinon® infusions are turned off and, if it is already in place, the rate of an IV infusion of Hartmann's solution is increased. Tocolysis with a drug such as terbutaline (Bricanyl®) has been used successfully to inhibit uterine contractions and thus further reduce compression on the umbilical cord. Even in a critical situation such as cord

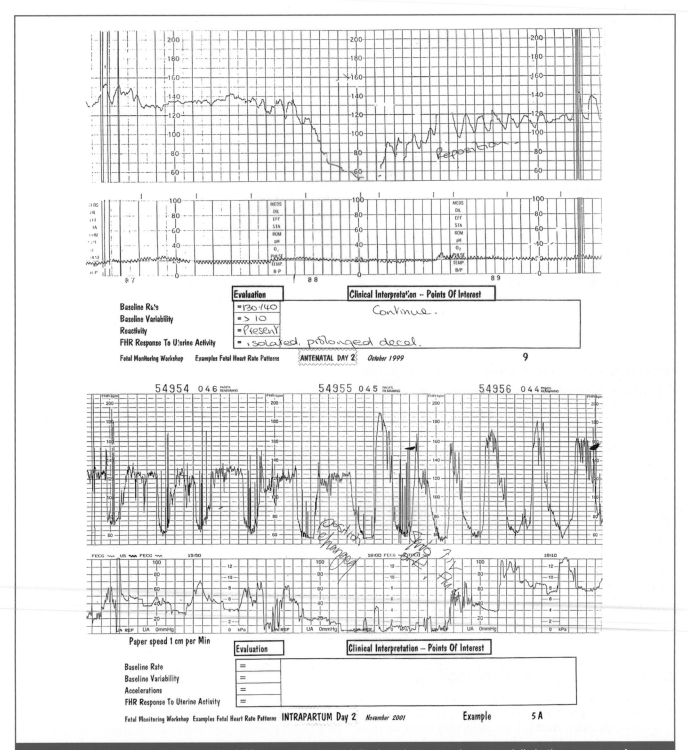

Figure 36.3 Variable decelerations on a CTG trace suggest umbilical cord compression, especially in the presence of oligohydramnios or amniotomy

BOX 36.2   Clinical review

The 'cardinal movements of labour' for a vertex presentation

▶ The bisacromial diameter of a term fetus is greater than the biparietal diameter.

▶ The pelvic inlet is wider in the oblique diameter than the anteroposterior diameter.

▶ Unless it has occurred already, during labour uterine contractions lead to flexion, descent of the fetal head and engagement.

▶ Usually the fetal head enters the pelvic inlet in the occipitolateral position, with the shoulders lying in the anteroposterior diameter.

▶ Internal rotation of the head occurs as the head reaches the level of the ischial spines and the shoulders rotate to the oblique position.

▶ The fetal head crowns and extends as it passes through the pelvic outlet.

▶ The shoulders now pass through the pelvic inlet in the oblique diameter of the pelvis. The posterior shoulder enters first, coming to rest in the sacral hollow or over the sacrosciatic notch, while the anterior shoulder follows it to lie over the obturator foramen.

▶ As further descent occurs, the anterior shoulder emerges from under the pubic ramus, and the shoulder girdle rotates to allow delivery in the anteroposterior position.

▶ The baby's body is born by lateral flexion.

prolapse, the midwife must still ensure that the woman gives her consent for the planned interventions.

Summary: cord prolapse

Umbilical cord prolapse is an infrequent obstetric emergency with a well-documented poor fetal prognosis. A high index of suspicion and recognition of predisposing factors may allow for early detection and timely delivery, thereby minimising perinatal morbidity and mortality. A multidisciplinary approach to management of this complication is essential to minimise maternal and fetal risks in such an emergency.

Shoulder dystocia

Shoulder dystocia is one of the most dramatic, anxiety-provoking emergencies encountered by midwives. It is unpredictable and has potentially catastrophic consequences for the neonate and often causes significant morbidity for the mother. This section discusses known risk factors, and provides guidance to the midwife regarding management in the antenatal and intrapartum periods. When shoulder dystocia occurs, it is best to have an action plan in place to guide clinicians as they manage this complication, and so one plan of action is described here.

Definition

Shoulder dystocia is best defined as a birth in which additional manoeuvres are required to deliver the fetal shoulders after normal gentle downward traction has failed.

Applied anatomy and physiology

Shoulder dystocia occurs as a result of disproportion between the bisacromial diameter of the fetus and the anteroposterior diameter of the pelvic inlet (11 cm) compared to the roomier oblique diameter of 13 cm. Usually the posterior shoulder has descended past the sacral promontory and entered the true pelvis. The fetal anterior shoulder begins its descent

into the pelvis but becomes impacted behind the symphysis pubis. Rarely, the posterior shoulder is also impacted above the sacral promontory. It is important to remember that the point of obstruction occurs at the inlet of the pelvis. Therefore no amount of tugging on the baby's head or cutting large episiotomies will release this bony obstruction.

Shoulder dystocia, 'bed' dystocia and 'mild' dystocia

Some clinicians confuse 'bed' dystocia or 'snug shoulders' with 'mild' shoulder dystocia. In none of these cases has the anterior fetal shoulder impacted behind the mother's symphysis pubis. Bed dystocia occurs when the woman is propped up in a semi-Fowler's position and the baby's head is born down into the mattress. There may be insufficient room for lateral (downward) flexion for delivery of the fetal anterior shoulder. In addition, because the weight of the mother is in part taken on the sacrum, it is pushed upwards, thus decreasing the anteroposterior diameter of the pelvic outlet. This problem is compounded if the woman has an epidural block and cannot assist the birth process. In most cases asking the woman to change her position—all fours, standing or rolling into a left lateral position—allows lateral flexion and easy birth.

Others fall into the trap of calling snug shoulders 'mild dystocia'—it is not. Delivery of 'snug' or tight fetal shoulders is more common in women who are obese. The fetal head may be larger than expected but the 'turtle' sign (slow extension of the head with the chin remaining tight against the maternal perineum) after delivery does not occur and the head still restitutes and goes through external rotation. Although the shoulders are 'tight', there is no need for the midwife to implement the steps used to manage shoulder dystocia, although sometimes supra-pubic pressure or asking the woman to birth in an 'all fours' position, standing or squatting, may prevent or alleviate the problem.

Incidence and risk factors

The incidence of 'true' shoulder dystocia is 0.2–2.8% of all births (Hope et al 1998). Most cases occur in fetuses of normal birthweight and are unanticipated, limiting the clinical usefulness of risk-factor identification. Approximately half occur without warning and in the absence of any known risk factors. However, most texts and hospital protocols list a number of antenatal and intrapartum factors believed to be associated with this complication. Box 36.3 lists these risk factors.

About half of all shoulder dystocias occur in macrosomic babies (Haram et al 2002; Rouse 1999). As birthweight increases, so does the occurrence of shoulder dystocia. However, even in the presence of macrosomia, the incidence of shoulder dystocia is approximately 8–20%, which means the majority occur in non-macrosomic babies.

Anecdotal, but not research-based, evidence suggests that women are increasingly choosing to have a caesarean section because they have been told by their lead caregiver that their baby is so big that they are at significant risk of shoulder dystocia. As yet medical science is unable to

---

Clinical point

True shoulder dystocia occurs when there is disproportion between the bisacromial diameter of the fetus and the anteroposterior diameter of the pelvic inlet. The anterior shoulder is impacted behind the symphysis pubis.

---

predict fetal weight with any certainty. Gonen and colleagues (1996) published the findings of a study aimed at testing the ability to detect macrosomic fetuses, and examining the relationships between antenatal diagnosis of macrosomia diagnosed by clinical assessment and by ultrasonography, and the incidence of shoulder dystocia and birth trauma. The authors (Gonen et al 1996) reported an overall frequency of shoulder dystocia of 2%, the majority (93%) occurring in infants weighing less than 4500 g. Moreover, the ability to predict macrosomia via clinical assessment and/or ultrasonography was limited. They concluded that because most cases of shoulder dystocia and birth trauma occur in non-macrosomic infants, this condition is almost impossible to prevent.

Maternal diabetes, macrosomia and shoulder dystocia

Currently, prevention of shoulder dystocia in diabetic women is based on quality antenatal care. Control of blood sugar levels reduces the incidence of fetal macrosomia (Wiznizer 1995). A review of the Cochrane Database (Boulvain et al 2000) reveals no firm evidence to support elective delivery, by induction of labour or by elective caesarean section, over expectant management at term for insulin-requiring diabetics. While induction of labour in women with gestational diabetes who require insulin may reduce the risk of macrosomia and shoulder dystocia, the actual risk of maternal or neonatal injury is not modified.

BOX 36.3 Risk factors

Risk factors for shoulder dystocia
Maternal:
▶ increasing maternal age
▶ maternal obesity
▶ maternal birthweight
▶ abnormal pelvic anatomy
▶ gestational diabetes
▶ prolonged pregnancy
▶ previous shoulder dystocia
▶ short stature.
Fetal:
▶ suspected macrosomia
▶ labour-related
▶ assisted vaginal delivery (forceps or vacuum)
▶ epidural block
▶ protracted active phase of first-stage labour
▶ protracted second-stage labour
▶ epidural analgesia—relaxes pelvic floor.

Research

Haram and colleagues (2002) conducted a literature search to explore the problems associated with diagnosing macrosomia and its relationship to shoulder dystocia. Approximately half of all cases of shoulder dystocia occurred in macrosomic babies when using 4000 g as the cut-off point, but only in about 25% of cases when 4500 g was used as the cut-off point. Further, the incidence of shoulder dystocia was only 8–20% of all macrosomic babies. Thus, most shoulder dystocias occurred in non-macrosomic babies, and contrary to popular medical opinion, most macrosomic babies do not suffer shoulder dystocia at birth.

Warning signs of shoulder dystocia

The single most common risk factor for shoulder dystocia is the use of a vacuum extractor or forceps during delivery (Sokol et al 2003). Instrumental vaginal deliveries carry a significant risk of shoulder dystocia due to the elongation of the head, extension of the neck and abduction of the shoulders. This increases the bisacromial diameter of the fetal shoulders, making entrapment of the fetal shoulder behind the symphysis more likely. A prolonged second stage of labour and 'bobbing' (recoil of the fetal head) up and down in second stage when the fetal head is in the vagina may be an indication that the fetal shoulders have not rotated and that the anterior shoulder is impacted behind the symphysis pubis. This is often followed by the appearance of the 'turtle' sign.

Management

Because most shoulder dystocias are unpredictable, birth attendants need to be skilled in the management of this condition when it occurs (Enkin et al 2000). Irrespective of the precise management plan, it is vital that each facility has a policy and training system so that all staff skilled in the manoeuvres are employed effectively and efficiently. The management of shoulder dystocia requires a focused and calm environment, with the midwife taking the lead to direct the team to ensure a coordinated approach. This section outlines one systematic set of manoeuvres (and a mnemonic) known to assist delivery of a baby with shoulder dystocia. While nomenclature of these manoeuvres (and mnemonics) may change within various textbooks, the principles of management remain the same. The HELPERR (ALSO©) mnemonic is a clinical tool that offers a structured framework for coping with shoulder dystocia.

Emergency manoeuvres for the management of shoulder dystocia are designed to do one of three things:

- increase the functional size of the bony pelvis through flattening of the lumbar lordosis and cephalad rotation of the symphysis. The McRoberts manoeuvre (Fig 36.4) is thought to alleviate approximately 40–50% of all shoulder dystocias (Gherman et al 1997). The woman lies in a supine position and her knees are lifted up to her nipples. This exaggerated knee–chest position can also be achieved by rolling the woman into an all fours position.
- decrease the bisacromial diameter of the fetus (i.e. the breadth of the shoulders) of the fetus through application of suprapubic pressure (i.e. internal pressure on the posterior aspect of the impacted shoulder)
- change the relationship of the bisacromial diameter within the bony pelvis through internal manoeuvres.

Whatever the resources available, it is vital that the midwife summons help. In a hospital, additional midwives, an obstetrician, neonatologist or other clinicians available to resuscitate the baby should be called. Allocating someone to document times and manoeuvres employed is very helpful. Managing shoulder dystocia is an extremely anxiety-provoking time, and if it is to be managed well, it needs cool minds and clear thinking. It is important to remember to talk to the mother and her support people and to explain what is happening, especially since their cooperation and assistance are required.

The HELPERR mnemonic

The HELPER® mnemonic has been developed by ALSO© (Advanced Life Support in Obstetrics). Each step of the mnemonic involves rotation of the shoulders using pressure on the scapula or clavicle, not the fetal head. Internal manoeuvres are more successful if combined with suprapubic pressure in a direction that facilitates rotation within the vagina.

The HELPERR mnemonic (ALSO©) works as follows:

H Call for help

Activate a prearranged protocol that summons the appropriate personnel to respond with necessary equipment to the birthing room.

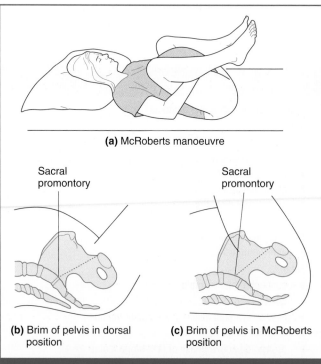

(a) McRoberts manoeuvre

(b) Brim of pelvis in dorsal position

(c) Brim of pelvis in McRoberts position

Figure 36.4 Shoulder dystocia (based on Henderson & Macdonald 2004)

> ### Clinical point
>
> Whenever the normal events and progress of labour are disturbed by obstetric intervention—epidural block, induction of labour or interfering with the normal progress of the second stage of labour with forceps and vacuum extraction—*think* about the increased risk of shoulder dystocia.

E Evaluate for episiotomy

Episiotomy should be considered throughout the management of shoulder dystocia but only because it makes more room if rotation manoeuvres are required. Shoulder dystocia is a bony impaction that occurs at the pelvic inlet, so episiotomy alone will not release the shoulder.

L Legs (McRoberts manoeuvre)

This procedure involves flexing and abducting the maternal hips, positioning the maternal thighs up onto the maternal abdomen (knees to nipples). This position flattens the sacral promontory and results in cephalad rotation of the pubic symphysis. The woman is placed in a recumbent position. Remove or lower the bottom of the bed and manipulate the woman's buttocks to the extreme edge of the bed. With an assistant on either side of the woman, the thighs are abducted and hyper-flexed onto the abdomen, while the midwife applies gentle traction to the baby's head.

P Suprapubic pressure

The hand of an assistant is placed suprapubically over the fetal anterior shoulder, applying continuous pressure in a cardiopulmonary resuscitation style with a downward and lateral motion on the posterior aspect of the anterior fetal shoulder, to disimpact the shoulder. It is important to identify the plane of the fetal back because the midwife is attempting to adduct the shoulders to decrease the bisacromial diameter. This manoeuvre should be attempted while continuing downward traction. If delivery is unsuccessful, a rocking motion may be applied. Initially the procedure should be continuous for 30 seconds, followed by a rocking motion for another 30 seconds. If delivery is still not possible, the midwife's hand must now enter the vagina in an attempt to expedite delivery.

E Enter manoeuvres (internal rotation)

The Rubin manoeuvre (Fig 36.7 (a)) attempts to manipulate the fetus to rotate the anterior shoulder into an oblique plane and under the maternal symphysis. They can be difficult to perform when the anterior shoulder is wedged beneath the symphysis. All internal manoeuvres must be effected with insertion of two fingers into the vagina posteriorly. They are then moved upwards to apply digital pressure to the posterior aspect of the anterior shoulder in a clockwise direction, pushing it towards the fetal chest for another 30 seconds. This motion will adduct the fetal shoulder girdle, reducing its diameter and rotating the shoulders forward into the oblique diameter. The midwife again attempts delivery.

Wood screw manoeuvre (the only manoeuvre using two hands) (Fig 36.7 (b))

While maintaining pressure on the posterior aspect of the anterior shoulder, the midwife now introduces two fingers of her second hand into the vagina, locating the anterior aspect of the posterior shoulder. Both hands apply pressure in an effort to rotate the posterior shoulder in the same direction as before. The midwife again attempts delivery once the shoulders move into the oblique diameter. If this does not work, the midwife moves to the next manoeuvre.

Reverse Wood screw manoeuvre

The fingers on the posterior shoulder (Fig 36.7 (c)) are removed from the vagina and the two fingers on the anterior shoulder moved down and along the fetal back to the posterior aspect of the posterior shoulder. The midwife attempts to rotate the shoulder in the opposite direction to the Wood screw manoeuvre for 30–60 seconds.

If these manoeuvres have not resulted in delivery of the baby, removal of the posterior arm may be possible.

R Remove the posterior arm

Removing the posterior arm from the birth canal (Figs 36.6, 36.7 (d)) aims to shorten the bisacromial diameter, allowing the fetus to drop into the sacral hollow, freeing the impaction. If the woman is not in the all-fours position, it may be helpful to do this first before attempting to remove the posterior arm. Repositioning the woman means the posterior arm is now lying anteriorly. Two fingers are inserted into the

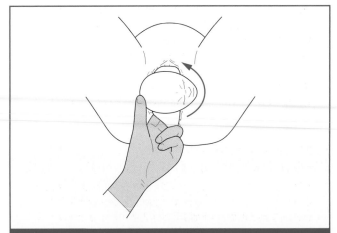

Figure 36.5 Shoulder dystocia: in the Rubin manoeuvre, the shoulders are adducted as the shoulder is rotated anteriorly (based on Henderson & Macdonald 2004)

vagina and passed down the front of the posterior arm as far as possible to flex the arm at the baby's elbow and the forearm delivered in a sweeping motion over the fetal anterior chest wall ('cat lick' manoeuvre). Grasping and pulling directly on the fetal arm may fracture the humerus.

R Roll the woman onto all fours (Gaskin manoeuvre)
The woman is rolled from her existing position to the all-fours position. Often, the shoulder will dislodge during the act of turning, so this movement alone may be sufficient to dislodge the impaction. Rotation of the woman may facilitate delivery by increasing the pelvic diameters and allowing better access to the posterior shoulder. In addition, the position change may affect gravitational forces, which further aid in the disimpaction of the fetal shoulders.

Some clinicians use this as their first-line management by asking the woman to move her knees to her nipples while in the all-fours position. The only manoeuvre that cannot be done in this position is the application of suprapubic pressure.

If at any time the midwife feels the shoulders move, delivery should be attempted without delay. Maternal effort is advisable but the midwife should not wait for contractions before proceeding through the steps. If, on the rare occasion that all these manoeuvres have been attempted, and birth has not been successful, the process is started again.

The complications associated with shoulder dystocia are listed in Box 36.5.

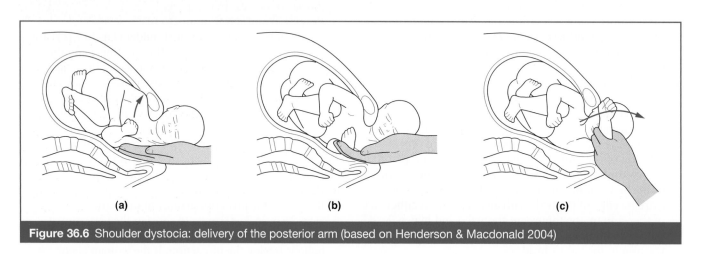

(a)   (b)   (c)

Figure 36.6 Shoulder dystocia: delivery of the posterior arm (based on Henderson & Macdonald 2004)

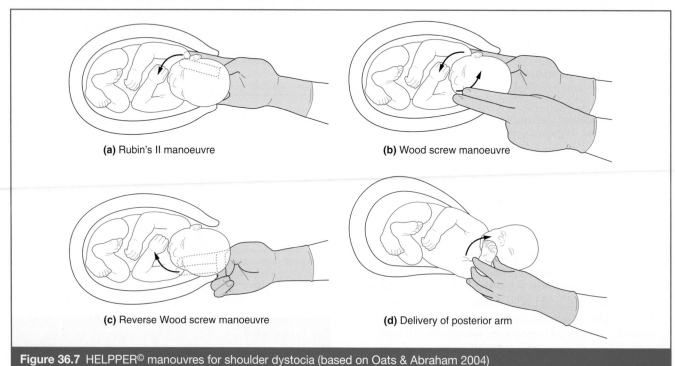

(a) Rubin's II manoeuvre

(b) Wood screw manoeuvre

(c) Reverse Wood screw manoeuvre

(d) Delivery of posterior arm

Figure 36.7 HELPPER© manouvres for shoulder dystocia (based on Oats & Abraham 2004)

> **BOX 36.5 Complications of dystocia**
>
> Maternal:
> ▸ postpartum haemorrhage
> ▸ rectovaginal fistula
> ▸ symphyseal separation or diastasis, with or without transient femoral neuropathy
> ▸ third or fourth degree episiotomy or tear
> ▸ uterine rupture.
>
> Fetal:
> ▸ brachial plexus palsy
> ▸ clavicle fracture
> ▸ death
> ▸ hypoxia, with or without permanent neurological damage
> ▸ fracture of the humerus.

Manoeuvres of last resort

A number of authors, such as Gobbo and Baxley (2000), Sandberg (1999) and Gherman et al (1998), describe a number of 'last-resort' manoeuvres. There is little or no evidence to support their use, except perhaps as a desperate last measure; they are briefly summarised below.

● *Deliberate clavicle fracture*—direct upward pressure on the mid-portion of the anterior fetal clavicle reduces the shoulder-to-shoulder distance. The danger of this procedure is that bone fragments may pierce the underlying lung or the subclavian blood vessels.

● *Zavanelli manoeuvre*—cephalic replacement is followed by caesarean delivery; it involves rotating the fetal head into a direct occiput anterior position, then flexing and pushing the fetal head back into the birth canal, while holding continuous upward pressure.

● *General anaesthesia*—musculoskeletal or uterine relaxation with halothane or another general anaesthetic may bring about enough uterine relaxation to effect delivery. Oral or intravenous nitroglycerine may be used as an alternative to general anaesthesia.

● *Symphysiotomy*—intentional division of the fibrous cartilage of the symphysis pubis under local anaesthesia is used more widely in developing than developed countries. It should be used only when all other manoeuvres have failed and caesarean delivery is unavailable.

Documentation

It is vital that the midwife attending a shoulder dystocia thoroughly document the manoeuvres employed and the time taken to deliver the baby. Midwives need to differentiate between 'difficult shoulders' and shoulder dystocia, to ensure that subsequent pregnancies are managed appropriately. Imprecise, subjective language such as 'mild or moderate' shoulder dystocia should never be used. Instead, documentation should clearly outline what procedures were used to expedite delivery, how long each one took and their effect. The woman

should also be fully informed about what happened and de-briefing or counselling offered.

Summary: shoulder dystocia

Sooner or later every midwife is confronted with a life-threatening and frightening complication such as shoulder dystocia. The key to management is that the team knows exactly what to do and, at a time of great tension, works calmly and without panic, and proceeds through a logical series of steps designed to disimpact the anterior shoulder from behind the symphysis pubis. Over-zealous techniques used to deliver the anterior shoulder frequently do more damage to the fetus than that caused by manoeuvres such as those described in the HELPERR© mnemonic.

Uterine inversion

Uterine inversion is a potentially life-threatening complication of childbirth in which, as Varney (2004, p 915) says, the uterus literally turns inside out (Fig 36.8), so that the inside of the fundus protrudes through the cervical os (incomplete), descends to the vaginal introitus (complete) or extrudes beyond the vulva (prolapsed). Uterine inversion may occur with the third stage of labour or, less frequently, post partum. Inversions are described as acute if they occur within the first 24 hours of birth, while those occurring more than 24 hours after birth are subacute. Mothers' survival rate is about 85%. The most frequent cause of death is intractable haemorrhage and associated shock. These complications are minimised by prompt recognition and management.

Incidence

The rate of uterine inversion is estimated at 1:2000 to 1:23,000 labours. This wide range reflects differences in recording methods and client populations.

Pathophysiology

Occasionally inversion is idiopathic, and it rarely occurs spontaneously, but most often it is due to 'mismanagement' of the third stage of labour. Nevertheless, for it to occur, a portion of the uterine wall either indents toward or prolapses through the dilated cervix. Thus, uterine relaxation combined with simultaneous downward additional traction force on the fundus of the uterus and/or with additional traction applied to the umbilical cord before it has separated, causes the fundus of the uterus to prolapse. Telling the mother to push to help expel the unseparated placenta increases the risk of uterine inversion.

Associated factors

According to Varney (2004, p 915), there are three circumstances that when combined create a situation favourable to uterine inversion:

● uterine atony, or flaccidity of the myometrium around the implantation site

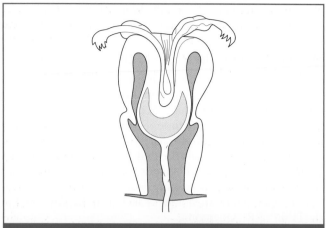

Figure 36.8 Inversion of the gravid uterus (based on Henderson & Macdonald 2004)

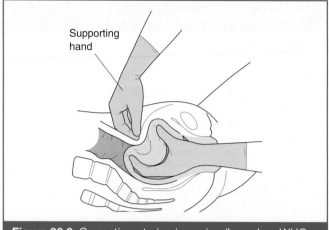

Supporting hand

Figure 36.9 Correcting uterine inversion (based on WHO n.d.)

- patulous dilated cervix
- fundal pressure (Credé's manoeuvre) or excessive traction on the umbilical cord, especially when the placenta has not separated from the uterine wall.

There are a number of other reported associations (not causations) with uterine inversion. In all likelihood, a number of common factors act in concert to result in an inversion. These include:

- a short umbilical cord
- multiparity
- sudden increase in abdominal pressure, as in coughing
- placenta accreta/increta/percreta
- fundal implantation of the placenta
- chronic endometritis
- fetal macrosomia
- use of $MgSO_4$
- 'trials' of vaginal birth following caesarean section
- myometrial weakness/uterine sacculation
- precipitate labour
- acute tocolysis with nitroglycerine or other potent agents.

Clinical presentation

The diagnosis of uterine inversion is usually established clinically when the midwife observes the uterus lying outside the vulva immediately after birth, or following vaginal examination—perhaps when the fundus of the uterus cannot be palpated after the delivery of the placenta. Uterine inversion should always be suspected if the woman becomes shocked immediately after birth without an obvious reason. However, if the inversion is not complete, PPH is usually the most striking sign that draws the attention of the clinician to suspect uterine inversion.

Management

Successful management of this rare but potentially life-threatening condition requires a collaborative effort. Skilled midwifery assistance, an accomplished obstetrician and anaesthestist, and immediate access to the operating room are important components of success. Treatment for inversion employs parenteral tocolytics to permit immediate uterine replacement, treatment of shock, fluid replacement and oxytocic drugs to maintain normal uterine positioning. The optimal technique for rapid uterine replacement is contentious. Theoretically, in the presence of neurological shock, further stretching of the pelvic viscera as the uterus is replaced has the potential to exacerbate shock. In practice, however, once the diagnosis is recognised, the best management is still immediate replacement, because the longer the delay, the more firmly contracted the lower uterine segment/cervix becomes, making the replacement increasingly difficult. In summary, reduction of the uterine inversion may be accomplished either by a conservative non-surgical approach or by a surgical procedure.

Non-surgical techniques

In 1945, O'Sullivan described a method for the correction of partial uterine inversion using hydrostatic pressure. Warm saline is rapidly instilled into the vagina via a Foley's catheter. The fluid pushes the uterine fundus upwards until it resumes its correct position. An oxytocic infusion is used to maintain uterine contraction.

Tocolytics, such as terbutaline or glyceryl trinitrate, make manual replacement less difficult. During this procedure, the clinician inserts a hand into the vagina and holds the inverted uterus so that the fundus is positioned in the palm of the hand (Fig 36.9). Pressure is then applied to lift the uterus upward and anteriorly through the pelvis into the abdominal cavity to the level of the umbilicus. If two or more attempts at this very painful procedure fail, surgery is indicated.

In most cases, as the placenta will not have separated before manual or surgical replacement is attempted, the best plan is not to try and remove it but to wait until the woman is transferred to the operating theatre with adequate personnel and resources to deal with the problem. Immediate placental removal without replacement simply increases blood loss. Furthermore, in the increasingly common event of a placenta accreta/increta/percreta, separation is very difficult, or impossible.

Surgical approaches

Occasionally, abdominal surgery is required to reposition the uterus. General anaesthesia, followed by laparotomy or incision of the contracted cervix may be necessary. Regardless of the procedure employed, after replacement, uterine atony and PPH is common. The prompt administration of 15-methyl prostaglandin $F_{2\alpha}$ (Hemabate®), high-dose oxytocin infusions and perhaps ergometrine (provided there are no contraindications), or misoprostol per rectum is recommended to control PPH. Many clinicians still prefer to administer a single prophylactic dose of a broad-spectrum first-generation cephalosporin or a similar drug at the time of repositioning. Reinversion may also occur.

Summary: uterine inversion

Puerperal uterine inversion is a rare but potentially life-threatening complication of the third stage of labour. It is often accompanied by massive haemorrhage and shock. Timely diagnosis, replacement of the inverted uterus, and prompt, expert management are mandatory. Judicious replacement of the inverted uterus by vaginal manipulation is recommended. Careful clinical observation following replacement and the administration of oxytocic drugs prevents most reinversions. In the rare case when the inversion is long-standing or if manual replacement fails, surgical replacement is required. The risk of recurrence of inversion in subsequent births is unknown.

Amniotic fluid embolism

Amniotic fluid embolism (AFE) is a poorly understood phenomenon usually occurring without warning, and perhaps because it is so rare its consequences are often catastrophic. It is unpredictable, unpreventable and rapidly progressive. AFE occurs in about 1:8000 to 1:30,000 pregnancies, with high maternal and fetal mortality and frequently permanent neurological damage in survivors. Women with AFE are critically ill and, if they survive the initial phase of this disorder,

will require admission to an intensive care unit (ICU). Most maternity hospitals in Australia and New Zealand do not have dedicated obstetric ICU units, so it is crucial that all maternity service providers are prepared to provide emergency care for these women until referral to an ICU can be effected.

Historical context

Steiner and Lushbaugh (1941) were the first researchers to use the term 'amniotic fluid embolism' to describe the signs and symptoms associated with sustained tachycardia, cardiovascular collapse, pulmonary oedema and shock that developed during labour in the absence of other illnesses. The authors postulated that powerful or tetanic uterine contractions caused an embolism of squamous cells, mucin and/or other amorphous debris, from the fetus, to lodge in the woman's pulmonary vessels. Benson (1993) was one of the first investigators to cast doubt on the belief that amniotic fluid leakage into the maternal circulation was the primary cause of AFE. He argued that the disease was probably associated with an immune response to a pregnancy-associated antigen, in part because the clinical features of AFE were more similar to anaphylaxis than to embolism. In the United States, Clark et al (1995) commenced a national registry of women with AFE. They reported a significant association between AFE and a male fetus. Moreover, 41% of women with this syndrome had a history of allergy or atopy (Clarke et al 1995). He and others recommended a new clinical definition, anaphylactoid syndrome of pregnancy, to describe the condition. More recently, Benson et al (2001) postulated that complement activation rather than anaphylaxis might play a role in the pathophysiology of AFE. Whatever the initial precipitating factor, there is little doubt that mechanical obstruction caused by emboli lodging in maternal blood vessels is a major feature in determining the severity of the condition and maternal and fetal outcomes.

Mortality/morbidity

Death rates from AFE vary between 26.4% and 61% (Clarke et al 1995). Most mortality occurs in the first few hours—50% within the first hour. More than half of those who develop AFE will experience coagulopathy, including disseminated intravascular coagulopathy (DIC). Less than 15% of women experiencing AFE survive without neurological impairment. Although 79% of neonates survive, 50% are neurologically impaired (Clarke et al 1995).

Pathophysiology

According to the *Maternal Deaths in Australia 1997–1999* report (Slaytor et al 2004), AFE was responsible for seven direct maternal deaths in Australia in the 1997–1999 triennium. In five of these cases, labour was induced. The authors note that drawing conclusions from analysis of such small numbers is problematic, but all clinicians should be aware that there may be an association between AFE and the induction of labour with Syntocinon® and/or ARM. However, it has been suggested that the uterine hypertonus sometimes observed prior to the onset of clinical signs of AFE occur because of an amniotic fluid embolism.

The precise pathophysiological pathway by which AFE occurs is still unknown. Under certain conditions, when amniotic fluid and its fetal components enter the maternal circulation, endogenous mediators (e.g. prostaglandins, leukotrienes, histamine, bradykinin, cytokines, thromboxane, complement-activating factors, and platelet-activating factor) are released and these trigger a two-phase response. In phase one, pulmonary artery vasospasm, pulmonary hypertension and elevated right ventricular pressure result in hypoxia, and myocardial and pulmonary capillary damage, resulting in left heart failure and adult respiratory distress syndrome. Phase two is characterised by haemodynamic instability and/or DIC.

Maternal clinical presentation

The onset of signs and symptoms associated with AFE are related to pulmonary vasospasm, pulmonary hypertension and ventricular dysfunction. According to Gei and Hankins (2000), the initial signs and symptoms have a typical chronology. Once the amniotic fluid enters the maternal systemic circulation:

- the amniotic fluid enters the pulmonary circulation, leading to respiratory distress and cyanosis occuring within 60 seconds
- pulmonary venous pressure increases, with a concomitant drop in cardiac output, pulmonary oedema, hypotension and shock
- neurological manifestations such as confusion, loss of consciousness and seizures occur
- the exposure of the circulatory system to amniotic fluid thromboplastin and other mediators induces DIC
- systemic hypotension and decreased uterine perfusion develop. Abnormalities of the FHR are apparent.
- more than 80% of cases end in cardiac arrest.

Fetal signs and symptoms

Profound fetal respiratory acidosis and associated FHR changes occur in response to maternal hypoxia and hypertonic uterine contractions. Prolonged late decelerations followed by baseline fetal bradycardia can result in neurological injury. A rate of 60 bpm or less for more than three minutes may indicate a terminal bradycardia. A short interval between cardiac arrest and delivery correlates positively with neonatal survival.

Diagnosis

The classic scenario of AFE involves an older multiparous woman in advanced labour who suddenly collapses, although it can occur following termination of pregnancy, amniocentesis, placental abruption and trauma, during caesarean section and without known risk factors within 30 minutes after birth (Box 36.6). There may be CTG abnormalities, uterine hypertonus and an obstetric intervention such as ARM. The

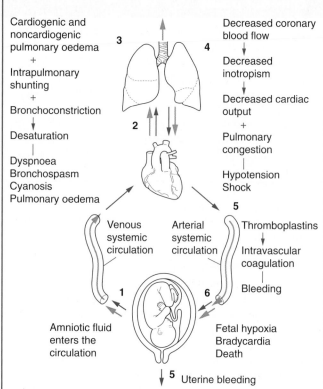

Sequence of events:

(1) For reasons not completely understood, amniotic fluid reaches the maternal intravascular compartment (systemic venous system).

(2) The amniotic fluid enters pulmonary circulation via the pulmonary artery. This contaminated blood crosses to the left atrium through a patent foramen and probably through intra-pulmonary shunts once the embolism is significant, as shown in cases of massive amniotic fluid embolism at autopsy.

(3) The exposure of the pulmonary vasculature to both soluble (leucotrines, surfactant, thromboxane A_2, endothelin, etc.) and insoluble components (squames, vernix, hair, mucin, etc.) of the amniotic fluid and possibly other mediators released locally induces capillary leak, negative inotropism, and bronchospasm. This results in sudden onset of respiratory distress and cyanosis.

(4) Within minutes, the negative inotropic effect becomes prevalent (probably due to myocardial ischaemia). Pulmonary venous pressure (congestion) increases and a drop in cardiac output are manifested by pulmonary oedema and hypotension to the point of shock.

(5) The exposure of the intravascular compartment to amniotic fluid thromboplastin and to other mediators freed in the circulation by the presence of amniotic fluid induces a consumptive coagulopathy in a large proportion of the first-phase survivors. This disseminated intravascular coagulation often results in severe uterine bleeding.

(6) The resultant systemic hypotension decreases the uterine perfusion. Abnormalities of the fetal heart tracing will rapidly follow and may result in fetal death.

Figure 36.10 Pathophysiology of amniotic fluid embolism (based on Perozzi & Englert 2004)

BOX 36.6 Diagnosis of AFE

The National Registry's criteria for diagnosis of Amniotic Fluid Embolism (Clarke et al 1995):

◗ acute hypotension or cardiac arrest
◗ acute hypoxia, defined as dyspnoea, cyanosis or respiratory arrest
◗ coagulopathy, defined as laboratory evidence of intravascular consumption or fibrinolysis (or severe clinical haemorrhage in the absence of other explanations)
◗ onset during cervical dilatation and curettage, labour, birth and caesarean delivery, or within 30 minutes post partum
◗ absence of any other significant confounding condition or potential explanation of symptoms and signs just listed.

Clinical point

Several clinical conditions (abruption, hydramnios, multiparity) are associated with AFE. There are no consistent clues, warning signs or associated complications to indicate an increased risk of AFE.

---

initial pulmonary symptoms may be minor but acute left ventricular failure usually develops and leads to cardiovascular collapse. This is followed by haemorrhage and DIC. Clarke and colleagues (1995) reported that 83% of cases documented in the national registry had either clinical or laboratory evidence of DIC. The remaining 17% died before clotting status could be determined. For a clinical diagnosis of AFE to be made, there needs to be evidence of:

● acute hypotension or cardiac arrest
● acute hypoxia (dyspnoea, cyanosis or respiratory arrest)
● coagulopathy (laboratory evidence of DIC or severe haemorrhage)
● onset of all of the above during labour or within 30 minutes of birth
● no other clinical conditions or potential explanations for the symptoms and signs.

There is no specific diagnostic test to confirm the diagnosis of AFE. The diagnosis is by exclusion. Any pregnant or labouring woman who exhibits signs associated with pulmonary embolus, septic shock, acute myocardial infarction, cardiomyopathy, anaphylaxis, cardiorespiratory collapse or intractable haemorrhage must be systematically evaluated to exclude the diagnosis of AFE. Laboratory investigations include:

● complete blood count
● coagulation parameters (FDP, fibrinogen)
● arterial blood gases
● chest X-ray
● ECG
● V/Q scan
● echocardiogram.

Management

Management of AFE depends on the following:
● oxygenation and ventilatory support:
  ● supplemental oxygen
  ● intubation
  ● ventilation
  ● diuretics

● correction of cardiovascular collapse and maintenance of normal cardiovascular function:
  ● CPR protocol
  ● delivery of the fetus
  ● volume
  ● inotropes
  ● after-load fluid reduction
● treatment of DIC with blood transfusion and replacement of clotting factors:
  ● fresh frozen plasma
  ● packed red blood cells
  ● platelets
  ● cryoprecipitate.
  Additional measures may include:
● high-dose corticosteroids
● adrenaline
● cardiopulmonary bypass
● nitric oxide
● inhaled prostacyclin.

Recognition of the condition followed by prompt and aggressive treatment of AFE is necessary to achieve better outcomes. All the cases described in the report on maternal deaths in Australia involved resuscitation and advanced life support (Slaytor et al 2004). Therefore it is crucial that all healthcare providers, irrespective of where they work, keep their basic and advanced life support skills up to date and be encouraged to attend appropriate courses, such as Advanced Life Support in Obstetrics (ALSO©) and Managing Obstetric Emergencies and Trauma (MOET©).

Dr Alex Tuffnell provides a valuable summary on the five maternal deaths caused by AFE in the *Report on Confidential Enquiries into Maternal Deaths in the United Kingdom* (CEMCH 2004). This summary helps us to understand this rare but often fatal complication and highlights the effects of treatment. Box 36.7 is derived from that analysis.

Summary: amniotic fluid embolism

Amniotic fluid embolism is not universally fatal but it is one of the most feared and devastating complications of pregnancy. It can be neither predicted nor prevented. Its presentation is variable and may mimic other embolic phenomena (pulmonary embolus). Medical management is essentially supportive. The primary goals of management are to provide oxygen, maintain cardiac output and organ perfusion, correct coagulopathy, and provide adjunctive therapies. Women with symptoms suspicious of AFE should be transferred to an ICU as soon as possible, as these women often have better outcomes.

Disseminated intravascular coagulation

Disseminated intravascular coagulation (DIC) is not a disease but a complex syndrome that is always secondary to an underlying disorder such as AFE. DIC occurs when the clotting cascade goes awry. It is characterised by systemic activation of the blood coagulation system, leading to the generation of intravascular fibrin, widespread fibrin deposition in the microcirculation, which contributes to the development of multi-organ failure. Consumption and subsequent exhaustion of coagulation proteins and platelets because of ongoing activation of the coagulation cascade may induce severe bleeding complications.

In obstetrics, DIC usually results from entrance into or generation within the blood of material with tissue factor activity (TFA), which initiates coagulation pathways. DIC usually arises in one of four clinical circumstances:

- obstetric calamities—where uterine material with TFA gains access to the maternal circulation (e.g. in abruptio placentae, retained dead fetus syndrome and following amniotic fluid embolism)
- shock—from any cause including PPH, probably because of the generation of TFA on monocytes and endothelial cells
- bacterial infection—particularly with Gram-negative organisms. Gram-negative endotoxins cause generation of TFA on the plasma membrane of monocytes and endothelial cells.
- malignancy—particularly mucin-secreting adenocarcinomas in which hypergranular, leucaemic cells are thought to release material from their granules with TFA.

Pathophysiology

The mechanisms by which DIC is triggered are not entirely understood and are too complex to be considered in detail in this chapter. In brief, several simultaneously occurring mechanisms play a role in the pathogenesis of DIC (Fig 36.11). For some reason, maternal blood is exposed to large amounts of the tissue factor FVIIa system. Two proteolytic enzymes, thrombin and plasmin, are activated and released into the systemic circulation. In normal circumstances the balance between these two substances determines a bleeding or thrombotic tendency. Thrombin cleaves fibrinogen to form fibrin monomers. The fibrin deposition is a result of tissue factor-mediated thrombin generation that is insufficiently balanced by physiological anticoagulant mechanisms such as the antithrombin system and the protein C system. In addition to enhanced fibrin formation, fibrin removal is impaired as a result of depression of the fibrinolytic system. This leads to small and large vessel thrombosis, with the end-result of multi-organ failure. As a result, large amounts of thrombin are generated, leading to a hypercoagulable state. In the normal physiological state, plasmin is responsible for breaking fibrin into fibrin split products, thereby limiting the formation of fibrin clots. In DIC, the quantity of plasmin is significantly increased, leading to the generation of significant quantities of fibrin degradation products. This results in the catastrophic bleeding seen in DIC.

Incidence and management

It is difficult to determine the exact incidence of DIC in obstetrics. If there is any suspicion of DIC arising from either clinical or laboratory findings, it is imperative to monitor the woman carefully with clinical and laboratory tests in order to identify the progression of the coagulopathy. In most cases the disease can be ameliorated in the early stages, for example in cases of DIC induced by abruptio placentae. Management

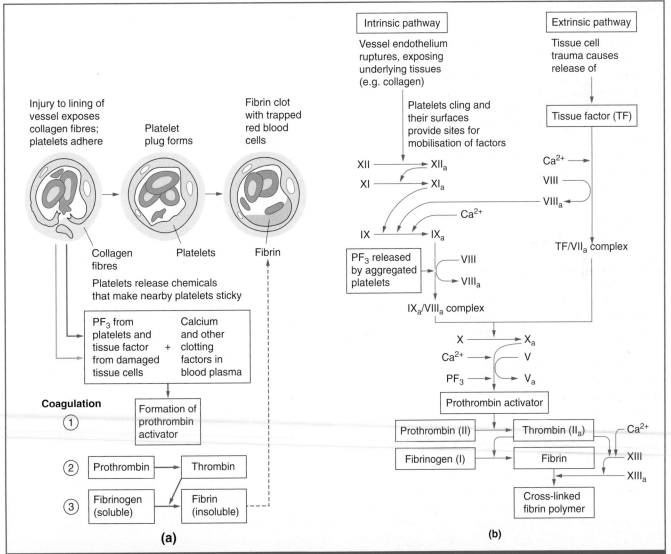

Figure 36.11 Platelet formation and blood clotting **(a)** Simplified overview of events. Steps 1 to 3 are the major events. **(b)** Detailed flow chart indicating intermediates and events involved in platelet plug formation and the intrinsic and extrinsic mechanisms of clotting (Note: subscript a: activated procoagulant) (based on Marien 2004)

is always individualised and supportive, and centred on treatment of the underlying disorder. Treatment includes:
- plasma and platelet substitution therapy
- anticoagulants
- restoration of anticoagulant pathways.

Eclampsia

Pre-eclampsia (PE) is a pregnancy-specific, multi-organ disorder usually associated with hypertension, thrombocytopenia and proteinuria. PE may progress to eclamptic seizures. Eclampsia, meaning literally to 'shine forth', complicates about 1:2000 pregnancies. In *Maternal Deaths in Australia 1997–1999*, Slaytor et al (2004) report six direct deaths where hypertension and/or eclampsia were identified. Seizures can occur before, during or after labour in roughly equal proportions (i.e. 30% antenatal, birth and postnatal). Women are at risk of eclampsia for about 48 to 72 hours after birth.

The Australasian Society for the Study of Hypertension in Pregnancy published its consensus statement on the detection, investigation and management of hypertension in pregnancy in 2000 (Brown et al 2000). The authors are unequivocal that prompt detection and treatment of eclampsia are the key to maternal and perinatal survival. Best practice recommendations are based on two international, multicentred trails. Both have shown that magnesium sulfate (MgSO$_4$) is the anticonvulsant agent of choice for the prevention and treatment of eclamptic seizures (Eclampsia Trial Collaborative Group 1995; Magpie Trial Collaborative Group 2002). This section focuses on identification and current management according to these recommendations.

Pathophysiology

Pre-eclampsia/eclampsia is part of a multi-system disorder of unknown aetiology characterised by vasoconstriction and hypercoagulability. Possible causes include a defect in placentation leading to uteroplacental hypoperfusion, immunological intolerance between mother and fetus, and genetic factors. Although the exact mechanism that leads to PE is not clear, several known factors are associated with the onset of the disease. Major pathological changes occur in the placental vascular bed, and trophoblastic implantation is abnormal, with reduced placental perfusion. An alteration in the ratio of prostacyclin and thromboxane occurs, along with platelet aggregation, thrombin activation and fibrin deposition in maternal vascular beds. Increased capillary permeability and hypoalbuminaemia also occur. The combination of profound vasospasm with consequent reduction of plasma volume and thrombosis causes dysfunction in almost all body systems. The latter triggers the coagulation cascade. Clotting times are often elevated in severe PE, although standard tests such as prothrombin time and partial thromboplastin time may be normal. The natural progression of the disease is from severe PE to eclampsia. Most women with

eclampsia present with a history of hypertension and seizures, although in about 20% of cases eclampsia may occur without warning in women who have no history of hypertension. It is believed that eclamptic seizures occur as the result of cerebral vasospasm and endothelial damage, which lead to cerebral ischaemia, microinfarcts and oedema.

Imminent eclampsia: signs and symptoms

Most women report premonitory symptoms of eclampsia:
- severe frontal headache—cerebral oedema
- diminished urinary output—renal failure: most important clinical feature
- visual disturbances—retinal oedema
- epigastric pain—haemorrhage of the subcapsular parts of the liver
- vomiting and nausea—related to cerebral oedema and liver damage
- hyper-reflexia—can signal impending eclampsia.

Management of severe pre-eclampsia and prevention of eclampsia

Early detection and prevention of severe PE is the key to prevention of eclampsia. The main aims of therapy centre on prevention or treatment of seizures, resuscitation, control of hypertension, treatment of complications, prompt consultation, and timely delivery of the infant and placenta. The only 'cure' for P-E/eclampsia is delivery of the placenta. The suppression of eclamptic seizures does not solve the underlying multi-system disease. It helps to protect the mother and baby from complications such as cerebral haemorrhage, antepartum haemorrhage, fetal asphyxia and death while the maternal condition is stabilised, and enables a multidisciplinary team to plan future care, including referral to a Level III hospital and the mode of delivery.

Prevention and control of seizures

Magnesium sulfate (MgSO$_4$) infusions for eclamptic seizure prophylaxis is now accepted as the gold standard of treatment of seizure-related complications of eclampsia and PE (Brown

---

Case study

Samantha, a primigravida at 38 weeks, attends a rural maternity centre with a severe headache. On assessment her BP is found to be 170/120. She has diminished urine output, a urine analysis of 3+ protein, epigastric pain and hyperreflexia. The FHR is within normal limits. Her lead carer is out of town and you are the only midwife on duty. You call the Emergency Retrieval Team for advice. They are now en route with an ETA of 45 mins. What will be your management of Samantha until the retrieval team arrives?

et al 2000; NSW Health Department 2002). Although the exact mechanism is unknown, $MgSO_4$ is thought to act as a physiological calcium antagonist, and may act by blocking calcium channels in smooth muscle, resulting in the reversal of cerebral vasospasm. Continuous infusion improves the maintenance of serum levels compared with intermittent bolus doses. Table 36.2 provides one example of a typical protocol for $MgSO_4$ used in the management of severe PE or eclampsia.

Side-effects of $MgSO_4$ (Magpie and Collaborative Eclampsia trials)

About 25% of women will experience one or more side-effects from the $MgSO_4$ infusion. The woman should be monitored carefully for clinical signs of magnesium toxicity, particularly:

- sensation of pain and warmth in arms
- disruption to sensation, particularly in extremities
- flushing of face, neck and hands
- thirst, headache, dizziness, itching
- nausea, vomiting
- loss of patellar reflexes—absent well before toxic serum levels are reached
- respiratory depression (rate < 10/min)
- slurring of speech, muscle weakness, drowsiness and double vision
- respiratory/cardiac arrest (Eclampsia Trial Collaborative Group 1995; Magpie Trial Collaborative Group 2002).

If toxicity is suspected, the infusion should be discontinued. If required, the antidote for maternal toxicity is an IV injection of calcium chloride or calcium gluconate (10 mL of 10% solution at a rate not exceeding 5 mL/min) over three minutes.

TABLE 36.2 Example of a protocol for $MgSO_4$ management of severe PE or eclampsia

Loading dose
Presentation is usually 50% solution in 5 mL H_2O
Undiluted, this = 10 mmol/5 mL = 2 mmol/mL
Ampoules: 2.47 g in 5 mL / 0.49 g in 1mL / 3.92 g in 8 mL
Recommended loading dose: 4 g (16 mmol) $MgSO_4$ over 15–30 mins

Infusion pump	Syringe pump
Loading dose	
4 g $MgSO_4$ (50% solution) diluted in normal saline via infusion pump over 20–30 min: • Using 500 mL flask normal saline, run 100 mL into burette. • Add 8 mL (4 g) $MgSO_4$ (50% solution) to 100 mL normal saline in burette. • Infuse over 20–30 min via infusion pump.	4 g $MgSO_4$ (50% solution) not diluted is given via syringe pump over 15 min: • Using 20 mL syringe, draw up 9 mL undiluted $MgSO_4$ (50% solution). • Prime line with 1 mL of solution. • Run the remaining 8 mL of 2 mmol/mL solution at 32 mL/hr for 15 min.
Maintenance infusion	
1 g $MgSO_4$ (50% solution) per hour via infusion pump: • Remove 20 mL normal saline from the remaining flask and discard. Add 20 mL (10 g) of $MgSO_4$ (50% solution) to the remaining 380 mL flask of normal saline. • Infuse at 40 mL/hr via infusion pump. • Run maintenance for at least 24 hrs.	1 g $MgSO_4$ per hour via syringe pump: • Using a 50 mL syringe, draw up 49 mL of undiluted $MgSO_4$ (50% solution). • Prime line with 1 mL of solution. • Run the remaining 48 mL of 2 mmol/mL at 2 mL/hr for at least 24 hrs.

Key points:
- Use an infusion pump or syringe.
- Do not use IV line to inject other drugs.
- Check serum levels 1 hour after administration and 6-hourly thereafter.

Contraindications include:
- renal failure—$MgSO_4$ is eliminated in the renal system, so can reach toxicity in the presence of oliguria
- hypocalcaemic states
- cardiac condition, e.g. conduction or myocardial damage.

Should be used cautiously with other drugs that cause respiratory depression, e.g. diazepam, narcotics.

Considerations:
- May lower BP due to vasodilatory effects.
- May have tocolytic effect.
- May decrease FHR variability as decompression of CNS.
- May cause loss of reflexes.

(Source: NSW Health Department 2002)

Control of hypertension

Anti-hypertensive therapy is an essential component in the treatment of severe PE/eclampsia. It controls severe hypertension and helps to protect the mother from cerebral haemorrhage. However, it is important not to decrease the blood pressure (BP) too quickly or by too much, as this may further reduce placental perfusion. Once the systolic BP reaches ≥ 170 mmHg and the diastolic BP ≥ 110 mmHg, antihypertensive therapy is begun. The aim is to decrease the systolic BP by about 20–30 mmHg and the diastolic BP by 10–15 mmHg. A rapid and precipitous decrease in the BP as result of antihypertensive drugs should be avoided because of the risks of further fetal compromise in babies that are often already growth-restricted. Hydralazine is known to be effective in controlling hypertension in severe PE/eclampsia. After an IV bolus dose of 10 mg over 20 minutes by slow IV infusion to a maximum of 60 mg, effects are seen by 10 minutes and reach maximum levels within a further 10 minutes. Its duration is six to eight hours. Side-effects include hypotension, tachycardia, tremor, headache, nausea and vomiting (often signs that herald the onset of eclampsia). In some countries, including New Zealand, labetalol is being used more frequently in the management of hypertension in pregnancy (the drug is not available for IV use in Australia). Its onset of action is more rapid than hydralazine, and reflex tachycardia does not occur. The typical regimen is: an initial dose of 50 mg IV (over two minutes). If necessary it is repeated every 10–20 minutes to a maximum of 300 mg. It can also be administered as an infusion at 2.0 mg/hr, increasing by 0.5 mg/hr as required (2–20 mg/hr is usually necessary).

Fluid balance

Severe PE/eclampsia is associated with high peripheral resistance, haemoconcentration, reduction and central distribution of plasma volume and oliguria. However, routine volume expansion is not recommended because of the danger of precipitating pulmonary oedema. Iatrogenic fluid overload is a common cause of maternal death in severe PE/eclampsia. Maintenance fluids should be given to prevent maternal hypotension and fetal compromise, especially in the presence of oliguria. Nevertheless, severe hypotension and fetal compromise have been reported in eclamptic women given epidural analgesia or hydralazine without prior infusion of solutions. The Australasian Society for the Study of Hypertension in Pregnancy (ASSHP 2000) recommends a 500 mL fluid load for severe pre-eclamptics prior to antihypertensive therapy, epidural therapy or immediate delivery, or as part of the initial management of oliguria.

Delivery

The timing and place of delivery depend on the maternal and fetal condition. Referral to a regional centre for advice and/or assistance is crucial in all cases of severe PE or eclampsia, but each case should be considered on its clinical merits. Delivery by caesarean section or induction of labour may be appropriate. In eclampsia the definitive 'cure' is delivery. Nevertheless, it is inappropriate to deliver a physiologically unstable mother even if there is evidence of severe fetal compromise. Once the seizures have been controlled and hypertension treated, delivery can be expedited. It is often necessary to admit the woman to an ICU. Best practice demands that a collaborative, multidisciplinary team, including obstetricians, midwives, anaesthetists and paediatrician, work with all women who have eclampsia.

Management of eclampsia

More than 50% of eclamptic seizures occur outside the hospital environment. It is therefore essential for all clinicians to be competent to deal with severe PE and eclampsia. The principles of management include the following:

- **ABCs—airway, breathing, circulation**
  - Do not leave the woman alone.
  - Protect from harm.
  - Obtain help.
  - Assess, maintain patency of airway.
  - Apply oxygen via Hudson mask (8 L/min).
  - Evaluate pulse and BP.
  - If absent, initiate CPR and call arrest team.
  - Secure IV access as soon as possible.
- **Control seizures**
  - $MgSO_4$—loading and maintenance dose
  - Monitor
    - urinary output
    - respiratory rate, oxygen saturation and patellar reflexes, initially every 10 mins, then 30 mins
    - Check serum magnesium levels at least daily if infusion is continued for > 24 hrs
  - Stop infusion: check $MgSO_4$ levels and review with specialist team if:
    - urine output < 100 mL in 4 hrs
    - *or* patellar reflexes are absent
    - *or* respiratory rate < 16 bpm
    - *or* oxygen saturation < 90%
    - Antidote 10% calcium gluconate 10 mL IV over 10 mins.
- **Control hypertension**
  - Treat hypertension if systolic BP ≥ 170 mmHg or diastolic BP ≥ 110 mmHg
    - hydralazine
    - labetalol
- **Deliver**
  - 'Stabilise' the mother before delivery.

Summary: eclampsia

Eclampsia remains a major, albeit rare, cause of maternal and perinatal morbidity and mortality in Australia and New Zealand. It is often associated with other morbidity, such as preterm birth. The relationship between the onset of pre-eclampsia and eclampsia is not fully understood. Despite successful identification of women at risk of PE or eclampsia during pregnancy, it is clear that not all cases can be prevented. Optimal emergency management of seizures, hypertension, fluid balance and subsequent safe transfer is essential to minimise morbidity and mortality. It is essential that midwives ensure that, irrespective of the place of birth, they are competent and confident to manage an eclamptic seizure until help arrives.

Critical thinking exercise

Significant findings from midwifery assessments
Midwives are in a good position to detect the early signs of obstetric risks. What might be the significance of the following findings from a midwifery assessment?

▶ oliguria < 30 mL/hr
▶ significant change in maternal vital signs
▶ diastolic BP 110 mmHg or higher
▶ seizure activity
▶ severe epigastric or upper right quadrant pain
▶ altered mental status
▶ signs of pulmonary oedema
▶ abnormal laboratory results.

- Delivery is a team effort.
- Ergometrine should not be used in the presence of PE or eclampsia.
- Consider prophylaxis against thromboembolism.
- Maintain vigilance, as most seizures occur after birth.
- **Ongoing care**
  - **Observations**
    - pulse oximeter, BP, respirations, temperature
    - ECG
    - test urine for protein
    - hourly urine output
    - strict fluid balance chart
    - continuous EFM
  - **Investigations**
    - FBP, platelets and urea and electrolytes
    - urate, liver function tests
    - coagulation screen
    - group, hold and serum
    - MSSU
    - 24-hour urine collection for total protein and creatinine clearance and catecholamines.

Further study

1 Visit sites designed for women with complications in pregnancy, such as:
   - Pre-eclampsia site, http://www.pre-eclampsia.co.uk/
   - Action On Pre-eclampsia http://www.apec.org.uk
2 Use a search engine such as PubMed, HighWire at: http://highwire.stanford.edu/ or Ovid, to study pre-eclampsia and eclampsia in more depth.
3 Compare and contrast clinical guidelines on management of pregnant women with hypertensive disorders.

Rupture of the uterus

Rupture of the uterus is one of the most serious complications of pregnancy, and can be fatal for the fetus. The incidence of uterine rupture is 1:1148 to 1:2250 deliveries (DeCherney & Nathan 2003). The term 'uterine rupture' is used to describe trauma to the uterus in a continuum of events, from a 'weak' spot in the uterine wall noticed by the obstetrician at the time of a caesarean section to the catastrophe of the uterus rupturing so that the fetus and placenta are expelled into the peritoneal cavity.

Classification

There are two types of uterine rupture, complete and incomplete, distinguished by whether or not the serosa is involved. In a complete rupture, the entire thickness of the uterine wall and usually the overlying broad ligament rupture, so the uterine contents, including fetus and occasionally the placenta, extrude into the peritoneal cavity. Occult or incomplete rupture refers to dehiscence of a surgical wound, where the visceral peritoneum stays intact and the fetus and placenta remain inside the uterine cavity. The complete variety is the rarer and more dangerous of the two. Uterine rupture most often occurs in the lower uterine segment, with the most common site of rupture being the anterior uterine wall. Longitudinal rupture of the lateral wall is also relatively common and may extend upwards into the fundus of the uterus or downwards into the vagina. Posterior ruptures are the least common and are usually transverse. Rupture of the uterus during labour is more dangerous than that occurring in pregnancy, because shock is greater and infection is almost inevitable.

Risk factors

Uterine rupture may develop as a result of pre-existing injury such as a scar from uterine surgery, perforation or anomaly. It is also associated with trauma, or it may complicate labour in a previously unscarred uterus. In developing countries, uterine rupture is most often caused by obstructed labour related to CPD, grandmultiparity and malpresentation. In contrast, in developed countries the most common cause of uterine rupture is dehiscence of a previous caesarean section scar. Injudicious use of oxytocin and traumatic rupture from obstetric manipulative procedures such as internal podalic version are also contributing factors.

Other associations include:
- caesarean section
- induction of labour
- uterine anomalies
- trauma (e.g. MVA)
- use of rotational forceps
- cervical laceration
- manual removal of the placenta (placenta percreta and increta)
- conditions causing overdistension of uterus:
  - hydramnios
  - macrosomia
  - multiple pregnancy
  - choriocarcinoma.

Presentation

In developing countries, where spontaneous rupture usually follows an obstructed labour, the clinical presentation is characterised by sudden, severe pain and vaginal bleeding (Ola & Olamijulo 1998). Cardiovascular collapse often occurs if the rupture involves major blood vessels. Cessation of uterine contractions accompanies the rupture. On clinical examination the contours of the uterus may change, especially if the fetus is only partially extruded. If it is completely extruded into the peritoneal cavity, the fetal parts are easily palpable but the fetal heart tones cannot be heard. Haematuria suggests that the bladder is also involved in the rupture.

In developed countries, the presentation may not be so dramatic because the rupture usually occurs during labour along a previous uterine scar. Moreover, it is most unlikely that the woman has had to endure many hours of obstructed labour before her uterus ruptures. There may, however, be no signs and symptoms associated with a rupture of a low cervical scar during labour.

When the uterus spontaneously ruptures during labour, the typical features are suprapubic pain and tenderness, cessation of uterine contractions, absence of fetal heart sounds, recession of presenting parts and vaginal haemorrhage. This may be followed by signs and symptoms of hypovolaemic shock

---

Clinical point

Following uterine rupture, in more than 75% of cases, signs of fetal distress will appear before pain or bleeding. Prolonged, late or variable decelerations and bradycardia seen on FHR monitoring are the most common—and often the only—manifestation of uterine rupture.

Clinical point

Intrapartum or postpartum collapse can occur because of uterine rupture, sepsis, uterine inversion and amniotic fluid embolism.

---

and haemoperitoneum. In some cases labour may progress to vaginal birth with a live neonate. Ultrasound may show abnormal fetal position or extension of fetal extremities or haemoperitoneum. If there is any doubt about the diagnosis, a laparotomy is essential, especially in the presence of persistent haemorrhage and shock that cannot be attributed to other causes and does not abate following the administration of oxytocics drugs and treatment for shock.

Management

In all cases of operative delivery, especially where there are significant risk factors for uterine rupture, there should be a careful examination of the uterus and birth canal for evidence of trauma. Once the diagnosis of a rupture is made, resuscitation following the guidelines described later in this chapter is the first priority. Provided the woman gives her consent, hysterectomy is the preferred treatment, especially if the rupture is extensive or in the presence of infection. However, where future childbearing is important, and depending on the facilities available, the skill of the surgeon and the extent of the rupture, a laparotomy and attempted rupture repair may be feasible. There is an increased risk of a repeat rupture in subsequent pregnancies.

Trauma in pregnancy

Major trauma in pregnancy is a relatively uncommon event. Management of the pregnant woman in trauma poses specific challenges often beyond the realm of midwifery or obstetric care. In part this is because it is such an uncommon experience for most midwives and obstetricians. Similarly, Emergency Department staff may not be aware of the normal maternal and fetal physiology and the woman's anatomical and physiological adaptations to pregnancy. These may mask or mimic injury or mean that physical signs are misinterpreted.

Normal clinical and laboratory findings in pregnant women may be suggestive of pathology in non-pregnant women. It is crucial for clinicians (trauma specialists, obstetric staff and midwives) to work collaboratively to establish safe and effective protocols for monitoring and treating the mother and the fetus. The following section provides an overview of the risks of trauma in pregnancy, its effects on the mother and fetus, and the management of trauma in pregnant women. It concludes with an overview of the skills required in cardiopulmonary resuscitation of pregnant women.

Trauma and maternal and neonatal mortality

Although it is a relatively uncommon event, occurring in less than 1% of all trauma admissions to Australian hospitals, trauma remains a leading cause of morbidity and mortality in young pregnant women and their babies (Sugrue et al 2004). According to the 2004 AIHW report, *Maternal Deaths in Australia 1997–1999* (Slaytor et al 2004), of the 90 deaths reported to the National Advisory Committee on maternal mortality, 28 deaths were classified as being from incidental causes. These are maternal deaths that result from a condition occurring during pregnancy, where the pregnancy is unlikely to have contributed significantly to the death, although it may be possible to postulate a distant association. Seven of these involved traffic accidents and two were the result of homicide (p 52). Of particular concern for midwives because of their role in parent education is that of the five deaths involving motor vehicles, alcohol and cannabis were contributing factors in three accidents; and three women were not wearing seatbelts at the time of the accident.

Fetal death associated with trauma in pregnancy affects about 0.03% to 0.09% of pregnancies (Warner et al 2004, p 125). Few studies provide data on pregnant women with trauma that can be used to direct management decisions. A 1991 US retrospective study (Esposito et al 1991) found that of 79 pregnant women who were admitted to a trauma centre during a nine-year period, the maternal mortality was 10%, which was similar to the rate for non-pregnant females. Overall, the rate of fetal death was 34%. These rates were no different between women with or without evidence of shock and/or hypoxia, or between women who were or were not wearing seat belts in motor vehicle accidents.

Trauma in pregnant women: morbidity, incidence and causes

In the United States (as in Australia and probably New Zealand), although less than 1% of admissions to hospital for trauma are pregnant, trauma complicates about 7% of all pregnancies and is the leading non-obstetric cause of maternal and fetal morbidity and death. Motor vehicle accidents, family violence and falls are the most common causes of blunt trauma in pregnancy (Shah et al 1998). Almost 60% of trauma in pregnant women is intentional (Shah et al 1998). It is difficult to ascertain precise rates of pregnant women who present to emergency departments following trauma. In Western Australia, Royal Perth Hospital, a tertiary-level hospital, maintains an electronic trauma registry (Warner et al 2004, p 126). From July 1994 until August 2002, 3383 women of reproductive age were entered in the register and 34 were known to be pregnant. The baseline characteristics of these women are listed in Table 36.3.

The clinical outcomes are listed in Table 36.4. None of the women had a ruptured uterus. The four women admitted following a motor vehicle accident and experiencing uterine contractions did not go on to have a preterm birth.

Risk of trauma in pregnancy

The pattern of major injuries in pregnant women is different from that in non-pregnant women: trauma to the abdomen is more common than injuries to the head and chest. Given that up to 24% of all pregnant women experience family violence (Commonwealth Fund 1999), the likelihood of domestic

TABLE 36.3 Characteristics of the 34 pregnant women listed in the Royal Perth Hospital trauma registry

Characteristic	Data*
Age (years)	29 (17–40)
Period of gestation (weeks)	19 (5–32)
First trimester	12 (35)
Second trimester	14 (41)
Third trimester	8 (24)
ISS	
Severe injury (ISS > 15)	5 (1–57)
Type of injury	
Blunt	28 (82)
Penetrating	6 (18)
Cause of injury	
Motor vehicle accident	18 (53)
Domestic violence	7 (21)
Falls	4 (12)
Laceration	2 (6)
Punch injury to MCP joint	1 (3)
Horseriding accident	1 (3)
Thermal injury	1 (3)

*Values are expressed either as an absolute number with the percentage in parenthesis, or as a median score with the range in parenthesis.
ISS: injury severity score. MCP: metacarpal joint.
(Source: Warner et al 2004, p 126)

TABLE 36.4 Summary of clinical outcomes for the 34 pregnant women listed in the Royal Perth Hospital trauma registry

Outcome	Number (%)
No complication	27 (79)
Contractions abated without intervention	4 (12)
Placental abruption (successful caesarean section)	1 (3)
Fetal death (maternal survival)	1 (3)
Maternal and fetal death	1 (3)

(Source: Warner et al 2004, p 126)

assault should always be borne in mind, especially when the observed injuries are inconsistent with their alleged cause. The rate of fetal mortality after blunt trauma is 3.8–38%, mostly from abruption, maternal shock and maternal death (Grossman 2004, p 1303). The risk to pregnancy in 'minor' or non-catastrophic trauma is still significant, with preterm labour occurring in 8%, placental abruption in 1%, and fetal death in 1%. For those with major trauma, maternal mortality is about 9% and the fetal death rate is 20% or greater (Sugrue et al 2004).

Fetal injury or death can still happen even if the mother has incurred no apparent abdominal injury. About 5% of fetal injuries occur without apparent trauma to the mother, often from complications associated with maternal hypoxia and shock. Irrespective of the apparent severity of the injury, all pregnant women should be evaluated in a medical setting.

Physiological changes in pregnancy

See Table 36.5. The non-pregnant uterus is thick-walled but loses this protection as it expands out of the pelvis during

pregnancy from about 12 weeks gestation. By the second trimester the growing fetus is protected somewhat by amniotic fluid. By the third trimester the uterus is thin-walled, and by the 36th week of pregnancy the head may engage in the pelvis. When full, the bladder also becomes an abdominal organ. An increase in heart rate and stroke volume leads to an increase in cardiac output by about 50% in pregnancy. Blood volume has increased by as much as 50% by the 28th week of gestation. The protective effects of hypervolaemia allow the woman to lose up to 30% (1500 mL) of her circulating blood volume before signs associated with hypotension appear. However, it is not uncommon for a pregnant woman to have what is often called 'low blood pressure'—perhaps 80/40 mmHg in early pregnancy, although late in the second trimester the blood pressure returns to 'normal levels'.

Maternal posture and haemodynamics

In the third trimester, the heavy gravid uterus compresses the descending aorta and the inferior vena cava. This results in a greater tendency for pooling of venous blood in the lower limbs, decreasing venous return from the heart, a fall in cardiac output and hypotension. One of the first signs of supine hypotension is often a non-reassuring FHR caused by decreased uteroplacental perfusion. If the woman is supine, cardiac return may be reduced by as much as 30% (Fig 36.12). This affects the mother's cardiac output. It is therefore important to tilt the pregnant woman to the left by about 30 degrees and it may be necessary to manually displace

---

BOX 36.8 Trauma in pregnancy

Unique problems of the pregnant woman with trauma

▸ The placenta is devoid of elastic tissue but the myometrium is very elastic, predisposing to shearing.

▸ From 16 weeks gestation, abruptio placenta is the most common result of blunt injury.

▸ Following trauma, the most common cause of preterm labour is abruptio placentae.

▸ Fetal skull injury is the most common fetal injury, with a mortality rate of 42%.

▸ After 12 weeks gestation, the bladder is displaced upward and forward by the enlarging uterus, leading to an increased risk of bladder injury from blunt or penetrating trauma.

▸ Because of the enlarging uterus, the diaphragm rises by about 4 cm and the diameter of the chest enlarges by about 2%. The trachea is displaced to the right. Upward displacement of the diaphragm and viscera decreases chest compliance and ventilation and makes chest compression in CPR more difficult.

▸ As pregnancy progresses, there is a decrease in the functional residual capacity of the lungs, coupled with a 20% increase in oxygen consumption, making women more prone to hypoxia. Further, 30% of pregnant women have airway closure during normal tidal ventilation if they are placed in a supine position. All these alterations predispose pregnant women to a rapid decrease in maternal PaO_2 during periods of apnoea or airway obstruction.

▸ Changes in the gastrointestinal tract and increased levels of progesterone make pregnant women more prone to regurgitation of gastric contents and Mendelson's syndrome.

▸ Enlarged breast tissue also makes chest compression more difficult.

TABLE 36.5 Physiological changes in pregnancy

	Non-pregnant	Pregnant
Cardiovascular		
Pulse	70–80 bpm	up by 10–15 bpm
Cardiac output	4.5 L/min	up to 6.7 L/min
Systolic blood pressure	110 mmHg	down by 5–15 mmHg
Haematological		
Blood volume	4000 mL	up by 30–50%
Plasma	2400 mL	up to 3700 mL
RBC volume	1600 mL	up to 1900 mL
Haemoglobin	120–160 g/L	down to 100–140 g/L
Respiratory		
Tidal volume	500 mL	up by 25%
Functional residual volume	1200 mL	down by 25%
Gastrointestinal		
Intra-abdominal pressure	normal	increased
Gastric emptying	normal	decreased

(Source: Sugrue et al 2004)

the uterine fundus to the woman's left. However, it should be remembered that airway control and efforts to reduce the risk of supine hypotension must be balanced against the need to stabilise the cervical spine. The woman should be tilted as an entire unit, maintaining stabilisation of the cervical spine (Sugrue et al 2004).

Management

When confronted with an injured pregnant woman, the mother is always attended to first. There are two patients with separate needs. The goals of management are to:
- identify and meet the needs of the pregnant woman
- identify and meet the needs of the fetus.

The important rule to remember is: 'What is good for the mother is good for the fetus'. Optimal care of the mother optimises fetal outcomes. However, an apparently stable mother may be compensating at the expense of the fetus.

Assessment

The following plan for maternal assessment follows guidelines set out by the Early Management of Severe Trauma (EMST®)/

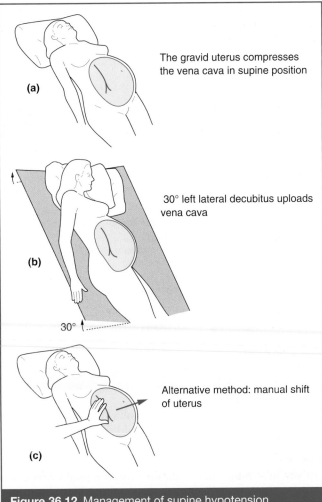

The gravid uterus compresses the vena cava in supine position

(a)

30° left lateral decubitus uploads vena cava

(b)

30°

Alternative method: manual shift of uterus

(c)

Figure 36.12 Management of supine hypotension

Advanced Trauma Life Support (ATLS®) approach to trauma, with detailed primary and secondary survey (assessments) (Fig 36.13). It outlines a systematic approach to initial stabilisation.

Primary survey

The purpose of the primary survey is to diagnose immediate life-threatening conditions. These should be treated as soon as they are discovered, before continuing the survey. As with any other injured person, the primary survey addresses the airway, cervical spine control, breathing and circulation, volume replacement/haemorrhage control, as well as assessment of conscious state and environmental injury. Once the ABCs have been achieved, an assessment of fetal wellbeing is conducted. An electronic trace of the FHR is usually started if the woman is more than 24 weeks pregnant, to detect fetal compromise and thus reduce the risk of unexpected fetal demise.

The survey is planned as follows:
- **A**irway control with cervical spine protection
- **B**reathing
- **C**irculation and control of haemorrhage
- **D**isorders of the central nervous system
- **E**xposure of the whole body.

During the course of the primary survey, any deterioration in the woman's clinical condition should be managed by reassessing from the start of the protocol, as a previously undiagnosed injury may become apparent. Supplemental oxygen is essential to prevent and treat maternal and fetal hypoxia. Severe trauma stimulates maternal catecholamine release, which causes uteroplacental vasoconstriction and compromised fetal circulation. Prevention of aortocaval compression (supine hypotension) optimises maternal and fetal haemodynamics. Hypovolaemia should be suspected before it becomes apparent, because relative pregnancy-induced hypervolaemia and haemodilution may mask significant blood loss. Aggressive volume resuscitation is encouraged even for normotensive women; however, care needs to be taken to ensure that the woman does not develop pulmonary oedema. A pneumatic anti-shock garment (PASG) may be used to stabilise lower extremity fractures and perhaps control

> ### Clinical point
>
> If the mother is haemodynamically compromised, so is the blood supply to the fetus, which rapidly becomes hypoxic and acidotic. Return of blood to the mother's heart may be impaired by the uterus pressing against the inferior vena cava and so circulation must be restored. Consequently, the key to resuscitation of the fetus is resuscitation of the mother. The mother cannot be resuscitated until blood flow to her right ventricle is restored, and therefore prevention of supine hypotension caused by the gravid uterus pressing on the mother's major blood vessels must be prevented.

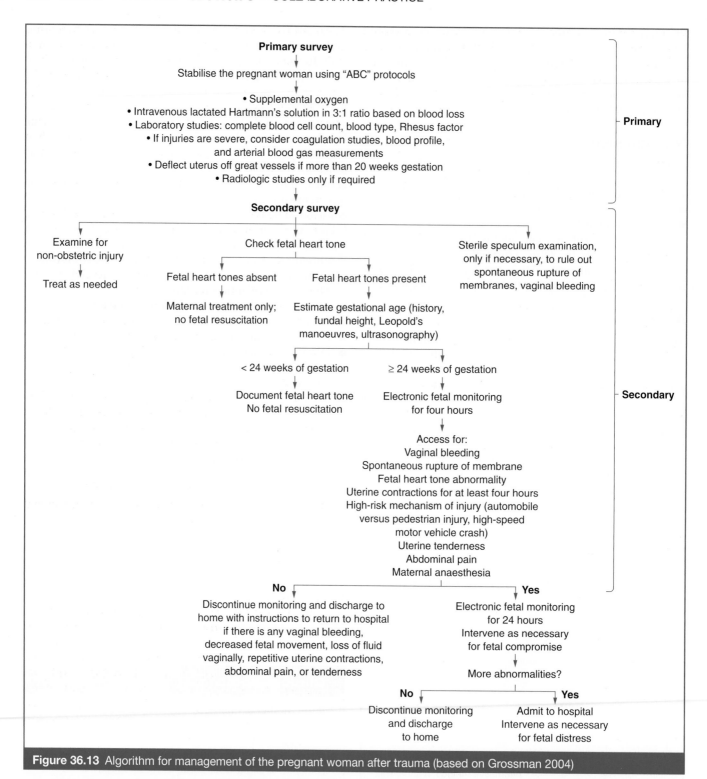

Figure 36.13 Algorithm for management of the pregnant woman after trauma (based on Grossman 2004)

haemorrhage; however, in the pregnant woman, inflation of the abdominal compartment of the PASG should be avoided because it compromises uteroplacental blood flow.

Secondary survey

The secondary survey—detailed assessment—only begins when the primary survey has been completed and immediate life-threatening injuries addressed. Following the initial survey and resuscitation, the woman should undergo a thorough secondary survey with the aim of documenting any other injuries. At the same time, the basics of the primary survey (airway, breathing and circulation) are continually reassessed to detect any unexpected deterioration. The secondary survey consists of obtaining a complete history, including an obstetric history, performing a physical examination, and evaluating and monitoring the fetus. It may be necessary at this stage to place the woman on her back for a short time to assess hidden injuries. The obstetric history is important because co-morbidities such as threatened preterm labour or antepartum haemorrhage predispose the woman to a recurrence of these complications. The obstetric history includes the date of the last menstruation, expected date of birth and any problems or complications of the current and previous pregnancies. Determination of the uterine size provides an approximation of gestational age—measurement of fundal height is a rapid method for estimating fetal age.

Determination of fetal viability, age and fetal maturity are important factors in decisions regarding the need for early delivery. Decisions about fetal viability are made on the basis of the best estimate of gestational age available. When estimating the fetal age in the resuscitation area or a non-obstetric setting, a rough guide might be that when the fundus of the uterus extends beyond the umbilicus, the fetus is potentially viable. Ultrasonography is the most accurate way of determining gestational age.

Aside from the usual secondary survey, assessment of the injured pregnant woman are performed to rule out vaginal bleeding, ruptured membranes and the presence of contractions or other signs of the onset of labour, and identify the FHR and rhythm. The physical examination includes assessment and reassessment of uterine size and tone. Provided there is no evidence of placenta praevia, a vaginal examination is performed to detect the presence of blood, liquor, cervical changes and the station of the fetus in the pelvis.

The AMPLE history is a good way to remember to ask the right questions during the secondary survey:

A History of allergies
M Medication history
P Past medical, surgical and obstetric history (including the current pregnancy)
L Time of the last meal
E Events leading up to injury and hospital admission.

Cardiotocographic monitoring

Controversy still exists about the ideal duration of fetal monitoring following a traumatic event needed to identify trauma-related fetal problems. A CTG is, however, the current standard of post-trauma care for all viable fetuses. The objectives of the monitoring period are to look for the onset of labour, placental abruption and fetal compromise. A combination of high-resolution real-time ultrasonography and CTG monitoring has the highest sensitivity and specificity. Both should be instituted as soon as possible without interfering with maternal resuscitative efforts. Fetal evaluation begins with checking FHR and noting fetal movement. This should be done late in the primary survey or early in the secondary survey and repeated regularly. CTG enables prompt identification of the fetus at greater risk for asphyxia and fetal death. A non-reassuring FHR pattern may be the first sign of maternal haemodynamic compromise.

Any viable fetus of 24 or more weeks gestation requires monitoring after a trauma event. This includes women with no obvious signs of abdominal injury, because direct impact is not necessary for feto-placental pathology to be present. Monitoring is commenced as soon as possible after initial stabilisation because most placental abruptions occur shortly after trauma. Continuous electronic fetal monitoring is more sensitive in detecting a placental abruption than ultrasonography, intermittent monitoring, Kleihauer Betke test or physical examination. The midwife assesses:

- FHR (baseline rate, pattern, variability, accelerations, decelerations)
- Uterine activity (tone, contractions). If after four hours of monitoring there is less than one contraction in 10 minutes, the risk of further complications drops to baseline. The occurrence of more than eight uterine contractions per hour over four hours is associated with a 20% increase in the risk of an APH.
  - A minimum of four hours monitoring is recommended, even after minor abdominal trauma. This is because clinical signs and symptoms of abruption, such as vaginal bleeding, abdominal pain and tenderness, and uterine tenderness, are often absent.
  - Monitoring for 24 hours is suggested following major trauma or signs of obstetric decompensation, such as regular uterine contractions, vaginal bleeding, premature rupture of the membranes, or a non-reassuring FHR pattern.

Procedures for evaluating abdominal trauma

The preferred diagnostic procedures for evaluating abdominal trauma are, in order of priority:

1 ultrasound
2 DPL (diagnostic peritoneal lavage)
3 CT scan
4 laparoscopy
5 laparotomy.

Diagnostic peritoneal lavage is a procedure most midwives will not be familiar with. During DPL, the peritoneum is visualised directly; it is safe and accurate in pregnancy, especially if a supraumbilical, open technique is used to avoid injury to the gravid uterus. If CT scan is necessary, both oral and IV contrast media should be administered. Ultrasound is also a useful method of assessing the abdomen. However, it misses 50–80% of placental abruptions but, as Grossman points out, it rapidly and safely determines fetal heart tones, placental location, gestational age and amniotic fluid index (Grossman 2004, p 1307).

Radiation exposure

Following maternal stabilisation and assessment, and fetal evaluation, the extent of maternal and fetal injury is further evaluated with the help of specific diagnostic modalities. With good reason, physicians and midwives are concerned about the risks to a pregnant woman and her fetus from radiation exposure. It may, however, be necessary to undertake comprehensive radiological assessment even though sensitivity to radiation is greater during intrauterine development than at any other time of life. The greatest risk to the fetus from radiation exposure (central nervous systems defects, microcephaly, growth restriction and childhood neoplasia, and death) is during the fourth and eighth weeks of gestation, a time of major organogenesis. Organs are less sensitive to radiation teratogenesis after the fifteenth week of gestation but growth restriction, central nervous system dysfunction and postnatal neoplasias may still occur.

Nevertheless, studies show that exposure of the fetus to less than 5–10 rad (radiation absorbed doses) causes no significant increase in the risk of congenital malformations, intrauterine growth restriction or miscarriage. Adverse effects from radiation exposure are unlikely at less than 5–10 rad. Grossman (2004, p 1308) quotes reports from some studies that indicate that the radiation dose from a plain AP chest X-ray is in general below 0.005 rad; a pelvic film < 0.2 rad, CT scan of the head < 0.05 rad; CT scan of the upper abdomen < 3.5 rad; and CT scan of the entire upper abdomen < 5.0 rad (depending on the trimester). Moreover, less than 1% of trauma patients are exposed to more than 3 rads (Grossman 2004).

Complications of trauma

The most common complication of trauma in pregnancy is uterine contractions and the onset of labour. Myometrial and decidual cells, damaged by contusion or placental separation, release prostaglandins, which stimulate uterine contractions. These may or may not be painful. Occasional uterine contractions are very common after trauma and in the vast majority of cases will resolve in a few hours, and therefore are not associated with adverse perinatal outcomes. Progression to true labour depends on the extent of uterine trauma, the amount of prostaglandins released, and the gestational age of the fetus.

Placental abruption

Grossman (2004, p 1309) comments that despite advances in trauma management, fetal and maternal mortality rates from traumatic injury have not declined. Prevention is therefore the key to increasing maternal and fetal survival. Both motor vehicle accidents and domestic assault are preventable causes of trauma in pregnancy. Even in countries where seatbelt use is compulsory, pregnant women have lower rates of seatbelt use than non-pregnant women.

Placental abruption after trauma occurs in 1% to 4% of 'minor' accidents and in up to 50% of 'major' injuries. Abruption can occur with little or no external signs of injury. Maternal mortality from abruption is less than 1%, but fetal death ranges from 20% to 35%. When present after trauma, vaginal bleeding is an ominous sign that is strongly suggestive of an abruption. The first-line test to confirm the presence of abruption is a transabdominal ultrasound, although it is less than 50% accurate. In general, CTG monitoring is more sensitive in picking up placental abruption by non-reassuring FHR pattern than ultrasound is by visualisation. Most cases of abruption become evident within several hours after trauma.

Feto-maternal haemorrhage

Feto-maternal haemorrhage (FMH), the transplacental haemorrhage of fetal blood into the normally separate maternal circulation, is a complication of trauma during pregnancy. The reported incidence of FMH after trauma is 8–30%. There is no real correlation between severity of trauma, gestational age and frequency and volume of FMH. Complications of FMH include Rh sensitisation in the mother, fetal anaemia, fetal atrial tachycardia and fetal death from exsanguination. FMH is most likely to occur after 12 weeks gestation, when the uterus rises above the pelvis and becomes more susceptible to direct trauma. FMH is detected by the Kleihauer Betke (KB) test. Estimation of the ratio of fetal to maternal cells enables calculation of the volume of fetal blood leaked into the maternal circulation. Unfortunately, the sensitivity of all the KB tests is relatively low. Therefore, all Rh-negative mothers who present with a history of abdominal trauma should receive one 300 μg prophylactic dose of Rh immunoglobulin within 72 hours of the trauma. As a general rule, 300 μg of Rh immunoglobulin should be given for every 30 mL of fetal blood found in the maternal circulation.

Perimortem caesarean delivery

If standard application of basic life support (BLS) and advanced cardiac life support (ACLS) fail and there is some chance that the fetus is viable, the goal is to deliver the fetus within four to five minutes after the onset of cardiac arrest. Perimortem caesarean delivery is rarely required, but is performed on the woman who has a viable fetus where maternal resuscitation is unsuccessful. A few cases of maternal survival after delivery of the fetus during unsuccessful cardiopulmonary resuscitation (CPR) have been reported, probably because delivery of the fetus increases maternal perfusion. It is also possible to commence trans-abdominal cardiac massage or, if the chest wall is opened, open-chest cardiac massage (OCM). Delivery improves thoracic compliance, which improves the efficacy

---

Clinical point

In an emergency, the simplest action may be the most often ignored. Many cardiovascular problems associated with pregnancy are due to nothing more than anatomy interacting with gravity. The pregnant woman's uterus may press down against the inferior vena cava, reducing or blocking blood flow. The ensuing failure of venous blood return can produce hypotension and even shock. These potentially catastrophic complications are often preventable or easily remedied by tilting the woman to the left (see Fig 36.12) (American Heart Association 2000).

of chest compressions and the ability to ventilate the lungs. According to the 'four-minute rule', if maternal resuscitation is unsuccessful after four minutes of CPR, the fetus should be delivered by the fifth minute. CPR is continued throughout the procedure and afterwards, in a final effort to improve the maternal and perinatal survival rate.

Resuscitation in pregnancy

Cardiac arrest occurs about once in every 30,000 pregnancies, and maternal and fetal survival from this catastrophic event is rare. The anatomical and physiological changes of pregnancy described earlier in this chapter militate against successful maternal resuscitation. Every maternity care provider, irrespective of their place of work, has a duty of care to the woman in need of resuscitation and should therefore be competent in BLS and ACLS.

Table 36.6 lists the recommendations for advanced life support from the American Heart Association (2000). The AHA paper states unequivocally that there are no changes to

TABLE 36.6   Recommendations for advanced life support in obstetrics

ACLS approach	Modifications to standard BLS and ACLS guidelines
Primary ABCD survey	**A**irway No modifications **B**reathing No modifications **C**irculation Chest compressions are ineffective when a woman in her last trimester lies on her back because the gravid uterus blocks the return of blood from the inferior vena cava. Start chest compressions after placing the woman on her left side with her back angled 30° to 45° from the floor. *or* Start chest compressions after placing a wedge under the woman's right side (so that she lies on her left side). *or* Have one rescuer kneel next to the woman on her left side and gently pull the gravid uterus laterally to relieve pressure on the inferior vena cava. **D**efibrillation No modifications. Defibrillatory shocks transfer no significant current to the fetus in utero.
Secondary ABCD survey	**A**irway No modifications to intubation techniques **B**reathing No modifications to secondary confirmation of successful intubation. A gravid uterus is known to push up the diaphragm and therefore decrease ventilatory volumes and make positive-pressure ventilation difficult. **C**irculation Follow standard ACLS recommendations for administration of all resuscitation medications. **D**ifferential diagnosis and decisions Decide whether to perform emergency caesarean section.

(Source: American Heart Association 2000)

Clinical scenario

At 0300 the ambulance brings a 35-year-old pregnant woman into the resuscitation room of the Emergency Department at your Level II hospital following cardiac arrest of almost four minutes duration. Full basic life support has been present since arrest; initial application of advanced protocols has not re-established circulation. You are the most experienced person on duty. You know that a perimortem emergency caesarean section could be life-saving for either fetus or mother. What are you going to do, when and why? What if you are unable to obtain consent from the next of kin in time?

BOX 36.9 Maternal death and PPH

The truth about maternal death and PPH
Worldwide:

▸ 515,000 women die during pregnancy and childbirth every year.
▸ 99% of maternal deaths occur in developing countries.
▸ 130,000 women bleed to death each year while giving birth.
▸ two-thirds of women with PPH have no identifiable risk factors.
▸ 90% of cases of PPH are due to uterine atony.

The majority of these deaths occur in:

▸ Sub-Saharan Africa (25%)
▸ West Africa (27%)
▸ Indonesia (45%).

(Source: JHPIEGO, http://www.jhpiego.org/scripts/pubs/category_detail. asp?category_id=24)

BOX 36.10 Definition of PPH

Definition of postpartum haemorrhage:

▸ Blood loss of ≥ 500 mL during and after childbirth.
▸ A primary PPH occurs within the first 24 hours after birth.
▸ A secondary (late) PPH occurs from 24 hours to the first six weeks after birth.
▸ A severe PPH is defined as blood loss of ≥ 1000 mL or more.

A more clinically useful definition is that a PPH is any amount of blood loss post partum that causes haemodynamic compromise.

the standard ACLS algorithms for medications, intubation and defibrillation. A pregnant woman in cardiac arrest is assessed and treated by using the Primary and Secondary ABCD Surveys of ACLS as modified for the pregnant woman. It is important that clinicians consider a wide variety of possible causes of arrest, such as amniotic fluid embolism, magnesium sulfate toxicity, and mishap in patients who have received spinal anaesthesia, as well as drug overdose, drug abuse, medication toxicity and iatrogenic events (American Heart Association 2000).

Postpartum haemorrhage

Postpartum haemorrhage (PPH) is defined as excessive blood loss occurring after the birth of the baby and is a potentially life-threatening emergency. Until recently, in Western countries, the incidence of maternal mortality caused by PPH has decreased due to improvements in early detection and treatment. In most cases PPH occurs in the immediate postpartum period (within 24 hours after birth and known as a primary PPH) and is due to uterine atony. Without immediate and proper medical attention, a woman with PPH may die.

Definition

There are numerous definitions of PPH in the literature. The most widely recognised is blood loss after childbirth in excess of 500 mL. Because it is often difficult to accurately measure blood loss, the true incidence of PPH may be underestimated by up to 50%. Consequently, the usefulness of 'traditional' definitions of PPH is now being questioned. Careful quantification of blood loss shows that many women bleed more than 500 mL and the blood loss following a caesarean section often exceeds 1000 mL (Shevell & Malone 2003). Clinical estimation of blood loss at childbirth is difficult because the blood mixes with amniotic fluid, urine and, if they are used, the solutions used to wash the vulval area before birth. In contrast to bleeding occurring after surgery, many clinicians in maternity settings do not routinely weigh pads, drapes and bed clothes in order to obtain an accurate estimation of blood loss. Further, the immediate post-birth period is a time when the parents want to be alone with their newly born infant and so it is difficult for the midwife to continue vigilant assessments without being intrusive. Analysis of 'avoidable factors' in reports such as *Maternal Deaths in Australia* (Slaytor et al 2004) and the UK *Confidential Enquiries into Maternal and Child Health* (RCOG 2002) show that midwives sometimes fail to appreciate the significance of slow, steady, blood loss over some hours until a massive PPH has occurred. When estimating the amount of postpartum blood loss, it is not sufficient to check the perineal pad; it is important that the midwife ask the woman to move or roll onto her side so that she can check for pooling of blood. As the amount of blood loss increases, estimates of the extent of the haemorrhage tend to be even less accurate. Given the relative hypervolaemia of pregnancy, the clinical signs of haemorrhage and shock, such as hypotension, tachycardia and oliguria, may not appear until the woman has lost over 1500 mL—that is, just before she becomes haemodynamically unstable.

Incidence

The incidence of PPH worldwide ranges from 5% to 15% of all births. However, there is evidence that the incidence of PPH is increasing, with both the United Kingdom and Australian reports on maternal deaths identifying a significant increase in direct maternal mortality from PPH, which is currently the leading cause of maternal deaths in Australia (CEMCH 2004; Slaytor et al 2004). According to Haynes et al (2004), in 2002 in Victoria, approximately 9.2% of women experienced a PPH. These rates are similar to those reported in published studies across Australia, in New Zealand, British Columbia and Nova Scotia. It is, however, higher than many North American centres (Haynes et al 2004).

In developed and developing countries, maternal mortality due to PPH is highest where there is inadequate access to skilled healthcare providers and transport and emergency services. Twenty-five per cent of all maternal deaths are caused by maternal haemorrhage. This is not surprising, considering that, on average, a woman will die within two hours after the onset of PPH if she does not receive proper treatment (e.g. appropriate drugs, blood transfusion or surgical intervention).

In 2004 the Victorian Government in Australia (Haynes et al 2004) initiated a review of morbidity caused by obstetric haemorrhage because it was so concerned about an alarming rise in the incidence of PPH (from 6.2% of all births in 1992–98 to 9.5% in 1999–2002). Between 1992 and 2002, nine Victorian women died as a direct result of obstetric haemorrhage and 132 women (0.05%) required hysterectomy as a life-saving measure (Haynes et al 2004).

Recently some possible risk factors have begun to emerge to explain the increase in PPH. These include the increased mean age of women in childbirth, advances in technology that enable women with complex medical problems to give birth, increasing multiple pregnancies with assisted reproductive technologies, and increased rates of Caesarean section leading to placenta praevia or accreta (CEMCH 2004). Nevertheless, as Haynes et al (2004) report, despite the identification of risk factors, PPH still occurs unpredictably in low-risk women. More than a quarter of women who experience an obstetric haemorrhage significant enough to require hysterectomy did not have any known risk factors (Haynes et al 2004).

The inclusion of haemodynamic compromise or shock is an important factor to consider in any definition of PPH, as some women will become compromised with a relatively small blood loss—for instance, women with pre-eclampsia or anaemia, women of small stature and those with socioeconomic disadvantage (Alexander et al 2002).

Haemorrhagic shock

Haemorrhagic shock can result in a combination of anaemic and ischaemic tissue hypoxia. Tissue hypoxia causes a progressive failure of cellular metabolism. Compensatory mechanisms and different oxygen requirements in various tissue beds cause a range of complications including organ damage, which may result in early or late multiple-organ dysfunction and death. Haemorrhagic shock may coexist with other types of shock; for example, after trauma septic shock

(most often from wound contamination or genital infection) may occur.

Prevention

Prevention of PPH is a key component of risk minimisation for women. Antenatal screening of previous history and risk is important so that a plan of care can be discussed with the woman before birth. Antepartum anaemia should be checked and corrected during pregnancy. The authors recommend that in the antenatal period, all women be fully informed of the current evidence related to the benefits and risks of physiological versus active management of the third stage of labour.

Causes of PPH

The four major causes of primary PPH are commonly known as the 4Ts:

- Tone—uterine atony
- Tissue—retained placental tissue
- Trauma—genital tract trauma
- Thrombin—coagulopathies.

Table 36.7 lists the aetiology and clinical risk factors associated with each of the 4Ts.

Early recognition of PPH

Once the placenta and membranes are delivered, they should be checked carefully for completeness. Even if vaginal blood loss is minimal, the vaginal vault and perineum must be thoroughly inspected for bleeding points, and sutured if necessary. Haematomas should be evaluated and treated. All women must be closely observed post birth, particularly in the first hour, when PPH is most likely to occur. Uterine tone and position are monitored frequently and maternal pulse and blood pressure recorded and documented. Mild shock is usually preceded by tachycardia and a fall in BP. However, the

---

Clinical point

An empty and contracted uterus will not bleed (except where coagulopathy occurs). The finding of a 'boggy' uterus indicates that it is not well contracted and the blood vessels or 'living ligatures' are not compressed, resulting in excessive postpartum bleeding. The midwife's first action is to massage or 'rub up the fundus' until it is firm and contracted and pooled blood or clots are expelled.

A uterus that is not centrally located suggests that a full bladder has pushed the uterus to one side.

If the woman continues to bleed vaginally even though the uterus is contracted and centrally located, the cause of the haemorrhage is due to other factors—trauma, retained placental fragments or coagulopathy.

TABLE 36.7 Antenatal and intrapartum risk factors for PPH

Cause	Process	Clinical risk factors
Abnormalities of uterine contraction (TONE) 70%	Atonic uterus	Prolonged 3rd stage (> 30 mins)
	Over distended uterus	Polyhydramnios Multiple gestation Macrosomia
	Uterine muscle exhaustion	Rapid labour Prolonged labour (1st/2nd stage) or augmented labour Labour dystocia or incoordinate labour High parity
	Intra amniotic infection	Pyrexia Prolonged ROM > 24 hrs
	Drug-induced hypertonia	Magnesium sulphate, nifedipine, Salbutamol, general anaesthetic
	Functional or anatomical distortion of the uterus	Fibroids Uterine anomalies
Genital tract trauma (TRAUMA) 20%	Episiotomy or lacerations (cervix, vagina or perineum)	Labour induced or augmented Labour dystocia Malposition Precipitous delivery Operative delivery (vacuum or forceps)
	Extensions, lacerations at caesarean section	Malposition Deep engagement
	Uterine rupture	Previous caesarean section
	Uterine inversion	Strong cord traction in 3rd stage, especially with fundal position Short umbilical cord High parity Relaxed uterus, lower segment and cervix Placental accreta, especially fundal insertion Congenital uterine weakness or anomalies Antepartum use of magnesium sulphate or oxytocin
Retained product of conception (TISSUE) 10%	Retained products of conception Abnormal placenta Retained cotyledon or succenturiate lobe	Incomplete placenta at birth Placenta accreta or percreta Previous caesarean section or uterine surgery High parity Abnormal placenta (succenturiate lobe)
Abnormalities of coagulation (THROMBIN) 1%	Retained blood clots	Atonic uterus
	Coagulation disorders acquired in pregnancy Idiopathic thrombocytopenic purpura (ITP) Von Willebrand's disease Haemophilia or carrier Thrombocytopenia with pre-eclampsia Disseminated Intravascular Coagulation (DIC) Pre-eclampsia Dead fetus in utero	Bruising Elevated BP, HELLP Fetal death Pyrexia, WBC Antepartum haemorrhage (previous or current) Sudden collapse

TABLE 36.7 Antenatal and intrapartum risk factors for PPH—cont'd

Cause	Process	Clinical risk factors
Abnormalities of coagulation (THROMBIN) 1%—cont'd	Severe infection Abruption Amniotic fluid embolism	
	Therapeutic anti-coagulation	History of blood clot such as DVT

(Sources: NSW Health 2002)

Research

Active versus expectant management in the third stage of labour (Cochrane Review, Prendiville et al 2000)

In 2000, Prendiville et al conducted a systematic review to assess the effects of active versus expectant management on blood loss, PPH and other maternal and perinatal complications of the third stage of labour. Expectant (physiological) management of the third stage of labour involves allowing the placenta to deliver spontaneously, or aiding it by gravity or nipple stimulation. Active management involves administration of a prophylactic oxytocic before delivery of the placenta, and usually early cord clamping and cutting, and controlled cord traction of the umbilical cord. 'Active management' is superior to 'expectant management' in terms of blood loss, PPH and other serious complications of the third stage of labour. Active management was, however, associated with an increased risk of side-effects such as nausea and vomiting, and hypertension, if ergometrine is used in the oxytocic. The authors concluded that 'active' management should be the routine management of choice for women expecting to deliver a baby by vaginal delivery in a maternity hospital. Of note is that the implications were less clear for other settings, including domiciliary practice (in developing and industrialised countries).

Reflective exercise

What would you say (and how would you say it) to a red-haired woman who is convinced that as a redhead she is much more likely to have a postpartum haemorrhage?

Clinical point

Retained placental fragments are a common cause of primary PPH and the most frequent cause of late haemorrhage. Retention of fragments is usually caused by partial separation of the placenta during massage of the uterine fundus prior to spontaneous placental separation. Following birth, the placenta and membranes should always be checked for completeness. Always look on the maternal side of the placenta for missing placental fragments or cotyledons. On the fetal side, blood vessels that traverse the edge of the placenta and then outwards into the membranes are suggestive of a succenturiate lobe.

Management

The cornerstones of management of resuscitation following a PPH are:

- restoration of the blood volume and oxygen-carrying capacity
- stopping the haemorrhage.

Each maternity setting should have a clear local plan of action to deal with PPH, and all grades of staff should participate in obstetric haemorrhage 'drills' (CEMCH 2002). The first priorities are to identify the cause, seek help, and control the haemorrhage. Given that the vast majority of PPHs are caused by atonia, the midwife's first action is to check the tone and position of the uterus and, if necessary, massage it or 'rub up the fundus' to promote uterine contractions and control of bleeding. Uterotonic agents are administered as required (see Box 36.11). In most cases these measures will expel any blood clots, and the uterus then contracts and the

altered haemodynamic state of pregnancy and immediately post birth can mask the signs of hypovolaemia even in the presence of large blood loss. Indeed, a woman may lose 1500 mL, almost a third of her total blood volume, before overt signs of shock become apparent. All women should be informed about the signs and symptoms of PPH and have strategies in place to detect primary and secondary PPH and to seek timely and appropriate assistance.

bleeding is controlled. If this is not the case, the midwife calls for help and commences resuscitation. Blood samples are taken for group and cross-match and two large-bore 14 G cannulae are sited. Crystalloid solutions (Hartmann's/normal saline) are infused at a rate of three times the measured blood loss. When estimating the required amount to infuse, it is important to remember that clinicians tend to underestimate blood loss at birth. Initial resuscitation with crystalloid and colloid infusions followed by blood transfusion is aimed at restoring systolic blood pressure and oxygen-carrying capacity. A urinary catheter is inserted into the bladder to ensure that a full bladder does not impede uterine contractions. A urine output of a minimum of 30 mL an hour indicates a functioning renal system and is a useful guide to the required amount of fluid to be infused. Some clinicians have suggested that if the baby is put to the breast this can stimulate the release of endogenous oxytocic; there is no evidence to support the efficacy of this intervention. If the uterus fails to contract, bimanual compression (Fig 36.14) is an effective method to initiate uterine contractions and stop PPH.

If on inspection there is no evidence of retained placental fragments or missing cotyledons, it may be necessary for a medical practitioner to perform a uterine exploration, preferably in an operating theatre and with adequate maternal analgesia. However, if the uterus is empty and well-contracted and there is no evidence of retained placental fragments, the most experienced clinician examines the genital tract and repairs cervical, vaginal and perineal lacerations. Uterine inversion and rupture are increasingly common causes of PPH. The former should always be suspected if the uterus is not palpable after the birth. This complication is dealt with later in the chapter. The diagnosis of uterine rupture is often only made when a well-contracted uterus does not stop bleeding. If bleeding persists despite the implementation of primary emergency measures, the woman's condition must be stabilised and then she is transferred to an operating theatre as soon as possible. Intractable haemorrhage requires a multidisciplinary team approach that focuses on the identification of cause, replacement of blood/clotting factors and surgery if all other

measures fail. Manual removal of placenta (Fig 36.15) is associated with an increase in PPH and infection. Other life-saving surgery such as hysterectomy may be required.

Following a PPH the woman may develop disseminated intravascular coagulation (DIC) a potentially catastrophic complication. The laboratory diagnosis of acute DIC is based on prolongation of the prothrombin time, activated partial thromboplastin time, and thrombin time, due to consumption of clotting factors and inhibition of their function. A condition of thrombocytopenia may also exist, caused by the consumption of platelets. Increased titres of fibrin degradation products can be measured due to resultant fibrinolysis. This topic is considered in more detail later in this chapter.

Special case: women who decline blood products

Some women faced with an objective, informed and clear explanation of the need to use blood products in the advent of massive obstetric haemorrhage will consent to their use as a life-saving measure. Others do not consent to blood transfusions because of religious or cultural beliefs. The UK Confidential Enquiry into Maternal Deaths report of 2002 provides guidance for maternity care providers faced with this ethical dilemma. Management begins at booking, with open discussion and identifying and remedying anaemia or other risk factors. Ultrasound can be used to locate the placental site. A senior obstetrician and anaesthetist are informed when labour is established. Caesarean section is only performed when there is a medical indication for this intervention. The third stage of labour is actively managed and the woman's wellbeing is closely monitored after birth. In the event of haemorrhage, the focus should be on pharmacological interventions such as the administration of vitamin K and early surgical intervention, as well as further discussion with the woman and her family if there is a medical indication for blood transfusion. Nevertheless, the woman's wishes must

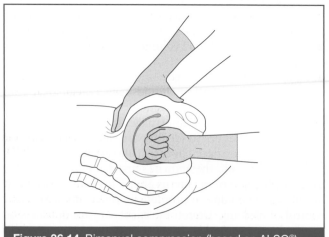

Figure 36.14 Bimanual compression (based on ALSO®)

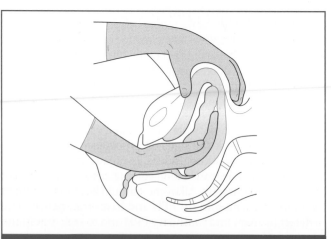

Figure 36.15 Manual removal of placenta (based on Henderson & MacDonald 2004)

BOX 36.11 Uterotonic drugs

Action, effect, dosage and route of uterotonic drugs

Syntocinon® (synthetic oxytocin) is the recommended drug to prevent PPH. It works rapidly, with minimal side-effects. Syntocinon® has an immediate onset and causes rhythmic uterine contractions for about an hour. It can be administered as an injection after birth of the anterior shoulder with no increase in the incidence of retained placenta or hypertension. The recommended prophylactic dose is 10 IU/mL intramuscularly or by **slow** intravenous (IV) injection of a bolus dose. Side-effects include mild, transient hypertension, water intoxication and hypertonic uterine action.

▸ **Syntocinon®** 40 IU/mL in 1000 mL Hartmann's (250 mL/hr) can be used as an infusion to maintain uterine contraction and can be left running for several hours after birth to ensure bleeding is controlled. The administration of 40 IU/mL has no demonstrable cardiovascular effect. However, even a small amount of Syntocinon® given as a bolus dose via IV push may elicit a pattern of hypotension and tachycardia

▸ **Syntometrine®** contains 5 units of Syntocinon® and 0.5 mg of ergometrine. Onset is 2–5 minutes and duration about 3 hours. Syntometrine® causes sustained tetanic uterine contraction. It is usually administered intramuscularly and is more effective than Syntocinon® in action. However, its routine use has declined in recent years due to its adverse effects, which include vomiting, dizziness, acute abdominal pain, headache, vasoconstriction, hypertension, chest pain and seizures. It should not be administered to a woman with a diastolic BP > 90 mmHg.

▸ **Ergometrine maleate** is available in a 500 µ/mL preparation that can be administered as an intramuscular or IV injection.

Onset is 7 minutes and duration 3 hours. It too causes sustained uterine contractions. It is not recommended as a first-line drug for prophylaxis but can be used for severe PPH. It is contraindicated in hypertensive women with diastolic BP > 90 mmHg.

▸ **Prostaglandin PGF$_2\alpha$** (Dinaprost® 5 mg/mL) is used to control refractory cases of PPH The dose is 0.5 mg (1 mL) of a 5 mg/mL solution. This is diluted with 9 mL normal saline and injected intramuscularly or transabdominally directly into the myometrium on each side of the fundus. The dose can be repeated up to a maximum of 3 mg. This is a life-saving measure and should always be carried out in the presence of an anaesthetist with resuscitation equipment available. All the prostaglandin drugs are contraindicated in women with active cardiovascular, renal, liver disease or asthma. Side-effects include nausea, vomiting, wheezing, pyrexia, uterine rupture and cardiac arrest.

▸ **Misoprostol** (Cytec®) is not approved for use in pregnancy but can be given rectally (800–1000 mg) if oxytocin has failed to work and PGF$_2$ is not available (NSW Health Department 2002). Side-effects include diarrhoea, fever and abdominal pain.

▸ **Carboprost** (Haemabate®, 14-methyl prostaglandin F$_2$) is a synthetic prostaglandin currently awaiting approval for use in Australia. It can be given IM (250 µg), and works within 5 minutes, lasting up to an hour. It can be repeated every 15 minutes to a total of 2 mg. Side-effects include hypertension, pulmonary oedema, nausea and dyspnoea due to vasoconstriction.

---

always be respected and family and staff supported in the event of her death.

Postnatal considerations

After any PPH the woman is observed closely for 24 to 48 hours. Blood pressure, pulse and vaginal loss are accurately documented and fundal tone and height checked regularly. A urinary indwelling catheter is usually left in situ to promote adequate drainage of the bladder and to further aid uterine contractions as well as providing a means to accurately measure and document urinary output. Women who have experienced an obstetric haemorrhage are predisposed to renal tubular necrosis and may become anuric.

Following a PPH the woman is at increased risk of infection and lactation may be delayed. It is important to discuss the events with the woman and her support people so that they can understand what has occurred and ask questions. Any subsequent pregnancies will require specialist care and counselling to prevent/manage recurrence. In developing countries, women who survive PPH are more likely to suffer

from long-term anaemia and other complications. Because their health is already compromised, such women often need blood transfusions but are susceptible to the associated risks of transfusion reactions or infection with HIV or hepatitis. Other possible morbidities include delayed healing and initiation of lactation, iron deficiency anaemia and exposure to blood products, haemorrhagic shock, coagulopathy, renal necrosis, and surgical intervention, which may result in hysterectomy and resultant sterilisation to control blood loss. Such procedures are costly and painful and may be emotionally devastating to the woman and her family. In addition, these procedures carry the risk of infection, reactions to anaesthesia and other complications.

Summary: postpartum haemorrhage

Catastrophic haemorrhage is a significant, life-threatening problem for some women. Midwives can be proactive in the prevention and early detection of PPH. Antenatal discussion of possible risk factors and careful management of the third stage are important components of midwifery care. Midwives

---

BOX 36.12 PPH management

Protocol for management of PPH

Diagnosis of PPH

▶ Blood loss > 500 mL, or

▶ Clinically abnormal bleeding with increase in pulse rate by 20 bpm or drop in systolic pressure by 20 mmHg

▶ If vital signs are worse than expected for observed blood loss, look for internal bleeding or uterine inversion.

▶ Monitor vital signs every five minutes as these may change rapidly.

▶ Consider calling emergency transport team.

General measures

▶ Call for help—notify senior obstetrician, anaesthetist and team leader. (Do not leave the woman alone.)

▶ Measure all blood loss (weigh pads, sheets etc).

▶ Massage uterine fundus, give slow injection of 10 IU/mL Syntocinon IV or intramuscularly.

▶ Take baseline vital assessments immediately and then every 5 minutes until the woman's condition is stable (document these).

▶ Continuous assessment of vaginal blood loss.

▶ Obtain IV access 14–16 G (x 2 if necessary)—collect blood for haemoglobin, coagulation studies, urgent cross-match.

▶ Commence normal saline infusion (Haemaccel if hypotensive) if blood loss >1000 mL.

▶ Administer oxygen 6–8 L/min by Hudson mask.

▶ Insert indwelling urinary catheter, hourly urine measurement, aiming to keep urine output > 30 mL/hr.

▶ Explain what is happening and reassure the woman and her support people.

▶ Call for assistance from emergency transport team if necessary.

Clinical point

Signs of disseminated intravascular coagulation
Bleeding from non-genital sites in the body, such as venous puncture sites, may suggest the development of disseminated intravascular coagulation (DIC).

---

should also be competent in managing active and physiological third stage, employing interventions as required. Before the midwife–woman relationship ends, it is important that the woman is able to identify abnormal changes that may occur at home and understands the importance of notifying her lead carer if they develop. Arrangements for follow-up care and tests such as haemoglobin tests should be made before discharge from hospital.

Neonatal resuscitation

The vast majority of newborn infants start to breathe without assistance and often cry almost immediately after birth. By one minute, most newly born infants are breathing spontaneously. These babies require little intervention immediately post birth. Caregivers should therefore practise from a philosophy of minimal invasiveness, coupled with maximal awareness and readiness. However, if the newly born infant fails to establish adequate, sustained respiration after birth, the infant is said to have neonatal asphyxia—an important cause of neonatal death if it is not managed quickly and correctly.

Effective resuscitation of the newly born infant requires: adequate training and preparation of staff involved in the care of women in labour; a knowledge of maternal, fetal and intrapartal risk factors that may influence the infant's ability to make the transition from fetus to neonate; and adequate and functioning equipment. The need for neonatal resuscitation may often be predicted but in many instances it is unexpected. For this reason, irrespective of the place of birth it is crucial that appropriate equipment and skilled personnel are available to resuscitate the newly born baby if necessary. Resuscitation involves much more than having an ordered list of skills and a resuscitation team on hand; it also requires excellent assessment skills and an in-depth knowledge of the physiological events triggering the transition from fetus to newly born infant.

Definition and purpose

The purpose of neonatal resuscitation is to establish or restore oxygenation, ventilation and circulation to depressed infants. Resuscitation is a series of actions taken to establish normal breathing, heart rate, colour, tone and activity in a newly born infant with depressed vital signs (i.e. low Apgar score). All babies who do not breathe well after birth (i.e. have neonatal asphyxia) or have a one-minute Apgar score below 7 need immediate resuscitation. Any newly born infant who has apnoea or who has depressed vital signs any time after birth also requires resuscitation. Guidelines have been established by various organisations such as the International Liaison Committee on Resuscitation (ILCOR). Australia and New Zealand are members of ILCOR. This section on neonatal resuscitation is based on two resources: ILCOR's Advisory Statement on Resuscitation of the Newly Born Infant (Kattwinkel et al 1999) and the Australian National Guidelines for the Resuscitation of the Newborn Infant (Draft 2, February 2004).

Unique physiology of the newly born

The transition from fetal to extrauterine life is characterised by a number of critical events, and these affect resuscitative interventions. After birth, for the lungs to operate as a functional respiratory unit providing adequate gas exchange, the airways must be cleared of fetal lung fluid; an increase in pulmonary blood flow must also occur. If the newborn infant's lungs do not rapidly become the site for gas exchange, cyanosis and hypoxia develop rapidly. The first breath must overcome the viscosity of the lung fluid and intra-alveolar tension. The initial breaths also generate high transpulmonary pressure, which helps to push the lung fluid across the alveolar epithelium and into the lymphatic circulation. Once this happens:

- The lungs change from fluid-filled to air-filled.
- Pulmonary blood flow increases dramatically and intracardiac and extracardiac shunts (foramen ovale and ductus arteriosus) initially reverse direction and subsequently close.
- Physical expansion of the lungs, with establishment of functional residual capacity and increase in alveolar oxygen tension, both mediate the critical decrease in pulmonary vascular resistance and result in an increase in pulmonary blood flow.

Developmental considerations at various gestational ages or additional pathology also influence resuscitative efforts. For instance, surfactant deficiency in the preterm lung alters compliance and resistance. Thus, in a preterm baby, for initial lung expansion to occur, higher pressures (peak inspiratory and/or expiratory) than those usually used during resuscitation of the term baby or in infancy may be required. Some experts state early prophylactic administration of surfactant is associated with better outcomes in extremely premature infants.

If the fetus passes meconium into the amniotic fluid, this irritating substance may be aspirated into the tracheobronchial tree in utero or during the first few breaths after birth, leading to airway obstruction and possibly meconium aspiration syndrome (MAS). Complications of MAS are particularly likely in infants who are small for their gestational age, or those born after term or with significant fetal compromise, perhaps after a long labour.

Response to asphyxia

The fetus or newly born infant who has been subjected to asphyxia begins a 'diving' reflex (so-called because of certain similarities to the physiology of diving seals) in an attempt to maintain perfusion and oxygen delivery to vital organs. The asphyxiated infant passes through a series of events that have been well described from experimental evidence in animal models.

Primary apnoea

After a few shallow breaths, the asphyxiated infant stops breathing. This phase is called primary apnoea and may last for as long as 10 minutes. Most infants with primary apnoea respond to stimulation alone. During this phase, heart rate and pH are maintained.

Secondary apnoea

Following this period, the infant begins to gasp. The period between the last gasp and cardiac arrest is known as secondary apnoea. In the phase of secondary or terminal apnoea, the newborn has a mixed acidosis, and active intervention is required to stimulate respiration. It is not possible to clinically distinguish primary from secondary apnoea, and for this reason

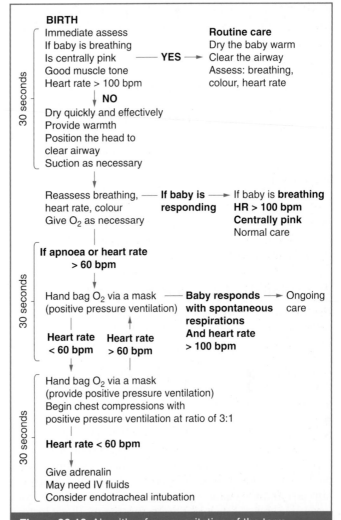

Figure 36.16 Algorithm for resuscitation of the term neonate at birth (based on Niermeyer et al 2000)

Clinical point

Definition of newborn, neonate and infant
In Australia and New Zealand, a fetus is viable if it weighs more than 400 g at birth or has a gestation of more than 20 weeks. However, a baby born at less than 23 weeks gestation is unlikely to survive. 'Newborn' refers to an infant in the first minutes to hours following birth. In contrast, the *neonatal* period is defined as the first 28 days of life. *Infancy* includes the neonatal period and extends through the first 12 months of life. In this section the term 'newly born' is used to prevent confusion with the other terms.

it is important to assume that the apnoeic infant is in secondary apnoea. If there is no response to simple interventions, active resuscitation is commenced immediately.

Incidence and risk factors

Approximately 5% of all newly born infants require some stimulation to breathe (Saugstad 1998), and about 1:100 infants born in hospital require assisted ventilation (Palme-Kilander 1992). Even though prenatal care is able to identify many potential fetal difficulties ante partum, poor cardiorespiratory adaptation at birth (low Apgar scores) cannot be predicted. Perinatal asphyxia and extreme prematurity (babies weighing less than 1000 g) are the two complications of pregnancy that most frequently require complex resuscitation. However, only 60% of asphyxiated newborns can be predicted ante partum and are often not identified until the time of birth. Also, approximately 80% of low birthweight infants (< 2500 g) require resuscitation and stabilisation immediately after birth. Effective, prompt resuscitation and management of asphyxia in the first few minutes of life may influence the long-term outcome for these infants.

Anticipation of resuscitation need

Anticipation and preparation are the key features of effective neonatal resuscitation. Anticipating those infants who may need resuscitation at birth begins in pregnancy, with careful screening of the maternal social, medical and obstetric health record. Each birth setting should establish criteria (see Table 36.8) that would indicate the need to:

● increase surveillance
● summon extra or expert help
● transfer to a centre that has the staff, equipment and resources readily available for immediate resuscitation.

Arranging for transfer should be initiated in a timely way, because maternal transfer is less risky than neonatal transfer. Support and consultation should always be available from Level III centres. Once labour begins, the mother's history and records often provide clues to the possibility that the newly born infant will require resuscitation. Therefore, it is important to ensure that:

● the maternal history is checked meticulously
● all events are documented in a systematic and orderly way
● personnel communicate effectively
● all equipment is present and functioning
● the environment is suitable for birth.

The following clinical situations often lead to the birth of an infant with birth asphyxia and a low Apgar score at one minute:

● signs of fetal compromise in labour
● depressed vital signs
● prematurity
● difficult or traumatic delivery
● meconium aspiration
● general anaesthesia or recent maternal analgesia (narcotics within the past four hours).

Personnel

At least two trained people are required for adequate resuscitation involving ventilation and cardiac compressions.

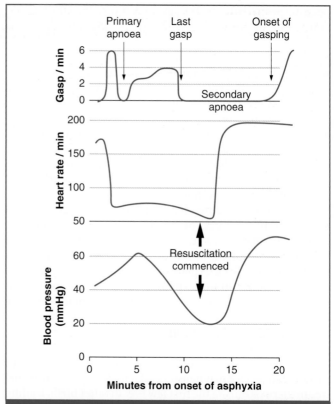

Figure 36.17 Physiological effect of acute asphyxia and the response to resuscitation (based on Levene et al 2000)

Therefore, it is important to always call for help. The most senior person available coordinates the resuscitation. Each person should have a dedicated job; for example, with three people, one is solely responsible for airway, one solely responsible for chest compressions and the third person coordinates the resuscitation and administers medication as necessary. If possible another person is responsible for recording events, including time of administration of drugs and the baby's response to resuscitation.

Equipment

Because it is not always possible to predict when resuscitation is required, emergency preparedness requires that a complete inventory of functioning resuscitation equipment and drugs be readily available for every birth. It is important that the care provider checks the resuscitation equipment at least daily and after each usage. When use is anticipated then the equipment is again rechecked.

● At every birth setting:
  ● radiant warmer or other heat source
  ● clock, timer
  ● light source
  ● warm towels, blankets, clothes
  ● resuscitation bag and masks (Laerdal™ or Neopuff™)
  ● oxygen source and tubing
  ● suction device and catheters

TABLE 36.8 Risk factors associated with the need for resuscitation in the newly born infant		
Maternal	**Fetal**	**Intrapartal**
Premature/prolonged rupture of the membranes	Multiple gestation	Fetal compromise
Bleeding in second or third trimester	Preterm gestation (especially < 35 wks)	Abnormal presentation
Severe hypertension (PE and chronic)	Post-dates gestation (≥ 42 wks)	Prolapsed cord
Substance abuse	Size–date discrepancy	Prolonged rupture of the membranes
Pharmacology therapy (lithium, magnesium sulphate, adrenergic blocking agents)	Intrauterine growth restriction	Prolonged labour (or prolonged second stage of labour)
Maternal diabetes mellitus	Rh isoimmunisation/ hydrops fetalis	Precipitous labour, hypertonic uterine action
Chronic illness (anaemia, cyanotic congenital heart disease)	Polyhydramnios and oligohydramnios	Antepartum haemorrhage (abruptio placenta, placenta praevia)
Maternal infection	Reduced fetal movement before the onset of labour	Thick meconium staining of the amniotic fluid
Heavy sedation	Congenital anomalies	Non-reassuring FHR patterns
Previous fetal or neonatal death	Intrauterine infection	Narcotic administration to mother within four hours of birth
No antenatal care		Operative delivery (caesarean, forceps, ventouse)

(Source: Kattwinkel et al 1999)

- oropharyngeal airways
- stethoscope
- syringes and needles
- polyethylene (or other equipment to keep the baby warm)
- Equipment in hospitals:
  - endotracheal tubes and introducers (sizes 2, 2.5, 3, 3.5 and 4 mmID)
  - laryngoscope and blades, batteries and bulbs
  - intravenous cannulae at various sites
  - umbilical vein catheterisation tray
  - pulse oximeter
- Drugs:
  - adrenaline 1:10,000 concentration (0.1 mg/mL)
  - volume expanders: normal saline, 4–5% albumin–saline, Hartmann's solution
  - naloxone hydrochloride: 400 µg/mL solution
  - sodium bicarbonate: 0.5 meq/mL solution (4.2% concentration)
  - dextrose: 5% and 10% solutions
  - sterile water for injection.

Communication

Effective communication is vital to smooth resuscitation. Preparation for an anticipated 'high-risk' birth and when arranging transfer requires effective communication between all members of the healthcare team. Communication among caregivers should include discussion of maternal condition, fetal condition and maternal therapies, including details of maternal social, medical and obstetric conditions and treatments that will affect the resuscitation and management of the newly born—for example, gestation, results of antenatal tests, ultrasonography and labour status, or the administration

of maternal analgesia, tocolytics and corticosteroids, all of which influence respiratory function. A description of the results of FHR monitoring may give information about fetal wellbeing. Whenever time permits, the team responsible for the resuscitation should introduce themselves to the woman and her family before the birth. If possible they should outline their plan of care and carefully respond to the family's questions and concerns. This is especially important in cases of potentially lethal fetal anomalies or extreme prematurity, when the family's values and beliefs may affect their wishes for resuscitation of their baby.

Environment

Prevention of heat loss is important for the newly born and reduces the mortality of low birthweight infants. Cold stress increases oxygen consumption and impedes effective resuscitation. Whenever possible the infant should be born into a warm, draft-free area. An excellent strategy to reduce heat loss is to place the newly born skin-to-skin on the mother's chest or abdomen to use her body as a heat source. It is essential to prevent further heat loss during resuscitation. Rapid drying of the skin, removing wet linens, placing the infant under a radiant warmer and wrapping the newly born in pre-warmed blankets are also ways to reduce heat loss.

Techniques of resuscitation

The techniques of ACLS described here are the same as those recommended by ILCOR (Kattwinkel et al 1999) and the Australian National Guidelines for the Resuscitation of the Newborn Infant (Draft 2, February 2004). Being properly prepared is the first step in successfully resuscitating the newly born.

Assessment

All newly born infants should be assessed immediately following birth for signs that indicate inadequate oxygenation, ventilation or circulation and thus the need to initiate resuscitative efforts. The steps of evaluation and intervention are often simultaneous processes. Evaluation begins immediately after birth and continues throughout the resuscitation process until the infant's vital signs have normalised. The complex of signs (initial cry, respirations, heart rate, colour, response to stimulation) should be evaluated simultaneously. It is crucial not to wait for the one-minute Apgar score to identify the newly born infant in need of resuscitation.

Initial steps

Infants who are blue, apnoeic, flaccid and cyanosed with a heart rate < 100 bpm (primary apnoea), and those who are white, apnoeic, flaccid and pallid with a heart rate < 100 bpm (secondary apnoea), can be recognised at or soon after birth and resuscitation should begin without delay. In addition, active resuscitation should be commenced for infants with persisting bradycardia, central cyanosis, poor respiratory effort, significant respiratory distress and/or low Apgar scores (< 6 at one minute). The clock is turned on and the umbilical cord is clamped and cut, and the baby is taken to a pre-warmed radiant source. The infant is dried with pre-warmed towels and all wet linen is removed. The infant's airway is opened, with positioning and clearing of secretions. The infant is placed on her or his back with the head in the 'neutral' or 'sniffing' position (see Fig 36.18). If respiratory efforts are present but not producing effective tidal ventilation, often the airway is obstructed; immediate efforts to reposition the head or clear the airway are warranted. There is, however, no evidence to support routine suctioning of the upper airway or stomach of newly born infants. If necessary, secretions should be cleared with a suction device (bulb syringe, suction catheter).

Oxygenation and ventilation

In all cases, the first priority is to ensure adequate inflation of the lungs, followed by close attention to the desired concentration of inspired oxygen, if required. The traditional management of central cyanosis is administration of 100% oxygen either by passive delivery via an oxygen mask or by positive pressure delivered by a resuscitation device. If the newly born infant's heart rate is > 100 bpm and the infant is breathing but is still cyanotic, 100% oxygen can easily be delivered at 5 L/min using oxygen tubing in the cupped hand over the baby's face (see Fig 36.19). Should supplemental oxygen be required for a prolonged period, then heated humidified oxygen is administered via head-box with the FiO_2 adjusted to result in a pulse oximetry saturation of 92–96% in the term infant and 88–92% in the preterm baby.

Although there is some clinical evidence to support resuscitation with lower oxygen concentrations or room air (21% oxygen), there is as yet insufficient evidence to support this as a routine practice (Ramji et al 1993, 2003; Saugstad et al 2003).

Drying and stimulation with or without suctioning is often enough to stimulate spontaneous respiration, and most infants do not require further intervention. If there is no response to stimulation, it may be assumed that the newly born is in secondary apnoea and positive pressure ventilation should be initiated. ILCOR guidelines recommend that the newly born infant's condition (respiratory rate, heart rate, colour, muscle tone, response to stimulation) be re-evaluated every 30 seconds until vital signs are stable.

Assisted ventilation

Assisted ventilation is initiated if the infant remains apnoeic after stimulation, or the heart rate remains < 100 bpm or is dropping. The rate for assisted ventilation is 40–60 breaths per minute. Effectiveness of ventilation is judged by watching the movement of the chest and upper abdomen with each inflation. Effective ventilation produces an increase in heart rate followed by the baby flushing pink. Few infants require immediate intubation. The majority can be managed with a 240 mL self-inflating bag and mask (e.g. Laerdal or a 'T piece' device such as Neopuff™) ventilation. Both require skill and continuous practice so that care providers can deliver a consistent peak inspiratory pressure (PIP). The PIP is usually limited by a pressure-release valve, which is set to activate at about 40 cmH₂O and can be overridden should higher PIP be required. As an added precaution, a pressure manometer limiting the positive pressure to 30–35 cmH₂O is attached to all Resuscitaires®. To provide adequate distending pressure, the infant must be positioned properly and the airway cleared of secretions; the mask must be the correct size and form a tight seal on the face. It should be remembered that during the baby's first breaths, the lungs are converting from a fetal, non-aerated status to the newly born state. Thus the first three to five 'rescue breaths' require

---

Clinical point

Signs that indicate an immediate need for intervention include:

▶ *absent or weak response to tactile stimulation*—drying the infant with a towel, rubbing the back, flicking the soles of the feet

▶ *respiratory effort absent or gasping*—the newly born infant should establish regular respirations in order to maintain HR > 100 bpm

▶ *heart rate < 100 bpm*—determined from direct palpation of cord, apex beat or with stethoscope. Peripheral pulses are often difficult to feel. If no pulsation is felt on palpation of the cord, auscultate the chest,

▶ *colour*—central cyanosis (blue trunk and oral mucosa). The well newly born infant should be able to maintain a central pink colour in room air.

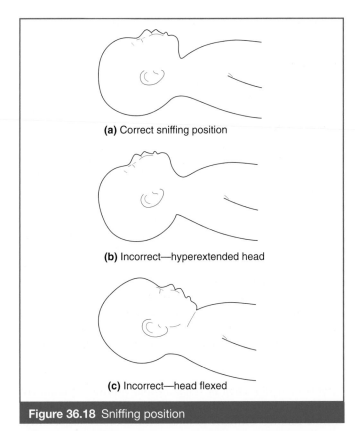

(a) Correct sniffing position

(b) Incorrect—hyperextended head

(c) Incorrect—head flexed

Figure 36.18 Sniffing position

Clinical point

Aggressive pharyngeal suction can cause laryngeal spasm, vagal bradycardia and delay the onset of spontaneous respiration. In the absence of meconium or blood, suction with a catheter should be limited to a depth of 5 cm for the lips for 5 seconds. Negative pressure of the suction apparatus should not exceed 100 mmHg (13.2 kPa). There is evidence that tracheal suctioning of the vigorous infant with meconium-stained fluid does not improve outcomes and may cause additional complications (Wiswell & Bent 1993).

higher inflation pressures and longer inflation times than subsequent breaths, particularly in infants who have not yet made any respiratory effort. For the first breaths, 30–40 cmH$_2$O is usually enough. For subsequent breaths, 15–20 cmH$_2$O is adequate. If appropriately skilled personnel are available, tracheal intubation may be considered if ventilation via face mask is ineffective or prolonged.

Cardiac compression

Chest compressions are started if, after 30 seconds of adequate, assisted ventilation with 100% oxygen, the heart rate is:
- absent
- < 60 bpm
- 60–80 bpm and falling.

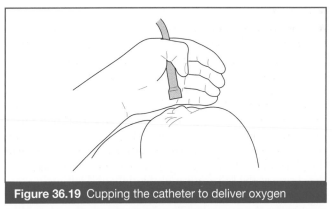

Figure 36.19 Cupping the catheter to deliver oxygen

Clinical point

Effective ventilation is the key to successful neonatal resuscitation.

Chest compressions may diminish the effectiveness of ventilation.

Procedure

The sternum is compressed one finger breadth below a line drawn between the nipples. No pressure should be applied to the xiphoid process or the chest margins, and it is important not to restrict chest re-expansion. Compressions should move the lower third of the anteroposterior diameter of the chest (1–2 cm) to generate a palpable pulse. Compressions and inflations are synchronised at a 3:1 ratio of compressions to inflations at a rate of 90 compressions and 30 inflations to achieve approximately 120 'events' per minute: count one-and-two-and-three-and-breath.

Specific techniques

Acceptable techniques are:
- two thumbs on the sternum, superimposed or adjacent to one another according to the size of the newly born infant, with fingers of both hands encircling the chest to support the back
- two fingers placed on the sternum at right angles to the chest (Fig 36.20).

Research suggests that the two-thumb technique may offer some advantage over the two-finger technique in generating higher blood pressure and better coronary perfusion pressure without introducing additional complications. Nevertheless, single operators find the 'two-finger technique' preferable.

Endotracheal intubation

Infants may require endotracheal intubation when:
- bag-and-mask ventilation and intermittent positive pressure ventilation (IPPV) is ineffective
- tracheal suction is required (in the presence of thick meconium)

● prolonged IPPV is necessary
● diaphragmatic hernia is suspected.

Endotracheal intubation is not a midwifery skill, and so only very brief details are included in this section. In summary, an appropriately sized blade and endotracheal tube (ETT) (depending on the size of the infant) are chosen. On insertion of the ETT, the tube is advanced until the vocal cord guide mark near the distal tip of the tube is visualised. This guide mark is positioned at a variable distance from the distal tip (depending on the ETT size) and is designed to result in the placement of the tube tip between the vocal cords and the carina at the bifurcation of the right and left main-stem bronchi. The ETT is secured with the appropriate centimetre marking at the upper lip. The depth of insertion should be recorded and maintained. Care providers should be aware that variation in head position alters the depth of insertion and may predispose to unintentional extubation or endobronchial intubation.

Medications in resuscitation

Drugs are rarely needed in resuscitation of the newly born infant and so they are dealt with only briefly here.

Possible routes of delivery

● umbilical venous catheter
● ETT—for either adrenaline or naloxone
● peripheral IV line—difficult to cannulate in the collapsed infant.

Umbilical arterial catheter should not be used for vasoactive substances and is not rapidly accessible.

Adrenaline

Adrenaline is recommended if the heart rate remains < 60 bpm for more than 30 seconds despite one minute of effective ventilation and compressions. The only exception to this rule may be newly born infants born without a detectable pulse or heart rate.
● *Dosage*: 0.1–0.3 mL/kg 1 in 10,000, repeated at 3–5 minute intervals

● *Volume* (preload) 10–15 mL/kg in normal saline and then repeated 2–3 times.

Sodium bicarbonate

Sodium bicarbonate has been recommended to reverse the effects of metabolic acidosis related to hypoxia and asphyxia. Currently there is insufficient evidence for routine use. Argument for correction of acidosis includes theoretical concerns about hypoxia and elevated pulmonary vascular bed pressure and poor cardiac contractility with acidosis. Argument against correction includes concerns regarding hyperosmolarity and carbon dioxide generation with intracellular acidosis from alkali infusion.

Dosage: 2 mL/kg of 4.2% sodium bicarbonate into the umbilical vein to correct acidosis and stimulate the cardiorespiratory system. It should only be given once adequate ventilation has been achieved. It is important to obtain early blood gases after resuscitation.

Dextrose: glucose has not been shown in animal models or adult humans to change the outcomes of CPR. No trial of glucose for resuscitation exists in neonates. Neonates requiring CPR should have an early blood sugar estimate after resuscitation and correction of hypoglycaemia if BSL < 3.0 mmol/L.

Volume replacement in resuscitation: volume replacement is not routine in neonatal resuscitation. Volume expanders (whole blood—difficult to obtain immediately after birth, 5% albumin, normal saline or Hartmann's solution) should be considered when there is suspected blood loss and/or the newly born infant appears to be in shock (pale, poor perfusion, weak pulse) and has not responded to other resuscitative measures. The initial dose is 10 mL/kg by slow IV push.

Post-resuscitation issues

After resuscitation with ACLS, ongoing supportive care, monitoring and appropriate diagnostic care must be provided. All newly born infants who require resuscitation must be

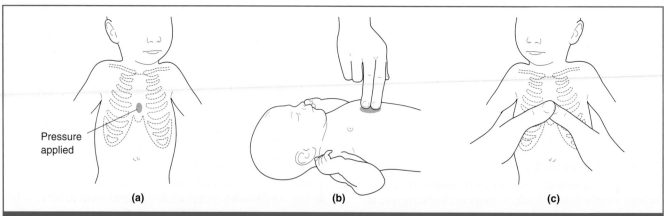

Figure 36.20 Cardiac compression **(a)** Position for applying pressure **(b)** Using two fingers **(c)** Using two thumbs with the hands encircling the chest (based on Henderson & MacDonald 2004)

Pressure applied

(a)   (b)   (c)

carefully observed for at least four hours. Temperature, pulse rate, colour and activity, and urinary output should be recorded. Hypoglycaemia may occur rapidly in critically ill or preterm infants. It is important to check blood glucose levels as soon as possible. These babies are often cold-stressed and so they must be kept warm, preferably in an isolette. A newly born infant who has required resuscitation, perhaps with ongoing respiratory compromise, may have experienced an insult to the gastrointestinal tract. It is important to provide fluids and energy; consideration should be given to parenteral versus oral hydration and nutrition for several days.

Preparation for transport

Medical transport of critically ill newly born infants requires skilled personnel and specialised equipment. Ideally, neonatal transport teams form a single component associated with a larger system of perinatal care composed of a tertiary care neonatal intensive care unit (NICU), and a neonatal outreach program. Preparation of the infant for transfer to a Level III nursery for subsequent care requires several considerations. First, it is important to complete all the routine care required for such ill infants. These basics may be neglected in the rush to prepare the newly born infant for transport. It is important to secure all lines, tubes, catheters and leads for transport. Monitoring en route to hospital is made more difficult if leads and lines are dislodged or do not function. Rapid and complete documentation of the resuscitation and subsequent therapies also is required for the receiving NICU.

Continuing care of the family

Irrespective of the outcome, witnessing the resuscitation of their baby is a distressing event for the family. While the resuscitation team is concentrating their efforts on the newly born infant and can often see that their efforts are achieving success, the parents cannot see what is happening. It is important that caregivers keep the family informed about what is going on and that the parents have contact with their baby as soon as possible. Most parents are unfamiliar with the complexities of care required for an extremely ill infant. It is often necessary to provide the information in small segments at frequent intervals to help the parents begin to comprehend the issues. The family needs clear and consistent explanations of the various supportive procedures that will likely be necessary after the infant's birth. Family members should also be provided with an overview of the potential complications of their infant's condition, including the possible need for prolonged intensive care. It is important to address the parents' needs and to be frank and honest in answering their questions.

Stopping resuscitation

It is difficult to accurately define a time beyond which active support worsens brain injury. However, it is reasonable to discontinue resuscitation after 10–15 minutes of appropriate resuscitative efforts for the infant with cardiorespiratory arrest who has not responded with spontaneous circulation

---

Clinical point

Naloxone

Naloxone is used to reverse respiratory depression in the newly born infant who is considered to be depressed by opiates given to the mother in labour (within four hours of birth), who require active resuscitation and/or continue to have inadequate spontaneous respiratory effort. It reverses narcotic-induced respiratory depression, analgesia, sedation, hypotension and pupillary constriction within 1–2 minutes. However, support with artificial ventilation remains the mainstay of treatment. The intramuscular administration of maloxone should not be used for other forms of vigorous stimulation.

Route, dose and frequency

Dose is 100 µg/kg solution for term or near-term infants. It can be given intramuscularly, intravenously or endotracheally. Naloxone acts more rapidly if it is injected into the umbilical vein, so all midwives should practise this technique. The dose can be repeated in 3–5 minutes if there is no improvement.

Contraindications

Infants of narcotic-dependent mothers (heroin, methadone) may experience abrupt withdrawal syndrome (increased heart rate and blood pressure, vomiting, seizures and tremors).

Neonatal side-effects

Excessive doses may result in irritability, increased crying and possible prolongation of partial thromboplastin time (PTT); tachycardia may occur. Some narcotics have a longer half-life in the newly born infant than naloxone, which may lead to respiratory depression in the postpartum unit. Therefore, any infant who has received naloxone should be closely monitored for the recurrence of respiratory depression for 12 hours. Naloxone acts more rapidly if it is injected into the umbilical vein, so all midwives should practise this technique.

Midwifery considerations

- Monitor respirations: rate and depth for improved respiratory effort.
- Assess for return of respiratory depression for 12 hours—when Naloxone's effects wear off and effects of longer-acting narcotics reappear.
- Monitor bleeding studies.
- Naloxone is incompatible with alkaline solutions such as sodium bicarbonate.
- Store at room temperatures and protect from light.
- Naloxone is compatible with heparin.

(measurable heart rate). Both survival and quality of life deteriorate precipitously at this point in term infants. Before resuscitation is stopped, a second opinion should be sought if possible.

> ### Reflective exercise
>
> Parents are often excluded from the room while their baby is being resuscitated or stabilised. Often, however, they are in an adjacent room and so they have some idea of what is going on and can often recall who said what to whom. Ask yourself:
>
> ▶ Is removing the parents to another room for the benefit of the parents, or for the comfort and benefit of the staff?
> ▶ If this was your baby, where would you want to be?
> ▶ How would you feel about a staff member who tried to prevent you from seeing your baby?
> ▶ Is it more frightening to see what is actually going on or to imagine what is going on?

Ethical issues

The birth of extremely immature babies and those with severe congenital anomalies raises questions among parents and care providers about the initiation of active resuscitation of the newly born infant. In such cases, initiation of resuscitation does not mandate continued support. Kattwinkel and colleagures (1999) point out that non-initiation of support and later withdrawal are usually considered to be ethically equivalent; however, the latter approach allows time to gather more complete clinical data and to provide counselling for the family. The authors (1999) comment that possible exceptions include infants with anencephaly or those who are extremely immature and for whom there is no possibility of survival.

Documentation

It is crucial for effective, quality care, and for medico-legal concerns, that all care providers attending a resuscitation of a newborn take responsibility for ensuring that assessments and the actions taken in the resuscitation are fully documented. Apgar scores quantify and summarise the response of a newly born infant to the extrauterine environment; they also provide an indication of the success of the resuscitation. Apgar scores should be recorded at one and five minutes, and sequentially after every five minutes until vital signs have normalised. However, Apgar scores should not be used to dictate appropriate resuscitative efforts (Kattwinkel et al 1999). A comprehensive, accurate narrative must also include a description of the events leading up to the birth of the infant, resuscitative efforts, and their timing and outcomes.

Review questions

1 Develop a plan of care for families at risk of complications in the postpartum period.

2 Identify the major causes of PPH, and for each one describe the appropriate strategies to prevent or manage it should it occur.

3 Do you think all parents should be taught the skills of neonatal resuscitation in pregnancy? If so, how would you go about doing this?

4 Describe the identification and assessment of a woman who has developed an amniotic fluid embolism.

5 What evidence-based strategies (if any) should be put in place for women at term with a macrosomic fetus?

6 Discuss the implications of trauma from accidents or battering for the pregnant woman and her fetus.

7 With colleagues and a torso and doll, practise using the HELPERR mnemonic during a 'mock' shoulder dystocia.

8 Practice neonatal resuscitation with colleagues during a 'fire drill'.

9 Name five interventions you would initiate for a woman who appears to have a cord prolapse.

10 Make a directory of the support networks available near you, for women who have had a traumatic pregnancy and birth.

Online resources

Reproline, Reproductive Health Online, http://www.reproline.jhu.edu.au

References

Alexander J, Thomas P et al 2002 Treatments for secondary postpartum haemorrhage (Cochrane Review). Cochrane Library. Update Software, Oxford

American Academy of Family Physicians 2000 Advanced life support in obstetrics (ALSO) course syllabus (4th edn). American Academy of Family Physicians, Kansas

American Heart Association 2000 Part 8: Advanced challenges in resuscitation. Section 3: Special challenges in ECC circulation 102(90001):229–252

Australasian Society for the Study of Hypertension in Pregnancy (ASSHP) 2000 The detection, investigation and management of hypertension in pregnancy: full consensus statement. Australian and New Zealand Journal of Obstetrics and Gynaecology 40(2):139–155

Australian College of Midwives Inc 2004 Australian College of Midwives' National Guidelines for Consultation and Referral. Australian College of Midwives Inc, Canberra

Australian Nursing and Midwifery Council (ANMC) 2006 National Competency Standards for the Midwife. Online: http://www.anmc.org.au/

Benson M 1993 Nonfatal amniotic fluid embolism. Archives of Family Medicine 2:989–994

Benson M, Kobabyashi H, Silver RK et al 2001 Immunologic studies in presumed amniotic fluid embolism. Obstetrics and Gynecology 97:510–514

Bonnar J 2000 Massive obstetric haemorrhage. Ballière's Clinical Obstetrics and Gynaecology 14:1–18

Boulvain M, Stan C, Irion O et al 2000 Elective delivery in diabetic pregnant women Cochrane Database of Systematic Reviews (2). Update Software, Oxford

Brown M, Hague W, Higgins J et al 2000 The detection, investigation and management of hypertension in pregnancy: full consensus statement. Australian and New Zealand Journal of Obstetrics and Gynaecology 40:139–155

CEMCH 2004 Confidential Enquiry into Maternal and Child Health. Improving the health of mothers, babies and children: why mothers die 2000–2002. RCOG Press, London

Clarke S, Hankins G, Dudley D et al 1995 Amniotic fluid embolism: analysis of the national registry. American Journal of Obstetrics and Gynaecology 172:1158–1169

Commonwealth Fund 1999 Health concerns across a woman's life span: The Commonwealth Fund 1998 survey of women's health. Online: http://www.cmwf.org.program/women/ksc_whsurvey99_332osp

Curran C 2003 Clinical issues: intrapartum emergencies. Journal of Obstetric, Gynecolog and Neonatal Nursing 32(6):802–813

DeCherney A, Nathan L 2003 Current obstetric and gynaecologic diagnosis and treatment. Lang Medical, London

Department of Health 2001 WO, Scottish Office. Why mothers die: report on confidential enquiries into maternal deaths in the United Kingdom 1997–1999. Stationery Office, London

Eclampsia Trial Collaborative Group 1995 Which anticonvulsant for women with eclampsia? Evidence from the Collaborative Eclampsia Trial. Lancet 345:1455–1463

Enkin M, Keirse J, Neilson J et al 2000 A guide to effective care in pregnancy and childbirth. Oxford University Press, London

Esposito TJ, Gens DR, Smith LG et al (1991) Trauma during pregnancy. A review of 79 cases. Archives of Surgery 126(9):1073–1078

Gabbe S, Niebyl J, Simpson J et al (Eds) 2002 Obstetrics: normal and problem pregnancies. Churchill Livingstone, New York

Gei G, Hankins G 2000 Amniotic fluid embolism: an update. Contemporary Obstetrics and Gynaecology 45:53–66

Gherman R, Ouzounian J, Incerpi M et al 1998 Symphyseal separation and transient femoral neuropathy associated with the McRoberts' manoevre. Journal of Obstetrics and Gynaecology 178:609–610

Gherman RB, Goodwin TM, Souter I et al 1997 The McRoberts' manoeuvre for the alleviation of shoulder dystocia: how successful is it? American Journal of Obstetrics and Gynaecology 176(3):656–661

Gobbo R, Baxley E (Eds) 2000 Shoulder dystocia. ALSO: advanced life support in obstetrics provider course syllabus. A Leawood, Kansas

Gonen R, Spiegel D, Abend M 1996 Is macrosomia predictable, and are shoulder dystocia and birth trauma preventable? Obstetrics and Gynaecology 88:526–529

Griese M, Prickett S 1993 Nursing management of umbilical cord prolapse. Journal of Obstetric and Gynaecologic Nursing 23: 311

Grossman NB 2004 Blunt trauma in pregnancy. American Family Physician 70(7):1303–1310. Online: www.afp.org/afp

Hannah WJ, Baskett TJ, Chance GW et al 1986 Indications for caesarean section: final statement of the panel of the National Consensus Conference on Aspects of Caesarean Birth. Canadian Medical Association Journal 134:1348–1352

Haram K, Pirhonen J, Bergsjo P 2002 Suspected big baby: a difficult clinical problem. Acta Obstetrica et Gynecologica Scandinavica 81:185–194

Haynes K, Stone C, King J 2004 Major morbidities associated with childbirth in Victoria: obstetric haemorrhage and associated hysterectomy. Public Health Group, Department of Human Services, Melbourne

Henderson C, Macdonald S 2004 Mayes' midwifery (13th edn). Baillière Tindall, London

Hope P, Breslin S, Lamont L et al 1998 Fatal shoulder dystocia: a review of 56 cases reported to the Confidential Enquiry into Stillbirths and Deaths in Infancy. British Journal of Gynaecology 195:1256–1261

Kattwinkel J, Niermeyer S, Nadkarni V et al 1999 ILCOR advisory statement: resuscitation of the newly born infant. An advisory statement from the Paediatric Working Group of the International Liaison Committee on Resuscitation Paediatrics. 103(4):e56

Landon MB, Hauth JC, Leveno K et al 2004 Maternal and perinatal outcomes associated with a trial of labour after prior caesarean delivery. New England Journal of Medicine 351:2581–2589

Levene MI, Tudehope DI, Thearle MJ 2000 Neonatal medicine (2nd edn). Blackwell, Oxford

MacKenzie IZ, Cooke I 2001 Prospective 12 month study of 30 minute decision to delivery intervals for 'emergency' caesarean section. British Medical Journal 322:1334–1335

Magpie Trial Collaborative Group 2002 Do women with pre-eclampsia, and their babies, benefit from magnesium sulphate? Lancet 359:1877–1890

Maine D, Wardlaw T, Ward V et al (1992) Guidelines for monitoring progress in reduction of maternal mortality. UNICEF, New York

Marien EN 2004 Human anatomy and physiology (6th edn). Pearson, New York

Midwifery Council of New Zealand (MCNZ) 2004 Competencies for Entry to the Register. Online: http://www.midwiferycouncil.org.nz/content/library/Competencies_for_Entry_to_the_Register1.pdf

Miras T, Collet F, Seffert P 2002 Acute puerperal uterine inversion: two cases. Journal of Gynecology, Obstetrics, Biology and Reproduction (Paris) 31(7):668–671

Morini A, Angelini R, Giardini G 1994 Acute puerperal uterine inversion: a report of 3 cases and an analysis of 358 cases in the literature. Minerva Ginecologica 46(3):115–1127

Niermeyer S, Kattwinkel J, Van Reempts P et al (contributors and reviewers) 2000 International Guidelines for Neonatal Resuscitation: an excerpt from the Guidelines 2000 for Cardiopulmonary Resuscitation and Emergency Cardiovascular

Care: International Consensus on Science. Pediatrics 106(3):e29. Online: http://www.pediatrics.org/cgi/content/full/106/3/e29

NSW Health Department 2002 Health circular 2002/99: framework for prevention, early recognition and management of postpartum haemorrhage (PPH). NSW Health Department, Sydney. Online: http://www.health.nsw.gov.au/policies/PD/2005/pdf/PD2005_264.pdf

Oats J, Abraham S 2004 Llewellyn-Jones Fundamentals of Obstetrics and Gynaecology (8th edn). Elsevier, Sydney

Ola E, Olamijulo J 1998 Rupture of the uterus at the Lagos University Teaching Hospital: Lagos, Nigeria. West African Medical Journal 17:188–193

Palme-Kilander C 1992 Methods of resuscitation in low-Apgar-score newborn infants—a national survey. Acta Paediatrica 81:739–744

Perozzi KJ, Englert NL 2004 Amniotic fluid embolism: an obstetric emergency. Critical Care Nurse 24(4):54–61

Prendiville WJ, Elbourne D, McDonald S 2000 Active versus expectant management in the third stage of labour. Cochrane Database of Systematic Reviews (3) Art No: CD000007 DOI: 101002/14651858

Ramji S, Ahuja S, Thirupuram S et al 1993 Resuscitation of asphyxiated newborn infants with room air or oxygen: an international controlled trial. The Resair2 Study. Journal of Paediatric Research 34:809–812

Ramji S, Rasaily R, Mishra P et al 2003 Resuscitation of asphyxiated newborns with room air or 100% oxygen at birth: a multicentre clinial trial. Indian Paediatrics 40:510–517

Rouse D 1999 Prophylactic caesarean delivery for fetal macrosomia diagnosed by means of ultrasonography—a Faustian bargain? American Journal of Obstetrics and Gynaecology 181: 332–335

Royal College of Obstetricians and Gynaecologists (RCOG) 2001 Confidential Enquiries into Maternal Deaths. Why mothers die 1997–1999. Fifth report of the Confidential Enquiries into Maternal Deaths in the United Kingdom. RCOG, London

Runnebaum I, Katz M 1999 Intrauterine resuscitation by rapid urinary bladder instillation in a case of occult prolapse of an excessively long umbilical cord. European Journal of Obstetrics, Gynaecology and Reprodroductice Biology 84(1):101–102

Sandberg E, 1999 The Zavanelli manoevre: 12 years of recorded experience. Obstetrics and Gynaecology 93:312–317

Saugstad K 1998 Practical aspects of resuscitating asphyxiated newborn infants. European Journal of Pediatrics 157(suppl): S11–S15

Saugstad O, Ramji S, Irani S et al 2003 Resuscitation of newborn infants with 21% or 100% oxygen: follow-up at 18–24 months. Paediatrics 112(2):296–300

Shah KH, Simons RK, Holbrook T et al 1998 Trauma in pregnancy: maternal and fetal outcomes. Journal of Trauma 45:83–86

Shevell T, Malone F 2003 Management of obstetric haemorrhage. Seminars in Perinatology 27(1):86–104

Slaytor E, Sullivan E, King F et al 2004 Maternal deaths in Australia 1997–1999. AIHW Cat. No. PER 24. AIHW National Perinatal Statistics Unit (Maternal Deaths Series No 1), Sydney

Sokol R, Blackwell S 2003 ACOG practice bulletin no 40: shoulder dystocia. International Journal of Gynaecology and Obstetrics 80:87–92

Steiner P, Lushbaugh C 1941 Maternal pulmonary embolism by amniotic fluid as a cause of obstetric shock and unexpected deaths in obstetrics. Journal of the American Medical Association 117:1245–1254

Sugrue M, O'Connor M, D'Amours S 2004 Trauma in pregnancy. ADF Health 5(1):24–28

Thomas J, Paranjothy S, James D 2004 National cross sectional survey to determine whether the decision to deliver interval is critical in emergency caesarean section. British Medical Journal 328:665

Usta I, Mercer B, Sibai B 1999 Current obstetric practice and umbilical cord prolapse. American Journal of Perinatology 16(9):479–484

Varney H 2004 Varney's midwifery. Jones & Bartlett, New York

Warner MW, Salfinger SG, Rao S et al 2004 Management of trauma in pregnancy Australia and New Zealand Journal of Surgery 74:125–128

Wiswell T, Bent R 1993 Meconium staining and the meconium aspiration syndrome: unresolved issues. Paediatric Clinics of North America 40:995–981

Wiznizer A 1995 Obstructed labour and shoulder dystocia. Current Opinion in Obstetrics and Gynaecology 7:486–491

World Health Organization (WHO) n.d. Correcting uterine inversion. Department of Reproductive Health and Research, WHO, Geneva. Online: http://who.int/reproductive-health/impac/Procedures/Correcting_P91_P94.html

Further reading

Jain L, Ferre C, Vidyasagar D et al 1991 Cardiopulmonary resuscitation of apparently stillborn infants: survival and long-term outcome. Paediatrics 118(5):778–782

Kecskes Z, Davies MW 2001 Rapid correction of early metabolic acidosis versus placebo, no intervention or slow correction in LBW infants. Cochrane Database of Systematic Reviews (1)

Lantos JD, Miles SH, Silverstein MD, Stocking CB 1988 Survival after cardiopulmonary resuscitation in babies of very low birth weight. Is CPR futile therapy? New England Journal of Medicine 318(2):91–95

Stable D, Rankin J 2004 Physiology in childbearing, with anatomy and related biosciences (2nd edn). Baillière Tindall, London

Tan A, Schulze A, Davis PG 2001 Air versus oxygen for resuscitation of infants at birth. Cochrane Database of Systematic Reviews (1)

Thoresen M 2000 Cooling the newborn after asphyxia—physiologic and experimental background and its clinical use. Seminars in Neonatology 5(1):61–73

Tucker Blackburn S 2003 Maternal, fetal and neonatal physiology (2nd edn). WB Saunders, St Louis

CHAPTER 37

Complications in the postnatal period

Jenny Gamble and Debra Creedy

Key terms

anxiety disorders, counselling, emotional support, endometritis, fatigue, pelvic floor dysfunction, postnatal depression, postpartum pain, post-traumatic stress disorder, psychological trauma, retained products of conception, secondary postpartum haemorrhage, sexual problems, thromboembolism, urinary incontinence

Chapter overview

This chapter describes and discusses physical and psychological morbidity following childbirth. The postnatal period has conventionally been defined as extending to six weeks following birth. After this time, women are presumed to have physically recovered from the birth and to be able to resume their roles. However, it is becoming clear that many women experience ongoing health problems related to the pregnancy and birth during the first year post partum. The considerable variety, duration and severity of morbidity is now being documented. In the past, health problems were narrowly defined as medical conditions requiring medical treatment, such as haemorrhage, thromboembolism and infection. More recently, researchers have broadened the scope of their work to incorporate women's perspectives on their health, which encompasses both physical and emotional dimensions, and other types of problems that are commonly experienced. This chapter commences with a review of physical complications and morbidity following childbirth. The second section relates to common emotional complications such as postnatal depression and anxiety disorders.

Learning outcomes

Learning outcomes for this chapter are:

1 To describe the range of physical health problems women may experience following childbirth

2 To discuss the factors associated with postpartum physical morbidity

3 To explain the assessment and treatment of secondary postpartum haemorrhage and infection

4 To discuss the various emotional responses to childbirth, and the factors that place women at risk for emotional distress

5 To apply the best available evidence to the care of postpartum women.

Postpartum physical morbidity

This section begins with a description of the extent of postpartum physical health problems and factors associated with poor postpartum physical health. Women's responses to their health concerns are outlined. Following this, specific postpartum health problems are described, along with associated factors, and research evidence on available treatment. Physical complications to be addressed include infection, vaginal bleeding, secondary postpartum haemorrhage, pelvic floor dysfunction, pain, thromboembolism and fatigue.

The extent of postpartum physical health problems warrants close attention. In a large questionnaire-based survey in the United Kingdom, 76% of women reported at least one health problem at eight weeks post partum (Bick & MacArthur 1995). An Australian study showed that 94% of surveyed mothers in Victoria reported ongoing health concerns up to six months post partum (Brown & Lumley 1998). In an Australian Capital Territory (ACT) study, 94% of new mothers reported health problems at eight weeks post partum. By 18–24 weeks post partum, this had declined only slightly to 81% (Thompson et al 2002). Recently, a study involving Queensland women found that although women's general health had largely been restored a year after birth, one-fifth of women continued to experience specific health concerns (Bogossian 2003). All studies (summarised in Table 37.1) highlight the extent of postpartum morbidity, with the percentage of postpartum women reporting health problems varying according to the types of problems measured, timing, and method of data collection.

Associated factors

There are several known factors consistently associated with poorer maternal health outcomes, such as obesity, poverty and smoking. Research has also predominantly examined factors associated with specific morbidities such as urinary incontinence. However, two recent studies (summarised below) investigated the association between general health status and type of birth. Women experiencing an operative birth generally have poorer postpartum health than women experiencing a spontaneous vaginal birth (Bogossian 2003; Lydon-Rochelle et al 2001).

A study by Lydon-Rochelle et al (2001) of 971 women in the United States found that primiparous women experiencing a caesarean section or operative vaginal birth reported significantly lower postpartum general health than women with spontaneous vaginal births. At seven weeks post partum, women experiencing a spontaneous birth reported better health status in terms of physical functioning, mental health, general health perception, bodily pain, social functioning and daily activity. These women also reported better physical, social, sexual, bowel and urinary functioning. Significant differences between groups were maintained even when the analysis was adjusted for maternal age, education, health insurance status, income, living situation, race/ethnicity and newborn length of stay (Lydon-Rochelle et al 2001).

TABLE 37.1 Selective summary of reported maternal morbidity

Study	Sample size (*n*)	Postnatal period (months)	Tiredness (%)	Perineal problems (%)	Backache (%)	Haemorrhoids (%)	Bowel problems (%)	Sexual problems (%)	Headache (%)	Vaginal bleeding (%)	Urinary incontinence (%)
Bick & MacArthur (1995)	1278	6–7 months	40	NM	46	NM	NM	NM	20	NM	22
Glazener et al (1995)	438	12–18 months	54	10	20	15	7	NM	15	13	14
Brown & Lumley (1998)	1336	6–7 months	69	21	43	25	NM	26	NM	NM	11
Thompson et al (2000)	1193	6 months	49	4	45	13	17	20	17	2	14
Bogossian (2003)	135	12 months	58	23	42	24	13	23	20		46

NM: not measured.
(Source: adapted from Bogossian 2003, pp 18, 169)

In an Australian study by Thompson et al (2002), women who had caesarean sections reported more exhaustion, lack of sleep and bowel problems, and were more likely to be readmitted to hospital within eight weeks of birth than women who had spontaneous vaginal births. In particular, women who had forceps or vacuum extraction reported more perineal pain and sexual problems than women who had had a spontaneous vaginal birth, after adjusting for parity, perineal trauma and length of labour.

Seeking healthcare for postpartum problems

Although many women experience a considerable burden of morbidity in the year following birth, they often do not seek any professional assistance for their health concerns (Bick & MacArthur 1995; Glazener 1997). In a study by Brown and Lumley (1998), one in seven women reporting a health problem had not talked to a health professional about their own health. Of women reporting health problems, 49% would have liked more help or advice. Similarly, Bogossian (2003) found that 47% of women did not seek any advice for prevalent health concerns. When women did seek advice, they most commonly consulted a GP (35%) or a medical specialist (12%). Only 3% of women sought advice from a nurse, midwife or other therapist.

Women may seem reluctant to seek professional help for ongoing postpartum health problems for several reasons. Some women may believe that their health concerns are minor, self-limiting or an expected consequence of having a baby. They may feel embarrassed or inadequate about their ability to get 'back to normal' as quickly as anticipated (Percival & McCourt 2000). Women may perceive that health professionals are unable to help or that there are limited options available to treat common postpartum problems such as extreme tiredness or musculoskeletal pain. Prescribing medication is a common response to women's postpartum health problems, and some women may find this unacceptable because they are breastfeeding or for other reasons (Bogossian 2003). When women do have contact with health professionals for routine care or for specific concerns, the focus by health professionals seems to be the wellbeing of the baby, not that of the mother. Women may perceive that health professionals lack interest in their wellbeing (Glazener 1997).

Postpartum infection

Postpartum infection can be a precursor to other postpartum problems such as secondary postpartum haemorrhage and pelvic pain. This section describes endometritis; however, infections of caesarean section and perineal wounds or urinary tract infections can hamper postpartum recovery and become a significant burden in women's lives.

Endometritis

Endometritis is inflammation of the lining of the uterus, usually caused by infection and causing pain. Caesarean section is the single most important risk factor for postpartum maternal

---

Case study

On day 10 post partum, following a normal birth of a 3570 g boy, Julie phones you, her midwife, and says, 'Last night, to my surprise, my husband took out the rubbish and washed out the bin. When my sister visited me this morning, she said, "You smell like road kill". I guess I need you to visit me.' You visit Julie at 12:30 pm. She is walking around and chatting but says she is feeling 'off-colour'. Her lochial loss has an offensive smell.

1 What does normal lochial loss smell like?
2 What additional assessment data would you seek? (Be specific.)
3 If you suspected endometritis, what would you do next?
4 How will you respond to Julie's comment about smelling like 'road kill'?

---

infection (Smaill & Hofmeyr 2002). Preterm labour (often associated with genital tract infection) is strongly associated with the development of postpartum sepsis (Kankuri et al 2003). Any procedure or event that introduces infection into the uterus or adversely affects women's ability to ward off infection predisposes them to endometritis. These include pre-labour rupture of membranes, blood loss, anaemia, operative vaginal birth, manual removal of placenta, repeated vaginal examinations, and internal electronic fetal monitoring. Although endometritis is frequently linked with uterine infection, it is not always the case. Sometimes the cause is unknown (Alexander et al 2002).

Women with endometritis may be febrile, with possibly only a low-grade temperature, and report abdominal/pelvic pain. On palpation, the uterus may be tender and sub-involuted. The lochial loss might be an unusual colour and frequently has an offensive smell. Bowel and bladder function may be disturbed and other possible infection or inflammation sites such as mastitis, or urinary tract or wound infections, need to be excluded. Treatment is with antibiotics. A risk of endometritis is septic shock.

Postnatal vaginal bleeding

Many women experience problems with postpartum vaginal loss that does not follow the expected course of lochial loss. Results from a UK survey showed that 20% of women had problems with postnatal loss occurring between 28 days and three months post partum. Only half of these women consulted a GP (Marchant et al 2002). A follow-up of GP data indicated that the common presenting symptoms were excessive bleeding (29/48; 66%) and prolonged bleeding (26/48; 54%). The most common form of treatment was antibiotics alone (15/48; 31%), however, 12 women (25%) were neither treated nor referred. Referral ($n = 19$) was for hospital admission, outpatient appointment, or direct referral for ultrasound scans.

Question

Is there a difference in the incidence of prolonged or excessive postpartum lochial loss between women who experienced physiological third stage labour and those who had actively managed third stage of labour?

Similarly, in an Australian study, 20% of women reported excessive or prolonged bleeding at eight weeks post partum, and although this problem resolved to a large extent by 24 weeks post partum, 2% of women continued to identify prolonged or excessive bleeding as a problem (Thompson et al 2002).

Secondary postpartum haemorrhage

Secondary postpartum haemorrhage (PPH) can be a life-threatening emergency, although in developed countries it is predominantly a problem of morbidity (Neill et al 2002). It has traditionally been defined as excessive bleeding from the genital tract that occurs after the first 24 hours following birth until the sixth postpartum week. However, many women bleed for longer than this period. Consequently, Marchant et al (2002) define it as any abnormal or excessive bleeding from the birth canal between 24 hours and 12 weeks post partum. This definition includes no reference to volume of blood loss or the woman's condition and, because normal lochial loss is poorly described, it is not very helpful in determining the incidence of secondary haemorrhage.

The incidence of secondary PPH determined by hospital admission is 1–2% (Alexander et al 2002; Hoveyda & Mackenzie 2001). In light of the findings from the study on postpartum vaginal loss described above (Marchant et al 2002), which showed that 'abnormal' bleeding is managed primarily in the community, calculating the incidence of secondary PPH from hospital admissions data results in under-reporting of the problem.

A history of primary PPH and manual removal of placenta are the only significant risk factors found to be associated with secondary PPH (Hoveyda & Mackenzie 2001). Other factors that may predispose women to secondary PPH include smoking, multiple pregnancy, threatened miscarriage, antepartum haemorrhage, hospital admission in the third trimester, precipitate labour of less than two hours, prolonged third stage, incomplete products of conception passed at birth, primary PPH, not breastfeeding and a history of previous secondary haemorrhage.

Assessment

Most women seek treatment for secondary PPH during the second week after the birth (Hoveyda & Mackenzie 2001). Because secondary haemorrhage and endometritis are not mutually exclusive conditions, some or all of the symptoms of endometritis may also be present for women who experience a secondary PPH. In addition, there must be abnormal bleeding. The blood loss varies in consistency and amount. Some women may have a highly offensive scant loss, while other women gush red blood or pass clots, some of which can be very large. Careful history-taking and clinical assessment of the woman is important, particularly in relation to the amount and duration of bleeding, signs of infection, and her current cardiovascular state.

Treatment

Women requiring admission to hospital for secondary PPH are treated with drug therapy and/or surgery. From UK figures, 1% of women undergo surgical uterine evacuation of retained products of conception and a further 1% of women are admitted to hospital and managed with drugs but not surgery (Alexander et al 2002). A study of 132 women with secondary PPH presenting to a hospital identified that 84% required hospital admission, 63% experienced surgical evacuation of the uterus, 17% received a blood transfusion, three women suffered uterine perforation, and a hysterectomy was performed on one woman (Hoveyda & Mackenzie 2001).

The rationale for these treatments appears to be that the uterus has failed to contract sufficiently to prevent bleeding from the placental site and that the underlying cause is retained products of conception and/or intrauterine infection (Alexander et al 2002). Previously undiagnosed genital tract tears may also be a cause of secondary PPH, especially in the presence of infection. Drug therapy consists of oxytocics and/or antibiotics to control the bleeding and treat the possible infection. Hormones such as prostaglandins may also be given to help control bleeding. Some women will require a blood transfusion. Surgery might involve evacuation of the products of conception, repair of cervical tear or uterine rupture and, rarely, hysterectomy (Alexander et al 2002).

In recent years, there has been an attempt to determine which women require surgical intervention to evacuate the uterus, because many women undergo this procedure with no resulting evidence of retained products of conception. The surgery itself has risks such as increasing haemorrhage by removing the placental site's clot, introducing infection, and uterine rupture. It was hoped that pelvic and/or abdominal ultrasound would assist in guiding treatment decisions about whether to intervene surgically. In a UK study, preoperative ultrasound examination did not provide better discrimination over clinical assessment about the likelihood of retained products of conception being removed during curettage (Hoveyda & Mackenzie 2001). It seems that retained products of conception can be over-diagnosed clinically and on ultrasound, as large clots produce a subinvoluted uterus and show echogenic material similar to retained products of conception.

A study conducted in Israel supports this finding. Histopathologic reports confirmed the diagnosis of retained products of conception in only 17 (48.5%) of the 35 postpartum women who underwent evacuation of the uterus for suspected retained products of conception. Since the false-positive rate for sonographic diagnosis of retained products of conception

Reflective exercise

1   Is there a role for alternative therapies such as reflexology, acupuncture and naturopathy in preventing secondary PPH?

2   What is the impact of secondary PPH on women's wellbeing?

3   How would women prefer to have this problem managed?

4   Are women informed of the benefits, risks and unknowns of various treatment options? (Explain how you would ensure that the woman had all the information she needed to make a decision about treatment options for secondary PPH.)

5   What are the implications of this complication for breastfeeding?

BOX 37.1   Summary: secondary PPH

> Secondary PPH is a significant cause of morbidity.

> Life-threatening secondary PPH in developed countries is rare.

> Secondary PPH is frequently associated with intrauterine infection.

> Treatment includes IV fluids, antibiotics, uterotonic medication, and surgical evacuation of the uterus.

> Prostaglandins or other drugs to control bleeding and/or hysterectomy and/or blood transfusion may be needed in extreme cases.

> Surgical evacuation of the uterus in cases of suspected retained products of conception carries risks and is possibly performed more often than warranted.

in postpartum women is high, the authors suggest a more conservative approach to the treatment of this condition (Sadan et al 2004). Similarly, Neill et al (2002) found that histology often failed to confirm retained placental tissue in women undergoing curettage for suspected retained products of conception.

Pelvic floor dysfunction

Pelvic floor dysfunction relates to urinary and faecal incontinence, perineal pain and dyspareunia. Previously a hidden burden associated with childbearing, pelvic floor dysfunction has recently received considerable media attention in Australia as part of a debate over the relative risks and benefits of different types of birth. While raising community awareness of the potential burden of pelvic floor dysfunction among childbearing women, the information provided was biased towards the protective effects of caesarean section in an attempt to justify the high caesarean section rates in Australia.

Urinary incontinence

The incidence of postpartum urinary incontinence is high. The most common type of incontinence suffered by postpartum women is stress incontinence, but urge incontinence is also common and many women experience a combination of different types of incontinence. Variable rates of urinary incontinence are reported in the literature as a result of different data collection methods, definitions of incontinence and the postpartum period in which incontinence was assessed.

A large population-based cohort study of women from the ACT (n = 1193) found that 19% of women reported incontinence at eight weeks post partum and 11% reported incontinence at 24 weeks post partum (Thompson et al 2002). Similarly, Burgio et al (2003) found that 11% of women reported some degree of incontinence at six weeks post partum. Other researchers have found higher rates of incontinence. Mason and colleagues (1999) reported that 31% of women had stress incontinence at eight weeks post partum. A New Zealand study on the prevalence, type, onset and frequency of urinary incontinence with over 1500 women reported that at three months post partum 34% of women experienced urinary incontinence, with 21% indicating that it occurred less than once per week (Wilson et al 1996).

Although problems with urinary incontinence often diminish in the weeks and months following birth, this is not always the case (Bogossian 2003; Burgio et al 2003). Importantly, urinary incontinence symptoms may worsen over the years (Continence Foundation of Australia 2003). A study by Grodstein et al (2003) reported that 34.1% of women (age range 50–75) had leaked urine at least once per month during the previous 12 months.

Factors associated with urinary incontinence

Childbearing per se has long been implicated in urinary incontinence. Parity is related to incontinence (e.g. Grodstein et al 2003; Thompson et al 2002) and the higher the parity the more likely the woman is to suffer from symptoms of incontinence (Mason et al 1999).

While parity has been found to be associated with urinary incontinence in a number of studies, the complete picture is far from clear. A longitudinal study involving 150 nuns (mean age 68 years, SD = 11.7) found that half had urinary incontinence and more than half of these women used sanitary pads for protection (Buchsbaum et al 2002). Stress incontinence was more common than urge incontinence. The authors concluded that the prevalence of incontinence in nulliparous, menopausal nuns was similar to rates reported in parous, postmenopausal women. While nuns differ from other women in a number of significant ways (due to their lifestyle), this study suggests that the effect of parity on urinary incontinence may contribute to differential morbidity in the premenopausal years.

Other variables associated with pregnancy and childbearing also affect pelvic floor function. It seems that some or all of the following factors may have a role to play in postpartum pelvic floor function:

- becoming pregnant
- antenatal pelvic floor exercises (Wilson et al 1996) and antenatal incontinence
- antenatal perineal massage (Heit et al 2001)
- gestation of pregnancy at birth
- age of mother at first birth (Grodstein et al 2003)
- commencing labour
- the nature of the labour (e.g. duration) (Brown & Lumley 1998)
- events and procedures during labour (e.g. type of birth, perineal trauma, type of pushing)
- birthweight of infant (Brown & Lumley 1998)
- length of breastfeeding (Burgio et al 2003).

There is conflicting evidence about a number of these variables (e.g. type of birth, infant birthweight), and the relative contribution of these factors to urinary incontinence requires further investigation. Other factors, not specific to pregnancy and childbirth, have been found to be associated with postpartum urinary incontinence. These include maternal obesity, smoking, pre-existing incontinence, race and lifestyle (Baessler & Schuessler 2003; Burgio et al 2003; Grodstein et al 2003; Hvidman et al 2003). The remainder of this section will examine the evidence relating to type of birth.

It seems that type of birth (elective caesarean section, emergency caesarean section, forceps, vacuum, spontaneous vaginal birth) is associated with differing rates of urinary incontinence. In the short-term, women having a caesarean section may have a lower incidence of incontinence (but not other urinary problems). Thompson et al (2002) found that compared with women having spontaneous vaginal birth, women having a caesarean section were significantly less likely to report urinary incontinence at eight weeks post partum, but this difference was not statistically significant at 16 and 24 weeks post partum. At 24 weeks post partum, women delivered by caesarean section were more likely to report other urinary problems, such as passing urine frequently or being unable to pass urine, than women having a spontaneous vaginal birth. Similar results were found in a population survey in South Australia, which reported that caesarean section may not be associated with significant reduction in long-term pelvic floor morbidity compared with spontaneous birth (MacLennan et al 2000).

A recent Israeli study, which excluded women with pre-existing stress incontinence, showed the prevalence of stress incontinence one year after the first birth to be 10.3% for women experiencing a spontaneous birth, 12% for women experiencing a caesarean for prolonged labour, and 3.4% for women experiencing a caesarean before the onset of labour (elective caesarean) (Groutz et al 2004). These rates support earlier findings of a New Zealand study (Wilson et al 1996). Similarly, an investigation of incontinence at six months post partum found that 9% of women who had a caesarean section reported incontinence, in contrast with 25% of other women (Hvidman et al 2003).

In their review, Baessler and Schuessler (2003) concluded that elective caesarean section might prevent trauma to the anal sphincter but not necessarily the urethral sphincter. The

development or presentation of defects in the endopelvic fascia leading to cystocele, rectocele, enterocele or loss of paravaginal support has not been investigated. Furthermore, prospective research is required on the impact of vaginal delivery and intrapartum management on the endopelvic fascia.

Inconclusive results are also evident on the effects of operative vaginal birth. The results of some studies have shown that women experiencing an operative vaginal birth are at higher risk of urinary incontinence than women following a spontaneous vaginal birth (Arya et al 2001; Brown & Lumley 1998). However, other studies have not demonstrated this association (Bogossian 2003; Hvidman et al 2003; Thompson et al 2002; Wilson et al 1996).

Urinary incontinence has a complex aetiology due in part to conflicting evidence. There are a large number of associated factors, lack of standardisation in categorising incontinence, and variable measures of duration and severity of symptoms. Rather than examine individual factors associated with the development of incontinence, predictive models of risk are required to promote prevention, early detection and effective treatment.

Postpartum pain

Compared with the intensity of the pain of labour, there has been little acknowledgement of postpartum pain except in the acute postoperative phase following caesarean section or perineal repair. After-birth pain and sore breasts/nipples also fit into the immediate aftermath of birth. Sources of ongoing postpartum pain include damage to the perineum, surgical wound pain following caesarean section, frequent headaches, shoulder, neck and back ache, and haemorrhoids.

The experience of ongoing pain is more common than realised. In a large Victorian survey, 43.5% of participants reported problems with backache 6–7 months post partum (Brown & Lumley 1998). The same study determined that 24.6% of women experienced problems with haemorrhoids 6–7 months post partum. Similar results were identified in a Queensland study, with 24% of women reporting pain from haemorrhoids one year after childbirth (Bogossian 2003).

Perineal pain and dyspareunia

Pain from perineal damage and associated dyspareunia can significantly affect the quality of life for postpartum women. A UK survey of 5404 women experiencing a spontaneous vaginal birth found that 7% of respondents reported perineal pain at three months post partum. Higher levels of pain were statistically associated with mid/upper vaginal lacerations and those women who had third- and fourth-degree perineal tears (Albers et al 1999). Brown and Lumley (1998) found that 21% of women reported problems with perineal pain 6–7 months post partum. Similarly, Bogossian (2003) found that 48% of women reported perineal pain at eight weeks, and 23% at one year post partum. Compared with women having a spontaneous vaginal birth, women who had a forceps or vacuum extraction consistently reported higher levels of postpartum perineal pain (Albers et al 1999; Thompson et al 2002).

Sexual problems and dyspareunia are commonly associated with perineal damage and operative vaginal birth. Brown and Lumley (1998) found that 26.3% of women reported sexual problems 6–7 months post partum. In a large UK study with over one thousand women, 53% of participants reported problems with intercourse at 8–12 weeks. These problems continued, with 49% of women still reporting difficulties in the subsequent year (Glazener 1997). Problems with intercourse were associated with perineal pain for 22% of women. Other concerns affecting sexual activity were tiredness, lack of interest, concerns about soreness or difficulty, worry about another pregnancy, or bleeding.

As with incontinence, prevention of perineal pain is aimed at maintaining perineal integrity during birth. Good general health in pregnancy, antenatal pelvic floor exercises, antenatal perineal massage, intrapartum midwifery care that maximises the chance of an intact perineum, early competent repair of the perineum if damaged, and postpartum pelvic floor exercises, should be part of routine practice. Women with persistent perineal pain or dyspareunia require further assessment and should be referred to a speciality service.

Thromboembolism

Pulmonary thromboembolism (PTE) is a leading cause of maternal death in Australia and New Zealand. PTE arises from deep vein thrombosis (DVT), which is frequently not recognised before PTE occurs. There were six maternal deaths from PTE in the 1997–1999 triennial report on maternal deaths in Australia (Slaytor et al 2004). Two of the six women who died from PTE were delivered by caesarean section; one woman had a spontaneous vaginal birth and the remaining three women died during pregnancy. Based on preliminary hospital discharge data, there is one case of PTE in every 1500 pregnancies and a case fatality rate of 1% (Slaytor et al 2004).

The major risk factors for venous thromboembolism include older age (35 years or older), caesarean section (particularly as an emergency in labour), operative vaginal birth, body mass index (BMI) greater than 29, heritable or acquired thrombophilia, a history of DVT or PTE, gross varicose veins, pre-eclampsia, immobility or a significant current medical problem (Greer 2002). Prophylaxis should be given when risk factors exist (Obstetric Medicine Group of Australasia (OMGA) 2001; Royal College of Obstetricians and Gynaecologists (RCOG) 2004). Postpartum women who have had a caesarean section should be assessed carefully for venous thrombosis.

Emerging issues

Fatigue

Sleep disruption during pregnancy and post partum is nearly universal and is often perceived as normal. However, when it leads to extreme tiredness, fatigue or exhaustion, it is a problem in itself. Sleep disruption may also contribute to other postpartum morbidities such as infection. Feeding and taking care of the newborn account for most sleep disturbances in the postpartum period and are greatest in the first postpartum months, especially for first-time mothers (Gay et al 2004; Moline et al 2003; Thompson et al 2002).

In one study, 60% of women reported problems of exhaustion/extreme tiredness at eight weeks post partum. At 24 weeks post partum this rate had dropped to 49% (Thompson et al 2002). Brown and Lumley (1998) measured problems with tiredness rather than exhaustion/extreme tiredness and found that 69% of women reported problems with tiredness 6–7 months post partum.

Postpartum fatigue is related to low levels of ferritin and haemoglobin (Lee & Zaffke 1999). Women who experienced a caesarean section are more likely to report exhaustion/extreme tiredness than women experiencing a spontaneous vaginal birth at eight weeks post partum (Thompson et al 2002), possibly because of the increase in postpartum pain or greater blood loss at the time of birth. Fatigue may also contribute to emotional distress. Reports of fatigue as early as seven days post partum have been found to be predictive of depression at day 28 post partum (Bozoky & Corwin 2002).

Emotional complications

Childbirth can be associated with a range of short- and long-term emotional consequences. Postnatal depression (PND) is the most prevalent psychological disorder associated with childbirth, but anxiety disorders are becoming increasingly prevalent. This section describes women's experiences of PND and postnatal anxiety disorders. This section also reviews research evidence on treatment of PND and outlines a midwifery model of emotional care.

Childbirth is a complex life event characterised by rapid biological, social and emotional transition. Many women experience significant somatic (physical) and cognitive–affective (thinking–feeling) changes following childbirth, but may not be clinically depressed. Changes in mood may be part of normal postpartum adjustment. The mildest and most common form of postpartum mood change is the baby blues, which occurs in the first few days post partum and lasts from 24 to 48 hours. Symptoms include weepiness, irritability, insomnia and anxiousness. Prevalence is thought to be around 80%, and so common as to be regarded as a normal reaction resulting from hormonal changes immediately following childbirth. For some women, however, the blues may represent the onset of clinical depression.

The most severe disturbance of mood is puerperal psychosis, which is extremely incapacitating, but relatively rare, occurring in one to two of every 1000 childbearing women (Buist 1996). It is characterised by severe depression with delusions (false ideas not based in reality). The severe disconnection from reality means that women with puerperal psychosis require hospitalisation.

Between the baby blues and puerperal psychosis is PND, affecting around 12% to 19% of childbearing women, and usually occurring within four to six weeks of childbirth (O'Hara 1997; Maternity Centre Association 2004). PND has a similar symptom pattern to that of depression, which can occur at any stage in life. There are differences, however, in the number, type and severity of depressive symptoms reported by postpartum women. In particular, PND is characterised by irritability, anger, low energy levels, loss of interest and feelings of guilt (Buist 1996).

PND often persists for many months but usually remits at around four to six months (O'Hara 1997); however, around 15% to 25% of cases continue for 12 months. A smaller proportion will continue for years, with inadequate treatment probably contributing to chronicity. Women with a first episode of depression following childbirth are less likely to experience depression at other times in their life but are more likely to experience PND with subsequent children. In contrast, women with a previous history of depression are more vulnerable to both childbearing and non-childbearing depressive episodes (Pope 2000).

Risk factors for postnatal depression

There has been considerable research on the factors that place women at risk of developing PND. Predictive risk factors for PND include a previous history of depression, psychological stress during pregnancy, young childbearing age (under 18 years), lack of social support (particularly partner support), stressful life events, and low socio-economic status (Pope 2000). This picture may be further complicated, however, if women experience difficult marital and parenting adjustments

---

> **BOX 37.2 Emotional complications**
>
> ▶ Baby blues is common, involves mild weeping and anxiety, and occurs between two and 10 days post partum.
> ▶ Depression has its onset around two weeks post partum. Enduring symptoms relate to anxiety, sleep and appetite disturbance at 4–6 weeks. Can last for up to 12 months.
> ▶ Common presenting symptoms include dysphoria, tearfulness, irritability, sleep disturbances and fatigue.

in the early postnatal period. Webster and colleagues (2003) completed a Brisbane-based study that identified that women in a violent relationship are at increased risk for PND.

There are significant associations between maternal depression and marital relationship, the partner's level of depression, and the infant's cognitive, emotional and social development. Depression associated with childbearing is particularly important, as the first year of childrearing brings additional responsibilities, personal disruptions and consequences in regards to relationships, loss of income and lifestyle changes.

Anxiety disorders and post-traumatic stress following childbirth

In addition to depressed mood, some women may experience symptoms of anxiety disorders. It has been proposed by some researchers that stress experienced around the time of birth can result in post-traumatic stress disorder (PTSD) (Wijma et al 1997). PTSD is a complex set of anxiety-related symptoms that result from and persist after exposure to extreme stress. According to the *Diagnostic and Statistical Manual of Mental Disorders* (4th edn) (DSM-IV-TR) (American Psychiatric Association 2000), there are explicit criteria that must be fulfilled for a specific time period in determining PTSD (as outlined in Box 37.3). First, the person must have experienced or witnessed an event that involves actual or threatened death or serious injury, or damage to self or others. Furthermore, the person's response should involve intense fear, helplessness or horror. The main symptoms of acute PTSD include persistent re-experiencing of the traumatic event, avoidance of stimuli associated with the event, and emotional numbing, as well as symptoms of increased physiological arousal. Symptoms must last for at least one month and cause impairment in daily life. A diagnosis of PTSD is made when at least one re-experiencing, three avoidance and two arousal symptoms are reported.

An Australian study found that one in three women (33%, n = 186) identified a stressful birthing event and reported the presence of at least three trauma symptoms. Twenty-eight women (5.6%) met DSM-IV criteria for acute PTSD (Creedy et al 2000). The findings from this study identified that obstetric intervention and a perception of poor care were

---

> **Reflective exercise**
>
> 1 How would you describe normal emotional reactions to early motherhood?
> 2 When would you become concerned about the emotional wellbeing of a new mother?
> 3 How comfortable would you be talking with a mother about her emotional response to childbirth?

BOX 37.3 PTSD

Diagnostic criteria for post-traumatic stress disorder

A The person has been exposed to a traumatic event in which both of the following were present:
1 the person experienced, witnessed, or was confronted with an event or events that involved actual or threatened death or serious injury, or threat to the physical integrity of self or others
2 the person's response involved intense fear, helplessness, or horror

B The traumatic event is persistently re-experienced in one (or more) of the following ways:
1 recurrent and intrusive distressing recollections of the event, including images, thoughts, or perceptions
2 recurrent distressing dreams of the event
3 acting or feeling as if the traumatic event were recurring (includes a sense of reliving the experience, illusions, hallucinations, and dissociative flashback episodes, including those that occur on wakening or when intoxicated
4 intense psychological distress at exposure to internal or external cues that symbolise or resemble an aspect of the traumatic event
5 physiological reactivity on exposure to internal or external cues that symbolise or resemble an aspect of the traumatic event

C Persistent avoidance of stimuli associated with the trauma and numbing of general responsiveness (not present before the trauma), as indicated by three or more of the following:
1 efforts to avoid thoughts, feelings or conversations associated with the trauma
2 efforts to avoid activities, places, or people that arouse recollections of the trauma
3 inability to recall an important aspect of the trauma
4 markedly diminished interest or participation in significant activities
5 feeling of detachment or estrangement from others
6 restricted range of affect (e.g. unable to have loving feelings)
7 sense of a foreshortened future (e.g. does not expect to have a career, marriage, children, or a normal lifespan)

D Persistent symptoms of increased arousal (not present before the trauma), as indicated by two (or more) of the following:
1 difficulty falling or staying asleep
2 irritability or outbursts of anger
3 difficulty concentrating
4 hypervigilance
5 exaggerated startle response

E Duration of the disturbance is more than one month.

F The disturbance causes clinically significant distress or impairment in social, occupational, or other important areas of functioning.

(Source: American Psychiatric Association 2000, p 468)

associated with the development of PTSD. Given the lifetime prevalence of PTSD for women in the general population of around 4% due to events such as assault, rape and natural disasters, Ayers and Pickering (2001) investigated whether PTSD following childbirth could be a continuation of the disorder in pregnancy. They screened and excluded women suffering from PTSD during pregnancy but still found that 3% of women suffered from PTSD following childbirth and that 1.5% continued to report significant symptoms six months later.

Anxiety disorders such as PTSD and mood disorders such as PND are commonly evoked by stressful events. Many of the anxiety-based symptoms reported by traumatised women, such as avoidance, sleep difficulties, trouble concentrating and preoccupation with the birth, may also be interpreted as symptoms of depression, and need to be delineated. Negative emotional states such as guilt, shame and anger are common in acute anxiety disorders and also associated with depression. After birth a woman may experience guilt or anger about the things she did or did not do. Women may also express feelings that they had let themselves down by not coping with the pain or by requiring more analgesia than anticipated. It is therefore particularly important to examine the symptoms of anxiety in order to understand possible ensuing depression and provide appropriate care and intervention. The case study of Maggie (on p 812) outlines the development of trauma responses in one young woman.

Consequences of postnatal emotional disorders

The consequences of postpartum emotional disorders can be debilitating at a time when a woman has to manage the extra demands of caring for her baby. Depressive symptoms may include impaired concentration and memory deficits, whereas anxious mothers may report unrealistic concern and worry about the baby. The effects of maternal anxiety on mothering are outlined in the case study of Gabrielle (on p 812).

The children of women who suffer from depression can have long-term disturbances to their emotional, behavioural and cognitive development (Righetti-Veltema et al 2003). For example, two-month-old infants of depressed mothers received less appropriate and responsive care, and more negative and rejecting care than babies of non-depressed mothers (Murray & Cooper 2003). Depression may also result in marital problems which, if unresolved, may lead to separation and divorce (Boyce & Stubbs 1994). Importantly, PND can progress to become a chronic condition that is disabling and difficult to treat successfully (Grace et al 2003).

Treatment of PND: review of the evidence

The following section reviews existing research evidence on treatment approaches to postpartum emotional disorders.

Psychological approaches to treatment

Counselling that involves emotional support and education by trained health professionals is a common and effective

Case study

Maggie, a primigravida, was induced using prostaglandin gel at 40 weeks gestation. She subsequently had a Syntocinon infusion, artificial rupture of membranes, epidural analgesia, continuous electronic monitoring and seven vaginal examinations. After a 14-hour labour the baby was delivered by vacuum extraction. Maggie said she needed 'loads of stitches'. Her baby needed resuscitation, had 'massive bruising on his head' and was admitted to the special care nursery. The baby was in a humidicrib for three days, developed jaundice and experienced feeding difficulties. A month later, Maggie still had difficulty sleeping. She experienced flashbacks, remembering 'every gruesome detail, all the fear and other emotions'. She reported being nervous and constantly on guard, especially about the baby, and described fearing that her baby would die or that she would die and her baby would be left motherless. She was anxious about the baby's health and insisted that visitors wash their hands before touching the baby, and sprayed the room with disinfectant when they left. She became so anxious following a news report of two cases of meningitis in another part of the city that she stayed with her mother out of town. Maggie described uncharacteristic angry outbursts and feeling detached or estranged from others for up to three months following the birth.

Case study

At six weeks post partum, Gabrielle reported 'difficulty caring for him [the baby]', and was 'slow to realise things like when he is crying for attention or when my older child is hitting the baby'. By three months she summed this up by saying, 'I am less responsive to him; I have a bonding problem'. She was experiencing symptoms of PTSD such as intense recollections of birth events, difficulty sleeping unrelated to the baby's needs, difficulty concentrating, feeling detached from others, and irritability.

approach to minimise the effects of depression. Women consistently respond positively to opportunities to talk about the birth with a supportive health professional. One study on women's postpartum needs found that 90% of nulliparous women and 79% of multiparous women wanted opportunities to express their feelings about the birth with a midwife (Cooke & Stacey 2003). Although many women want to discuss their feelings about the birth with a midwife, it seems that few women are offered this opportunity. Cooke and Stacey (2003) found that only 42% of primiparous and 20% of multiparous

women were offered an opportunity to discuss the birth. Similarly, recent Australian studies reported that only 13.5% of postpartum women were offered an opportunity to express how they felt about the birth to health professionals prior to discharge (Creedy et al 2000; Gamble 2003).

Well-controlled research trials report that PND responds well to treatment in the short term, almost doubling the spontaneous recovery rate (O'Hara et al 2000). In a landmark British study, women in the intervention group received eight weekly, one-hour counselling visits in their own homes by nurses who had received very brief training on non-directive counselling, and who had been told that the women were depressed (Holden et al 1989). The women in the control group received standard care from the same group of health visitors, who had not been told that these women were also depressed. At the end of the intervention, 69% of women were no longer depressed compared with 38% of women in the control group.

The long-term effects of psychological approaches are less clear. In one longitudinal study, nulliparous women were randomly allocated to one of four conditions: routine care, non-directive counselling, cognitive-behavioural therapy and psychodynamic therapy (Cooper et al 2003). Women received a one-hour home visit each week for 10 weeks. Although all therapeutic approaches were initially effective in reducing depressive symptoms (as measured by the Edinburgh Postnatal Depression Scale), by nine months post partum there were no apparent benefits between any treatment group and the control group. Similarly, a 12-month Australian study did not find statistically significant differences between mothers in a counselling intervention and those in control groups (Morse et al 2004).

Given the geographic distances faced by many health services in Australia and New Zealand, other methods of support need to be investigated. Telephone interventions have been used to deliver a range of community health services including the provision of health information, anticipatory guidance and crisis intervention. Increasingly, studies are investigating the effectiveness of telephone intervention as a means of postpartum follow-up. One Canadian study found that women from disadvantaged backgrounds who received a 'telephone visit' by a midwife were more likely to utilise parent–baby support groups than women who received mailed information or a reminder call by a ward clerk (Edwards & Sims-Jones 1997).

Debriefing

Debriefing describes a structured intervention intended to act as primary prevention to mitigate, or at least inhibit, acute stress reactions. There is insufficient evidence at present to draw conclusions about the effectiveness of debriefing following childbirth, primarily because it is unclear whether a standardised debriefing intervention was used in many of the studies (Lavender & Walkinshaw 1998; Priest et al 2003; Small et al 2000). The extent of training or therapeutic skills of the person providing the counselling is not often explained in the literature (Gamble & Creedy 2004). The idea that one simply 'allows the woman to talk' belies the depth of skill involved in facilitating such disclosure. The woman may have very good reasons not to talk; mistrust, lack of rapport, previous experience of being patronised, silenced or disregarded by health professionals may all adversely hinder the therapeutic process. Midwives providing counselling may be effective if the model of care provides time to develop a meaningful relationship with women throughout the pregnancy, birth and recovery, and training to understand and develop these 'listening' skills.

Although there is consensus in the literature about the importance of providing counselling for postpartum women, this does not seem to have been translated into practice. Many studies have been critical of the poor postpartum emotional care provided, and yet women consistently report that the intervention facilitated their postpartum adjustment/recovery (Lavender & Walkinshaw 1998; Priest et al 2003; Small et al 2000). Consumer groups such as Trauma and Birth Support (TABS), based in New Zealand, and Birth Experience Stress and Trauma support group (BEST), in Australia, continue to advocate for women to be provided with opportunities to talk with a supportive person about their birth experience (www.tabs.org.nz/; Yee, BEST Coordinator, personal communication, July 2003).

Response

Little is known about the specific skills of midwives in counselling postpartum women, and it may be that midwives are unsure about exactly what to do in providing counselling in the aftermath of a negative or distressing birth experience (Alexander 1998; Hunter 2001). Several published papers advocate postpartum counselling, but descriptions of how to engage with women in this way are general and non-specific (Gamble & Creedy 2004). Midwives may also be concerned that providing counselling about the birth is ineffective or potentially harmful. Hammett (1997) argued, however, that such concerns may be a reflection of midwives' anxieties in providing debriefing rather than substantiated misadventures.

Pharmacological approaches

There is a paucity of evidence for the treatment of PND using antidepressant medication. In a small, double-blind, randomised controlled trial (RCT) of antidepressant treatment (using nortriptyline or sertaline for eight weeks), depressive symptoms and most measures of functional status of women improved; however, improvement in one dimension did not imply improvement in the other (Logsdon et al 2003). Although participants were assessed after eight weeks of antidepressant treatment, clinical guidelines

recommend continuation of antidepressants for six to nine months after remission of symptoms (Wisner et al 2002). Given that most psychotropic drugs are excreted into breast milk, many women suffering from PND prefer not to take them (Whitton et al 1996). Furthermore, there is little available evidence on adverse effects of psychotropic drugs on the infant, and long-term effects are not known (Austin & Mitchell 1998).

Combined pharmacological and psychological approaches

There is limited research on different combinations of pharmacological and psychological therapies for PND. Appleby and colleagues (1997) conducted a double-blind RCT of fluoxetine and a psychoeducational program. CREST (Childcare advice, Reassurance, Enjoyment, Support from others, Targets) is an intervention program based on cognitive behavioural counselling and designed for health workers who are not specialists in mental health. Women were randomised to receive either fluoxetine or a placebo, plus either one session or six sessions of counselling for three months. There was significant improvement in all four groups but improvement was greater in women receiving six group sessions as opposed to one, and women receiving fluoxetine showed greater improvement than those receiving a placebo. It is important to note that of the 188 eligible women, 101 refused to participate because they did not wish to take medication, and a further nine women dropped out of the study due to adverse drug effects.

Social support

Social support has long been recognised as playing an important role in the prevention and treatment of depression. Misri and colleagues (2000), in a small Canadian study, offered women a support group of women alone ($n = 13$) or a group with partners ($n = 16$) in comparison with women and their partners in a control group. The intervention groups consisted of seven sessions and partners attended four sessions. In comparison to women who received standard care, women attending either support group had decreased symptoms of depression. Both women and their partners in the intervention groups perceived their relationship more positively, and ratings of general health improved, while those of the control group deteriorated.

An eight-week support program by Morgan et al (1997) offered women ($n = 34$) the opportunity to explore the myths of motherhood, receive information on PND, and challenge negative beliefs through the use of cognitive-behavioural exercises. Partners attended one session and opportunities were provided for women to explain their difficulties, for partners to add their perceptions, couples to discuss issues together, and for group discussion. There was a significant improvement in women's scores for depression, general health and couple satisfaction.

Hormonal approaches to treatment

Currently there is limited evidence of a link between hormones and PND. Lawrie and colleagues (2000) conducted a Cochrane

---

Reflective exercise

What are some of the possible reasons that midwives may not provide women with opportunities to discuss their birth experiences?

Review of the role of progesterone and oestrogen in the treatment and prevention of PND. They included only one RCT double-blind study, by Gregoire et al (1996) with women who had severe and chronic PND. The women received either treatment with oestradiol skin patches or placebo patches. Ten out of 35 women dropped out of the study. Although a positive effect was reported, no consideration was given to the influence of the women's menstrual cycle and whether any of the women suffered from premenstrual syndrome. Furthermore, 47% of women in the treatment group and 37% of women in the control group were already taking antidepressant medication, and this was not considered in the analysis.

Critical reflection on the evidence

Despite the relatively high prevalence and negative impact of PND on the mother, her infant, and her social and marital relationship, the quantity and quality of research on the treatment of PND is surprisingly limited. Indeed, a comprehensive review by Boath and Henshaw (2001) identified only 30 studies. While there are good theoretical justifications for many of these treatment approaches, the methodological limitations of these studies means that the efficacy of these approaches have not been clearly established, and there is very little good evidence available on which to make policy and practice recommendations.

Despite the intuitive appeal of a link between a hormonal trigger and PND, there is no evidence to support this. The limitations of the only RCT that has been carried out (Gregoire et al 1996) mean that many questions remain unanswered. There has been no study that has reported the use of only oestrogen on mood. Inevitably, women in such studies have received some form of antidepressant medication or counselling in addition to hormonal treatment.

Antidepressant medication is the most common form of treatment for depression in primary care and there is extensive evidence to support its use in the general population (Clinical Evidence 2000). There are no RCTs of antidepressants alone in the treatment of PND, and clinicians must rely on general recommendations for depression occurring at other times. In the absence of any evidence specifically for women with PND, the ethics of continuing to prescribe antidepressants to postnatal women, particularly in light of the range of unpleasant side-effects such as sedation, weight gain and dry mouth, needs to be considered. These drugs are known to pass through breast milk, and the long-term effects on infants are unknown.

The evidence suggests that cognitive and interpersonal therapy are as effective as antidepressants in treating depression. There is no evidence of a difference between these treatments in terms of long-term benefits, and combining drug and psychological treatments may be more effective in severe, but not mild to moderate depression (Clinical Evidence 2000). Further research is required on whether antidepressants should be prescribed only when counselling interventions have proved ineffective. Clinical trials on the treatment of depression suggest that continuing antidepressant drug treatment for four to six months after recovery reduces the risk of relapse, but we do not know whether this continuation treatment is the same for women with PND.

Implications for practice

Unlike New Zealand, childbirth practices in Australia remain predominantly hospital-centered and highly medicalised. The adverse psychological consequences for birthing women demand changes to maternity care. In particular, there needs to be a continued review to reduce the use of invasive obstetric procedures during labour and birth. It is also necessary to inform women of the incidence of obstetric interventions and associated risks so they can participate more effectively in decision-making.

There is evidence that depression and anxiety disorders are often overlooked in routine clinical practice. If trauma symptoms are not recognised in women with depression then it is likely that counselling approaches will not be provided. Psychological trauma that is not acknowledged and dealt with will manifest in a variety of destructive and negative ways. Women who have not processed the trauma associated with childbirth may experience depression, helplessness, self-destructive behaviours, marital difficulties, anger and hostility.

There is a strong association between women's perception of the helpfulness of the midwife and emotional wellbeing. Having the care of a midwife who is kind, respectful, informative and 'on-side' may be emotionally protective. The relationship may also be enhanced if the woman and midwife come to know and trust each other, as occurs in woman-centred midwifery (where the woman has the same midwife throughout the pregnancy).

The incidence and severity of postpartum emotional distress is of grave concern. Traumatised women may experience emotional numbing and dissociation as a result of the delivery that hinders their ability to engage with the baby and others. Alternatively, women may experience intense emotions that result in feelings of uncontrollable anxiety and an inability to make sense of what has happened. Accordingly, staff should provide opportunities to discuss the birth and try to bring structure to the experiences of the woman in an adaptive, reality-oriented manner. The discussion should involve reviewing the chronology of events, providing an explanation for interventions and procedures, and acknowledging feelings. It may also be necessary for staff to acknowledge issues of poor management and poor affective care. Robinson (1999) claims that women's fears in relation to childbirth are iatrogenic in

Reflective exercise

Given the number of questions surrounding the use of antidepressants and the fact that many women prefer not to take antidepressants, or may refuse medication if it requires stopping breastfeeding, should research concentrate on psychological interventions?

origin and result in women feeling unsafe and powerless. Health professionals need to reflect on their own practices and the service provided to women, and aim to engender more choice and control. As the woman begins to understand the sequence of events during labour and birth, and makes sense of her feelings, she may be able to recapture a sense of fundamental safety and control.

Effective follow-up in the community following discharge is important, as emotional distress is debilitating and may have long-term consequences for the mother, the child and the family. Women at risk of developing acute and/or chronic depression and anxiety can be readily identified prior to discharge from hospital and it is therefore feasible to organise for targeted follow-up of these women. Appropriate referral mechanisms to mental health services should be instituted so that women experiencing emotional distress, which cannot be effectively addressed by a midwife or child health nurse, can receive appropriate care (e.g. psychiatric liaison linked to maternity services).

Meaningful consultation with consumers is still in its infancy (Chambers 2000). Interventions for PND are more likely to be appropriate and effective if they are based on needs identified together with women. Logically, the people who should be involved and consulted are those for whom the interventions are destined. None of the studies reviewed included service users. Women with postnatal depression, together with their partners, should be involved in designing studies and interventions.

Summary: emotional support

Midwives need to acknowledge the unique nature of childbirth for each woman and attend to the emotional aspects of care in order to promote wellbeing.

Review questions

1   What are some of the factors associated with poorer postpartum health?

2   List some of the barriers women face in accessing professional assistance for healthcare.

3   Describe the symptoms and treatment of endometritis.

4   What assessment data would you need to determine whether a woman was experiencing a secondary postpartum haemorrhage?

5   Describe the initial treatment for a woman admitted to hospital via ambulance reporting that she is 12 days postpartum and bleeding heavily.

6   What are the factors that place women at risk for postpartum emotional distress?

7   How would you respond to a woman who seems to have the 'baby blues'?

8   Identify the symptoms of depression.

9   Briefly describe the effect of social support in relation to postnatal depression.

10 Describe best practice in maternity care to specifically prevent emotional distress for postpartum women.

Online resources

Australian Institute of Health and Welfare, perinatal statistics and maternal deaths, http://www.aihw.gov.au

Chartered Society of Physiotherapy (for information on incontinence), http://www.csp.org.uk/

Medical Journal of Australia, 'Anticoagulation in pregnancy and the puerperium', http://www.mja.com.au/public/issues/175_05_030901/omga/omga.html

New Zealand Health Information Service, 'Report on Maternity: Maternal and Newborn Information 2002', http://www.nzhis.govt.nz/publications/maternityreport.html

New Zealand Ministry of Health, http://www.moh.govt.nz

RCOG, http://www.rcog.org.uk

Safe Motherhood website (pregnancy-related complications for women in developing countries), http://www.safemotherhood.org

TABS (Trauma and Birth Stress) website, 'PTSD after childbirth', http://www.tabs.org.nz

References

Albers L, Garcia J, Renfrew M et al 1999 Distribution of genital tract trauma in childbirth and related postpartum pain. Birth 26(1):11–15

Alexander J 1998 Confusing debriefing and defusing postnatally: the need for clarity of terms, purpose and value. Midwifery 13:122–124

Alexander J, Thomas P, Sanghera A 2002 Treatments for secondary postpartum haemorrhage (Cochrane Review). Cochrane Library (1). Update Software, Oxford

American Psychiatric Association 2000 Diagnosis and statistical manual of mental disorders TR (4th edn). APA, Washington DC

Appleby L, Warner R, Whitton A et al 1997 A controlled study of fluoxetine and cognitive-behavioural counselling in the treatment of PND. British Medical Journal 314:932–936

Arya L, Jackson N, Myers D et al 2001 Risk of new-onset incontinence after forceps and vacuum delivery in primiparous women. American Journal of Obstetrics and Gynecology 185(6):1318–1324

Austin M, Mitchell P 1998 The use of psychotropic medications in breastfeeding women. Australian and New Zealand Journal of Psychiatry 32:561–569

Ayers S, Pickering AD 2001 Do women get posttraumatic stress disorder as a result of childbirth? A prospective study of incidence. Birth 28(2):111–118

Baessler K, Schuessler B 2003 Childhood-induced trauma to the urethral continence mechanism: Review and recommendations. Urology 62(Suppl 4A):39–44

Bick D, MacArthur C 1995 The extent, severity and effect of health problems after childbirth. British Journal of Midwifery 3(1):27–31

Boath E, Henshaw C 2001 The treatment of postnatal depression: a comprehensive literature review. Journal of Reproductive and Infant Psychology 19(3):215–248

Bogossian F 2003 The Mothers' Health Study: a randomised controlled trial of a social support intervention on the health of mothers in the year after birth. University of Queensland, Brisbane

Boyce PM, Stubbs JM 1994 The importance of postnatal depression [editorial]. Medical Journal of Australia 161:471–472

Bozoky I, Corwin E 2002 Fatigue as a predictor of postpartum depression. Journal of Obstetric, Gynaecological and Neonatal Nursing 31(4):436–443

Brown S, Lumley J 1998 Maternal health after childbirth: results of an Australian population based survey. British Journal of Obstetrics and Gynaecology 105(2):156–161

Buchsbaum G, Chin M, Guzick D 2002 Prevalence of urinary incontinence and associated risk factors in a cohort of nuns. Obstetrics and Gynecology 100(2):226–229

Buist A 1996 Psychiatric disorders associated with childbirth: a guide to management. McGraw-Hill, Sydney

Burgio K, Zyczynski H, Locher JL et al 2003 Urinary incontinence in the 12-month postpartum period. Obstetrics and Gynecology 102(6):1291–1298

Chambers R 2000 Involving patients and the public: how to do it better. Radcliffe Medical Press, Abingdon

Clinical Evidence 2000 BMJ Publishing, June

Continence Foundation of Australia 2003 New mothers and incontinence. Online: http://www.continence.org.au, accessed August 2003

Cooke M, Stacey T 2003 Differences in the evaluation of postnatal midwifery support by multiparous and primiparous women in the first two weeks after birth. Australian Midwifery 16(3):18–24

Cooper P, Murray L, Wilson A et al 2003 Controlled trials of the short- and long-term effect of psychological treatment of postpartum depression. British Journal of Psychiatry 182: 412–419

Creedy D, Shochet I, Horsfall J 2000 Childbirth and the development of acute trauma symptoms: Incidence and contributing factors. Birth 27(2):104–111

Edwards NC, Sims-Jones N 1997 A randomized controlled trial of alternate approaches to community follow-up for postpartum women. Canadian Journal of Public Health 88(2):123–128

Gamble JA 2003 Improving emotional care for childbearing women: an intervention study. Unpublished doctoral dissertation, Griffith University, Brisbane

Gamble J, Creedy D 2004 Content and processes of postpartum counseling after a distressing birth experience: A review. Birth 31(3):213–218

Gay C, Lee K, Lee S 2004 Sleep patterns and fatigue in new mothers and fathers. Biological Research for Nursing 5(4):311–318

Glazener CM 1997 Sexual function after childbirth: women's experiences, persistent morbidity and lack of professional recognition. British Journal of Obstetrics and Gynaecology 104(March):330–335

Grace SL, Evindar A, Stewart D 2003 The effect of postpartum depression on child cognitive development and behaviour: a review and critical analysis of the literature. Archives of Women's Mental Health 6:263–274

Greer I 2002 Venous thromboembolism and thrombophilia. In: AB MacLean, J Neilson (Eds) Maternal morbidity and mortality. RCOG Press, London, pp 173–189

Gregoire A, Kumar R, Everett B et al 1996 Transdermal oestrogen for treatment of severe PND. Lancet 347:930–933

Grodstein F, Fretts R, Lifford K et al 2003 Association of age, race, and obstetric history and urinary symptoms among women in the Nurses' Health Study. American Journal of Obstetrics and Gynecology 189(2):428–434

Groutz A, Rimon E, Peled S et al 2004 Cesarean section: does it really prevent the development of postpartum stress urinary incontinence? A prospective study of 363 women one year after their first delivery. Neurourology and Urodynamics 23:2–6

Hammett PL 1997 Midwives and debriefing. In: MJ Kirkham, ER Perkins (Eds) Reflections on midwifery. Baillière Tindall, London, pp 135–159

Heit M, Mudd K, Culligan P 2001 Prevention of childbirth injuries to the pelvic floor. Current Women's Health and Reproduction 1(1):72–80

Holden J, Sagovsky R, Cox J 1989 Counselling in a general practice setting: a controlled study of health visitor intervention in the treatment of postnatal depression. British Medical Journal 298:223–226

Hoveyda F, Mackenzie I 2001 Secondary postpartum haemorrhage: incidence, morbidity and current management. British Journal of Obstetrics and Gynaecology 108(9):927–930

Hunter B 2001 Emotion work in midwifery: a review of current knowledge. Journal of Advanced Nursing 34(4):436–444

Hvidman L, Foldspang A, Mommsen S et al 2003 Postpartum urinary incontinence. Acta Obstetricia et Gynecologica Scandinavica 82(6):556–563

Kankuri E, Kurki T, Carlson P et al 2003 Incidence, treatment and outcome of peripartum sepsis. Acta Obstetricia et Gynecologica Scandinavica 82(8):730–735

Lavender T, Walkinshaw SA 1998 Can midwives reduce postpartum psychological morbidity? A randomized trial. Birth 25:215–219

Lawrie T, Herxheimer A, Dalton K 2000 Oestrogens and progestogens for preventing and treating postnatal depresion. Cochrane Database of Systematic Reviews (2). Update Software, Oxford

Lee K, Zaffke M 1999 Longitudinal changes in fatigue and energy during pregnancy and the postpartum period. Journal of Obstetric, Gynecological and Neonatal Nursing 28(2):183–191

Logsdon M, Wisner K, Hanusa B et al 2003 Role functioning and symptom remission in women with postpartum depression after antidepressant treatment. Archives of Psychiatric Nursing 27(6):276–283

Lydon-Rochelle M, Holt VL, Martin DP 2001 Delivery method and self-reported postpartum general health status among primiparous women. Paediatric and Perinatal Epidemiology 15(3):232–240

MacArthur C, Winter H, Bick D et al 2003 Redesigning postnatal care: a randomised controlled trial of protoco-based midwifery-led care focused on individual women's physical and psychological health needs. Health Technology Assessment 7(37):1–98

MacLennan AH, Taylor AW, Wilson DH et al 2000 The prevalence of pelvic floor disorders and their relationship to gender, age, parity and mode of delivery. British Journal of Obstetrics and Gynaecology 107:1460–1470

Marchant S, Alexander J, Garcia J 2002 Postnatal vaginal bleeding problems and general practice. Midwifery 18:21–24

Mason L, Glenn S, Walton I et al 1999 The prevalence of stress incontinence during pregnancy and following delivery. Midwifery 15:120–128

Maternity Centre Association 2004 Recommendations from listening to mothers: report of the first national US survey of women's childbearing experiences. New York: Maternity Centre Association. Birth 31:61–65

Misri S, Kostaras X, Fox D et al 2000 The impact of partner support in the treatment of PND. Canadian Journal of Psychiatry 45:554–558

Moline M, Broch L, Zak R et al 2003 Clinical review: sleep in women across the life cycle from adulthood through menopause. Sleep Medicine Reviews 7(2):155–177

Morgan M, Matthew S, Barnett E et al 1997 A group program for postnatally distressed women and their partners. Journal of Advanced Nursing 26:913–920

Morse C, Durkin S, Buist A et al 2004 Improving the postnatal outcomes of new mothers. Journal of Advanced Nursing 45:465–474

Murray L, Cooper P 2003 The impact of postpartum depression on infant development. In: I Goodyear (Ed) Aetiological mechanisms in developmental psychopathology. Oxford University Press, Oxford

Neill A, Nixon R, Thornton S 2002 A comparison of clinical assessment with ultrasound in the management of secondary postpartum haemorrhage. European Journal of Obstetrics and Gynaecology and Reproductive Biology 104:113–115

Obstetric Medicine Group of Australasia (OMGA) 2001 Anticoagulation in pregnancy and puerperium. Medical Journal of Australia 175:258–263

O'Hara M 1997 The nature of postpartum depressive disorders. In: L Murray, PJ Cooper (Eds) Postpartum depression and child development. Guilford, New York, pp 3–31

O'Hara M, Stuart S, Gorman LL et al 2000 Efficacy of interpersonal psychotherapy for postpartum depression. Archives of General Psychiatry 57(11):1039–1045

Percival P, McCourt C 2000 Becoming a parent. In: LA Page (Ed)The new midwifery—science and sensitivity in practice. Churchill Livingstone, Sydney, pp 185–222

Pope S 2000 Postnatal depression: a systematic review of published scientific literature to 1999. National Health and Medical Research Council, Commonwealth of Australia

Priest S, Henderson J, Evans S et al 2003 Stress debriefing after

childbirth: a randomised controlled trial. Medical Journal of Australia 178:542–545

Righetti-Veltema VM, Bousquet A, Manzano J 2003 Impact of postpartum depression on mother and her 18-month-old infant. European Child and Adolescent Psychiatry 12:75–83

Robinson J 1999 The demand for caesareans: fact or fiction? British Journal of Midwifery 7(5):306

Royal College of Obstetricians and Gynaecologists (RCOG) 2004 Thromboprophylaxis during pregnancy, labour and after vaginal delivery. Guideline No. 37. RCOG, London

Sadan O, Golan A, Girtler O et al 2004 Role of sonority in the diagnosis of retained products on conception. Journal of Ultrasound Medicine 23(3):371–374

Slaytor EK, Sullivan EA, King JF 2004 Maternal deaths in Australia 1997–1999. Online: www.aihw.gov.au, accessed 16 August 2004

Smaill F, Hofmeyr GJ 2002 Antibiotic prophylaxis for caesarean section (Cochrane Review). Cochrane Library (3). Update Software, Oxford

Small R, Lumley J, Donohue L et al 2000 Randomised controlled trial of midwife led debriefing to reduce maternal depression after operative childbirth. British Medical Journal 321:1043–1047

Thompson JF, Roberts CL, Currie M et al 2002 Prevalence and persistence of health problems after birth: associations with parity and method of birth. Birth 29(2):83–94

Webster J, Pritchard M, Creedy D et al 2003 A simplified predictive index for the detection of women at risk for postnatal depression. Birth 30(2):102–108

Whitton A, Warner R, Appleby I 1996 The pathway to care in PND: women's attitudes to PND and its treatment. British Journal of General Practice 46:427–428

Wijma K, Soderquist MA, Wijma B 1997 Posttraumatic stress disorder after childbirth: a cross sectional study. Journal of Anxiety Disorders 11:587–597

Wilson PD, Herbison RM, Herbison GP 1996 Obstetric practice and the prevalence of urinary incontinence three months after delivery. British Journal of Obstetrics and Gynaecology 103:154–161

Wisner KL, Parry BL, Piontek CM 2002 Postpartum depression. New England Journal of Medicine 347:194–199

Further reading

Chiarelli P 2004 Women's waterworks: curing incontinence. Online: http://www.womenswaterworks.com

Gamble J, Creedy D, Webster J et al 2002 A review of the literature on debriefing or non-directive counselling to prevent postpartum emotional distress. Midwifery 18(1):72–79

Pope S 2000 Postnatal depression: a systematic review of published scientific literature to 1999. National Health and Medical Research Council, Commonwealth of Australia

CHAPTER 38

Complications of the newborn

Linda Jones and Annette Wright

Key terms

apnoea, birth asphyxia, cephalhaematoma, chromosomal abnormalities, cleft palate, coagulopathies, congenital abnormalities, congenital dislocation of the hip, cystic fibrosis, cytomegalovirus, exomphalos, galactosaemia, gastroschisis, Group B haemolytic streptococcus, hepatitis, hypoglycaemia, imperforate anus, listeriosis, meconium aspiration syndrome, neonatal jaundice, neural tube defects, oesophageal fistula, phenylketonuria, physiological jaundice, pneumothorax, preterm neonate, rubella, SIDS, sticky eyes, subarachnoid haemorrhage, subdural haemorrhage, talipes, thermal instability, transient tachypnoea of the newborn, undescended testes, vitamin K

Chapter overview

This chapter outlines the common complications of the newborn; it includes preterm birth, jaundice, infections and bleeding in the neonate. In addition, this chapter discusses congenital, cardiorespiratory, metabolic and endocrine disorders that could affect the neonate, and sudden infant death syndrome. It is not within the scope of this chapter to discuss all the neonatal disorders in detail—a brief outline of conditions is given. It is important to remember that, when caring for neonates, midwives must always be prepared for the unexpected in this fragile population.

Learning outcomes

Learning outcomes for this chapter are:

1 To outline the common causes of preterm births and the characteristics of the neonate

2 To describe the problems faced by preterm neonates and give an overview of management

3 To explain the normal physiology of bilirubin metabolism and identify common causes of hyperbilirubinaemia

4 To describe the assessment and management of jaundice

5 To explain the neonatal immune system and its role in preventing infection in the neonate

6 To discuss common neonatal infections

7 To identify the common causes of bleeding in the neonate

8 To explain the aetiology and risk factors for congenital abnormalities, and identify some common congenital abnormalities

9 To describe the most common types of cardiac lesions and their prognosis

10 To discuss some common neonatal respiratory disorders and the various respiratory support measures for a neonate

11 To describe the features of the common metabolic and endocrine disorders

12 To identify the risk factors for sudden infant death syndrome (SIDS), and discuss how to provide clear and accurate information to parents and families on reducing the risk of SIDS.

Preterm neonate

The role of the midwife regarding preterm neonates is in prevention and in assisting parents in identifying the potential risk factors. In the event of a preterm birth, the midwife plays a crucial role in supporting the parents. This section outlines the causes and characteristics of a preterm neonate. The emphasis of this section is on neonatal care, highlighting some of the major problems encountered in the preterm neonate.

Definition and causes

Preterm birth is defined as the birth of a newborn before 37 weeks gestation, occurring either spontaneously or after being induced for maternal or fetal health problems. This group of neonates provide the majority of work in neonatal units. The incidence of preterm birth varies from one part of the country to another and depending on the ethnic group. In 2000, the rate of neonates born at less than 32 weeks gestation was 2.23% of live births in Australia, and 3.43% of live births in New Zealand. Overall survival for preterm neonates at more than 28 weeks gestation is 92%, a figure that has remained constant since 1998 (ANZNN 2002).

The gestational age at which a preterm neonate is considered viable has been falling in recent years. Current technology and care offer considerable hope for neonates born at 24 to 25 weeks gestation. Neonates as young as 22 to 23 weeks gestation can now be saved by the intensive care facilities currently available. Obviously, the earlier the gestational age at birth, the greater the risk of neurological deficits in those neonates who survive. Current evidence indicates that 90% of neonates born at 26 to 28 weeks gestation will develop into normal, healthy children (Johnston et al 2003).

The cause of spontaneous preterm births is unknown in 40% of cases; however, there are certain predisposing antenatal factors, including:

- poor socio-economic status
- pre-eclampsia
- infection
- smoking, substance abuse or alcoholism in pregnancy
- antepartum haemorrhage
- overdistension of the uterus—multiple pregnancies, polyhydramnios
- fetal development abnormalities
- maternal age < 20 years or > 35 years
- serious maternal diseases—acute or chronic, such as pyelonephritis, chronic nephritis or essential hypertension
- cervical incompetence
- poor obstetric history
- short maternal stature
- primiparity (Henderson & Macdonald 2004; Johnston et al 2003).

Characteristics

Preterm neonatal characteristics will depend on the gestational age at birth. Generally speaking, preterm neonates have a head circumference that exceeds that of the chest. In turn, the chest tends to be relatively small and narrow, with no breast tissue. The face of the preterm neonate is triangular, with a pointed chin, and the fontanelles and sutures are widely spaced due to poor ossification. Ears in the preterm are easily folded, lacking firmed cartilage. Also, the length of the trunk in proportion to the limbs is greater in the preterm than in the term neonate. The skin in the preterm is pinkish red with prominent surface veins due to the absence of subcutaneous fat. Fine hair, or lanugo, on the face and trunk is more plentiful in the preterm, as is the protective creamy white substance known as vernix. The limbs are thin, with decreased muscle tone, and the nails are soft. With neonates of less than 34 weeks gestation, the creases in the feet are almost absent. In the preterm female, the labia minora are prominent and gaping, and the male usually has incompletely descended testes. In addition, the suck-and-swallow reflex is uncoordinated in preterm neonates.

Assessment

Many scoring systems have been developed over the years in order to estimate the gestational age of the neonate. These scoring systems require a complete and careful examination of the neonate. The scoring system examines characteristics such as appearance, and reflexes that give an indication of whether the neonate is small or preterm. The two most commonly used scoring systems are the Dubowitz and, more recently, the Ballard, an adaptation of the former.

Labour and birth care

In most cases it should be possible to diagnose the onset of preterm labour early enough to ensure that the birth occurs in a maternity unit containing the necessary neonatal services and thus avoid the greater hazard of transfer after birth. During a preterm labour, the midwife should avoid giving narcotics to the woman, in order to prevent respiratory depression in the neonate at birth. All resuscitation equipment must be checked and ready before the birth. It is important that an experienced neonatologist and midwife be present at the birth of the preterm to ensure immediate and expert resuscitation. Cold stress at birth must be prevented, as this increases neonatal oxygen requirements. The neonate, therefore, must be dried quickly and thoroughly with warm towels and placed under a radiant heater immediately after birth.

Specific preterm problems

The preterm neonate is unable to adequately perform many physiological functions, due to immaturity. The aim of neonatal care is, therefore, to compensate and support these deficiencies until support is no longer needed. The main problems are:

- *birth asphyxia*—can occur if there is any disruption to the oxygen supply prior to or during birth, due to reduced energy reserves of the preterm neonate
- *thermal instability*—preterm neonates have little or no

brown fat stores to maintain their core temperature. In addition, preterm neonates have a larger surface area relative to their size, with thin skin, which facilitates rapid heat loss. Those born at less than 30 weeks gestation also have porous skin, allowing evaporation of fluids. The aim of care, therefore, is to maintain body temperature within the thermoneutral range, thus reducing energy and oxygen requirements.

- *diminished primitive survival reflexes*—these include the suck, swallow and gag reflex
- *jaundice*—physiological jaundice in preterm neonates is exacerbated due to an immature liver, resulting in delayed conjugation of bilirubin. This will be discussed in more detail later in the chapter.
- *respiratory diseases*—this is the most common problem experienced by preterm neonates, and is exacerbated by younger gestation. Preterm neonates have weak muscles and immature respiratory control. It is not uncommon for the preterm neonate to breathe well initially, later developing expiratory grunt, apnoeic episodes and cyanosis, requiring respiratory support. Respiratory conditions experienced by preterm neonates are discussed later in this chapter; they include apnoea, hyaline membrane disease, transient tachypnoea of the newborn, pneumothorax, pneumonia and bronchopulmonary dysplasia.
- *metabolic disturbances*—these include hypoglycaemia, hypocalcaemia, hypomagnesaemia, hyponatraemia and hypokalaemia
- *patent ductus arteriosus*—the ductus arteriosus fails to close in very preterm neonates due to immaturity and as a consequence of the chemical imbalance that results from hypoxia and ventilation perfusion mismatching. Closure of the ductus is usually achieved by a course of indomethacin, with surgical ligation sometimes being necessary.
- *neurological problems*—these include intracranial haemorrhage, the risk factors for which include poor skull ossification, fragile blood vessels and episodes of hypotension, hypertension or hypoxia
- *susceptibility to infection*—this is increased due to low maternal IgG levels, less efficient skin barrier, fewer immune cells, and being subjected to more invasive procedures and multiple caregivers
- *gastrointestinal intolerance and necrotising enterocolitis (NEC)*—NEC is an inflammatory disease of the bowel usually associated with septicaemia
- *ophthalmic problems*—these include retinopathy of prematurity, with the major risk factor being excessive oxygen exposure or fluctuating quantities; myopia; and strabismus
- *surgical lesions*—including the possibility of undescended testes, inguinal and umbilical herniae
- *haematological problems*—this includes haemorrhagic disease of prematurity due to accentuation of the normal neonatal deficiency of vitamin K-dependent clotting factors; and iron deficiency anaemia resulting from

Clinical point

There is a growing body of evidence regarding management of painful procedures in neonates with use of breastfeeding (Carbajal et al 2003) and sucrose (Gibbins et al 2002; Gradin et al 2002) to help reduce the pain experienced by the neonate during these procedures.

frequent blood sampling, often requiring a transfusion of packed red blood cells
- *renal immaturity*—inability to concentrate urine and excrete an acid load, resulting in late metabolic acidosis (Henderson & Macdonald 2004; Levene et al 2000).

Nutrition

Fetal sucking is seen as early as 13 weeks gestation (Hafstrom & Kjellmer 2000). Suck-swallow coordination, however, is not efficient until nearer term. Preterm neonates of less than 34 weeks gestation are, therefore, usually fed via an orogastric or nasogastric tube (Levene et al 2000). Breast, cup or bottle feeds may be tried, depending on the gestational age and the responses of the preterm. Feeding is usually necessary every one, two or three hours, as preterm neonates have small gastric capacity and to prevent respiratory compromise from a full stomach. Whenever possible, breast milk is the feed of choice, as it is tailor made to the neonate's requirements (Blackburn 2003). A very preterm, ventilated or sick neonate may require parenteral fluids, as milk in the stomach increases the respiratory effort (Henderson & Macdonald 2004).

Neonatal intensive care environment

The neonatal intensive care environment is busy, bright, noisy and harsh for the preterm neonate. In recent times, developmental care programs have been initiated in many neonatal units in an attempt to minimise many of these insults on the preterm neonate. This includes such measures as clustering of nursing activities or minimal handling, positioning, creating a night pattern in the day, and minimising noise (Johnson 2003), and the involvement of parents in the care of their neonate as much as possible (Israel 2003), including the use of massage (Yellott 2001). The aim of developmental care is to decrease respiratory effort, achieve acceptable growth patterns, decrease length of hospital stay and improve neurological outcomes. All these objectives appear to have been achieved (Symington & Pinelli 2003).

Neonatal jaundice

Jaundice can potentially affect a large number of term as well as preterm infants and its management therefore is an important part of the day-to-day role of the midwife. This section examines only the main causes of jaundice in the neonate as well as the assessment and management of these.

Physiology of bilirubin metabolism

When red blood cells age, or are immature or malformed, they are removed from the circulation and broken down in the reticuloendothelial system (liver, spleen and macrophages). Haemoglobin is broken down to form:

- *haem*, which is converted to unconjugated bilirubin
- *globin*, which is broken down into amino acids, and then used by the body to make proteins
- *iron*, which in turn is either stored by the body or recycled to make new red blood cells.

Two forms of bilirubin are found in the body.

- *Unconjugated bilirubin* cannot be excreted easily from the body via urine or bile, as it is fat-soluble. The fat-soluble unconjugated bilirubin is deposited in the connective tissue of the skin, with excess levels giving rise to the characteristic skin yellowing. Unconjugated bilirubin is transported to the liver, linked to albumin for processing. Being fat-soluble means that unconjugated bilirubin has the potential to cross the blood–brain barrier and enter the brain cells to cause kernicterus (discussed in detail later in this section).
- *Conjugated bilirubin* has been processed by the liver to become water-soluble, and can then be easily excreted from the body, through faeces mainly, and urine. Some conjugated bilirubin is hydrolysed back to unconjugated bilirubin in the colon. This unconjugated bilirubin is then absorbed across the intestinal mucosa into the capillaries.

Physiological jaundice

Physiological jaundice is a normal state that occurs in 50% of term neonates as a consequence of the transition from intrauterine to extrauterine life (Fraser & Cooper 2003) and 80% of preterm neonates (Levene et al 2000). Hypoxia is the stimulus for red blood cell (RBC) production. Hypoxia leads to release of erythropoietin, which stimulates RBC production. At birth, the neonate is exposed to air breathing, with a higher oxygen level, and therefore the stimulus to release erythropoietin is reduced. Neonatal RBCs have a shorter lifespan than adult RBCs, and preterm neonates even shorter. During the first three to four months following birth, destruction of RBCs exceeds production. This increased destruction leads to increased bilirubin load on the immature liver. Characteristically, physiological jaundice never appears before 24 hours of age, peaks on day 3, and usually resolves by one week, with serum bilirubin levels not exceeding 200–215 µmol/L. The neonate with physiological jaundice is usually well, though not as alert as normal. Physiological jaundice may be exacerbated by:

- increased bilirubin production—polycythaemia, bruising
- decreased albumin-binding capacity—acidotic neonate, competition from some drugs (e.g. gentamycin)
- decreased bilirubin excretion—delayed feeding or poor feeding, resulting in delayed intestinal transit and delayed stooling
- sepsis in the neonate.

Unconjugated hyperbilirubinaemia

Increased red cell breakdown, or haemolytic disease of the newborn, describes the immune-mediated red cell breakdown that occurs in Rhesus disease and ABO incompatability. The maternal immune system can become sensitised to fetal RBC. Usually this sensitisation process occurs in a previous pregnancy, during which fetal blood cells entered the maternal circulation; or it can occur following a blood transfusion and ABO incompatability.

Rhesus disease can occur when an Rh-negative woman is pregnant with an Rh-positive fetus. During pregnancy or birth, small amounts of fetal Rh-positive blood may cross the placenta and enter the maternal circulation. This triggers a reaction by the women's immune system to produce anti-D antibodies, resulting in sensitisation. Then, in a subsequent pregnancy, the antibodies cross the placenta and destroy fetal RBCs.

At-risk women and neonates can be identified by assessing maternal and cord blood after birth in order to identify the blood group and perform a Coombs' test on the neonate. The Coombs' test identifies the level of maternal antibodies in the neonate's blood. A Kleihauer test is also undertaken to identify the number of fetal cells in the maternal blood.

The overall aim of care with Rh-negative women is to prevent Rh isoimmunisation from occurring, by administering anti-D immunoglobulin to women at risk. This prevention process has changed considerably in recent years, following the results of a Cochrane Review (Crowther & Keirse 1999). The current regimen recommended by CSL (2002) is that all primigravida Rh-negative women should receive Rh D immunoglobulin injections at 28 and 34 weeks gestation and within 72 hours following the birth of an Rh-positive neonate. In addition, Rh D immunoglobulin should be given to Rh-negative women following any sensitising events, such as miscarriage, termination of pregnancy, ectopic pregnancy, amniocentesis or chorion villus sampling, external cephalic version, abdominal trauma, antepartum haemorrhage or fetal death in utero.

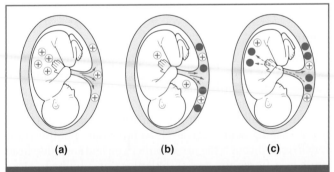

Figure 38.1 Antibody formation. **(a)** Transfer of Rhesus antigen (+) to the maternal circulation. **(b)** Antibody formation (●) in the Rhesus-negative mother. **(c)** Transfer of Rhesus antibody to the fetus (based on Henderson & Macdonald 2004)

Other causes of unconjugated hyperbilirubinaemia include:

- glucose-6-phosphate dehydrogenase (G6PD) deficiency—x-linked (male-affected); increased incidence in people of Mediterranean and Asian descent; strong correlation between maternal infection, taking a variety of drugs, and eating fava beans; possible trigger is G6PD deficiency (Henderson & Macdonald 2004)
- hereditary spherocytosis
- septicaemia and TORCH infection
- twin-to-twin transfusion
- dehydration
- delayed passage of meconium
- hypothyroidism
- galactosaemia
- infant of a diabetic mother (Merenstein & Gardner 2002)
- breast milk jaundice.

Kernicterus is a complication that may result from excessive levels of serum unconjugated hyperbilirubinaemia in the neonate. The term 'kernicterus' describes the yellow staining of the basal ganglia noted on postmortem. This condition presents in the affected neonate as a progressive development over 24 hours of lethargy, rigidity, opisthotonos, high-pitched cry, fever and convulsions. Fifty per cent of affected neonates will die, with survivors developing some level of brain damage, resulting in cerebral palsy, deafness, developmental delay and paralysis of upward gaze (Henderson & Macdonald 2004; Levene et al 2000). The development of kernicterus is influenced by the rate at which the unconjugated bilirubin level rises, as well as the level it reaches.

Assessment of jaundice

Jaundice is defined as levels of serum bilirubin of 85–100 μmol/L. The most common method of determining the level of jaundice is to use Kramer's rule (Kramer 1969). This technique involves assessing the skin of the neonate to determine how much of the body is jaundiced. The more zones of the neonate's skin that are affected, the greater the level of jaundice (Fig 38.2).

The Kramer's rule assessment may be undertaken in conjunction with transcutaneous measuring devices. Transcutaneous measuring devices have been shown to correlate well with serum bilirubin measurements (Rubaltelli et al 2001), which is the next level of total bilirubin measurement. Further investigations to establish the cause of the jaundice should be undertaken in the following circumstances:

- neonate who is visibly jaundiced in the first 24 hours
- jaundiced neonate whose mother has Rhesus antibodies
- preterm neonate whose serum bilirubin exceeds 200 μmol/L
- neonate who has clinical signs of obstructive jaundice
- prolonged hyperbilirubinaemia of greater than one week in term and two weeks in preterm neonates.

A thorough investigation of the jaundiced neonate would also take into consideration the pregnancy history, and the gestational and neonatal age. In addition, it is important to

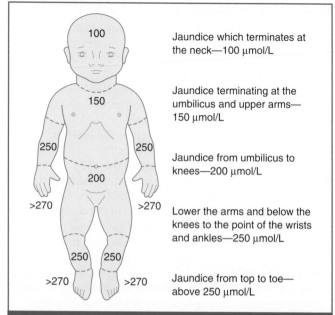

Jaundice which terminates at the neck—100 μmol/L

Jaundice terminating at the umbilicus and upper arms—150 μmol/L

Jaundice from umbilicus to knees—200 μmol/L

Lower the arms and below the knees to the point of the wrists and ankles—250 μmol/L

Jaundice from top to toe—above 250 μmol/L

Figure 38.2 Kramer's rule (based on Henderson & Macdonald 2004)

note the racial origins of the parents (see G6PD deficiency above) and the use of medications. The assessment would also include a physical examination of the neonate and laboratory investigations.

Management

Effective, frequent and early breastfeeding assists the neonate by providing hydration, supplying glucose to the liver, encouraging normal bowel colonisation and increasing bowel motility. Supplying glucose to the liver assists in the production of enzymes needed for conjugation. Increasing the bowel motility in turn decreases the time that bilirubin stays in the gut and thereby decreases enterohepatic reabsorption. General supportive measures in the treatment of jaundice may include the correction of dehydration and the administration of antibiotics if septicaemia or TORCH infections are noted to be the cause.

Phototherapy

Phototherapy is the use of blue light to enhance bilirubin excretion by photochemically converting unconjugated bilirubin into water-soluble bilirubin, which can be excreted through the kidneys. Phototherapy may be intermittent or continuous, and aims to prevent unconjugated bilirubin from reaching neurotoxic levels in the blood. Phototherapy is delivered through the use of either conventional overhead units or a fibreoptic pad (biliblanket) or a bilibed placed around the neonate. In all instances, the entire skin surface of the neonate must be exposed to the light. There are a number of considerations of care in the use of overhead phototherapy units:

- temperature control of the environment

- loose stools due to decreased intestinal transit time, resulting in increased fluid loss
- risk of dehydration
- eye protection—risk of retinal damage from high-intensity light
- disruption of maternal–neonatal interaction
- maternal anxiety.

The use of phototherapy makes it impossible to assess the level of jaundice by examining the skin alone, and therefore serum bilirubin measurement should occur, usually twice daily. If phototherapy fails to reduce the serum bilirubin levels sufficiently, an exchange transfusion may be performed in order to prevent kernicterus. An exchange transfusion involves removing the blood of the neonate, which contains maternal antibodies and bilirubin, and replacing it with fresh, Rhesus-negative blood.

Neonatal infections

The potential impact of a neonatal infection cannot be overstated, as it can very quickly affect the neonate and be fatal. The midwife's role is in prevention, early detection and prompt management of neonatal infections, and in providing support for the parents. This section gives an overview of neonatal defences, followed by a discussion of the main prenatal, perinatal and postnatal infections.

Neonatal defences

Neonates are prone to a higher incidence of infection, due to their immunodeficiency compared with older children. Maternal immunoglobulin (IgG) is able to cross the placenta from 32 weeks gestation, and this confers limited passive immunity to the neonate against specific viral infections. Neonates born before 32 weeks, therefore, are more susceptible to infection. Breast milk, particularly colostrum, is rich in IgA and interferon, enhancing resistance to enteric infections in the neonate through passive immunity. In addition, breast milk may actively stimulate the immune system of the neonate (Oddy 2001) as well as providing passive immunity through IgD, lactoferrin, *Lactobacillus bifidus* and lysozyme, an anti-infective agent (Henderson & Macdonald 2004). Neonates have limited passive and active immunity—prevention, early detection and prompt treatment of neonatal infection are crucial.

Prevention of infections

In utero

The first line of defence that midwives can direct to women is the use of vaccinations known to prevent conditions that can affect the fetus, such as hepatitis B and rubella. The next level of prevention is the sensitive screening and identification of risk factors for infections in women, such as sexually transmitted infections and HIV. The final line of defence is through health education of women to decrease the risk of infection by avoiding: high-risk foods (e.g. soft cheeses); high-risk lifestyle/behaviour (e.g. not using condoms, needle sharing); countries or areas with high prevalence of some infections; and contact with people who have infectious diseases. When an infection does occur, timely and appropriate management of the women is crucial.

Handwashing

The most important means of preventing infection in the neonate is careful and frequent handwashing with soap. The impact of handwashing alone should not be underestimated. Carers should wash their hands with soap before and after handling each baby, particularly after nappy changes, to reduce the incidence of cross-infection. Use of alcohol-based hand-rub solutions has been shown to also be effective in preventing infection and to increase compliance in busy units (Fraser & Cooper 2003; Girou et al 2002). Recent work has examined the increased risk of infection with carers who wear rings, watches, false nails and nail polish.

Equipment

Equipment should be provided for each neonate. Any shared equipment should be thoroughly cleaned between uses. Feeding equipment should be effectively sterilised before use and milk should be appropriately prepared and stored.

Environment

Strategies to significantly reduce cross-infection risks in neonatal units include adequate spacing of cots and rooming-in with the mother. Neonates or mothers with a known contagious disease should be isolated. Likewise, visitors who have infections should be discouraged from entering the unit.

Invasive procedures

Keeping invasive procedures to a minimum can further reduce the risk of infection in the neonate. When invasive procedures are undertaken, strict aseptic techniques and gloves should be used. Strict attention given to wound care following the invasive procedure will also help reduce the risk. Undertaking the procedure with great care will help prevent the necessity for a repeated attempt.

Prenatal infections

Certain protozoa and viruses are small enough to cross the placenta and cause teratogenic effects and infection. The acronym TORCH (toxoplasmosis, other, rubella, cytomegalovirus and hepatitis) lists some of these.

Toxoplasmosis

Toxoplasmosis is caused by a protozoan found in uncooked meat, and in cat and dog faeces. Risk factors include eating uncooked meat, having a pet cat or dog, poor hand hygiene, contact with soil, travel outside Western countries, and frequent consumption of raw vegetables outside the home (Cook et al 2000). Congenital infection with toxoplasmosis is rare in Australia (Levene et al 2000). Preventative advice to women by the midwife is essential, including advice on hygiene and safe preparation of food.

Adults with toxoplasmosis are usually asymptomatic or experience flu-like symptoms. Anti-toxoplasmosis IgM antibodies would be detected in the blood of infected women. Transmitting the infection to the fetus between 10 and 24 weeks gestation can result in intrauterine death and subsequent miscarriage. Infections in the third trimester are more likely to be transmitted to the fetus. The infected neonate may present with low birthweight, hepatosplenomegaly, jaundice, anaemia, blindness, intercranial calcifications, cerebral ventricular dilation and deafness.

Other infections

Syphilis

Syphilis rates are increasing worldwide, with antenatal screening of all women recommended to detect, treat and prevent congenital syphilis (WHO 1991). Fetal infections occur in the second trimester of pregnancy (never before 16 weeks gestation) and can result in miscarriage, stillbirth, preterm birth or congenital syphilis. Infected neonates may present with hepatosplenomegaly, skin lesions, maculopapular rashes, eye infection, persistent snuffles, jaundice and widespread metaphysical bony lesions.

Varicella zoster

Varicella zoster is a highly contagious virus that is responsible for chickenpox infection. If contracted during the first trimester of pregnancy, congenital varicella syndrome occurs in 2–5% of neonates, resulting in possible neurological damage and skeletal abnormalities. Maternal infection between seven days prior and 28 days after the birth is more serious, with up to 25% of neonates developing the infection, with possible complications of renal disorders and pneumonia (Henderson & Macdonald 2004; Levene et al 2000).

Listeriosis

Listeriosis is caused by a Gram-positive bacterium found in certain foods. It causes non-specific, flu-like symptoms in the woman if contracted. Intrauterine infection results in spontaneous miscarriage or stillbirth in 20% of cases, and preterm labour and amnionitis may occur in the remainder. Neonatal infections result in severe pneumonia, general sepsis and meningitis, accounting for a 50% mortality rate. Those neonates who survive have significant handicaps (Henderson & Macdonald 2004).

Rubella

Rubella vaccination programs for infants and women of childbearing age are readily available. All women are screened antenatally for rubella antibodies. Infections in the first trimester of pregnancy have the most effect, with the fetus developing viraemia. The earlier the gestation (< 8 weeks), the more likely it is that the fetus will be affected (Levene et al 2000). Viraemia inhibits cell division and causes defects of the developing organs, specifically the eyes, ears, and cardiovascular and nervous systems. Spontaneous miscarriage may occur. Women in this situation require a great deal of information and support, and some may request a termination. Infected neonates are highly infectious, excreting rubella virus in the urine for up to 12 months. Isolation of these neonates is therefore crucial. Preventative advice from the midwife is essential, emphasising the importance of the women avoiding contact with rubella during pregnancy. After 20 weeks gestation, congenital infection of rubella does not occur.

Cytomegalovirus

Cytomegalovirus is a common perinatal infection, occurring in 0.4–2.3% of all births (Witters et al 2000), the rate of in-utero transmission increasing with gestational age. The risk of transmission during birth or breastfeeding is minimal. Infection in the woman results in flu-like symptoms and possible severe abnormalities in the fetus, including eye and ear defects, hepatitis, thrombocytopenia and meningoencephalitis. Neonatal mortality of 20–30% results from disseminated intravascular coagulation, sepsis or liver problems, with survivors having severe neurological deficits. Isolation of these neonates is crucial as they remain infectious for many months, secreting the virus in the urine.

Hepatitis

Hepatitis infections in the neonate may occur from in-utero transfer or during birth. The currently identified hepatitis viruses are A, B, C, D, E and G. In-utero transfer of A and E are rare but can result in fetal abnormalities. Pregnant women who are chronically infected with hepatitis B may have a neonate who is positive for the hepatitis B e antigen. This neonate will in turn have an 80–90% risk of being chronically infected with hepatitis B (Shiraki 2000). The midwife's role is in antenatal education, screening and ensuring that the neonate receives a hepatitis B vaccination within 12 hours of birth. Currently, all women receive information on hepatitis B vaccinations, including the follow-up injections at six weeks and three months of age. All women are then offered the vaccination following birth.

Hepatitis C is common among intravenous drug users and in-utero transfer rates are approximately 5%, and higher if also HIV-positive (10%), resulting in liver cirrhosis, carcinoma, failure and death. The midwife's role is in antenatal education and screening of all women. During labour and birth, transmission can be minimised by avoiding invasive procedures such as artificial rupture of membranes.

Perinatal infections

It is often difficult to decide at birth whether a neonate is infected or not. Important points to consider are:

- evidence of maternal sepsis
- membranes ruptured for longer than 18 hours
- length of labour greater than 12 hours
- number of vaginal examinations undertaken
- instrumental birth
- presence of fetal distress or birth asphyxia.

All these factors increase the risk of a neonatal infection. Signs of neonatal infection include lethargy, vomiting, diarrhoea, jaundice, mild respiratory difficulty, pyrexia, hypothermia, hypotonia, irritability, poor feeding, weak cry, abdominal distension, failure to thrive, rashes, purpura, respiratory distress, shock and renal failure.

Group B haemolytic Streptococcus

Group B haemolytic Streptococcus (GBS) is one of the most common causes of early-onset perinatal infection in industrialised countries, affecting 1–4:1000 births and fatal in 20% of cases. Approximately 12–15% of Australian women are asymptomatic vaginal carriers of GBS (NSW Health Department 2002). Vertical transmission at birth is the process by which neonates acquire the infection, occurring in approximately 10% (Levene et al 2000). The neonate then suffers from either early or late onset of disease. Early onset typically presents with symptoms of septicaemia, respiratory distress and septic shock, which will rapidly detoriate to be fatal if untreated. Late onset presents as meningitis after five to seven days.

Postnatal infections

Mild eye infection

Mild eye infections (sticky eyes) are common in neonates and can be treated with routine eye care, colostrum and antibiotics, if required for aggressive infections. Eye care involves the use of cool, boiled water or sterile saline and cotton wool

---

Clinical point

The incidence of early-onset Group B streptococcal disease in the neonate was found to be reduced from 3.5 to 0.6 per 1000 live births following universal screening and intrapartum antibiotics for all maternal carriers (Jeffery & Moses 1998). This is supported by later work (Gilbert 2004; Oddie & Embleton 2002), which emphasised the importance of the use of prophylaxic antibiotics with women who have identified risk factors, such as prolonged rupture of membranes, rupture of membranes before the onset of labour and intrapartum fever. A conclusion reached from another study indicated that routine screening for GBS during pregnancy prevents more cases of early-onset disease in the neonate than the risk-based approach (Schrag et al 2002).

---

swabs, cleaning the eye from inner to outer aspect once, and discarding the swab. Hand washing before and after eye care is also important.

Skin infections

Skin infections are mostly caused by *S. aureus*, resulting in septic spots or pustules, located either as solitary lesions or clustered in the umbilical or buttock regions. Treatment involves regular cleaning and antibiotics if more extensive.

Umbilical infections

Umbilical infections are rare, and with good standards of hygiene can be prevented. Signs of infection include inflammation, a moist, offensive-smelling cord, and delay in separation. The most common organism responsible is *S. aureus*. Antibiotics are required as there is a risk of transportation through the umbilical vein to the liver, causing hepatitis and septicaemia. Prevention with good care and monitoring is best.

Urinary tract infections

Urinary tract infections can be caused by *E. coli* or may result from a congenital abnormality obstructing the flow of urine. Signs of infection include non-specific symptoms such as feeding difficulties, failure to thrive, occasionally pyrexia and jaundice. Management involves undertaking a urine culture and administering appropriate antibiotics.

Neonatal bleeding

This section discusses the main causes of neonatal bleeding, including those due to trauma, coagulopathies and other causes.

Bleeding due to trauma

Cephalhaematoma

Cephalhaematoma is bleeding that occurs between the periosteum and the skull bone as a result of friction, usually between the skull and the pelvis. A cephalhaematoma may also occur during a forceps or vacuum birth. The bleeding results in a separation of the periosteum from the underlying bone and subsequent bleeding. This bleeding is therefore confined to the area of the skull bone contained by the periosteum layer (see Fig 38.3).

A cephalhaematoma:

- appears 12–72 hours after birth
- tends to enlarge after birth
- usually affects the parietal bone
- is circumscribed, firm and does not pit on pressure
- may be bilateral
- may contribute to jaundice
- can persist for weeks, slowly subsiding.

Subdural haemorrhage

Subdural haemorrhage occurs due to excessive compression or abnormal stretching of the fetal head. This results in

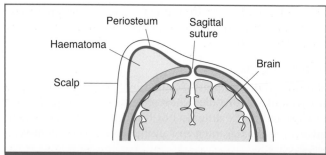

Figure 38.3 Cephalhaematoma (based on Henderson & Macdonald 2004)

tearing of the dura, and rupture of the venous sinuses. Predisposing factors for a subdural haemorrhage include situations in which the moulding is rapid, abnormal or excessive, such as from precipitate labour or rapid birth, malpositions, malpresentations, cephalo-pelvic disproportion or undue pressure from forceps application. Tearing of the tentorium (tentorial tear) results from these events, followed by cerebral haemorrhage. The neonate presents with signs of cerebral irritation and raised intracranial pressure, such as tense, expanded fontanelle, asphyxia, abnormal eye movements, vomiting, non-responsiveness and convulsions. Its incidence has decreased somewhat owing to a reduced use of high and mid-cavity forceps, prolonged labours and a simultaneous increase in caesarean births.

Bleeding due to disruptions in blood flow

Subarachnoid haemorrhage

A primary subarachnoid haemorrhage is bleeding directly into the subarachnoid space. This occurs in response to hypoxia or trauma in preterm or term neonates and is a common, benign condition. A secondary subarachnoid haemorrhage, however, is caused by leakage of blood from an intraventricular haemorrhage into the subarachnoid space. The neonate with subarachnoid haemorrhage is usually asymptomatic, but may present with convulsions and apnoea, and is neurologically normal.

Bleeding due to coagulopathies

Vitamin K deficiency bleeding

Vitamin K deficiency bleeding was previously termed 'haemorrhagic disease of the newborn' and occurs in 0.4–1.7% of neonates in the first week of life (Merenstein et al 1993). This bleeding is due to an accentuated deficiency of normal neonatal vitamin K dependent clotting factors. Vitamin K is poorly transferred across the placenta, resulting in low fetal levels that are quickly depleted after birth. Synthesis of vitamin K occurs in the bowel flora, which is restricted until colonisation occurs, as the neonate's bowel is sterile. Colonisation does not occur until feeding has been established, making neonates susceptible to vitamin K deficiency bleeding. The amount of vitamin K in breast milk is low, though colostrum and hind milk contain the highest amounts (Enkin

et al 2000). Milk from cows has a higher, though still low, level of vitamin K. Formula milk is fortified with vitamin K, offering some protection.

Vitamin K deficiency bleeding is classified according to its onset:

● Early-onset occurs within the first 24 hours. It is rare, seen in neonates of women prescribed certain medications, including vitamin K antagonist anticoagulants (warfarin) and some anticonvulsants (phenobarbital or phenytoin). Women should be asked antenatally if they are taking these medications and alternatives prescribed if possible. Otherwise, women require vitamin K supplementation towards the end of pregnancy. Administering neonatal vitamin K will not prevent it.

● Classic occurs one to seven days after birth. It is preventable by the administration of the recommended schedule of vitamin K at birth (Puckett & Offringa 2002).

● Late-onset occurs 8–12 months after birth. This type of bleeding presents as intraventricular or pulmonary haemorrhage in mostly exclusively breastfed neonates. The morbidity rate is reported to be as high as 33% (Bor et al 2000).

The recommendation is that all neonates at birth receive prophylactic vitamin K, although the optimal route, dosage and frequency of administration are still subject to great debate (Autret-Leca & Jonville-Bera 2001). Such is the debate that some question whether vitamin K is needed. This may be because of the evidence indicating that neonates who do not breastfeed effectively, frequently and early are at increased risk of bleeding (Hey 2003). The areas of contention are the efficacy of prophylaxis for the different categories (described above), the most efficient administration for at-risk neonates, and the possible link between intramuscular administration and a potential increased risk of childhood leukaemia (Roman et al 2002). Subsequent studies have disputed this link (Hull 1992; Merenstein et al 1993; Puckett and Offringa 2002). It is the role of the midwife to discuss this issue with parents, giving them all the information and gaining their consent.

The alternatives available to parents are: no prophylactic administration of vitamin K at birth; oral vitamin K at birth, repeated at 3–5 days and again at 4–6 weeks for breastfed neonates; or a single intramuscular dose of vitamin K at birth. Oral administration has compliance issues and has not yet undergone randomised controlled trials to assess its efficacy (Puckett & Offringa 2002). It is recommended that all high-risk neonates receive intramuscular vitamin K at birth. This group includes preterm, hypoxic neonates and those who have had a difficult or instrumental birth. Neonates who are artificially fed do not require prophylactic vitamin K (Hey 2003).

Bleeding due to other causes

Vaginal

Vaginal discharge consisting of bloodstained mucus in the first days after birth in the female neonate is termed pseudomenstruation. It is due to the withdrawal of maternal oestrogen and is normal, and self-limiting. Midwives need to reassure women that this is a possibility and that it is normal.

Haematemesis

Haematemeis occurs when the neonate has swallowed maternal blood, either during birth or from cracked nipples while breastfeeding. This needs investigating to ensure that the underlying cause is not something more sinister, such as oesophageal, gastric or duodenal ulceration. Cracked nipples need to be appropriately managed by checking positioning and attachment. The woman needs reassuring that this is self-limiting and no cause for alarm.

Congenital conditions

Parents expect to have a normal, healthy neonate, which predominantly is the case. There is no guarantee, however, that this will happen. When a neonate is found at birth to have an abnormality, it can be devasting for the parents. The role of the midwife in such circumstances is to assist in early detection and then to provide support and sensitivity for the parents. This section outlines some of the potential causes of congenital abnormalities, and the main conditions.

Causes

A congenital abnormality, by definition, is a defect present at birth; it can be either a malformation or a deformation. The incidence is believed to be around 2–3% of neonates, with more malformations than deformations. A malformation is a defect in the development of an organ or tissue in the fetus, whereas a deformation is damage that occurs to normal structure as a result of external factors. The specific cause of up to 80% of abnormalities is unknown, with the remainder occurring because of the following factors (Henderson & Macdonald 2004):

- genetic—a fault occurs either during the formation of the gametes or following fertilisation, resulting in an excess or deficit of chromosomal material
- teratogenic—refers to agents that increase the incidence of congenital abnormalities. These include: prescribed medications (such as anticonvulsants, anticoagulants, thalidomide); substance abuse (such as heroin, nicotine, alcohol, cocaine); environmental factors (such as radiation, pesticides); infective agents (such as rubella, cytomegalovirus); sustained hyperthermia (saunas during pregnancy are discouraged, as is exercise that is likely to raise maternal temperature); and maternal disease (such as poorly controlled diabetes mellitus).
- iatrogenic—includes such things as congenital constriction band syndrome, occurring when early amniotic rupture results in a constriction band forming and occluding some part of the fetal body.

The role of the midwife is in giving preconceptual advice to would-be parents about maximising their health prior to conception. Unfortunately, most of the damage may have been done by the time the woman sees the midwife during her first antenatal visit. There is, therefore, a need to increase awareness regarding preconceptual health in the general community.

Early detection of abnormalities through antenatal screening is the next line of defence. Early detection results in some families making the decision to terminate the pregnancy, or allows families time to accept the news that their baby will be born with a particular problem. Great sensitivity and understanding are required at this time, to help support the family in making their decision.

Congenital conditions can affect any part of the fetus; the main conditions only are outlined here.

Central nervous system

Spina bifida

Spina bifida and anencephaly are the most common neural tube defects, affecting up to 1:1000 pregnancies (Henderson & Macdonald 2004). The recurrence rate in subsequent pregnancies is 1 in 25 (Fraser & Cooper 2003). Routine use of folic acid daily for one month preconceptually and during the first trimester has been shown to result in a dramatic drop in the incidence of these conditions (Hasenau 2002). Spina bifida results from a failure of the vertebral column to fuse, with a number of levels of involvement. This defect can occur anywhere between the head and the sacrum, most commonly affecting the lumbosacral region. There are a number of types. Spina bifida occulta involves a defect of the bone and is without symptoms. It is noticed by a tuft of hair or sinus at the base of the spine. Spina bifida meningocele is where there is no skin covering the spinal defect, allowing the protrusion of the meninges. This sac may contain cerebrospinal fluid but does not contain neural tissue. Spina bifida myelomeningocele does include the spinal cord and is therefore more serious. There may be leakage of cerebrospinal fluid, giving rise to the risk of meningitis.

Hydrocephalus

Hydrocephalus occurs when there is a blockage in the circulation or impaired absorption of the cerebrospinal fluid, resulting in an accumulation in the lateral ventricles and an increase in the size of the ventricle. This accumulation can eventually lead to compression of the brain tissue. Cerebrospinal fluid is produced in the lateral ventricles of the brain, and hence the effect. Diagnosis is usually by the midwife possibly feeling an enlarged head, or there may be CNS depression evident on cardiotocography (decreased variability and reactivity) or during an antenatal ultrasound.

Microcephalus

Microcephalus is defined by a head circumference of more than two standard deviations below normal for gestational age. This can result either from a brain that has not grown, or from prematurely ossified sutures constricting the growth of the brain.

Respiratory system

Diaphragmatic hernia

Diaphragmatic hernia is a defect in the formation of the diaphragm that allows herniation of the abdominal contents into the thoracic cavity. Lung development may be impaired due to compression or hypoplasia. The amount of compression that occurs depends on the gestational age at which herniation occurred and on the size of the defect, ranging from very small to complete agenesis of the diaphragm. Usually the left side is affected, though it may be unilateral or bilateral, and it is more common in males, with an overall incidence of 1:1000 to 10,000 births (Braby 2001). The true incidence is unknown, however, as the fetus or neonate often dies before being diagnosed. There is a high mortality and morbidity rate, with an approximate survival rate of 50% (Henderson & Macdonald 2004). This condition is often associated with other abnormalities, usually cardiac. The main aim of care is to avoid filling the gastrointestinal tract with air, as this may impede lung expansion. Immediate management involves free-flowing oxygen, insertion of a gastric tube and then endotracheal intubation and mechanical ventilation (Braby 2001; Juretschke 2001).

Choanal atresia

Choanal atresia involves the unilateral or bilateral narrowing of the nasal passage(s) by a membranous or bony septum, resulting in occlusion of the nasopharynx. Neonates will suffer from acute respiratory distress from birth, as they are predominantly nose breathers. These neonates find feeding impossible without cyanosis. Dyspnoea and cyanosis are improved by crying.

Alimentary system

Cleft lip and palate

Cleft lip and palate are one of the most common structural birth defects. Cleft lip may occur with or without a cleft palate, and can be unilateral or bilateral, involving the soft palate, hard palate or both. Incidence of cleft lip is 1:700 and cleft palate is 1:2000 births, being more common in Asian families (Henderson & Macdonald 2004). A thorough examination in good light is essential for accurate diagnosis.

Oesophageal atresia and tracheo-oesophageal fistula

Incomplete canalisation of the oesophagus in early fetal development results in oesophageal atresia, or a blind end. The condition affects 1:4000 neonates (Henderson & Maconald 2004). Tracheo-oesophageal fistulas are commonly associated with this condition, and involve one or two connections between the oesophagus and the trachea. The fetus is therefore unable to swallow amniotic fluid, and polyhydramnios results. After birth, the neonate has copious amounts of oral mucus. Aspiration in the presence of a fistula will cause cyanotic episodes. Patency of the oesophagus must be assured prior to commencing oral feeding.

Imperforate anus

Imperforate anus occurs in 1–3:5000 births and can be easily detected by visually examining the anus for patency (Henderson & Macdonald 2004). No object should be inserted into the anus in order to check for patency. A paediatric referral should be made if there is any doubt. There is a high association of imperforate anus with other abnormalities. A thorough examination of the neonate should therefore be undertaken.

Exomphalos and gastroschisis

Exomphalos and gastroschisis both occur late in first trimester, with an incidence of 1–2:10,000 neonates. The incidence has increased significantly over the past several decades (King & Askin 2003). Essentially these conditions are a herniation of the abdominal contents through either the base of the umbilical cord (exomphalos), or through a defect in the anterior abdominal wall (gastroschisis). With exomphalos there is a covering of fused peritoneum and amnion over the abdominal contents, which may rupture at birth. There is also a strong association with other abnormalities, more males being affected than females. In gastroschisis there is no protected covering of the abdominal contents, which may appear oedematous and have disrupted blood supply. The main aim of care is to avoid over-handling of abdominal contents, prevent infection, and reduce heat and fluid loss by covering with clear plastic. Proper diagnosis and treatment are crucial to achieve a satisfactory outcome.

Genitourinary

Undescended testes

By 36 weeks gestation, the testis would normally be present in the scrotum. Undescended testes may be unilateral or bilateral and occurs in 1–2% of male neonates. On examination at birth, if the testes are not felt in the scrotum, they may be felt in the inguinal pouch. This should be documented and checked again at six weeks. If the testes are not detected by four months, a paediatric referral is necessary (Henderson & Macdonald 2004).

Hypospadias

Hypospadias occurs when the urethral meatus opens on the under-surface of the penis. The meatus may be placed at any point along the penis, even the perineum. Circumcision should not be performed until repair has been undertaken. The further the meatus is from the tip of the penis, the more urgent the surgery.

Renal agenesis

Renal agensis is a fatal condition characterised by the failure of the development of the kidneys. Incidence is 1:1500, found during antenatal ultrasounds (Henderson & Macdonald 2004). There is a high association with other abnormalities.

Ambiguous genitalia

Great sensitivity and support for the parents are required in cases of ambiguous genitalia. Any doubt as to the sex of the neonate should be further investigated by chromosome analysis before gender is defined. A physical examination may reveal any of the following: a small hypoplastic penis, chordee, bifid scrotum, undescended testis, enlarged clitoris, incompletely separated or poorly differentiated labia.

Limbs

Talipes

In talipes equinovarus, or club foot, the ankle is bent downwards (plantarflexed) and the front part of the foot is turned inwards (inverted) (see Fig 38.4). This is the most common type of talipes. In talipes calcaneovalgus, the foot is dorsiflexed and everted (see Fig 38.4). In talipes metatarsus varus, the forefoot is turned inwards. This deformity occurs due to contraction of certain muscles or tendons related to a restriction of movement in utero. It may also have a genetic origin if more severe.

Syndactyly and polydactyly

Syndactyly means webbing and polydactyly means extra digits (see Fig 38.5). Webbing is more commonly identified in the hands. This deformity may be hereditary or genetic. Extra digits may be fully formed, including bone, or simply extra tissue attached to a digit. The latter is usually ligated, causing necrosis, with the extra digit then falling off.

Congenital dislocation of the hip

Congenital dislocation of the hip is the abnormal development of one or both hips, with the head of femur being partially or wholly displaced from the acetabulum. It is more common in females, in the left hip, with breech presentation, fetal restriction in utero, and where there is a family history. The incidence is 1:1500 births. Early detection is important to prevent long-term problems. The hip may present as either dislocated, dislocatable or with subluxation of the joint. Treatment requires an abduction device and follow-up ultrasounds to assess progress (Wilkinson 2003).

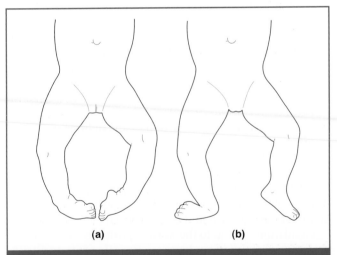

Figure 38.4 (a) Talipes equinovarus **(b)** Talipes calcaneovalgus (based on Henderson & Macdonald 2004)

Skin

Capillary haemangiomas

Capillary haemangiomas, or strawberry marks, are red, raised lesions that appear in the first few weeks of life, and are caused by dilated capillaries in the skin. These lesions can appear anywhere on the body. The lesions usually increase in size in the first few months and then regress, usually disappearing completely by five to six years of age.

Capillary malformations

Capillary malformations, or port wine stains, are purple-blue, flat, well-defined and dense lesions affecting the face. They occur in 1:3000 births. They occur more commonly in females and do not regress with time. Laser treatment has been fairly successful at removing the lesions (Sheehan-Dare 2001).

Pigmented naevi

Pigmented naevi are brown marks, or moles, on the skin that vary in size and may be flat or raised, or hairy. They are present at birth, can be anywhere on the body and do not usually require treatment, though they can become malignant (melanoma).

Chromosomal

Down syndrome

Down syndrome, or trisomy 21, occurs in 1:700 live births (Henderson & Macdonald 2004) and consists of a number of well-recognised characteristics, including:

- varying degrees of intellectual disability
- widely set and obliquely slanted eyes
- white flecks in the iris (Brushfield's spots)
- small head with a flattened occipital region
- increased fat pad on the neck
- small, droopy mouth
- protruding tongue
- broad, flat nose
- generalised hypotonia
- short, broad hands with an incurving little finger
- deep single palmar (simian) crease
- short, broad feet with a wide deviation of the great toe.

Not all these characteristics need be present and any of them can occur without implying a chromosomal

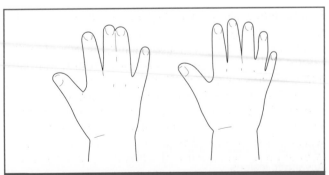

Figure 38.5 Syndactyly (left) and polydactyly (right) (based on Henderson & Macdonald 2004)

abnormality. Family resemblance alone may explain some neonates' appearance. Down syndrome neonates also have an increased incidence of cardiac abnormalities, leukaemia and hypothyroidism.

Potter syndrome

Potter syndrome is a condition characteristised by dysmorphic clinical features and renal agenesis. A consequence of the renal agenesis is oligohydramnios and severe hypoplastic lungs. Incidence is 1:4000 births, predominantly in males (Levene et al 2000). Other features include low-set ears, furrows under wide-set eyes, a beaked nose, two umbilical cord vessels and pulmonary hypoplasia resulting in severe respiratory failure. This condition is incompatible with life.

Turner syndrome

Turner syndrome, in which one of the X chromosomes is missing or abnormal, affects only females. The sex chromosomes are therefore defined as XO. These neonates are characterised by a short, webbed neck, widely spaced nipples, oedematous feet, short stature, low birthweight, under-developed ovaries and infertility. Many will be miscarried, with those surviving having a decreased life expectancy due to related heart defects.

Cardiorespiratory conditions

This section discusses some of the cardiorespiratory conditions the midwife may encounter in the neonate after birth. It is important that the midwife is able to recognise these conditions, as they can fatal. A brief overview of each condition is given. Various respiratory support mechanisms are also discussed at the end of this section.

Cardiac

Diagnosis

Routine antenatal ultrasound screening fails to diagnose 60–80% of cardiac abnormalities (Grandjean et al 1999). Approximately 50% of these abnormalities are missed at birth and more than 33% are missed at the six-week check (Ainsworth et al 1999). This highlights the fact that obvious clinical signs of cardiac abnormalities are not always present in the early neonatal period, often being picked up only when early signs of cardiac failure occur. The signs of cardiac failure include tachypnoea, tachycardia, hepatomegaly, dyspnoea, feeding difficulties and vomiting. A key to early diagnosis is the feeding pattern of the neonate. If the neonate is not feeding well, a full cardiac assessment should be undertaken.

Types of cardiac conditions

Acyanotic lesions

Acyanotic lesions are cardiac lesions where there is no cyanosis present in the neonate at birth:

- *Patent ductus arteriosus*—from 25 weeks gestation, specialised contractile tissue is formed. This enables spontaneous closure of the ductus arteriosus 15–24 hours after birth. The ductus is, however, not fully mature and functional until approximately three months. Preterm neonates therefore have a higher incidence of patent ductus. Any preterm neonate who sustains birth asphyxia or hypoxia after birth will commonly have a patent ductus arteriosus. This is the most common congenital heart abnormality and cause of congestive cardiac failure. The symptoms are tachypnoea, dyspnoea, lethargy, bounding pulses and audible systolic and diastolic murmurs occurring at around 3–10 days of age. Patent ductus results in reduced pulmonary resistance with reversed blood flow through the ductus from left to right. This results in oxygenated blood being shunted back into the pulmonary circulation. Management involves restricting fluid (though this is controversial), preventing hypoxia, administering indomethacin and ibuprofen, and, rarely, surgical ligation (Wyllie 2004).
- *Ventricular septal defect*—a hole in the ventricular septum permitting a left-to-right flow of blood. The size of the hole varies, as do the corresponding symptoms. This is often one component of an array of cardiac abnormalities.
- *Coarctation of the aorta*—a narrowing of the aorta at the entry point with the ductus arteriosus. If this narrowing is small, symptoms may not appear for several years. When severe, the neonate on day 2 to 10 suddenly becomes dyspnoeic and tachypnoeic with hepatomegaly, and signs of renal and cardiac failure. These neonates are given prostaglandins to maintain the ductus arteriosus. This condition is associated with other cardiac abnormalities in 50% of cases.
- *Aortic valve stenosis*—narrowing of the aortic valve, causing restricted blood flow through from the left ventricle to the aorta. It is commonly associated with coarctation of the aorta or other cardiac abnormalities. If mild to moderate, apart from a murmur, the neonate is usually asymptomatic. If severe, it may cause a sudden collapse, with a replacement valve being necessary.

Cyanotic lesions

Cyanotic lesions are cardiac lesions where there is cyanosis at birth.

- *Transposition of the great arteries*—the pulmonary artery exits the left ventricle and the aorta exits the right ventricle, creating two separate circulations. As the ductus arteriosus closes, severe cyanosis occurs, with dyspnoea and cardiac failure resulting. The ductus needs to be maintained urgently with prostaglandins, and surgery undertaken in the next few days to switch the circulation around to the normal positions.
- *Tetralogy of Fallot*—pulmonary stenosis, ventral septal defect, right ventricular hypertrophy and an overriding aorta across the ventricular septal defect. The neonate

presents as pink at birth, gradually becoming cyanosed when crying. As the pulmonary stenosis worsens at four to six months of age, the infant presents with cyanotic episodes in the morning, resulting in a loss of consciousness. Timing of the surgery depends on the severity of the symptoms.

- *Hypoplastic left heart syndrome*—underdevelopment of the left side of the heart, a hypoplastic ascending aorta and coronary arteries, and blood passing into the aorta through the patent ductus arteriosus. With closure of the ductus arteriosus, cyanosis and dyspnoea worsen. Unless a heart transplant is available, most neonates will die within the first week.

Respiratory

Asphyxia

Asphyxia results from impaired gas exchange leading to a depletion of oxygen (hypoxaemia) and accumulation of carbon dioxide (hypercapnia) and acidosis in the blood. Asphyxia may occur in utero, during labour or birth, or the neonatal period. The asphyxia will worsen unless respiratory function is established quickly. Immediate resuscitation is therefore necessary. Mild asphyxia may result in no neurological injury in the neonate, whereas severe asphyxia will result in significant neurological sequelae. The causes of birth asphyxia include:

- preterm birth
- obstruction of the trachea
- drugs that depress respirations
- congenital abnormalities
- cerebral damage
- infection
- haemorrhage
- pneumothorax.

Pharyngeal suctioning may cause a reflex apnoea.

The Apgar score performed at one minute after birth gives some indication of the level of birth asphyxia. A score of 7–10 indicates no asphyxia; 4–6 indicates mild to moderate birth asphyxia; and 3 or less indicates severe birth asphyxia with the need for immediate resuscitative measures.

Meconium aspiration syndrome

Fetal asphyxia results in the passage of meconium into the liquor, because hypoxia causes increased gut paralysis and relaxes the anal sphincter. This is normally unproblematic unless the neonate gasps or breathes in the amniotic fluid and, hence, meconium. The meconium becomes trapped in the airways, allowing air in but not out of the airways. This results in air accumulating behind the blockage. This in turn can cause the alveoli to rupture, resulting in a pneumothorax (discussed later in this chapter). Once the meconium touches the lung tissue, a pneumonitis develops, creating a fertile site for infection. In addition, the surfactant is broken down in the presence of meconium. This all culminates in a severe disease state, with gas exchange at the alveoli level inhibited, areas of hypoxic lung bypassed as blood is shunted away, and

> ### Clinical point
>
> Mild brain hypothermia is proving promising in the management of neonates with asphyxia to prevent further neurological damage (Flavin 2001). Hypothermia reduces the infant's metabolic rate.

fetal circulation maintained due to increasing pulmonary resistance. These neonates need intensive care and ventilation to prevent further detoriation. Use of surfactant has been found to reduce the severity of respiratory distress in these babies (Merrell & Ballard 2003).

In approximately 10–15% of labours there is meconium-stained liquor, but only in approximately 1–5% of neonates will meconium aspiration syndrome occur (Henderson & Macdonald 2004). The majority of these neonates will suffer a mild respiratory distress, resolving over 24–48 hours. In the reminder of neonates, the respiratory distress initially may be mild, moderate or severe, with a gradual detoriation over 12–24 hours, the neonate becoming acutely ill.

Transient tachypnoea of the newborn

Transient tachypnoea of the newborn is thought to result from mild surfactant deficiency or failure to adequately absorb lung fluid following birth. Hence this condition is typically seen in neonates post caesarean birth, due to lack of chest compression. The neonate presents with a tachypnoea of up 120 breaths per minute, plus flaring of nostrils, sternal recession, expiratory grunting and cyanosis. These neonates may need oxygen and observation in an incubator. Symptoms usually resolve within 24 hours.

Respiratory distress syndrome

Respiratory distress syndrome occurs as a result of insufficient surfactant production. It is seen predominantly in preterm (less than 34 weeks) neonates, but is occasionally evident in infants of mothers with diabetes and infants with meconium aspiration syndrome. Surfactant reduces the surface tension in the alveoli, preventing complete collapse during expiration and facilitating lung expansion. A deficiency of surfactant means that more respiratory effort is required to inflate the lungs, and the neonate quickly becomes exhausted, the alveoli collapse and hypoxaemia results. This results in stimulation of prostaglandins from the wall of the ductus arteriosus, preventing its closure. Blood then continues to be shunted away from the lungs, further reducing the oxygenation. Hypoxaemia then further impedes the production of surfactant, and a vicious cycle ensues unless appropriate respiratory support is commenced immediately. The neonate will need to be ventilated for some time but should be gradually weaned off as soon as possible to prevent further lung damage. Long-term ventilation, particularly with the use of high pressure, may cause damage to the lungs, resulting in chronic lung disease or pneumothoraces. Respiratory distress syndrome occurs within four hours of birth.

Clinical point

Prevention of aspiration of the meconium previously involved routinely suctioning the oropharynx and nasopharynx before birth of the shoulders. Some work undertaken recently indicates that this in fact makes no difference to the incidence of meconium aspiration syndrome (Vain et al 2004).

Apnoeas

Apnoea is the cessation of respiratory effort for 20 seconds or more, and requires constant monitoring. It occurs commonly in preterm neonates, the incidence increasing with decreasing gestational age. Apnoeas are a consequence of the immature respiratory centre and immaturity of chemoreceptor response to hypoxia and acidosis. This tends to resolve as the neonate matures. Apnoea can also occur at the conclusion of increasing respiratory fatigue in term infants. In addition, apnoea can often be the first sign of sepsis, pneumonia, necrotising enterocolitis or meningitis in a neonate. There are three types of apnoea, depending on whether there is respiratory effort: central (no respiratory effort), obstructive (ineffective effort) and mixed (both). Factors affecting the respiratory centre include prematurity, hypoxia, maternal drug taking (narcotics, magnesium sulfate), metabolic (hypoglycaemia), sepsis, intercranial haemorrhage, necrotising enterocolitis, patent ductus, and temperature instability. Neonates with apnoea require cardiac/apnoea monitors and continual assessment of status, including the amount of stimulation required with an apnoea episode. Methylxanthines, such as theophylline, may be prescribed to help reduce the number of apnoeic episodes (Theobald et al 2000). These drugs work by stimulating the central respiratory control centre.

Chronic lung disease

In chronic lung disease, the preterm neonate continues to require supplemented oxygen supply at 36 weeks postconceptual age. Risk factors for chronic lung disease include:
- prematurity
- endotracheal intubation
- high-level ventilator peak inspiratory pressures
- oxygen toxicity
- low birthweight neonates with mild respiratory distress syndrome with patent ductus arteriosus and nosocomial infections.

It is clear that severe initial lung disease is not a prerequisite for developing chronic lung disease in the preterm neonate (Cole & Fiascone 2000). The aim of treatment of chronic lung disease is to reduce the requirements for supplementary oxygen and high ventilatory pressures in the neonate as soon as possible. Use of surfactant therapy and new ventilation techniques have helped to reduce the severity of the condition (Henderson & Macdonald 2004). The neonate with chronic lung disease will require low-flow oxygen therapy for several months, until the lung tissue has regenerated enough to support adequate oxygenation.

Pneumothorax

Pneumothorax occurs when the alveoli rupture, causing air to enter the pleural cavity. This may occur spontaneously at birth, due to the large pressures generated by the first breath, following meconium aspiration, or as a consequence of high ventilator pressures. The neonate's condition will suddenly deteriorate, with signs of respiratory distress indicating a possible pneumothorax. Mild cases will resolve spontaneously within a few days. It may be necessary to aspirate the air by inserting a needle into the pleural cavity. An underwater drain will need to be inserted for larger cases.

Respiratory support

For the parents of a neonate suffering from respiratory problems, a great deal of support, reassurance and explanation of what is happening to their baby, will be required. As much as possible, and at the earliest possible moment, women should be prepared for what might happen to their baby. If the woman is deemed at high risk antenatally of having a neonate who will need respiratory support, she should be prepared at that time, with visits to the nursery and explanation.

Oxygen therapy

Oxygen therapy needs to be administered carefully and monitored closely, to prevent hyperoxaemia and hypoxaemia in the neonate and the long-term disabilities that would result. The aim of care is to provide sufficient oxygen to maintain arterial oxygenation within normal limits, and avoid excessive or fluctuating concentrations of oxygen, which has been implicated in the cause of retinopathy of prematurity (Whitfill & Drack 2000). Previously termed 'retrolental fibroplasia', this condition causes various levels of retinal vascular changes, often resulting in blindness (Merenstein & Gardener 2002). The use of oxygen therapy therefore requires a skilful practitioner together with saturation monitors, transcutaneous monitors and arterial catheter readings. Regular eye examinations are undertaken on neonates of less than 32 weeks gestation until term to assess for early signs of retinal damage.

Intermittent positive-pressure ventilation

Intermittent positive-pressure ventilation (IPPV) involves the use of a ventilator that is preset for the pressures generated from a non-cuffed endotracheal tube. A non-cuffed endotracheal tube results in unavoidable and variable leak around the tube. The flow through the neonatal ventilator circuit is constant, with the pressure in the circuit being controlled at a valve in the gas return port. This means that the pressure required to open this valve varies with the ventilator settings, and in turn determines the pressure generated through the endotracheal tube. This is necessary as neonates with respiratory distress syndrome have small airways, which collapse at the end of each breath, taking considerable effort to reinflate.

Continuous positive airway pressure

Continuous positive airway pressure (CPAP) is administered through nasal prongs and prevents collapse of the alveoli on expiration by maintaining a positive pressure in the airway while the neonate breathes spontaneously. This effectively keeps the airway open, reducing the respiratory oxygen required. It is important to leave a gastric tube in place at all times to prevent air accumulating in the stomach, causing distension and compromising respiratory effort. The use of CPAP in New Zealand and Australia has increased fourfold in the past decade. The technique is being used with increasing success as an alternative to intubation and ventilation of respiratory distress syndrome (De Paoli et al 2002).

Synchronous intermittent mandatory ventilation

Synchronous intermittent mandatory ventilation (SIMV) is helpful when weaning a neonate off a ventilator. During prolonged apnoea periods, for example, this system triggers ventilation, responding to pressure changes in the neonate's airway and causing the ventilator to produce an inspiration in time with the neonate's breathing pattern.

Nitric oxide

Nitric oxide is used as a vasodilator of the pulmonary circulation in neonates with persistent pulmonary hypertension associated with respiratory diseases. This technique improves arterial oxygenation, reducing the amount of ventilatory support required, and reducing mortality rates (Merenstein & Glicken 2002; Sadiq et al 2003).

Extracorporeal membrane oxygenation

Extracorporeal membrane oxygenation (ECMO) is used in severe cases of meconium aspiration syndrome, persistent pulmonary hypertension or respiratory distress syndrome that do not respond to other methods of ventilation. Basically, the right internal jugular vein is cannulated with blood which then circulates into an oxygenator and returns via the right common carotid artery. The benefits of ECMO have been well documented (Merenstein & Glicken 2002). There is great debate about the increase in risk of neurological damage from

---

Clinical point

Surfactant can be given prophylactically to all preterm neonates at birth, or as a rescue treatment to neonates following a diagnosis of respiratory distress syndrome. It has been shown, however, that not all preterm neonates need prophylactic surfactant, especially with increased rates of antenatal steroid use. A rapid bedside test, called a *click test*, has been developed to diagnose surfactant deficiency in the neonate. The click test is performed on a specimen of endotracheal aspirate taken immediately after intubation. Clicking occurs when air diffuses rapidly out of bubbles suspended in air-free water, and depends on the presence of surfactant. This test enables more appropriately targeted administration of surfactant with improved clinical outcomes and contained costs (Osborn et al 2000).

---

respiratory disorders with this technique, which has been shown to be minimised by inducing hypothermia (Ichiba et al 2003).

Exogenous surfactant

Surfactant deficiency has been shown to be the primary abnormality in respiratory distress syndrome, and hence the use of exogenous surfactant administered through an endotracheal tube (Levene et al 2000). The indications are that this results in an improved lung compliance and volume, improved gas exchange and a decrease in the need for high levels of oxygen and ventilatory support. Surfactant therapy also reduces the incidence of pneumothorax and increases survival rates (Merenstein & Glicken 2002).

Metabolic and endocrine disorders

Screening

Screening consists of genetic counselling following gene mapping from collected blood samples of parents in situations of high-risk. Assessing the individual fetus for specific risk can be undertaken through amniocentesis or chorionic villus sampling. Parents need to be fully informed of the risks of each procedure and the options available to them. The role of the midwife is in supporting the parents through this decision-making process by providing the necessary information.

Inborn errors of metabolism

Phenylketonuria

Phenylketonuria (PKU) can be successfully screened for and is a treatable cause of brain injury, occurring in 1:10,000 births (Henderson & Macdonald 2004). This condition is due to a deficiency in the enzyme phenylalanine hydroxylase, which converts the amino acid found in most foods, phenylalanine, into tyrosine. On establishing milk feeds, the levels of phenylalanine, together with the by-product of its metabolism, phenylpyruvic acid, start to rise. Phenylpyruvic acid is toxic to the neonatal brain, causing irreversible neurological damage, manifesting at three months of age as persistent vomiting, eczema and a characteristic musty smell in the urine. Early detection through the newborn screening test, and placing the neonate on a phenylalanine-restricted diet, have led to excellent outcomes.

Galactosaemia

Galactosaemia is a disorder of carbohydrate metabolism occurring in 1:60,000 neonates (Henderson & Macdonald 2004). The cause is absence, or severe deficiency, of the enzyme galactose-1-phosphate uridyltransferase, important for converting galactose into glucose in the intestine. The result is an accumulation of galactose and galactose-1-phosphate in erythrocytes, causing liver cirrhosis, neurological damage and cataract formation. The neonate presents with failure to thrive, hypoglycaemia, vomiting, bleeding, persistent jaundice, hypotonia, sepsis and signs of hepatosplenomegaly within the first week. Early detection through the newborn screening test and a galactose-free diet through use of soya milk, results in an improved prognosis.

Acquired errors of metabolism

Hypoglycaemia

The definition of hypoglycaemia is controversial, as is what constitutes a normal plasma glucose level in the neonate (Cornblath et al 2000; Cowett & Loughead 2002). It is well accepted that hypoglycaemia does cause damage to the newborn brain, but the severity and duration of hypoglycaemia required to cause this damage is unclear (Cowett & Loughead 2002). In addition, neonates with hypoglycaemia do not exhibit obvious signs of impairment (Cowett & Loughead 2002). The consensus appears to be that a glucose level of 2.6 mmol/L should be the lower limit (Henderson & Macdonald 2004). Levels lower than this should be treated in neonates who may be asymptomatic or show signs of lethargy, poor feeding, hypotonia and jitteriness. If hypoglycaemia is untreated, the neonate may suffer from convulsions, cyanosis and apnoea leading to possible neurological damage, coma and even death.

The causes of hypoglycaemia include the following:
- Preterm neonates lack energy stores, as the bulk of glycogen and fat stores are laid down in the last trimester.
- Small for gestational age neonates use up their energy reserves because of intrauterine malnutrition.
- Large for gestational age neonates rapidly use up their energy stores unless fed regularly.
- Neonates of diabetic mothers suffer from an overproduction of insulin, which quickly uses up glycogen stores.
- Inborn errors of metabolism
- Specific abnormalities such as pancreatic tumours or pituitary insufficiency
- Miscellaneous situations such as feeding difficulties, hypothermia, cerebral damage, infection and severe Rhesus isoimmunisation.

Mild cases of hypoglycaemia should be fed immediately, and regularly thereafter. A repeat blood glucose level should be undertaken one hour after feeding and, if still low, may warrant intravenous fluids with dextrose, and further investigation.

Exocrine disorders

Cystic fibrosis

Cystic fibrosis is the most common serious genetic disorder in Caucasian people, with an incidence of 1:2500–3500 neonates (Henderson & Macdonald 2004). It is an autosomal recessive disorder associated with chromosome 7, and as carriers are common (1:40), preconceptual or antenatal testing is available for parents. A newborn screening test indicates raised levels of immunoreactive trypsinogen, which is followed by a sweat test, measuring the salt content, before diagnosis is confirmed.

Early diagnosis and treatment may greatly improve the prognosis.

Cystic fibrosis is a condition in which there is an abnormality of the exocrine mucus-secreting glands throughout the body, specifically the intestine, lungs and pancreas. The protein required to carry chloride ions across cell membranes is absent. This results in the formation of thick mucus with abnormal electrolyte concentrations, distending and dilating the affected area, leading to obstruction and fibrosis. Pulmonary disease is the primary cause of morbidity and mortality. Management includes chest physiotherapy, antibiotics, pancreatic enzyme supplementation, improved nutrition, use of DNase (a synthetic protein) to break down mucus and a heart–lung transplantation. Fertility tends to be reduced due to an alteration in the chemical constitution of the cervical mucus (Bolyard 2001). There is no cure for this condition, and management is aimed at preventing complications and maintaining optimal growth and development. Currently, the life expectancy is around 30 years (Chini 2002).

Endocrine disorders

Congenital adrenal hypoplasia

Congenital adrenal hypoplasia refers to a group of inherited disorders that result from a deficiency of the enzymes responsible for hormone production within the adrenal glands. This deficiency can result in, most commonly, an excess of androgenic hormones, or glucocorticoid, and mineralocorticoids less frequently. These disorders cause abnormalities in the formation of the genitalia, leading to ambiguous genitalia and symptoms of adrenal insufficiency (vomiting, diarrhoea, vascular collapse, hypoglycaemia, hyponatraemia or hyperkalaemia). Diagnosis is through the newborn screening test and chromosomal analysis may be necessary to ascertain the sex of the neonate.

Congenital hypothyroidism

Congenital hypothyroidism is detected through the newborn screening test and has an incidence of 1:3500 neonates. There are several possible causes, including abnormalities in gland formation, defects in hormone synthesis and secondary pituitary causes (rare). The affected neonate tends to be large, post mature and have a large posterior fontanelle, with coarse features and often an umbilical hernia. Untreated neonates develop impaired motor development, growth failure, a low IQ, impaired hearing and language problems. Neurological prognosis is poor unless treated early with thyroxine sodium.

Sudden infant death syndrome

(This section on SIDS was written by Sally Baddock.)
To make a diagnosis of sudden infant death syndrome (SIDS) requires exclusion of all other possibilities of a sudden death in an infant aged less than 12 months. In other words, where

death is unexplained following a postmortem examination, review of the clinical history and examination of the death scene are required. For the parents, this can be a very distressing process and requires an immense amount of support.

Incidence

The incidence of SIDS in Australia has fallen from 1.89 per 1000 live births in 1986 to 0.81 per 1000 live births in 1996, to 0.3 per 1000 live births in 2003. Despite this dramatic fall in incidence, SIDS remains the major cause of death in infants aged from one month to one year of age. The peak incidence is at four months of age, with the majority occurring under six months of age (80%). Winter remains a peak period, with the incidence being higher for Aboriginal infants, and boys in general (Mitchell 2000).

SIDS rates in industrialised countries have decreased more than 50% from their peak in the late 1980s but SIDS remains the leading single cause of post-neonatal death. In 2000 the rate in Australia was 0.6 deaths/1000 live births and in New Zealand, 1.1 deaths/1000 live births (NZHIS n.d.). New Zealand still has the highest rate in the industrialised world. Despite the decrease in national rates, Australian Aborigines and New Zealand Maori remain over-represented in the SIDS statistics. Effective strategies are needed to reduce risk factors in these groups.

Reducing the risk factors

No single cause of SIDS has been identified, and the cause of death is likely to be multifactorial. Mechanisms that have been explored include: asphyxiation due to rebreathing of expired air, hyperthermia (directly or leading to respiratory compromise), airways obstruction, impaired arousal, cardiovascular mechanisms and infection. One hypothesis is that SIDS may result from a vulnerable infant (e.g. of a smoking mother), during a vulnerable developmental period (three months of age), unable to respond to an environmental stress (e.g. accumulation of carbon dioxide due to inadvertent covering of the head by bedding) (Filiano & Kinney 1995).

Epidemiological studies have identified several infant and maternal risk factors that are largely unchangeable. These include lower socio-economic status, unmarried or young mother, lower level of education, non-attendance at antenatal classes, Indigenous ethnicity, increased parity, low birthweight, short gestation, male infant, and admission to a baby care unit (Mitchell et al 1991; Ponsonby et al 1992b). The presence of these factors should alert a midwife to an increased risk of SIDS.

There is also another group of factors that are potentially open to change This includes prone sleep position, smoking, bed sharing with a mother who smoked in pregnancy, solitary infant sleeping, not breastfeeding, infant head covering and over-wrapping (Mitchell et al 1991; Ponsonby et al 1992b; Scragg et al 1996). Midwives are in a key position to discuss these factors with families.

It was not until a successful prevention campaign in New Zealand that the potential for reducing the risk by modifying the risk factors was recognised in Australia. This campaign, in conjunction with Red Nose Day, commenced in 1991 in Australia. The risk factors targeted for change in Australia and New Zealand include:

- sleeping position
- position of bed covering
- smoking.

The infant sleeping position still accounts for many SIDS deaths. A large European study reported that 48% of SIDS cases were attributable to sleeping in the side or prone position (Carpenter et al 2004). The prone position often results from infants rolling from the side position. In the prone position babies sleep for longer (Kahn et al 1993) and are more difficult to rouse (Galland et al 1998), resulting in vulnerability to physiological stressors such as rebreathing or overheating. Autonomic nervous system function is reduced in the prone position (Galland et al 1998) and this may impair cardiovascular control. There has been concern that aspiration of vomit is more likely when infants sleep on their back, but evidence does not support this. One study showed that aspiration of vomit was more common in infants lying face down into bedding (Bajanowski et al 1996). Prone sleep may have contributed to overheating in cold climates, particularly if infants were over-wrapped and face down into bedding (Nelson et al 1989). With the reduction in prone sleep, SIDS

TABLE 38.1 Sudden unexpected death in infancy (SUDI) ethnicity by age group, 2002 and 2003

Ethnicity	4–52 weeks					1–4 years			Total
	2002	Per 1000 live births	2003	Per 1000 live births	Total	2002	2003	Total	
Māori	20	1.34	34	2.17	54	1	2	3	57
Pacific Island	3	0.52	2	0.33	5		1	1	6
Other	10	0.30	14	0.41	24	1	1	2	26
Total	33	0.61	50	0.89	83	2	4	6	89

Source: Child and Youth Mortality Review Committee 2005.

is no longer more common in colder climates. Identification of prone (front) sleeping as a risk factor for SIDS, and the subsequent education programs encouraging families to sleep babies on their back, have been credited with the decrease in SIDS (Ponsonby et al 2002).

All infants should be placed in a supine position for sleeping (Mitchell 2000). Healthy infants placed in a supine position for sleeping are not at an increased risk of choking, provided that swallowing and arousal mechanisms are intact and are therefore able to protect the airway (Page & Jeffery 1997).

Smoking is now the most important risk factor for SIDS, and has proved very resistant to change. Smoking is associated with over 80% of all SIDS cases (Blair et al 1999). Exposure to smoke in utero compromises the baby in many ways: placental blood flow is reduced, carbon monoxide is transported on haemoglobin at the expense of oxygen, and nicotine influences development of respiratory receptors in the brainstem and increases the risk of a small baby, of impaired lung development and impaired cardiorespiratory and thermal control. This may compromise responses to rebreathing or overheating situations. Exposure to smoking after birth, by mothers or other household members, poses a further risk. Components from cigarette smoke are shown to be re-emitted into the air from walls and furniture for hours to months after smoking (Daisey 1999). Babies are more likely to be hospitalised with a respiratory infection if the mother smokes in the same room compared with a separate room, and the effect is even greater for smoking while holding baby, and greater again while breastfeeding (Blizzard et al 2003).

It has been shown that infants of mothers who smoke are at a five-fold increased risk of SIDS. Where the fathers smoke around the infant there has been shown to be an independent additive risk. Bed sharing with a mother who smoked in pregnancy and after birth should be avoided. The recommendation is therefore to keep the infant in a smoke-free environment before and after birth (Mitchell 2000; SIDS and Kids Victoria 2004).

Another risk factor for SIDS is the covering of infants' head by bedding. The use of quilts has been shown to increase the risk, whereas firm tucking of the bedding around the infant had been shown to decrease the risk in New Zealand. Being found with head covered is a significant risk for SIDS. In a study of 30 cot-sleep infants it was demonstrated that only 23% at two months of age and 60% at five months could remove a duvet from their head when sleeping supine. When sleeping prone, only one five-month infant could clear the duvet from his face (Skadberg & Markestad 1997). Evidence supports both rebreathing and hyperthermia as potential mechanisms. Overwrapping and excess bedding is also associated with SIDS (Ponsonby et al 1992a), particularly in response to infant illness. The recommendation therefore is that infants be placed to the bottom of the infant bed or cot, and tucked in securely with the bedding. Quilts, pillows, soft toys and cot bumpers should not be used.

There is now strong evidence that sleeping baby in the same room as the parents is protective against SIDS. Infants sleeping prone in a separate room face a 17-fold increase in risk, but this reduces to a three-fold risk if sharing the room with parents. This suggests some protection from increased maternal interactions. Room sharing with siblings is not protective (Scragg et al 1996). Room sharing meets with resistance from many families, but it is calculated that 36% of SIDS could be prevented by infant–parent room sharing (Carpenter et al 2004).

Breastfeeding is targeted in many education campaigns. The evidence for a direct protective effect against SIDS is equivocal, but other health benefits to the infant are important. Protection from SIDS may be via reduced infections. Fleming and colleagues (1996) suggest that breastfeeding is simply associated with higher socio-economic level. Pacifier use has long been shown to be associated with a small decreased risk of SIDS (Carpenter et al 2004; Mitchell et al 1993) but it is also linked with decreased breastfeeding (Pollard et al 1999; Vogel et al 2001). Consequently, there is little support for pacifier use as a means of reducing SIDS.

While bed sharing is often a valued practice, it carries a high risk if the baby is exposed to smoking. The combination of bed sharing and maternal smoking has consistently been identified as a risk for SIDS and largely accounts for the high SIDS rates within Maori and Aboriginal communities. The risk to a two-week-old baby, bed sharing with a mother who smoked during pregnancy, is 27 times that of a baby without smoke exposure and sleeping in a cot. The risk decreases with age but is still 10-fold greater by six months (Carpenter et al 2004). Increased risk is also associated with factors that impair a parent's ability to respond to the baby (e.g. alcohol consumption). Unsafe sleeping places include bed sharing on a couch (50-fold increase in risk) (Blair et al 1999), and sleeping on waterbeds or surfaces other than firm mattresses.

The above factors have been the focus of 'reduce the risks' campaigns around the world. Since the decrease in prone sleep there has been a shift in the demographics of SIDS families to more deprived social groupings (Leach et al 1999). Midwives can play an important role in educating families to avoid known risk factors such as prone position, smoking, bed sharing if the baby has been exposed to smoking, head covering and over-wrapping. Circumstances often make change difficult for these families, but evidence suggests that choosing a messenger and medium appropriate to the family does have more effect (Abel et al 2001). Midwives may be well placed to deliver safe sleeping messages to families in a positive and trusting environment. More information is available from a number of websites, including the SIDS and kids website (see the online resources list at the end of this chapter).

Apnoea alarms

There are many issues regarding the use of apnoea alarms for monitoring normal, healthy neonates. First, apnoea monitors are impractical and undesirable, with a high rate of false alarms, which only serves to increase the parents' anxiety. In addition, parents may become too reliant on the apnoea monitors and ignore subtle signs of pending illness in the neonate. The evidence indicates that the use of apnoea monitors at home does not decrease the incidence of SIDS, and they are therefore not recommended.

Neonatal abstinence syndrome

As drugs of addiction cross the placenta readily, the fetus of a drug-addicted mother becomes passively dependent on the drugs from conception. The main concern, then, is the withdrawal effects after the birth, when the neonate is deprived of the regular supply of drugs previously ingested by the mother. A wide variety of drugs may be consumed by the mother during pregnancy, with neonatal withdrawal symptoms being reported with alcohol, amphetamines, barbiturates, codeine, ethchlorvynol, heroin, pethidine, methadone, morphine and pentazocine. It should be remembered that a neonate will take longer to metabolise drugs than an adult, and that withdrawal may occur up to a week or more after birth.

Heroin and methadone are the drugs most commonly abused by women during pregnancy. The neonates of these women will exhibit withdrawal in 70% of cases, with symptoms appearing within 48 hours of birth (Levene et al 2000). It is important, therefore, to monitor all neonates of mothers who took opioids for prolonged periods of time during pregnancy. These neonates will exhibit extreme jitteriness, tachycardia, vomiting, diarrhoea and fever. Various assessment tools have been devised in order to fully assess these neonates for withdrawal or for neonatal abstinence syndrome. These neonates are often difficult to care for as they are usually irritable and difficult to feed. Added to this are the social issues that may occur as a consequence. The midwife plays a large role in supporting these families and monitoring the neonate.

Conclusion

This chapter has outlined the common complications of the newborn, which include preterm birth, neonatal jaundice, neonatal infections and neonatal bleeding. In addition, congenital conditions, cardiorespiratory conditions, metabolic and endocrine disorders and SIDS were discussed. It is important to emphasise that midwives must always be prepared for the unexpected when caring for this fragile population.

Review questions

1 While caring for a neonate who is 123 hours old, the midwife notices a yellow tint on the skin and sclera. What laboratory test should she consider ordering?

2 Describe the process of physiological jaundice.

3 A newborn is admitted to the nursery with transient tachypnoea of the newborn. In planning care for this neonate, what would be the goal?

4 While caring for a neonate receiving phototherapy, what assessment would warrant further investigation?

5 Describe the role of vaccination in preventing infection in the neonate.

6 Discuss the main causes of bleeding in the neonate.

7 Outline the process that midwives might follow for detecting an imperforate anus in a newborn infant.

8 Discuss four types of cardiac conditions that midwives might encounter in the neonate.

9 Discuss the risk factors associated with SIDS.

10 Briefly describe early signs and symptoms exhibited by neonates with a mother addicted to opioids.

Online resources

SIDS Australia, http://www.sidsandkids.org/research.html
SIDS International: the Global Strategy Task Force, http://www.sidsglobal.org/

References

Abel S, Park J, Tipene-Leach D et al 2001 Infant care practices in New Zealand: a cross-cultural qualitative study. Social Science and Medicine 53(9):1135–1148

Ainsworth S, Wyllie JP, Wren C 1999 Prevalence and clinical significance of cardiac murmurs in neonates. Archives of Disease in Childhood 80(1):F43–F45

Autret-Leca E, Jonville-Bera AP 2001 Vitamin K in neonates: how to administer, when and to whom. Paediatric Drugs 3(1):1–8

Bajanowski T, Ott A, Jorch G et al 1996 Frequency and type of aspiration in cases of sudden infant death (SID) in correlation with the body position at the time of discovery. Journal of Sudden Infant Death Syndrome and Infant Mortality 1(4):271–279

Beckwith JB 1970 Discussion of terminology and definition of the sudden infant death syndrome. Paper presented at the Second International Conference on the Causes of Sudden Deaths in Infants. Seattle

Blair P, Fleming P, Smith I et al 1999 Babies sleeping with parents: case-control study of factors influencing the risk of the sudden infant death syndrome. British Medical Journal 319:1457–1462

Blackburn ST 2003 Maternal, fetal and neonatal physiology: a clinical perspective. WB Saunders, Philadelphia

Blizzard L, Ponsonby AL, Dwyer T et al 2003 Parental smoking and infant respiratory infection: how important is not smoking in the same room with the baby? American Journal of Public Health 93(3):482–488

Bolyard DR 2001 Sexuality and cystic fibrosis. Maternal Child Health Nursing 26(1):39–41

Bor O, Akgun N, Yakut A et al 2000 Late haemorrhagic disease of the newborn. Pediatrics International 42(1):64–66

Braby J 2001 Current and emerging treatment for congenital diaphragmatic hernia. Neonatal Network 20(2):5–13

Carbajal R, Veerapen S, Couderc S et al 2003 Analgesic effect of breastfeeding in term neonates: randomised controlled trial. British Medical Journal 326(4):13–15

Carpenter RG, Irgens LM, Blair PS et al 2004 Sudden unexplained infant death in 20 regions in Europe: case control study. Lancet 363(9404):185–191

Child and Youth Mortality Review Committee 2005 Second Report to the Minister of Health, 1 July 2003 to 31 December 2004, Table A12, p 43. CYMRC, Wellington. Online: http://www.newhealth. govt.nz/cymrc

Chini BA 2002 Update on cystic fibrosis. Current Opinion in Otolaryngology and Head and Neck Surgery 10(6):431–434

Cole CH, Fiascone JM 2000 Strategies for prevention of neonatal chronic lung disease. Seminars in Perinatology 24(6):445–462

Cook AJC, Gilbert RE, Buffolano W et al 2000 Sources of Toxoplasma infection in pregnant women: European multicentre case-control study. British Medical Journal 321(7254):142–147

Cornblath M, Hawdon JM, Williams AF et al 2000 Controversies regarding the definition of neonatal hypoglycaemia: suggested operational thresholds. Paediatrics 105(5):1141–1145

Cowett RM, Loughead JL 2002 Neonatal glucose metabolism: differential diagnosis, evaluation, treatment of hypogylcaemia. Neonatal Network 21(4):9–19

Crowther CA, Kierse MJNC 1999 Anti-D administration during pregnancy for preventing Rhesus issoimmunisation (Cochrane Review). Cochrane Library (2). Update Software, Oxford

CSL 2002 WinRho SDF approved production information. Bioplasma Products, Bioplasma Division, CSL Ltd, Broadmeadows, Victoria

Daisey JM 1999 Tracers for assessing exposure to environmental tobacco smoke: what are they tracing? Environmental Health Perspectives 2:319–327

De Paoli G, Morley C, Davis PG 2002 Nasal CPAP for neonates: what do we know in 2003? Archives of Disease in Childhood Fetal and Neonatal Edition 88:F168–172

Enkin M, Keirse MJ, Renfrew M et al 2000 A guide to effective care in pregnancy and childbirth (2nd edn). Oxford University Press, Oxford

Filiano JJ, Kinney HC 1995 Sudden infant death syndrome and brainstem research. Pediatric Annals 24(7):379–383

Flavin NE 2001 Perinatal asphyxia: a clinical review, including research with brain hypothermia. Neonatal Network 20(3):31–40

Fleming PJ, Blair PS, Bacon C et al 1996 Environment of infants during sleep and risk of the sudden infant death syndrome: results of 1993–5 case-control study for confidential inquiry into stillbirths and deaths in infancy. British Medical Journal 313(7051):191–195

Fraser DM, Cooper MA 2003 Myles textbook for midwives (14th edn). Churchill Livingstone, Sydney

Galland BC, Reeves G, Taylor BJ et al 1998 Sleep position, autonomic function, and arousal. Archives of Disease in Childhood Fetal and Neonatal Edition 78(3):189–194

Gibbins S, Stevens B, Hodnett E et al 2002 Efficacy and safety of sucrose for procedural pain relief in preterm and term neonates. Nursing Research 51(6):375–382

Gilbert R 2004 Prenatal screening for group B streptococcal infection: gaps in the evidence. International Journal of Epidemiology 33(1):2–8

Girou E, Loyeau S, Oppein F et al 2002 Efficacy of handwashing with alcohol based solution versus standard handwashing with antiseptic soap: randomised clinical trial. British Medical Journal 325(7360):362

Gradin M, Eriksson M, Holmqvist G et al 2002 Pain reduction at venepuncture in newborns: oral glucose compared with local anaesthetic cream. Pediatrics 110(6):1053–1057

Grandjean H, Larroque D, Levi S 1999 The performance of routine ultrasonographic screening of pregnancies in the Eurofetus Study. American Journal of Obstetrics and Gynecology 181(2):446–454

Hafstrom M, Kjellmer I 2000 Non-nutritive sucking in the healthy pre-term infant. Early Human Development 60(1):13–24

Harahan KS, Lofgren M 2004 Evidence-based practice: examining the risk of toys in the micro environment of infants in the neonatal intensive care unit. Advances in Neonatal Care 4(4):184–201

Hasenau SM 2002 Neural tube defects: prevention and folic acid. American Journal of Maternal and Child Nursing 27(2):87–91

Henderson C, Macdonald S 2004 Mayes' midwifery. A textbook for midwives (13th edn). Baillière Tindall, Sydney

Hey E 2003 Vitamin K—can we improve on nature? MIDIRS Midwifery Digest 13(1):7–12

Hull D 1992 Vitamin K and childhood cancer: the risk of haemorrhagic disease is certain; that of cancer is not. British Medical Journal 305:326–327

Ichiba S, Killer HM, Firmin RK et al 2003 Pilot investigation of hypothermia in neonates receiving extracorporeal membrane oxygenation. Archives of Disease of Childhood 88(2):F128–F133

Israel C 2003 The preterm infant parenting study. MIDIRS Midwifery Digest 13(2):239–241

Jeffery HE, Moses LM 1998 Eight-year outcome of universal screening and intrapartum antibiotics for maternal group B streptococcal carriers. Pediatrics 101(1):2–8

Johnson AN 2003 Adapting the neonatal intensive care environment to decrease noise. Journal of Perinatal and Neonatal Nursing 17(4):280–288

Johnston PGB, Flood K, Spinks K 2003 The Newborn Child (9th edn). Churchill Livingstone, Sydney

Juretschke LJ 2001 Congenital diaphragmatic hernia: update and review. Journal of Obstetric, Gynaecological and Neonatal Nurses 30(3):259–268

Kahn A, Groswasser J, Sottiaux M et al 1993 Prone or supine body position and sleep characteristics in infants. Pediatrics 91(6):1112–1115

King J, Askin DF 2003 Gastroschisis: etiology, diagnosis, delivery options, and care. Neonatal Network 22(4):7–12

Kramer LI 1969 Advancement of dermal icterus in the jaundiced newborn. American Journal of Diseases of Children 118:454–459

Leach CEA, Blair PS, Fleming P and the CESDI SUDI Research Group

1999 Epidemiology of SIDS and explained sudden infant deaths. Pediatrics 104(4):e43

Levene M, Tudehope DI, Thearle MJ 2000 Essentials of neonatal medicine (3rd edn). Blackwell Science, Oxford

Merenstein GB, Gardner SL 2002 Handbook of neonatal intensive care (5th edn). Mosby, St Loius

Merenstein GB, Glicken AD 2002 Best evidence-based practices: a history perspective. Neonatal Network 21(5):31–35

Merenstein K, Hathaway WE, Miller RW et al 1993 Controversies concerning vitamin K and the newborn. Pediatrics 91:1001–1002

Merrell JD, Ballard RA 2003 Pulmonary surfactant for neonatal respiratory disorders. Current Opinion in Pediatrics 15(2):149–154

Mitchell EA 2000 SIDS: facts and controversies. Medical Journal of Australia 173:175–176

Mitchell EA, Scragg R, Stewart AW et al 1991 Results from the first year of the New Zealand cot death study. New Zealand Medical Journal 104(906):71–76

Mitchell EA, Taylor BJ, Ford RP et al 1993 Dummies and the sudden infant death syndrome. Archives of Disease in Childhood 68(4):501–504

Nelson EA, Taylor BJ, Weatherall IL 1989 Sleeping position and infant bedding may predispose to hyperthermia and the sudden infant death syndrome. Lancet 1(8631):199–201

New Zealand Health Information Service (n.d.) Mortality statistics for 2000 and 2001. Online: http://www.nzhis.govt.nz/stats/mortstats.html#03, accessed 5 April 2005

NSW Health Department 2002 Circular 2002/28. Minimisation of neonatal early onset of group B streptococcal infection. NSW Health Department, Sydney

Oddie S, Embleton N 2002 Risk factors for early onset neonatal group B streptococcal sepsis: case-control study. British Medical Journal 325(7359):308–311

Oddy WH 2001 Breastfeeding protects against illness and infection in infants and children: a review of the evidence. Breastfeeding Review 9(2):11–18

Osborn DA, Jeffery HE et al 2000 Targeted early rescue surfactant in ventilated preterm infants using the click test. Pediatrics 106(3):30–42

Page M, Jeffery HE 1997 Airway protection in sleeping infants in response to pharyngeal fluid stimulation in the supine position. Paediatric Research 44:691–698

Pollard K, Fleming P, Young J et al 1999 Night-time non-nutritive sucking in infants aged 1 to 5 months: relationship with infant state, breastfeeding, and bed-sharing versus room-sharing. Early Human Development 56(2/3):185–204

Ponsonby AL, Dwyer T, Gibbons LE et al 1992a Thermal environment and sudden infant death syndrome: case-control study. British Medical Journal 304(6822):277–282

Ponsonby AL, Jones ME, Lumley J et al 1992b Climatic temperature and variation in the incidence of sudden infant death syndrome between the Australian states. Medical Journal of Australia 156(4):246–248, 251

Ponsonby AL, Dwyer T, Cochrane J 2002 Population trends in sudden infant death syndrome. Seminars in Perinatology 26(4):296–305

Puckett RM, Offringa M 2002 Prophylactic vitamin K for vitamin K deficiency bleeding in neonates. Cochrane Database of Systematic Reviews (4). Update Software, Oxford

Rubaltelli FF, Gourley GR, Lockamp N et al 2001 Transcutaneous bilirubin measurement: a multicentre evaluation of a new device. Pediatrics 107(6):1264–1271

Roman E, Fear NT, Ansell P et al 2002 Vitamin K and childhood cancer: analysis of individual patient data from six case-controlled studies. British Journal of Cancer 86(1):63–69

Sadiq HF, Mantych G, Benawra RS et al 2003 Inhaled nitric oxide in the treatment of moderate persistent pulmonary hypertension of the newborn: a randomised controlled, multicentre trial. Journal of Perinatology 23(2):98–103

Schrag SJ, Zell ER, Lynfield R et al 2002 Early onset neonatal group B streptococcal disease. A population-based comparison of strategies to prevent early-onset group B streptococcal disease in neonates. 347(4):233–239

Scragg RK, Mitchell EA, Stewart AW et al 1996 Infant room-sharing and prone sleep position in sudden infant death syndrome. New Zealand Cot Death Study Group. Lancet 347(8993):7–12

Sheehan-Dare RA 2001 The use of lasers in dermatology. Hospital Medicine 62(1):14–17

Sherman TI, Blackson T, Touch SM et al 2003 Physiologic effects of CPAP: application and monitoring. Neonatal Network 22(6):7–15

Shiraki K 2000 Perinatal transmission of hepatitis B virus and its prevention. Journal of Gastroenterology and Hepatology 15(Suppl.):E11–15

Stables D, Rankin J 2005 Physiology in childbearing: with anatomy and related biosciences (2nd edn). Elsevier, Edinburgh

SIDS and Kids Victoria 2004 SIDS and Kids Safe Sleeping Program guidelines. SIDS and Kids Victoria, Malvern

Skadberg BT, Markestad T 1997 Consequences of getting the head covered during sleep in infancy. Pediatrics 100(2):E61–E67

Symington A, Pinelli J 2003 Developmental care for promoting development and preventing morbidity in preterm infants. Cochrane Database of Systematic Reviews (2). Update Software, Oxford

Theobald K, Botwinski C, Albanna S et al 2000 Apnea of prematurity: diagnosis, implications for care, and pharmacologic management. Neonatal Network 19(6):17–21

Vain NE, Szyld EG, Prudent LM et al 2004 Oropharyngeal and nasopharyngeal suctioning of meconium-stained neonates before delivery of their shoulders: a multicentre, randomised controlled trial. Lancet 364(9434):597–602

Vogel AM, Hutchison BL, Mitchell EA 2001 The impact of pacifier use on breastfeeding: a prospective cohort study. Journal of Paediatrics and Child Health 37(1):58–63

Whitfill CR, Drack AV 2000 Avoidance and treatment of retinopathy of prematurity. Seminars in Pediatric Surgery 9(2):103–105

Wilkinson S 2003 Pressure on the next generation. Journal of the Association of Physiotherapists in Women's Health 92(8):42–44

Witters I, van Ranst M, Fryns JP 2000 Cytomegalovirus reactivation in pregnancy and subsequent isolated hearing loss in the infant. Genetic Counseling 11(4):375–378

World Health Organization (WHO) 1991 Maternal and perinatal infection: report of a WHO consultation. WHO, Geneva

Wyllie J 2003 Treatment of patent ductus arteriosus. Seminars in Neonatology 8(9):425–432

Yellott G 2001 The loving touch: more than just a therapy. Journal of Neonatal Nursing 7(6):207–208

Acknowledgement

The authors wish to acknowledge Sally Baddock's valuable contribution to the 'Sudden Infant Death Syndrome' section of the chapter.

CHAPTER 39

Grief and bereavement

Chris Stanbridge

Key terms

blighted ovum, complete miscarriage, early neonatal death, ectopic pregnancy, hydatidiform mole, incomplete miscarriage, inevitable miscarriage, infant death, late neonatal death, miscarriage, missed miscarriage, neonatal death, perinatal death, post neonatal death, recurrent miscarriage, spontaneous miscarriage, stillbirth, stillborn child, termination of pregnancy, threatened miscarriage

Chapter overview

Loss experienced anywhere along the reproductive continuum inevitably leaves the woman and her family with a sense of loss and deprivation that needs to be addressed through the painful process of grief. Death, like birth, is part of human experience, and as midwives we have a unique opportunity to support women and their families in times of unexpected loss, in order to assist and enhance their ability to grieve.

This chapter focuses on grief, how it may present, and how it may be explained and understood. It offers strategies for midwives to develop their skills in recognising grief and working with women experiencing grief in order to offer support and help them to grieve.

Learning outcomes

Learning outcomes for this chapter are:

1 To recognise grief situations related to women before pregnancy, and through pregnancy and childbirth

2 To discuss aspects of grief and how they may present

3 To describe several theories of grief

4 To describe options for supporting women in their grief

5 To identify appropriate legal requirements related to death of a baby

6 To list some sources of support in the community

7 To develop awareness of your own grief issues

8 To establish a strategy for self-care.

Potential for loss and grief

When a woman enters her childbearing years, there are many times when she may experience grief because of a loss, either actual or potential. Infertility brings grief for the loss of anticipated fertility and the consequence of no children or a smaller family than planned or hoped for. For some women, the experience of pregnancy is different from their expectations, because of, for example, sickness, tiredness, altered appearance or discomfort, and they can grieve for the loss of those expectations. Some women experience violence in the home, which may begin or escalate during pregnancy, causing fear and perhaps grief for the loss of the hoped-for relationship with their partner (Espinosa & Osborne 2002; Ministry of Health 2001). Sexual abuse experienced by a woman during her own childhood may surface when she becomes pregnant, and as well as grieving for her own loss of innocence it may affect her pregnancy and raise fears for her baby's safety in the future (Stojadinovic 2003; Brewis et al 2004). Screening tests may raise the possibility of complications for the baby, such as a genetic abnormality, and alongside the worry and uncertainty a woman will then experience, she may also begin to grieve for the baby in anticipation that her fears will turn out to be real. A premature, abnormal or sick baby, or one that is the 'wrong' sex, can evoke grief. A decision to undergo a therapeutic abortion often leads to feelings of guilt and grief regardless of the reason for the decision. Miscarriage, ectopic pregnancy, blighted ovum, hydatidiform mole, stillbirth and neonatal death all mean the death of an anticipated baby and grief for the actual loss of the baby as well as loss of dreams of family life with that child in its midst.

The experience of labour is often different from women's expectations. When labour is assisted or altered through technological intervention, women may feel a loss of control and grieve for their unmet expectations. Separation from her baby for whatever reason, such as illness in the mother or baby, is usually distressing for a mother. Even when adoption is seen as a positive choice, there is still a sense of loss for the birth mother and her family, and possibly grief for the adoptive family in that they have not been able to bear their own child. Some women experience a sense of loss in no longer being pregnant even after birthing a healthy baby. They may miss their baby's movements or the positive feelings they had while carrying their babies. The experience of motherhood or breastfeeding is not always as one envisages, and women may grieve for the loss of the 'ideal' baby who feeds, sleeps and is 'easy' to care for.

There may be losses brought about by pregnancy that are not recognised as grief, such as loss of status, loss of employment and loss of income. Pregnancy and birth may rekindle or intensify distress and grief for the death of someone important to the woman, no matter how much time has elapsed since the death. The physical or emotional absence of her mother to share her childbearing time can be painful for a woman as she takes on her own mothering role. Similarly, being away from their own country or locality, or important people, may leave women feeling alone and isolated, grieving for the familiar and for the support of family and friends. Families may also experience grief when confronted by the loss of the woman they knew through postnatal depression or psychosis or post-traumatic distress disorder (PTSD), or through the rare but still possible occurrence of maternal death.

All these scenarios may leave a woman and her family grieving for what is lost or for what might have been.

Grief can be a response to many and varied losses. Often the experience of grief is not recognised as such and that which is mourned is unacknowledged. While this chapter deals primarily with pregnancy loss at various stages, much of it is equally relevant to grief experienced as a result of any kind of loss, as the same principles apply. Nor is there a timeframe for grief. It is a lifelong journey of adaptation, and many years later the feelings associated with a loss can resurface, especially if there is a new grief situation.

Grief

Like birth, 'grief is not a pathological state, it is a normal life event' (Golden 2000, p 30). Grief can be defined as 'mental pain, distress, or sorrow; deep or violent sorrow, caused by loss or trouble; a keen or bitter feeling of regret for something lost; remorse for something done; or sorrow for mishap to oneself or others' (*Oxford English Dictionary*). Bereaved means 'deprived or robbed; taken away by force; deprived by death of a near relative, or of one connected by some endearing tie' (*Oxford English Dictionary*).

Elisabeth Kübler-Ross (1969) brought grief issues to greater public awareness in her seminal text, *On Death and Dying*. She identified the stages of grief that people experience when they are facing their impending death. Figure 39.1 shows these stages, identified by Kübler-Ross as denial, anger, depression, bargaining and acceptance. The stages are not sequential and 'these stages do not replace each other but can exist next to each other and overlap at times' (Kübler-Ross 1969, p 264). The experience of grief is not a timely progression from one stage to another, but rather a roller coaster of feelings and thoughts occurring over a period of time, possibly many months, or years. The various stages of grief may occur intermittently and with no set pattern.

Other theorists also offer perspectives that can increase midwives' understandings of experiences of loss and grief. Worden (1997) identifies five 'tasks' of grieving as: accepting the reality of the loss, working through the pain of grief, adjusting to living without the deceased, 'relocating' the dead emotionally, and moving on with life.

After any major loss, such as a death, there is often a sense that it hasn't happened, and the first task is 'to come full face with the reality that the person is dead, that the person is gone and will not return' (Worden 1997, p 10). This generally begins with denial of the facts, then denial of the meaning of the loss, and finally denial of the irreversibility of the loss. Coming to terms with the reality of the loss involves searching

The stages of grief

- Denial
- Anger
- Depression
- Bargaining
- Acceptance

Figure 39.1 The stages of grief (based on Kübler-Ross 1969)

for the deceased or that which is lost, and it is common to swing between belief and disbelief. It is particularly difficult to accept the reality when the death is sudden, and especially if the griever does not see the body. The funeral helps, as does the common need to initially retain things (e.g. the baby's room) as they were before the death. Any formal recognition of that which is lost helps reinforce the reality, such as talking about the baby or acknowledging other, more hidden losses such as loss of fertility. Acceptance of the reality may take a long time and involves intellectual and emotional acceptance.

Working through the pain of grief requires effort. Freud used the term 'grief work' to describe this (cited in Worden 1997, p 10). Another theorist, Parkes (1972, p 173), said 'it is necessary for the bereaved person to go through the pain of grief to get the grief work done'. Not everyone experiences the same intensity of pain, or feels it in the same way, and it will vary for the individual depending on the significance of the loss to them. Worden (1997) identifies different expressions of pain as physical, emotional and behavioural pain. Some try to avoid the pain by idealising the dead (or their dream of what would have been), avoiding reminders, using alcohol or drugs (prescription or recreational), or physically moving away.

Worden's (1997) third task is adjusting to living without the deceased. In other words, adjusting to life without that person or without whatever it is they have lost. When a baby dies, the parents have to adjust not only to life without their child, but also to an alteration in their roles. No longer are they a new mother or new father, and the loss of these roles can be deeply tied to their sense of self or may challenge their femininity or masculinity. Sometimes people regress to more dependent behaviour such as withdrawing, being helpless, inadequate, incapable or childlike, as they learn new ways to deal with their world. There is often a challenge to fundamental life values and philosophical beliefs, bringing with it a loss of direction, and a search for meaning in order to make sense of the loss and regain some control of their life. Part of this task is to learn to live without an answer, to understand the fragility of life and the limits of human control. Sometimes this task needs to be addressed again at a later time. For example, parents who lose a baby may not be aware of all they have lost until a later time, such as when a subsequent baby is born and grows and develops new skills, and they realise the joy and work they have missed with the death of their previous baby.

Worden's fourth task involves a shift from thinking that the dead person is still here, to thinking about what the person would have done had they lived, to planning the future without them. It involves acknowledging one's ability to love others without loving the person who has died any less. Warden describes the feelings involved with this task as numbness, shock, sadness, fatigue, guilt, helplessness, loneliness, anger, anxiety, yearning, emancipation and relief. He also describes these emotions as physical sensations such as hollowness, depersonalisation (nothing seems real, including oneself), weakness, lack of energy, dry mouth, tightness of chest or throat, over-sensitivity to noise, shortness of breath, and headaches. Thoughts include disbelief, confusion, and preoccupation with the dead person, a sense of (their) presence, and hallucinations. Behaviours include crying, appetite and sleep disturbances, loss of interest in the outside world, sighing, social withdrawal, restless over-activity, absentmindedness, searching or calling out, nightmares or dreams of the deceased, avoiding reminders of the deceased or visiting places of significance, and carrying or treasuring objects that are reminders.

Worden's fifth task is related to moving on without the overwhelming sense of grief. As Mary, the mother of a stillborn baby said, 'I was really down for so long, you wonder if things are ever going to be normal again—but what is normal? I felt so empty' (Mary, in letter to author).

Rando's (1996) work identifies six patterns in the grief process:

- recognising the loss, which includes acknowledging and understanding the death
- reaction to separation by experiencing the pain and expressing reactions to the loss
- remembering the deceased and the relationship realistically, and re-experiencing the feelings
- relinquishing old attachments and one's old life
- readjusting and adapting to the new world (without forgetting the old), and developing a new relationship with the deceased as a new identity and new ways of being in the world are formed
- reinvesting in life again (Rando 1996).

Golden (2000, p 7) describes grief as a part of life that 'is the physical, emotional and mental responses we have to a loss of any kind'. He depicts joy and grief as inseparable emotions; however, joy is inevitably temporary and, once gone, one is left with a sense of loss. Golden (2000) describes our reactions to small losses being intensified and of longer duration with major grief. He likens grief to a beast, severe grief being like a dragon: 'their size is unreal to us, and they are so powerful', which draws us out of our normal functioning and into an inner world that feels fraught with danger and unknowns (Golden 2000, p 11). Golden identifies five common grief reactions as: getting in touch with the loss, holding on, letting go, making new attachments, and observing one's growth through the loss. He describes the experience of grief as being 'all consuming' and emotions such as anger, sadness, helplessness, fear, guilt and loneliness can be overwhelming, chaotic and unpredictable (Golden 2000). People in grief can feel confined by their loss and surrounded by grief, and so they can feel cut off from everyday life. In this unfamiliar and dark environment, people's coping skills can be less effective and they have to find and draw on their strengths to find ways to get through their grief.

Greenspan (2003) concurs with Golden's belief that each person grieves uniquely; that each person needs to affirm their need to grieve; that grieving is a demanding physical and emotional process; that there is a need to find a safe place to grieve for periods of time to allow 'sorrow to be sorrow' (Greenspan 2003, p 113); and that there are both active and quiet ways to grieve.

As midwives we are mostly involved with loss that occurs during the childbearing cycle and we will not usually be part of the long-term grief experience of women and their families. So let us look at how we can assist women to begin to work through their grief and loss, and help them on the journey to understanding and living with their loss. Our role is to provide support, to share our knowledge, to open opportunities, to bring in other caregivers with specific expertise, and encourage the woman to have faith in herself to 'do' what she needs to do, to make good decisions for herself, to seek the support she needs, to recognise her strengths and to reinforce that she will survive the tragedy she is involved in.

What women need, ideally, is to be cared for by health professionals who are comfortable with death, who are in tune with women as people, who are empowering, and who can step back and work at the woman's pace (Tonkin 1998).

When midwives and women establish relationships of partnership, they are able to share power and control and make decisions together (Pairman 1998). Shared decision-making relies on midwives sharing knowledge and information and accessing resources, but consciously encouraging women to make the final decision on the basis of information and their personal feelings and circumstances. When women feel in control of decisions they feel empowered, and it is important for midwives to understand the link between a sense of control and later emotional wellbeing (Pairman 1998). This is particularly important for women inevitably debilitated by grief. They may need information offered at times when they are ready to hear it and may need to have it repeated a number of times. It is useful to provide information in written form (either in the midwifery notes, or as handouts, articles, books or leaflets) as well as talking it through. All decisions need time and women who are grieving particularly need time to assimilate options, relate them to their personal circumstances, make decisions, and be enabled to change their minds if necessary.

There is a sense of timelessness in grief. A woman may need longer than she would normally take to make good decisions for herself. It is very important that the time is taken to allow her to make the decisions herself. She may well have significant input from family and friends as well as midwifery, medical, religious and funeral professionals. Care must be taken to allow her the freedom (both in time, options and with lack of pressure) to make these decisions. It is then essential that we respect her choices regardless of our own beliefs (Hughes et al 2002; NZCOM 2005).

Midwives know the importance of telling the story of each birth and recording the context and feelings of the important events. Midwives know that the midwifery or hospital notes 'will become precious reminders of the pregnancy and birth once the immediate memories fade' (Pairman 1998, p 141). An important role for the midwife is to record the story of a baby's death, including the hours, days and weeks that follow. This can be demanding, and often we are more comfortable with recording physical aspects of midwifery care than in recording emotions. However, we need to write more—to record who was with the woman, the support she received, experiences shared, and her progression through coming to terms with her baby's birth, death and parting. The woman's story is very precious to her and will become a treasured part of her baby's being. Enabling women to carry their own notes ensures that they can refer back to written information and revisit their experiences as recorded. No information is hidden and as well as enhancing the relationship between a midwife and a woman, providing a woman with her clinical notes is 'a positive way of shifting power to the

WOMAN'S STORY

Bev's story of the death of her baby at term. This was Bev's second perinatal baby death.

On Monday about midnight, after I felt better and stronger in myself, it was time once again to focus on the baby. The paediatric registrar came down at 3 to 4 am to say things like liver dysfunction, profound hypotension, so I guess then I knew the writing was on the wall. We went to see Gemma again at six o'clock, when all I could say was, 'She is going to die' and refused to bond. Gordon, as you know, bonded beautifully and was then going into a real down. Finally, by midday, I realised that if I maintained this attitude I would suffer the long-term consequences so next visit I gave her a wee kiss and cuddle. By mid-afternoon the paediatrician talked about taking extra specimens and then turning the ventilator off, which was fine by me. A bit disappointed when I heard she would have to be cool overnight but obviously finding answers is especially important so if refrigeration gave better specimens then I was willing to compromise.

By Tuesday afternoon I had decided to let Gemma die at my breast and indicated so. Gordon had said he didn't want to see it but I gave him a ring and asked him if he wanted to reconsider, which he did of his own volition, which was great. At 8.30 pm or so I switched off the ventilator and she was removed and given to us.

We then had a magic moment which even got through my shell of numbness. Gemma actually opened her eyes and took a couple of small sucks from my breast. Whenever I want to think of this baby I shall think of that—the absolute sadness and joy as we had a wonderful moment of communication. She then died very peacefully over the next quarter hour and Gordon found it a very peaceful thing as it dispelled a lot of his fears (Bev Taylor, in letter to author, 1998).

woman and promoting self-responsibility' (Pairman 1998, p 143).

A woman's confidence in the decisions she has made is often strongly challenged when her baby dies. She has made the decisions to date and the outcome has been disastrous. She may well blame herself and lose confidence in her ability to make wise choices. Guilt is a normal aspect of grief and will probably see her searching for the 'what ifs?', looking to see what she could (or commonly 'should') have done differently. Our work as midwives is in listening to her explore these thoughts, often accompanied by distress, and helping her to be realistic about her control over what happened. Verbally, and in her notes, reinforcing the positive decisions she has made, and gently encouraging her to 'risk' making decisions again is one way of helping her to re-establish a sense of control and empowerment. As described elsewhere in this text, partnership with women is central to midwifery care and is particularly important in helping restore a sense of power and control for those women who have experienced a loss.

Early pregnancy loss

Although often almost dismissed as a common and relatively unimportant physical event because it is usually followed, sooner or later, by a successful pregnancy, a miscarriage still marks the death of a baby and can have a major emotional impact. It is estimated that 30% of pregnancies are lost to miscarriage (N Hung, personal communication, 2004). Grieving following the loss of a baby at this stage may be overwhelming, often with no or minimal acknowledgement from family or friends or sometimes even health professionals (Dent & Stewart 2004; Worden 1997).

It is important to always refer to the *baby*, not an embryo, fetus or product of conception (POC), for the mother has a *baby* from the moment she knows she is pregnant.

Women with bleeding or pain in early pregnancy need emotional support and acknowledgement of their feelings as well as physical care. A threatened miscarriage is often associated with feelings of uncertainty and fear. There is no known treatment for threatened miscarriage that ensures a term pregnancy, and while about 25% of threatened miscarriages may miscarry, there is also the probability that the rest can continue as pregnancies with no other adverse effects (Collier et al 2003).

It may be most appropriate for women with a threatened miscarriage, but who are not clinically compromised, to stay at home with close support from their midwives. Women should not be left unattended, and family and friends should be encouraged to provide emotional and physical support. Mild analgesia (e.g. paracetamol) or warmth (shower, hot water bottle or wheat pack) may help alleviate discomfort. Remember to administer Rh D immunoglobulin if the woman is Rhesus-negative.

Women need information about the possible course of events. A threatened miscarriage may settle and bleeding may cease. Or the bleeding may continue and clots may be passed

---

> ### WOMAN'S STORY
>
> **Kate**
>
> Kate miscarried at six weeks. For the children, her husband Jules, and Kate, a warm bond already existed for the unborn child she carried. They felt it was important for them to grieve and ritualise the death. They buried the remains at the end of the garden, preceded by a small procession, prayers and song. The immediate family attended (cited in Groufsky 1991, p 13).

followed by passage of the embryo and placenta. Sometimes, especially when the pregnancy is earlier than 12 weeks, it may be difficult to recognise that the embryo and placenta have been passed. The baby is not always recognised because of its small size and it is often accompanied by clot. Sometimes it is the marked decrease in cramping and blood loss that marks the completion of the miscarriage.

If women are at home waiting to see what happens, they should be informed to seek assistance if their condition changes. Hospital care may be more appropriate if they feel faint or unwell, as these changes may indicate heavy blood loss, an ectopic pregnancy, or an embryo that is lodged in the cervical os. Increasing or ongoing blood loss or signs of infection may indicate an incomplete miscarriage or retained products. This may need to be diagnosed by ultrasound scan. Women need to be informed that scans may be performed via the vagina (endovaginal scans) in early pregnancy. If the miscarriage is incomplete, a dilatation and curettage (D&C) may need to be performed in hospital.

Women should have the option of seeing and holding their baby if possible, including tissue from D&C, as it can give them a physical focus for their grief (Worden 1997). As with all options, it is an individual choice—for some women it may be undesirable, and for others very helpful.

Sometimes an embryo may be passed into a toilet unnoticed. Hospitals often dispose of remains through incineration. Women should be offered options and their desires respected regarding the disposal of their baby's remains. There is no legal requirement for burial or cremation at this stage of pregnancy; however, women may wish to do so and a ceremony of some kind may help acknowledge their baby and their loss. Giving their baby a name, perhaps a unisex name, helps provide a clear way to refer to their baby, and helps personalise their loss. Physical mementos may be impossible, although positive pregnancy test results, any scans, and measurements (weight, length) will all help. Planting a tree in memory of their baby, or having a special bush or vase or picture, are other ways of having a symbolic memorial.

Later pregnancy loss

When babies die later in pregnancy and are stillborn, women have to undergo labour and birth, often knowing that their baby is dead. To assist a woman to accept the reality of the baby's death, midwives should encourage the woman to spend time with her baby in order to establish memories to reminisce over later. Women can experience a compounding sense of loss when they look back at the time of their baby's death and regret not having had the opportunity to see their baby, or be part of the baby's physical presence and care (Tonkin 1998).

There is considerable evidence to suggest that parents should be encouraged to spend as much time as possible with their baby, as this not only assists with dealing with grief but also acknowledges their role as parents (Trulsson & Radestad 2004). However, a study by Hughes et al (2002) suggests that women who saw and held their stillborn babies were more likely to be depressed, have greater anxiety, have higher symptoms of PTSD, and disorganisation of mother–infant attachment in the next-born child. While there are some concerns about aspects of the study (Lovett 2001; Sheehan 2001), it highlights the importance of women making decisions for themselves about what is the right thing for them to do, and their need for ongoing support and care, including through subsequent pregnancies.

It is common and normal for women to want to see their baby. Some will be afraid—they may never have seen a dead person before, or may have had an earlier unpleasant experience with death. Support a woman to share any fears, whether from the past or anticipatory, to think about the options, and to take time to do what she needs to do. Women need to be prepared for the silence of their stillborn babies (Trulsson & Radestad 2004). When women have time between the diagnosis of the baby's death and the baby's birth, whether spontaneous or induced, they have time to begin to come to terms with the death of their child, to rest, to learn about or reappraise their plans for their forthcoming labour, to know what to expect at birth, and to prepare themselves for the coming days.

Women need time to gather information and think through what they want for themselves, and their families, around the time of the birth of their babies. This may include delaying an induction of labour to enable time at home before the birth. Women need to be informed of options regarding how any induction of labour might be carried out, what to expect of the labour and birth, the baby's possible appearance (see Clinical box below), how time may be spent with baby after the birth, possible investigations that may need to be done, and funeral and legal requirements. They should be encouraged to

think about who they want to share this time with and what mementos they wish to keep. Most of all they need plenty of time to try and think about what they want while coping with the impact of acknowledging their baby's death. It is a complex time, with overwhelming emotions of celebrating the birth while also grieving the death of their infant, and being mindful of how we work with women at this extremely vulnerable time can all improve the care (Trulsson & Radestad 2004).

WOMAN'S STORY

Lisa

I'm really pleased I continued with my plan and made it through without an epidural—it made me reach right into myself for a strength I didn't know I had and it made me reach out to my faith and trust in God for the mental and spiritual strength to see it through (comments made to author by Lisa, after her second son was stillborn).

Clinical point

Appearance of a stillborn baby

After death, changes can occur while the baby is still in utero. Known as maceration (to soften), this process of aseptic autolysis begins within 12 to 24 hours after death. Maceration causes the following changes in the baby:

▶ colour—pink, pale, livid
▶ blisters, eventually breaking and skin slippage, exposing red/livid subcutaneous tissue
▶ skull collapse
▶ papyraceous—flattened, paper-like fetus born long after its death.

After birth, further changes occur:

▶ increasing paleness
▶ darkening of lips, abdomen, dependent areas
▶ increasing skin fragility
▶ fluid leakage—may be bloodstained; from mouth, nose, umbilicus, skin.

Other support and advice

As midwives we are expected to consult and refer and work collaboratively with other health professionals when we reach the limit of our expertise (NZCOM 2005). It is appropriate to seek advice from midwifery colleagues and other professionals with more knowledge and experience, particularly if our experiences are limited. Because grief lasts well beyond the six-week postnatal period, it is important to ensure that the woman has networks in place that will continue to

---

WOMAN'S STORY

Margaret

As everything happened very quickly and he did not survive, we were not able to think clearly and we found your suggestions, such as taking photos and footprints, of great value. Some things were not easy at the time but we now appreciate that we did them, as it has since made it easier to accept that our son really existed (letter to author from Margaret after her baby's death).

Clinical point

Ways to create memories
Support the family to do as much as they can in their own time. Allow time for them to reach the stage where they are ready to move on to the next step. Offer options:

▶ take lots of photos, videos
▶ footprints and hand prints, plaster feet / hands, a snip of hair
▶ talk to baby, sing songs to baby, read stories to baby
▶ bathe baby (as many times as they like if baby's skin is sound)
▶ dress baby
▶ take baby home
▶ bath or shower with baby (especially for Dad)
▶ sleep with baby
▶ take baby for a walk in their garden, in pram, along the beach
▶ put baby in his or her own crib
▶ play baby their favourite or baby's own special music
▶ lots of cuddles
▶ share baby with siblings, grandparents, family and friends
▶ encourage the woman or family members to keep a diary of events, thoughts, feelings and activities
▶ keep mementos such as cot card with name, weight, measurements, time and date of birth; baby's name bracelet; copies of records, scans; clothing or wraps used with baby.

Clinical point

Tips on taking photos/videos
'The photos taken are so precious. We took piles of others at each stage but probably the Polaroid ones of Simon nearest to life are the most precious' (Bev Taylor, in letter to author).

▶ Use a camera that can focus well on close-up images.
▶ Be aware of backgrounds.
▶ Consider lighting.
▶ Try and have the baby held or with someone (e.g. a hand close by).
▶ Ensure that some photos show close-up of face, ears, hands and feet clearly.
▶ Take some photos as soon as possible after birth without impinging on the parents' needs.
▶ Take photos with each member of the family including children and grandparents.
▶ Take photos of the baby undressed, including abnormalities.
▶ Consider using a professional photographer.
▶ Polaroid photos may need to be copied as they tend to deteriorate with time.
▶ Provide prints of digital photos as well as electronic storage.

WOMAN'S STORY

Judy

Thank you for going into everything so thoroughly and clearly with us. It gave us a clear insight into what was going to happen, settled all our doubts, and enabled us to make the decision that was the right one for us. Those moments after delivery would have been very confusing and upsetting, whereas thanks to your efforts we found them very relaxed and loving. The memories we have of the time we spent with Kim are going to be a great comfort over the next few weeks and months, and the photo will always be there to look back at (Judy, letter to author).

support her through the months ahead. Midwives may suggest accessing a stillbirth support group, such as Stillbirth and Newborn Death Support (SANDS), a social worker, or grief or counsellor services; her GP and/or religious or lay spiritual support.

Midwives should be aware of local support agencies for women and the contact details for such organisations. There are many support groups available, such as:

● Bereaved Parents
● Compassionate Friends
● Trauma And Birth Stress (for those suffering from PTSD)
● Miscarriage Support
● Parent to Parent
● Action on Pre-eclampsia (NZApec)
● Heart Children
● Sudden Infant Death Syndrome (SIDS) Support
● Neonatal Unity for Mothers and Babies (NUMB)
● Citizens Advice Bureau
● National Association for Loss and Grief

● local counselling and church social services
● relationship services
● Barnadoes
● parents' centres
● women's refuges
● infertility support groups
● cultural support groups.

Establishing personal contact with these organisations means that midwives can be more aware of what they offer, and it is often easier for a woman to accept referral to someone who is known to the midwife.

Farewelling the baby

Trulsson and Radestad (2004, p 194) say that a woman needs to 'bond to her baby, recognise her pride in the baby, progress to the unavoidable fact that she and her baby must separate, and finally, say goodbye'. Different women will have different needs and different timeframes for what they need to do to achieve this. Remember, there is no hurry. The midwife can assist by providing information and options, helping to create

---

Clinical point

Post mortem examination

Making a decision may involve consideration of the following factors:

▶ the need to know what may have caused the death
▶ may identify or eliminate abnormalities and/or disease
▶ religious and cultural considerations
▶ may provide information that affects future pregnancies
▶ may not find cause of death
▶ generally performed within a few days of birth
▶ full or partial examination
▶ consent required, unless ordered by a Coroner if baby was born alive and cause of death is not certain.

Post mortem examination includes the following:

▶ consideration of maternal information and investigations (e.g. family, medical and obstetric history; pregnancy history; amniocentesis/CVS results; ultrasound scan results; microbiology, virology, cytogenesis, biochemistry, autoimmune, coagulopathy, haematology results)
▶ consideration of baby's investigations (e.g. microbiology, virology, cytogenesis)
▶ possible photographs and X-rays
▶ external measurements and examination
▶ surgical-type procedure requiring incisions to examine internal organs and repair by suturing
▶ incisions generally behind the head and Y on chest to abdomen
▶ internal examination of organs both macroscopically and microscopically
▶ histology of placenta even if baby not for post mortem.

After post mortem:

▶ Baby should be returned to the family or funeral director.
▶ Provisional results may be available shortly after the examination, but full results may be some weeks later.
▶ Results to be shared with the family, preferably by a health professional they know and who can help explain terminology and findings.

---

memories and encouraging parents to trust and express their feelings. As Susan said in a letter to the author, 'We are forever grateful for the information so Jack could be buried the way we wanted'.

Instead of enjoying their newborn baby, couples whose baby has died must face death and the decisions that are required at such a time. It is important to encourage new parents to make decisions about funerals themselves and to advise those close to the couple not to 'take over' in an effort to spare them pain. Parents can make all funeral arrangements themselves, with the help of family and friends, or they can engage the services of a funeral director. The funeral or Tangi is one of the last physical parenting roles for the baby, and it is appropriate for them to plan and participate in this as they did for the baby's birth. Cultural mores and religious customs may provide significant guidance. Options to consider include:

● post mortem (see Clinical box)
● burial or cremation
● a service—where (e.g. home, hospital, park, beach, church, hall, graveside); time of day; religious or not; who will lead the service (e.g. themselves, family member, friend, hospital chaplain or own clergy, Justice of the Peace, funeral celebrant); what songs, hymns, music, poems, readings
● place they want baby buried or cremated (some cemeteries have special baby areas; baby may be able to be buried at the head of a relative's plot)
● wording of birth/death/funeral notice(s)
● coffin; what baby will wear; what will go in coffin (e.g. toys, mementos, letters, photos, flowers, siblings, drawings)
● digging the grave (needs to be with sexton's guidance)
● flowers from their own, family's or friends' gardens
● use their own car or funeral director's hearse for transport for baby
● carry baby's coffin themselves
● someone to photograph/video/record service
● lower the coffin themselves
● fill in the grave themselves
● pre- or post-service get-together
● make their own memorial headstone
● if using a funeral director, compare fees.

WOMAN'S STORY

Bev

We had Simon here the last night and it felt okay. He watched his sister have a bath and slept the last night in a coffin at the end of the bed where he was conceived, which felt good. We think he began to smell—both Gordon and I could feel ourselves dissociating from his physical body and were very ready to bury him. We couldn't give our son life but we tried to give him respect, dignity and an identity with love, the best we could do. I feel very, very good about that (Bev Taylor, letter to author, 1998).

Subsequent pregnancy

Women approaching another pregnancy after the loss of a baby, or who have had to cope with a significant grief in a previous pregnancy, will inevitably bring anxieties to the new pregnancy. They may express ambivalence, fear of a recurrence, or uncertainty about their competence to make good decisions or to cope. They may have lost faith in their bodies, or in the normalcy of pregnancy and birthing, or in their caregivers. Subsequent pregnancies often bring the previous loss to mind and emotions may be raw again, often for protracted periods of time. Support, knowledge and reassurance are important to help women and their families through what may be a difficult time. Extra time may be needed to help women recognise their concerns and find ways to address them. Women may need acknowledgement that their apprehensions and fears are valid, and the reassurance of more frequent visits and baby checks, particularly around anniversary times. Support from family members (although they will have anxieties of their own) and support groups can play a major role in helping them through the months, and referral to other health professionals may be appropriate.

Men and grief

Men may grieve in ways that are different from women's. Golden (2000) describes feminine ways of grieving that often involve a community of support where the woman verbally shares and openly expresses her pain and relieves her pain through intimacy with others. Masculine ways of grieving are structured with the need for the man to know his own strength, know how he is going to use it and linking action to his pain (Golden 2000). Some men have difficulty expressing their sadness with tears, particularly when they may have been discouraged from crying when young. For some men their self-image involves being seen as the provider and protector who is independent, autonomous and strong, rather than vulnerable (Golden 2000). The sense of powerlessness involved in grief is another difficult aspect that conflicts with his sense of mastery and power and doesn't respond to his normal problem-solving methods (Golden 2000). Often 'the husband feels powerless and his need to act strong and to be supportive may be misinterpreted by the woman as not caring' (Worden 1997, p 104). Men are more likely to be action-orientated and may see grief as a 'problem' they should be able to manage themselves, rather than share with others. Some men may consciously acknowledge grief through activity such as making a coffin for their baby, preparing a funeral service, writing and giving an address at the funeral, gathering mementos for the baby's memory box, or fundraising for a cause related to their baby's death. Creative activities may help give meaning to his child's life and death (Golden 2000).

Although Western society has few rituals for grieving after the time of the death and funeral, personal or societal rituals can help people to put time and energy aside to be

Clinical point

Legal definitions and requirements in New Zealand
If a baby's death meets the legal definition of a miscarriage, the baby may be cremated or buried, or disposed of by the hospital (may be incinerated or cremated). If the baby is being buried at a cemetery or being cremated, the family will require a letter from the midwife (or nurse or doctor) confirming that the baby's death was defined as a miscarriage.

If a baby's death was defined as stillborn, a Notice of Birth (BDM9) must be completed by the occupier of the hospital (may be electronic) or midwife within five working days; a Medical Certificate of Cause of Fetal and Neonatal Death (BDM167) must be completed by a midwife or doctor, or a Coroner's Order be issued; the baby must be buried in a cemetery or cremated at a crematorium (complete an application form and a written statement confirming the baby was stillborn); and have a Notification of Birth for Registration (BDM27) which includes acknowledgement of the baby's death (stillbirth) completed by the parents.

If a baby is born alive (breathes or shows any sign of life such as beating of the heart, pulsation of the umbilical cord, or definite movement of the voluntary muscles after issuing completely from the mother, whether or not the umbilical cord has been severed or placenta detached) at any gestation (including termination), a Notice of Birth (BDM9) must be completed by the occupier of the hospital (may be electronically) or midwife within five working days, and a Notification of Birth for Registration (BDM27) must be completed by the parents.

If the baby subsequently dies, a Medical Certificate of Cause of Fetal and Neonatal Death (BDM167) must be completed; the baby must be buried in a cemetery or cremated at a crematorium (if for cremation have an application form and medical referee's certificate) and have a Notification of Death for Registration (BDM28) completed by the parents (or their representative, may be a funeral director) within three working days after the disposal of the body.
(*Births, Deaths and Marriages Registration Act 1995; Burial and Cremation Act 1964*).

aware of and work with their grief. For example, unveilings of headstones, shared memorial services or annual candle lighting ceremonies can provide a focus for ongoing grief.

In Western societies, death, like birth, has also become a process of medicalisation that has moved the experience from the community to hospitals, funeral homes and crematoria. Media portrayals are often graphic and traumatic rather than gentle. Society has become insulated from death and our experiences of it are limited and mediated by these external processes. It is now rare for families lay out the dead where they died in their homes, or make their coffins, or dig their graves. These changes have deprived men, in particular, of active roles in addressing their grief (Golden 2000).

Self-care

The loss of a loved person is one of the most intensely painful experiences any human being can suffer, and not only is it painful to experience, but it is also painful to witness, if only because we're so impotent to help (Bowlby 1980, p 7).

Facing loss and death in our work as midwives can bring up unresolved issues of our personal experiences of death and grief, and we may identify with the woman (or her relatives) and consequently expose ourselves to anxiety, anger, fear and other manifestations of loss. We may become more aware of our own health and mortality. We may project our own needs onto the women we work with, and we may feel guilty or disillusioned at not having coped as well as we expected of ourselves, or not having met the expectations of the women or their families, or our peers.

Blame is a common grief reaction, and both parents and midwives may express this. Blaming others allows individuals to shift responsibility from themselves and avoid painful introspection, and it may be a mechanism that is used to gain a sense of control. For midwives it is important to face what has occurred and to reflect on it, particularly in relation to the midwifery care we have provided and midwifery judgements we have made. Midwives need to explore the 'what ifs', to face any mistakes or poor judgement, to acknowledge the role of others, and learn from what has happened. There may well be the opportunity to also review the care given by the multi-disciplinary team in a morbidity and mortality review that allows for a critical analysis of the systems and processes as a core component of any service quality plan (Ministry of Health 2002).

Loss experienced by someone we are caring for challenges our need to be helpful as well as making us aware of our own losses, whether actual or feared, and increases our awareness of our own health and mortality, or that of those close to us. Coping with our own responses to grief as well as assisting a woman to cope can be stressful and exhausting, and the care may feel difficult and be tiring because of the emotional work involved. Practice colleagues may help by sharing workloads. Just as we support a woman to establish supports for herself for birthing and parenting, and for grieving, so we need supports for ourselves when dealing with unexpected outcomes in our work. Sharing our experiences and seeking support is a normal need, not a personal or professional inadequacy. We need someone to return the gift of listening and caring that we have given the parents; someone who listens as we explore our thoughts and feelings associated with the experiences we have been involved with and the midwifery care we have given. McDrury and Alterio (2002, p 52) describe 'response dialogue', in which the listener(s) 'remain focused on the original story and dialogue centres on the elements of the experience being related, which helps the teller explore their experience in depth'. Response dialogue provides an opportunity for the

teller to explore in more depth and detail, to be heard, and for both the teller and the listener to learn from the teller's experience. This type of interaction could be undertaken with other midwifery colleagues or with someone outside midwifery. Other strategies for coming to terms with grief in our work as midwives include writing, reflective journaling, relaxation activities, creative activities, physical activities, contemplation, and putting energy into relevant political activities or causes.

As midwives we owe it to ourselves as well as the women we care for to have a good support system established for ourselves, and to care for ourselves.

Critical thinking exercise

Immediately before Susan started to labour at 35 weeks, her husband was killed in a car crash.
1 As a midwife, what can you offer as you support Susan with her labour, birthing, early parenting and grief?
2 How would you recognise that she was grieving?

Reflective exercise

1 Reflecting on your own experiences of grief, what were your feelings, thoughts, actions, other responses? How did your family and friends react? What helped you most? How might this affect your support of women confronted with grief?
2 Think about a grief situation you have encountered as a midwife. How did you feel? What did you think? How did you help the woman? How did you help yourself to cope?
3 Identify six ways you can receive support for yourself when dealing with the grief of women you are caring for as a midwife.

Conclusion

In our practice as midwives we will inevitably work with grieving women. We may not be able to prevent their losses but we can support them with caring, knowledge, information and choices that can enhance their ability to cope with their grief and facilitate their chance of making the best of the experience. To do this, we need awareness of how our own experiences affect our care; we need to recognise grief situations and reactions, and understand the ways in which people work through their grief over time. Midwives need to know what options are available for women and families, and to support them to make choices that will meet their needs. Grief is a lifelong process but one that midwives can support women and their families to begin positively.

Review questions

1 List the kinds of grief situations experienced by women you have cared for.

2 Identify two theories of grief, and explain these.

3 Discuss how one theory of grief could relate to a non-death loss being experienced by a woman you have cared for.

4 How might men express their grief differently to women?

5 What are the legal requirements for registration and disposal of a dead baby at each stage of pregnancy?

6 How can you help women establish memories of their stillborn babies?

7 What local organisations could you recommend to women who have grief issues?

8 Name three strategies you can implement in your care to help women deal with grief.

9 Identify six ways in which you can assist women and their families to grieve for their stillborn child.

10 Identify three strategies for self-care when working with women and families experiencing loss and grief.

Online resources

For women suffering from PTSD related to birthing:
http://www.tabs.org.nz, and www.twinloss.org.nz
http://www.miscarriagesupport.org.nz
http://www.miscarriage.org.nz

Information and support for parents of children with special needs,
http://www.parent2parent.org.nz

Resources for children and those caring for them in dealing with loss and grief, http://www.skylight.org.nz

References

Australian Bureau of Statistics (ABS) 2005 Causes of death, Australia, 2003. ABS Cat. No. 3303.0. ABS, Canberra

Bowlby J 1980 Attachment and loss: loss, sadness and depression, vol III. Basic Books, New York

Brewis K, Touffet M, Wihongi J 2004 Disturbing the silence: childhood sexual abuse and the implications for midwifery care. Proceedings of NZCOM Conference, Wellington, pp 249–255, CD-ROM

Collier J, Longmore M, Scally P (Eds) 2003 Oxford handbook of clinical specialties (6th edn). Oxford University Press, Oxford

Dent A, Stewart A 2004 Sudden death in childhood. Butterworth-Heinemann, Edinburgh

Espinosa L, Osborne K 2002 Domestic violence during pregnancy: implications for practice. Journal of Midwifery and Women's Health 47(5):305–317

Golden R 2000 Swallowed by a snake (2nd edn). Golden Healing, Maryland

Greenspan M 2003 Healing through the dark emotions. Shambhala, Boston

Groufsky P 1991 A dignified choice. Ploughshares, Christchurch

Hughes P, Turton P, Hopper E et al 2002 Assessment of guidelines for good practice in psychosocial care of mothers after stillbirth. Lancet 360:114–118

Kübler-Ross E 1970 On death and dying. Tavistock, London

Lovett K 2001 PTSD and stillbirth. British Journal of Psychiatry 179:367

McDrury J, Alterio M 2002 Learning through storytelling. Dunmore Press, Palmerston North

Ministry of Health 2001 Interpersonal violence. New Zealand Health Strategy. MOH, Wellington

Ministry of Health 2002, Towards clinical excellence. MOH, Wellington

National Health Data Committee (NHDC) 2003 National health data dictionary, Version 12. AIHW Cat. No. HWI 43. AIHW, Canberra

New Zealand College of Midwives (NZCOM) 2005 Midwives handbook for practice. NZCOM, Christchurch

Pairman S 1998 The midwifery partnership: an exploration of the midwife/woman relationship. Unpublished master's thesis. Victoria University of Wellington

Parkes C 1972 Bereavement: studies of grief in adult life. International Universities Press, New York

Rando T 1996 Complications in mourning traumatic death. In: K Doka (Ed) Living with grief after sudden loss. Taylor and Francis, Philadelphia, pp 139–159

Sheehan J 2001 PTSD and stillbirth. British Journal of Psychiatry 179:368

Stojadinovic T 2003 For the first time somebody wants to hear. Women's Health Statewide, Adelaide

Tonkin L 1998 Still life. Hazard Press, Christchurch

Trulsson O, Radestad I 2004 The silent child—mothers' experiences before, during and after stillbirth. Birth 31(3):189–195

Worden J 1997 Grief counseling and grief therapy (2nd edn). Springer, London

Statutes

Births, Deaths, and Marriages Registration Act 1951 (NZ)

Burial and Cremation Act 1964 (NZ)

Further reading

Dent A, Stewart A 2004 Sudden death in childhood. Butterworth-Heinemann, Edinburgh

DeSpelder L, Strickland A 1996 The last dance (4th edn). Mayfield, California

Miller-Clendon N 2003 Life after baby loss. Tandem, Auckland

Tonkin L 1998 Still life. Hazard, Christchurch

APPENDIX: Definitions

- *miscarriage*—the issue from its mother, before the 21st week of pregnancy, of a dead fetus* weighing less than 400 g (*Births, Deaths and Marriages Act 1951* NZ and 1953 Australia):
  - *spontaneous*—the natural complete expulsion of a dead embryo or fetus from the uterus
  - *threatened*—abdominal pain and bleeding with the embryo/fetus still alive, cervical os is closed
  - *incomplete*—most but not all the products of conception (POC) have been passed
  - *complete*—complete expulsion of a dead embryo or fetus from the uterus
  - *inevitable*—cervical os open, usually bleeding and pain
  - *missed*—the fetus has died but is retained
  - *induced, termination of pregnancy* (TOP)—legal medical or surgical procedure to terminate a pregnancy and empty the uterus
  - *recurrent*—loss of three or more consecutive pregnancies
- *blighted ovum, anembryonic pregnancy*—the fertilised egg develops the placental tissue but the embryo doesn't develop or dies very early (Collier et al 2003)
- *ectopic pregnancy*—the fertilised ovum implants outside the uterine cavity (Collier et al 2003)
- *stillbirth*—NZ: the issue from its mother of a stillborn child (*Births, Deaths and Marriages Act 1951* NZ); Australia: death prior to the complete expulsion or extraction from its mother (ABS 2005; NHDC 2003)

of the products of conception of 20 or more completed weeks of gestation or of 400 grams or more birthweight: the death is indicated by the fact that after such separation the fetus does not breathe or show any other signs of life, such as heartbeat, pulsation of the umbilical cord, or definite movement of voluntary muscles

- *stillborn child*—a dead fetus born after the 20th completed week of pregnancy or weighing 400 grams or more (*Births, Deaths and Marriages Registration Act 1951* NZ)
- *perinatal death*—NZ: stillbirth or death of the baby in the first week of life; Australia: fetal or neonatal death (ABS 2005; NHDC 2003)**
- *neonatal death*—NZ: death in the first 28 days of life (*Births, Deaths and Marriages Act 1995*); Australia: death of a live-born infant within 28 days (ABS 2005; NHDC 2003)
  - *early neonatal death*—death of a live-born infant within seven completed days after birth
  - *late neonatal death*—death of a live-born infant after seven completed days and before 28 completed days after birth
  - *post-neonatal death*—death of a live-born infant after the first completed 28 days after birth and before the end of the first year after birth
- *infant death*—death in the first year of life
- *hydatidiform mole*—multivesicular mass as result of degeneration of chorionic villi at early stage of pregnancy.

---

* Legislation uses terms such as 'fetus' and 'embryo', but most women refer to the loss of their baby, and midwives should acknowledge this by referring to 'the baby'.

** There are different definitions in Australia for reporting and registering *perinatal deaths*. The *National Health Data Dictionary* specifies a definition of perinatal deaths to include all fetal and neonatal deaths of at least 400 grams birthweight or at least 20 weeks gestation (NHDC 2003). The Australian Bureau of Statistics (ABS) definition of perinatal deaths includes birthweight of at least 400 grams or, where birthweight is unknown, a gestational age of at least 20 weeks (ABS 2005). The data on perinatal deaths published by the ABS are based on the year of registration rather than on the year of birth. In Australia, the states all have different regulations concerning registration and burial. For example, under the NSW *Births, Deaths and Marriages Registration* Act 1995, all deaths that occur in New South Wales must be registered within seven days after the burial or cremation.

Index